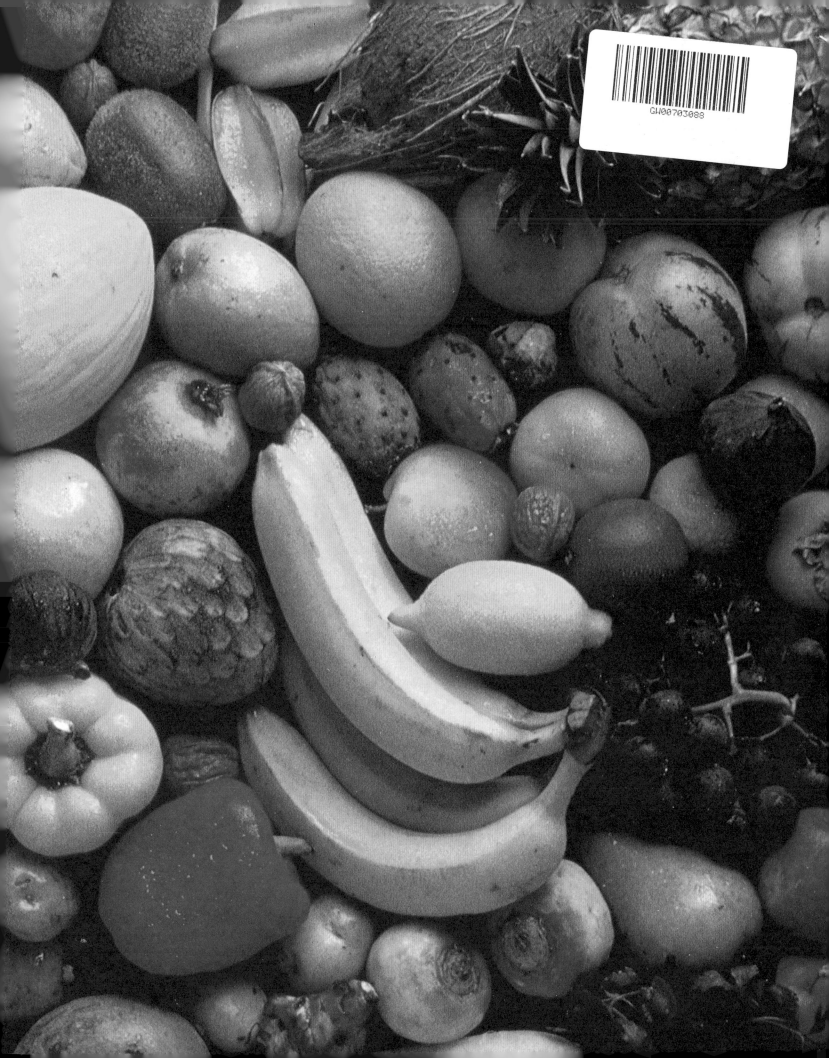

What Food Is That?

and How Healthy Is It?

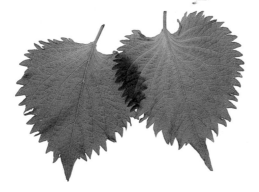

What Food Is That?

and How Healthy Is It?

JO ROGERS
CHIEF NUTRITIONIST

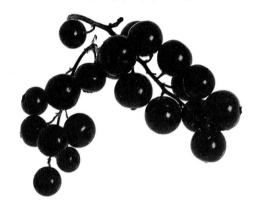

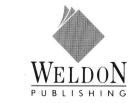

WELDON
PUBLISHING

SYDNEY · HONG KONG · CHICAGO · LONDON

ACKNOWLEDGEMENTS

The publisher would like to thank a number of people for supplying additional photographs (the column number is given after the page number). ANT Photo Library 84(2); Vic Cherikoff 57(1), 69(3), 76(2), 93(3), 96(1), 103(2), 104(1), 108(2), 314(2), 321(2); CSIRO 60(1,3); R. Cusack 153(2); Russell Frances 55(3), 64(3); Garry Gleason 83(1,3); NSW Department of Agriculture and Fisheries 70(3); NSW Department of Primary Industries 150(3), 152(1,2), 154(3), 156(2), 160(2); W & C Steptoe 149(3); Weldon Trannies (Ray Joyce) 151(1), 152(1), 156(2), 156(3), 157(1,2) 159(3), 163(2,3), 164(3), (Ray Joyce) 166(3), 167(1); B Wilson 154(1). Thanks are also due to food buyers Michelle Gorry, Vicki Finch and Dianne Bedford, to Tony Bishop for help with the text, and to all the authors for their assistance throughout the preparation of this book. The illustrations on pages 21 and 62 were drawn by Eamon Taylor. Those on pages 88, 97, 101 and 106 were drawn by Rod Scott. The Index was compiled by Jo Rudd.

A Kevin Weldon Production
Published by Weldon Publishing
a division of Kevin Weldon & Associates Pty Ltd
372 Eastern Valley Way, Willoughby, NSW 2068, Australia

Designer: Susan Kinealy
Photographer: Per Ericson, Twilight Studios
Production Manager: Dianne Leddy
Project Editor: Cheryl Hingley

National Library of Australia Cataloguing-in-Publication Data

What food is that? and how healthy is it?

Includes index.
ISBN 1 86302 091 8.

1. Food. 2. Nutrition. I. Rogers, Josephine F. (Josephine Frances).

641.3

Typeset in 10 pt Garamond by Savage Type Pty Ltd, Brisbane, Queensland
Printed by Griffin Press Ltd, Adelaide, S.A.
Distributed by Child & Associates Pty Ltd

CONTENTS

Contributors 6

Foreword 7

How To Use This Book 8

Introduction 10

Vegetables 14

Fruits 46

Fungi 81

Meats 87

Sausages & Preserved Meats 109

Poultry & Eggs 139

Fish & Shellfish 148

Breads 187

Grains and Cereals 200

Pasta & Noodles 220

Salt & Baking Agents 233

Cakes & Pastries 243

Desserts & Puddings 252

Milk Products 262

Cheeses 273

Pulses 301

Seeds & Nuts 312

Fats & Oils 323

Herbs & Spices 338

Sugars, Syrups & Sweeteners 364

Confectionery 370

Jams, Spreads & Dips 381

Sauces, Mustards & Pastes 385

Pickles & Preserves 404

Extracts, Essences & Colourings 412

Dressings & Vinegars 421

Fast Foods 429

Canned & Packaged Foods 441

Drinks 454

Tables 468

Index 474

CONTRIBUTORS

Josephine Frances Rogers, AM, BSc, MDAA, FCIA

Jo Rogers brings to this book a strong interest in all aspects of food and food preparation, a deep knowledge of nutrition and dietetics, and a lifelong connection with scientific research into food, the human diet, and nutrition.

For twenty-one years, Jo Rogers was Chief Dietitian and Food Service Manager of the Royal Prince Alfred Hospital in Sydney. She lectured concurrently at the University of Sydney, where she was a member of the Board of Studies and of the Examiners' Committee for the Graduate Diploma in Nutrition and Dietetics. In the field of national health and medical research, she served on the Nutrition Committee and the Food Services Committee, besides being part of several Working Parties from 1980–1988. Being a member of the Council on Overseas Professional Qualifications, she was also responsible for the screening examination for overseas dietitians applying to work in Australia, a position she resigned in 1989.

Having been a foundation member of the Australian Nutrition Foundation in 1981, Jo Rogers is now its National and NSW Chairperson, and Convenor of its Editorial Committee. In addition, she is a member of the Council of the Nutrition Research Foundation; a member of the Research Advisory Committee of the CSIRO Division of Food Processing; and a member of the councils of both the Dental Health Foundation and the School Canteen Committee of the NSW Department of Education.

She is co-author of five books on nutrition, and several scientific papers and articles. Her book, *You and Your Food*, has run to six editions and is used in schools and tertiary colleges throughout Australia.

Jo Rogers was made a Member of the Order of Australia in the Australia Day Honours of 1980.

CONTRIBUTORS ON FOOD

Doreen Badger

With a background in teaching Home Sciences in schools, Doreen Badger is Food Adviser with the Consumer Information Division of the Bread Research Institute of Australia. She has contributed to a number of recipe books and textbooks for Home Economics students.

Elena Barry

With an interest in retailing and food services and special knowledge of poultry, smallgoods and processed meats, Elena Barry is a food marketing consultant who works for a catering service. After studying at Canterbury University in New Zealand she gained a Diploma of Marketing at the University of NSW and studied at the Ryde Food School.

Vic Cherikoff, BAppSc

Vic Cherikoff has worked in the field of Australian bush foods for seven years, as a research scientist and consultant. He is Managing Director of Bush Tucker Supply Pty Ltd.

Dian Coffey

With a background in Home Economics, Dian Coffey spent nine years with the home management team of the Sydney County Council. She has also worked on food styling, product development and testing, television programmes and cookbooks.

Diana Dasey

Diana Dasey has taught cooking at home and in technical colleges, prepared foods for television commercials and catered for film crews, edited a foodservice journal, and devised and tested recipes for publishers and manufacturers. Her latest venture is as editor of a cake decorating magazine.

Cheryl Goodman

With particular interests in seafood and in natural and vegetarian cooking, Cheryl Goodman is a qualified Home Economist who instituted the Market Development section of the NSW Fish Marketing Authority. She has written a range of literature on seafood, including the NSW High School Seafood education programme.

Elizabeth Hemphill

An expert on culinary herbs, Elizabeth Hemphill wrote *Your First Book of Herb Gardening* in 1978. Since then, along with her husband Ian Hemphill, she has continued a freelance writing career.

Ian Hemphill

Ian Hemphill is managing director of his own management and marketing consultancy business. He has extensive experience in the production and marketing of herbs and spices.

Patricia Hoad

With fifteen years in the dairy industry, Tricia is MD of Auscheese Promotions and a newspaper, television and radio contributor on cheese, also lecturing on dairy foods at tertiary level.

Jennifer Isaacs, BA, DipEd

A writer and consultant with fifteen years' experience in the study of Aboriginal traditional culture, Jennifer Isaacs has a special interest in writing about Australian native plants and foods.

Barbara Kozak, BSc (Hons)

Barbara Kozak has spent ten years working for a major industrial company, chiefly with the edible oils division, as a chemist and product development officer. She is now a senior food development chemist in the cereals industry.

Marie McDonald

Trained in commercial cookery and with a background of Home Economics, Marie McDonald was for seven years the senior home economist in a leading advertising agency. She has handled public relations for the NSW Egg Marketing Board and the Mushroom Growers' Association. She has spent six years as food writer for two major magazines, and published four books on food and cooking.

Tess Mallos

Tess Mallos has specialised as a writer on food. Her cookbooks, including particularly successful ones on Greek and Middle Eastern food, and the cooking of pulses, have had worldwide sales and been translated into other languages. She places great value on extensive research, including first-hand information on food and cooking from people of many nationalities.

Anne Elizabeth Marshall, DipEd

Now Senior Home Economist with a major industrial company, Anne Marshall has published extensively on food, with sixteen cookbooks to her name and years of professional experience in education, food marketing and promotion, television and radio. She has been cookery editor for a number of national magazines in Australia and has a particular interest in food research and travel.

Jacki Passmore, DipModDietNut

A qualified cooking teacher in Asian and cordon bleu cuisines, Jacqueline Passmore is the author of twelve cookbooks. In addition to professional cooking certificates, Jacqueline also holds a Diploma in Modern Dietetics and Nutrition. She manages her own company, specialising in restaurant and general food consultancy, food styling and publication.

Mary-Louise Phillips

With certificates in cookery, home economics, hospitality and catering, teaching, interior design and marketing, Mary-Louise Phillips has built up years of experience in all facets of food service. She has written many cookbooks, and writes regular columns for magazines on food and wine.

Jennifer Wells

Jennifer Wells has worked for fifteen years in the advertising industry, both in production and as a stylist. She has written a number of articles for magazines and other publications, and works as a freelance food stylist for stills photography and television.

CONTRIBUTORS ON THERAPEUTIC VALUES

Gillian Marshall

With twenty-five years as a general nurse in public hospitals, Gillian has also spent four years as a specialist in herbal medicine.

Christine Muir

An accredited member of the Australian Traditional Medicine Society and the Australian Flower Essence Society, Christine Muir is a graduate of the Dorothy Hall College of Herbal Medicine.

CONTRIBUTORS ON NUTRITION

Soumela Amanatidis, BSc (Hons), DipNutDiet

Soumela Amanatidis worked for three years as a clinical dietitian at the Royal Prince Alfred Hospital, dealing particularly with patients of Greek origin. She now works as a nutritionist with the Australian Nutrition Foundation.

Jane Barnes, BSc (Hons), DipNutDiet, MDAA

In addition to her training as a biochemist, Jane Barnes is a qualified nutritionist. Irish born, she has worked as a consultant to major food industries and manufacturers in Australia. She runs her own freelance consultancy.

Janette Brand, BSc (Hons), PhD, FAIFST

A senior lecturer in Human Nutrition at the University of Sydney, Janette Brand has specialised in the nutritional analysis of Australian Aboriginal bush foods.

Sarah Garnett, BSc, DipNut Diet

After a year of research Sarah began as Clinical Dietitian at St Vincent's Hospital in Sydney, then spent three years as Administrative Dietitian at the Royal Prince Alfred Hospital. During this time she also acted as a consultant dietitian with a range of organisations, including lecturing at the Sydney College of Advanced Education and other centres.

Jill Gosper, MDAA

Jill Gosper is a Dietitian Nutritionist trained in New Zealand and qualified in Australia. She is also a certified fitness leader and qualified Home Economist, and has recently acquired a growing practice with private and corporate clients.

Judith Nichols, BAgSc, DipNutDiet

Judith Nichols has worked for the National Heart Foundation, on the National Dietary Survey of Adults, with the South Australian Health Commission, and at Newcastle University, as Research Dietitian to the Professor of Paediatrics.

Marina Pang, BSc, MDAA

With a specialised interest in ethnic food habits, Marina Pang has worked as a qualified dietitian in both the clinical and educational fields.

Sylvia MacKay Pomeroy, BSc, MDAA

Sylvia Pomeroy has worked as a hospital dietitian and a community nutritionist, besides being co-author of four cookbooks on diet and heart disease, and writing articles on food preparation and nutrition for magazines. Sylvia has a regular radio programme and gives lectures at the Royal Melbourne Institute of Technology.

Louise Spencer, BSc, DipNut Diet

While studying for a Graduate Diploma in Communication from the NSW University of Technology, Louise Spencer is also writing a cookbook for sportspeople. With experience as a researcher, a hospital dietitian and a community dietitian for the NSW Department of Health, she also runs a private practice.

Judy Walker, BSc, DipDietet, MDAA

Judy Walker has had a wide and varied career in nutrition: as Consultant Dietitian for the Australian National Heart Foundation, as a food and nutrition consultant in Brisbane, and as a lecturer to bodies such as the Australian Sports Medicine Foundation. She is co-author of three books on foods.

Jane Whatnall, BSc, DipNutDiet

The co-author of two books on food and cooking published by the National Heart Foundation, Jane has worked with the latter organisation, and in the area of community nutrition. She acts as a consultant dietitian.

FOREWORD

I am pleased to introduce this new book, *What Food Is That?*, designed to help consumers in their choices for healthy and pleasant eating.

A great deal has now been learned about the role of food in our general health. We know that for good health it is best to choose a varied diet with the right balance of nutrients — in other words, a balance which contains the energy, proteins and vitamins we need, but which is not too high in factors like fat and salt. Nowhere is this more important than in the case of heart health, where poor eating patterns have contributed to so much unnecessary suffering and so many deaths through heart attacks.

But to eat a balanced diet we still need to choose the individual foods which are part of it. We need to know how easily a food or product can fit into a healthy diet, and we need simple ways of finding out. There are several ways of achieving this, and *What Food Is That?* can be part of this vital educational process.

What Food Is That? is attractive, well organised and full of accurate information. I commend this book to readers as part of the healthy diet of information on foods that we all deserve.

DR R. L. HODGE
DIRECTOR
NATIONAL HEART FOUNDATION OF AUSTRALIA

How To Use This Book

IDENTIFYING A FOOD

If you have on hand a food which no one can name but everyone describes as a 'fruit', for instance: look up the appropriate chapter and see whether the clear, detailed photograph above each food name, or the paragraph headed DESCRIPTION, can help identify it.

FINDING A FOOD ENTRY

There are two methods:

1. Check the appropriate chapter in the Contents, turn to that chapter and run through the alphabetical listing to locate the entry. For instance, knowing Salami is a type of sausage, it is possible to turn to the chapter on Sausages and Preserved Meats, and locate Salami in the section on Sausages: Salami is in fact a long entry, containing many varieties.

2. Look up the food in the Index. This gives the page numbers of *every* reference to the item which occurs in the book. For instance, Chicken, besides having its own entry in Poultry and Eggs, also appears as Smoked Chicken in the chapter on Sausages and Pre-

served Meats and as Barbecue Chicken and Fried Chicken in Fast Foods, besides numerous other references throughout the text. If the food you seek is listed as a variety of another (for instance Custard-apple, which is in fact a variety of Cherimoya in the Fruits chapter), the Index is the best guide.

LEARNING ABOUT A FOOD

Each chapter begins with an introduction examining one category of food: dealing with its main features, discussing it clearly from the nutritional point of view, elaborating on important dietary considerations. After each introduction, the food entries are arranged in alphabetical order. In some chapters containing more than one section, the entries are listed alphabetically within sections: for instance, in the chapter on Fish and Shellfish, which finishes with a section on Preserved Seafood. Each entry is accompanied by a photograph of the food. The most commonly known name of the food is used, followed by the scientific name where appropriate. Any other names by which the food is known are also given.

NUTRITIONAL INFORMATION

For every food in this book, there is a commentary on its nutritional value. The quantities of MAJOR NUTRIENTS are discussed, along with any other significant nutrients present. In addition, a food may be described as an excellent, good or moderate source of a nutrient. This does **not** define any food as 'excellent' or 'good' overall; it specifies only the amount of a certain nutrient contained in a food, as seen in relation to the Recommended Dietary Intake of the nutrient for the average adult.

Excellent source: 15% or over
Good source: 10–15%
Moderate source: 5–10%
of the Recommended Dietary Intake.

Each entry is organised under some or all of the following headings, conveying a valuable range of information.

MAJOR NUTRIENTS Here the amounts are given of the important nutrients present in any given SERVE SIZE of a food. The serve size itself has been chosen by the team of dietitians as a representative quantity of the food, appropriate to a normal meal. Note that not all the elements present in a food item are recorded: only those which the nutritionists considered significant, and which allowed the tables to be consistent throughout the volume.

Where a nutrient is absent from a particular serve size of a food, or present in a negligible quantity, the figure zero is given. Other figures have been rounded off. Wherever possible, the Commonwealth Department of Community Services and Health Nutrient Data Tables for use in Australia (1987) have been referred to. Other tables include the A.A. Paul and D.A.T. Southgate figures from *McCance and Widdowson's Composition of Foods* (1978). Other sources were figures from the United States Department of Agriculture, and where necessary those from other countries and from industry sources.

The following are the nutrients which may appear:

Energy	Phosphorus
Protein	Magnesium
Fat	Iron
Cholesterol	Zinc
Carbohydrate	Thiamin
Total Sugars	Riboflavin
Dietary Fibre	Niacin Equivalent
Sodium	Vitamin A
Potassium	Vitamin C

These are all discussed in the Introduction, and, where relevant, in the introduction to chapters.

NUTRITIONAL INFORMATION This is the commentary on the major nutrients, a guide to the food's effect on diet and the body. It helps interpret the facts, and can provide warnings about such things as sodium levels, or the nature of fat content. It may mention the effects processing or cooking have on the food's nutritional value. If a significant nutrient, which does not appear in the table (such as folate, for instance, or vitamin B12) is present in the food, this information will be given. In addition, a food may be defined as a source of a particular nutrient, measured against the percentage it supplies of the Recommended Daily Intake. An excellent source provides 15% or over; a good source provides 10–15%; a moderate source provides 5–10%.

DESCRIPTION Along with the photograph, this is a valuable guide to identification.

ORIGIN AND HISTORY For some, these are the most fascinating aspects of any food. Knowing where a plant, for instance, first grew, or how it influenced the cuisines of the known world, can add a lot to our enjoyment when we come to eat its fruit, seeds, flowers, roots or leaves. The food writers' research adds colour and interest to the information on each food in the volume.

BUYING AND STORAGE Going on a food expedition is a pleasant experience when we know where both the favourite and the less familiar foods can best be obtained. And it is equally important to know how long they will keep before consumption.

PREPARATION AND USE Although this volume is not a cookbook, it is nonetheless a fund of delights for those who value the culinary skills. This section pinpoints the main ways in which a food may be used, describing the preparation before serving, often naming and sometimes giving basic recipes for popular dishes.

PROCESSING For some food, the way it is processed is as vital as the raw material: the soya bean, for instance, gives rise to foods which are listed under chapters as diverse as Drinks, or Sauces, Mustards and Pastes.

In chapters dealing with already refined foods, the processing discussed is that of the item itself: the extraction and refining of many oils is interestingly described in Fats and Oils, for example.

VARIETIES If a food has one or more varieties, they are mentioned in this section.

In some cases, the varieties are so numerous that a full list is impracticable.

In others, detailed information and some illustration are possible. If a photograph is used, it appears *above* the variety illustrated. The rest of the variety may contain a sentence or two about the item — or it may be a full entry, under the usual headings: DESCRIPTION, ORIGIN AND HISTORY, etc. This is the case, for instance, with the Cabbage entry in the Vegetables chapter: no less than ten varieties are listed, with illustrations and extended entries given wherever they are of value to the reader.

SEE ALSO This section is added to an entry where the food itself, or different forms of it, appear in the same or other chapters of the volume. It is best to consult the listed foods in the Index, for easy location of each reference.

TABLES There are a number of tables at the end of the volume designed as a quick reference for those with further interest in nutrition.

INDEX As mentioned, the index is the most valuable guide when using this book.

INTRODUCTION

This book provides the answers to a host of questions about food and nutrition.

A talented team of specialists, food consultants, dietitians and nutritionists have combined their knowledge and expertise to assemble a comprehensive list of nearly two thousand foods known and available to consumers today.

The separate entry for each item contains a photograph, for easy identification, followed by the nutritional facts and comments which help to define the food's function in a healthy diet, plus a full and informative description and history, including valuable advice about buying, storage, preparation and use.

This book is timely, coinciding with a growing community interest in food and nutrition. The division into chapters allows the reader to understand such staple items in the diet as vegetables, for instance, by reading the short nutritional introduction to the subject, and then looking up the specific food entries, which are listed alphabetically within the chapter.

Living in a multicultural society and enjoying an abundant food supply, we are constantly encouraged to extend our knowledge of food and food cultures, as well as appreciating old favourites. Among the sources examined in this book are some which are known as 'bush foods' — gathered in the wild and part of the traditional diet of Australian Aborigines and New Zealand Maoris. Since space does not permit all of these foods to be included, those represented have been selected mainly in terms of their availability. Many of the foods appearing in this book are those of Asian origin whose use has become widespread throughout the Pacific region. The foods and cuisines of Greece, Italy, North African and Middle Eastern countries have stocked the shelves of grocery and fruit stores, and delicatessens, with an even wider range of products. Shopping for unfamiliar food can be a fascinating experience — provided we have a reliable handbook to help identify and prepare what is purchased. And sharing information about food with people from other countries is an important means of building understanding and friendship.

To help in research, the two previous pages explain how to use this book. The rest of this introduction provides a basic guide to the nutrients that food contains, and to a sensible, healthy selection of those nutrients within the modern diet.

THE ROLE OF FOOD IN HISTORY
Our health is dependent on the bodily features we have inherited, but is also affected by the environment and by behavioural factors. Important amongst these are the foods we eat and the food habits we adopt.

The more we know about food, what it is, where it comes from, how it is used, its nutritional value and its place in a reasonable diet, the easier it is to eat for both pleasure and health.

Food has played a major role in the evolution and history of the human race. Great voyages of discovery have been made in search of food, wars have been fought for it, and it is linked with the rise and fall of empires.

The early humans were hunter/gatherers eating a variety of plant foods and the flesh from animals. Often they were also nomads, using the foods that were available in different regions. In times of extreme food shortage they perished. Anthropologists comment on the evidence that the collecting and sharing of food was a characteristic that separated early humans from other animals, and helped in their survival.

When the hunter/gatherers turned to agriculture and settled long enough to cultivate plants and domesticate animals, a significant cultural evolution began. This was between 10 000 and 20 000 years ago, a very short time in the 2 000 000 years or more covering the evolution of modern humans.

Whole civilisations were founded on the cultivation of cereals. Wheat and barley spread from the Middle East to Egypt, Rome and Greece and to India, China and Asia. Rye and oats grew in the colder northern and western zones of Europe, while rice and millet were cultivated in India, China and South-East Asia and maize in Central America. The cereals provided the staple foods in the various regional diets. These cereal crops have survived and they are an important ingredient in many of the foods included in this book. Many of the regional dishes discussed began to emerge early in the history of the human race.

EARLY FOOD PROCESSING
Food processing began in the home and the small community or village. The aims of processing were to prolong the life of the food and stabilise the supply of food throughout the seasons and to add palatability and variety to the diet.

Fire was used to cook or to smoke food. Other early forms of processing were sun-drying, salting and fermentation and in cold climates foods were packed in ice.

Cereals were ground to produce meal, which was made into gruel and later bread. Milk was fermented to produce cheese, buttermilk, sour cream and yoghurtlike products. Vegetables were salted and fermented, meat was stored in brine. Yeast, leavened bread and beer were made by the Egyptians as long ago as 2500 BC. They were probably first made when wild yeasts in the atmosphere contaminated foods, and would have been very different from the products we enjoy today.

Many of the products discussed in this book which are manufactured today in factories and sold in our supermarkets, were traditional foods first produced in these agricultural societies. Some have already been mentioned; others include vinegar, sauerkraut, salami, soya sauce, fish sauce, tempeh (soya bean paste) and tofu (soya bean curd).

THE BEGINNING OF MODERN
FOOD PRODUCTION AND PROCESSING
The Industrial Revolution in the late 18th and in the 19th centuries brought about dramatic changes in the lifestyle and the eating habits of people in the Western world. Fewer people were involved in agriculture and more people lived in towns and cities

where they depended on the food produced by others. Gradually some of the processing of food moved from the home into the factory.

Methods of animal husbandry changed and food production and processing were mechanised. In the latter half of the 19th century, steel rollers were introduced for milling, and white flour, previously only available to the wealthy, was enjoyed by the majority. White flour and white bread remained the foods of choice for the large majority in Europe and in countries like Australia until the 1980s, but since then there has been a return to wholemeal and wholegrain products.

Sugar had been known and highly prized for hundreds of years: it was brought back to Europe by the early explorers who had gone to the East seeking spices and perfumes. It was expensive and mainly restricted to use in medicines, so only the very wealthy could afford to use it as a food.

Sugar was first produced from beets in Europe in the late 18th century and the sugar bounties offered by Napoleon in 1806 led to the development of improved varieties of beet and improved extraction rates. Gradually sugar became available at a price which most people could afford. In the UK the annual sugar consumption per head between 1800 and 1900 went from less than 10 kg to between 40 and 50 kg. This is typical of the change which took place in the Western world.

Since the Industrial Revolution there have been some major changes in the nutritional characteristics of the diet in the Western world.

The use of more refined cereal products and the fall in the amount of cereal foods eaten has led to a decline in the amount of complex carbohydrate (starch) and dietary fibre consumed. Some of the complex carbohydrate in the diet has been replaced by added sugar.

The breeding of animals with fatter carcasses, and the availability of fats extracted from animal products — e.g. butter, dripping, lard and tallow — has led to an increase in the amount of saturated fat consumed.

THE MODERN DIET AND HEALTH

These changes gained momentum in the Western world after World War II. The increase in affluence, and in the number of wives and mothers working outside the home, coincided with developments in the food industry. More foods were produced and eaten outside the home. Ready-to-eat foods, fast foods restaurants and takeaway food gained popularity.

Many of these foods were high in fat, particularly saturated fat. They were often low in dietary fibre and high in salt.

Other foods high in fat and/or sugar gained popularity: commercial biscuits, pies, pastries, potato crisps and similar snack foods, confectionery, soft drinks and cordials are only a few examples.

Between 1968 and 1978 fat consumption in Australia for instance, increased by more than 19 per cent. Sugar consumption remained steady but more sugar was used by the food manufacturer and less was added to food in the home.

Alcohol consumption has increased: for example, between 1938–39 and 1985–86 consumption per head of beer, wine and spirits increased by 105, 617, 144 per cent respectively.

At the same time as the fat and alcohol intake of the average person has been increasing, people have become more sedentary. Mechanisation in the workplace and the home, improved transport, the family car, spectator sports . . . these are some of the factors accounting for the drop in energy output. More kilojoules consumed and fewer kilojoules used in the human body will result in overweight and obesity, which are major public health problems. Obesity is not only a problem for aesthetic reasons, it increases the risk of developing a number of problems including heart disease, high blood pressure and non-insulin-dependent diabetes.

Almost 60 per cent of the deaths in Australia, for instance, are linked with nutrition-related diseases, and 25 per cent of these deaths are premature: that is, occurring in people under the age of 65 years. The causes include heart disease, high blood pressure, stroke, non-insulin-dependent diabetes, certain types of cancer (breast, womb, colon), gallbladder disease and cirrhosis of the liver. Many of these premature deaths are preventable.

This is the unfortunate side of the story and it needs to be balanced against the improvements in health. Over the last hundred years, life expectancy in the Western world has increased by about 24 years for males and about 28 years for females. The infectious diseases, which were the major cause of death for our grandparents and great-grandparents, account for few deaths today. These have been replaced by the lifestyle diseases, many of which are related to the nutrition excesses discussed previously. The diseases associated with nutritional deficiencies such as protein/energy malnutrition, scurvy, beri beri, pellagra and night blindness are rare in the Western world, occasionally occurring in minority groups or in association with terminal illnesses.

THE NUTRIENTS

Food consists of hundreds of different chemicals, and amongst these are the nutrients which are essential for the growth, development and reproduction of humans. Other chemicals provide flavour and colour, or have pharmacological properties, such as caffeine; while still others are compounds, which are not essential nutrients, and may be toxic if consumed in sufficient quantities. It is a mistake to believe that because something is 'natural' it contains no harmful substances.

There are approximately 50 essential nutrients in food, which can be grouped into the following categories: *Proteins, Carbohydrates, Fats, Vitamins, Minerals* and *Water. Dietary Fibre* is another important nutrient, consisting of complex carbohydrate molecules and lignin. It is not, however, essential for survival.

Proteins consist of amino acids linked together, and their quality varies depending on the amino acids they contain. Eight amino acids must be supplied by food. They are referred to as the essential or indispensable amino acids: isoleucine, leucine, lysine, methionine, phenylalanine, threonine, tryptophan, valine. For children, a ninth amino acid, histidine, is added to the list. The other 14 amino acids can be produced in the body from the indispensable amino acids.

With the exception of gelatine, animal proteins contain all the indispensable amino acids. Vegetable proteins lack one or more of them, but when they are taken in a mixed diet the amino acids in one food can complement those in another.

Good combinations are:
Cereals (e.g. rice, bread, pasta) *plus* pulses (e.g. chickpeas, kidney beans, baked beans, lentils).
Pulses *plus* nuts (e.g. pine nuts, walnuts).
Cereals *plus* milk products (e.g. milk, cheese, yoghurt).

Proteins build and repair tissue, and are used in the production of enzymes, hormones and antibodies, all essential in regulating body metabolism and protecting against disease. Protein can also be metabolised to release energy, yielding 17 kilojoules (kJ) or 4 Calories per gram.

Carbohydrates are the major source of food energy occurring in all plant foods, where they are produced from carbon dioxide and water by photosynthesis. The starches in cereal crops and in the starchy vegetables are the main carbohydrates which occur naturally. The naturally occurring sugars, which are part of carbohydrate content, are in fruits, honey and in milk (where the sugar is called lactose). Carbohydrates yield 16 kJ (4 Calories) per gram.

Most of the carbohydrate which is not used for energy is converted to fat in the body, while a small amount is stored as glycogen in the liver and muscles. Glycogen is a complex carbohydrate consisting of a number of glucose units linked together. The glycogen stores are used during exercise and glycogen is broken down to glucose and used as a source of energy.

Fats are found in most natural foods. In plant foods they are usually in low concentration (although some nuts are more than 60 per cent fat), while in animal foods they are often in higher concentrations.

Fats are combinations of glycerol (commonly known as glycerine) and fatty acids, and their chemical, physical and physiological properties vary according to each combination. Fatty acids are made up of long chains of carbon atoms. If all the carbon atoms along the chain are saturated with hydrogen, the fatty acid is said to be saturated. If two adjoining carbon atoms have one, instead of two, hydrogen atoms attached, they share a double bond and are said to be monounsaturated. If there are two or more carbon atoms sharing double bonds, the fatty acid is said to be polyunsaturated.

The polyunsaturated fatty acids and the monounsaturated fatty acids have important properties in the body. They help to lower blood cholesterol levels, some help to lower the level of triglycerides (another fat in the blood), some of them support the body's immune system and protect the body against infection and inflammatory conditions, some help to prevent blood clots. Safflower, sunflower, maize, grapeseed, soya bean oil and some fish are good sources of polyunsaturated fatty acids.

Olive oil is the most important source of monounsaturated fatty acids, but peanut oil and rapeseed oil are also good sources. Meat and eggs also contain significant amounts of monounsaturated fatty acids.

Three specific polyunsaturated fatty acids are referred to as essential fatty acids because they must be available to the body.

In the 1980s studies of fish oils, which contain two further polyunsaturated fatty acids, have been widely discussed because of the apparent protection against heart disease which the consumption of seafoods has bestowed on groups like the Inuit and other dwellers in the far north of North America.

Although reduced fat intake is recommended for a healthy diet, it is also recommended that some of the saturated fats be replaced by polyunsaturated and monounsaturated fats.

Fats are the most concentrated source of energy, which is why reducing fat intake is the first important step to controlling body weight. Fat provides 37 kJ (9 Calories) per gram.

Vitamins are organic compounds required in very small amounts (i.e. milligrams or micrograms) for the normal functioning of the body. Along with the minerals, they are often known as micronutrients, in contrast to the macronutrients — protein, carbohydrate and fat — which make up the bulk of the nutrients in foods. Vitamins are usually obtained from food, but most of the vitamin D used by the body is produced in the skin by the action of ultraviolet rays or 7-dehydrocholesterol, and some vitamin K is synthesised in the gut.

There are 13 essential vitamins:

Vitamin A (and beta carotene, which is converted to vitamin A in the body)	Vitamin B6 (pyridoxine)
	Vitamin B12
	Vitamin C (ascorbic acid)
Thiamin (vitamin B1)	Biotin
Riboflavin (vitamin B2)	Vitamin D
Niacin (vitamin B3)	Vitamin E
Pantothenic acid (vitamin B5)	Vitamin K

The vitamins act mainly as enzymes and coenzymes, facilitating metabolic processes in the body: for example, the metabolism of carbohydrates, fats and protein to produce energy; the building up of body proteins; the absorption of calcium from the gut and its deposition in the bones; the multiplication of body cells and the formation of blood cells. Without the presence of the vitamins, these processes cannot take place.

Not all of these vitamins are listed in the nutrition information relating to the various foods, because it is difficult to obtain reliable nutrition data. When a food is known, however, to be an important source of a particular vitamin, this will be mentioned in the text.

Minerals are the inorganic chemical elements in the diet and body. If organic material, either vegetable or animal, is burnt, the ash which remains consists of the minerals.

Calcium and phosphorus, and to a lesser extent magnesium, are used in building up the skeleton and teeth. Because phosphorus is widespread in foods, most diets provide adequate quantities, but calcium and magnesium occur in a more limited range of foods.

Iron is needed for the formation of haemoglobin in red blood cells, and myoglobin in muscles. Haemoglobin and myoglobin act to transport oxygen around the body and inside the muscles.

Many of the minerals occur in enzymes, which are the organic catalysts which facilitate the chemical processes in body metabolism.

When minerals occur as ions or electrically charged particles in the body fluids, they help control muscle contraction and relaxation, including the heartbeat. They also carry electrical impulses along nerve pathways.

Fluorine is an essential nutrient which strengthens the teeth and bones.

Chromium is part of the Glucose Tolerance Factor, which enhances the action of insulin in carbohydrate metabolism.

Zinc, as well as occurring in a number of body enzymes, is essential for normal sexual maturation, and for the healing of wounds.

Copper works with iron in the formation of haemoglobin and occurs in melanin pigments in skin and hair.

Sodium is an essential nutrient, important in the regulation of fluid balance in the body, but eating habits worldwide promote overconsumption of sodium chloride (salt), which has been linked with the prevalence of high blood pressure.

Potassium acts in conjunction with sodium in the transmission of nerve impulses, and is involved in many enzyme systems.

The minerals in foods and in the body are usually measured in milligrams (a milligram is one thousandth of a gram). For some of the minerals the range between a recommended intake and a harmful or toxic level of intake is relatively small.

Water makes up about 60 per cent of the human body. The body fluids have important functions in maintaining the body temperature, transporting nutrients around the body, transporting waste products for elimination and providing the medium for a number of essential metabolic processes to take place. This water is continuously being lost from the body as urine, in excretions from the bowel, and as sweat. It must therefore be replaced through the diet, as we can only survive for a very short period without water.

Dietary fibre occurs only in plant foods (cereals and foods made from grains, vegetables, fruit and nuts) and it is defined as that part of the food which is not broken down by enzymes in the small intestine. However, fibres are partly broken down by bacteria in the large bowel and some are then absorbed and used for energy.

There are many different types of fibre, each with different chemical, physical and physiological properties. Fibre adds bulk to the diet, and normalises the flow of food through the gut. Fibre attracts water in the bowel, producing bulky soft stools which are easily excreted, so lessening the risk of constipation.

The soluble fibres in oatmeal, barley, pulses (dried peas, beans, lentils) and fruits have a role in reducing the level of cholesterol in the blood and some fibres have been linked with the control of blood sugar levels, as they slow down the absorption of carbohydrates from food.

The best way to have an adequate intake of dietary fibre is to eat wholemeal bread, wholegrain cereals, vegetables and fruit regularly.

RECOMMENDED DIETARY INTAKES (RDI)

In Australia the National Health and Medical Research Council has established a table of recommended daily intakes for many of the nutrients available in food. This table, which is relevant to a healthy diet in any country, gives levels of nutrient intakes for males and females of various age groups. It is the first of the tables reproduced in a special section at the back of this book.

There are wide individual variations in the need for nutrients, but the further an individual's intake falls below the RDI, the greater is the likelihood that his or her diet will be deficient. The exception is the RDI for sodium, which is given as a 'desirable' range. Problems are likely to arise when the upper level of the range for sodium is exceeded, because of the link between sodium intake and high blood pressure.

Throughout this book, the RDI have been used for comparison with the nutrients in a serving of food, to establish whether that food is an 'excellent', 'good' or 'moderate' source of a particular nutrient.

THE CONDITION OF FOOD

People purchasing or consuming food may harbour concerns over a range of issues including its composition, strength, purity and safety. In respect of labelling and advertising, those issues may also include the potential for deception and fraud. To address these concerns, food laws have evolved over many years. Irradiation of fruit and vegetables, for instance, is permitted in some countries but not in others.

From a public health perspective, the major priority is microbiological food poisoning, usually associated with poor conditions of handling, processing and storage. The second priority is the metallic contamination of foods, particularly by the heavy metals such as arsenic, mercury, lead and cadmium. Residues of pesticides will remain a priority for many years, despite the move away from persistent organochlorides to the less stable organophosphates. Even foods grown without the use of agricultural chemicals can pick up significant levels of pesticides from the soil. As noted, in addition, many foods in their natural state contain highly toxic components. The range of plants suitable for human consumption is surprisingly narrow, as anyone who has taken jonquil stems from the garden instead of green onions can tell.

Food additive safety tends to fall behind these other health concerns, largely because of the rigorous testing and approval required before an additive is cleared for use. Nonetheless, many individuals find they experience allergic responses to specific additives and components in food. A combination of public education and ingredient declaration is the best means of assisting and protecting these sensitive individuals.

A HEALTHY DIET

A healthy diet is one which satisfies the physiological, psychological and social needs of a consumer or group of consumers. The preparation and eating of food, besides being vital and pleasurable, are also amongst the more complex of human activities. The range of information in this book reflects that complexity, and the text discusses the cultural aspects of the foods included, which are enjoyed in many nations and regions.

It is possible to plan a healthy diet along many different lines, using a very wide range of foods. The following are two model plans which have been developed to guide food selection.

The first divides food into five groups:
- Bread and cereals
- Vegetables and fruit
- Meat and meat alternatives (fish, eggs, pulses, dried peas, beans, lentils, nuts)
- Milk, cheese and yoghurt
- Butter and table margarine

Each of these groups contributes different nutrients, and by selecting a diet to include a variety of foods from each group each day, a person can ensure that the diet will meet all his or her nutritional needs.

The second model is a food pyramid, first devised by the Australian Nutrition Foundation, which puts together the five food groups while giving some guidance to the proportions of these which should be included in the diet.

Bread and cereals, vegetables and fruits form the foundation of this diet. Next come the foods rich in protein: meat, poultry, fish, pulses, nuts, eggs, milk, cheese and yoghurt. As the pyramid narrows it takes in the fats, butter, margarine and oil. Finally, small amounts of sugar form the point of the pyramid, which is shown in the tables at the end of this book.

CONCLUSION

Selecting and enjoying a healthy diet is up to each family and individual. Amongst an abundant food supply, it is possible for most people to promote their nutritional health by following a few simple guidelines. Health is more than the absence of disease: it is a positive state of physical, psychological and social well-being, which rewards those who choose the healthy pathways.

VEGETABLES

Vegetables provide a wonderful array of foods, bringing variety in flavour, texture, colour and appearance to the diet. Their seasonal nature, and the regional variations in these interesting plants, add further dimensions and interest.

There are hundreds of different vegetables eaten in countries around the world. This book includes as wide a range as possible, with particular thoroughness concerning vegetables available in the southern Pacific region — including those imported into this part of the world from Europe, America, Asia and the Middle East.

For some families and individuals vegetables make up a major part of the diet and for others they are a minor accompaniment to meat, poultry or fish. The imaginative cook can make a variety of vegetable dishes including soups, salads, entrées and main courses. These culinary opportunities are touched on in this book. Many recipes have come from peasant communities where vegetables and cereals were the main foods available.

Botanically, vegetables are varied, since they include: the starchy root vegetables such as potatoes and yams; the other root vegetables like onions, carrots, parsnips and radishes; the leafy vegetables such as spinach and lettuce; the fruits like aubergine, zucchini, squash; the stalks such as celery; and the flowers like cauliflower and broccoli. Another important botanical group is formed by the pulses or legumes; a separate chapter has been devoted to the dried form of these nutritious foods, while the fresh plants such as green beans and peas are discussed here.

In epidemiological studies, which compare the relationship between disease patterns and environmental factors such as diet, the prevalence of cancer has been found to be lower in populations where the intake of vegetables is higher. This particularly applies to the carotene-rich vegetables (yellow, orange and green) and the cruciferous vegetables (broccoli, cauliflower, Brussels sprouts and cabbage).

It is not known exactly why vegetables may be protective against cancer. Dietary fibre, beta carotene and vitamin C have been suggested as protective, but the effects may also be due to non-nutritional components such as other carotenoids which are not converted to vitamin A.

It is wise to add more vegetables to the diet, because they are low in fat and rich in fibre and essential nutrients. Their high fibre and high water content means that they are bulky, and satisfy the appetite without adding a lot of food energy (kilojoules or calories). This means that they are a valuable food for people wishing to keep in the healthy weight range and those who want to reduce their fat intake. The nutrient-to-energy balance of vegetables is upset when they are prepared with a lot of fat, either by frying or roasting in fat or oil, or by serving the vegetables with fatty sauces.

As a group of foods, vegetables make a valuable contribution to our diet. The individual nutrient tables in this chapter give an opportunity to see how much they may also differ from one another. Generally speaking, they all contain dietary fibre. The legumes are a good source of protein, and potatoes, sweet potatoes and taro provide significant amounts of protein in diets where they are used as a staple. It is as a source of beta carotene (which is converted to vitamin A in the body), and of vitamin C, that vegetables are particularly important.

Vegetables are also an important source of folate, particularly the green vegetables. Vitamin E is another nutrient occurring in significant amounts. Both these are mentioned under the heading Nutritional Information.

Unless otherwise stated, the major nutrients listed in each entry of this chapter are those for the raw vegetable. It should be noted that cooking often reduces the content of some nutrients in food: such information is given where necessary in individual entries.

The vegetables chosen for discussion in this chapter are those most readily available, but many others may appear in greengrocers' shops from time to time, such as amaranth, matrimony vine, swamp cabbage or water spinach. Plants commonly considered as weeds, such as nettle or the peppery-flavoured purslane, can give an added taste to soups and stews, and unusual vegetables like the ridged gourd, or the hairy gourd (which looks rather like furry zucchini) can sometimes be bought fresh from specialist shops. Some vegetables are available for short periods only, such as the unusual winter melon, a large, white vegetable which Chinese chefs carve into fantastic soup bowls for traditional banquets, and whose flesh tastes similar to the chayote, or choko.

Fresh vegetables, either home grown or from well run markets or supermarkets, are most people's first choice, but the alternatives of frozen and canned vegetables offer convenience, reliability of supply and a more stable price throughout the year. Fortunately, a high proportion of the nutrients remain in these processed foods. Dehydrated vegetables are also useful, but much of the vitamin C and folate are lost. The losses are smaller with the freeze-dried varieties.

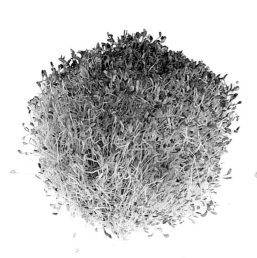

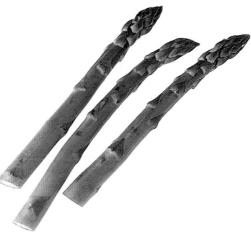

Alfalfa Sprouts *Medicago sativa*

also called Lucerne sprouts

MAJOR NUTRIENTS — SERVE SIZE 3 G

Energy	4 kJ	Cholesterol	0
Protein	0	Sodium	0
Fat	0	Dietary Fibre	0
Carbohydrate	0		

NUTRITIONAL INFORMATION In a small serving, nutrients are not significant.

DESCRIPTION A very fine, short sprout with a pale green stalk and fresh green tip.

ORIGIN AND HISTORY Any whole seed is capable of sprouting and is then known as a bean sprout or grain sprout. The bean sprout is produced from certain legumes (or pulses) such as mung bean, soya bean, lentil, fenugreek, and alfalfa bean, whereas the grain sprout can be produced from wheat, barley, corn, maize, and oats. The alfalfa legume is also known as lucerne or buffalo herb. It was first grown by the Arabs for their horses, as its high protein content helped develop remarkable strength in the animals. The alfalfa plant is used as a food supplement in third-world countries in the form of powder, cereal, and flour. The leaves make a beneficial tea, rich in manganese. In a larger serving than above, they are a good source of vitamin C and riboflavin. The fat and starch content is converted into easily digestible vitamins, proteins and simpler starches.

BUYING AND STORAGE Choose springy alfalfa sprouts with a fresh smell. Avoid slimy, wet sprouts with brown stains.

Store in a well-ventilated container in the refrigerator for up to 4 days.

PREPARATION AND USE Rinse sprouts in cold water and drain well if liked or use as bought if hygienically packaged.

Use in salads, sandwiches and for garnishing. Serve with eggs, seafood and Chinese dishes.

Asparagus *Asparagus officinalis*

MAJOR NUTRIENTS — BOILED SERVE SIZE 50 G

Energy	20 kJ	Sodium	0
Protein	0	Dietary Fibre	0
Fat	0	Vitamin C	5 mg
Carbohydrate	0	Vitamin E	1 mg
Cholesterol	0		

NUTRITIONAL INFORMATION This is a good source of vitamin C; moderate source of vitamin E.

DESCRIPTION The young shoot of a green plant with feathery leaves.

ORIGIN AND HISTORY This plant is thought to have originated in the eastern Mediterranean region and Asia Minor. The Greeks ate it wild and the Romans ate it both wild and cultivated, in 200 BC, according to precise growing instructions recorded by Cato at that time. Asparagus came into vogue in France under Louis XIV and it was introduced to the other courts of Europe, which looked to France in matters of culinary fashion. Asparagus has often been served with rich sauces, in contrast to its delicate shape and unique flavour, which may be one of the reasons why it is a symbol of epicurean taste. Asparagus has also been valued for over 2 000 years for its medicinal properties as a diuretic, a laxative, to restore eyesight, ease toothache, and cure a bee's sting. It is an important member of the lily family and has brought fame to restaurants in Argenteuil in France, Malines in Belgium, and Heidelberg in Germany, which serve it in dozens of delicious ways, during the asparagus season in spring.

BUYING AND STORAGE Available from spring to summer. Choose straight spears with a fresh green or fresh white colour, with large but tightly compressed pointed tips.

Very perishable so store as bought, without washing, in the vegetable crisper or in a plastic bag with a kitchen paper towel inside, in a refrigerator. Stores for 2–3 days only. Canning does not significantly affect nutrients.

PREPARATION AND USE Snap off coarse base or cut off at a point where the stalk is tender. Trim scales off stalk from the base to the buds at the top. Wash in cold water and drain. Cook asparagus spears whole by boiling briefly in a frying pan or tie in a bunch and boil upright in a special asparagus pan, or cook in a microwave oven. If serving cold, plunge into iced water after cooking, to retain fresh colour.

Serve cold with French or vinaigrette dressing or add to a salad. Serve hot as a vegetable or with a classic hollandaise sauce, or use in soups, quiches, Chinese stir-fry and savoury dishes.

PROCESSING Can be canned.

VARIETIES

Green and white (or blanched green) asparagus, each type with many sub-varieties. The green is cut as soon as the tips of the stalks are 20 cm above the ground. The blanched white is the same variety as the green but is cut while the stalk is still below the ground.

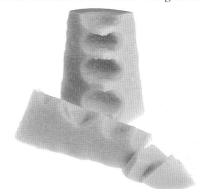

Bamboo Shoot *Phyllostachys edulis*

also called Juk soon, Rebung, Takenoko

MAJOR NUTRIENTS — SERVE SIZE 50 G

Energy	60 kJ	Dietary Fibre	0.5 g
Protein	1 g	Potassium	270 mg
Fat	0	Thiamin	0.1 mg
Carbohydrate	3 g	Vitamin C	2 mg
Cholesterol	0		

NUTRITIONAL INFORMATION A moderate source of potassium, thiamin and vitamin C. Good for weight-watchers.

DESCRIPTION The tender young shoot of an edible bamboo plant, cream-coloured, and fibrous in texture. The shoot has a round base which tapers in layers to a point, and the interior is interspersed with graduated cavities. Raw shoots are covered with layers of brown husk which must be removed before cooking. The spring bamboo shoot is small, sweet-tasting, and pale in colour, while the winter bamboo shoot is of a different type, being thinner, longer, and of a creamy-yellow colour. It has a more pronounced flavour than the spring bamboo shoot which is enjoyed throughout Asia for its unique delicate taste and crunchy texture.

ORIGIN AND HISTORY The bamboo plant is native to Asia, growing in almost every Asian country. However, it was in ancient China that the delicately flavoured root was discovered as a food, while its almost indestructible stems had many uses in the kitchen and as utensils, cooking vessels and furniture. Slips of bamboo were used as the first writing paper, for fortune-telling, and for scaffolding in construction. Some 6th century records name a 'bamboo leaf wine', but this was most probably a rice or millet wine coloured by an infusion of the leaves. In this same period the Imperial Bamboo Gardens provided the tender shoot for the emperor's table. An excellent variety was sent from the Yangtze Estuary and a fine quality winter variety from southern Shensi province.

BUYING AND STORAGE Generally sold canned in water as whole shoots or slices. This form will keep indefinitely. Once opened, the canned bamboo shoots should be transferred to a non-metal container and can be stored for up to 1 week. Change the water several times.

The fresh bamboo shoot can sometimes be purchased, and will keep for several weeks in the refrigerator. Some Chinese greengrocers stock it preboiled.

Store in the refrigerator in plain or lightly salted water for up to 10 days, changing the water several times.

PREPARATION AND USE The fresh bamboo shoot should be peeled to remove the husk, trimmed across the base of the shoot, and boiled in lightly salted water or starch water (water used to wash rice) until tender. Use whole, cubed or sliced in stir-fried, braised and simmered dishes. Particularly favoured in Chinese cooking.

PROCESSING Peeled and left whole, cut into chunks, or sliced, the shoot is boiled in water and canned in unsalted water. Some companies pack it processed in glass jars.

For salted bamboo shoot, strips of the fresh bamboo shoot are salt pickled, turning it a light brown colour with a soft, pliable texture. This is used mainly in soups and braised dishes for its strong flavour. Rinse well to remove salt before cooking. Sold in cellophane or plastic packs, the shoot will keep indefinitely in a covered jar.

VARIETIES
Winter bamboo shoot, spring bamboo shoot.

Bean, Green *Phaseolus coccineus, P. vulgaris*

DESCRIPTION The green, succulent bean is valued for the crisp flesh of its pod and the flavour of the seed inside.

ORIGIN AND HISTORY The green bean is the best known of all the edible pod vegetables. It is thought to have originated in tropical Central America and spread to North and South America before white settlers arrived. There is evidence that the green bean was cultivated in the Americas in the 7th century and early explorers later found the climbing bean planted with the sweet corn. The green bean was taken to Europe in the 16th century and to England from France in 1594. It became known as the French bean. The scarlet-flowered runner bean was introduced into England during the early 17th century as a decorative plant. By the end of the 19th century the green bean was established as a popular vegetable in Europe and, although it is a perennial, it is cultivated as an annual. Some varieties produce a yellow wax bean, some produce a purple bean which turns green when cooked. Some plants that are not *Phaseolus* are also known as beans, such as the winged asparagus bean or pea, sometimes found in Asian foodstores.

BUYING AND STORAGE Available all year round, peaking in spring and summer. Choose the young, firm, fresh-coloured beans, free from blemishes, which snap easily and contain small seeds (beans).

Store in the vegetable crisper or in a plastic bag in a refrigerator. Will store for up to 5 days.

PREPARATION AND USE Wash the beans, cut or snap off tops and tails and remove any strings. Leave whole or cut into short lengths or slice thinly with a special bean slicer.

Cook until just tender, in a microwave oven or by steaming, boiling or stir-frying. If serving cold, plunge into iced water after cooking, to retain fresh colour.

Serve hot as a vegetable, plain or dressed, or serve cold in a salad.

PROCESSING Can be frozen.

VARIETIES

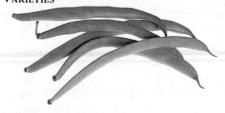

French/Haricot Bean **Phaseolus vulgaris** is a bush bean, small, tender and stringless.

MAJOR NUTRIENTS			BOILED SERVE SIZE 60 G
Energy	80 kJ	Sodium	0
Protein	0	Dietary Fibre	2 g
Fat	0	Iron	0.4 mg
Carbohydrate	4 g	Vitamin A	38 µg
Cholesterol	0	Vitamin C	3 mg

NUTRITIONAL INFORMATION This is a good source of vitamin C; moderate source of vitamin A (beta carotene), iron, fibre and folate.

Runner Bean **Phaseolus coccineus** is a climbing bean, larger and coarser than the French, with tough strings (some varieties are stringless).

MAJOR NUTRIENTS			BOILED SERVE SIZE 60 G
Energy	50 kJ	Sodium	0
Protein	0	Dietary Fibre	2 g
Fat	0	Iron	0.4 mg
Carbohydrate	2 g	Vitamin A	40 µg
Cholesterol	0	Vitamin C	3 mg

NUTRITIONAL INFORMATION This is a good source of vitamin C; moderate source of fibre, folate and vitamin A. The raw runner bean has three times as much vitamin C as the cooked.

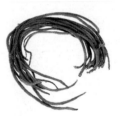

Snake Bean

MAJOR NUTRIENTS		YOUNG PODS WITH SEEDS SERVE SIZE 100 G	
Energy	180 kJ	Calcium	65 mg
Protein	3 g	Phosphorus	65 mg
Fat	0	Iron	1 mg
Carbohydrate	10 g	Vitamin A	480 µg
Cholesterol	0	Thiamin	0.15 mg
Dietary Fibre	2 g	Riboflavin	0.1 mg
Sodium	5 mg	Niacin Equiv.	1 mg
Potassium	215 mg	Vitamin C	33 mg

NUTRITIONAL INFORMATION An excellent source of vitamin C, vitamin A, iron and potassium and a good source of thiamin. Only a moderate source of calcium, phosphorus, riboflavin and niacin.

DESCRIPTION *Vigna unguiculata; V sinensis* var. *sesquipedalis*, is the haricot baguette of France, a long, round-bodied thin bean which is used throughout South-East Asia. It grows to at least 40 cm and has earned the various names: long-podded cow bean or cow pea; yard long bean; snake bean. It has a taste and texture similar to a green bean. In colour, it varies from a very deep to a pale green.

ORIGIN AND HISTORY This is an ancient Chinese vegetable, it is in the same genus as cow pea and black-eyed pea. The southern Chinese eat the young bean whole, the northerners patiently await seed maturation and use the vegetable dried. It is known in China as doh gok and in Indonesia as kalang panjang.

BUYING AND STORAGE Sold fresh tied in loops of 6 or more beans.

Store unwrapped or loosely wrapped in plastic in the vegetable compartment of the refrigerator for up to 1 week.

PREPARATION AND USE Cut crossways into lengths and use as other green beans, in stir-fried dishes, as a vegetable, in curries or soups.

Bean Sprout *Phaseolus aureus; Glycine max*

also called **Bean shoot**

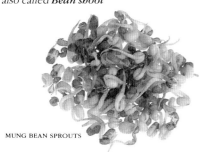

MUNG BEAN SPROUTS

MAJOR NUTRIENTS		MUNG BEAN SPROUTS SERVE SIZE 100 G	
Energy	150 kJ	Potassium	225 mg
Protein	4 g	Iron	1.3 mg
Fat	0	Thiamin	0.15 mg
Carbohydrate	6 g	Riboflavin	0.15 mg
Cholesterol	0	Vitamin C	19 mg
Sodium	5 mg		

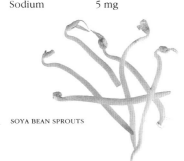

SOYA BEAN SPROUTS

MAJOR NUTRIENTS		SOYA BEAN SPROUTS SERVE SIZE 100 G	
Energy	190 kJ	Phosphorus	70 mg
Protein	6 g	Iron	1 mg
Fat	1 g	Thiamin	0.2 mg
Carbohydrate	5 g	Riboflavin	0.2 mg
Cholesterol	0	Niacin Equiv.	1 mg
Dietary Fibre	1 g	Vitamin C	13 mg
Calcium	50 mg		

NUTRITIONAL INFORMATION Mung bean sprouts are an excellent source of vitamin C and iron; a good source of thiamin; a moderate source of potassium and riboflavin.

Soya bean sprouts are an excellent source of iron, thiamin and vitamin C; a good source of riboflavin; a moderate source of calcium, phosphorus and niacin.

DESCRIPTION The sprouted mung bean is about 5 cm long, a translucent white colour and with a short tapering root at one end and a green-sheathed small, pale yellow pod at the other. The soya bean sprout is up to double the size of a mung bean sprout, and with long roots and a large oval-shaped yellow bean on top. The flavour is stronger, the texture coarser. The fresh soya bean has a nutty flavour and crisp texture.

ORIGIN AND HISTORY The most commonly sprouted bean is the small, round lemon-green mung bean, so to many people bean sprout means mung bean sprout, but many other legumes are capable of sprouting (see Alfalfa Sprout). The mung bean is a native of tropical Asia and has been cultivated in China and India for thousands of years where it is still very popular. The whole dried bean is used in stews and savoury dishes, and in a porridge. The mung bean is also known as the green gram, golden gram or Oregon pea and the green-seeded bean is generally used for sprouting or cooking. The processes used in the commercial bean sprout industry are protected with great secrecy but it is very easy to grow bean sprouts at home. Place the dried seeds inside a large glass jar, cover with muslin and secure with a rubber band. Rinse several times a day with warm water, then leave the jar on its side to drain. The seeds should sprout within 6 days but keep the jar in a warm place out of direct sunlight.

BUYING AND STORAGE Bean sprouts are readily available in the refrigerated section of most supermarkets. Avoid buying sprouts with a greyish tinge or limp feel as they are not fresh.

Store in the refrigerator for up to one week. It is preferable that bean sprouts be eaten while very fresh as toxic substances can build up in older sprouts.

PREPARATION AND USE Both the mung and the soya bean are used extensively in eastern Asia. Rinse and drain sprouts. Use whole in Chinese stir-fried dishes, or pick off roots and beanpods and use just the silvery-white sprout (silver sprouts) in stir-fried dishes, soups and raw in salads. If using canned sprouts, drain, then soak in iced water for 30 minutes to improve their crispness.

PROCESSING The bean sprout is available canned, but the sprouts lose their crispness and much of their flavour.

SEE ALSO Mung bean, Soya bean.

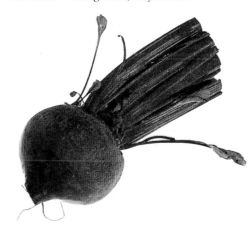

Beetroot *Beta vulgaris*

also called **Beet**

MAJOR NUTRIENTS		SERVE SIZE 25 G	
Energy	30 kJ	Cholesterol	0
Protein	0	Sodium	0
Fat	0	Dietary Fibre	0
Carbohydrate	2 g		

NUTRITIONAL INFORMATION An excellent source of folate although boiling reduces this by nearly half.

DESCRIPTION A rounded root vegetable with dark brown-purple skin and distinctive purple flesh.

ORIGIN AND HISTORY In the Middle Ages the beetroot was developed from a sprawling plant which grew from the seashores of the Mediterranean to the Caspian Sea. Originally the leaves only were eaten in pre-Christian times as the roots of the wild varieties were much smaller than those of the cultivated varieties. There is a reference in Roman literature of AD200 to cooking the small roots but the next reference to cooking beetroot is not found until in 15th century English recipes. An improved variety, Roman beet, was recorded in Italy, France, and Germany in the 16th century. Today the root is used far more than the leaves as it stays fresh longer and is easily stored.

BUYING AND STORAGE Available all year. Choose firm, clean, smooth, globe-shaped, rich red-coloured beetroot without soft, wet areas, and with fresh, clean, young leaves, if still attached.

To store, cut leaves off 50 mm above the beetroot and store leaves and beetroot in the vegetable crisper of a refrigerator. Leaves store for 1–2 days but beetroot stores for 4–5 days.

PREPARATION AND USE To prepare beetroot, wash in cold water with a soft vegetable brush, then cook whole in boiling water or bake in the oven or cook in a microwave oven. Peel and use according to recipe. Alternatively peel raw beetroot, then grate or dice and sauté in butter.

To prepare beetroot leaves, trim leaves from stalks, wash in cold water, drain lightly and boil rapidly as for spinach.

Use beetroot hot as a vegetable, in orange or sweet and sour sauce, grated in the classic Russian borsch soup, or use cold in salads and pickled. Use beetroot leaves as for spinach.

PROCESSING Can be canned and pickled.

VARIETIES

Three other beets have been developed from the same seashore plant, namely the leaf beet or chard, used as a green vegetable, the larger sugar beet, used to manufacture sugar not eaten as a vegetable, and the mangold or mangel-wurzel which is now grown for feeding livestock.

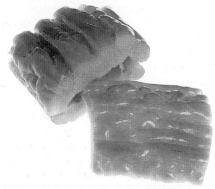

Bitter Melon Momordica charantia

also called **Bitter gourd, Balsam pear, Fu kwa, Karela, Peria, Pare**

MAJOR NUTRIENTS			SERVE SIZE 100 G
Energy	40 kJ	Potassium	260 mg
Protein	2 g	Magnesium	15 mg
Fat	0	Iron	1 mg
Carbohydrate	1 g	Vitamin A	65 µg
Cholesterol	0	Thiamin	0.1 mg
Dietary Fibre	4 g	Riboflavin	0.4 mg
Sodium	5 mg	Vitamin C	50 mg

NUTRITIONAL INFORMATION An excellent source of vitamin C, iron, riboflavin and folate; a moderate source of vitamin A. It also contains copper. Canned bitter melon has a high sodium content.

DESCRIPTION A mid-green, cucumberlike vegetable with a knobbly, wrinkled skin. Usually about 18 cm long, it has a fibrous melonlike core containing numerous white seeds when in its unripe stage, which is when it is eaten. On ripening it turns a deep orange

to red colour. The flesh is bitter tasting, although this partially dissipates during cooking.

ORIGIN AND HISTORY Native to South-East Asia, it was originally used as a medicinal food to purify the blood, as it has a cooling, cleansing effect on the system. It has been an important pickling ingredient in India for many centuries.

PREPARATION AND USE Indonesians enjoy it in cooked salads. To the Indians the karela makes a palate-stimulating tart pickle. The Chinese use it in stir-fries, and when sliced, filled with minced pork and steamed with a black bean sauce it is incomparable in its subtle blending of flavours. Although its bitterness makes it one of the less frequently used Asian vegetables it holds a place in the cuisines of South-East Asia which no other vegetable can fill.

BUYING AND STORAGE Choose when young, unripe and firm.

It can be kept unwrapped for several weeks in the vegetable compartment of the refrigerator.

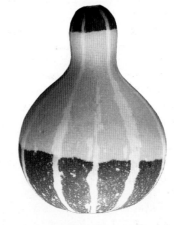

Bottle Gourd Lagenaria siceraria

also called **Bu thei, Hu gwa, Labu air, Upo, Woo la gua**

MAJOR NUTRIENTS			SERVE SIZE 100 G
Energy	70 kJ	Sodium	5 mg
Protein	1 g	Potassium	150 mg
Fat	0	Iron	0.5 mg
Carbohydrate	3 g	Zinc	0.7 mg
Cholesterol	0	Vitamin C	10 mg

NUTRITIONAL INFORMATION An excellent source of vitamin C; a moderate source of potassium, iron and zinc.

DESCRIPTION A green squash with a smooth tough skin. Gourds come in many shapes and sizes, the more familiar being bottle-shaped. Similar to zucchini in taste and texture.

ORIGIN AND HISTORY The bottle gourd or squash has a long and colourful history, beginning life well over 5 000 years BC in Africa from where it is said to have floated to South America. There it readily took root, and was then carried on to Asia where it now grows prolifically. Its name comes not from its bottlelike shape, but from the fact that for many centuries, the hardened dried skin of the gourd was one of the only receptacles for carrying liquids. In South America an ancient tradition of trace-carving intricate patterns and scenes into the shell of these gourds still continues today. In China, carvings in wood, jade and precious metals, and art through the ages, celebrate its attractive shapes.

BUYING AND STORAGE Choose the gourd which is firm and with an unblemished skin. It will keep for many weeks.

PREPARATION AND USE It is used extensively throughout China, Burma, the Philippines, and Malaysia. Peel, rinse, and slice. Stir-fry or add to braised dishes and soups. Zucchini, fuzzy melon or winter melon and other squash can be substituted.

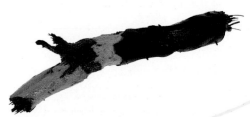

Bracken Root Pteridium esculentum

MAJOR NUTRIENTS			SERVE SIZE 50 G
Energy	200 kJ	Cholesterol	0
Protein	1 g	Dietary Fibre	17 g
Fat	0	Sodium	5 mg
Carbohydrate	11 g	Iron	2 mg

NUTRITIONAL INFORMATION This is a low energy fibrous food. The iron content is high but may not be well absorbed.

DESCRIPTION The edible portion of bracken root is the starch extracted from the underground stem or rhizome.

ORIGIN AND HISTORY Bracken and fern roots were important sources of starch for a number of peoples.

The New Zealand Maoris pounded fern root and made a flour-like substance from it. The North American Indians ate the bracken rhizome to treat intestinal worms. The rhizomes were an important food for many Aboriginal groups in south-eastern Australia and could be considered a staple at times.

BUYING AND STORAGE Not commercially available. If harvested, extract the starch and store dried.

PREPARATION AND USE Roast the rhizome and peel away the outer bark. Hammer the fibrous stem with a wooden mallet to remove the starch from between the fibres and discard the fibre residue. Collect the starch, sieve it and dry for storage or mix with water to a dough and bake as for bread or damper.

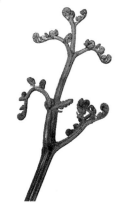

Bracken Tip *Pteridium esculentum*

also called Fiddlehead fern

MAJOR NUTRIENTS		SERVE SIZE 50 G	
Energy	210 kJ	Cholesterol	0
Protein	6 g	Dietary Fibre	7 g
Fat	1 g	Sodium	5 mg
Carbohydrate	4 g		

NUTRITIONAL INFORMATION Like many green leafy vegetables, this bush food is a low energy food that supplies important nutrients such as protein and fibre. It also contributes iron (1 mg/100 g) and zinc (2 mg/100 g) to the diet.

DESCRIPTION The new, uncurled, bracken fern frond tip while at the fiddlehead or crozier stage.

ORIGIN AND HISTORY The bracken's related species *P. aquilinum* has a long history of use as a vegetable in Japan, where it is used raw like lettuce or cooked and served like broccoli.

BUYING AND STORAGE Not widely available as a market product in Australia but Asian food outlets occasionally stock imported bracken tips boiled and tinned. For domestic use, bracken is best picked fresh.

PREPARATION AND USE Tips *must* be well roasted in order to heat-degrade a carcinogenic component. Once roasted the tips can be lightly pan fried with tamari or soya sauce for a traditional Japanese dish or used as a low energy substitute for nuts in casseroles, curries, and stir-fry dishes.

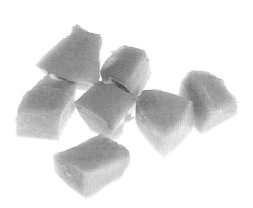

Breadfruit *Artocarpus communis*

MAJOR NUTRIENTS		SERVE SIZE 100 G	
Energy	430 kJ	Sodium	15 mg
Protein	2 g	Potassium	440 mg
Fat	0	Iron	1.2 mg
Carbohydrate	26 g	Thiamin	0.1 mg
Cholesterol	0	Niacin Equiv.	1 mg
Dietary Fibre	1 g	Vitamin C	29 mg

NUTRITIONAL INFORMATION An excellent source of vitamin C and iron; a good source of potassium; a moderate source of thiamin and niacin.

DESCRIPTION The large ovoid fruit of a tree native to Polynesia. It has a knobby, green skin separated into small 5-sided segments. The fibrous flesh when cooked, tastes like a yam or potato.

ORIGIN AND HISTORY There are about 40 species grown in Polynesia. The fruit has been a staple food of most of the Pacific Islands throughout their history. It was introduced to Hawaii by Tahitian settlers who made the hazardous journey across thousands of kilometres of ocean in their massive canoes. Captain Bligh in his infamous *Bounty* was transporting breadfruit trees from Tahiti to Jamaica when Fletcher Christian and his shipmates began the mutiny. Breadfruit is rarely eaten in Asia, but may be served in remote parts of Indonesia, and the Philippines.

BUYING AND STORAGE Sold fresh in markets where West Indian or Pacific Island foods are stocked. It should be green and hard for cooking as a vegetable. When yellow-brown and soft, it can be used for desserts.

PREPARATION AND USE Cut breadfruit in half, scoop out the white pulpy flesh and remove seeds. Boil flesh and use in place of potato or add sugar and milk and serve for a dessert. Seeds may be roasted like chestnuts. Also ground to a pastelike consistency it can be sweetened with fruit or sugar, or seasoned with savoury spices.

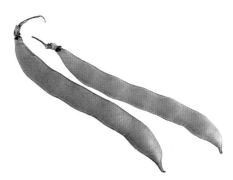

Broad Bean *Vicia faba*

also called Fava bean

MAJOR NUTRIENTS		BOILED SERVE SIZE 180 G	
Energy	370 kJ	Magnesium	50 mg
Protein	7 g	Phosphorus	178 mg
Fat	0	Iron	1.8 mg
Carbohydrate	13 g	Niacin Equiv.	4 mg
Cholesterol	0	Vitamin C	15 mg
Dietary Fibre	7 g	Vitamin A	75 µg
Sodium	0		

NUTRITIONAL INFORMATION High in carbohydrate. An excellent source of fibre, phosphorus, iron, niacin, vitamin C, pantothenic acid; good source of vitamin A.

An unusual bean as it contains beta carotene (the plant form of vitamin A), vitamin C and pantothenic acid, which are not typical nutrients of legumes.

DESCRIPTION A bean with a large flat green pod and large seeds.

ORIGIN AND HISTORY The broad bean is one of the oldest vegetables cultivated in the Western world. It has grown in Europe since prehistoric times, but the ancient bean was a small-seeded variety. Cultivated in England as early as the Iron Age it can be traced back to Swiss lake dwellings of the Bronze Age. It became a staple food for the poorer masses in Egypt and for the Greeks and Romans, in spite of strange beliefs concerning them. Egyptian priests thought the broad bean unclean, Pythagoras, the Greek, loathed it and in Italy it was known as a funeral plant as a bean feast traditionally ended a funeral there. The broad bean was also used as counters when voting in Roman elections. Today the bean is cultivated worldwide in temperate regions.

BUYING AND STORAGE It is available in spring and summer. Choose young tender pods with a fresh green colour and no blemishes. Avoid large, puffy broad beans.

Store in the vegetable crisper or in a plastic bag in the refrigerator for up to 7 days.

PREPARATION AND USE If the broad bean is very young, the pod is edible. Wash the beans, trim ends and remove any string. Cut each into 3 pieces. Boil, steam or cook in a microwave oven. Serve as for the green bean.

If mature, remove from pod, then boil, steam or cook in a microwave oven until tender. Serve hot with a sauce or pureed with hot boiled ham or use cold in a salad.

PROCESSING Can be canned, frozen and dried.

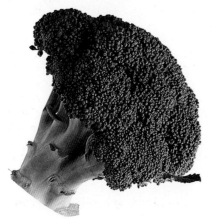

Broccoli *Brassica oleracea*

MAJOR NUTRIENTS			BOILED SERVE SIZE 60 G
Energy	45 kJ	Dietary Fibre	3 g
Protein	0	Vitamin A	250 µg
Fat	0	Iron	0.6 mg
Carbohydrate	1 g	Calcium	46 mg
Cholesterol	0	Vitamin E	1 mg
Sodium	0	Vitamin C	34 mg

NUTRITIONAL INFORMATION An excellent source of vitamin A, vitamin C, folate; good source of vitamin E; moderate source of fibre, calcium, iron. Boiling reduces the vitamin C content of raw broccoli by two-thirds but the vegetable remains a good source of vitamin C. It is a good source of vitamins for vegetarians.

DESCRIPTION Broccoli is a member of the cabbage and cauliflower family — a green vegetable with light clusters of green flowers which form a head.

ORIGIN AND HISTORY Originated in the Mediterranean and Asia Minor; cultivated in Italy in the 16th century. The word comes from the Italian word brocco meaning branch or arm.

BUYING AND STORAGE Available all year. Choose fresh-coloured, compact heads with tender stalks. Avoid yellow broccoli with tough hollow stalks.

Store, unwashed, in the vegetable crisper in a refrigerator for only 1 or 2 days.

PREPARATION AND USE Cut the broccoli florets off stalks in equal-sized pieces. Wash in cold, salted water to kill any insects. Steam or boil or stir-fry or cook in a microwave oven until just tender. Refresh in iced water if serving cold. Use cold in salads or hot as a vegetable, in soups, omelettes, stir-fries and with pasta.

PROCESSING Can be frozen.

VARIETIES

Apart from Chinese broccoli there are two main varieties, the green sprouting or 'heading' broccoli or Calabrese, and the purple 'hearting' broccoli which resembles a cauliflower in shape.

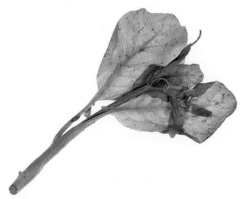

Chinese Broccoli *Brassica alboglabra*

NUTRITIONAL INFORMATION No reliable data are available.

DESCRIPTION A Chinese stem vegetable resembling flowering white cabbage, but with small white flowers and slightly darker green stems and leaves. It has a slightly bitter taste and crisp texture. Both leaves and stem are eaten.

ORIGIN AND HISTORY A native of southern China, until recently it was only known to have been cultivated in the southern states, in particular Guangzhou (Canton).

It is one of the world's most nutritious vegetables having the highest calcium content of any food, as well as iron, and vitamins A and C. It is said that a Chinese could survive indefinitely on a diet of unpolished rice and Chinese broccoli. It may also be known as Chinese kale, gai laarn, guy lan, kai laarn.

BUYING AND STORAGE Now available in Chinese fresh-food stores. Select vegetables with crisp, unmarked leaves and firm stems.

It will keep for up to 1 week in the vegetable compartment of the refrigerator, in plastic wrap.

PREPARATION AND USE Cut longer stems in half and cook them in boiling stock or water until crisp-tender. Serve Canton-style with oyster sauce. Cut into shorter lengths and use in stir-fried dishes, with noodles, and in soups. Broccoli, Chinese flowering white cabbage and cauliflower can be substituted.

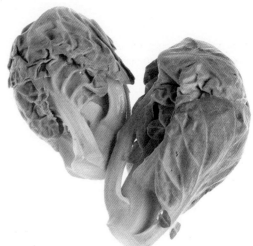

Brussels Sprout *Brassica oleracea* var. *gemmifera*

also called **Baby cabbage**

MAJOR NUTRIENTS			BOILED SERVE SIZE 70 G
Energy	113 kJ	Dietary Fibre	2 g
Protein	2 g	Phosphorus	50 mg
Fat	0	Iron	0.7 mg
Carbohydrate	3 g	Vitamin C	58 mg
Cholesterol	0	Vitamin A	67 µg
Sodium	0		

NUTRITIONAL INFORMATION An excellent source of vitamin C; moderate source of fibre, phosphorus, iron, vitamin A.

DESCRIPTION The plant is a member of the cabbage family which, instead of producing one large head, produces many tiny heads at the bases of the leaves along the stem.

ORIGIN AND HISTORY This vegetable has an obscure history. It is thought to have been cultivated in the market gardens of Brussels, Belgium, in the 13th century, according to discoveries in archaeological sites there. It became better known when it spread to French and English vegetable gardens between 1800 and 1850. A luxury vegetable in the British Isles, especially when picked small, where the cold climate is particularly suitable for cultivation. It is still served today with a traditional English Christmas dinner. The Brussels sprout is a perennial green vegetable now grown in Europe, America and Australia, but all too often is allowed to grow too big, which coarsens its flavour and texture.

BUYING AND STORAGE Available all year but at its best in winter. Choose firm, compact, crisp, bright green sprouts. The small ones have the best flavour.

Store in the vegetable crisper, or in a plastic bag with a paper towel in the refrigerator for up to 7 days.

PREPARATION AND USE Wash in cold water, remove any loose or damaged leaves, trim the stem end, then score stem with a cross to allow heat to penetrate. Cook by boiling, steaming, stir-frying or in a microwave oven until just tender. Do not overcook or a sulphur smell develops.

Use as a dressed vegetable, in soups, savoury dishes, and casseroles. Shred raw into salads.

PROCESSING Can be frozen.

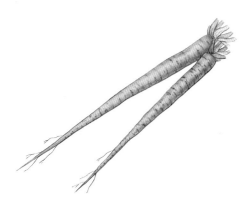

Burdock Root *Arctium lappa*

also called **Gobo**

NUTRITIONAL INFORMATION No reliable data are available, but carbohydrate content is high.

DESCRIPTION A slender root vegetable with white flesh and a brown covering. It has an earthy flavour and crunchy texture.

ORIGIN AND HISTORY A member of the aster family, this biennial plant grows wild in China and Japan. One of the world's cheapest natural medicines, Chinese in the past ate it for health, attributing it with great medicinal value. Even in Japan, it was eaten as early as the 10th century as a source of energy and to speed recovery from illness.

BUYING AND STORAGE Available fresh in specialist Asian greengrocers. Choose long thin roots, no thicker than 2 cm and about 40 cm long. Scrub thoroughly, although it is not necessary to remove the skin which is edible. Cut into pieces by using the tip of a sharp knife to shave off points, in the same way as sharpening a pencil. Immediately submerge in cold water, with a few drops of vinegar or lemon juice added, to prevent discoloration.

The fresh burdock root can be kept in the refrigerator for up to 1–3 weeks. Also available in cans, but the vegetable loses much of its characteristic taste and texture.

PREPARATION AND USE Use in stir-fried and simmered dishes. It has no distinct flavour but absorbs and retains the flavour of seasonings and other ingredients. It can be made into a strong-tasting pickle.

Cabbage *Brassica oleracea*

MAJOR NUTRIENTS			STEAMED SERVE SIZE 50 G
Energy	50 kJ	Sodium	0
Protein	0	Dietary Fibre	0
Fat	0	Vitamin C	24 mg
Carbohydrate	3 g	Vitamin A	variable
Cholesterol	0		

NUTRITIONAL INFORMATION An excellent source of vitamin C; good source of folate; moderate source of vitamin A. Cabbage is high in vitamin C and may also contain some beta carotene, but this depends on the amount of chlorophyll and the outer leaves of the cabbage may contain 50 times as much beta carotene as the inner white ones. Raw cabbage has a higher level of vitamin C and folate.

DESCRIPTION A green leaf vegetable forming a tightly folded head. Cabbage is a member of the *Brassica* genus and is related to broccoli, Brussels sprout, cauliflower, kale, and kohlrabi.

ORIGIN AND HISTORY There is some evidence that the cabbage may have originated in the eastern Mediterranean and Asia Minor and there are references to cultivated cabbage plants in Roman writings. Yet a leafy wild variety also grew for centuries on the British and European coasts. The Celts are thought to have introduced the cabbage into northern Europe in 600 BC where it has since become the national vegetable. The word cabbage in the English, French, German, Norwegian, and Swedish languages can be traced to Celtic root words. The smooth, hard-head cabbage of today, however, was unknown until AD 800. Later, reference was made to the difference between the hard head and the non-heading cabbage, called colewarts, in 13th-century writings. Gradually the hard-head variety developed by Celtic and Nordic peoples became popular as the vegetable of the masses. The sauerkraut process was introduced to Germany by the Slavs. The French introduced the cabbage to Canada; the Dutch settlers took it to North America; and the early white settlers took it to Australia. Chinese cabbage is native to China.

BUYING AND STORAGE Available all year with more varieties available in winter. Choose firm, crisp cabbage, heavy for its size, with crackling fresh, bright-coloured leaves.

Store in a vegetable crisper, or in a plastic bag with a paper towel, in the refrigerator.

PREPARATION AND USE Remove any discoloured leaves. Cut off amount of cabbage to be used and wash in cold water. Slice thinly and use according to recipe. Steam, boil or cook in a microwave oven with a walnut added to reduce odour. Do not overcook or a sulphur smell and flavour develops. The round smooth head is used for stuffed cabbage leaves and served as a cooked vegetable in soups and casseroles, the pointed head variety likewise. Savoy is good raw, sliced into salad. Red cabbage is stewed with apple and onion or pickled. White cabbage is used for coleslaw and sauerkraut. Chinese cabbage is used in Chinese cuisine, particularly in stir-fries.

PROCESSING Used to make sauerkraut, which may be canned.

VARIETIES

Chinese Flowering White Cabbage

NUTRITIONAL INFORMATION Similar to Chinese white cabbage.

DESCRIPTION *Brassica chinensis* var. *parachinensis* has long pale to mid-green stems with rounded pale to mid-green leaves. The small yellow flowers at the tips of the inner stems resemble those of the central stem of the Chinese white cabbage when it is in bud. It is commonly believed that the two are closely related. Its Chinese name choy sum means vegetable heart, which is possibly a reference to the heart of the white cabbage.

This cabbage has a distinct flavour with a characteristic mild bitterness. The stems are preferred to the leaves.

ORIGIN AND HISTORY There is no exact knowledge of how this vegetable developed in China, but until recently, it was unique to that country.

BUYING AND STORAGE Select vegetables with crisp unmarked stems. Leaves may be trimmed back. Most well-stocked Asian food stores now sell fresh Chinese cabbage of several types.

Wrap in plastic and store in the vegetable compartment of the refrigerator for up to 1 week.

PREPARATION AND USE Cut in halves, poach until crisp-tender in unsalted water and serve with oyster sauce. Cut into 5 cm lengths and use in stir-fries and other Chinese dishes, or as a substitute for common broccoli.

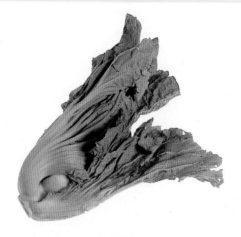

Chinese Mustard Cabbage

MAJOR NUTRIENTS		SERVE SIZE 100 G	
Energy	130 kJ	Calcium	180 mg
Protein	3 g	Phosphorus	50 mg
Fat	0	Iron	1 mg
Carbohydrate	6 g	Thiamin	0.1 mg
Cholesterol	0	Riboflavin	0.2 mg
Dietary Fibre	1 g	Niacin Equiv.	1 mg
Sodium	30 mg	Vitamin C	97 mg
Potassium	380 mg	Vitamin A	2100 µg

NUTRITIONAL INFORMATION An excellent source of vitamin A, vitamin C and calcium; good source of thiamin, iron and riboflavin; moderate source of phosphorus and niacin. Also a good source of potassium.

DESCRIPTION Dai gai choy or Swatow mustard cabbage (*Brassica alba*) has thick, pale green, grooved, curving stems with a small fringe of deeper green leaf along the edges and across the top of the stems. They curve inwards into a head and somewhat resemble a loose-leafed lettuce. Chuk gai choy or bamboo mustard cabbage (*Brassica cernua*) has ribbed mid- to bright-green stalks with the leaves extending along the stalks almost to the base. It grows in length to about 30 cm.

ORIGIN AND HISTORY Known to grow wild in China from neolithic times. Mustard cabbage is cultivated extensively, particularly in central China, with the best bamboo mustard cabbage growing near the Yangtze River. Marco Polo observed that the wealthy Chinese of Hangchow had a passion for obtaining the very first vegetables of the season, among these the mustard cabbage, eggplants, and cucumbers. Mustard cabbage has a pungent flavour. The Swatow type is rarely eaten fresh, being made into a salty pickle which is the backbone of flavourings in many central Chinese dishes. The bamboo type, though unpleasantly strong in taste when raw, becomes subtle and delicate after parboiling. Yang Fang noted in the Sung dynasty that sons of officials 'were unwilling to eat vegetables, looking on greens and broth as coarse fare'. The Chinese gourmet has a long history.

BUYING AND STORAGE Swatow mustard cabbage is very occasionally available fresh in select Asian food stores. Pickled mustard cabbage is sold by the piece from large pottery storage jars, or is packed into plastic bags or tubs.

It will keep indefinitely in the refrigerator in a sealed container.

PREPARATION AND USE Swatow mustard cabbage is best used in moderation in braised dishes and soups as its flavour is rather too astringent to use as a plain vegetable. Bamboo mustard cabbage can be chopped and added to soups, or parboiled, drained and served dressed with vegetable oil and oyster sauce. Its strong flavour also marries well with garlic, ginger and black beans.

Chinese White Cabbage

MAJOR NUTRIENTS		SERVE SIZE 100 G	
Energy	70 kJ	Iron	0.8 mg
Protein	2 g	Sodium	25 mg
Fat	0	Potassium	305 mg
Carbohydrate	3 g	Riboflavin	0.1 mg
Dietary Fibre	0.5 g	Niacin Equiv.	1 mg
Cholesterol	0	Vitamin C	25 mg
Calcium	165 mg	Vitamin A	930 µg

NUTRITIONAL INFORMATION An excellent source of vitamin C, vitamin A and calcium; good source of iron and potassium; moderate source of riboflavin and niacin.

DESCRIPTION *Brassica chinensis* is a vegetable of the *Brassica* family, with long, fleshy, thick white stems and mid-green leaves similar in shape to spinach. It can grow to 65 cm, but is at its best when young, about 18 cm. A mild cabbagelike flavour, and crisp texture.

ORIGIN AND HISTORY Native to southern China, it is believed to have been cultivated for over 3000 years. The ancient Chou text *Shih ching* lists no fewer than 46 plants that may be called vegetables, of which *Brassica chinensis* is one. Along with taro and yams, these vegetables antedated rice as the staple foods of China. The Cantonese regard it as the pinnacle of perfection in the vegetable world, while northerners prefer their own Peking cabbage. It is also called bok choy, pak chai, pau t'sai, Chinese chard, and white mustard cabbage. It remained unknown in the Western world until the Chinese gold rush to the USA and later to Australia. It was first grown in these countries by Chinese market gardeners, for sale in oriental markets only, however, nowadays it is found more and more in other markets.

BUYING AND STORAGE Choose young cabbages with firm unmarked stems and leaves.

Store in a plastic bag in the vegetable compartment of the refrigerator for up to 1 week.

PREPARATION AND USE Cut in halves and cook in water or stock to serve as a vegetable. Slice across the stems and roughly chop the leaves, and use in stir-fries, braised and simmered dishes or soups. In China white cabbage, halved lengthways and quickly poached, is served with a crabmeat or shrimp roe sauce. The small and tender young heart is much prized for its tenderness and delicate flavour.

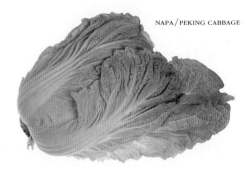

NAPA / PEKING CABBAGE

Napa/Peking Cabbage

MAJOR NUTRIENTS		SERVE SIZE 100 G	
Energy	60 kJ	Calcium	45 mg
Protein	1 g	Iron	0.6 mg
Fat	0	Sodium	25 mg
Carbohydrate	3 g	Potassium	255 mg
Cholesterol	0	Vitamin A	45 µg
Dietary Fibre	0.5 g	Vitamin C	25 mg

NUTRITIONAL INFORMATION An excellent source of vitamin C; good source of iron; moderate source of calcium, vitamin A and potassium.

DESCRIPTION *Brassica pekinensis* is the large, cylindrical-shaped, tightly packed Chinese cabbage which looks very much like a cos (romaine) lettuce. It has a mild but distinct flavour. The ribs are thick and wide, light cream-white in colour, the leaves long and narrow attaching the full length of the ribs, and of a pale green colour.

ORIGIN AND HISTORY Like its relatives, the Peking cabbage is a native of China, growing in most provinces and particularly in the north, hence its common name of Peking or Tientsin cabbage. In winter a familiar sight on Beijing roadsides is stacks of fresh cabbage brought in from nearby market gardens, protected from winter chills by a covering of blankets. As a prime source of vitamins, when fresh cabbage cannot be served, a meal in the north must include a dish of crunchy, chilli-impregnated pickled cabbage. It is also known as wombok/wong ngabok, Chinese white cabbage, giant white cabbage, celery cabbage.

BUYING AND STORAGE Inspect the cabbage for rust marks and insect holes, otherwise all but the very large ones (45 cm) should be tender and mildly flavoured.

Can be stored for up to 2 weeks in the vegetable compartment of the refrigerator, the leaves protected from drying out by plastic wrap.

PREPARATION AND USE The thicker parts of the stems should be cut into narrow strips, the smaller stems and leaves can be roughly chopped to stir-fry or braise, to use in hot-pots, soups, and in noodle dishes. It can be used as a substitute for cabbage in coleslaw and other dishes, but common cabbage does not make an ideal substitute for napa cabbage, having a much stronger taste and smell. Braised cabbage is often served with a creamy sauce which may contain crab or shrimp.

Pointed Head Cabbage A spring cabbage.

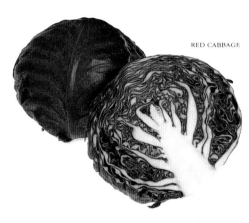
RED CABBAGE

Red Cabbage Round, smooth and purple-red in colour.

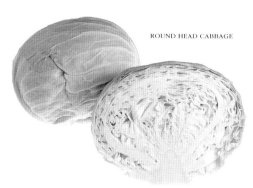
ROUND HEAD CABBAGE

Round, Smooth Head Cabbage The common cabbage.

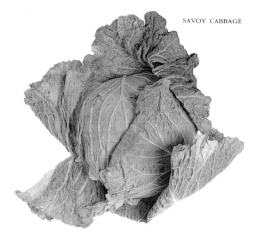
SAVOY CABBAGE

Savoy Cabbage Similar to a round head, with wrinkled leaves.

Spring Greens Young cabbages with no hearts, native to Europe and western Asia and harvested when young cabbages are being thinned. Buy in spring.

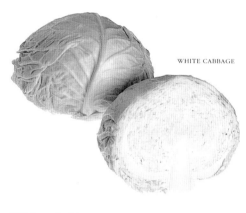
WHITE CABBAGE

White Cabbage This has a round, tight head.

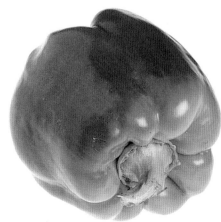

Capsicum *Capsicum annuum*

*also called **Green, Red or Yellow pepper***

MAJOR NUTRIENTS		SERVE SIZE 15 G	
Energy	16 kJ	Cholesterol	0
Protein	0	Sodium	0
Fat	0	Dietary Fibre	0
Carbohydrate	1 g	Vitamin C	32 mg

NUTRITIONAL INFORMATION An excellent source of vitamin C and baking whole does not significantly affect the vitamin C level; 15 g of capsicum contains three-quarters of the total daily requirements for this vitamin.

DESCRIPTION A shiny green, red or yellow vegetable with crisp, moist flesh.

ORIGIN AND HISTORY The sweet capsicum pepper is the fruit of a tropical South American shrub. Evidence of different types of capsicum were found in Peruvian ruins, more than 2000 years old, and illustrations have been found dating back to AD 100. The Aztecs used and cultivated it and explorers later discovered many other varieties on visits to Mexico, Chile, Peru, and the West Indies in the 16th century. The use of the name pepper was derived when Columbus discovered the many fiery hot varieties of capsicum used by the Indians in the West Indies and South America, and must not be confused with the pepper spice.

Capsicums were taken to Spain in 1493 and 100 years later the capsicum was growing in central Europe and the Balkans. The Portuguese traders introduced it to India and South-East Asia in the 17th century where it now flourishes.

BUYING AND STORAGE Available all year. Choose well-shaped, firm, thick peppers with a shiny colour and no blemishes. Avoid peppers with wet stems.

Store in the crisper of the refrigerator for up to 12 days.

PREPARATION AND USE To prepare sweet capsicum pepper, wash and dry, remove stem top and seeds and rinse again. Leave whole or cut in half lengthways for stuffing, or cut in rings, slices, chunky pieces or dice according to recipe. Use in salads, cook in casseroles and omelettes.

PROCESSING Capsicum peppers are used to make paprika pepper and can be canned or bottled as pimento. Chilli peppers are used to make cayenne, chilli powder, and tabasco sauce.

VARIETIES

There are hundreds of varieties with a range of size, shape, colour and flavour but the two main types are: large, sweet, yellow, green and red bell capsicum; small, hot, green and red chilli peppers, which are dealt with in Herbs and Spices.

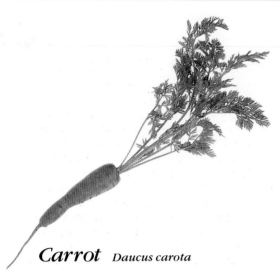

Carrot *Daucus carota*

MAJOR NUTRIENTS
SERVE SIZE 60 G

Energy	92 kJ	Sodium	0
Protein	0	Dietary Fibre	2 g
Fat	0	Vitamin A	765 µg
Carbohydrate	5 g	Vitamin C	3 mg
Cholesterol	0		

NUTRITIONAL INFORMATION This is an excellent source of vitamin A; moderate source of vitamin C and fibre. Vitamin C is reduced by about 1 mg in cooking. Carrots have by far the highest beta carotene level of any vegetable.

DESCRIPTION A crisp root vegetable with orange flesh.

ORIGIN AND HISTORY It is thought that the wild carrot originated in Afghanistan, but the fleshy orange carrot of today differs from the small, tough, pale-fleshed, acrid wild ancestor. Carrot seeds from 2000–3000 BC were found in the remains of the Bronze Age lake dwellings of Switzerland, but there were no signs of cultivation. The wild carrot spread throughout Europe as the lovely weed Queen Anne's lace and was gradually improved in the Mediterranean countries, but how and when is not documented. Then in the 12th century, an Arab writer in Spain recorded a description of red, juicy and tasty carrots and green-yellow carrots eaten with oil, vinegar and salt.

The carrot was known in Italy in the 13th century, and in France, Germany, and Holland in the 14th century. In fact in Holland the feathery green leaves were also used by ladies of fashion as hair decorations. Flemish refugees took up carrot-growing in Kent and Surrey, in England, during the reign of Elizabeth I and today the sweet juicy orange carrot has superseded all the past colours as a most popular vegetable.

BUYING AND STORAGE Available all year, but best in spring. Choose firm, smooth, well-shaped, bright orange carrots. Avoid those with cracks or soft, wet areas. Occasionally the young spring carrot is available with the green top still attached; this should be light, feathery, and a fresh green colour.

Store unwashed in the vegetable crisper or in a plastic bag with a paper towel in the refrigerator. Will store for up to 7 days.

PREPARATION AND USE Wash in cold water, brushing well with a vegetable brush, then cut off top and tail. Cook with skin on or peel very thinly. Leave carrot whole or slice into rings or obliquely or into julienne strips for cooking. Grate to serve raw in salads and sandwiches or cut into sticks for dips.

The carrot is a foundation vegetable in stews, casseroles, sauces and soups, and grated carrot may be added to pancakes, cakes and plum puddings.

PROCESSING May be canned, frozen and juiced.

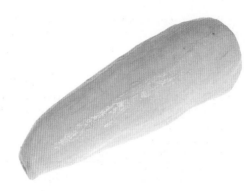

Cassava *Manihot utilissima*

also called **Kamoteng kahoy, Manioc, Ubi kayu**

MAJOR NUTRIENTS
SERVE SIZE 100 G

Energy	504 kJ	Calcium	91 mg
Protein	0	Iron	3.6 mg
Fat	0	Magnesium	66 mg
Carbohydrate	27 g	Phosphorus	70 mg
Cholesterol	0	Potassium	764 mg
Sodium	0	Vitamin C	48 mg
Dietary Fibre	3 g	Niacin Equiv.	1.6 mg

NUTRITIONAL INFORMATION High carbohydrate food. An excellent source of iron, magnesium, vitamin C; good source of fibre, calcium, phosphorus, potassium; moderate source of niacin. Quite a nutritious vegetable, but individuals on low potassium intakes should consult their dietitian.

DESCRIPTION The name given to a number of plants of the genus *Manihot*, of which the oriental species is *M. utilissima*. The plant has long, coarse brown tubers which when peeled reveal a fibrous white flesh. It is tasteless.

ORIGIN AND HISTORY Because it grows prolifically, it became a staple throughout the Pacific Islands and in Indonesia and the Philippines. It is a staple food in New Guinea. The dessert ingredient tapioca is derived from cassava, the roots being pounded and the tapioca extracted and formed into small 'pearls', for use in a variety of South-East Asian desserts, usually combined with coconut milk and sweet brown palm sugar. Tapioca starch is one of the earliest known forms of flour used for thickening Chinese foods, particularly in subtropical southern China.

BUYING AND STORAGE Sold in dried form, by weight in cellophane packs. It can be kept indefinitely in dry conditions. Grated or pounded fresh cassava root is available in some specialist food stores and where Pacific Island provisions are sold.

PREPARATION AND USE Use the powdered dried cassava or paste as a thickener for curry sauces and stewed dishes. Use tapioca pearls or fresh-grated cassava, commonly mixed with palm sugar and coconut milk, in making desserts. The attractive, almost star-shaped leaf of the cassava plant is eaten in Indonesia and other parts of South-East Asia as a vegetable, when young. When older it is used to wrap food for steaming, baking or grilling.

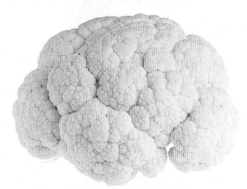

Cauliflower *Brassica oleracea*

MAJOR NUTRIENTS
BOILED
SERVE SIZE 60 G

Energy	58 kJ	Sodium	0
Protein	0	Dietary Fibre	2 g
Fat	0	Iron	0.4 mg
Carbohydrate	3 g	Vitamin C	30 mg
Cholesterol	0		

NUTRITIONAL INFORMATION An excellent source of vitamin C; good source of folate; moderate source of iron, fibre. Boiling reduces the vitamin C content in cauliflower but it is still classed as an excellent source of this vitamin. The other predominant nutrient is folate. Cauliflower is recommended for vegetarians.

DESCRIPTION Cauliflower is sometimes called the aristocrat of the cabbage family because of its impressive, tight head of white flower buds.

ORIGIN AND HISTORY There is some confusion concerning the origin of the cauliflower. Some references claim it originated in the Mediterranean and Asia Minor, others in Turkey and Egypt, others in the Orient, travelling to Europe via Cyprus. Records show it has been used since the 6th century BC and grown in Egypt and Turkey since 400 BC and in Syria since 200 BC. English records mention it was known there in 1586 as Cyprus colewarts, meaning a non-heading cabbage, and the seeds continued to be supplied from Cyprus for many years. The name was later changed to coleflower, then again to cauliflower. The cauliflower is botanically similar to broccoli and is a member of the *Brassica* family.

BUYING AND STORAGE Available all year but most seasonal in winter. Choose cauliflower with a head of white or creamy, tightly packed mass of flower buds, known as 'curd', surrounded by fresh green leaves. Avoid cauliflower with a ricy appearance, open flower clusters, spots and bruises. Large cauliflowers do not necessarily indicate quality.

To store, remove tough, coarse leaves and place cauliflower in the vegetable crisper in the refrigerator. Use within 5 days.

PREPARATION AND USE Wash whole or in equal-sized florets, in cold salt water to remove any insects. Steam or boil whole cauliflower, steam, boil, stir-fry, deep-fry or microwave florets. Serve raw for dips or in salads. Serve cooked, coated with a classic sauce, or use in soups, casseroles, savoury dishes, pickles and relishes.

PROCESSING May be frozen, pickled or made into relish.

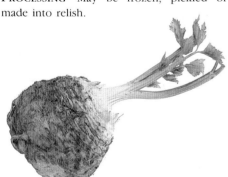

Celeriac *Apium graveolens* var. *rapaceum*

also called **Celery root**

MAJOR NUTRIENTS | | | BOILED
| | | SERVE SIZE 60 G

Energy	36 kJ	Sodium	0
Protein	0	Dietary Fibre	3 g
Fat	0	Iron	0.5 mg
Carbohydrate	2 g	Vitamin C	3 mg
Cholesterol	0		

NUTRITIONAL INFORMATION Very low in kilojoules. A good source of dietary fibre; moderate source of vitamin C and iron.

DESCRIPTION A thick tuberous root, subglobose in shape, with brown skin and white internal flesh, with a celerylike flavour.

ORIGIN AND HISTORY The plant came from the Mediterranean region. It is a special hybrid celery, which is grown for its enlarged roots, unlike celery which is grown for its stalks. It is known by many names such as celery root, celery knob, and turnip-rooted celery. Celeriac was first described by a Neapolitan and a Swiss writer in the early 17th century and had become popular in Italy, France, and Germany 100 years later. It became known in England by the mid-18th century and is now grown in Australia in limited supplies.

BUYING AND STORAGE Available in winter. Choose small to medium-sized firm roots.

Store in the vegetable crisper or in a plastic bag in the refrigerator. Use within 7 days.

PREPARATION AND USE Peel carefully, cut into segments or slices and remove any soft centre flesh. Serve fresh, grated and mixed with French dressing or added to a mixed salad. Boil, steam or microwave and serve coated with a sauce, or use in soups, stews and casseroles.

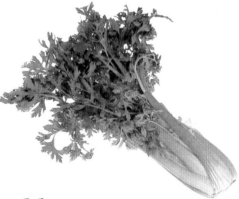

Celery *Apium graveolens*

MAJOR NUTRIENTS | | | SERVE SIZE 30 G

Energy	25 kJ	Carbohydrate	1 g
Protein	0	Sodium	0
Fat	0	Dietary Fibre	0
Cholesterol	0	Vitamin C	2 mg

NUTRITIONAL INFORMATION A moderate source of vitamin C only.

DESCRIPTION A leafy, upright vegetable with an edible stem.

ORIGIN AND HISTORY Leaf celery or bunch celery, as we know it, is the cultivated version of wild celery which is one of the oldest plants used by people. It was first recorded in 850 BC in Homer's *Odyssey*. Wild celery originated in the Mediterranean, native to wet places throughout Europe. It was not eaten as a food but used as a medicine throughout the Middle Ages to settle over-acid digestion and relieve arthritis. Celery began to be cultivated for eating in the 16th century, in Italy, and in 1623 the French started to use it as a flavour for soups, meats, and stews. By the mid-17th century, celery was being eaten fresh in Italy and France, with an oil dressing. 'Blanching' or covering up the growing stalks with soil produced a whiter, milder flavoured celery which was introduced into England in the late 17th century. The refreshing, crunchy, stringless celery of today was developed in Utah, USA and is very popular as a salad vegetable.

BUYING AND STORAGE Available all year. Choose a compact bunch or 'head' of celery with clean, undamaged stalks or 'sticks' that snap easily and are not too thick. Avoid soft stalks and limp leaves.

Wrap celery in a plastic bag and store, unwashed, in the vegetable crisper, or on a low shelf, in the refrigerator for up to 7 days.

PREPARATION AND USE Snap required stalks off the bunch, cut base and leaves off and wash well. Remove any strings or damaged areas, then cut according to recipe. Inner tender stalks can be served whole with cheese. Use raw in salads, cook in soups, casseroles, stir-fries, or braise or microwave and serve as a vegetable accompaniment. Celery curls and leaves may be used as an edible garnish.

PROCESSING May be canned; used to flavour celery salt.

VARIETIES
Pascal is a heavy green-ribbed celery with large leaves. Golden is blanched with white stalks and yellow leaves.

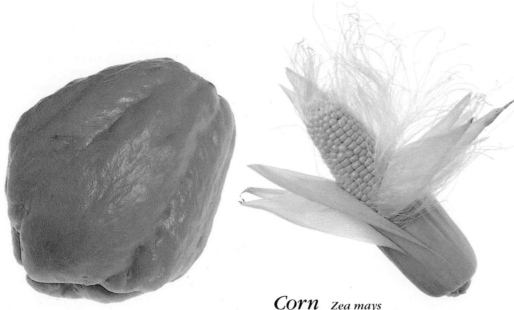

Chayote Sechium edule

also called **Choko, Mango squash, Mirliton, Vegetable pear**

MAJOR NUTRIENTS			SERVE SIZE 80 G
Energy	79 kJ	Cholesterol	0
Protein	0 ·	Sodium	0
Fat	0	Dietary Fibre	0
Carbohydrate	4 g	Vitamin C	6 mg

NUTRITIONAL INFORMATION An excellent source of vitamin C.

DESCRIPTION A pear-shaped green vegetable which grows on a vine, has a single soft seed and pear-textured pale green flesh.

ORIGIN AND HISTORY The chayote is a perennial rooted vine of the gourd or cucurbit family. It is native to Central America, Mexico, and the West Indies. It is believed to have originated in Central America in prehistoric times, and it has also grown in Mexico and the West Indies for hundreds of years. The Aztecs called it chayote and it was introduced into the Mediterranean region by the early traders. It flourishes well in Algeria from where it is exported to Europe. The early white settlers introduced the chayote to Australia where it is commonly known as the choko.

BUYING AND STORAGE Available all year, with the season peaking in summer and autumn. Choose firm, small, fresh green chayotes with no brown spots or sprouting.

Store in the vegetable crisper of the refrigerator.

PREPARATION AND USE Cut into quarter segments, remove peel and seed, then slice or cut into chunky pieces. Steam, boil or microwave and serve with a sauce as a vegetable, or use in soups and casseroles, stuff halves and bake, or poach as for pears for a dessert.

PROCESSING Can be used in chutney.

Corn Zea mays

also called **Indian corn, Maize, Sweet corn**

MAJOR NUTRIENTS			BOILED
			SERVE SIZE 70 G
Energy	242 kJ	Dietary Fibre	3 g
Protein	2g	Phosphorus	62 mg
Fat	0	Thiamin	0.10 mg
Carbohydrate	13 g	Niacin Equiv.	1.3 mg
Cholesterol	0	Vitamin C	5 mg
Sodium	0		

NUTRITIONAL INFORMATION An excellent source of vitamin C; good source of fibre, phosphorus, folate; moderate source of thiamin and niacin. Canning reduces thiamin content to an insignificant amount. As corn is actually the seed of a type of grass, it is also classed as a cereal. It has therefore a higher protein and vitamin B content compared to other vegetables.

DESCRIPTION The round, yellow kernels of maize formed on an ear which is surrounded by a green husk, growing on a tall plant.

ORIGIN AND HISTORY Corn is the only cereal known to have originated in the Americas. Tiny husks of wild corn were found by the natives of South America thousands of years ago and pictures of the wild grass, from which corn descends, have been found in pre-Inca tombs, suggesting that the Peruvian Indians first cultivated corn in the Andes. Its correct name, maize, is an Indian word. Later this primitive maize went north and was hybridised with another type of corn in Central America. Further hybridisation produced other types of corn such as flint corn for animal fodder, dent corn for meal and flour, flour corn and popcorn as well as sweet corn. These varieties travelled to North America and were cultivated by some of the Indian tribes. It was the Indians who showed the early English settlers how to plant and use corn. Columbus saw it growing in Central America in 1492 and took the first corn back to Europe. However, the vegetable sweet corn as we know it now has been developed by mutation and is the most popular.

BUYING AND STORAGE Available all year, peaking in season in summer and autumn. Always buy corn with the fresh green husk still attached. The silk threads between the husk and corn should feel damp and the corn kernels should spurt out milk when burst. Once the husk is removed, the sugar content in corn changes to starch resulting in a poor starchy flavour. Avoid dry, yellow husks, small shrinking kernels and excessively large, firm kernels.

Store briefly as corn should be eaten as soon as possible after picking to enjoy the sweetness. If it must be stored, wrap damp paper towels around husks and store in the coldest part of the refrigerator.

PREPARATION AND USE Peel all but the last 4 husks off the ears of corn and pull off all the silk threads. Cut base off, then plunge into iced water for 1 hour. Cook by boiling briefly, barbecuing or microwaving. Serve corn on the cob topped with butter and pepper, or use in chowders, casseroles, fritters and hominy.

PROCESSING May be canned cream-style, frozen, preserved in brine, used in relish and ground to make cornmeal.

SEE ALSO The chapter on Grains and Cereals.

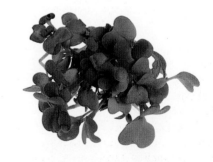

Cress Lepidium sativum

MAJOR NUTRIENTS			SERVE SIZE 30 G
Energy	12 kJ	Cholesterol	0
Protein	0	Sodium	0
Fat	0	Dietary Fibre	1 g
Carbohydrate	0	Vitamin C	12 mg

NUTRITIONAL INFORMATION An excellent source of vitamin C.

DESCRIPTION A seedling with small bright green leaves on tender white stalks.

ORIGIN AND HISTORY Cress is the sprouts produced from the seeds of a plant native to Europe and related to pepperwort. It tastes hot and peppery and is often bought in combination with the sprouts of mustard seeds. Together they are sold as 'mustard cress'.

BUYING AND STORAGE Available all year. Select fresh, upright, springy seedlings. Avoid limp, dull, discoloured cress.

Store, covered, in a refrigerator. Use as soon as possible.

PREPARATION AND USE Snip seedlings off roots with kitchen scissors. Use in salads, sandwiches, with eggs and as a garnish.

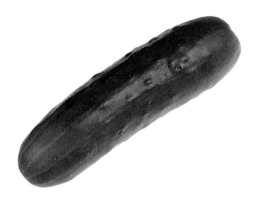

Cucumber *Cucumis sativus*

MAJOR NUTRIENTS		SERVE SIZE 30 G	
Energy	16 kJ	Cholesterol	0
Protein	0	Sodium	0
Fat	0	Dietary Fibre	0
Carbohydrate	1 g	Vitamin C	3 mg

NUTRITIONAL INFORMATION A moderate source of vitamin C.

DESCRIPTION A vegetable with dark green to pale skin, with mild-flavoured flesh that has a high water content.

ORIGIN AND HISTORY An ancient plant, possibly cultivated in Burma and India around 9000 BC. A member of the Cucurbitaceae family, to which pumpkins and marrows belong.

BUYING AND STORAGE Available all year, but season peaks in summer and autumn. Choose firm, fresh, bright green cucumbers. Avoid dull-coloured cucumbers with damaged skin.

Wash cucumber and dry well, then store in the vegetable crisper in the refrigerator.

PREPARATION AND USE Peel, if liked, then slice thinly or cut into sticks, dice or cubes according to recipe. Use fresh in salads, sandwiches, with dips, in cold sauces and chilled soups. May be steamed, sautéed or microwaved and served as a vegetable accompaniment.

PROCESSING May be pickled, particularly the gherkin variety, and used in relish and chutney.

VARIETIES

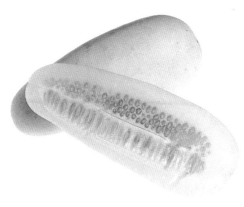

Apple Cucumber Short, round, stubby and light green.

European/Lebanese/Burpless Cucumber Long, slender and dark green.

Gherkin Cucumber Short, slim, rough-skinned and green.

Green Ridge Cucumber Smooth-skinned and dark green.

Italian Cucumber Dark green, long, slender with a hook at the top.

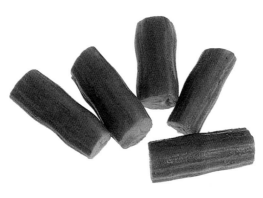

Drumstick Vegetable
Moringa pterygosperma

*also called **Seeng***

MAJOR NUTRIENTS		SERVE SIZE 100 G	
Energy	180 kJ	Calcium	60 mg
Protein	3 g	Iron	0.8 mg
Fat	0	Niacin Equiv.	1 mg
Carbohydrate	10 g	Vitamin C	159 mg
Cholesterol	0		

NUTRITIONAL INFORMATION An excellent source of vitamin C; good source of iron; moderate source of calcium and niacin.

DESCRIPTION A long, round, beanlike Indian vegetable with a hard, deep green skin, slightly ridged and showing regularly spaced indentations along its length. Akin to a marrow, it grows on a tree, and has, in size and shape, a rough resemblance to a drumstick, hence the name. Its flavour is subtle, its texture somewhat like a zucchini.

ORIGIN AND HISTORY India has the honour of being the country from which these unusual vegetables originate. Indians in Malaysia now cultivate it and it has been adopted in some Western countries with sizeable Indian populations. Little is known of it, except that it is an intrinsic part of the Indian cuisine.

BUYING AND STORAGE Sometimes available in Asian food stores. Choose those with deep green, unmarked skin and a firm feel.

It can be kept for up to 2 weeks in the vegetable compartment of the refrigerator.

PREPARATION AND USE Cut into equal lengths, trimming the ends, tie in bunches in the same way as asparagus and simmer gently until tender. Drain and serve with a sauce or butter, or add to curries.

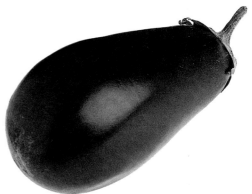

Eggplant *Solanum melongena*
*also called **Aubergine***

MAJOR NUTRIENTS		RAW SERVE SIZE 100 G	
Energy	60 kJ	Sodium	5 mg
Protein	1 g	Potassium	240 mg
Fat	0	Iron	0.5 mg
Carbohydrate	3 g	Niacin Equiv.	1 mg
Cholesterol	0	Vitamin C	15 mg
Dietary Fibre	2.5 g		

NUTRITIONAL INFORMATION An excellent source of vitamin C; moderate source of potassium, iron, niacin and folate.

DESCRIPTION A smooth and shiny-skinned vegetable with a creamy-white, pithy interior with many small light brown seeds dispersed through the flesh. Colours range depending on variety from a deep purplish-black, through pale green to yellow and white.

ORIGIN AND HISTORY It probably originated in India. Grown for many centuries in South-East Asia and Turkey, it was also noted as a common food in China as far back as 600 BC, and its Chinese name k'un-lun tzu kua translated as Malayan purple melon. It was eaten cooked or raw, and ladies of fashion used a black dye made from the skins to stain their teeth. In the 13th century it was offered to the shrine of imperial ancestors on the Fifth Month. The French have cultivated it from the 17th century, but it is a relative newcomer to the Americas and Australia.

BUYING AND STORAGE Available all year. Choose a firm eggplant with a smooth satinlike skin, free from dark brown spots and scars, heavy in relation to its size.

It can be stored for up to 2 weeks unwrapped in the vegetable compartment of the refrigerator but does not require refrigeration except in hot climates. Cut eggplant will discolour quickly and should be wrapped tightly in plastic. The discoloured part can be cut away.

PREPARATION AND USE Remove the stem with a sharp knife. Cook whole, sliced or cubed. It can have a bitter taste, which can be extracted by sprinkling the cut vegetable with salt and allowing about 15 minutes for the salt to draw juices to the surface where they can be rinsed away. Dry on paper towels before use. It will discolour if not cooked a short time after preparation. Avoid carbon steel knives as they leave a dark stain and metallic aftertaste.

Eggplant is used as a vegetable in Indian and Malaysian curries, and elsewhere in Asia it may be braised, fried, stir-fried or grilled. Some varieties are thinly sliced and eaten raw in salads.

Pea aubergine is an essential ingredient in Thai curries, and is used raw in the Thai sauce nam prik to give a sour taste. The hairy orange aubergine is ground to a paste to add a sharp, tart flavour to Thai sauces.

VARIETIES

There are many varieties, shaped like globes, eggs or sausages, and the colour varies from white through to dark purple.

Brinjal A Malaysian and Indian aubergine which can vary in size and shape and is usually deep purple in colour.

Globe Eggplant A readily available variety.

Hairy Orange Aubergine Medium-sized with bright orange skin and a covering of fine dark hairs.

Japanese Aubergine Small in size, about 7 cm long, deep purple, and may be round, oval or pear-shaped.

Thai Aubergine Ma khua comes in the globe category. A Thai aubergine which is similar to that used in China, Malaysia, and India. It is slender and long, about 20 cm, and may be cream, pale green, or deep purple.

The smaller variety known as ma khua khun is pale green, white or yellow.

Thai Pea Aubergine Makua phuong is a little larger than the green pea and of a similar shape and colour.

Terung Engkol A small rounded variety from Indonesia, it has a bitter taste and is eaten, raw or cooked, before it is ripe.

Endive *Cichorium* spp.

DESCRIPTION Belgian endive, also called witloof, is a shoot vegetable with elongated, blanched white leaves wrapped tightly around each other, approximately 15 cm tall.

Curly endive is a salad leaf vegetable made up of a rosette of green curly leaves, darker at the tips and lighter in the centre.

Broadleaf Batavian endive is similar to curly endive but the leaves are toothed and wavy rather than curly.

ORIGIN AND HISTORY Endive originated in China and other parts of Asia, but it is also native to the Mediterranean and still grows wild in some parts of Europe. Wild or cultivated, it has been used for centuries for human food and animal fodder.

Curly endive and Batavian endive have been described as a salad green and a pot herb in Roman writings. They were popular in England in the 16th century and the English Navy grew them in pierced barrels, on board ship, to use in salads to help to prevent scurvy.

Belgian endive was first discovered by accident in the middle of the 19th century, when some coffee chicory roots that had been left lying in the dark were found to have sprouted white leaves. A horticulturist from Brussels

Botanical Gardens, inspired by this discovery, cultivated the first crop of Belgian endive (chicory or witloof), in the cellars of the botanical gardens, along with mushrooms. By 1872 it was being produced for the Paris market and although still exported from Belgium, it is now grown successfully in other countries.

There is much confusion about the endive family owing to its variety of names.

BUYING AND STORAGE Belgian endive is available from autumn to spring. Choose fresh-coloured, crisp, tender-leaved shoots. Avoid shoots with brown marks at the top of the leaves.

Store in the vegetable crisper in the refrigerator and use as soon as possible.

Curly endive and broadleaf Batavian endive are available from midsummer to midwinter. Choose crisp, tender, firm, bright green bunches of endive which are heavy for their size. Avoid those with soft, moist curves.

To store, remove damaged leaves, wrap in paper towels and store in the vegetable crisper in the refrigerator.

PREPARATION AND USE Wash Belgian endive in cold water, pat dry and cut off base. Serve raw whole leaves or thinly sliced in salads. Cook by steaming, boiling or in a microwave oven and serve traditionally topped with cooked ham and cheese au gratin sauce.

Wash curly endive and broadleaf Batavian endive as for lettuce. Use in green salads or cook and serve as for spinach.

VARIETIES

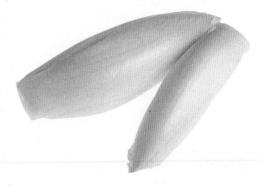

Belgian Endive Chicory (*Cichorium intybus*), also called witloof, Flemish for white leaf, known as chicory in England.

MAJOR NUTRIENTS		SERVE SIZE 50 G	
Energy	13 kJ	Sodium	0
Protein	0	Dietary Fibre	0
Fat	0	Vitamin C	3 mg
Carbohydrate	1 g		
Cholesterol	0		

NUTRITIONAL INFORMATION This is a good source of folate; moderate source of vitamin C.

Broadleaf Batavian Endive Also called escarole, this variety has deeply indented leaves, giving it a frilled appearance.

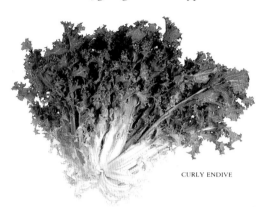

CURLY ENDIVE

Curly Endive *Cichorium endivia*, also known as chicory in England.

MAJOR NUTRIENTS		SERVE SIZE 30 G	
Energy	14 kJ	Sodium	0
Protein	0	Dietary Fibre	1 g
Fat	0	Iron	0.5 mg
Carbohydrate	1 g	Vitamin C	5 mg
Cholesterol	0		

NUTRITIONAL INFORMATION A good source of vitamin C; moderate source of iron.

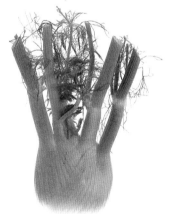

Fennel *Foeniculum vulgare* var. *dulce*

DESCRIPTION A celery-like shoot, short and bulbous with the flavour of aniseed. The feathery green leaves are used as a herb. The seeds which follow the flowers are also used in cuisine, particularly in bread, pastries, pasta and pickles.

ORIGIN AND HISTORY A native of the Mediterranean region, which thrives well on sea cliffs, and is often found by the roadside.

Florence fennel is very popular. Now grown in many countries in temperate climate areas.

BUYING AND STORAGE Available during autumn, winter, and spring. Buy crisp, well-shaped, clean, fresh-looking fennel. Avoid fennel with withered outer stalks.

Store in a crisper or in a plastic bag in the refrigerator.

PREPARATION AND USE Cut base off head (or bulb) and cut leaves off the top. Remove any damaged outer stalks, then wash and dry. Slice fennel across into thin rings or lengthways into thin strips and use raw in salad, or cut in half lengthways, steam or microwave and serve with a cheese sauce as a dressed vegetable.

SEE ALSO Fennel in the chapter on Herbs and Spices.

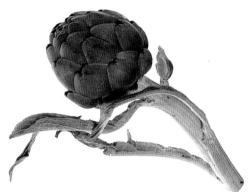

Globe Artichoke *Cynara scolymus*

also called **French artichoke**

MAJOR NUTRIENTS			BOILED SERVE SIZE 100 G
Energy	62 kJ	Calcium	44 mg
Protein	0	Phosphorus	40 mg
Fat	0	Iron	0.5 mg
Carbohydrate	2.7 g	Thiamin	0.07 mg
Cholesterol	0	Niacin Equiv.	1.1 mg
Sodium	0	Vitamin C	8 mg
Dietary Fibre	4g		

NUTRITIONAL INFORMATION An excellent source of fibre and vitamin C; moderate calcium, phosphorus, iron, thiamin and niacin.

DESCRIPTION Resembles an unopened, round flower bud, with green, purple or bronze-coloured tightly wrapped leaves, ranging from 30–500 g in weight. The large artichoke grows at the top of the main stem, while the baby artichoke is found near the ground.

ORIGIN AND HISTORY The artichoke is believed to be native to the western and cen-

tral Mediterranean region and grew wild in Italy 3000 years ago. It was taken to Egypt and further east over 2000 years ago. It was first recorded in Naples in AD 1400. It is a perennial thistlelike plant, belonging to the daisy family and related to the sunflower, chrysanthemum, and the Italian cardoon. This prickly vegetable has not always enjoyed popularity, probably owing to the method of roasting it on an open fire. This was used by the Romans who charred the leaves and made the tender artichoke heart smoky. However, Catherine de Medici of Florence introduced the artichoke to France in 1533, when she married the heir to the French throne. From France it was introduced to England, where Henry VIII fancied it because it was alleged to be an aphrodisiac. Its original name, al-kharshuf, is of Arabic origin; it became artichaut in French, carciofo in Italian, alcachofa in Spanish and artichoke in English. It was introduced to North America in the 18th century.

BUYING AND STORAGE Available in the spring. Choose the compact, heavy, plump globe, with large tightly clinging leaves which yield slightly when pressed.

Store, unwashed, in the vegetable crisper or in a plastic bag in the refrigerator for up to 1 week.

PREPARATION AND USE Slice stem off, remove lower coarse leaves, then cut 25 mm off top of globe and trim the sharp tips from the remaining leaves. Brush cut surface with lemon juice to prevent darkening. Gently press the top leaves apart to expose the centre, pull out the prickly lavender-tipped leaves from the centre and scrape out the fuzzy, hairy choke with a sharp vegetable knife or a metal teaspoon. If liked, the trimmed artichoke may be cooked first so the centre can be removed more easily. Artichokes may be steamed, boiled in water with lemon juice or microwaved, and served classically with French dressing or hollandaise sauce. Stuffed artichokes may be baked, braised or microwaved. Use also in salads, sauces and soups.

PROCESSING The artichoke heart may be canned and preserved in French dressing.

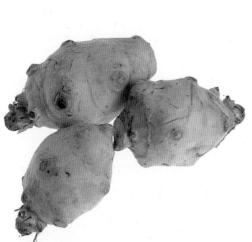

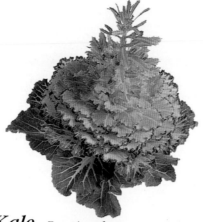

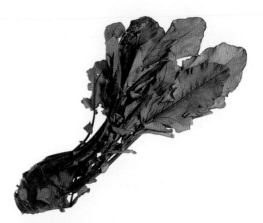

Jerusalem Artichoke

Helianthus tuberosus

also called Sunchoke

MAJOR NUTRIENTS

		BOILED SERVE SIZE 100 G	
Energy	78 kJ	Sodium	0
Protein	0	Dietary Fibre	no data
Fat	0	Potassium	420 mg
Carbohydrate	3 g	Iron	0.4 mg
Cholesterol	0	Thiamin	0.10 mg

NUTRITIONAL INFORMATION A moderate source of potassium, iron and thiamin.

DESCRIPTION A gnarled tuber or root, yellow-beige or pink tinged in colour, 100 mm long and 50 mm across, with short, knobbly, club-shaped branches.

ORIGIN AND HISTORY The Jerusalem artichoke is the edible root or tuber of a special sunflower plant, belonging to the daisy family and native to North America. It resembles knobbly potatoes or root ginger and is no relation whatsoever to the globe/French artichoke. Nor is it related to Jerusalem, because its name is an adaptation of the Italian word girasole meaning sunflower which when literally translated means turn to the sun. It was cultivated for centuries by the North American Indians when Columbus arrived there. Columbus introduced it into Italy and the French explorers took the plant to France from Canada, calling it the potato of Canada. It is now cultivated throughout the Western world.

BUYING AND STORAGE In season from autumn to spring. Choose the large, firm, clean, crisp tuber.

Store unwashed, in the vegetable crisper in the refrigerator or in a cool, dry place.

PREPARATION AND USE Peel and cook as for a potato. Use as a vegetable, in soups, sauces, stews and casseroles. May be used raw in salad.

Kale *Brassica oleracea*

also called Curly kale, Collard, Borecole

MAJOR NUTRIENTS

		BOILED SERVE SIZE 50 G	
Energy	84 kJ	Dietary Fibre	0
Protein	0	Calcium	102 mg
Fat	0	Phosphorus	38 mg
Carbohydrate	3 g	Iron	0.6 mg
Cholesterol	0	Vitamin A	276 µg
Sodium	0	Vitamin C	25 mg

NUTRITIONAL INFORMATION An excellent source of vitamins A and C; good source of calcium; moderate source of phosphorus and iron. In the vegetable family kale has the highest levels of calcium per serve. It is recommended as a good source of calcium for non-dairy eating people. This vegetable is also high in beta carotene.

DESCRIPTION A coarse green leaf, very curly or smooth, resembling cabbage, on an upright stem, with a strong flavour.

ORIGIN AND HISTORY Kale is native to the eastern Mediterranean region, where it has been cultivated for 2000 years. It was taken throughout Europe and became popular in the cool northern countries such as Germany. Curly kale was first recorded in England in the early 18th century but used the name bore cole, which was derived from the Dutch boerenkool meaning peasant's cabbage. Kale is a member of the cabbage family and resembles cabbage in its wild form. The names kale and collard are derived from the old English word cole, originally the generic name for the cabbage family.

BUYING AND STORAGE Buy in winter. Choose dark green, crisp, clean leaves free from damage, brown spots and bruising.

Store in a vegetable crisper in the refrigerator. Use as soon as possible.

PREPARATION AND USE Trim leaves off stalks, then wash in cold, salt water and drain well. Cook and use as for silverbeet. Collard greens are traditional with pork in the south of the USA.

VARIETIES

There are many varieties of both curly and smooth-leaved types.

Kohlrabi *Brassica oleracea* var. *gongyloides*

MAJOR NUTRIENTS

		BOILED SERVE SIZE 50 G	
Energy	50 kJ	Cholesterol	0
Protein	0	Sodium	0
Fat	0	Dietary Fibre	1g
Carbohydrate	3 g	Vitamin C	22 mg

NUTRITIONAL INFORMATION An excellent source of vitamin C.

DESCRIPTION A round, turniplike, purple or light green globe, with several stalks all sprouting green leaves. Kohlrabi is a swollen stem, not a root.

ORIGIN AND HISTORY Kohlrabi, a cabbage mutant, was probably developed in northern Europe. Some references claim it travelled to China via the silk route, others suggest it came to Europe from Asia along with Attila the Hun. However, these references probably refer to another member of the cabbage family in view of the kohlrabi's name which, translated from the German, means cabbage turnip and describes it well as it is a turnip-rooted cabbage. The kohlrabi was first described by a European botanist in the mid-16th century. It was well known in Germany and also in the Mediterranean, and known but not very popular in England by the end of the 1500s. The first record of it being used in the USA was in 1806. Farmers in the south planted it as a rotation crop with cotton as 'vittles' for the slave quarters.

BUYING AND STORAGE Available in winter. Choose firm globes, no larger than a large apple for the best, sweetest flavour.

Store in a vegetable crisper in the refrigerator for up to 7 days.

PREPARATION AND USE Cut base off and trim stalks. Wash and drain, then cook whole, with skin on, by baking or microwaving. Scoop out centre, stuff with a savoury filling and bake, or peel and use in a salad. Alternatively, peel, then steam or boil, or use in soups, stews and casseroles.

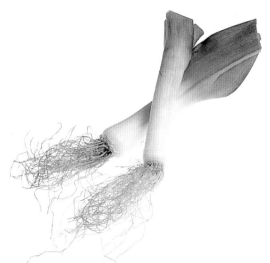

Leek *Allium ampeloprasum* var. *porrum*

MAJOR NUTRIENTS		BOILED SERVE SIZE 75 G	
Energy	78 kJ	Sodium	0
Protein	0	Dietary Fibre	3 g
Fat	0	Iron	1 mg
Carbohydrate	4 g	Vitamin C	11 mg
Cholesterol	0		

NUTRITIONAL INFORMATION An excellent source of vitamin C; good source of iron and fibre.

DESCRIPTION A member of the onion family, the leek resembles the green onion (spring onion), but is larger and cylindrical in shape. The lower part is blanched by drawing up the soil to cover it and exclude the light.

ORIGIN AND HISTORY The leek probably originated in the eastern Mediterranean region where the wild leek still grows. It is documented that it has been cultivated in the Middle East for 3000 years and the Greeks and Romans prized it as a delicacy. The name leek is a corruption of loch, a word the Romans used to describe any medicine that could be licked to cure a sore throat. The Roman emperor, Nero, apparently ate large quantities of leeks to improve his voice. The Romans spread the leek throughout Europe and introduced it to Britain. When the Welsh went into battle against the Saxons in AD 640, King Cadwallader's soldiers wore a leek as a distinguishing emblem. The leek became the national emblem of Wales, the victor in that battle, and is still worn traditionally on St David's day.

BUYING AND STORAGE Buy in winter. Choose the firm white leek with crisp undamaged green tops. Select small to medium size for a good sweet flavour and tender texture.

Trim tough green leaves off and store in a crisper or a plastic bag in the refrigerator.

PREPARATION AND USE Remove outer layer if dirty or damaged. Trim off the roots and coarse tops of the green leaves. Fan the leaves open and wash under cold running water. Boil, steam, microwave, braise and serve as a vegetable entrée, in dressing or cream sauce, or use in classical vichysoisse, other soups, tarts, chicken pie and stir-fries.

PROCESSING May be frozen as a dressed vegetable.

Lettuce *Lactuca sativa*

MAJOR NUTRIENTS		SERVE SIZE 20 G	
Energy	16 kJ	Cholesterol	0
Protein	0	Sodium	0
Fat	0	Dietary Fibre	0
Carbohydrate	1 g	Vitamin C	3 mg

NUTRITIONAL INFORMATION A moderate source of vitamin C. It is also a favourite with weight-watchers because of the low kJ content.

DESCRIPTION A green-leafed vegetable.

ORIGIN AND HISTORY The lettuce is descended from wild, loose-leaved plants which are native to the Mediterranean region and the Near East. It was recorded that Persian kings ate lettuce around 550 BC and Hippocrates informed the Greeks that it was good for them. Garden lettuce was known in China in the 5th century. Chaucer wrote about lettuce in England in 1387 in his Prologue to *The Canterbury Tales*. The cos lettuce travelled from Italy to the rest of Europe in the 16th century. Crisphead lettuce appeared at the same time, and oak-leaved lettuce and curly-leaved lettuce soon after. Columbus took lettuce to the New World and today it is the most popular salad plant in the world.

BUYING AND STORAGE It is available in spring, summer, and autumn. Choose crisp, fresh, firm lettuce, heavy for their size. Avoid any damp or brown-edged leaves and soft wet cores.

Remove any coarse damaged outer leaves, and store in the vegetable crisper, or in a plastic bag with a paper towel, in the refrigerator for up to 5 days.

PREPARATION AND USE Remove the core from crisphead varieties, hold hollow core under a cold running tap to wash well, then drain and dry by shaking in a clean dry tea towel.

To wash other varieties, remove leaves individually from stalk and wash in cold water, drain, then dry well in a clean dry tea towel.

Use in salads, sandwiches, soups, around fish en papillote, as a garnish and a base for cold buffet platters.

VARIETIES

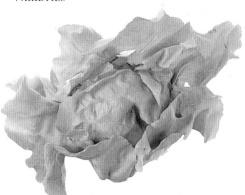

Butterhead With soft, buttery leaves, loosely packed like an opening rose, varying in size from large to tiny, for example, mignonette, butterleaf, bibb and cabbage lettuce.

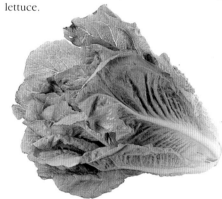

Cos This has crisp, elongated leaves, tightly wrapped to form an enlongated head, for example, romaine.

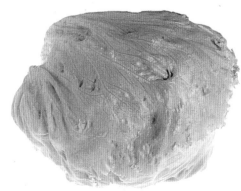

Crisphead Heavy, firm, round, tightly packed and crisp texture, for example, Iceberg.

Leaf Lettuce This has loose, crisp leaves branching from a stalk and does not form a head, for example, lambs' lettuce or salade de mâche.

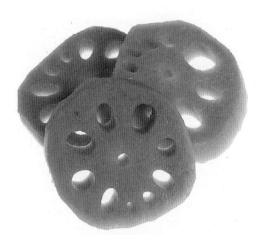

Lotus *Nelumbo nuciferum*

also called **Ito, Renkon**

MAJOR NUTRIENTS			CANNED SERVE SIZE 100 G
Energy	60 kJ	Carbohydrate	3 g
Protein	1 g	Sodium	20 mg
Fat	0	Iron	0.6 mg

NUTRITIONAL INFORMATION A moderate source of iron. There are no data for magnesium, copper, zinc, vitamin A, vitamin C and fibre.

DESCRIPTION A rhizome with horizontal, bottom growing stems from which shoots the thick edible root which is a light brown in colour. It is segmented at intervals like a string of sausages. When cut in cross-section, it shows a series of evenly spaced, round holes running the length of the root. It has a fibrous texture, a delicate nutty flavour, and exudes a sticky gum when cut.

ORIGIN AND HISTORY An ancient plant, lotus flowers are depicted in the art of ancient Egypt, China, and India, the soft-textured perfect petals, and the full rounded shape of the flower equated with the womanly curves as a symbol of purist beauty. It has been represented as the symbol of Buddhism, and so appears on most depictions of Buddhist deities and in many religious symbols and artefacts. From the earliest times both roots and seeds have been eaten in China, and the leaves used as food wrappers.

BUYING AND STORAGE Lotus root is available fresh in specialist Asian food stores. It should be thoroughly scrubbed with a brush to remove mud. Canned lotus root, either sliced or in lengths, is packed in water, usually unsalted. Its flavour and texture are inferior to the fresh product. Lotus seeds are sometimes available fresh, but are more usually sold canned or dried.

PREPARATION AND USE Soak fresh lotus root in cold water for 15 minutes, drain and slice to cook by stir-frying or braising; coat with batter and deep-fry, or simmer in stock. Canned lotus root should be drained and rinsed in clean cold water before use.

Dried lotus seeds are soaked for several hours, then simmered until tender. Use a needle to remove the bitter-tasting core. Canned lotus seeds can be used straight from the can. Sweetened, cooked lotus seeds are mashed to make a thick sweet puree used as a filling for Chinese and Japanese cakes and pastries.

Lotus leaves are not strictly a food, but the leaves of the plant are used, dried or fresh, as a wrapper for various Chinese dishes, particularly 'sticky' rice. It imparts a delicate, unique flavour to the food.

PROCESSING The stems may be canned, pickled and made into starch.

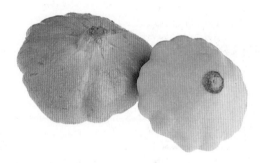

Marrow *Cucurbita pepo*

also called **Summer Squash**

MAJOR NUTRIENTS			BOILED SERVE SIZE 50 G
Energy	15 kJ	Cholesterol	0
Protein	0	Sodium	0
Fat	0	Dietary Fibre	0
Carbohydrate	1 g		

NUTRITIONAL INFORMATION No nutrients present in a significant quantity. This vegetable is good for weight-watchers as it contains so few kilojoules.

DESCRIPTION The marrow or summer squash is a member of the gourd family.

ORIGIN AND HISTORY It probably originated in the north of South America, like the rest of the squash family, but it was developed in England as a garden vegetable in the early 19th century and became very popular in Victorian times. The marrow was grown to giant sizes, to be exhibited at country fairs, but small or medium-sized marrows have a superior taste and texture.

BUYING AND STORAGE The marrow is best eaten soon after purchase, as it easily softens and shrivels.

PREPARATION AND USE The larger the marrow, the blander its taste; one way to enhance this vegetable is to hollow out some of the central portion and bake the halves with a savoury stuffing. Smaller marrows can be cooked whole, with flavourings like garlic and tomato and sautéed in a pan.

VARIETIES

There are many popular varieties of marrow, including the snake squash, so called because of its snakelike neck, the large custard squash, and the small, attractive patty pan squash and decorative scallopine.

SEE ALSO Zucchini.

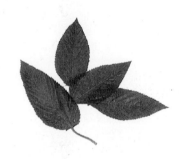

Melokhia *Chorchorus olitorius*

also called **Jews' mallow**

MAJOR NUTRIENTS			SERVE SIZE 100 G
Energy	300 kJ	Iron	11 mg
Protein	4 g	Magnesium	55 mg
Fat	1 g	Phosphorus	60 mg
Carbohydrate	17 g	Vitamin C	64 mg
Cholesterol	0	Vitamin A	6400 μg
Calcium	300 mg		

NUTRITIONAL INFORMATION An excellent source of magnesium, calcium, iron, vitamin C and vitamin A; moderate source of phosphorus and protein.

DESCRIPTION The plant is a source of inferior jute. The younger stalks are harvested for the oval leaves, which are about 4–8 cm long, for culinary use. When cooked, melokhia has the viscous properties of okra, with a spinachlike flavour. Melokhia is widely regarded as an Egyptian pot herb.

ORIGIN AND HISTORY Native to tropical regions, melokhia was probably first used in Egypt as a fibre plant. From the times of the Pharaohs, the peasants found the young leaves made a pleasant potherb, and soon discovered that its viscous properties and green colour enhanced the appearance and palatability of soups based on vegetable, meat, game or poultry stock. The leaves are dried during their season and stored for use throughout the year.

The plant was grown for the table by the Jews of Aleppo, Syria, and became known as Jews' mallow. It is also used in India and Jamaica as a spinach substitute.

BUYING AND STORAGE Bunches of fresh melokhia can be found in some city vegetable markets from late spring, available for some two months in its season. They can be stored in the refrigerator and used while fresh. Dried melokhia leaves are available year round at Middle Eastern and Greek food stores. Store in a sealed container in a cool, dry place and use within a year.

PREPARATION AND USE To prepare fresh melokhia, wash well then strip leaves from stalks. Drain leaves and allow to dry, then chop finely with a sharp knife. About 500 g fresh leaves is required for the average soup quantity, added during the last 10–15 minutes of cooking. Use a quarter of this amount of dried melokhia, rubbed to a powder and soaked with a little hot water before adding to the stock. The melokhia should remain suspended in the soup. Flavour with a mixture of chopped garlic fried in a little butter with ground coriander, salt and a pinch of chilli powder.

Melokhia can also be used as a green vegetable — prepare as for spinach and serve dressed with olive oil and lemon juice.

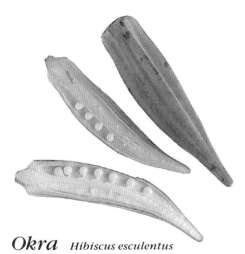

Okra *Hibiscus esculentus*

also called Lady's fingers, Gumbo

MAJOR NUTRIENTS			STEAMED SERVE SIZE 100 G
Energy	140 kJ	Iron	0.7 mg
Protein	2 g	Magnesium	60 mg
Fat	0	Thiamin	0.15 mg
Carbohydrate	8 g	Niacin Equiv.	1.5 mg
Dietary Fibre	3 g	Riboflavin	0.50 mg
Cholesterol	0	Vitamin C	30 mg
Sodium	0	Vitamin A	60 mg
Calcium	90 mg		

NUTRITIONAL INFORMATION An excellent source of folate, vitamin C and magnesium; a good source of thiamin, vitamin A, riboflavin, niacin, iron, zinc and dietary fibre.

DESCRIPTION A green, ridged, immature seed pod, pointed at one end, 5–10 cm long.

ORIGIN AND HISTORY Okra is the fruit pod of a plant native to tropical Africa. It is said to have originated in Abyssinia (now Ethiopia) and the east of the Sudan, although little has been recorded about its history. The first record was written in 1216, by a Spanish Moor, who saw it when visiting Egypt. Okra was taken to Egypt and other Arab countries by slave-raiders and it is still very popular in Arab cookery. Okra was taken further to North Africa and the Mediterranean countries, then to South-east Asia. It was taken to the new world from the Gold Coast, along with the African slaves, and was known as slave fruit in the deep South where the crops of okra flourished like wild flowers.

BUYING AND STORAGE Available in summer and autumn. Choose tender pods which snap easily or burst when lightly pressed. Avoid okra with dull dry skins.

Store in the crisper in the refrigerator. Will keep for up to 2 weeks.

PREPARATION AND USE Wash okra before using. Trim stalk end, then leave whole or slice according to recipe. Boil, microwave, bake or fry, use in soups, stews and casseroles, in a traditional chicken or seafood gumbo, or cold in salad.

In Middle Eastern and Greek cooking, the pod is left intact. Trim the stem end, and if you have the patience, pare the thick skin covering the remnant of stem so that the whole pod is edible. Do not remove the stem or puncture the pod. It is then ready for the pot, but further preparation can reduce the viscosity. To do this, put the prepared okra in a bowl with a half cup of white vinegar for each 500 g okra. Toss gently with the hand, to coat with vinegar, leave for 30 minutes, drain and rinse well. Dry if okra is to be fried.

Add prepared okra to Greek and Middle Eastern lamb or vegetable stews towards the end of cooking. Fry them in olive oil, covering with a lid to steam-cook at the same time, turning the okra carefully to lightly brown, then serve with lemon (they taste like asparagus cooked this way). For Creole gumbos, remove stems and leave whole, or cut pods into thick slices.

PROCESSING Dried okra, and canned okra in brine or tomato sauce, are available from Greek and Middle Eastern food stores.

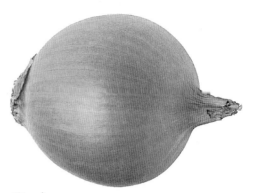

Onion *Allium cepa*

MAJOR NUTRIENTS			BOILED SERVE SIZE 40 G
Energy	40 kJ	Cholesterol	0
Protein	0	Sodium	0
Fat	0	Dietary Fibre	0
Carbohydrate	2 g	Vitamin C	4 mg

NUTRITIONAL INFORMATION This is a good source of vitamin C if not cut. Frying increases the kJ content of onions, because of the addition of the fat.

DESCRIPTION A bulb with white, pungent flesh and thin outer layers closely wrapped together.

ORIGIN AND HISTORY The onion is a native of central and western Asia and has been cultivated for centuries in the Mediterranean region. The slaves who built the pyramids in Egypt ate it along with garlic and radishes. The Children of Israel, fleeing from Egypt, longed for it during their wanderings in the desert. Hippocrates, the Greek physician, known as the father of medicine, declared it as being bad for the body but good for the sight. Like garlic, the onion developed myths such as being a cure for colds, warts, earache, and bad complexion, an aphrodisiac, and a defence against evil. Without this important member of the lily family, most cuisines would be tasteless.

BUYING AND STORAGE The best time to buy is summer and autumn. Choose dry, firm, well-shaped onions with thin skin. Avoid sprouting onions and excessively dry, crackling skin.

Store in a cool, dry, dark, well-ventilated place. Store purple-red Spanish onions in the crisper in the refrigerator.

PREPARATION AND USE Peel onions under water, using a sharp vegetable knife, to avoid tears from the odour. Alternatively, peel all but the root end of the onion, leaving this until last, since the cut root releases the irritating fumes. Use whole, sliced into rings, cut into quarters or segments, diced or chopped.

Gently fry, boil, braise, bake (roast), stuff and bake, deep-fry in batter, use in French onion soup, onion tart, in cream sauce, bread sauce and add to soups, sauces and casseroles. Use purple-red onions raw in salads and sandwiches.

PROCESSING Small white and brown onions are pickled or processed as frozen dressed vegetables.

VARIETIES

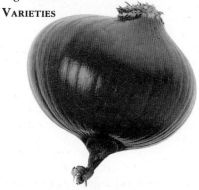

Dry Onion Left in the ground to mature and produce an onion with a tougher, dry outer skin suitable for long storage. The varieties include white, brown, large yellow Spanish, large red Spanish, red globe and pickling onions.

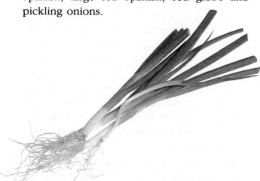

Green Onion Properly known as scallion, it is long and slender with a white, slim, cylindrical bulb and dark green, bitter-flavoured top.

The green onion is an immature onion pulled when the top is still green and before the bulb has formed. In China today, it is still used more than the dry mature onion.

Choose dry, firm, crisp green onion with undamaged, clean green tops. Trim the coarse green tops off and untie the twine binding the bunch to prevent bruising.

Store in a crisper or in a plastic bag in the refrigerator.

To use, wash and dry green onions, then either use whole or thinly sliced, in salads and as a garnish, gently stir-fried or steamed, or in soups, sauces, stuffings and savoury tarts.

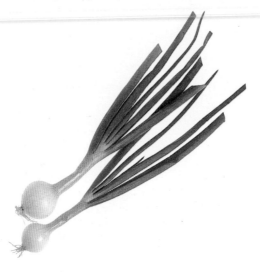

Spring Onion

NUTRITIONAL INFORMATION The nutrients of the spring onion are the same as those of the mature onion.

DESCRIPTION *Allium cepa* is long, with a definite small bulb formation having the same concentric layers as a dry, mature onion.

ORIGIN AND HISTORY The spring onion is an immature onion that is pulled when the top is still green and the bulb has started to form. It is at a more advanced stage than the green onion or scallion. Its history and origin is of course that of the onion. It is very popular in China.

BUYING AND STORAGE Buy the young, tender, clean spring onion with firm, well-trimmed bulb and fresh green stalk. Untie the twine binding if sold in bunches and store in a crisper in a refrigerator.

PREPARATION AND USE Trim the root and top, then wash and dry before use. Cook whole as a delicate vegetable, or slice or chop and use in Chinese cuisine or in salads.

SEE ALSO Shallot.

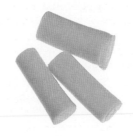

Palm Heart   *Sabal palmetto*

DESCRIPTION Palm hearts, better known as hearts of palm, are the inner portion of the sabal palm tree which grows wild in tropical areas and enjoys a beach environment.

ORIGIN AND HISTORY Brazil and Florida (USA) have developed orchards for the commercial production of hearts of palm. The young palm trees are cut down, the outer husks are stripped off and the inner layers chopped off until the edible heart is reached. This is placed in cold water immediately to prevent discoloration.

BUYING AND STORAGE Choose the crisp, clean, conical palm shoots about 15 cm long. Store in the refrigerator.

PREPARATION AND USE Wash well, then peel off the outer skin. Cook lightly by steaming, sautéeing or stir-frying but best used fresh, thinly sliced, in salad.

PROCESSING May be canned.

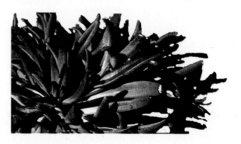

Parakeelya   *Calandrinia balonensis*

NUTRITIONAL INFORMATION Leaves provide water and minerals, the roots are significant sources of complex carbohydrate and minerals, and the seeds are high in fat, protein, dietary fibre and energy. Parakeelya leaves should not be consumed in large amounts because of the possible presence of oxalates. Roots and seeds can be eaten as desired.

DESCRIPTION Parakeelya is a low growing herb with a single stem and radiating succulent leaves. It flowers in winter with bright purple daisylike flowers. Leaves, root and seeds are edible.

ORIGIN AND HISTORY Parakeelya was used by Aborigines in Central Australia as a standby or emergency food. It was therefore significant in contributing to the diet when the range of nutrients was limited owing to food scarcity.

BUYING AND STORAGE If the whole plant is pulled up the leaves and roots maintain their freshness for up to 1 week stored in the refrigerator. Seeds keep well for years if stored dry.

PREPARATION AND USE The leaves must be well blanched for several minutes to dissolve any oxalates. They can then be used as a substitute for conventional leafy vegetables.

The small root can be eaten after cooking as for turnip or carrot. The seeds can be treated similarly to those of cereals and milled to a flour or boiled whole and used as a decorative sprinkle in the same manner as sesame or poppy seeds.

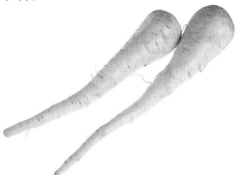

Parsnip *Pastinaca sativa*

MAJOR NUTRIENTS			BOILED SERVE SIZE 60 G
Energy	150 kJ	Sodium	0
Protein	0	Dietary Fibre	2 g
Fat	0	Vitamin C	5 mg
Carbohydrate	9 g	Vitamin E	1 mg
Cholesterol	0		

NUTRITIONAL INFORMATION An excellent source of vitamin C; moderate source of vitamin E and folate which is reduced to a moderate source if the parsnip is boiled.

DESCRIPTION A white root vegetable similar in shape to a carrot.

ORIGIN AND HISTORY The parsnip originated in eastern Europe, around the Mediterranean and the Caucasus. Known in Roman times, Emperor Tiberius is said to have imported it from Germany, where it grew along the Rhine. The parsnip can be described as an ordinary vegetable with an appropriate botanical name — from the Latin pastus meaning food and sativa meaning cultivated. Developed in Germany, it was the vegetable of the poor in northern Europe for many centuries. In Tudor times it was added to bread. At some stage the parsnip escaped from cultivation in Europe and now grows wild in England and some parts of Asia. The English settlers took the parsnip to North America where it was first recorded as growing in Virginia in 1609. It took second place in the Old World when the potato was introduced but it still enjoys great popularity in North America.

BUYING AND STORAGE Available all year, but at its seasonal best in winter. Choose the clean, firm, small-medium sized root of parsnip. Avoid the large parsnip as it has a woody core.

Store in a vegetable crisper in the refrigerator for 1–2 weeks.

PREPARATION AND USE Brush the parsnip in cold water, trim off the top and root end, then peel thinly. Cut into round slices, segments, chunky pieces, julienne strips or dice. Boil, steam, microwave, braise or bake (roast). Serve as a vegetable accompaniment, or use in soups, stews and casseroles. Candied parsnip is popular in North America.

PROCESSING May be used to make wine.

Pea *Pisum sativum*

MAJOR NUTRIENTS			SERVE SIZE 60 G
Energy	170 kJ	Dietary Fibre	3 g
Protein	0	Phosphorus	60 mg
Fat	0	Iron	1.1 mg
Carbohydrate	6 g	Thiamin	0.2 mg
Cholesterol	0	Niacin Equiv.	3 mg
Sodium	0	Vitamin C	15 mg

NUTRITIONAL INFORMATION An excellent source of thiamin, niacin, vitamin C; good source of fibre, phosphorus, iron; moderate source of pantothenic acid.

It is important to eat it *fresh* or else the thiamin, niacin and pantothenic acid content will be much lower.

Boiling peas reduces the amount of all nutrients. Thiamin and niacin drop from an excellent level in raw peas to a good level in the boiled equivalent. Boiling also reduces phosphorus and iron from a good to a moderate level. Vitamin C is affected but not significantly. The amount of pantothenic acid is diminished to an insignificant amount. Boiled frozen peas are similar nutritionally to boiled fresh peas. Canning peas reduces their vitamin C content, thiamin and niacin to moderate amounts. The sodium is significantly increased but is still present only at a moderate level. Fibre is also increased.

DESCRIPTION The tiny, round pea has a delightful flavour which is shared by its sometimes edible pod.

ORIGIN AND HISTORY The popular pea is possibly the first of all cultivars. The wild pea is said to have originated in the Near East, the middle of Asia and in Africa near Ethiopia, and to have been domesticated in the Middle East. It is also possible that it was cultivated near the Burma-Thailand border 2000 years before cultivation began in the Middle East. Seeds of primitive varieties have been found among the remains of the Bronze Age lake dwellers of Switzerland, dated at 5000 BC, and in caves in Hungary and in the ruins of Troy. The Greeks and Romans grew peas before the Christian era and the Romans probably introduced it to England. A small vegetable, it was used dried. The green pea, eaten fresh, came as a later development in the 16th century. It took a French gardener to develop a hybrid pod that climbed on trellises and produced the green, smooth, sweet, tender pea, which became fashionable at the court of Louis XIV. The French refined the pea to the tiny petit pois. In 1602, the Mayflower colony log book records that the pea planted by Captain Bartholomew Gosnold grew successfully on the island of Cuttyhunk. Much later the sugar snap pea was developed in North America and the snow pea was developed in China.

BUYING AND STORAGE Available in the spring, summer, and autumn. Choose shiny, bright green, well-filled, undamaged pods for the garden pea and sugar snap pea. Choose the very tiny petit pois pea. Select the flat, small–medium snow pea. Avoid swollen, withered yellowish pea pods. If the raw pea tastes sweet, it will still taste sweet when cooked.

Store peas in the pod in the crisper in the refrigerator.

PREPARATION AND USE Shell or 'pod' the vegetable just before use by pressing with a thumb on the rounded edge. The pod will split and the peas may be pushed out in one movement. Peas with edible pods, sugar snap and snow peas, should be topped, tailed, strung and washed in cold water, then drained. Boil, steam, braise, microwave and serve as a vegetable accompaniment or use in soups, casseroles and salads. Use the snow pea in oriental dishes.

PROCESSING The garden pea and petit pois may be canned or frozen.

VARIETIES

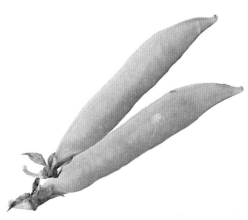

Garden Pea Also called the green pea and is the fresh seed of the green pea pod.

Petit Pois A young, small-seeded garden pea, popular in France.

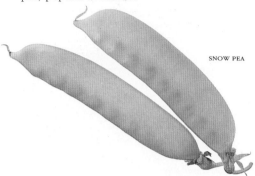

SNOW PEA

Snow Pea Also called mangetout (French for eat everything), sugar pea and Chinese pea, all flat, edible pea pods containing tiny peas.

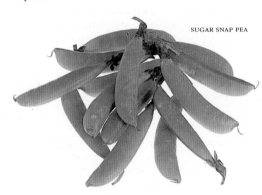

SUGAR SNAP PEA

Sugar Snap Pea A young tender spring pea with edible pod.

Potato *Solanum tuberosum*

MAJOR NUTRIENTS		SERVE SIZE 90 G	
Energy	300 kJ	Phosphorus	60 mg
Protein	0	Iron	0.6 mg
Fat	0	Potassium	470 mg
Carbohydrate	17 g	Thiamin	0.1 mg
Cholesterol	0	Niacin Equiv	1 mg
Sodium	0	Vitamin C	10 mg
Dietary Fibre	0	Vitamin B6	0.18 mg

NUTRITIONAL INFORMATION An excellent source of vitamin C; moderate source of phosphorus, iron, thiamin, niacin and vitamin B6; moderate in potassium. Compared to most other vegetables, the potato is higher in kJ. Individuals on low potassium diets should consult their dietitians if potato is restricted in the diet. Baking makes potato very high in kJs, but it has a slightly higher potassium level than the boiled equivalent as boiling potato leaches some potassium out into the water. Individuals on a low potassium diet should consult their dietitians to determine if baked potato is restricted. Though frying potato increases the level of a number of the nutrients, the actual nutrient density (i.e. the ratio of nutrients to kJ content) is lower, as chips are extremely high in kJs because of the addition of the fat. Therefore it is not recommended as a good cooking method to provide these nutrients. Potato chips are also high in potassium and individuals on low potassium diets should definitely avoid such food.

DESCRIPTION The thin-skinned potato, harvested from underground, has an unpleasant taste and watery texture when raw. Cooked, its floury insides and nutty-tasting skin make it one of the most widely used of vegetables.

ORIGIN AND HISTORY This very important and popular vegetable probably originated in Chile. It is thought that prehistoric tribes took the potato from Chile into the Andes region of Bolivia, Ecuador and Peru, because a wild species still grows in this area. The South Americans had been cultivating the potato for centuries when the Spanish conquerors arrived. In 1537, an expedition led by Gonzalo Jimenez de Quesada first discovered the potato growing in a deserted village, high up in the Andes in Peru, along with corn and beans. It is probable that the Spanish sailors took the potato back to Spain and Portugal in the mid-16th century although Sir Francis Drake is credited as discovering it in Chile and introducing it to England in 1577, while Sir Walter Raleigh first grew it in Ireland in 1585. The Indian name of pappas became batata in Spanish, then potato in English. The Irish economy became dependent on the potato but, when blight attacked the crops of 1845–6, a dreadful famine was the result with many deaths. The survivors emigrated to North America and Australia. German peasants were encouraged to cultivate potato in the mid-17th century. The French adopted it in the 18th century. The English were also slow to accept it as the Puritans distrusted a crop not mentioned in the Bible, however, by the 18th century it had become an important vegetable for the masses.

BUYING AND STORAGE With new potato, choose the small, even-sized, thin-skinned potato, free from dirt and bruises.

With mature potato, choose the firm, smooth, well-shaped potato, free from blemishes, cuts and sprouts, with few 'eyes'. Avoid the damp or green potato.

Store in a cool, dry, fairly dark place with good ventilation. New potatoes may be stored in the refrigerator for a short time.

PREPARATION AND USE With the new potato, wash, then scrape or scrub clean and boil or microwave. With the mature potato, wash, then scrub clean and remove eyes for baking and boiling. Peel thinly and cut into chunky pieces for boiling, microwaving, roasting (baking), or for cooking chips.

Serve the new potato boiled, scalloped, sauteed and in salads. Use the mature potato mashed and creamed, in soups, as pie toppings, for piping, and in patties.

PROCESSING Potato, particularly small new types, may be canned. Mature potato is processed as chips (French fries) or croquettes and frozen. May also be dehydrated, flaked and made into flour.

VARIETIES

There are several varieties of potato, each country favouring different ones which are best suited to the soil, climate and use, such as Idaho in USA, King Edward in Britain and Pontiac in Australia. However, the potato is classified into two basic types: early crop or new, which is marketed before maturity; late crop or mature/old, which is fully grown.

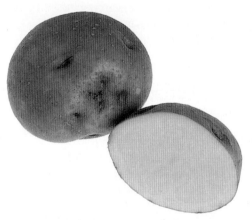

Pontiac Potato

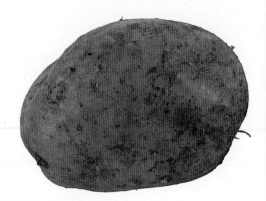

Robinson Potato

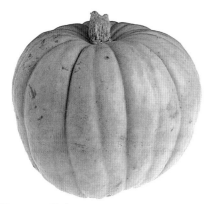

Pumpkin *Cucurbita maxima*

also called **Winter squash**

MAJOR NUTRIENTS

		BOILED SERVE SIZE 60 G
Energy	80 kJ	Sodium	0
Protein	0	Dietary Fibre	0
Fat	0	Vitamin A	330 µg
Carbohydrate	4 g	Vitamin C	3 mg
Cholesterol	0		

NUTRITIONAL INFORMATION An excellent source of vitamin A; moderate source of vitamin C, folate and pantothenic acid.

DESCRIPTION Pumpkins are the fruit of trailing vines. They are usually round and large with grey-blue to yellow-orange hard skin and deep yellow flesh, with flat oval seeds in a central cavity.

ORIGIN AND HISTORY The large, hard-skinned pumpkin originated in northern Argentina, near the Andes. Although a South American native vegetable, it remained isolated in the Andean valleys until the discovery of the New World, when it was introduced into Central and North America, and to Europe in the 16th century. It did not flourish there, as it needs a hot climate. Some other long-vined species of pumpkin originated in Mexico and were cultivated by the Indians throughout North America before the arrival of the white settlers. Archaeological discoveries in Mexico found pumpkin fragments dating back to 2000 BC. Pumpkin pie is served traditionally at Thanksgiving dinner in the USA. The pumpkin was transported to Australia by the early white settlers, where it is now a very popular vegetable.

BUYING AND STORAGE Most varieties of pumpkin are available all year round, but for the smaller varieties the season is wintertime.

Select clean, unblemished pumpkins which are heavy for their size. Whole pumpkin will keep longer than cut pumpkin.

Store whole pumpkin on a rack in a cool, well-ventilated, dry place. Store cut pumpkin wrapped in clear plastic film in the crisper of the refrigerator for up to 5 days.

PREPARATION AND USE Cut the amount required off the whole pumpkin, then remove the seeds and a thick layer of peel.

Large pumpkin may be cut into chunky pieces and boiled, steamed, microwaved or baked (roasted) and served as a vegetable or added to casseroles. It may also be pureed and used in soups, sauces, as a vegetable or in a dessert pie. Mashed pumpkin is used in stuffed pasta. Small pumpkins may be hollowed out and refilled with pumpkin soup or a savoury stuffing. Pumpkin puree may also be used in scones and cakes.

PROCESSING Pumpkin seeds are dried and sold in health food stores as a snack or for sprinkling over vegetarian dishes. Pumpkin shells may be hollowed out and used for jack o'lanterns for Halloween. Used commercially in canned soup and canned pie filling.

VARIETIES

Baby Blue Small and spherical with a slightly pointed stem end; has thick blue-grey skin with pale orange flesh and weighs 1.5–2 kg.

Banana Pumpkin A large cylindrical pumpkin with pointed ends; it has a blue-grey fairly soft skin and weighs about 10 kg.

Blue Max An Australian hybrid. It is round and indented at the blossom and stalk ends, thick skinned, blue-grey in colour, with bright orange flesh. Weighs about 4 kg.

BUTTERNUT

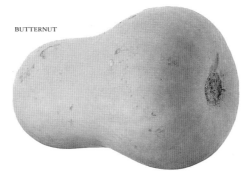

Butternut This vegetable is shaped like an elongated pear or a church bell, with a golden brown, hard skin and deep orange flesh, weighing about 2 kg.

Butter Pumpkin Spherical with a flattened top; has a fairly soft, orange-pink skin with deep yellow flesh and weighs 6–11 kg.

Cattle Pumpkin A very large, thin-skinned variety, about 100 kg in weight, grown mainly for pig feed.

Crown Prince A flattened drum shape; thin-skinned, creamy-grey with rich red-orange flesh; weighs about 6 kg.

GOLDEN NUGGET

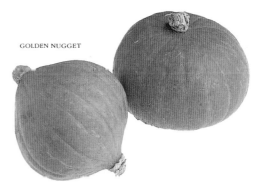

Golden Nugget A small, round orange-red variety with bright orange flesh, weighing up to 1.5 kg. It is a bush variety (not a trailing vine) with the small pumpkins growing in a cluster around the central stem.

Hubbard A pear-shaped pumpkin weighing about 4.5–5.5 kg; popular with home gardeners.

Jarrahdale A large, round pumpkin, 25 cm in diameter and 12 cm deep, with hard, ribbed, slate-blue to grey skin and bright orange flesh.

Queensland Blue A medium-sized pumpkin with blossom and stem ends flattened; it has a deeply ribbed, hard slate-grey skin with yellow-orange flesh and weighs 5.5–7.5 kg.

Trombone Another gramma, long and curved like a horse's collar, with a bulbous blossom end, golden brown in colour with sweet yellow flesh.

WINDSOR BLACK

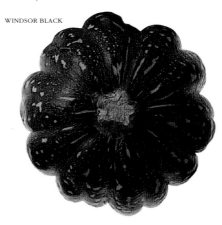

Windsor Black A round, flattened, multiribbed, dark green pumpkin with deep orange flesh; weighs 8–9 kg.

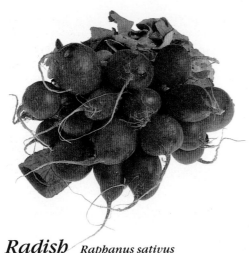

Radish *Raphanus sativus*

MAJOR NUTRIENTS		SERVE SIZE 30 G	
Energy	16 kJ	Cholesterol	0
Protein	0	Sodium	0
Fat	0	Dietary Fibre	0
Carbohydrate	1 g	Vitamin C	7 mg

NUTRITIONAL INFORMATION An excellent source of vitamin C.

DESCRIPTION A root vegetable with very peppery white flesh.

ORIGIN AND HISTORY The red radish was known to be cultivated in Egypt 2000 years ago, but its origin is believed to be in China or Middle Asia. The wild radish still grows in China and was introduced by the Chinese to Middle Asia in prehistoric times. The Greeks valued it highly around the 3rd century BC and the Romans recorded several varieties of shape and colour growing during the Christian era. The Romans took the radish north and cultivation was established in Germany by the 13th century. It was one of the first European crops to be taken to the Americas and was growing well in Mexico and Haiti before it became established in England in 1548. In Western cuisine it is used fresh in salads and hors d'oeuvres but in China and Japan, where it makes up about one-third of the vegetable crops grown, radish is pickled in brine.

BUYING AND STORAGE Available all year. Choose the firm, clean, undamaged, bright radish with fresh green leaves.

Remove leaves and store in a plastic bag in the vegetable crisper of the refrigerator. Will keep for up to 7 days.

PREPARATION AND USE Trim root and stalks from the red radish, wash in cold water, then drain and dry well. Wash the daikon radish, then peel thinly before use.

Use the red radish in salads and sandwiches, with dips and for garnishing.

VARIETIES

Giant White Radish

MAJOR NUTRIENTS		SERVE SIZE 100 G	
Energy	100 kJ	Sodium	30 mg
Protein	1 g	Potassium	230 mg
Fat	0	Iron	0.5 mg
Carbohydrate	4 g	Vitamin C	42 mg
Cholesterol	0		

NUTRITIONAL INFORMATION An excellent source of vitamin C and a moderate source of iron. It also contains copper and a moderate amount of potassium.

DESCRIPTION This radish, also called icicle radish, is a large, white-skinned mild radish which is a native to southern Asia, and a vegetable of the turnip family. The Chinese variety, known as loh bok, is thick at the top, shorter, 22 cm in length, and comes to a point at the end; the Japanese variety known as daikon, grows to about twice that length and is almost cylindrical.

ORIGIN AND HISTORY One of the best of the root vegetables because of its delicate taste and fine texture, the giant radish has been used in Chinese cooking for centuries. In earlier times the radish from Hupei province was considered the best, and its tender shoots were also eaten. A steamed dough cake made with mashed radish and rice flour is vital to the proper celebration of Chinese New Year. The Chinese did not regard it with the same reverence as do the Japanese who have devised a multiplicity of uses for its clean fresh flavour and crisp, crunchy texture. Grated it is used as a dip; cut into tissue-fine slices, shredded and crisped in iced water, it is an appealing garnish, and is cut into fanciful shapes when simply being used as a vegetable. It is pickled to serve with almost every meal, shaved and salted as a preserved vegetable, and the delicate peppery hot sprouts are enjoyed as a summer salad vegetable and garnish.

PREPARATION AND USE In Chinese cooking, the white radish is grated and made into a steamed savoury pudding, or is used in braised dishes and soups as a vegetable. Japanese use daikon extensively as a garnish. It is peeled and cut into 10–13 cm pieces, trimmed to a perfect cylinder, then cut paper-thin in a continuous sheet which is then rolled and cut crossways into fine shreds. It can be peeled and cut into fine shreds, grated or sliced for use in salads. Finely grated daikon is added to various Japanese dips as daikon-oroshi, particularly those accompanying tempura and fried foods.

BUYING AND STORAGE It is extensively cultivated and is now available almost year round in better Asian food stores.

When buying, choose the radish which is white and firm, smaller ones will have a better flavour and be more moist, very large ones can become woody.

It can be kept, wrapped in plastic, in the vegetable compartment of the refrigerator for several weeks.

Young giant white radish leaves can be used as a green vegetable, steamed, stir-fried or used raw in salads. Use in place of pickled/salted mustard greens.

In Japan, daikon is preserved to make the crunchy yellow pickle takuan.

Kiriboshi daikon, shavings of dried giant white radish are used to give its flavour to many Japanese braised and simmered dishes, and soups.

Daikon sprouts, kaiware in Japanese, are peppery hot sprouted daikon seeds, used in salads and as a garnish.

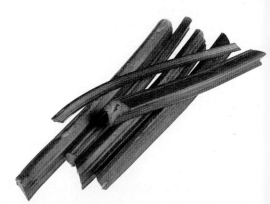

Rhubarb *Rheum rhaponticum*

MAJOR NUTRIENTS		SERVE SIZE 100 G	
Energy	80 kJ	Sodium	0
Protein	2g	Dietary Fibre	2.4 g
Fat	0	Calcium	30 mg
Carbohydrate	1 g	Iron	0.4 mg
Cholesterol	0	Vitamin C	8 mg

NUTRITIONAL INFORMATION Rhubarb is very low in kJ compared to most fruits, though sweetening rhubarb increases the kJ content. Rhubarb is most noted for its high level of calcium, which would contribute significantly to a non-dairy diet; moderate fibre, iron.

DESCRIPTION Rhubarb is a vegetable related to wild dock and sorrel, of which only the pinkish stems are eaten. Because rhubarb is normally sweetened and eaten as a dessert, many people think of it as 'fruit'.

ORIGIN AND HISTORY Native to China, Siberia, and the Himalayas, rhubarb was brought to the West by travelling caravans, from Baghdad, which were commissioned to bring foods from afar. Records of cultivation go back 2000 years BC. It was cultivated for many centuries for its medicinal properties, often prescribed for looseness of the bowels, but in the 18th century it was discovered that it could be eaten as a fruit in the diet. The leaves *must not* be eaten as they contain oxalic acid.

BUYING AND STORAGE Available all year, peaking in autumn and winter. Choose firm, crisp yet tender, long, plump, bright pink stalks or stems of rhubarb. Avoid wilted, flabby stems. Cut off the leaves, and remove the cord tying the bunch together to stop bruising.

Store in the crisper or in a plastic bag in the refrigerator, but use within 3–5 days.

PREPARATION AND USE Trim white root ends off stems of rhubarb, then wash well. Drain and dry well. Remove any marks with a small sharp knife. Cut into short lengths, then stew, poach or bake in a sugar syrup until tender. Serve warm or cold, puree for a fool, mousse, sauce, sorbet or ice cream. Use in pies, crumbles, charlottes, tarts, muffins, and wine.

PROCESSING May be canned.

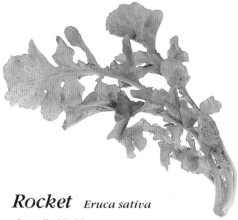

Rocket *Eruca sativa*

also called *Rokka*

NUTRITIONAL INFORMATION No reliable data are available.

DESCRIPTION An unusual green salad plant with pinnately lobed leaves and white or yellow flowers with violet-red veins.

ORIGIN AND HISTORY Native to the Mediterranean region and now an annual plant grown in Britain, Australia, and North America.

BUYING AND STORAGE Choose fresh, firm, bright green leaves. Avoid limp, damaged, damp leaves.

Store as for lettuce.

PREPARATION AND USE Wash in cold water, drain well, then pat dry in a clean tea towel. Use in salads or shred and use to garnish soup.

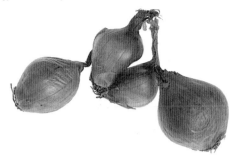

Shallot *Allium ascalonicum*

also called *French shallot*

MAJOR NUTRIENTS		SERVE SIZE 25 G	
Energy	38 kJ	Cholesterol	0
Protein	0	Sodium	0
Fat	0	Dietary Fibre	0
Carbohydrate	2 g	Vitamin C	6 mg

NUTRITIONAL INFORMATION This is a good source of vitamin C; moderate source of folate.

DESCRIPTION The shallot is a very hard, small onion with a reddish-brown tough skin which grows in a cluster of bulbs with 'pods' similar to garlic 'cloves' in formation. The flavour is strong, being a cross between onion and garlic.

ORIGIN AND HISTORY The shallot is a bulb, native of the eastern Mediterranean region. Its botanical name comes from the city of Ascalon and the Ascalonicum onion was noted as being good for sauce. The French knights, returning from the Crusades in the Middle East, brought the shallot back to France, where it is now an essential ingredient. Charlemagne grew it in his garden near Aix-la-Chapelle. Earlier, in the 9th century, the shallot was claimed to be one of 18 herbs grown in the kitchen gardens of the Monastery of St Gall, in Switzerland, then one of the centres of early European civilisation. It is often called the 'aristocrat of the onion family' and is now cultivated in California and recently in Australia, as well as in Europe. The word shallot is sometimes incorrectly used to mean a spring onion or green onion.

BUYING AND STORAGE Choose the dry, firm shallot with undamaged skin.

Store in a cool, dry, well-ventilated place as for the (dry) onion.

PREPARATION AND USE Peel the shallot with a sharp vegetable knife. Blanch first if the skin is very tough and proves difficult to remove. Peel under water or cut root end off last to avoid crying. Use whole, sliced or finely chopped according to recipe. Gently fry, use in marinades, soups, sauces and casseroles.

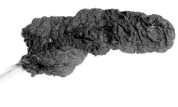

Silverbeet *Beta vulgaris*

also called *Seakale, Spinach, Swiss chard*

MAJOR NUTRIENTS			BOILED SERVE SIZE 60 G
Energy	75 kJ	Sodium	429 mg
Protein	0	Iron	1.9 mg
Fat	0	Dietary Fibre	2g
Carbohydrate	3 g	Vitamin A	576 µg
Cholesterol	0	Vitamin C	10 mg

NUTRITIONAL INFORMATION An excellent source of vitamins A and C and iron; high in sodium. Like most green leafy vegetables, silverbeet is high in iron (for oxygen transport in the blood) plus vitamin C and vitamin A. However it is also high in sodium and individuals on low salt diets should be conscious of this. If the low salt diet is for medical reasons consult the dietitian to check if silverbeet is to be restricted. The high iron content makes the vegetable extremely suitable for vegetarians.

DESCRIPTION A vegetable with attractive dark green, glossy leaves and white stems.

ORIGIN AND HISTORY Silverbeet is the oldest type of beet known to be used as a vegetable and was noted in Roman writings in the 3rd and 4th centuries BC. Since then the leaves have been developed in size. It was not cultivated in Britain until the 18th century, being far more popular in Europe. It is misnamed spinach in Australia, where it is a popular green leaf vegetable. It is also cultivated in America.

BUYING AND STORAGE Available all year, but best in winter. Choose crisp, fresh, undamaged leaves with crisp creamy-white stalks. Remove string from bunched stalks, trim off bruised stalks and remove damaged leaves.

Store in a crisper or in a plastic bag in the refrigerator, but use as soon as possible.

PREPARATION AND USE Wash leaves and stalks in cold salted water, then drain well. Trim green leaves from stalks, cutting down from thick base to top of leaf. Place leaves with only the water that clings to them, in a stainless steel or aluminium-lined pan and cook, covered, for 2–3 minutes, just until silverbeet has wilted, stirring if necessary to cook evenly. Drain thoroughly by pressing in a sieve with a large spoon or saucer, then serve chopped or pureed as a vegetable or use according to recipe. If cooking stalks, boil, steam or microwave and serve together. Use cooked in soup, pies and quiche. Shred raw tender silverbeet leaves and use in salads.

PROCESSING May be frozen, used in commercial pie fillings.

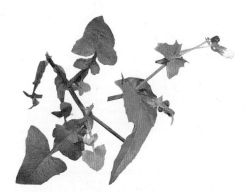

Sow Thistle   *Sonchus oleraceus*

also called **Hare's lettuce, Milkweed, Puha**

NUTRITIONAL INFORMATION Data are not available except that sow thistle is a very good source of vitamin C.

DESCRIPTION This leafy herb grows to 1 m with soft, smooth almost velvety leaves, milky sap and dandelionlike flowers. The leaves are the edible portion.

ORIGIN AND HISTORY Sow thistle leaves have a history of use in northern Europe, the Pacific Islands and South Africa. Aborigines of south eastern Victoria and southern South Australia ate the leaves as well as the tap root.

There are three varieties of puha in New Zealand, and the shore-growing one (*Sonchus littoralis*) is believed to be the one used by Captain Cook and the French Captain de Surville to cure crew members of scurvy.

BUYING AND STORAGE Tender young leaves are best foraged.

Keeps well both frozen and refrigerated. However, refrigerated storage should be minimised if the plants harvested are from high nitrate soils such as vegetable gardens. Storage of these leaves may lead to a high intake of harmful nitrites.

PREPARATION AND USE When washing the leaves, squeeze some of the white juice from the stalks, as some find the juice imparts a bitter taste. Blanch the leaves and use in salads, soup or pies, as a substitute for spinach.

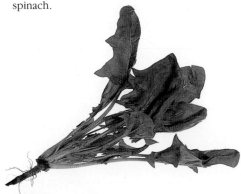

Spinach   *Spinacea oleracea*

MAJOR NUTRIENTS			BOILED SERVE SIZE 60 G
Energy	63 kJ	Iron	1.9 mg
Protein	0	Vitamin A	656 μg
Fat	0	Thiamin	0.1 mg
Carbohydrate	2 g	Vitamin C	19 mg
Cholesterol	0	Vitamin B6	0.18 mg
Sodium	0	Vitamin E	2 mg
Dietary Fibre	2 g		

NUTRITIONAL INFORMATION An excellent source of fibre, iron, vitamins A, C, E, folate; moderate source of thiamin, vitamin B6. Spinach is one of the most nutritious vegetables known. It is high in most vitamins and minerals normally found in meats and therefore is highly recommended for vegetarians.

DESCRIPTION Spinach has vivid green, slightly crinkled leaves on fine stems.

ORIGIN AND HISTORY Spinach probably originated in Persia (now Iran) where it was cultivated at the time of the Graeco-Roman civilisation. It was first recorded by the Chinese in AD 647 as 'the herb of Persia'. It was introduced into North Africa via Syria and Arabia and the Moors took it to Spain in 1100. By the 14th century, prickly seeded spinach was growing in monastery gardens throughout Europe and spinach recipes were included in a cookbook used by King Richard II in 1390. Smooth seeded spinach was first documented in England in 1551. Spinach as a body builder was identified with Popeye the Sailorman and today is recommended to young girls and women suffering from anaemia because of its high iron content.

BUYING AND STORAGE Available almost all year. Choose fresh, clean, good quality, bright green leaves. Avoid wilted, yellow,

wet, damaged leaves.

Remove string from bunched stalks, trim off roots, place in the crisper or in a plastic bag in the refrigerator. Use as soon as possible.

PREPARATION AND USE Trim the delicate spinach leaves from stalks, cutting down from stalk end to tip. Wash well in cold, salted water to kill any bugs, drain well. Place in a stainless steel or ceramic-lined pan with the water that clings to its leaves, cover and cook just until spinach has wilted, about 1–2 minutes, stirring once if necessary to complete cooking. Drain well in a sieve pressing excess water out with a large spoon or saucer. Chop and puree spinach, then serve with butter, cream or lemon juice and pepper as a vegetable accompaniment. May be used in soup, with poached fish and eggs, in soufflés, stuffed vegetables, pies, and quiches. Use raw spinach in salads, to line terrines and enclose fish en papillote.

PROCESSING May be canned, preserved in glass jars, frozen, used in commercial pie and quiche fillings.

VARIETIES Curly leaf or summer spinach, and flat leaf or winter spinach.

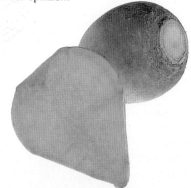

Swede   *Brassica napobrassica*

also called **Rutabaga**

MAJOR NUTRIENTS			BOILED SERVE SIZE 60 G
Energy	84 kJ	Carbohydrate	4 g
Protein	0	Sodium	0
Fat	0	Dietary Fibre	1 g
Cholesterol	0	Vitamin C	15 mg

NUTRITIONAL INFORMATION An excellent source of vitamin C.

DESCRIPTION The swede is a root vegetable with yellow flesh and a pale yellow skin.

ORIGIN AND HISTORY It is believed to be a hybrid of the cabbage and the turnip and was probably developed in Bohemia in the 17th century, first described by a Swiss botanist in 1620, then later documented as growing

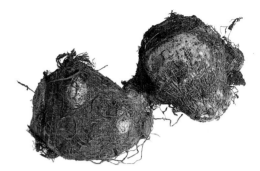

in England in 1664. The North American name rutabaga is derived from the Swedish word rotabagge. It has become a staple vegetable in the colder climate countries of north Europe and was a staple food during World War II. It is a traditional accompaniment to haggis in Scotland, where it is known as neeps.

BUYING AND STORAGE At its peak in winter although available all year. Choose the firm, clean swede, heavy for its size.

Trim and store in the crisper in the refrigerator.

PREPARATION AND USE Wash first then peel thickly. Cut into chunky pieces, then boil or microwave and serve mashed as a vegetable. May be used in soups, stews and casseroles, fritters and pancakes and in a traditional Finnish baked, savoury pudding.

Sweet Potato *Ipomoea batatas*

MAJOR NUTRIENTS		BOILED, FLESH ONLY SERVE SIZE 60 G	
Energy	313 kJ	Sodium	0
Protein	0	Dietary Fibre	2 g
Fat	0	Vitamin C	12 mg
Carbohydrate	20 g	Thiamin	0.1 mg
Cholesterol	0		

NUTRITIONAL INFORMATION An excellent source of vitamins C and E; moderate source of thiamin, folate and pantothenic acid. Sweet potato is similar to potato for the kJ count but contains more vitamins.

DESCRIPTION A long, large tuberous vegetable weighing 500 g–1 kg, which is not botanically related to the common potato.

ORIGIN AND HISTORY The sweet potato is the tuberous root of a vine, related to morning glory, and a native of the New World where it has been used for thousands of years. It was grown by the Incas of Peru and the Mayans of Central America but could be native to other tropical areas. Columbus noted it in his diaries in 1493 and de Soto later discovered it growing in Indian gardens in 1540 in what is now Louisiana. It was taken to Africa by the Portuguese traders around that time, then introduced into the East Indies, and the Philippines by the Spanish explorers. Portuguese traders took it to India, Malaya, and China. It is still a staple food in all these countries. It was introduced into Europe, via Spain, in 1526, but has never become as popular there, even though Henry VIII is said to have adored it.

BUYING AND STORAGE Choose the firm, clean, undamaged sweet potato.

Store in a cool, dry place.

PREPARATION AND USE Brush clean, then peel thickly and cut into chunky pieces. Use as for potato, mashed, roasted, chipped or added to casseroles. May also be cooked and pureed and added to cakes, scones or savoury soufflés, or used to make traditional Hawaiian poi.

VARIETIES

Red has red skin with orange flesh. The New Zealand red-skinned variety, called kumara, has yellow flesh. So-called white sweet potato has yellow skin with yellow flesh and is smaller than the red variety.

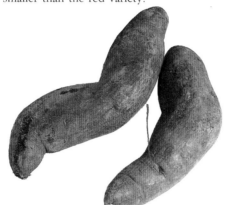

Red Sweet Potato

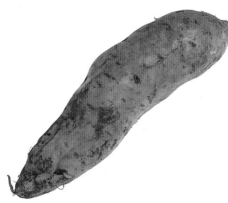

White Sweet Potato

Taro *Colocasia antiquorum*

also called **Dalo, Dasheen, Talo**

MAJOR NUTRIENTS		COOKED SERVE SIZE 60 G	
Energy	392 kJ	Sodium	0
Protein	0	Dietary Fibre	2 g
Fat	0	Iron	0.5 mg
Carbohydrate	23 g	Phosphorus	50 mg
Cholesterol	0		

NUTRITIONAL INFORMATION An excellent source of vitamin C; moderate source of phosphorus and iron. Like most root vegetables, taro is high in kJ owing to an increase in carbohydrate content.

DESCRIPTION A large tuber vegetable which grows just below the soil on a tropical plant which has pointed, almost triangular-shaped leaves and is of the species of decorative plant commonly known as the elephant ear. It is similar to certain yams, and has a flavour akin to sweet potato, though with a drier texture. The skin is light brown and rough in appearance, resembling thin bark. The flesh is dry in texture and ranges from cream to pink in colour, often with distinct pink-coloured veins. Taro has a bitter flavour if eaten raw.

ORIGIN AND HISTORY Taro is one of the world's oldest vegetables and is a vital staple food in many tropical countries, particularly in the Pacific Islands. It has been grown as food in China since the Han dynasty (206 BC–AD 220). It is still cultivated in Egypt, where it is known as kolkas, and grown in Cyprus as kolokassi. In Hawaii, taro is pounded to a thick paste with water to make poi which is allowed to ferment to various stages of flavour. Lavender in colour, it is served thick or thin as 'one, two or three finger' poi depending on how many fingers are needed to transport this delicacy to the mouth. Taro, and consequently poi, came to Hawaii from Tahiti where the same dish is called poe and contains mashed and simmered banana and breadfruit. Captain Bligh probably found poe more appetising than the breadfruit he was to transport from Tahiti to the West Indies.

BUYING AND STORAGE Sold by weight at Asian and Pacific food stores or those frequented by Egyptians and Cypriots, it should be thickly peeled before use.

It can be kept for several weeks in the vegetable compartment of the refrigerator. Cut surfaces will turn grey in storage; this does not affect the vegetable, and grey parts can be cut away. If the raw flesh irritates one's skin, rubber gloves can be worn while peeling and preparing.

PREPARATION AND USE Use as an alternative to potato or sweet potato. After peeling, cut into 2.5 cm cubes and boil or steam until tender, then drain off starchy cooking liquid. A versatile vegetable which can be used to make dessert or vegetable dishes.

Peel corms, leave whole, rub with lemon juice and fry slowly in oil until tender. The Cypriot way to prepare taro is to scrub it well and wipe dry, then peel and slice without wetting it further. To cut it into wedges, the knife should slice upwards at an angle, and then the slice broken off. It is claimed this prevents the taro becoming viscous in cooking. Slices are cooked in a tomato-flavoured pork stew. Egyptians prepare it similarly but simply slice the taro and cook it in a garlic-flavoured beef stew with silverbeet and fresh coriander.

Taro starch is a greyish-coloured flour made from ground taro, which is used as a thickener in some Asian dishes. In Chinese cooking it is used to make a popular snack woo kok, which has an oval-shaped outer casing of taro dough filled with diced meat. When deep-fried the surface turns golden brown and takes on the appearance of being covered in fine, feathery breadcrumbs. Taro starch is also used in Chinese cooking to make sweet hot soups.

Taro leaves are deep green, and triangular or heart-shaped. They are available fresh from Pacific Island and speciality Asian foodstores.

Wipe with a damp cloth, roll up and keep for several days in the vegetable compartment of the refrigerator. Throughout the Pacific Islands, taro leaves are cooked in the same way as spinach. Otherwise the leaves are used as a wrapping for foods which will be cooked in underground ovens.

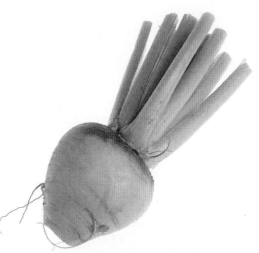

Turnip *Brassica rapa*

MAJOR NUTRIENTS			BOILED SERVE SIZE 60 G
Energy	58 kJ	Cholesterol	0
Protein	0	Sodium	0
Fat	0	Dietary Fibre	2 g
Carbohydrate	3 g	Vitamin C	9 mg

NUTRITIONAL INFORMATION An excellent source of vitamin C.

DESCRIPTION A white-fleshed root vegetable valued for its distinctive flavour.

ORIGIN AND HISTORY The turnip is a prehistoric vegetable which was grown in the Near East and South-East Asia around 10 000 BC. It used to be cultivated for medicinal purposes as well as food. When the Greeks and Romans discovered it, they cooked it for several hours, then pounded it with honey, vinegar, grapes, and oil. It became popular in Flanders in the 15th century, and during the time of Henry VIII the roots were roasted in the fire ashes and the leaves served in salad or cooked as vegetable greens. This root vegetable is a member of the mustard family and is still used extensively in China and Japan as well as in Europe.

BUYING AND STORAGE Available all year. Choose the firm, clean, unblemished turnip, heavy for its size with fresh green leaves, if still attached.

Trim off green leaves and store root and leaves in vegetable crisper in refrigerator. The turnip root will keep for a few weeks but the turnip greens for only 2 days.

PREPARATION AND USE Wash then peel turnip root, leave small turnips whole, cut larger ones into segments, chunky pieces, slices or sticks. May be boiled or microwaved then mashed or baked (roasted) or used in soups, stews and casseroles. The young tender turnip can be used in salad. Wash and cook turnip tops as for spinach.

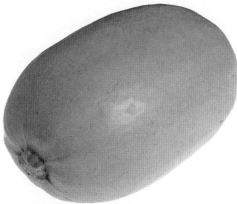

Vegetable Spaghetti
Cucurbita pepo

also called Spaghetti squash

NUTRITIONAL INFORMATION Similar to pumpkin: an excellent source of vitamin A; moderate source of vitamin C, folate and panthothenic acid.

DESCRIPTION A large, oval, deep yellow squash.

ORIGIN AND HISTORY The vegetable spaghetti is a winter squash, grown by the Indians of the USA for many centuries. Its other name is related to the fact that the cooked flesh may be forked out in thin strands similar to spaghetti. It is rich in natural fibre and has recently been introduced into Australia, where it is becoming popular as a vegetable and as an alternative to pasta spaghetti.

BUYING AND STORAGE It stores well, but not as long as pumpkin.

PREPARATION AND USE This vegetable is usually boiled in its skin, and the flesh is forked out and served with other foods. It can also be stuffed and roasted.

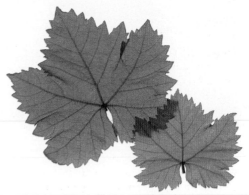

Vine Leaf *Vitis vinifera*

NUTRITIONAL INFORMATION No reliable data are available.

DESCRIPTION The young, tender, attractively shaped leaves of the grape vine.

ORIGIN AND HISTORY Native to the Mediterranean area and now grown worldwide, particularly in wine-producing countries.

BUYING AND STORAGE Available fresh in summer and autumn. Buy fresh ones if possible or pick your own.

Store flat in a clean plastic bag, with a paper towel, in the refrigerator. Use as soon as possible.

PREPARATION AND USE Blanch leaves, then drain on a clean tea towel. Use in salads, to stuff and roll up as for traditional dolmas, to wrap around small game birds before braising, or to decorate cheese platters and fruit bowls.

PROCESSING May be processed in brine and canned.

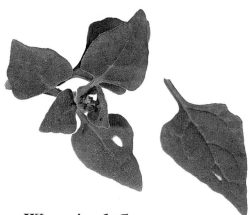

Warrigal Greens
Tetragonia tetragonoides

also called Botany Bay spinach, New Zealand spinach

NUTRITIONAL INFORMATION No detailed analysis is available.

DESCRIPTION A low, leafy green plant whose new shoots, young leaves and last 4–5 cm of the growing stem are edible.

ORIGIN AND HISTORY Warrigal greens were not eaten by Aborigines but were used by Maoris in New Zealand and by Australia's first white settlers. The plant is native to the Pacific Islands, Japan, South America, New Zealand, and Australia. It is cultivated as a vegetable in Indonesia.

BUYING AND STORAGE The edible parts should be fresh and not wilted.

Store warrigal greens in an open bag in the refrigerator where they will keep for up to 1 week. If longer storage is required prepare for consumption and freeze in usable portions.

PREPARATION AND USE Warrigal greens must be blanched for at least 3 minutes to reduce the level of saponins and oxalates pres-

ent. As a vegetable warrigal greens can substitute for English spinach and make an excellent cooked salad with nuts and dressing.

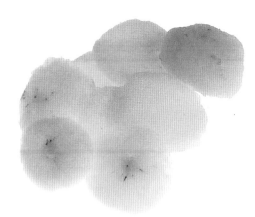

Water Chestnut *Eleocharis dulcis, Scirpus tuberosa, Trapa* spp., *Sagittaria sinensis*

also called Arrowhead, Calthrop, Haew, Kuwai, Ling gok, Ma t'ai, Sha gu

MAJOR NUTRIENTS		CANNED, DRAINED SERVE SIZE 50 G	
Energy	210 kJ	Sodium	15 mg
Protein	1 g	Potassium	155 mg
Fat	0	Iron	0.5 mg
Carbohydrate	13 g	Vitamin C	6 mg
Cholesterol	0		

NUTRITIONAL INFORMATION These are a good source of vitamin C and a moderate source of iron and potassium.

DESCRIPTION The name 'water chestnut' is applied to several different plants. The one most commonly known, the Chinese water chestnut, is the round corm of a tule or other bulrush, which has a shiny, dark brown, thick skin plus a paperlike outer skin, with crisp, sweet white flesh. Another type of water chestnut is *Trapa bicornis* or two-horned water calthrop, which may be poisonous if eaten raw. It grows on a floating water plant. The third type, arrowhead, resembles Chinese water chestnuts but is a pale yellow in colour with thin husklike leaves. The flesh is somewhat similar to that of Mexican jicoma.

ORIGIN AND HISTORY These are all ancient foods. There are three species of the genus *Trapa*. The two-horned water chestnut is one of China's important foods used since ancient times. *T. bispinosa* or the singhara nut was eaten in Kashmir, a land where water plants are traditionally important food sources. *T. natans*, otherwise known as the Jesuit's nut, has four horns and was a common food in ancient Europe.

The Chinese water chestnut is known as ma t'ai or horse's hoof after the appearance of its outer shell. It was first used in China medicinally for its yin or cooling characteristics. It is still used in this way, eaten raw to dispel summer heat and indisposition. A tonic soup is made by boiling water chestnuts with pig's intestines.

The water chestnut grows readily in natural or artificial waterways where the water is too deep for rice and too shallow for fish.

BUYING AND STORAGE Chinese water chestnut is sometimes available fresh. Look for full firm ones without brown soft spots. Peel with a sharp knife and trim root and stem flat to give a thick round disc. Soak the chestnut in iced or salted water when serving raw as a fruit. More commonly, it is available in cans, either as whole or sliced pieces, packed in water. Drain and rinse.

Canned water chestnut will keep for up to a week in the refrigerator if the water is changed daily. The two-horned water chestnut (calthrop) should have a hard, firm almost black shell.

It can keep for several weeks in the refrigerator, unpeeled.

PREPARATION AND USE Use in sweet dishes and in salads, vegetable dishes and spicy stir-fries for its crunchy texture and sweet taste. Often finely diced and added to stuffings and fillings. A good substitute is the Mexican jicoma or Malaysian bangkuang (yam bean). Calthrop should be boiled for at least 1 hour before using, to destroy bacteria and parasites. Arrowhead is used, particularly in northern China and in Japan, much like a potato. Unlike the Chinese water chestnut, arrowhead is never eaten raw.

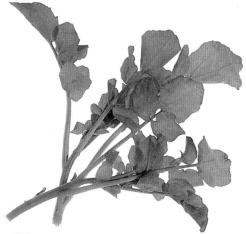

Watercress *Nasturtium officinale*

also called Kong syin ts'ai

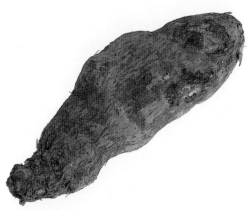

MAJOR NUTRIENTS		SERVE SIZE 100 G	
Energy	60 kJ	Calcium	80 mg
Protein	3 g	Magnesium	17 mg
Fat	0	Iron	3 mg
Carbohydrate	1 g	Thiamin	0.1 mg
Cholesterol	0	Riboflavin	0.1 mg
Dietary Fibre	3.5 g	Niacin Equiv.	1 mg
Sodium	60 mg	Vitamin C	100 mg
Potassium	500 mg	Vitamin A	500 µg

NUTRITIONAL INFORMATION An excellent source of vitamin C, vitamin A, calcium and iron; moderate source of magnesium, thiamin, riboflavin and niacin. It also provides a good source of potassium.

DESCRIPTION A vegetable with small, deep green, rounded leaves and a peppery flavour.

ORIGIN AND HISTORY Watercress is a perennial green leafy plant of the mustard family. It is found growing wild in clear streams and springs in many countries, and in winter in South-East Asia it favours very wet fields and the edges of waterways. It used to be gathered wild until its cultivation was begun as a salad plant in the early 19th century. Watercress is thought to be native to the eastern Mediterranean region: the Persians, Romans and Greeks all ate it for its health properties. Xerxes, a Persian king, recommended it to keep his soldiers healthy, and the Greeks thought it was good for the brain. Its cultivation has only recently been introduced to Canada, the USA, West Indies, South America, and Australia although street vendors sold it in London and in Sydney from baskets on top of their heads in the mid-19th century. It was taken to southern China, where it complements the native ong choy or weng ts'ai, water spinach, which grows in summer, by occupying the same waterlogged soil during winter months. It shares with other aquatic vegetables the quality of yin or cooling.

BUYING AND STORAGE Select the short sprigs, no more than 20 cm long, with crisp, deep green stems and firm, well-coloured leaves. Yellowing of the leaves indicates age and loss of flavour. It should be thoroughly washed, then shaken to remove excess water.

Wrap in paper towel and store in a plastic container in the refrigerator for up to 5 days. In cool climates, it can be kept in a jar of water, changing the water daily.

PREPARATION AND USE Remove leaves from stems. Use only leaves in salads and soups, or puree stems for more intense flavour. As a garnish for Japanese dishes, select the small attractive ends of the sprig.

Yam *Dioscorea batatas, D. esculenta*

also called Shu yu

MAJOR NUTRIENTS		SERVE SIZE 100 G	
Energy	560 kJ	Potassium	500 mg
Protein	2 g	Magnesium	40 mg
Fat	0	Iron	0.3 mg
Carbohydrate	32 g	Thiamin	0.1 mg
Cholesterol	0	Vitamin C	10 mg
Dietary Fibre	4 g		

NUTRITIONAL INFORMATION An excellent source of vitamin C and potassium; good source of magnesium; moderate source of iron and thiamin. It is high in carbohydrate, providing a good source of energy.

DESCRIPTION The edible root of a climbing plant of which there are many species. The root has a rough, papery, thick skin which varies in colour depending on the variety, from black to a pinkish-brown. The yam is similar to the sweet potato, although the flesh tends to be drier and more floury. The Japanese field yam is the common yam given the name sato imo to differentiate it from the native mountain yam, yama no imo. The most commonly used yam in China (*D. batatas*) is coated in a rough grey-brown skin, and is about the size and shape of a tennis ball. Others range from small elongated shapes to quite large roots, resembling the taro.

ORIGIN AND HISTORY The yam has been eaten as a staple by peasants in China since its early history, although some varieties are thought to be native to Central America. Under the reign of Emperor Ch'eng (32 to 7 BC), a political upheaval caused a major breakdown to an irrigation dam which seriously affected agriculture, and gave birth to a song which the people of Ju-nan in Honan sang, 'It was Chai Tzu-wei who destroyed our dam, Now all we have for food is soy beans and yam.' The yam grows readily in tropical and subtropical climates and provides an inexpensive source of carbohydrate, making it a secondary staple in the Asian diet. In Japan the small field yam is known as ko-imo, and the larger one, yatsugshira.

The yam is found growing in tropical countries. The most commonly cultivated variety is a native of southern Asia. A white yam grows in the monsoon zone of west Africa. There is also a New Zealand yam, *Oxalis crenata*, with pink skin and a tuber up to 15 cm long. The yam resembles sweet potato and has become confused with it because early black African slaves used their word nyam for the sweet potato in North America.

BUYING AND STORAGE Choose the firm, undamaged yam with a regular shape.

Store as for potato.

PREPARATION AND USE Remove the outer bark and cook and use as for potato, boiled, mashed, baked (roasted), and chipped.

In the islands of the Pacific there are many delicious ways of serving yam, such as yam soup, which also contains banana, pawpaw and sweet potato; or rissoles, made with pureed yam, flaked cooked fish and coconut cream, rolled in grated coconut and fried.

Mashed yam moistened with vegetable oil is used to make certain snack dishes in Malaysian, Indian, and Chinese cooking, and is also made into sweet snacks and desserts.

VARIETIES

Mountain Yam

also called Nago imo, Yama no imo

NUTRITIONAL INFORMATION No nutritional data are available.

DESCRIPTION A beige-coloured, hairy, Japanese root vegetable, yama no imo is unlike other forms of yam. The mountain yam comes in several varieties and has inconsistent shapes and sizes, ranging from small rocklike shapes of about 5 cm diameter, to irregularly formed spearlike shapes which grow to as long as 38 cm. The Japanese name nago imo, which describes the long yam, translates as long potato. It has a gluey texture when peeled and grated, and is an acquired taste.

ORIGIN AND HISTORY The mountain yam has been part of Japanese peasant cooking for centuries. It is considered to be good for the digestion. When served with various other foods, mountain yam is known as tororo.

BUYING AND STORAGE Larger Japanese food specialists may stock the yam fresh as it lasts many weeks and can be easily transported.

PREPARATION AND USE Peeled and cut into pieces, the yam is cooked as a root vegetable, and in Japan it is also grated to use as a thickener and binder. Taro can be substituted.

Zucchini *Cucurbita pepo*

also called **Courgette**

MAJOR NUTRIENTS

SERVE SIZE 60 G

Energy	40 kJ	Dietary Fibre	1 g
Protein	1 g	Iron	0.3 mg
Fat	0	Vitamin C	10 mg
Carbohydrate	1 g		

NUTRITIONAL INFORMATION Zucchini are an excellent source of vitamin C.

DESCRIPTION Zucchini are a variety of marrow or summer squash, picked when small.

ORIGIN AND HISTORY This vegetable with a thin edible skin was first developed in Italy, hence its name, which is a derivative of the word 'sweetness'. Christopher Columbus brought the seeds to North America where it became established. Internationally, it was well known only to people of Mediterranean descent for hundreds of years, but it is now a very fashionable vegetable in the Western world.

BUYING AND STORAGE Zucchini are best eaten soon after purchase, or they may become soft or shrivelled.

PREPARATION AND USE Zucchini are a very versatile vegetable. The small ones can be cooked whole with a sauce, and larger ones can be stuffed, or cut into various shapes for stir-fries and stews. Zucchini are a traditional ingredient of such dishes as ratatouille, and combine well with the flavour of tomatoes. The flowers of the plant are also edible.

VARIETIES

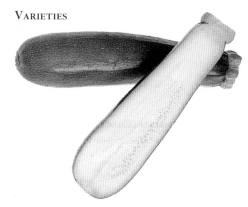

Green Zucchini

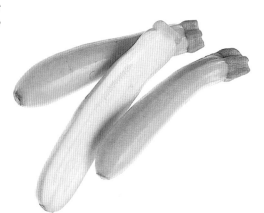

Yellow Zucchini

FRUITS

People today enjoy an abundant supply of a wide variety of fruits including tropical fruits, the fruits from temperate zones and those from colder climates. As transport and marketing have improved, the range of fresh fruits available throughout the year has increased. Fruits such as grapes and strawberries, which were once only on sale for a relatively short season, now appear during most months of the year in large cities. The seasons for specialty fruits such as raspberries are lengthening.

Although there are fluctuations in the per capita consumption of fruit there has been a general increase since the late 1950s. The use of fresh fruits has increased, while the use of dried fruits and processed fruits is gradually declining. Much of the increase is due to the growing popularity of fruit juices and fruit juice drinks and to improved marketing.

The popularity of a 'lighter' style of eating and the search for quickly prepared meals and snacks, combined with a growing interest in healthy eating, have also contributed to the increasing use of fruit.

Fruits are closely related to vegetables, and some foods we refer to as vegetables are botanically fruits: for example, eggplant and zucchini. In daily usage the term 'fruit' is used to describe the plant foods in which the carbohydrate occurs mainly as sugars, while vegetables are those plant foods in which the carbohydrate occurs mainly as starch.

It is said that in the evolution of humans the innate liking of sweet foods came from the fact that sweet fruits were safer foods than other plant foods, since the latter were more likely to contain alkaloids and other naturally occurring toxins which betrayed themselves by their bitter taste.

Fruits provide us with a variety of flavours, colours and textures, and with sweet foods which are not energy dense. This means that per unit of weight their kilojoule or calorie value is relatively low. Fructose, or fruit sugar, which is one of the sweetest of the sugars, is found in many fruits and contributes to their sweet taste.

With the exception of the avocado, which contains monounsaturated fats, fruits contain very little fat. This means that fruits are a valuable food for all those wishing to reduce fat intake and keep in the healthy weight range.

Fruits are a valuable source of vitamin C and of dietary fibre. Some fruits, such as the citrus fruits and apples, contain the soluble fibres which are helpful in controlling cholesterol levels in the blood.

The orange and yellow fruits such as yellow peaches, apricots, rockmelon and prunes, are excellent sources of beta carotene (converted to vitamin A in the body). Fruits generally, however, do not match vegetables as a source of beta carotene.

Oranges, mandarins, bananas, avocados and rockmelons are excellent sources of folate, and bananas are an excellent source of pyridoxine (vitamin B6).

Fruits contain very little sodium and many of them are an excellent source of potassium. This high potassium-to-sodium ratio is a plus in the public health strategy to reduce the prevalence of high blood pressure by lowering sodium intake and increasing potassium intake.

Unless otherwise stated, the major nutrients listed in this chapter are for the raw fruit.

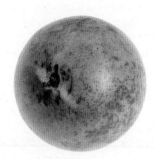

Abiu *Pouteria caimito*

also called **Abi, Caimo**

MAJOR NUTRIENTS   SERVE SIZE 100 G

Energy	590 kJ	Dietary Fibre	0
Protein	1.8 g	Vitamin C	50 mg
Fat	0	Niacin Equiv.	3.5 mg
Carbohydrate	36 g		

NUTRITIONAL INFORMATION Abiu is an excellent source of Vitamin C and niacin.

DESCRIPTION A bright yellow, 5–10 cm almost round fruit with a point at the blossom end and gelatinous, translucent, white, sweet caramel-flavoured flesh with 1–5 seeds.

ORIGIN AND HISTORY The delicious abiu is thought to have originated in Peru. It is now cultivated extensively in the tropical basin of the Amazon River where it grows to an enormous height. There are also some orchard plantings in Florida (USA) and Australia where this evergreen tree is pruned to a height of 4–8 metres. The abiu can bear as many as 3 crops a year. It should be picked when absolutely ripe or when it falls off the branches because the immature fruit contains an unpleasant latex which sticks to the lips.

BUYING AND STORAGE Available in summer and autumn. Choose firm, shiny well-shaped fruit with no damaged skin. Store at room temperature until soft, which indicates fruit is fully ripe, then store in the refrigerator until required.

PREPARATION AND USE Eat fresh in the hand, or dice, remove stones and serve fresh or add to fruit salad. Puree and use in sorbet, ice cream or drinks.

Apple *Malus communis*

MAJOR NUTRIENTS   SERVE SIZE 125 G

Energy	270 kJ	Cholesterol	0
Protein	0	Sodium	0
Fat	0	Vitamin C	4 mg
Carbohydrate	17 g	Dietary Fibre	2 g

NUTRITIONAL INFORMATION The energy content is provided by carbohydrate. A good source of vitamin C and moderate in fibre.

Unsweetened canned apple is unaffected nutritionally. Sweetened canned apple has a marginally higher energy content owing to the addition of sugar.

'An apple a day keeps the doctor away' may well be true, as it is relatively low in kilojoules, contains fibre, and is an excellent source of vitamin C.

DESCRIPTION The apple is a plump fruit with a shiny skin which varies according to type from green, through yellow to deep red. It has a firm, crisp, juicy white flesh.

ORIGIN AND HISTORY The apple is known to have been gathered, eaten fresh, dried and stored as far back as the Stone Age. The wild crab-apple, from which the modern apple was cultivated, still grows in Europe, western Asia and the Himalayas, but the direct history of the apple is difficult to trace as various peoples have moved around Europe, taking the fruit with them. Once it was the only fresh fruit available in winter in northern Europe, and has continuously been improved on its travels. The apple was cultivated by the Egyptians along the Nile in the 12th century BC. The Greeks and Romans cultivated it as a symbol of love and beauty. The Persians valued it as the fruit of immortality. At the beginning of the 17th century, apple varieties were sent to North America from England and France. The apple was later taken to South Africa and Australia by the white settlers and today this pome fruit is cultivated extensively. The apple is popularly believed to ease stomach acidity and constipation.

BUYING AND STORAGE Autumn is the best time to buy new season's fruit, but apples are available all year, owing to controlled atmosphere storage which halts their respiration and normal enzyme ripening. Choose firm apples of a bright colour and undamaged skin.

Store in the refrigerator to retain crisp texture for up to 2 weeks.

PREPARATION AND USE Wash and dry the apple if serving fresh. Use sliced in salad, sliced into segments or rings with cheese boards and fruit platters, or eat fresh in the hand. Wash or peel and remove core if cooking it. Leave whole and bake or microwave, or slice into segments for stewing or using in pies, puddings, and apple sauce. Brush peeled and cut apple with lemon juice to prevent discoloration.

PROCESSING May be canned, juiced, preserved as puree, dried, used in chutney, processed and frozen.

VARIETIES
Apart from the wild, tart crab-apple, there are many delicious varieties of apple.

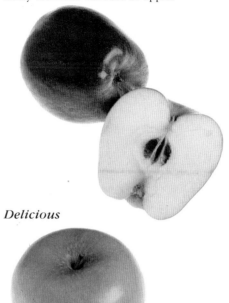

Delicious

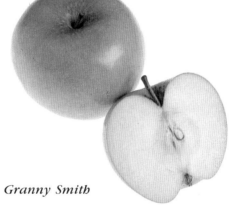

Granny Smith

SEE ALSO Dried Apple.

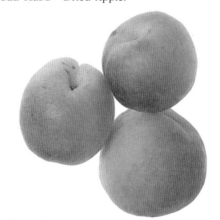

Apricot **Prunus armeniaca**

MAJOR NUTRIENTS SERVE SIZE 100 G

Energy	190 kJ	Sodium	0
Protein	0	Dietary Fibre	3 g
Fat	0	Vitamin A	111 µg
Carbohydrate	11 g	Vitamin C	7 mg
Cholesterol	0		

NUTRITIONAL INFORMATION The energy comes from carbohydrate. An excellent source of beta carotene (the plant form of vitamin A) and vitamin C; good source of fibre.

If apricot is canned with added sugar, this doubles the kilojoule content. Apricot is very high in beta carotene. However the kernel contains a substance called laetrile, a cyanide compound that may cause death if taken in repeated doses.

DESCRIPTION A plump and rounded fruit with soft, yellow to orange skin and juicy, fragrant flesh.

ORIGIN AND HISTORY The apricot is a stone fruit, native to China, and was documented in Chinese writings 2000 BC. The tree was first introduced through eastern Asia, then the Arabs introduced it into the Mediterranean. The Romans took it into Europe, where it later became popular in monastery gardens, the prerunner to orchards. In 1570 it was seen to be an attractive addition to noblemen's gardens in England. In the 18th century, it was equally popular in gardens in the USA. Early white settlers and immigrants introduced apricot cultivation into South Africa, New Zealand, and Australia. Intensively cultivated in the Mediterranean region, North Africa and Zambia, it is also grown in India and Turkey. It is the fruit most prized by confectioners and pastry cooks and has given its name to the French verb abricoter, meaning to make a glaze by reducing jam by boiling, then straining and flavouring with a liqueur.

BUYING AND STORAGE Available in early summer. Choose ripe, soft, plump fruit with a bright yellow colour and avoid very firm, dull fruit.

Keep in the crisper or in a plastic bag in the refrigerator. To ripen, place in a brown paper bag at room temperature.

PREPARATION AND USE Wash and dry thoroughly. Eat fresh in the hand or use pureed, or halve, remove the stone and serve stuffed. Stew, poach, microwave, use in tarts, pies, pastries, pancakes, soups, soufflés, ice creams and sorbets.

PROCESSING May be canned, used dried, glacéed, brandied, used in chutney and jam, to make wine and brandy, processed and frozen.

SEE ALSO Dried Apricot.

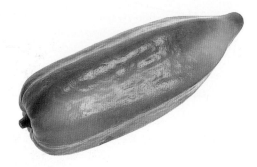

Avocado Persea americana

also called **Aguacate**

MAJOR NUTRIENTS		SERVE SIZE 100 G	
Energy	890 kJ	Potassium	470 mg
Protein	0	Thiamin	0.08 mg
Fat	23 g	Vitamin A	100 µg
Carbohydrate	0	Riboflavin	0.10 mg
Cholesterol	0	Vitamin C	9 mg
Sodium	0	Niacin Equiv	2 mg
Iron	0.6 mg	Dietary Fibre	1.5 g

NUTRITIONAL INFORMATION An excellent source of folate and vitamin C. High source of fat, predominantly mono-unsaturated. Good source of riboflavin, niacin and vitamin A. Moderate source of iron, potassium and thiamin. The avocado is the only fruit that contains fat, and is high in calorific value. Weight-conscious people or those on low fat diets need to restrict their intake of avocado.

DESCRIPTION The avocado is the shape of a large pear, with shiny skin or rind which is green or almost black depending on type. The flesh is a delicate yellow with a characteristic green outer hue.

ORIGIN AND HISTORY The history of the avocado fruit goes back to 7000 BC according to evidence found in Mexican excavations. It was also recorded by the Aztecs in South America nearly 300 BC, and was known to be an important part of the diet of the Aztecs and Incas when the Spanish conquistadors invaded their lands in the 16th century. It is also native to Guatemala and the Mexicans call it aguacate. It has also been called alligator pear because of its alligatorlike skin and its pear shape. Some varieties are indigenous to the Canary Isles and the Azores, others to South-East Asia. It is now an important cultivated crop in Florida, Israel, South Africa, Australia and New Zealand and it flourishes in California. It has enjoyed increased popularity since the arrival of modern air transport to reach the world market.

BUYING AND STORAGE Buy well-shaped fruit with no bruises or blemishes. Look for 'ripe' labels or test for ripeness by pressing around the neck which should yield softly, otherwise buy firm fruit and ripen with a banana in a brown paper bag at room temperature.

Store at room temperature until fully ripe, then store in refrigerator for up to 3 days.

PREPARATION AND USE Cut avocado in half lengthways, using a stainless steel knife. Twist halves gently to separate. Press the knife into the seed and twist gently to remove. Serve avocado halves in the skin, topped with French dressing, seafood or salad. Avocado may be peeled and sliced or cubed and used in salads and sandwiches, or pureed for traditional guacamole dip, soup or ice cream or spread on toast. Do not cook for it turns bitter.

PROCESSING May be processed and preserved as guacamole or used in commercial pâtés.

VARIETIES

There are hundreds of varieties, the most popular are listed.

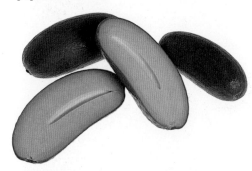

Cocktail Small, seedless, unfertilised fruit about 5 cm long.

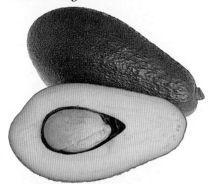

Fuerte Pear-shaped with a thin green skin, a large seed and creamy-yellow-green, smooth, buttery flesh.

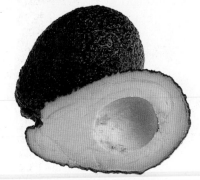

Hass Has a pebbly skin which turns from green to purple-black when ripe.

Sharwil Similar to Fuerte but with a thicker neck.

SEE ALSO Guacamole.

Babaco Carica pentagona

MAJOR NUTRIENTS		SERVE SIZE 90 G	
Energy	80 kJ	Cholesterol	0
Protein	1 g	Sodium	0
Fat	0	Dietary Fibre	0
Carbohydrate	3 g	Vitamin C	18 mg

NUTRITIONAL INFORMATION An excellent source of vitamin C. Babaco is very low in kilojoules and the only major nutrient is vitamin C.

DESCRIPTION Looks like a long five-sided pawpaw (papaya) with a thin, waxy, yellow, edible skin. Flesh is yellow with a white fibrous centre and tastes of strawberries, pineapple, and pawpaw.

ORIGIN AND HISTORY The babaco is a member of the pawpaw family, the fruit of a tropical tree, native to Ecuador. It is now grown commercially in New Zealand and Australia, where it is promoted as 'the fruit with the champagne taste'. It is important that it is eaten fully ripe to be appreciated. Like the pawpaw, the babaco also contains the enzyme papain, which has the quality of tenderising meat and aiding digestion.

BUYING AND STORAGE Available during autumn. Select fruit with shiny, yellow, undamaged skin.

Store in the refrigerator.

PREPARATION AND USE Wash and dry, slice into rings or lengths, then cut into cubes. Serve fresh, in fruit salad, pureed in drinks, with cheese, or barbecued. Will tenderise tough meat.

PROCESSING May be juiced, used in jam.

Banana *Musa paradisiaca*

Major Nutrients		Serve Size 100 g	
Energy	350 kJ	Sodium	0
Protein	1 g	Dietary Fibre	4 g
Fat	0	Iron	0.5 mg
Carbohydrate	2 g	Vitamin C	11 mg
Cholesterol	0		

Nutritional Information The energy comes from carbohydrate; excellent source of vitamin C; moderate in fibre and iron. Sometimes people who need to avoid potassium are advised against eating bananas and conversely many sportspeople consume bananas to replace potassium. Either way it would be necessary to eat many bananas each day. If in doubt consult your dietitian.

Description The banana grows on the main stalk of the tree in half spiral branches, called 'hands', each bunch containing a varying number of bananas called 'fingers'.

Origin and History The banana family is native to tropical regions throughout the world. The genus itself is thought to have originated in the region from India to New Guinea. Alexander the Great is said to have enjoyed the fruit on his travels through India. The banana was probably introduced into Africa by the Arabs and then taken later into North America and other colonies by the Spanish and Portuguese. It is thought to be one of the first fruits gathered and cultivated. Joseph Banks, who accompanied Captain Cook on his early voyage to Australia, found wild bananas in north Queensland and described them as scarcely edible, being filled with bitter black seeds. Careful selection over the years has led to a sweet, soft-textured banana which is rich in food value. The Canary Isles once supplied bananas to Europe exclusively, but now the banana travels long distances by sea from the tropical producers to the northern markets of the world.

Buying and Storage Available all year, peaking in autumn. Choose firm, plump, brightly coloured yellow fruit, free from damage. Green tips indicate fruit is not ripe, solid yellow fruit is riper and fruit with brown specks is at prime ripeness.

Store at room temperature but when fully ripe store wrapped in newspaper, in the refrigerator, for up to 5 days. Skins turn black when bananas are stored in a refrigerator but the flesh remains unchanged.

Preparation and Use The banana is valued throughout the South Pacific region and forms a major part of the diet of many island nations. It can be served in a multitude of ways at any meal of the day.

Peel banana and eat fresh in the hand, or slice for fruit salad, banana cake, or mash for toddlers. May be flambéed, baked, barbecued or used in drinks. Brush peeled banana with lemon juice to prevent discoloration.

Processing May be dried.

Varieties

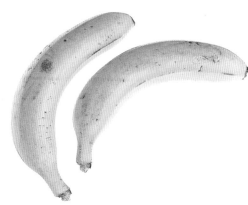

Cavendish A large, long variety.

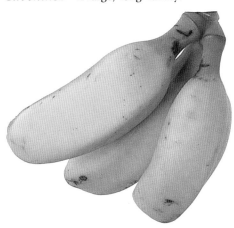

Lady Fingers Short bananas.

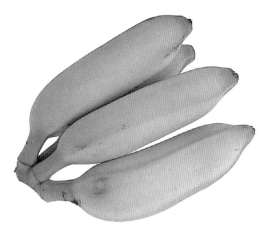

Sugar Bananas Short bananas.

See Also Dried Banana, Plantain.

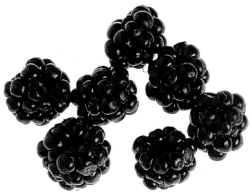

Blackberry *Rubus fruticosus*

also called ***Bramble***

Major Nutrients		Serve Size 100 g	
Energy	125 kJ	Dietary Fibre	8 g
Protein	1 g	Calcium	60 mg
Fat	0	Iron	1 mg
Carbohydrate	6 g	Vitamin C	22 mg
Cholesterol	0	Magnesium	30 mg
Sodium	0		

Nutritional Information An excellent source of iron, vitamin C, fibre, vitamin E; high in carbohydrate, a good source of magnesium, and a moderate source of calcium.

Canning has little effect on nutrients.

As the nutritional information shows, the blackberry is quite a nutritious fruit. The unusual nutrients not normally found in any great quantities in fruit are calcium, magnesium and vitamin E. Blackberries also contain iron which could be a valuable source for vegetarians; 1 cup of blackberries would also provide the recommended daily amount of vitamin C necessary for an individual.

Description A collection of tiny, shiny black drupelets around a central white core.

Origin and History Native to Britain, North America and Africa, and introduced to Australia. A member of the rose family, a climber which is cultivated on trellises in America and is still gathered wild from hedgerows in England and Australia.

Buying and Storage Available in late summer and autumn. Choose fresh, dry berries with a bright appearance and uniform black colour which indicates ripeness.

Store unwashed, but covered, in the refrigerator.

Preparation and Use Pick over the blackberries, remove any insects, and hull. Rinse in a colander if liked and dry by draining on kitchen paper towels. Use fresh, in fruit salad, in traditional summer pudding, in pies and tarts or pureed in ice cream, sorbet and drinks.

Processing Used for jam, jelly, and for cordial.

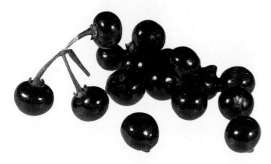

Black Nightshade *Solanum nigrum*

also called **Woderberry**

NUTRITIONAL INFORMATION There is no detailed nutritional information available on this fruit. It is thought the underripe berry could be used as an abortogenic agent owing to its content of the alkaloid solanine.

DESCRIPTION Black nightshade is a small branching shrub up to 1 m with clusters of shiny black berries about 6 mm in diameter.

ORIGIN AND HISTORY Botanists are now unable to differentiate between native and introduced *S. nigrum* owing to the weedlike spread of the species. This spread is now aided by soil disturbance and the plant is often found around vacant urban blocks. The black nightshade berry has a history of use by many people throughout China, Malaysia, India, Africa, the Americas, and New Zealand. Aborigines almost certainly ate the native fruits. In many of these countries the leaves and shoots were also used as a green vegetable.

BUYING AND STORAGE The berry is not available commercially in Australia and so must be foraged or cultivated domestically. Only fully ripe berries should be selected.

Store refrigerated for up to a week.

PREPARATION AND USE The ripe berry can be eaten raw or made into jams, pickles, preserves or used in pies.

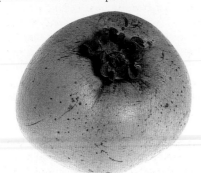

Black Sapote *Diospyros digyna*

also called **Chocolate pudding fruit**

MAJOR NUTRIENTS		SERVE SIZE 100 G	
Energy	280 kJ	Vitamin A	45 µg
Protein	2 g	Vitamin C	20 mg
Carbohydrate	15 g	Dietary Fibre	0
Fat	0		

NUTRITIONAL INFORMATION This is an excellent source of vitamin C and a moderate source of vitamin A.

DESCRIPTION Similar to a persimmon in shape and size but with a green skin and full of soft, pasty, sweet, dark chocolate-coloured flesh when ripe, with no aroma.

ORIGIN AND HISTORY The black sapote is native to Central America where it was known in Mexico around 5000 BC. It is the fruit of an evergreen tree and is related to the oriental persimmon. In Hawaii it is called black persimmon, in the Philippines it is known as zapote negro and the West Indians call it guayabote. It is now cultivated in Florida (USA) and Australia. Although sweet, its bland flavour can be enhanced by adding fresh lime juice, liqueur or a little rum. Its most interesting characteristic is its chocolate brown colour. It is related to the mamey sapote and the white sapote.

BUYING AND STORAGE Available in winter. Buy well-shaped undamaged fruit. Store at room temperature until skin turns dark green and is soft to the touch.

Store in refrigerator once ripe.

PREPARATION AND USE Cut fruit in half and serve fresh in the hand with a teaspoon for eating. The flesh may be scooped out and pureed for a sauce, or served with or added to ice cream, used in mousse or mixed with other fruit and a little rum.

PROCESSING Used in commercial ice cream.

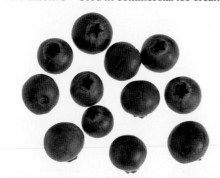

Blueberry *Vaccinium* spp.

MAJOR NUTRIENTS		SERVE SIZE 100 G	
Energy	240 kJ	Sodium	0
Protein	1 g	Dietary Fibre	2.5 g
Fat	0	Iron	0.5 mg
Carbohydrate	14 g	Vitamin C	16 mg
Cholesterol	0		

NUTRITIONAL INFORMATION The energy source is carbohydrate; excellent vitamin C; moderate iron, fibre.

DESCRIPTION A small, very dark blue berry with an attractive bloom on the skin.

ORIGIN AND HISTORY The blueberry is a member of the heather family, growing on deciduous and evergreen shrubs. It is a native of North America and east Asia. There is also a native British blueberry which grows wild on moorlands. The true blueberry, suitable for cultivation, is a result of complex hybridisation of several species in North America. A commercial advantage of blueberry is that it grows well on otherwise barren land. It has recently been introduced successfully into Australia on a large cluster-farm project, where the variety of bushes produce blueberries every month of the year. Blueberry, once a favourite fruit with North Americans only, is gaining popularity worldwide.

BUYING AND STORAGE Available during most of the year, blueberries should be kept dry, in the refrigerator.

PREPARATION AND USE Traditionally used in pies, blueberries also make a magnificent dessert on their own, or incorporated into fruit salads.

VARIETIES

Blueberry Highbush (*Vaccinium corymbosum*) and Blueberry Lowbush (*V. angustifolium*).

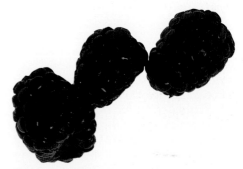

Boysenberry *Rubus*

MAJOR NUTRIENTS		SERVE SIZE 50 G	
Energy	53 kJ	Sodium	0
Protein	0	Dietary Fibre	3.7 g
Fat	0	Iron	0.6 mg
Carbohydrate	3 g	Vitamin C	13 mg
Cholesterol	0		

NUTRITIONAL INFORMATION An excellent source of vitamin C; good fibre; moderate iron.

As with most berry fruit, the boysenberry is an excellent source of vitamin C. Weight-conscious individuals should also note the fruit's low kilojoule content.

Canning reduces the vitamin C by two-thirds. The kilojoule content of canned sweetened boysenberry is three times higher than that of the raw fruit.

DESCRIPTION A collection of small, purple-red drupelets, the boysenberry is the fruit of a trailing plant.

ORIGIN AND HISTORY Thought to be a combination of the blackberry, loganberry, and raspberry. Produced by Rudolph Boysen in California in the 1930s and now grown in temperate climate areas of the USA. Now cultivated in Australia and New Zealand.

BUYING AND STORAGE Available in late summer and autumn. Choose berries with a bright appearance and store unwashed, but covered, in the refrigerator.

PREPARATION AND USE Rinse in a colander and dry by draining gently. Use fresh, in pies or tarts, or pureed in ice cream, sorbet and drinks. Avoid dishes where the dark juice will spoil the colours of other ingredients.

PROCESSING May be canned and used for jam.

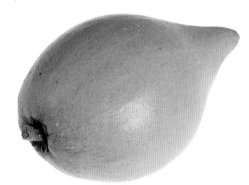

Canistel Pouteria campechiana

also called *Egg fruit, Marmalade fruit*

MAJOR NUTRIENTS		SERVE SIZE 100 G	
Energy	640 kJ	Dietary Fibre	7.5 g
Protein	2 g	Niacin Equiv.	2.5 mg
Fat	1 g	Vitamin C	40 mg
Carbohydrate	39 g		

NUTRITIONAL INFORMATION This is an excellent source of fibre, retinol equivalents, vitamin C; a good source of niacin.

DESCRIPTION An egg-shaped berry, from 7–18 cm long, with a smooth yellow-orange skin enclosing mealy yellow pulp with several large shiny seeds.

ORIGIN AND HISTORY The canistel is a tropical tree native to Central America and the West Indies. The fruit is closely related to the abiu. It also grows in New Caledonia and cultivation has recently been introduced into northern Australia in the frost-free tropics. It has not been marketed in commercial quantities to date.

BUYING AND STORAGE Available most of the year. Select firm, undamaged fruit, well developed in size. Leave to ripen at room temperature, out of direct sunlight until soft to the touch, then store in refrigerator.

PREPARATION AND USE Cut fruit in half and eat fresh in the hand with a teaspoon to scoop out the flesh. Peel fruit and remove seeds, mash or puree the fruit flesh with lime or lemon juice and serve with ice cream, pancakes, waffles, or mix with mayonnaise and serve as a dip.

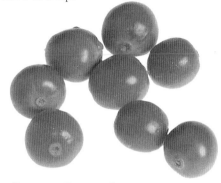

Cape Gooseberry Physalis peruviana

also called *Golden berry, Strawberry tomato, Tomatillo, Ground cherry*

NUTRITIONAL INFORMATION No reliable analysis is available.

DESCRIPTION A round, yellow-green, globose, tart-flavoured berry, similar in size and shape to a small cherry tomato, with internal texture similar to a gooseberry, enclosed in a green husk.

ORIGIN AND HISTORY The Cape gooseberry is mainly native to South America, Mexico, and the southern states of USA, although it takes its name from the Cape of Good Hope in South Africa where it has been cultivated extensively since the 19th century. It is also native to a region stretching from the Caucasus to China where it is known as Chinese lanterns and grown only in flower gardens for winter floral arrangements. The tough outer husk is inedible but the fruit, which belongs to the tomato family, is refreshing and delicious. The first white settlers introduced the Cape gooseberry to Australian gardens and its commercial cultivation has been introduced recently so it is becoming available to all consumers.

BUYING AND STORAGE Available in summer. Choose firm, large, evenly coloured berries with a fragrant smell. If sold in the husk, it turns from a soft texture to a brittle texture when the berries are ripe.

Store in refrigerator.

PREPARATION AND USE Wash and dry in a clean tea towel. Serve as a fresh fruit, like grapes or cherries, or with cheese; or cut in half and add to fruit salad or green salad; poach or puree, use in ice cream, sorbet or jam.

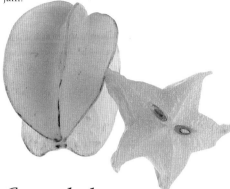

Carambola Averrhoa carambola

also called *Belimbing asam, Belimbing manis, Bilimbi, Five corners fruit, Mafueng, Star apple, Star fruit*

MAJOR NUTRIENTS		SERVE SIZE 100 G	
Energy	150 kJ	Sodium	5 mg
Protein	1 g	Iron	1.5 mg
Fat	1 g	Potassium	195 mg
Carbohydrate	8 g	Vitamin A	360 μg
Cholesterol	0	Vitamin C	35 mg
Dietary Fibre	1 g		

NUTRITIONAL INFORMATION An excellent source of vitamin C, vitamin A and iron; contains a moderate amount of potassium.

DESCRIPTION There are two species of this attractive fruit. The carambola is slightly larger than the bilimbi, at about 10 cm in length, with five prominent angles, producing a star shape when cut. It is yellow in colour with a waxy skin and crisp, juicy flesh, and is eaten raw as a fruit or used in desserts. The bilimbi is greener in colour, slightly smaller and sour-tasting. It is used in cooking for its high acidity and tart flavour. It is known in Indonesian as belimbing asam (asam referring to the tart fruit tamarind), while the former is belimbing manis, or sweet belimbing. Another kind of carambola, known as the sour finger carambola, does not have the characteristic star shape.

ORIGIN AND HISTORY This fruit is a true star of the east. The carambola is said to have originated in Indonesia and Malaysia and has spread to South-East Asia, the southern Philippines, and India. The Portuguese and Spanish traders introduced carambola to South America and today it is cultivated from China, southwards across Asia, to Australia.

The Portuguese name carambola originated from the Sanskrit word kamara. The fruit was introduced into Europe towards the end of the 18th century as a novelty for the ostentatious hothouses then becoming fashionable among the rich. The tree is very pretty as it bears small lilac-coloured flowers throughout the year. The fruit is high in oxalic acid, particularly under the corner edges, which makes it good for cleaning copper and brass.

BUYING AND STORAGE Choose firm fruit without bruises. Mature fruit turns yellow or orange when ripe but some varieties remain green, however the translucent thin skin turns waxy in appearance when fruit is fully ripe.

Store in the crisper or in a plastic bag in the refrigerator. It will store for up to 3 weeks.

Dried sliced star fruit is available in some Asian food stores. It can be kept indefinitely in an airtight jar in dry conditions.

PREPARATION AND USE Wash, then slice the top and bottom off the carambola and trim the skin off the corner of each rib. Eat the fruit fresh in the hand, like an apple, or slice into star shapes and use in fruit salad, on fruit platters, on cheese boards, with savoury salads, to garnish and decorate food, or puree to use in drinks or sorbets.

Use the sour kind in curries and soups requiring a tart flavour, and in freshly made tart sauces.

VARIETIES

Sour Finger Carambola

NUTRITIONAL INFORMATION Similar to carambola.

DESCRIPTION This is *Averrhoa bilimbi*, also called belimbing wuluh, a light green, acidic fruit which is finger-shaped and about 9 cm in length. It has firm, slightly rough skin and looks something like a small, underripe mango.

ORIGIN AND HISTORY It is of the same family as the elegant star-shaped carambola and is probably also a native of India, although it is known more for its use in Indonesian cooking.

BUYING AND STORAGE Occasionally sold in specialist Indonesian stores, it should feel firm and have unwrinkled, clear green skin. If unobtainable the green gooseberry has a very similar taste and texture and could be substituted.

PREPARATION AND USE Used in Indonesian cooking in soups, sauces, and pickles for its sharp tang. It is also occasionally used as a vegetable.

Cherimoya *Annona* spp.

NUTRITIONAL INFORMATION No reliable analysis available.

DESCRIPTION A fleshy, round, green-skinned fruit, made up of a number of carpels joined together, containing smooth creamy flesh, with a flavour of pineapple and strawberries, and several large brown stones. Reminiscent of a globe artichoke at first glance.

ORIGIN AND HISTORY The cherimoya plant originated in Peru. Many hybrids have been developed as commercial crops, including the soursop and the custard-apple. The genus is native to the Andes in Peru and Ecuador and to tropical America. It was taken from Mexico to the West Indies. More recently it has been introduced to tropical Asia, Australia, and Israel, as the cherimoya thrives best in a warm climate outside the tropics. The cherimoya was introduced to Europe in 1690 where it still grows in hothouses or greenhouses.

BUYING AND STORAGE Available during autumn and winter. Choose fruit which is evenly coloured, turning a dull yellow-brown, with a bloom on the skin and no dark spots. Fruit is picked firm for transportation and is fully mature after about 5 days when the carpels start to separate.

Store at room temperature until fully ripe, then in the refrigerator for up to 4 days.

PREPARATION AND USE Cut fruit in half or twist open in half, then serve fresh in the hand with a teaspoon for eating. Or scoop pulp out, discard seeds and use in fruit salad, with ice cream, in soufflés, crumbles or curries, or puree and use in ice cream, drinks, desserts, and cakes.

PROCESSING Canning and freezing of the pulp is being developed currently.

VARIETIES
There are several species, the best commercially known being the custard-apple and the soursop.

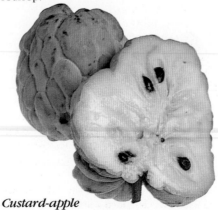

Custard-apple

MAJOR NUTRIENTS		SERVE SIZE 100 G	
Energy	300 kJ	Cholesterol	0
Protein	1 g	Sodium	0
Fat	0	Dietary Fibre	2.5 g
Carbohydrate	15 g	Vitamin C	32 mg

NUTRITIONAL INFORMATION The energy comes from carbohydrate; excellent source of vitamin C.

Half a medium-sized custard-apple provides the body with the total recommended daily intake of vitamin C.

DESCRIPTION This is *Annona reticulata*, a large, round fruit with a greenish-yellow, lumpy skin. The African Pride has lots of stones, and the Pink's Mammoth is larger, and more knobbly, with fewer stones.

ORIGIN AND HISTORY The custard-apple is probably the best-known species of the cherimoya family. It is also known as bullock's heart, because of the shape. It was introduced to Europe in 1690 where it is grown in hothouses.

BUYING AND STORAGE Readily available. Choose evenly coloured fruit.

PREPARATION AND USE As for cherimoya in general.

Soursop *Annona muricata*

MAJOR NUTRIENTS		SERVE SIZE 100 G	
Energy	270 kJ	Sodium	15 mg
Protein	1 g	Potassium	265 mg
Fat	0	Iron	0.6 mg
Carbohydrate	16 g	Thiamin	0.1 mg
Dietary Fibre	1 g	Niacin Equiv.	1 mg
Cholesterol	0	Vitamin C	20 mg

NUTRITIONAL INFORMATION An excellent source of vitamin C; moderate source of iron, thiamin, niacin and potassium.

DESCRIPTION A large green, spiny or wart-covered, heart-shaped tropical fruit from a small tree, *Annona muricata*. Each fruit can weigh at least 1 kg and its fragrant white flesh has a unique taste, somewhat similar to the durian. The flesh separates into segments, containing large black seeds which must not be eaten as they contain a toxic substance.

ORIGIN AND HISTORY The soursop or prickly custard-apple is a native of tropical America. It grows well in tropical lowlands and thrives near the ocean. It is popular in the Philippines, tropical Asia, and the north of Queensland, but unfortunately does not travel well to non-tropical markets.

It is well known in the Latin American countries where it is called guanabana fruit. In Asia it is known as sirsak or durian belanda.

BUYING AND STORAGE Rarely available fresh. The flesh is canned, for use as a dessert, but more usually in Western countries, it is the canned or bottled juice which is available.

PREPARATION AND USE Use the pulp, as for custard-apple and cherimoya. The juice makes a refreshing summer drink and can be used in desserts and ices.

PROCESSING It has become popular for its pulp and juice in drinks, cocktails, mousses and sorbets.

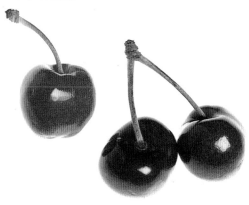

Cherry *Prunus* spp.

MAJOR NUTRIENTS		SERVE SIZE 100 G	
Energy	220 kJ	Sodium	0
Protein	1 g	Dietary Fibre	1.5 g
Fat	0	Iron	0.4 mg
Carbohydrate	12 g	Vitamin C	18 mg
Cholesterol	0		

NUTRITIONAL INFORMATION The energy comes from carbohydrate; excellent vitamin C, moderate iron. If canned cherries are sweetened the kilojoule content is higher.

DESCRIPTION The cherry tree has bunches of beautiful flowers hanging on slender stems, which are delightful harbingers of the fruit itself: the small, round cherry with a shiny skin that matures to a deep purple-red.

ORIGIN AND HISTORY The cherry is a stone fruit related to the plum and is native to the temperate regions of the northern hemisphere. The sweet cherry is believed to be native to Europe and areas across to western Asia, while the sour cherry originated in southeast Europe and western Asia. During the Roman occupation of Britain in AD100, the Romans imported and cultivated their own cherries. Owing to careful selection and good cultivation, there are some fine varieties of cherries grown today. The cherry is an important crop in Italy, forming part of the Italian export crop, likewise in Australia. The cherry was first planted in Young in Australia in 1878, and today it is known as the cherry capital of Australia. However, the French still serve the cherry with more flair than any other nationality and apparently consume

2.5 kg per head during the short cherry season.

BUYING AND STORAGE Available in early summer for a short season. Select plump, firm, brightly and evenly coloured, undamaged cherries with fresh green stalks. Avoid soft, dull cherries as these are overripe. Small, hard, poorly coloured cherries are underripe and lack juice and flavour.

Store unwashed in the vegetable crisper or in a plastic bag in the refrigerator for up to 3 days as the cherry is highly perishable.

PREPARATION AND USE Wash, remove the stems and dry well, then remove stones with a special cherry stoner. Serve fresh in fruit salad, with a cheese board, or poach (stew), then puree and use in ice cream, sorbet or soup, with duck and chicken, in pies and tarts.

PROCESSING The Morello (sour) cherry is preserved and canned. Sweet cherries may be canned, glacéed, preserved in maraschino, used in brandy, liqueur and confectionery.

VARIETIES
There are many varieties but they are divided into sweet cherries, such as Ron Seedlings, Regina, Williams, Napoleon; and sour cherries such as Morello, Kentish, Driotte.

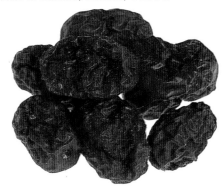

Chinese Red Date *Zizyphus jujuba*

also called **Hoong joh, Jujube, Red Date, Tsao**

NUTRITIONAL INFORMATION No reliable analysis is available.

DESCRIPTION A small, red, wrinkled fruit with firm skin and soft, pulpy, datelike flesh with a semisweet prunelike flavour.

ORIGIN AND HISTORY These are not exactly dates, but the fruit of the ancient Chinese jujube tree, known from earliest recorded times. There are several edible varieties, grown in the northern provinces. An aromatic type which became known as the Persian jujube was imported from Turkestan, along with black dates, in the 7th century. The jujube was included amongst shrine offer-

ings. The Nangking author of the chen-wu essay 'Precious Things' wrote 'The fruit is crisp and soft. Its skin red as blood, its flesh whiter than gleaming snow.' The red jujube is also cultivated in India.

BUYING AND STORAGE Usually sold by weight in their dried form, they will keep indefinitely in a sealed jar in a dark, dry store cupboard. Occasionally sold fresh, when they are a brownish colour, they should be dried in a warm oven.

PREPARATION AND USE Soak dates to be used in desserts in cold water to soften. Add dried dates directly to soups, steamed and braised dishes to give a subtle sweet taste. Excellent in a soup with watercress. Usually one date per serving is sufficient.

Citron *Citrus medica*

also called **Kitron**

MAJOR NUTRIENTS		CANDIED SERVE SIZE 28 G	
Energy	370 kJ	Cholesterol	0
Protein	0	Sodium	0
Fat	0	Dietary Fibre	0
Carbohydrate	22.5 g		

NUTRITIONAL INFORMATION High in carbohydrate.

DESCRIPTION A large lemon-shaped citrus fruit with a thick, tough, fragrant green-lemon rind, covering a thick inner white skin or pith.

ORIGIN AND HISTORY Citron is a native of China and a member of the citrus family. It is thought to be the first citrus to be introduced to the Mediterranean region from China, around 500 BC. It was probably first brought to Israel from Babylonia after the exile and since then the citron has been used in the Jewish festival of Sukhot to celebrate the harvest of fruit in particular. The Jews identify the citron with the forbidden fruit in the Garden of Eden. They also have a superstition that if a pregnant woman bites it, she will bear a son. The citron is grown commercially in Corsica, Greece and Sicily.

BUYING AND STORAGE Buy for its peel only, and if storing fresh, keep in the refrigerator after one week.

PREPARATION AND USE Wash and dry the citron, then remove peel and pith neatly using a small, sharp, serrated knife. Use in cakes, biscuits, lemon desserts, and confectionery, for glacéed citron peel and for making liqueur. Also used to perfume rooms in China and Japan.

PROCESSING Used to make glacéed and candied citron peel.

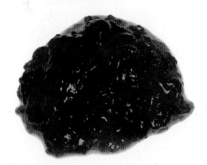

Cranberry *Vaccinium macrocarpum*

also called **Bounce berry, Craneberry**

MAJOR NUTRIENTS		SERVE SIZE 100 G	
Energy	60 kJ	Cholesterol	0
Protein	0	Dietary Fibre	4.5 g
Fat	0	Iron	1.1 mg
Carbohydrate	4 g	Vitamin C	12 mg

NUTRITIONAL INFORMATION All energy comes from carbohydrate; excellent source of iron, vitamin C, fibre. The amount of iron would provide a valuable contribution in a vegetarian diet.

DESCRIPTION The cranberry is a small fruit related to the blueberry, but tart in flavour; it is a member of the heather family.

ORIGIN AND HISTORY The large cranberry is native to North America, the small cranberry is native to Europe, particularly Finland, and North Asia. The Indians in North America taught the English settlers how to boil it and serve as a sauce with turkey. Cultivation was started in the early 1800s at Cape Cod and is now extensive in the east of the USA.

BUYING AND STORAGE Available in summer and autumn. Choose plump, firm, shiny red to reddish-brown berries which will bounce when ripe.

Store in a cool dry place, in the crisper, or in a plastic bag in the refrigerator for several weeks.

PREPARATION AND USE Wash and drain the fruit, discard soft ones and remove stems. Dry on kitchen paper towels. Use whole, chopped or crushed according to recipe, in sauce, relish, bread, cakes, pies, tarts, salads, desserts and stuffings.

PROCESSING May be used in sauce, jelly or liqueur or preserved in jars.

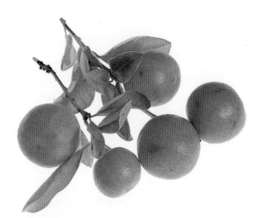

Cumquat *Fortunella* spp.

also called **Kumquat**

MAJOR NUTRIENTS		SERVE SIZE 20 G	
Energy	50 kJ	Sodium	0
Protein	0	Dietary Fibre	0
Fat	0	Iron	0
Carbohydrate	3 g	Vitamin C	7 mg
Cholesterol	0		

NUTRITIONAL INFORMATION An excellent source of vitamin C only.

DESCRIPTION Botanically a berry like the orange, tiny, oval, miniaturelike orange fruit with edible, sweet, thin skin and bitter flesh.

ORIGIN AND HISTORY Native to China and now cultivated there and in Japan and Malaysia. Introduced to Europe in 1846 and to the USA in 1850. Now grown commercially in Mediterranean climatic regions, including Australia, often as an ornamental bush in private gardens.

BUYING AND STORAGE Available during autumn and winter. Select firm, evenly coloured, bright orange, undamaged fruit. Store in the refrigerator.

PREPARATION AND USE Wash and dry the fruit and serve fresh if quite ripe, peeled or unpeeled. Use for garnishing fish or meat platters, serve with duck, game birds or Chinese food, use for marmalade or preserve in brandy and serve with ice cream.

PROCESSING May be preserved in glass or as brandied fruit or in marmalade.

Currant *Ribes* spp.

DESCRIPTION A small, thin-skinned, juicy, many-seeded rather sour berry.

ORIGIN AND HISTORY Currants grow wild in the northern hemisphere across the whole of Europe, across Russia as far as the northern Himalayas, all the way to Siberia. They are a popular garden bush in Britain. They have been cultivated since the 15th century and during this century have been the subject of much research in order to improve the strain of currants, both black and red. The juicy currant is cultivated in New Zealand where most of the crop is used in processed cordial. Cultivation of blackcurrants and redcurrants has been recently introduced into Australia, but they have a very short season of fruiting.

BUYING AND STORAGE Available in midsummer for a short season. Choose firm, plump, shiny, juicy ripe currants.

Store in the refrigerator. Red and white currants keep longer than blackcurrants.

PREPARATION AND USE Rinse in a colander, then drain well. Remove currants from stems by pulling stems upwards through the tines (prongs) of a fork. Serve fresh sprinkled with sugar, or use in a fruit salad or a traditional summer pudding; poach, then puree if liked and use in ice cream and sorbet; serve with chicken, lamb or veal; or use in tarts and pancakes.

PROCESSING May be used to make jelly, jam and cordial, and frozen commercially. Blackcurrants are used to make cassis liqueur. The dried fruits also known and sold as currants are actually very small, dried grapes, unrelated to *Ribes*.

VARIETIES

Blackcurrant

MAJOR NUTRIENTS		SERVE SIZE 100 G	
Energy	120 kJ	Dietary Fibre	8.5 g
Protein	1 g	Calcium	60 mg
Fat	0	Vitamin C	188 mg
Carbohydrate	7 g	Magnesium	22 mg
Cholesterol	0		
Sodium	0		

NUTRITIONAL INFORMATION The energy from *Ribes nigrum* comes from carbohydrate; excellent fibre and vitamin C; good vitamin E; and moderate calcium and magnesium.

The currant is unusual in that it contains three other nutrients not normally found in any appreciable amount in fruit — calcium, magnesium and vitamin E.

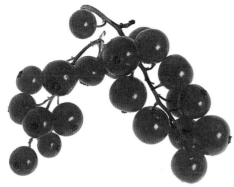

Redcurrant, White Currant

MAJOR NUTRIENTS   SERVE SIZE 100 G

Energy	90 kJ	Sodium	0
Protein	1 g	Dietary Fibre	9 g
Fat	0	Iron	1.2 mg
Carbohydrate	4 g	Vitamin C	32 mg
Cholesterol	0		

NUTRITIONAL INFORMATION The energy comes from carbohydrate; excellent source of vitamin C; excellent source of fibre; good source of iron.

Like the raw blackcurrant, red and white currants (*Ribes sativum*) are an excellent source of fibre. Red and white currants have one-fifth of the vitamin C content but this amount still supplies the body with the total recommended daily intake for that vitamin. These currants are different from the black variety in that they contain a good source of iron.

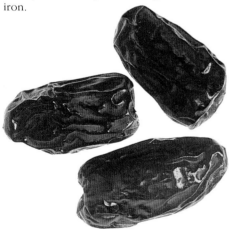

Date *Phoenix dactylifera*

MAJOR NUTRIENTS   SERVE SIZE 33 G

Energy	380 kJ	Dietary Fibre	8.5 g
Protein	0	Magnesium	20 mg
Fat	0	Iron	0.7 mg
Carbohydrate	25.3 g	Niacin Equiv.	0.7 mg
Cholesterol	0	Vitamin B6	0.15 mg
Sodium	0		

NUTRITIONAL INFORMATION The energy comes from carbohydrate; good source of folic acid, iron; moderate vitamin B6, magnesium, niacin; high in carbohydrate.

The date is an excellent source of fibre and a good source of iron. What makes the date slightly unusual is that it also contains folic acid and niacin.

DESCRIPTION The oval, fleshy fruit of a palm, dates range in colour from pale golden to a dark brown. Dates for drying are firm-fleshed with a tender skin, brown in colour and high in sugar content. Those which are eaten fresh can be a firm-skinned black date with flesh that melts in the mouth, or a golden date with a tender skin and stringy sweet flesh with peppery undertones; both are frozen and exported, to be sold as 'fresh' dates.

ORIGIN AND HISTORY Native to Arabia and North Africa, the date palm has served the people of these regions for thousands of years. It was cultivated in southern Mesopotamia, between the Euphrates and Tigris Rivers, from 3500 BC, and is as important to present day Iraqis as it was to this early civilisation of their region. Not only did the date palm provide a valuable food, the palm itself provided building materials, household and personal articles and fuel. The seeds were used as camel fodder as well as fuel. In many regions of the Middle East and North Africa, such uses are still found for the palm, its fronds and seeds.

BUYING AND STORAGE Available all year. Iraq remains the main exporter of dried dates: those varieties unsuitable for drying are frozen. Dates found in Western markets come from Israel, Lebanon and from the United States (grown in California and Arizona). Because of the high sugar content of the date, it is excellent for freezing, and when thawed tastes exactly like freshly picked fruit. Choose large, soft, plump, shiny fresh dates with a smooth, undamaged skin.

Store covered in the refrigerator.

PREPARATION AND USE Cooking dates only need to be chopped; serve dessert dates as they are, or remove seeds and fill with a stuffing. Rinse fresh dates and drain well just before serving.

Use dried dates in puddings, cakes, muffins and scones, add to chutneys and curry dishes. Make dessert dates into sweetmeats by replacing the seed with cream cheese, nuts or marzipan. Add dessert or fresh dates to the morning cereal, to fruit salads and to the cheese board, or enjoy them au naturel.

Chop dried dates and use in cakes, scones and pastries or add to dried fruit salad.

PROCESSING As dates are being dried, they exude a thick molasseslike syrup. It is used in the cooking pot, as a beverage base and for date vinegar.

VARIETIES

There are many varieties of date palm trees but for consumption the fruit may be grouped simply as soft and fresh, or dried.

SEE ALSO Dried Date.

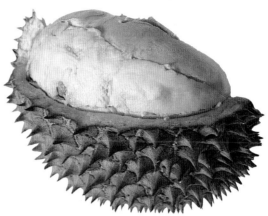

Durian *Durio zibethinus*

MAJOR NUTRIENTS   SERVE SIZE 100 G

Energy	130 kJ	Carbohydrate	7 g
Protein	1 g	Cholesterol	0
Fat	0		

NUTRITIONAL INFORMATION No information available for other nutrients.

DESCRIPTION The fruit which earns the saying 'Tastes like heaven but smells like hell!' A very large, oval tropical fruit, approximately 10 kg in weight, with a thick, rough, green-yellow skin, covered with spines and containing delicious white, creamy, pulpy flesh.

ORIGIN AND HISTORY The durian is the tropical fruit of a native Malayan tree, which still grows wild in South-East Asia. Known as the 'king of fruit' it is much sought after by Asian people and is very expensive. Prestigious competitions are held in Thailand to decide who has grown the best fruit of the year and some commercial growers employ armed guards to protect their durian orchards at night as stealing is not uncommon. The sharp spines on the fruit make it hard to carry, so it is usually trussed with string to carry it home from the market. However, because of its pungent smell it is not allowed into hotel rooms or on aeroplanes. There are now many hybrids of durian grown in Asia. It is best to serve this rich, buttery-textured fruit chilled as chilling reduces the smell.

In Malaysia and Indonesia, where the durian is most commonly found, the foul smell of this fruit has been blamed for marital breakups and family feuds, and for loss of business in nearby shops during the height of its season.

BUYING AND STORAGE A yellowing of the skin indicates the fruit is ripe. It should be stored away from other fruits, vegetables and packaged goods. Canned durian is packed in water or syrup, and may be jellied with agar agar.

PREPARATION AND USE Cut fruit open at the segment joints, scoop out flesh and separate seeds. Eat flesh fresh or with ice cream, cook with rice or use in cakes. Seeds may be roasted and eaten like nuts.

PROCESSING May be canned.

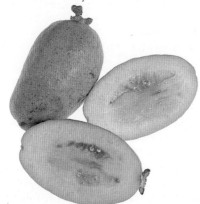

Feijoa *Feijoa sellowiana*

*also called **Pineapple guava, Brazilian guava***

MAJOR NUTRIENTS		SERVE SIZE 100 G	
Energy	200 g	Dietary Fibre	3 g
Protein	1 g	Niacin Equiv.	1.8 mg
Carbohydrate	13 g	Vitamin C	30 mg
Fat	0		

NUTRITIONAL INFORMATION This is an excellent source of vitamin C; a good source of fibre and niacin.

DESCRIPTION A dull green ovoid berry, the size of a duck's egg, with yellow-green slightly grainy flesh around a jellylike centre, and a scented fragrance of pineapple and strawberry.

ORIGIN AND HISTORY Native of Brazil, Uruguay, and other parts of South America. Feijoa was named after a botanist called Don da Silva Feijoa. Now cultivated in New Zealand and Australia.

BUYING AND STORAGE Available during autumn. Select plump fruit with undamaged skin. When ripe skin turns greenish-yellow and fruit yields if pressed.

Store at room temperature until ripe, then in refrigerator.

PREPARATION AND USE Cut fruit in half and eat fresh from the skin with a teaspoon, or cut into quarters and serve with cheese boards and fruit platters. Feijoa can be peeled and sliced. It is a good fruit for salad, jam, puree, ice cream and sorbet.

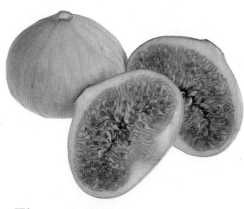

Fig *Ficus carica*

MAJOR NUTRIENTS		SERVE SIZE 100 G	
Energy	160 kJ	Sodium	40 mg
Protein	1 g	Dietary Fibre	2.5 g
Fat	0	Vitamin C	2 mg
Carbohydrate	8 g	Calcium	40 mg
Cholesterol	0		

NUTRITIONAL INFORMATION The energy comes from carbohydrate; moderate fibre, vitamin C.

DESCRIPTION The bulbous fig grows on a tree with dark green, distinctively indented leaves. The pulpy, sweet flesh has a pleasant, characteristic fragrance.

ORIGIN AND HISTORY The fig is one of the oldest known plants. It is probably a native of Syria in western Asia and was an important food in the staple diet in many countries in the Old World. Its food value improves with drying as it also does with dates. The Phoenician trade caravans introduced it, along the silk route, into India and China. The Romans introduced it into other countries in Europe. The fig has recently been planted on a commercial scale in Madagascar, South Africa, and Australia. It also grows commercially in Turkey, Greece, Italy, Portugal, Algeria, and California.

BUYING AND STORAGE Select the soft, plump, sweet-smelling fig with a bright-coloured, undamaged skin. Avoid fruit with a sour smell as this indicates it is overripe.

Store covered in the refrigerator.

PREPARATION AND USE Wash and dry, peel if liked, and serve fresh as a dessert fruit, on cheese boards and fruit platters, stuffed with a sweet filling, poached or added to ice cream or cakes.

PROCESSING May be dried, canned and glacéed.

VARIETIES There are 700 varieties, the Smyrna fig being the most well known, but the fruit is generally classified by colour: white, purple, black, and red.

SEE ALSO Dried Fig.

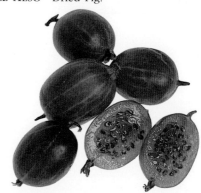

Gooseberry *Ribes grossularia*

MAJOR NUTRIENTS		SERVE SIZE 100 G	
Energy	160 kJ	Sodium	0
Protein	0	Dietary Fibre	3.5 g
Fat	0	Iron	0.6 mg
Carbohydrate	9.2 g	Vitamin C	40 mg
Cholesterol	0		

NUTRITIONAL INFORMATION Like most berries, the gooseberry is an excellent source of vitamin C — ¾ cup providing over the total daily recommended intake of this vitamin. The fruit contains fibre and iron.

DESCRIPTION Small oval berries with green, yellow or red-black tough skins, some hairy, containing fleshy, tart-flavoured juicy seeds.

ORIGIN AND HISTORY The gooseberry probably originated in the mountainous and the northern regions of Europe and also in North Africa. It still grows wild in some areas but the bush is thought to be a descendant of cultivars as it is usually close to populated settlements. It has been cultivated since the 16th century in England, and was enormously popular at one time, but went into decline, possibly because its spiny stems make it difficult to harvest, and also because of the competitive appeal of newer fruits coming into season. There used to be a Gooseberry Club in many English villages and the members aimed to grow the largest gooseberry. The North American gooseberry is derived from a native species found in the east of North America. Gooseberry-growing was introduced into Australia by the early white settlers, with some nurseries now offering over 100 varieties. However, the berry of greatest culinary value comes from the varieties cultivated today.

BUYING AND STORAGE The gooseberry is fairly readily available.

PREPARATION AND USE Like other berries, gooseberries are popular in desserts.

PROCESSING May be canned or made into jam.

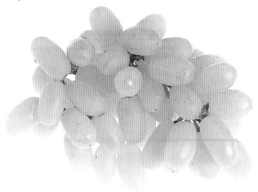

Grape *Vitis vinifera*

MAJOR NUTRIENTS		SERVE SIZE 100 G	
Energy	280 kJ	Cholesterol	0
Protein	1 g	Sodium	0
Fat	0	Dietary Fibre	3 g
Carbohydrate	16.8 g	Vitamin C	5 mg

NUTRITIONAL INFORMATION The energy comes from carbohydrate. Nutritionally the grape does not contain a great deal besides vitamin C and fibre.

DESCRIPTION The small, round fruits of the grapevine grow in tight bunches and ripen to a range of colours varying from green to pinkish-grey through to a deep purple, depending on variety.

ORIGIN AND HISTORY The common wild grapevine probably originated in the Caucasus, and in western Asia. It is also found growing wild in southern Europe and northern Africa and there is another variety native to North America. The grape was valued as a refreshing, nourishing food in hot climates. Viticulture, or the cultivation of the grape, probably began around the Caspian Sea. The first wine was probably made by accident by allowing a container of grapes to ferment naturally. Wine was first recorded in Mesopotamia and Egypt, 3000 BC, where it was used in temple ceremonies. During the same period the Chinese were making wine from grapes in areas where vine rootstocks have been found which date back to before the great ice age. In Europe the Greeks and Romans made wine a popular drink and the Romans introduced it to Britain in AD 10. With the fall of the Roman Empire, and the Roman withdrawal back to Rome, monasteries maintained the vineyards and produced the wine.

Grapes are cultivated for eating fresh and for wine making throughout the world.

BUYING AND STORAGE In season in late summer and autumn, though available nearly all year. Choose bunches with firm stalks and well-shaped, plump, undamaged fruit. Green grapes have an amber yellow tinge when ripe, black grapes should be totally dark with no green tinge. Avoid split, wet grapes. Taste to test flavour as they will not continue to ripen once picked.

Store, unwashed, in the refrigerator and keep for up to 5 days only.

PREPARATION AND USE Wash by rinsing in a colander, dry gently with kitchen paper towels. Serve small bunches fresh as a dessert fruit, with cheese boards, to garnish savoury fish or meat platters, or remove from stem and add to fruit salad, tarts or fruit cup. Serve with traditional chicken or fish, or chilled and frosted as a petit four.

PROCESSING Use to make wine, or grape juice. May be dried as currants, sultanas or raisins, or canned.

VARIETIES

There are several varieties of grape, differing in size and colour, but these may be put into four groups: wine grapes; table or dessert, with and without seeds; dried, for currants, sultanas and raisins; juice grapes.

However, the same grape may be in more than one or in all these groups.

Grapes are also divided into two colours, black and green, with a wide range of each colour.

Eating grape varieties are listed below.

Cardinal A purple-red, large, round, soft-skinned, firm-fleshed grape.

Cornichon A purple-blue, very large, olive-shaped, thick-skinned, soft-fleshed grape.

Muscat A blue-black, large, oval, firm-skinned, muscat-flavoured grape.

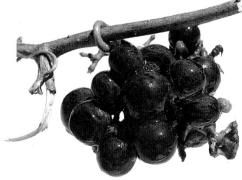

Native grape

MAJOR NUTRIENTS		SERVE SIZE 50 G	
Energy	150 kJ	Carbohydrate	8 g
Protein	less than 1 g	Dietary Fibre	6 g
Fat	0		

NUTRITIONAL INFORMATION Is lower in energy and sugar compared to the cultivated grape.

DESCRIPTION Native grapes (*Cissus antarctica, C. hypoglauca*) are of a similar size and taste to conventional dark grapes but have pale white spots on the skin.

ORIGIN AND HISTORY The native grapes were a popular forage food for Aborigines on the east coast of Australia.

BUYING AND STORAGE As for conventional grapes.

PREPARATION AND USE The skins of native grapes are often astringent and can be discarded, however, fully ripe fruit from vines growing in filtered sunlight do set fruit which are not astringent. Discard the seeds in either case. The grapes can be used for wine making and yield an excellent jam. The pectin content of some fruit is very high, making them a good source of dietary fibre and also enabling them to be used as a natural source of jam-setting agent.

Sultana Grape A very popular green-gold, small, oval, soft-skinned, sweet grape.

Waltham Cross A golden-green, large, long, oval, firm-skinned, juicy grape.

SEE ALSO Dried Currant, Raisin, Sultana.

Grapefruit *Citrus paradisi*

MAJOR NUTRIENTS		SERVE SIZE 100 G	
Energy	110 kJ	Cholesterol	0
Protein	1 g	Sodium	0
Fat	0	Dietary Fibre	2.5 g
Carbohydrate	5 g	Vitamin C	36 mg

NUTRITIONAL INFORMATION The energy comes from carbohydrate; excellent vitamin C. A good food for the weight-conscious as grapefruit is not very high in kilojoules. Grapefruit also contains nearly 1½ times the daily recommended intake of vitamin C.

DESCRIPTION Large citrus fruit, with yellow to golden skin.

ORIGIN AND HISTORY The grapefruit is believed to have originated in the West Indies and is either a sport of the pomelo or a hybrid of the pomelo and an orange. After growing for centuries, it was eventually cultivated commercially in Florida (USA) in 1880 by a French surgeon from Napoleon's army. Apparently he was captured at Trafalgar by the British and sent as a prisoner to the Bahamas, where the grapefruit grew in abundance. After his release, he practised medicine in South Carolina but dreamed of the Bahamas, so eventually moved to Florida and established the first citrus plantation there. Other plantations were developed in Texas, Arizona, and California. In 1914 the grapefruit was introduced to Palestine. Today it is also produced in Israel, Greece, Spain, South Africa, Australia, Brazil, and Central America.

BUYING AND STORAGE Choose evenly coloured fruit without brown or soft patches. In dry conditions, grapefruit keep well because of their thick skin.

PREPARATION AND USE Wipe or wash clean, cut in half crossways, loosen segments from membrane with a special serrated knife and serve in the skin with a teaspoon for eating, or remove peel, cut into segments and add to green salad, seafood salad or fruit salad. May be juiced and used in cheesecake, mousse, sorbet or marmalade.

PROCESSING May be juiced, canned and used in marmalade.

VARIETIES
The most common varieties are listed.

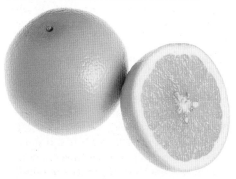

Marsh Lemon-coloured with few seeds.

Thompson Lemon-coloured skin with pinkish-yellow fruit.

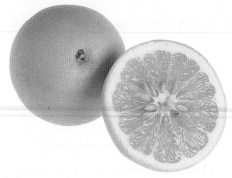

Wheeney Lemon-green with lots of seeds.

Texan pink Lemon skin with sweeter pink fruit.

Green Plum *Terminalia ferdinandiana*

also called Billy goat plum

MAJOR NUTRIENTS		SERVE SIZE 50 G	
Energy	430 kJ	Dietary Fibre	n/a
Protein	1 g	Sodium	20 mg
Fat	0	Vitamin C	2565 mg
Carbohydrate	26 g		

NUTRITIONAL INFORMATION The billy goat plum is the world's highest known source of vitamin C with levels of up to 4000 mg/100 g (80 times that of an orange).

DESCRIPTION An olive-sized green fruit with a fibrous flesh and a large seed.

ORIGIN AND HISTORY The green plum is found in Australia, north of the Tropic of Capricorn, and west of Katherine. Aborigines ate the fruit throughout its distribution and regarded it as a tonic food.

BUYING AND STORAGE Eat fresh.

PREPARATION AND USE To gain the most benefit from the vitamin C level the fruit should be eaten when fully ripe and picked fresh. The plums can be used to make a jelly or sliced as a substitute for lemon in garnishing fish.

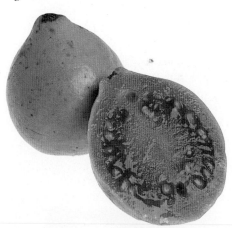

Guava *Psidium guajava*

MAJOR NUTRIENTS		SERVE SIZE 100 G	
Energy	100 kJ	Dietary Fibre	5 g
Protein	1 g	Vitamin A	44 µg
Fat	0	Vitamin C	240 mg
Carbohydrate	3 g	Niacin Equiv.	1 mg
Cholesterol	0		

NUTRITIONAL INFORMATION The energy comes from carbohydrate; excellent vitamin C, fibre; moderate vitamin A. Guava has the highest vitamin C content of the commonly available fruits, containing seven times the daily recommended intake for this vitamin. It is also high in fibre and contains vitamin A.

DESCRIPTION Small, round, green-skinned tropical fruit, which turns yellow when ripe, with white to salmon pink, juicy, 'seedy' flesh with a fragrant perfume.

ORIGIN AND HISTORY The guava is a native of Mexico, Brazil, and other tropical areas of South America. Birds love the fruit and have spread the seeds over large areas so that the guava has almost become a weed in some areas. The Portuguese traders took it to India and the Spanish traders took it to the Philippines. It is a fast-growing tree which bears fruit within two years and is now cultivated commercially in Hawaii, where guava juice is very popular, also in California, Florida (USA), and recently Australia. It bears fruit year-round in the tropics and seasonally in the subtropics. Some varieties of guava, particularly the white and strawberry, are best for eating fresh, while others are very acidic and are more suitable for processing into jam and jelly. Orchid lovers who are familiar with the genus *Cattleya* may be interested to learn that William Cattley, after whom it was named, also discovered and promoted the strawberry guava.

BUYING AND STORAGE Available during autumn Select firm, undamaged fruit with a greenish-yellow skin.

Store at room temperature until ripe, when the fruit yields to gentle pressure, and then store in a refrigerator. Stores well for several days.

PREPARATION AND USE Wash guava, cut in half lengthways and serve fresh in the skin with a teaspoon for eating. Use on fruit platters and with cheese boards; peel, slice or dice and add to fruit salad or fruit tart, or puree to use in ice cream, sorbets, and drinks.

PROCESSING May be juiced, canned or made into jam.

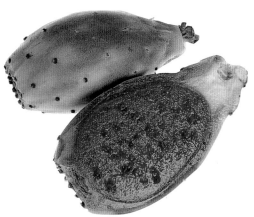

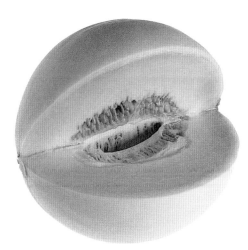

Honeydew Melon

Major Nutrients

Energy	135 kJ	Cholesterol	0
Protein	1 g	Sodium	0
Fat	0	Dietary Fibre	1 g
Carbohydrate	6.2 g	Vitamin C	18 mg

NUTRITIONAL INFORMATION The energy comes from carbohydrate; excellent source of vitamin C and folate; moderate source of vitamin A; good source of iron. Honeydew melon is slightly unusual as it contains folate, which is not normally found in many fruits in a significant amount.

DESCRIPTION The honeydew melon is oval in shape, with a clear, thick, creamy-white to creamy-yellow skin and with pale to dark green flesh containing white seeds. It is the fruit of a trailing vine.

ORIGIN AND HISTORY Honeydew melons and winter melon varieties are probably native to Asia. They have been cultivated since ancient times in the Nile Valley and were introduced to Europe through Italy at the beginning of the 15th century. Charles VIII took them to France after campaigning in Naples in 1495. The new fruit became so popular among gourmands that many are reputed to have died from eating too much melon — including Pope Paul II. More recently, the Israelis have cultivated new varieties such as the Ogen melon, which is named after a kibbutz. The hard-skinned honeydew and casaba varieties are excellent for the export market. Melons are now grown extensively in America, Europe, Africa, Asia and Australia.

BUYING AND STORAGE Available all year, peaking in late summer.

Melons do not ripen further once picked, so select a melon with a good colour and unblemished skin, and, in particular, one which gives off a sweet odour at the stalk end. The skin changes to a creamy-white colour on ripening.

Store at room temperature for 1–2 weeks. Once cut, cover with clear plastic wrap and store in the refrigerator. Use cut melons within a few days.

PREPARATION AND USE Cut melon in half and remove seeds. Cut into wedges and serve fresh in the hand; with prosciutto or powdered ginger for a fruit course; or with a fruit platter, with ice cream or with cheese. Cut fruit into balls with a melon-ball scoop and add to fruit and savoury salads or use as a garnish. Puree fruit and use in drinks or sorbets.

VARIETIES

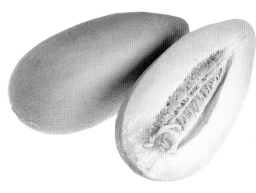

Casaba Round or ovoid in shape with smooth or wrinkled, non-netted, lemon to orange skin and creamy gold-peachy pink flesh.

Charentais Similar to Ogen with hard, pale green skin with dark green ribs and deep golden orange flesh.

Crenshaw A cross between casaba and Persian melon. It is pointed at the stem end, smoothly rounded at the blossom end. The skin is smooth, non-netted, mottled dark green and gold in colour, and flesh is salmon-coloured.

Ogen melon A small, round melon with a hard, mottled yellow-green skin with green ribs and a deep pink to red flesh.

Santa Claus or Christmas melon Looks like a small watermelon but has the flesh of a honeydew melon.

Spanish melon Resembles a casaba but has green skin and pale yellow-green flesh.

Indian Fig Opuntia ficus-indica

also called **Prickly pear**

Major Nutrients

Energy	170 kJ	Sodium	0
Protein	0	Dietary Fibre	5 g
Fat	0	Calcium	48 mg
Carbohydrate	9 g	Magnesium	29 mg
Cholesterol	0	Vitamin C	18 mg

NUTRITIONAL INFORMATION An interesting fruit in that it contains calcium and magnesium, neither of which is commonly found in fruits in a significant amount. It is also an excellent source of fibre and vitamin C.

DESCRIPTION Botanically a berry fruit of the cactus family, it is cylindrical and can vary from 4–8 cm in length. It is yellow-orange or brick red-purple in colour, according to variety, and the skin is covered with bristles or prickles. The fruit flesh is white, pink, yellow, orange or red, tastes sweet and usually encloses several edible seeds, but some fruits are seedless.

ORIGIN AND HISTORY Possibly native to South America, it was introduced to California by the Franciscan monks, and is now abundant there. Believed to have been introduced to Europe by Christopher Columbus. Now cultivated in Italy, Sicily, Malta and India. Grows wild in Australia where it was introduced to nurture the cochineal insect used by the early white settlers to produce red dye.

BUYING AND STORAGE Available in winter. Select well-coloured fruit without bruises. Tongs should be supplied by the retailer to protect customers from prickles.

Store in refrigerator in a paper bag.

PREPARATION AND USE Take care to avoid prickles when preparing Indian figs and wear rubber gloves for protection. Firstly wash the fruit with a stiff vegetable brush under running water to remove the prickles; cut a slice from the top and the base of the fruit, then slice the remaining skin off, cutting downwards. Slice the fruit and serve fresh with lime or lemon juice, or add to dried fruit compote, or Indian or Mexican dishes. Can be pureed and sieved and used in ice cream and other desserts or in marmalade and jam.

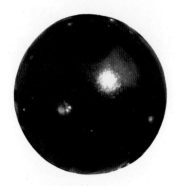

Jaboticaba *Myrciaria* spp.

also called Brazilian tree grape

NUTRITIONAL INFORMATION No reliable analysis is available.

DESCRIPTION A 1.5–4 cm round fruit with a tough, black or dark purple skin enclosing white or pale pink, sweet juicy flesh with 1–4 seeds. Looks like a black grape or olive, at first glance. Flesh tastes like a combination of grape and lychee, but skin has a blackcurrant flavour.

ORIGIN AND HISTORY The jaboticaba is a tropical tree which originated in southern Brazil. Although the fruit looks like a grape it grows in true tropical tree style directly on the trunk of the tree. Most trees bear fruit twice a year in the summer and have some fruit throughout the whole year. It has recently been introduced into the subtropical areas of Australia.

BUYING AND STORAGE Available in summer. Choose large, firm, shiny, dry fruit with undamaged skin.

Store in the refrigerator in a covered container. Will store for up to 2 weeks.

PREPARATION AND USE Rinse, then dry and eat fresh in the hand like grapes, or add to fruit salad, fruit platters or a cheese board. Use to make wine.

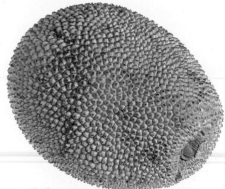

Jackfruit *Artocarpus heterophyllus*

also called Kathal, Khanun, Nangka

MAJOR NUTRIENTS		SERVE SIZE 100 G	
Energy	330 kJ	Dietary Fibre	3 g
Protein	0	Iron	0.8 mg
Fat	0	Zinc	0.8 mg
Carbohydrate	17 g	Vitamin A	115 µg
Cholesterol	0	Vitamin C	8 mg
Sodium	0		

NUTRITIONAL INFORMATION The energy source is carbohydrate; excellent vitamin A, vitamin C; good fibre, iron; moderate zinc.

Like star fruit (carambola), jackfruit is relatively high in kilojoules. Interestingly this fruit contains a moderate amount of zinc, which is not commonly found in fruit in a significant amount. Jackfruit also contains iron.

DESCRIPTION A very large, ovoid-oblong fruit weighing 4–25 kg, with a rough green skin made of hexagonal fleshy spines, containing soft white, juicy flesh with 100–500 large white seeds. The flesh comprises 30%, the seeds 5%; the remainder is rubbery latex.

ORIGIN AND HISTORY The jackfruit originated in the rainforests and mountainous regions of tropical India and Malaysia. It is now cultivated throughout the tropical lowlands particularly in Indo-China, Singapore, parts of Africa, and the West Indies. When Christopher Columbus sailed past Trinidad on his third journey to the New World, he was so impressed by all the palm trees and the jackfruit trees, that he decided he must be in the Garden of Eden, thought to be in eastern Asia at that time. This giant fruit is grown experimentally in northern Australia. There are two main kinds of jackfruit, a soft-skinned, soft type and a firm-skinned, crunchy type.

Nowhere in South-East Asia is jackfruit given more importance as an ingredient than in Central Java where they have devised gudeg, a creamy, spicy curry-like dish sweetened with palm sugar and local spices. It must be cooked in an earthenware pot as cooks believe metal pots do not bring out the 'warmth' of the dish. In a Javanese Rijstafel banquet, gudeg may be fancied up with chicken, beancurd and hard-boiled eggs, as well as its prime ingredient, jackfruit.

BUYING AND STORAGE Choose jackfruit with undamaged skin.

Store in a cool, dry place if whole, but if cut, cover with clear plastic and store in refrigerator.

PREPARATION AND USE Cut fruit in half, with an oiled knife to prevent the latex sticking to it. With oiled fingers and knife, remove the arils, or pouches of flesh, which surround the seeds; then, by turning the arils inside out, it is possible to remove the seeds, leaving you with the flesh only. Store the flesh in a covered container in the refrigerator until required. The soft flesh may be eaten fresh, stuffed with seafood, in fruit salad, in ice cream or juiced. The crunchy flesh is good cooked in curries, boiled, deep-fried as chips, or eaten raw and crunchy chilled on ice. The seeds may be boiled, roasted and used like chestnuts, or sliced and used in desserts and sweet drinks — usually mixed with coconut milk. They are also boiled and used as a vegetable. The flowers, too, are used as a vegetable, in salads and curries. Canned jackfruit segments can be used in the same way as the fresh fruit.

PROCESSING May be dried or preserved in syrup.

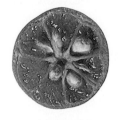 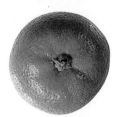

Kalamansi *Citrus mandarensis*

also called Calamansi, Calamondin

MAJOR NUTRIENTS		SERVE SIZE 100 G	
Energy	40 kJ	Carbohydrate	8 g
Protein	1 g	Cholesterol	0
Fat	0		

NUTRITIONAL INFORMATION No reliable data are available for the remaining nutrients.

DESCRIPTION A small citrus fruit similar to the cumquat, with yellow-orange flesh. The flavour is tart-sweet when ripe.

ORIGIN AND HISTORY A native fruit of the Philippines, kalamansi is used extensively in cooking and its juice is a popular, refreshing drink. Kalamansi juice is the base of some of the most exotic and refreshing cocktails sold in Asian bars. Kalamansi and various other sour local fruits such as carambola, santol and green guavas provide the basic acid content of one of the most important Philippine dishes, sinigang.

BUYING AND STORAGE As an ornamental garden fruit tree, the plant is often sold as the calamondin in nurseries. The juice is now sold in most Asian stores in cans or jars. Unfortunately, it is almost always sweetened.

Store opened kalamansi juice no longer than 24 hours as its flavour dissipates.

PREPARATION AND USE Juice is used as a drink. Concentrated juice, when available, can be used in cooking.

PREPARATION AND USE Juice is used as a drink. Concentrated juice, when available, can be used in cooking.

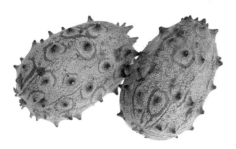

Kiwano Cucumis sp.

also called African horned melon

NUTRITIONAL INFORMATION No specific information is available.

DESCRIPTION Looks like a short, fat cucumber covered with spikes on the yellow-gold-green skin. When cut open it is full of refreshing lime green, edible seeds, resembling those of a cucumber.

ORIGIN AND HISTORY This fruit from Africa now grows on the fringe of the Australian desert and is cultivated in New Zealand.

BUYING AND STORAGE Available during autumn. Select firm, good-sized kiwanos with undamaged golden skin.

Store in the refrigerator.

PREPARATION AND USE Rinse, dry in a clean tea towel, then slice or cube and use in green salad, fish salad, and fruit salad, serve with smoked salmon or trout, or puree and serve in a chilled soup or sauce with salmon or tuna.

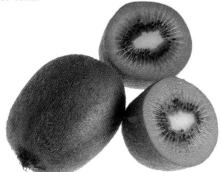

Kiwifruit Actinidia chinensis

also called Chinese gooseberry

MAJOR NUTRIENTS		SERVE SIZE 100 G	
Energy	205 kJ	Sodium	0
Protein	1 g	Dietary Fibre	3.3 g
Fat	0	Vitamin C	72 mg
Carbohydrate	10 g	Iron	0.5 mg
Cholesterol	0		

NUTRITIONAL INFORMATION An excellent source of vitamin C — one kiwifruit contains the total recommended daily intake; moderate source of iron. Low in kilojoules.

DESCRIPTION An ovoid fruit, as big as a plum, with a thin brown, rough, hairy skin enclosing bright green refreshing flesh with black seeds.

ORIGIN AND HISTORY The fruit is a native of China, where it grows on the edge of the forests in the Yangtze Valley. Cultivation is extensive in China and USSR. It is said to have been discovered in China by a European botanist, Robert Fortune, in 1845, who introduced it into Europe, where it became popular in gardens. More recently it was introduced for cultivation into New Zealand, Australia, Israel, France, Italy, Spain, and the USA. The New Zealand vines have all been developed from plants brought in from China in 1910 and now produce excellent quality fruit for the export market. In spite of its ugly external appearance — the French describe 'le kiwi' as a mouse hanging by its tail — the kiwifruit now enjoys world popularity.

BUYING AND STORAGE The season peaks in autumn and winter. Choose large, well-shaped, undamaged, firm fruit. The ripe fruit yields slightly when pressed.

Ripen at room temperature, then store in a refrigerator. Will keep for several weeks.

PREPARATION AND USE Rub fruit with a paper towel to remove hairs. Cut fruit in half and eat fresh from skin with a teaspoon, or peel, then halve, quarter, slice or dice. Add to fruit salad, use in tarts, on cheese boards or on fruit platters, or puree and serve with a dessert, or in ice cream or sorbets.

PROCESSING May be used in liqueur.

Lemon Citrus limon

MAJOR NUTRIENTS		SERVE SIZE 50 G	
Energy	50 kJ	Cholesterol	0
Protein	0	Sodium	0
Fat	0	Dietary Fibre	1.5 g
Carbohydrate	1 g	Vitamin C	24 mg

NUTRITIONAL INFORMATION Contains excellent vitamin C and very few kilojoules. Vitamin C is the only significant nutrient.

DESCRIPTION The ovoid lemon, with one pointed tip, has a hard, gleaming rind whose yellow can vary from a light, acidic hue to a bright gold.

ORIGIN AND HISTORY The lemon's origin is not definite but it is thought to have originated in South China, India, and Burma. The English word lemon and the French limon are thought to be derived from the Hindi word lemoen. The Arabs were responsible for the lemon's cultivation in the 14th century, and it was taken to Greece by Alexander the Great's armies. The returning Crusaders spread the fruit throughout Europe. It was first recorded growing in Britain in 1577, outdoors in summer but indoors in winter. Christopher Columbus took lemons from Spain, across the Atlantic to Haiti in 1493. The North American lemon is thought to have originated from a seed from a box of lemons that travelled from Sicily to Los Angeles in 1858. The best lemons are now cultivated in the Mediterranean, Italy, Sicily, Cyprus, Israel and North Africa, California, Florida, Texas, and Australia. Botanically, the lemon is a spherical berry, the fruit of a deciduous citrus tree.

BUYING AND STORAGE Available all year, with season peaking in autumn. Choose lemons that are brightly coloured and heavy for their size with a thin, undamaged skin. The lemon does not ripen further after picking. Avoid soft, shrivelled, discoloured lemons.

Store at room temperature for up to a week, then store in a refrigerator.

PREPARATION AND USE Wash and dry lemon, then grate zest off finely, squeeze out juice and use according to recipes. Use in drinks, soups, marinades, sauces, icings, savoury and sweet dishes, or cut into segments or slices and use to garnish fish and decorate desserts and drinks.

PROCESSING May be juiced or used to make commercial sorbets and dried lemon peel.

VARIETIES

Eureka Suitable for cooking and juicing.

LISBON

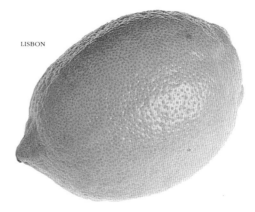

Lisbon Suitable for cooking and juicing.

Villa Franca Suitable for cooking and juicing.

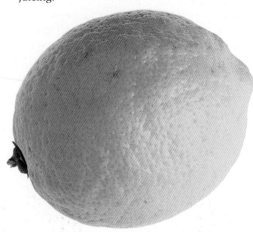

Meyer Suitable to use fresh for garnishing and decorating food and drinks.

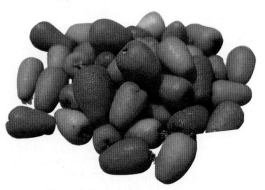

Lillypilly *Syzygium* spp.

MAJOR NUTRIENTS SERVE SIZE 100 G

Energy	105 kJ	Dietary Fibre	5 g
Protein	1 g	Sodium	35 mg
Fat	0	Vitamin C	15 mg
Carbohydrate	5 g		

NUTRITIONAL INFORMATION The lillypilly not only has the texture of crisp watermelon, its composition is also very similar. It is a source of vitamin C.

DESCRIPTION The fruit of lillypilly trees varies from white to cherry red in colour and has a crisp acid taste.

ORIGIN AND HISTORY Lillypilly fruit is eagerly eaten by Aboriginal children and was used by white settlers in country areas of Australia.

BUYING AND STORAGE Not commercially available except in jams and chutneys, but can be foraged from urban street trees.

Store refrigerated or frozen.

PREPARATION AND USE A good thirst-quenching fruit. Eat raw, discarding the seed, or use to prepare jellies, jams and preserves.

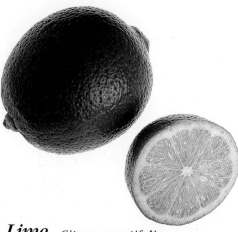

Lime *Citrus aurantifolia*

MAJOR NUTRIENTS SERVE SIZE 50 G

Energy	45 kJ	Cholesterol	0
Protein	0	Sodium	0
Fat	0	Dietary Fibre	2 g
Carbohydrate	1 g	Vitamin C	20 mg

NUTRITIONAL INFORMATION An excellent source of vitamin C.

DESCRIPTION A small citrus fruit with a distinctive flavour.

ORIGIN AND HISTORY Probably it originated in India, Persia, China, and the East Indies. Now grown commercially in Florida, Mexico, West Indies, Israel, and Australia.

BUYING AND STORAGE Available during spring and autumn. Choose a firm lime with thin skin, heavy for its size. Avoid small shrivelled fruit.

Store at room temperature for a week, then keep in the refrigerator.

PREPARATION AND USE Wash and dry in a clean tea towel, then slice to use in drinks or for garnishing fish. Grate zest of rind finely and squeeze juice and use in savoury and sweet recipes as a substitute for lemon. Use to marinade fish for traditional Tahitian fish and in Key lime pie.

PROCESSING Used for marmalade and cordial; also dried.

VARIETIES
Tahiti, also called Persian — larger, lime green-coloured, oval with acidic fragrant flavour. Mexican, also called West Indian or Key lime — smaller, lemon yellow-coloured, round-oval with very acidic strong flavour.

SEE ALSO Dried Lime

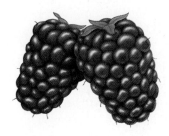

Loganberry *Rubus loganobaccus*

MAJOR NUTRIENTS SERVE SIZE 100 G

Energy	75 kJ	Sodium	0
Protein	1 g	Dietary Fibre	6 g
Fat	0	Iron	1.3 mg
Carbohydrate	3 g	Vitamin C	35 mg
Cholesterol	0	Magnesium	30 mg

NUTRITIONAL INFORMATION The energy comes from carbohydrate; excellent fibre, vitamin C; moderate magnesium; ¾ cup of loganberries would contribute significantly to the total iron intake.

DESCRIPTION Resembles a large raspberry, but is pink-burgundy in colour.

ORIGIN AND HISTORY The loganberry is a hybrid between a blackberry and a raspberry. It was accidentally developed in a Californian garden in 1881 by Judge J. H. Logan, a Scotsman. It was first exhibited in England by a well-known nurseryman in 1897 and is now widely grown in English gardens. The loganberry is grown commercially on the Pacific coast of the USA and in temperate climate areas of Europe and Australia.

BUYING AND STORAGE Available in midsummer. Buy and store as for blackberries and raspberries.

PREPARATION AND USE Pick over for grubs, then serve fresh with cream, liqueur or ice cream. May be pureed for sauce, used in ice cream, sorbets, soufflés and mousses or in fruit tarts and pies.

PROCESSING May be canned or bottled in glass jars.

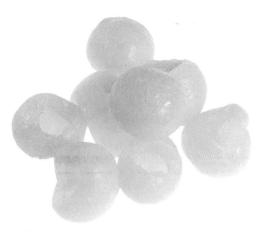

Longan *Euphoria longan*

also called Dragon's eyes, Lungan

MAJOR NUTRIENTS		SERVE SIZE 33 G	
Energy	80 kJ	Cholesterol	0
Protein	0	Sodium	0
Fat	0	Dietary Fibre	1 g
Carbohydrate	5 g		

NUTRITIONAL INFORMATION Contains no significant nutrients.

DESCRIPTION Similar to the lychee but smaller with a dull, yellow-brown, thin, leathery skin, sweet, juicy, translucent white flesh and a small, round, brown seed.

ORIGIN AND HISTORY The longan is known as the little brother of the lychee and is also related to the rambutan. In fact there is a wonderful Asian description: 'The rambutan is the long-haired old man, the lychee is closely cropped and the longan is shaved like a Buddhist monk.' It is thought to be native to many Asian countries including Sri Lanka, India, Burma, Thailand, and China. Dragon's eyes is its Chinese name. Today it grows in Vietnam, Taiwan, Hong Kong, and Malaysia and cultivation has been introduced into the tropical north of Australia.

In Canton in the ninth and tenth months of the lunar year, festivals are held to herald the arrival of the longan season.

BUYING AND STORAGE Available during autumn. Choose evenly coloured fruit with undamaged skin, still attached to the branch if possible. Should yield to gentle pressure when ripe.

Store in the crisper of the refrigerator.

The longan is available in cans, and unless specifically needed, canned lychees are a better buy. Transfer canned fruit to a non-metal container and refrigerate for up to 5 days.

Dried longans will keep indefinitely in an airtight jar.

PREPARATION AND USE Prepare as for lychee. Eat fresh, add to fruit salad or savoury salad, poach, or use in Chinese dishes.

Dried longan is commonly available. It is used to add flavour to sweet soups, certain simmered and braised Chinese dishes, and in some sweet and sour sauces.

PROCESSING May be canned, bottled in syrup, and dried.

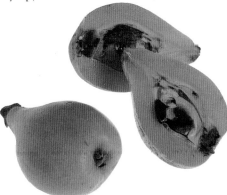

Loquat *Eriobotrya japonica*

also called Japanese loquat, Japanese medlar, Pai pah guor

MAJOR NUTRIENTS		SERVE SIZE 100 G	
Energy	100 kJ	Sodium	0
Protein	0	Dietary Fibre	1.7 g
Fat	0	Vitamin C	3 mg
Carbohydrate	5 g	Vitamin A	85 µg
Cholesterol	0		

NUTRITIONAL INFORMATION The energy comes from carbohydrate; good source of vitamin A; moderate vitamin C. The major contributing nutrient from this fruit is the non-animal form of vitamin A, called beta carotene.

DESCRIPTION A yellow, oval, subtropical fruit with juicy tart-sweet yellow flesh with a delicate flavour and crisp texture. It contains large brown seeds.

ORIGIN AND HISTORY Native to Asia, this delicate fruit was revered during the Ming dynasty (1368–1644). Elaborate ritual surrounded the transportation of delicacies from the Yangtze region to the palace in Peking. The Grand Canal fleet of barges was used, and the 'directorate of foodstuffs' had priority of canal facilities, next only to the 'directorate of ceremonials'. Even in these early times, ice was used to keep perishables fresh.

Introduced into Europe in 1787 for its foliage. Now cultivated in parts of Australia, California, and in some Mediterranean countries. A member of the Rosaceae family, the same botanical family as the apple and the pear.

BUYING AND STORAGE Available during spring. Select firm, bright-coloured fruit, still attached to the stem if possible.

Store in the refrigerator.

PREPARATION AND USE The loquat is peeled and eaten fresh or used to make desserts. In Thailand, China, and Japan, it is often set in an agar agar jelly.

In China the loquat is dried and used to add flavour to braised dishes and desserts. Dried loquats will keep indefinitely in an airtight container in the refrigerator.

PROCESSING May be candied, or jellied. Made into a liqueur in Bermuda.

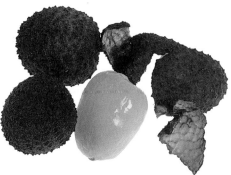

Lychee *Litchi chinensis*

also called Chinese cherry, lichee, litchee, litchi, litchie

MAJOR NUTRIENTS		SERVE SIZE 100 G	
Energy	290 kJ	Sodium	0
Protein	0	Dietary Fibre	1.3 g
Fat	0	Iron	0.5 mg
Carbohydrate	16 g	Vitamin C	49 mg
Cholesterol	0		

NUTRITIONAL INFORMATION The energy comes from carbohydrate. The lychee is extremely high in vitamin C — 1 cup provides 1½ times the daily recommended intake. It also contains a moderate amount of iron.

Canning reduces the vitamin C content by three-quarters.

DESCRIPTION A small, oval fruit, pointed at one end, with a rough, leathery, scaly skin, which is bright red, orange or yellow in colour, depending on variety. The flesh is translucent pearly white, sweet and juicy, with a flavour similar to a grape, around a large, shiny brown seed or stone.

ORIGIN AND HISTORY The lychee is a native of China, where it has been cultivated as far back as 1700 BC. Chinese literature records that the lychee was taken on horseback from southern China to the imperial court in the north during the Han dynasty. This delicious fruit has been the subject of many Chinese poems. One poet, who was exiled from the imperial court in the north to Kwangtung in the south, is said to have taken comfort by eating 300 lychees a day. It is now grown in India, throughout South-East Asia, the Philippines, Japan, Florida (USA), and Africa. It was introduced to Australia by the Chinese goldminers in the 1870s. Lychees marketed attached to their branch are valued for their decorative value as well as their fruit.

BUYING AND STORAGE Available in summer. Select bright, evenly coloured fruit with moist-looking, undamaged skin, still attached to the branch if possible, as it will last longer. The skin turns dull red-brown and the scaly texture becomes flattened when the lychee is fully ripe. Store in the crisper of the refrigerator. Will keep for up to 3 months.

PREPARATION AND USE With a small, sharp, stainless steel vegetable knife, cut the skin crossways across the pointed end of the fruit, then peel back and serve lychee fresh in the hand. Or remove peel and add to fruit salad, savoury salads or serve with liqueur, cream or ice cream. May be poached, stuffed and served as a savoury or added to Chinese dishes, particularly sweet and sour fish, pork and chicken.

PROCESSING May be canned or dried.

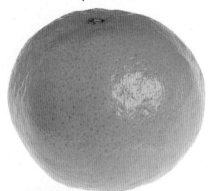

Mandarin *Citrus reticulata*

also called *Tangerine*

MAJOR NUTRIENTS		SERVE SIZE 100 G	
Energy	160 kJ	Cholesterol	0
Protein	0	Sodium	0
Fat	0	Dietary Fibre	2 g
Carbohydrate	8 g	Vitamin C	31 mg

NUTRITIONAL INFORMATION The energy source is carbohydrate; excellent vitamin C.

DESCRIPTION A sweet orange-coloured citrus fruit, smaller and flatter than a standard-sized orange, with a thin, loose skin.

ORIGIN AND HISTORY This fruit originated in the East, in China and Indo-China in particular, and it is also found in the Philippines. There is no difference between the mandarin and the tangerine — mandarin is the older name. The clementine is also a variety of mandarin. The mandarin crosses easily and has been crossed with the grapefruit to give us the tangelo, which is gaining popularity, and the ugli fruit. The mandarin has more resistance to cold than the orange and so can be grown farther north in China, Japan,

and Spain. It is cultivated commercially in the USA, South Africa, France, Algeria, and Australia.

BUYING AND STORAGE Available in winter. Choose a fruit with a thin, fairly loose, undamaged, evenly coloured orange skin. A mandarin should feel heavy in relation to its size.

Store at room temperature for up to a week, then keep in refrigerator until ready to use.

PREPARATION AND USE Peel a mandarin and eat fresh in the hand. Or peel, slice and use as for an orange, or for marmalade.

PROCESSING May be canned, glacéed or candied, or used to make liqueur or marmalade.

VARIETIES

The mandarin, which has lots of pips; the satsuma, which has none; the clementine, grown in the northern hemisphere.

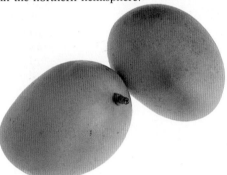

Mango *Mangifera indica*

also called *Manga*

MAJOR NUTRIENTS		SERVE SIZE 120 G	
Energy	300 kJ	Sodium	0
Protein	0	Dietary Fibre	2 g
Fat	0	Vitamin C	36 mg
Carbohydrate	15 g	Vitamin A	200 µg
Cholesterol	0	Iron	0.6 mg

NUTRITIONAL INFORMATION High levels of vitamin A, moderate iron. Major contributing nutrient is from beta carotene, the plant form of vitamin A. A mango provides the recommended daily intake of vitamin C.

DESCRIPTION A plump, soft fruit which may be very large or small and rounded depending on the variety. The skin is usually green, and the flesh a pleasant, fragrant light orange.

ORIGIN AND HISTORY The mango is one of the earliest known tropical fruits and the favourite fruit of many people. It is native to India and Burma where it has been cultivated for more than 4000 years. Wild mangoes are found growing in forests in Vietnam, Thailand, Burma, and India. Indian legends make many references to the mango. There

are also references to the mango being cultivated in China in the 7th century. The Spanish introduced the mango into the Philippines and the Portuguese traders introduced its cultivation into east and South Africa, then into Brazil, and the West Indies. The mango was introduced to Australia by the early white settlers and excellent quality fruit is produced in Queensland and the Northern Territory. This 'king of fruits' belongs to the same family as the luxurious cashew nut.

BUYING AND STORAGE Available in summer. Choose fruit that has a smooth, firm but soft skin. When ripe, it will yield if pressed gently and will have a perfumed aroma. The colour can vary from green-yellow to orange with a pink blush, according to variety. Avoid fruit which has wrinkled skin or black spots as this is a sign of age and decay.

Ripen mangoes at room temperature until soft when pressed, then store in the crisper or in a plastic bag in the refrigerator until required. Use as soon as possible.

PREPARATION AND USE Score the skin downwards from the stem end into quarter segments, peel the skin back and eat the fruit fresh in the hand. The most attractive way to serve fresh mango is in the porcupine style; cut the two fleshy cheeks off, as near to the large flat stone as possible, then score each half into small squares and push the skin inwards so that the fruit pops up like a porcupine.

PROCESSING May be canned, or used in Indian pickles and chutneys.

VARIETIES

The varieties fall into two groups: those from India, considered to be the better fruit, and those from the Philippines and the Americas — a smaller fruit.

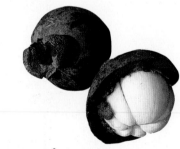

Mangosteen *Garcinia mangostana*

MAJOR NUTRIENTS		SERVE SIZE 100 G	
Energy	320 kJ	Dietary Fibre	1 g
Protein	1 g	Thiamin	0.05 mg
Fat	1 g	Vitamin C	2 mg
Carbohydrate	18 g		

NUTRITIONAL INFORMATION This is a

moderate source of thiamin and vitamin C.

DESCRIPTION A round fruit with a thick, smooth, leathery purple skin, which contains 4 or 6 segments of delicious, soft, treacly ivory-white flesh surrounded by a fine pink membrane and containing 1 or 2 brown seeds.

ORIGIN AND HISTORY The mangosteen is native to the Malay Peninsula, the East Indies, and the Philippines. It has been cultivated in South-East Asia and India for many centuries and is now growing in the humid north of Queensland, Australia. It is, however, a slow-growing tree and takes from 8–15 years to bear fruit. The mangosteen is often referred to as the 'Queen of Tropical Fruits'. Eaten straight from the tree or from an Asian market, it tastes delicious and it will travel well if carefully packaged.

BUYING AND STORAGE The mangosteen is picked when ripe. Store in the refrigerator, and eat as soon as possible.

PREPARATION AND USE Peel fruit, divide into segments and eat fresh like an orange. Use in fruit salad or compote, serve with ice cream or puree for a sauce or sorbet.

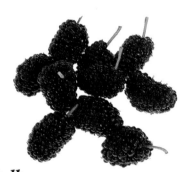

Mulberry Morus nigra

MAJOR NUTRIENTS		SERVE SIZE 100 G	
Energy	120 kJ	Sodium	0
Protein	2 g	Dietary Fibre	2 g
Fat	0	Vitamin C	10 mg
Carbohydrate	4 g	Phosphorus	48 mg
Cholesterol	0		

NUTRITIONAL INFORMATION The energy comes from carbohydrate; excellent vitamin C, which is the major nutrient; moderate phosphorus, fibre.

DESCRIPTION A shiny, deep purple, juicy fruit which resembles a large berry fruit in appearance but grows on a small tree.

ORIGIN AND HISTORY A native of either Persia (now Iran) and the southern Caucasus or the Nepal mountains. The Greeks introduced it into Europe in ancient times. Taken to England in the 1500s where it was valued for its leaves (fed to silkworms) as well as its fruit. Grown in domestic gardens as well as under cultivation.

BUYING AND STORAGE Available in summer. Choose firm, well-shaped, even-coloured, dry fruit. Mulberries are picked when ripe, so store in the refrigerator and use as soon as possible — they are very soft and perishable.

PREPARATION AND USE Like the blackberry, boysenberry, loganberry, and raspberry, this soft fruit may be served alone with a little cream, or used to fill pies or tarts, and also to flavour ice cream. Also pulped and strained to make juice.

PROCESSING Not applicable but may be frozen.

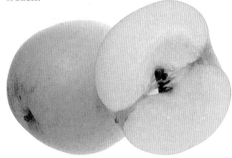

Nashi

NUTRITIONAL INFORMATION No specific information is available.

DESCRIPTION Technically a member of the pear family, the nashi fruit has the round shape and size of an apple and the flavour of a pear, with a smooth, green-yellow or brownish-russet skin according to variety, and a crisp, crystal-like texture. It has a delicate flavour and lots of refreshing clear juice.

ORIGIN AND HISTORY A native of Japan, China, and Korea. Originally introduced to Australia in the mid-1800s by Chinese goldminers. Cultivation of the nashi fruit was later introduced extensively into the temperate fruit-growing areas of Australia around 1980.

BUYING AND STORAGE Available in the autumn and early winter. Look for unblemished, firm fruit which weighs heavily for its size to ensure a good juice content. Nashi are picked when ready to eat.

Store in a fruit bowl, out of direct sunlight, as fruit will remain crisp for 2 weeks, then store in the crisper in the refrigerator to keep longer.

PREPARATION AND USE Wash fruit and eat fresh in the hand, like an apple or a pear. The fruit can be cut into quarters, the core removed and the fruit sliced into thin wedges to serve on fruit platters or with cheese.

Nectarine Prunus persica var. nectarina

MAJOR NUTRIENTS		SERVE SIZE 100 G	
Energy	160 kJ	Cholesterol	0
Protein	0	Sodium	0
Fat	0	Dietary Fibre	2.5 g
Carbohydrate	8 g	Vitamin C	13 mg

NUTRITIONAL INFORMATION The energy comes from carbohydrate; excellent vitamin C; moderate fibre. Canned nectarine has a slightly reduced vitamin C and fibre content, and the sweetened canned fruit has twice as many kilojoules as its raw counterpart.

The dried nectarine contains no vitamin C but has a high fibre content of 3.5 g.

DESCRIPTION Similar to a peach in shape and colour but smaller and with a smooth, shiny red-yellow skin.

ORIGIN AND HISTORY Originally from China. Was taken to Britain via Persia and Europe in the 16th century. Botanically a one-seeded drupe, a member of the rose family, related to the peach and almond. The nectarine used to be totally white-fleshed, but since crossing with the peach it has become yellow or pink-fleshed, larger and firmer.

BUYING AND STORAGE Available in the late spring and summer. Choose bright, undamaged, even-coloured fruit which yields slightly to pressure along the 'seam'. The nectarine stops ripening once picked.

Store at room temperature until soft enough to eat, then in refrigerator until served.

PREPARATION AND USE Wash, dry and leave whole, then eat fresh in the hand or serve as dessert fruit in a bowl of iced water. Stew or poach, use in ice cream, sorbets and sauces, puddings, tarts, stuffed, or as a substitute for peaches.

PROCESSING May be canned.

VARIETIES

There are several varieties with white, yellow or pink flesh, but two main types: freestone, where stone separates easily from the flesh, and clingstone.

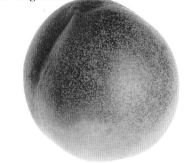

Clingstone Nectarine

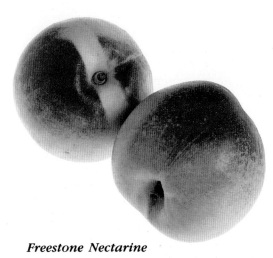

Freestone Nectarine

Orange *Citrus sinensis*

MAJOR NUTRIENTS		SERVE SIZE 150 G	
Energy	160 kJ	Sodium	0
Protein	1 g	Dietary Fibre	3 g
Fat	0	Iron	0.5 mg
Carbohydrate	8 g	Thiamin	0.10 mg
Cholesterol	0	Vitamin C	70 mg

NUTRITIONAL INFORMATION The energy comes from carbohydrate; excellent vitamin C; good folic acid, fibre, thiamin; moderate iron. Compared to many other fruits, the orange is very nutritious, containing a wide variety of nutrients.

NUTRITIONAL INFORMATION The vitamin C content can reach 35 mg/100 g, so this is a useful source of the vitamin. This fruit is higher in energy and a more concentrated source of nutrients than most fresh cultivated fruit.

ORIGIN AND HISTORY Thought to have originated in China and maybe in India and Siam (Thailand), oranges were cultivated around the Mediterranean Sea during the domination of the Arab empire. Now cultivated in California, Florida (USA), South America, Israel, Spain, Italy, South Africa, and Australia. The orange, lemon and lime were valued by the early sailors on their long journeys to guard against scurvy. A member of the citrus family and one of the most important and extensively cultivated fruits of the tropical and subtropical regions of the world.

BUYING AND STORAGE Navel oranges available in autumn, winter and spring. Valencia oranges available in spring and summer. Seville oranges available in winter. Choose the orange with a thin skin which is heavy for its size. The orange does not ripen further after picking, so a spongy-skinned orange, light for its size, will be poor quality

and not very juicy. Avoid fruit with soft areas which are water-soaked as this indicates decay. Wilted shrivelled skin is a sign of an old orange.

Store oranges in a cool, dry place for 1 week, then transfer to a refrigerator to keep longer.

PREPARATION AND USE Peel fruit and eat fresh in the hand, or remove peel and pith with a small serrated knife, then cut into slices or segments and serve with liqueur, in fruit or green salads, with duck, ham, chicken and veal, or in fruit cup. Squeeze juice from oranges and serve fresh for breakfast, add to fruit punch, fruit salad, milkshakes, eggnogs and salad dressings, or use in sorbets, soufflés, with pancakes or French toast, or in cakes, puddings, biscuits and icing. Use for marmalade.

PROCESSING May be juiced, used for marmalade, candied orange peel, glacéed orange, orange liqueurs and orange flower water.

VARIETIES

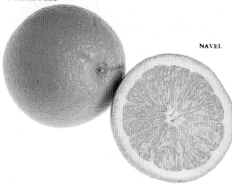

NAVEL

Navel (winter) orange Seedless with a pebbly skin and usually has a circular mark at the blossom end resembling a navel. It is ideal for eating and for serving in round slices or segments.

Sweet/Jaffa/Spanish (all year) orange Sweet and juicy, ranging from small to large, smooth-skinned with few seeds.

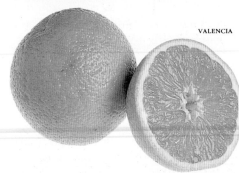

VALENCIA

Valencia (summer) orange This variety has seeds and a smooth skin. It is ideal for juicing.

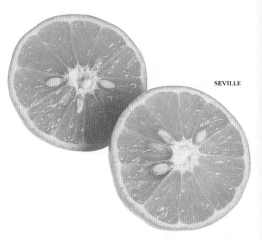

SEVILLE

Seville (winter) orange Large, with seeds and a strong, bitter flavour. It is ideal for making marmalade.

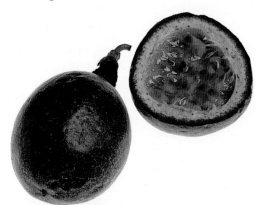

Passionfruit *Passiflora* spp.

also called Granadilla

MAJOR NUTRIENTS		SERVE SIZE 30 G	
Energy	60 kJ	Cholesterol	0
Protein	0	Sodium	0
Fat	0	Dietary Fibre	4 g
Carbohydrate	3 g	Vitamin C	5 mg

NUTRITIONAL INFORMATION The energy source is carbohydrate; good source of vitamin C, the main nutrient; and good fibre.

DESCRIPTION The round fruit of a vine, which may have a variety of skin colours, containing sweet pulp and a large number of small, edible seeds.

ORIGIN AND HISTORY The passionfruit comes from a large family of several hundred species. Most passionfruit are native to the South American tropics, Brazil, Mexico, Central America and the West Indies, in particular, but there are also several native species in Australia. The flower of the vine was named passion flower (flor passionis) by the Spanish Jesuit priests, when colonising South America. They used it to explain the Passion and Crucifixion of Christ, because it showed the Three Nails, the Five Wounds, the Crown of Thorns, and the Apostles. The priests believed God had created the flower to help them save the American Indians. The Spanish explorers called the fruit granadilla, meaning little pomegranate, but it became known as the passionfruit. It is now cultivated extensively in Australia and New Zealand and is known in all the major cities of the world.

BUYING AND STORAGE Available all year, but the season peaks in autumn. Choose large, heavy passionfruit with undamaged slightly wrinkled skin. Wrinkling of the skin indicates peak of ripeness.

Store at room temperature but transfer to a refrigerator when the skin becomes densely wrinkled. Will keep in refrigerator for a few weeks.

PREPARATION AND USE Wash passionfruit and dry, then cut in half and serve with a teaspoon for eating fresh. Passionfruit pulp may be scooped out of the skin and added to fresh berries, fruit salad, and drinks. It can also be used in sorbets, ice cream, icing, sauce, flummery, soufflés, and mousses, or to decorate pavlovas or sponge cakes. Freeze in ice cubes. Use also for passionfruit butter, a variation of lemon butter.

PROCESSING May be canned or used in commercial juice, to flavour yoghurt and in passionfruit butter.

VARIETIES

Banana passionfruit A long egg-shaped fruit, 8 cm long, with a tough, yellow-green, slightly downy skin containing thick orange pulp inseparable from numerous small black edible seeds.

Giant granadilla This is 30 cm long, and shaped like a marrow. It has a thick, leathery yellow-green skin containing thick, purple pulp with seeds similar to those of a canteloupe melon.

Golden/Hawaiian/sweet granadilla This has a tough, leathery orange to orange-brown skin containing sweet, translucent white pulp.

Purple granadilla/passionfruit This is a small round fruit the size of a large egg, with a tough, leathery, purple-black skin containing fragrant juicy yellow pulp which is inseparable from the small black edible seeds.

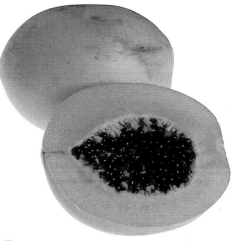

Pawpaw Carica papaya

also called *Papaya, Papaw*

MAJOR NUTRIENTS		SERVE SIZE 100 G	
Energy	120 kJ	Sodium	0
Protein	0	Dietary Fibre	2 g
Fat	0	Iron	0.5 mg
Carbohydrate	7 g	Vitamin A	153 µg
Cholesterol	0	Vitamin C	60 mg

NUTRITIONAL INFORMATION Along with most yellow/orange fruits, pawpaw is high in vitamin A and vitamin C. In addition it supplies iron. Pawpaw is also a good weight-watcher's food, as it is low in kilojoules and supplies moderate fibre.

DESCRIPTION The pawpaw is a large, soft fruit with thin greenish skin and very juicy flesh which has a distinctive aroma when ripe.

ORIGIN AND HISTORY The pawpaw is a tropical herbaceous plant, native to the Americas. It is closely related to the babaco, which is native to the Andes mountains of South America. The name comes from the Caribbean word ababai. It is thought that the Portuguese explorers took it home to Europe and it then travelled with traders to other hot tropical countries, such as Malaysia and the East Indies and eventually to Australia. Marco Polo was apparently the first European to discover pawpaw and he fed it to his sailors to cure their scurvy, as the fruit is rich in vitamin C. It grows fast, producing fruit in the first year, so has never been too expensive. It contains papain, a protein-splitting enzyme, which helps both to tenderise and digest meat. The papain is extracted from the skin of the unripe pawpaw or from the tree trunk and is used in the manufacture of chewing gum.

BUYING AND STORAGE Available all year, peaking in spring.

Choose evenly coloured, bright yellow, firm, undamaged fruit with a sweet perfume. Avoid fruit which is dull or has damp dark spots on the skin.

Pawpaw may be stored at room temperature for a few days, until soft to the touch, which indicates peak ripeness, and then stored, well wrapped, in the refrigerator for up to a week.

PREPARATION AND USE Cut pawpaw in half lengthways and remove seeds. Slice into segments and eat fresh in the hand or serve for breakfast with lime or lemon juice. Or peel and slice, dice or puree and use in fruit salad, sorbets, ice cream, serve with chicken, pork or scallops, or use in a marinade to tenderise meat. Pawpaw may be halved, stuffed with a savoury filling and baked. Green pawpaw may be grated and dressed with French dressing as a salad or an accompaniment to curry, or cooked as a vegetable. Pawpaw seeds may be pureed and added to French dressing or used in a marinade. Fresh pawpaw will not set in gelatine desserts.

VARIETIES

The most popular South American variety has a bright yellow flesh, and the Fijian variety has a peachy pink flesh.

Peach Prunus persica

MAJOR NUTRIENTS		SERVE SIZE 100 G	
Energy	140 kJ	Sodium	0
Protein	1 g	Dietary Fibre	2 g
Fat	0	Vitamin C	8 mg
Carbohydrate	6 g	Vitamin A	150 µg
Cholesterol	0		

NUTRITIONAL INFORMATION Like most yellow or orange fruits, the peach contains the plant form of vitamin A, called beta carotene, and vitamin C. Canning produces no significant changes in nutrient levels.

DESCRIPTION Often called the queen of fruits, the plump, round peach with its soft skin and juicy yellow, orange or white flesh provides delicious eating. It grows on a deciduous tree belonging to the rose family and related to the almond.

ORIGIN AND HISTORY The peach originated in China and was recorded in Chinese literature in 551 BC. It was transported along the silk route to Persia then into Europe 2000 years ago. Alexander the Great is thought to have transported it to Greece and Rome where it is pictured being enjoyed on many ancient frescoes.

The peach was known to the Anglo-Saxons, and by the time of Queen Elizabeth I it was being cultivated in England. Spanish voyagers introduced the peach to Latin America during the 16th century and it was brought to Australia by the early white settlers. Italy and the USA are the largest peach producers, followed by Canada, China, Japan, Australia, Israel, South Africa, and New Zealand. There is local production in Spain, France, Greece, and Yugoslavia.

BUYING AND STORAGE Available in late spring and summer. Choose peaches which are firm but will yield when pressed gently. This indicates ripeness; at this stage the skin has an even colour ranging from whitish-yellow to golden-yellow with a red 'blush'. The peach stops ripening once picked, so it is important to select ripe fruit.

Store at room temperature out of sunlight until soft, then store in a refrigerator and use as soon as possible as peaches are very perishable.

PREPARATION AND USE Wash, then dry and serve fresh in the hand, or serve as dessert fruit in a large bowl of iced water. Use halved, quartered or in segments, in fruit and savoury salads; stew, poach or bake; serve stuffed or in traditional 'Peach Melba'; use to make jam or brandied peaches.

PROCESSING May be canned, juiced or used in commercial yoghurt or jam.

VARIETIES
There are many varieties but the two main types are: freestone, where the stone separates easily from the flesh; and clingstone.

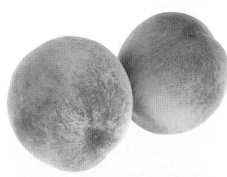

Clingstone Peach

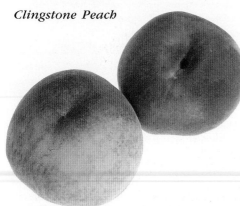

Freestone Peach

SEE ALSO Dried Peach.

Pear *Pyrus communis*

MAJOR NUTRIENTS		SERVE SIZE 150 G	
Energy	225 kJ	Cholesterol	0
Protein	0	Sodium	0
Fat	0	Dietary Fibre	4 g
Carbohydrate	14 g	Vitamin C	5 mg

NUTRITIONAL INFORMATION The energy source is carbohydrate. Good fibre and folic acid. This fruit is quite high in kilojoules compared to most other fruit. Its other major contributing nutrient is vitamin C of which it is a good source. Canning reduces the vitamin C content to an insignificant amount.

DESCRIPTION The pear has a green or yellow skin and juicy, white flesh.

ORIGIN AND HISTORY It is thought that the wild pear originated in west Asia and the ancient Greeks introduced it to Europe from where it spread to Britain. The pear is botanically a pome fruit, a member of the rose family; it is now cultivated in temperate climatic regions throughout the world. One of the world's most popular pears was first produced in Australia in 1896 by Charles Henry Packham, when he crossed a Williams (Bartlett) pear with an Yvedale St Germain, resulting in the Packham Triumph variety.

BUYING AND STORAGE Available all year, owing to the technique of controlled atmospheric storage, but the season peaks in late summer and autumn. The pear is fully developed but firm when picked, and it continues to ripen from the inside out after picking. It is therefore important to choose well-shaped, plump, firm pears with undamaged skin. Avoid fruit with dull, wilted skin and with spots near the blossom end as these indicate corky areas in the flesh.

Ripen the pear at room temperature until the skin starts to change colour, then store in refrigerator, but use as soon as possible.

PREPARATION AND USE Wash and dry pear and eat fresh in the hand, or cut into halves or quarters, remove core and serve with cheese or with fruit platters. Peel and bake or poach whole in wine for dessert, or peel, core and slice into a savoury salad or dice for a fruit salad. Puree for a sauce or sorbet. Use in crumbles, charlottes, pies, tarts and cakes. Preserve in bottles.

PROCESSING May be canned, juiced, dried, glacéed, crystallised or used in commercial sorbet. Used in a commercial mustard relish in Italy.

VARIETIES
There are thousands of types of wild pear to be found, but the following are the popular cultivated varieties.

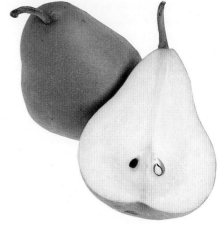

Beurre Bosc A dessert pear with a long, tapering neck; has a russet brown skin which turns dark cinnamon brown when fully ripe, and an aromatic, juicy, white flesh.

Cornice A large rounded dessert pear with a short neck; has a greenish-yellow skin which turns to yellow, often with a pink blush and russet patches when fully ripe, and a perfumed, very juicy, yellow-white flesh.

Conference A long, elegantly-shaped dessert pear; has a green and brown dull scaly skin, and a creamy-white, juicy, sweet flesh.

Corella A miniature dessert pear approximately 5 cm long; has a green skin with a pink blush (turns light green-gold when fully ripe) and a juicy white flesh.

Josephine A medium, conical dessert pear; has light green skin which turns to yellow with a pink blush when ripe, and aromatic juicy, yellow flesh.

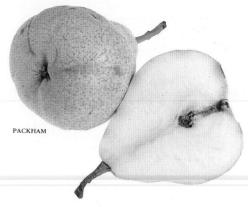

PACKHAM

Packham A popular large, rounded pear with a short neck; has a green skin which turns to light green-gold when ripe, and a juicy, sweet, white flesh.

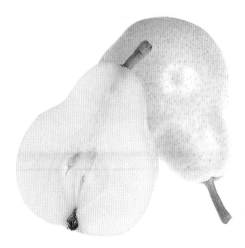

Williams, or Bartlett A good cooking pear with a regular shape; has a light green skin which turns to clear yellow when ripe, and a buttery-textured, sweet, white flesh.

SEE ALSO Dried Pear.

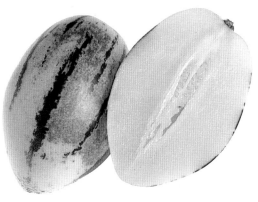

Pepino Solanum muricatum

also called ***Tree melon, Mellowfruit***

MAJOR NUTRIENTS		SERVE SIZE 100 G	
Energy	90 kJ	Cholesterol	0
Protein	0	Sodium	0
Fat	0	Dietary Fibre	1 g
Carbohydrate	5 g	Vitamin C	31 mg

NUTRITIONAL INFORMATION The energy source is carbohydrate; excellent source of vitamin C, which is the only significant nutrient in this fruit.

DESCRIPTION The small melon-shaped fruit of a vine, the size of an apple, with a creamy-green satinlike skin with purple stripes. The juicy flesh is pale yellow with edible soft seeds in the centre. The flavour is a delicate mixture of melon, lemon, and pineapple.

ORIGIN AND HISTORY The pepino originated in Peru and Chile. The plant was introduced into Florida about 100 years ago and now flourishes there. Cultivation tests are being conducted currently in Australia. Botanically, the pepino is a berry with no fertile seeds, so the plants must be raised from cut-

tings and grow somewhat like a tomato. The pepino has a lovely violet flower which is popular in flower arrangements.

BUYING AND STORAGE Available during autumn, winter and spring. Select firm fruit with no bruises. Pepinos continue to ripen after picking and the skin turns creamy-yellow when fully mature. Should have a fragrant aroma when ripe.

Store at room temperature until ripe, then in the crisper of a refrigerator.

PREPARATION AND USE Wash and dry gently, cut fruit in half, then into segments and serve fresh. Serve for breakfast. Add to fruit salad, fruit platters, cheese boards or chicken salad. Macerate in a liqueur, or puree to use in sorbets or drinks.

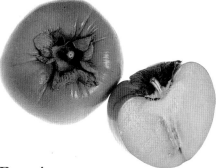

Persimmon Diospyros spp.

also called ***Date plum, Kakee, Kaki***

MAJOR NUTRIENTS		SERVE SIZE 150 G	
Energy	420 kJ	Sodium	0
Protein	0	Dietary Fibre	4 g
Fat	0	Iron	1 mg
Carbohydrate	24 g	Vitamin A	206 µg
Cholesterol	0	Vitamin C	14 mg

NUTRITIONAL INFORMATION The energy source is carbohydrate; excellent source of vitamin C, vitamin A; good source of fibre. When comparing standard serving sizes, the persimmon is higher in kilojoules than most fruits. However it is also higher in the plant form of vitamin A known as beta carotene, and in iron.

DESCRIPTION A round fruit with a smooth, brightly coloured, shiny skin with a large, dry green calyx at the stem end. When fully ripe, the hard astringent flesh softens to a delicious sweet jelly texture in some varieties.

ORIGIN AND HISTORY The persimmon is a native of China, Japan, the Himalayas, western Asia, and North America. It was known in the days of the Chinese dynasties and inspired many Chinese poets. The name means 'food of the gods'. It is also known as 'apple of the Orient'. It belongs to the same family as the ebony tree and is related to the sapote tropical fruits. It is a winter fruit which still hangs dra-

matically from the tree after all the leaves have fallen. The North American variety often grows wild as far north as the Great Lakes. It also grows in the olive-producing zones of Spain, France, and Italy, often as a garden fruit. The Israelis have developed a non-astringent fruit that can be eaten while still firm and crunchy, and they call it Sharon. This variety has been recently introduced into Australia where it is called Kaki which leads to some confusion.

BUYING AND STORAGE Available during autumn and early winter. Choose plump fruit with smooth, brightly coloured, undamaged skin. Ripen at room temperature until as soft as jelly; kaki fruit should be ripened just until soft. When ripe, serve as soon as possible.

Wrap securely and store in the refrigerator, but use as soon as possible.

PREPARATION AND USE Cut persimmon in half and serve fresh with a teaspoon for eating the jellylike fruit. Or scoop fruit out and add to fruit salad, or puree for a sauce, sorbet or jelly. Often an unripe persimmon is unpalatable until jellylike in texture, but the firmer kaki variety is not as astringent and may be cut into segments and served fresh with cheese or on a fruit platter. May also be poached in wine or used in pies, cakes or jam.

PROCESSING May be used in jams and jellies. Dried in Japan.

VARIETIES

There are three main varieties.

Chinese/Japanese (*D. kaki*) is the most popular. The fruit are 5–7.5 cm in diameter and are a rich yellow-orange colour. The North American (*D. virginia*) fruit is smaller and is dark red-maroon in colour. *D. lotus*, or date plum, is 1–2 cm in diameter and yellow turning to purple-black with a datelike flesh.

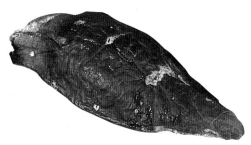

Pigface Carpobrotus spp.

MAJOR NUTRIENTS		SERVE SIZE 50 G	
Energy	150 kJ	Dietary Fibre	7 g
Protein	1 g	Vitamin A	0
Fat	1 g	Calcium	220 mg
Carbohydrate	7 g	Iron	3 mg
Cholesterol	0		

NUTRITIONAL INFORMATION The mineral content is higher than usually found in a fruit. Calcium and iron content are particularly high for a fruit. There is no scientific evidence for a nutritional therapeutic effect apart from the food value.

DESCRIPTION Pigface has succulent, angular leaves and forms a horned, globular fruit which is purple when ripe. The leaves and fruit pulp are edible.

ORIGIN AND HISTORY Pigface is a ground creeper widespread on coastal dunes and in inland areas. The fruits were harvested by Aborigines and the leaves were used to salt meat. Juice from the leaves of a Chilean species is known to cure dysentery and that of an Australian species can help to relieve pain from insect stings.

BUYING AND STORAGE Pigface is not commercially available and must be harvested wild or cultivated domestically. The leaves can be harvested at any time but are best while actively growing. The fruit should be picked when not fully ripe and can be stored frozen.

PREPARATION AND USE Peel the outer succulent skin and eat the inner pulp and seed mass raw. Use could parallel that of kiwifruit (Chinese gooseberry), which pigface resembles in taste. The leaves can be used dried or fresh to dress meats and impart a salty flavour.

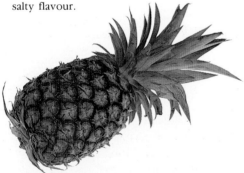

Pineapple *Ananas comosus*

MAJOR NUTRIENTS		SERVE SIZE 80 G	
Energy	130 kJ	Cholesterol	0
Protein	0	Sodium	0
Fat	0	Dietary Fibre	2 g
Carbohydrate	9 g	Vitamin C	17 mg

NUTRITIONAL INFORMATION Has excellent vitamin C, which canning reduces by half.

DESCRIPTION The pineapple is a cylindrical fruit which grows upright on a low bush with a thick, blue-green bunch of cactuslike leaves. The skin is divided into an attractive pattern with prickly spines growing from each 'eye'.

The flesh is yellow and juicy with a characteristic fragrance.

ORIGIN AND HISTORY A native fruit of Brazil and tropical South America. Columbus enjoyed the pineapple with the natives when he landed in the West Indies, where offering it later became a traditional symbol of hospitality. It was introduced to many other countries including Spain and India in the 15th century, and in 1838 Lutheran missionaries in Australia imported the first plant from India. Hawaii is the most important pineapple producer and Australia is also a leading producer. Botanically, the pineapple is a multiple fruit formed by the coalescence of the fruits of 100-odd individual flowers.

BUYING AND STORAGE Available all year. Pineapples do not ripen further after harvesting, so select one that is at the peak of ripeness and has a sweet aroma. The varieties with yellow and golden flesh have the best flavour. Choose one that is plump and heavy in relation to its size, with fresh-looking skin and fresh green leaves. Green pineapples can be fully ripe, and a high colour in fruit may be due to respiration and mean it is overmature.

Store in the refrigerator but use as soon as possible. Cut pineapple will store for 3–4 days in the refrigerator if in a tightly sealed container.

PREPARATION AND USE Cut leaves off pineapple and slice bottom off. Stand fruit upright and slice all skin off, cutting downwards, then remove all eyes carefully, cutting diagonally with a small, sharp stainless steel knife. Lay peeled fruit on its side and slice into rings, then remove core with a small sharp knife or apple corer. You can also use a special pineapple peeler and a large serrated knife for preparing pineapple rings.

Alternatively, cut the pineapple in half lengthways, then loosen the fruit from the skin, remove it, cut out the core and cut fruit into wedges or chunky cubes.

Serve pineapple fresh in rings or cubes; add to fruit salad, tarts, fruit cup, savoury salad or sweet and sour Chinese dishes; serve grilled or fried with ham or chicken. Use to glaze and decorate a leg of ham. Chop and use in cakes and pies; puree for drinks or sorbets.

PROCESSING Pineapple is canned, juiced, glacéed, made into jam or added to commercial yoghurt.

VARIETIES
Usually identified as the summer variety, Smooth Cayenne, which is better, and the winter variety, Red Spanish.

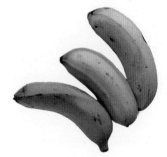

Plantain *Musa paradisiaca*

MAJOR NUTRIENTS		SERVE SIZE 80 G	
Energy	370 kJ	Dietary Fibre	0
Protein	0	Iron	0.9 mg
Fat	0	Magnesium	49 mg
Carbohydrate	24 g	Phosphorus	43 mg
Cholesterol	0	Vitamin A	70 µg
Sodium	0	Vitamin C	8 mg

NUTRITIONAL INFORMATION An excellent source of iron, magnesium and vitamin C; moderate source of phosphorus and vitamin A. This fruit is also a good source of folate, which is essential for blood formation.

Raw plantains are indigestible and therefore must be cooked to be eaten.

DESCRIPTION Looks like a banana but is plumper and longer with a green-yellow skin.

ORIGIN AND HISTORY A native of the tropics and of Central America, where it is used as a vegetable. Related to the banana and now cultivated in north Queensland, Australia.

BUYING AND STORAGE Available all year. Choose firm undamaged fruit.

Store at room temperature out of direct sunlight until skin turns yellow.

PREPARATION AND USE Not suitable for eating raw so must be cooked. Barbecue in the skin or remove peel and bake, grill or deep fry and serve as a vegetable, or add to a curry, soup or casserole.

PROCESSING Not applicable.

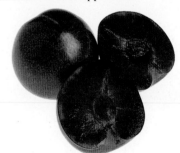

Plum *Prunus* spp.

MAJOR NUTRIENTS		SERVE SIZE 100 G	
Energy	160 kJ	Sodium	0
Protein	0	Dietary Fibre	2 g
Fat	0	Vitamin C	3 mg
Carbohydrate	10 g	Vitamin E	0.7 mg
Cholesterol	0		

NUTRITIONAL INFORMATION   Moderate fibre, vitamin C. The plum is a slightly uncommon fruit in that it contains a moderate amount of vitamin E.

DESCRIPTION   The plum is a round fruit with a shiny skin that varies from green through to deep red when ripe, and pulpy, sweet flesh.

ORIGIN AND HISTORY   This fruit is thought to have originated in west Asia, south of the Caucasus Mountains, over 2000 years ago, although the wild plum can still be found today in Japan and on the Pacific coast of North America. The plum is now cultivated in many temperate regions, California producing three-quarters of the world's annual product. It is also cultivated in Australia. The plum is the stone fruit of a deciduous tree belonging to the rose family.

BUYING AND STORAGE   Available in late summer and autumn. Choose plump, fully coloured, undamaged plums that range from fairly firm to slightly soft and have a sweet aroma. Avoid hard, shrivelled fruit and soft, moist fruit with brown marks.

Store in the refrigerator and use as soon as possible.

PREPARATION AND USE   Wash and dry plums and eat fresh in the hand. Cut in half, remove stone and add to fruit salad and compote, use on a fruit platter, puree and use for sauces, sorbets, ice cream and desserts. Stew or poach; use in pies, tarts, cakes and puddings; use for jam or bottling.

PROCESSING   May be canned, bottled, used in jam and sauces. The sugar plum variety are dried commercially to make prunes. Sloe plums are used to make sloe gin.

VARIETIES

There are over 2000 varieties but three main types: Japanese (*P. triflora*), European and British (*P. spinosa*) and west Asian (*Prunus cerasifera*).

They can also be classified as cooking and dessert plums. In general plums with dark flesh are the best for cooking and all varieties with a high sugar content, whether light or dark-fleshed, are delicious eaten fresh.

The small sugar plum with a small stone is dried to produce a prune. It can be eaten to give energy.

SEE ALSO   Prune.

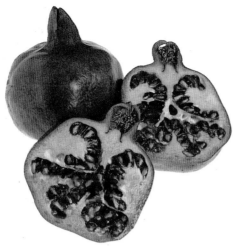

Pomegranate   *Punica granatum*

MAJOR NUTRIENTS		SERVE SIZE 100 G	
Energy	276 kJ	Sodium	0
Protein	0	Dietary Fibre	6 g
Fat	0	Vitamin C	14 mg
Carbohydrate	14 g	Iron	0.5 mg
Cholesterol	0		

NUTRITIONAL INFORMATION   Has excellent vitamin C, fibre; moderate iron. The pomegranate is slightly higher in kilojoules than most fruit but contains a wealth of fibre. One pomegranate supplies a quarter of the daily recommended requirement.

DESCRIPTION   A round fruit, the size of an orange, with a thick leathery red skin, crowned with a hard calyx. Inside, it is divided into large segments by walls of pith, and each contains several large white seeds in small sacs of pinkish-red juicy sweet pulp.

ORIGIN AND HISTORY   For centuries the pomegranate has been associated with religious ceremonies and buildings. It is found on temple carvings in Egypt, Persia and Rhodes, and in ancient Chinese paintings. It was the fruit given by Venus to Paris, being a symbol of fertility. There are also several references to the pomegranate in the Bible. Moses promised the wandering Israelites a land of wheat, barley, vines, fig trees, and pomegranates. The prophet Mohammed recommended eating the pomegranate to purge the body of envy. In Solomon's time pomegranate juice was a refreshment. The pomegranate is both native and cultivated in the whole of the Mediterranean region. It is often called 'the apple with many seeds'. The Moors planted an avenue of pomegranates in Granada in Spain where it is incorporated into the city's coat of arms. It is also cultivated in India, South America, and more recently in Australia.

BUYING AND STORAGE   Available in late autumn. Choose large fruit with a shiny, bright red skin which looks fresh. Avoid shrivelled fruit.

Store at room temperature until it splits open, which indicates the peak of ripeness. Once ripe, store in the refrigerator.

PREPARATION AND USE   If fruit has split, then break open. If not, cut the fruit in half, scoop out the seeds in their sacs of juice and discard the bitter membrane. Eat fresh in the hand by sucking the juice away from the seeds. The numerous seeds are edible. Add to fruit salad, fruit drinks, sauces, chicken, fish, and Turkish dishes. Also used as a decorative fruit in floral arrangements.

To extract juice, warm the fruit, then roll firmly in the hand to burst the sacks of juice. Make a hole in the bottom of the pomegranate, stand it on a glass and allow the juice to drain out. Use in drinks, sweet soup, sauce, sorbet and jelly.

PROCESSING   Used to make grenadine, a sweet, pink syrup used in cocktails and pink lemonade.

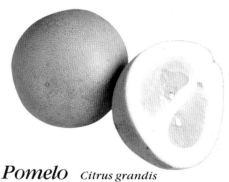

Pomelo   *Citrus grandis*

also called *Shaddock*

MAJOR NUTRIENTS		SERVE SIZE 100 G	
Energy	190 kJ	Dietary Fibre	0
Protein	1 g	Carbohydrate	11 g
Fat	0	Vitamin C	45 mg

NUTRITIONAL INFORMATION   This is an excellent source of Vitamin C.

DESCRIPTION   Looks like an oversized grapefruit, 20 cm in diameter, with a thick skin and pinkish-yellow flesh.

ORIGIN AND HISTORY   The pomelo is a very large citrus fruit but its origin is obscure. Wild pomelo seedlings grow in Indonesia and Malaysia and yet it is recorded in Chinese literature in 2200 BC. It was discovered in Palestine in AD 1187, and also in Spain. In the 17th century, a British captain, Shaddock, on an East India Company ship, took a pomelo on board in Polynesia and took it to Barbados, where it was planted and produced abundant pomelo trees. Years later botanists crossed this shaddock with a sweet orange and produced the grapefruit. The pomelo is now overshadowed by grapefruit cultivation in the

Western world, but improved varieties are now cultivated in northern Australia which are valued for their superior flavour and texture.

BUYING AND STORAGE Buy fruit which has an evenly coloured skin and no brown or soft patches. Like grapefruit, this fruit stores for a long time because of its thick skin.

PREPARATION AND USE Segment as for grapefruit, and use alone or in salads.

PROCESSING Canning, juicing and candied peel are potentially possible.

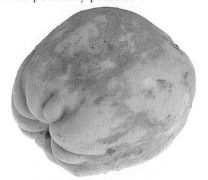

Quince *Cydonia oblonga*

MAJOR NUTRIENTS		SERVE SIZE 100 G	
Energy	200 kJ	Cholesterol	0
Protein	0	Sodium	0
Fat	0	Dietary Fibre	6 g
Carbohydrate	11 g	Vitamin C	40 mg

NUTRITIONAL INFORMATION The major contributing nutrient is vitamin C, of which quince is an excellent source. The quinine extracted from quince has an antimalarial action.

DESCRIPTION Looks like a large green apple with a peak at the blossom end, and has a similar apple texture but a very sour taste.

ORIGIN AND HISTORY The quince was known in Greece in Homer's time and was sacred to Aphrodite, the goddess of love, as a symbol of love, happiness and fertility. It probably travelled from western Asia via Persia (now Iran). Botanically a pome fruit, related to the apple and the pear and a member of the rose family. Grows in temperate climate areas, in the Mediterranean, Australia, East Africa, Israel, Turkey, USA, and South America.

BUYING AND STORAGE Available during autumn. Choose plump, well-shaped, evenly coloured bright green fruit with undamaged skin.

Store in the crisper or in a plastic bag in the refrigerator.

PREPARATION AND USE Peel and core quince, then cut into quarters, slice or chop

according to recipe. Quinces are usually cooked to improve their flavour. Use as for apples in pies and puddings, stew, poach or bake, or use for jam, jelly or paste.

PROCESSING Used in the manufacture of ratafia.

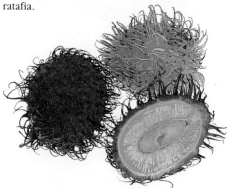

Rambutan *Nephelium lappaceum*

also called Hairy lychee

MAJOR NUTRIENTS		SERVE SIZE 50 G	
Energy	150 kJ	Cholesterol	0
Protein	0	Sodium	0
Fat	0	Dietary Fibre	2 g
Carbohydrate	8 g	Vitamin C	35 mg

NUTRITIONAL INFORMATION The major contributing nutrient in this fruit is vitamin C.

DESCRIPTION Botanically the rambutan is a drupe. The fruit is ovoid, 5–8 cm long, and is borne on the tree in clusters of 10 or 12. It usually has a bright red skin when ripe, but some varieties are orange; the skin is covered with soft fleshy spines or hairs. The flesh is translucent, white to dark grey in colour, clinging to a large flattened brown seed, with a refreshing flavour similar to a grape.

ORIGIN AND HISTORY The rambutan, related to the longan and the lychee, originated in the Malay Archipelago and Sumatra and still grows wild on the Malay Peninsula. Its name comes from the Indonesian word rambut, meaning hair. It is a tropical fruit suited to equatorial lowlands with a high rainfall, and is now cultivated in the Philippines, Thailand, Vietnam, Burma, and Central America. Fifty varieties of rambutan were imported from Asia to north Queensland in the 1970s and its cultivation is now well established in Australia. It is a very attractive, eye-catching fruit which displays well and tastes delicious, but it is still little known beyond the Asian equatorial countries.

BUYING AND STORAGE Available in summer, autumn and winter.

Select firm, dry, undamaged, brightly coloured fruit. Store in a single layer in the refrigerator.

Will store for 7–10 days in the refrigerator.

PREPARATION AND USE Cut the skin in half or in quarter segments with a sharp, stainless steel knife, peel skin back and eat fresh in the hand. The fruit can be peeled and stoned and used in fruit salad, green salad or fish salad, or added to sautéed chicken and Asian dishes. Serve on fruit platters and with cheese boards.

PROCESSING Drying, bottling and canning is carried out commercially in Asia.

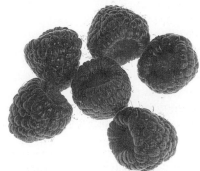

Raspberry *Rubus idaeus*

MAJOR NUTRIENTS		SERVE SIZE 100 G	
Energy	105 kJ	Sodium	0
Protein	0	Dietary Fibre	8 g
Fat	0	Iron	1.1 mg
Carbohydrate	6 g	Vitamin C	23 mg
Cholesterol	0	Magnesium	20 mg

NUTRITIONAL INFORMATION The raspberry contributes a significant amount of fibre and vitamin C. It is also high in iron, which would contribute significantly to the diet of vegetarians. There is a moderate amount of magnesium present.

DESCRIPTION Known as the king of berries, the raspberry grows on climbing canes, the soft red fruits looking like jewels amongst the leaves.

ORIGIN AND HISTORY The wild red raspberry is a native of Europe stretching from Britain, through Scandinavia to northeast Asia. It requires a cool climate and still grows wild, even in the hilly country of Italy and Greece. In most European countries, however, it has been transferred to the gardens and the better plants were selected for cultivation in the mid-16th century. The native raspberries of North America are black or yellow and suited to a warmer, drier climate. They have been cultivated in Canada and the USA since the beginning of the 19th century, but still grow wild at the edge of some woodland areas. Some hybrids have been developed between the red and black berries. Raspberry cultivation has developed recently in the south of Australia including Tasmania, and in New

Zealand. Botanically it is a member of the rose family.

BUYING AND STORAGE Choose plump, brightly coloured fruit which has no brown or squashy patches. Store dry, but covered, in the refrigerator.

PREPARATION AND USE Rinse carefully and drain on paper towels, then serve fresh with cream, ice cream or a liqueur, add to fruit salad, use in fruit tarts and meringue fillings, or puree for sorbet, ice cream, mousse, soufflé and the classic Peach Melba dessert. Add to champagne.

PROCESSING May be canned, made into jam, or used for raspberry liqueur.

VARIETIES
There are three varieties classified by colour. The red raspberry grows in North Canada, the northern states of the USA, Britain, and in European countries stretching from Scandinavia to east Asia. The black raspberry and the yellow variety grow in the woodlands in the southern coastal provinces of Canada and the USA.

Rockmelon *Cucumis melo*

also called **Musk melon**

MAJOR NUTRIENTS		SERVE SIZE 100 G	
Energy	90 kJ	Dietary Fibre	1 g
Carbohydrate	5 g	Vitamin C	30 mg
Fat	0		

NUTRITIONAL INFORMATION Rockmelon is an excellent source of vitamin C and retinol equivalents.

DESCRIPTION The rockmelon is a round, medium-sized fruit with a corky, netted surface on a golden brown skin. The flesh is golden orange in colour with flat white seeds. It is the fruit of a trailing vine.

ORIGIN AND HISTORY The canteloupe was first cultivated near the city of Cantelupe in Italy, in the mid-18th century.

BUYING AND STORAGE Available all year, peaking in summer. Melons do not ripen further once picked, so it is important to select a ripe, sweet melon at purchase time. Choose a rockmelon which has a sweet odour at the stalk end and is slightly soft at the blossom end.

Store all netted melons in the refrigerator. Once cut, cover with clear plastic wrap, return to the refrigerator and use within a few days.

PREPARATION AND USE Cut in half and remove seeds. Cut fruit into segments or into cubes or melon balls with a melon-ball scoop and serve with ice cream, in a fruit salad, or with breakfast cereal. Serve melon balls in port wine for a first course. Use to garnish meat and seafood. Puree for sorbet.

VARIETIES

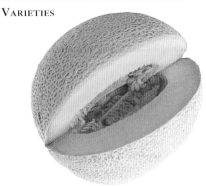

Canteloupe A small, round melon with a hard, scaly, yellow-green skin and a deep orange-yellow flesh.

Gallia Melon A finely netted, green-skinned, small, round melon with pale green flesh.

Persian Melon A round melon, similar to canteloupe, with a fine, flatter netting on a deeper green skin.

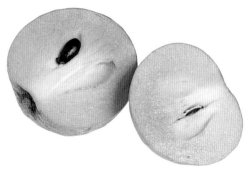

Sapodilla *Manilkara zapota*

also called **Chiku**

MAJOR NUTRIENTS		SERVE SIZE 170 G	
Energy	400 kJ	Cholesterol	0
Protein	0	Sodium	0
Fat	0	Iron	1.4 mg
Carbohydrate	24 g	Vitamin C	25 mg

NUTRITIONAL INFORMATION An excellent source of vitamin C; moderate source of pantothenic acid (an unusual component in fruits) and retinol equivalents.

DESCRIPTION A round or oval fruit, 5–8 cm in diameter, with a thin, green skin which turns to a rough corky, russet brown, containing honey-coloured, sweet, juicy, translucent but sometimes gritty flesh with shiny black hooked seeds.

ORIGIN AND HISTORY The sapodilla tree is a native of the West Indies and Central America. The Aztecs knew the tree and called it 'chick'. The Spanish discovered it in Central America and took it to the Philippines, where it is known as 'chiko'. It is commercially important, not only for its fruit, but also for the milky latex or chicle gum, which is obtained by tapping the bark, and used as a basis for chewing gum. The sapodilla is cultivated for its gum in Mexico, British Honduras and other countries in Central America. It is cultivated primarily for its fruit in other Central American countries, India, California, and recently in north Australia. When ripe it tastes like brown sugar, when unripe it has an unpleasant high tannin content.

BUYING AND STORAGE Available in winter, spring and summer. Select firm, well-shaped, undamaged fruit.

Ripen at room temperature until soft, then store in refrigerator until ready to use.

PREPARATION AND USE Cut fruit in half and eat fresh in the hand with a teaspoon for eating. Scoop out fruit, remove seeds, puree flesh and add to fruit salad, use in ice cream or serve as a sauce.

PROCESSING Fruit not processed but the latex from the tree is used in chewing gum.

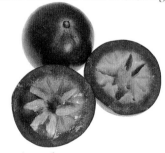

Star Apple *Chrysophyllum cainito*

also known as **Caimito**

MAJOR NUTRIENTS		SERVE SIZE 100 G	
Energy	280 kJ	Niacin Equiv.	10 mg
Protein	1 g	Vitamin C	7 mg
Fat	1 g	Dietary Fibre	0
Carbohydrate	15 g		

NUTRITIONAL INFORMATION This is an excellent source of vitamin C and niacin.

DESCRIPTION A round fruit, up to 10 cm in diameter with a flat bottom and top on which appears the pattern of the calyx in a star shape. Skin turns from green-yellow-rose to purple-brown (like a ripe fig) and contains 8 segments of white translucent flesh inside a layer of thicker flesh.

ORIGIN AND HISTORY The star apple originated in the West Indies and Central America. It is grown in Cuba, Jamaica, Florida,

Hawaii and Sri Lanka, and cultivated in South-East Asia and northern Australia. The name comes from the Greek chrysos meaning gold and phyllon meaning leaf, referring to the golden underside of the leaves. The star apple is related to the sapodilla and the black sapote. It was introduced into Britain in 1727 and became popular as a hothouse plant because of its handsome appearance.

BUYING AND STORAGE Available winter and spring. Select fruit with a firm, purple-brown, undamaged skin.

Allow to ripen at room temperature until soft, then store in refrigerator until required.

PREPARATION AND USE Cut fruit in half and serve on fruit platters or cheese boards, or in the hand with a teaspoon for eating. Or scoop out flesh and add to fruit salad — good with citrus fruit — or puree for drinks, sorbets, ice cream or sauces.

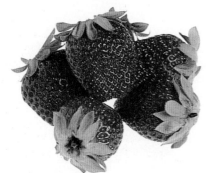

Strawberry *Fragaria virginiana, F. chiloensis*

MAJOR NUTRIENTS		SERVE SIZE 100 G	
Energy	80 kJ	Sodium	0
Protein	2 g	Dietary Fibre	2 g
Fat	0	Iron	0.6 mg
Carbohydrate	3 g	Vitamin C	58 mg
Cholesterol	0		

NUTRITIONAL INFORMATION Like most berries, the strawberry is high in vitamin C. The above amount contains one and a half times the recommended daily intake of this vitamin. It is also a good source of folic acid, and a moderate source of iron.

DESCRIPTION The cultivated strawberry is big and smooth-skinned. The wild strawberry is smaller and more aromatic and does not require hulling.

ORIGIN AND HISTORY Native to North America and a member of the rose family. The Virginian species was discovered there on the eastern seaboard by the explorers around 1600 and introduced to Europe soon after. One hundred years later the West Coast pine strawberry, *F. chiloensis*, was taken to Europe. The cultivated species were intro-

duced to Australia by the first white settlers. It is possible that the name originated when the berries were strung on pieces of straw to carry them to the market. In the past the strawberry was recommended for pregnancy because it was believed it strengthened the pelvic floor.

BUYING AND STORAGE The cultivated strawberry is available all year but the season peaks in summer. The wild strawberry is available in summer and autumn. Choose brightly coloured, firm, well-shaped, medium-sized cultivated strawberries and small wild strawberries, with undamaged skin and the stem still attached. Very large and badly shaped berries are often poor in flavour. Dull, soft, moist berries are often overripe.

To store, remove top from container of strawberries and store unwashed in refrigerator, but use as soon as possible.

PREPARATION AND USE Wash the strawberries, drain, then remove stem (or hull) if liked. Leave whole or cut in halves, quarters or slices and serve fresh sprinkled with icing sugar or caster sugar. Serve with cream, yoghurt, ice cream or liqueur; add to fruit salad, fruit platters or cheese boards; use in mousses, soufflés, tarts, shortcakes and cheesecakes, to decorate gateaux, in ice cream, sorbets and sauces. Make into jam.

PROCESSING May be used for jam or liqueur, canned, frozen or used in commercial frozen products and yoghurt.

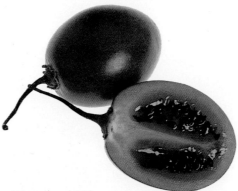

Tamarillo *Cyphomandra betacea*

also called **Tree tomato**

MAJOR NUTRIENTS		SERVE SIZE 100 G	
Energy	110 kJ	Dietary Fibre	5 g
Protein	0	Phosphorus	40 mg
Fat	0	Iron	0.7 mg
Carbohydrate	4 g	Vitamin A	155 µg
Cholesterol	0	Vitamin C	15 mg
Sodium	0		

NUTRITIONAL INFORMATION The tamarillo is a quite nutritious fruit, as it contains a number of nutrients in significant quantities

for correspondingly few kilojoules. Like most fruit, it contains vitamin C but also provides a high level of fibre; vitamin A in the plant form known as beta carotene; a moderate amount of phosphorus and iron.

DESCRIPTION An oval, large egg-sized, burgundy-coloured fruit containing red flesh and tangy flavoured seeds. A yellow variety is also grown.

ORIGIN AND HISTORY Native to Peru and Brazil. The tropical fruit of a tree which, like the tomato, belongs to the nightshade family. It is grown commercially in New Zealand and Australia and other tropical regions with a medium-high altitude.

BUYING AND STORAGE Available in winter. Choose large, firm, shiny, deeply coloured fruit with undamaged skin.

Store in the refrigerator.

PREPARATION AND USE Slice the top and bottom off the fruit, then remove peel with a fine peeler. Slice fruit and add to sweet and savoury salads, or use in tarts and hot puddings, compotes, mousses or soufflés. Puree and use for sauces, sorbets, ice cream or drinks. May be poached or baked whole and served as for tomatoes with lamb, veal or chicken. Use in jam, jelly or chutney.

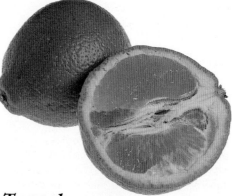

Tangelo *Citrus*

NUTRITIONAL INFORMATION No specific information is available.

DESCRIPTION A large, juicy citrus fruit with a loose, orange skin and a sharp, refreshing flavour.

ORIGIN AND HISTORY The tangelo is a hybrid produced by crossing a grapefruit with a tangerine. Grown in citrus-producing areas.

BUYING AND STORAGE Choose evenly coloured fruit. In dry conditions, tangelos keep well because of their thick skin.

PREPARATION AND USE Peel and eat fresh in the hand; peel and cut into segments and use as for orange; or squeeze juice and use in fruit cups, marinades or salad dressings.

Tomato Lycopersicon esculentum

also called Love apple

MAJOR NUTRIENTS

		SERVE SIZE 100 G	
Energy	60 kJ	Sodium	0
Protein	0	Dietary Fibre	1.5 g
Fat	0	Vitamin A	350 µg
Carbohydrate	3 g	Vitamin C	20 mg
Cholesterol	0		

NUTRITIONAL INFORMATION Two major contributing nutrients in the tomato are the excellent vitamin C and vitamin A. Canning has no significant effect on nutrients.

DESCRIPTION The plump, bright red tomato has pulp with a high water content and a thin, shiny skin.

ORIGIN AND HISTORY The versatile tomato originated in South America where it grew wild like a weed in the time of the Incas in Peru and the Indian Aztecs in Mexico. The Spanish explorers took the seeds of the yellow 'tomatl', as it was called, from Mexico to Europe and it became popular in Italy where it was called pomo d'oro or apple of gold. The Moors called it pomo dei mori and the French translated this to pomme d'amour or apple of love. The English grew the plant out of curiosity for decoration, thinking it poisonous — it is a member of the nightshade family. Later the red tomato was introduced and it became a popular salad vegetable. Botanically it is a berry. The tomato is now cultivated extensively in warm temperate and subtropical climates and enjoys world popularity.

BUYING AND STORAGE Available all year, but season peaks in late summer. Choose well-shaped, uniformly red, firm tomatoes, heavy for their size and free from damaged skin. Light, puffy tomatoes usually have a poor texture and taste.

Do not store tomatoes in the refrigerator. Store them at room temperature, out of direct sunshine, to allow the natural ripening process to continue. If not used within 5 days, store in the crisper of the refrigerator for up to 5 days only, as texture starts to deteriorate with prolonged chilling.

PREPARATION AND USE Best eaten at room temperature for a good flavour. Rinse and dry, then use halved, quartered, cut in segments or slices, or pureed. Skins may be removed by blanching. Use fresh in salads, sandwiches, hamburgers as an edible garnish, in fresh or cooked sauces, or grill, bake, stuff, fry or microwave. Use in soup, casseroles or chutney, or preserve in glass jars.

PROCESSING May be canned, concentrated as paste, used in commercial tomato sauce and sun-dried.

VARIETIES

There are several varieties but these are generally categorised according to shape and size.

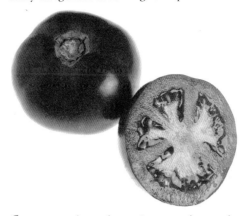

Common tomatoes Large and round, with several varieties.

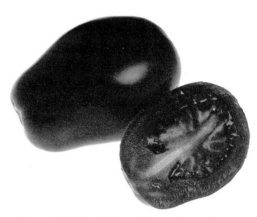

Roma/Italian/Plum/Egg tomatoes Similar to a plum or egg in size and shape.

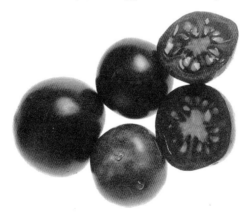

Tom Thumb or Cherry tomatoes Very small and round.

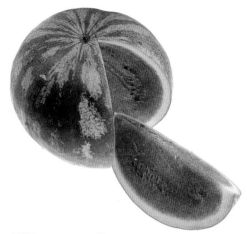

Watermelon Cucumis citrullus

MAJOR NUTRIENTS

		SERVE SIZE 100 G	
Energy	100 kJ	Cholesterol	0
Protein	0	Sodium	0
Fat	0	Dietary Fibre	0
Carbohydrate	5 g	Vitamin C	7 mg

NUTRITIONAL INFORMATION An excellent source of vitamin C. Watermelon, despite its very sweet taste, is quite low in kilojoules, making it a good filling food for weight-conscious individuals. The major contributing nutrient is vitamin C.

DESCRIPTION Watermelon is the large, smooth, barrel-shaped or round, dark green, hard-skinned fruit of a trailing vine. The flesh is usually bright pink to bright red with black seeds when ripe.

ORIGIN AND HISTORY Melons belong to the same family as squash, pumpkin and marrow. They are the fruit of an annual trailing vine and grow on the ground. They are indigenous to tropical Africa, but now grow all over the world in areas of subtropical climate.

BUYING AND STORAGE Available almost all year round, peaking in summertime. Watermelons do not ripen any further once picked, so select a melon with a good colour which gives off a sweet odour at the stalk end and is slightly soft at the blossom end. The watermelon will have a creamy area on its underside when ripe and its seeds turn black as a further guide to ripeness.

Store watermelon at room temperature but, after cutting, wrap the watermelon in clear plastic wrap and store in the refrigerator. Use within a few days once cut and refrigerated.

PREPARATION AND USE Wash or wipe watermelon skin clean. Cut fruit into thick slices or segments and eat flesh in the hand, or cut flesh into melon balls with a melon-ball scoop, or into cubes. Add melon balls or cubes to fruit salad or mix with other varieties of melon, or breakfast cereal. Puree fruit and use for a sorbet or for drinks. Skin may be pickled and a whole watermelon skin may be carved into a melon basket to hold fruit salad.

VARIETIES

The main varieties are the large pink-fleshed watermelon and the smaller, round, yellow-fleshed type.

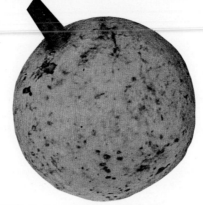

Wild Orange *Capparis* *mitchellii, C. umbonata* and others

also called **Native capers**

MAJOR NUTRIENTS		SERVE SIZE 50 G	
Energy	470 kJ	Dietary Fibre	12.5 g
Protein	7 g	Vitamin C	35 mg
Fat	3 g	Sodium	5 mg
Carbohydrate	19 g	Iron	1.5 mg
Cholesterol	0		

NUTRITIONAL INFORMATION The average vitamin C content is 35 mg/100 g, a useful source of the vitamin. This fruit is higher in energy and a more concentrated source of nutrients than most fresh cultivated fruit.

DESCRIPTION A fleshy berry up to 7 cm in diameter, purple-green to orange-brown in colour, with large seeds embedded in the fruit pulp.

ORIGIN AND HISTORY Wild orange is a member of the caper family. The tall bushy shrubs are widespread in drier parts of Australia and the fruits are keenly sought by Aborigines of the area.

BUYING AND STORAGE The fruits keep well even at room temperature.

PREPARATION AND USE Wild oranges are eaten raw by Aborigines and have not been cultivated commercially. The skin and seeds are discarded. Overseas, the buds of *Capparis spinosa* (which is also found in Australia) are pickled and used as flavourings. Other Australian species could also be used similarly.

DRIED FRUITS

There is a wide variety of dried and candied fruit available to consumers today, the most ancient and most popular being cherry, date, prune, fig, and grape, which make raisin, sultana and currant. Dried and candied fruit available more recently include apricot, peach, nectarine, apple, pear, and banana.

Candied fruit is discussed under its own heading in the chapter on Confectionery.

Drying is the oldest known method of preservation. Long before the pyramids were built, the Egyptians discovered that dry fruit clinging to the vines and branches of trees had a pleasant flavour, owing to the evaporation of the natural moisture content. Dried fruit was placed in the tombs of the ancient kings of Egypt to help on the journey to the after-life. The Mesopotamians bartered their dried fruit for other necessities. The Romans valued the cultivation of dried fruit and imported it into Rome to enjoy at their banquets. Later, the Crusaders took gifts of dried fruit from Palestine and the Holy Land back to Europe. From South Africa in 1775 dried fruit was sold to passing ships as it could counteract scurvy. Today dried fruit is processed in many countries and is a food of great value to sports people, athletes and even astronauts.

Buy dried fruit from a reputable store that has a good turnover of stock, to ensure that it is as fresh as possible. Choose fruit that is either sold in clear packaging or displayed in glass jars or has a reputable brand name on the packaging.

Store in an airtight container, preferably glass or transparent material, in a cool, dry cupboard or pantry. Dried fruit usually stores well for 6 months up to 1 year depending on variety. It also freezes well.

Those who live in climates where there is hot sunshine and a dry atmosphere, can dry their own fruit naturally in the sun in the open air. If this is impossible, select fully ripe, good quality fruit and prepare accordingly. Lay the fruit on wire cooling trays or baking trays in a single layer and dry out in a low oven at 60°C (140°F) for 6–24 hours until soft and leathery.

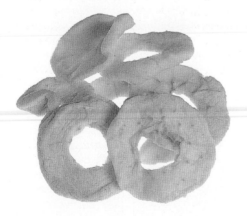

Dried Apple

MAJOR NUTRIENTS		SERVE SIZE 30 G	
Energy	397 kJ	Sodium	0
Protein	0	Iron	0.5 mg
Fat	0	Dietary Fibre	4 g
Carbohydrate	24 g	Vitamin C	3 mg
Cholesterol	0		

NUTRITIONAL INFORMATION An excellent source of dietary fibre; the energy content is provided by carbohydrate; moderate source of vitamin C and iron, though note that drying reduces the content of a raw apple by half. As water is removed in the drying process, the nutrients are effectively concentrated. Consequently the kilojoule content is higher in dried fruit and weight-watchers should be conscious of this.

DESCRIPTION Dried apple is usually available in slices.

ORIGIN AND HISTORY In medieval times, people in Europe peeled the apple, cut it into rings, then hung it from strings in the kitchen to dry. Today the slices of apple are laid on wire trays and dried in sulphur houses for 18 hours, then the trays are placed in the sun to complete the drying process. The apple feels like chamois leather when the process is complete. Produced in Australia and California.

BUYING AND STORAGE Dried apples can store for up to 6 months.

PREPARATION AND USE Soak the apples in cold water for 8 hours or in boiling water for 30 minutes, then stew gently until tender, or drain and use according to recipe.

Use in dried fruit salad, serve as a dessert, or with breakfast cereal or muesli. Puree stewed apple and use as apple sauce. Chop drained soaked apple and add to stuffing for roast pork and goose.

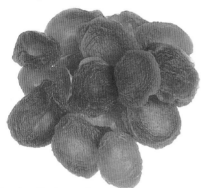

Dried Apricot

MAJOR NUTRIENTS		SERVE SIZE 25 G	
Energy	276 kJ	Sodium	0
Protein	0	Dietary Fibre	6 g
Fat	0	Vitamin A	220 μg
Carbohydrate	17 g	Vitamin C	2 mg
Cholesterol	0	Iron	1.1 g

NUTRITIONAL INFORMATION The energy content comes from carbohydrate; excellent source of fibre, vitamin A and iron; moderate source of vitamin C. Though drying reduces vitamin C, other nutrients become more concentrated, for example fibre and iron. When you compare standard serving sizes, dried apricot is a better source of dietary fibre than the usual favourite, the prune.

DESCRIPTION Dried apricot is usually available whole, but can be diced in dried mixtures.

ORIGIN AND HISTORY Although the apricot tree is thought to have been first cultivated in China, it was the Californians who first perfected the art of drying apricots. The apricots are picked at a certain stage of ripeness, halved and stoned, then placed in wooden trays with mesh bases. The trays are dampened and stacked in sulphur houses, which help retain colour and flavour. The trays are later placed in the sun to dry the fruit in natural sunshine. Today most of the world's apricots are produced in Australia (from the Riverland district of the Murray Irrigation Arca) and in California, Iran, and Turkey.

BUYING AND STORAGE Dried apricots will keep for up to 1 year. They also freeze well.

PREPARATION AND USE Soak in cold water overnight or for 6 hours; alternatively, soak in boiling water for 30 minutes. Stew the apricots or drain and use according to recipe. Serve as a compote; puree and serve as a sauce or use in ice cream; chop and add to stuffing; or use in cakes and desserts. May be eaten dry as a nourishing snack or added to a school lunch box.

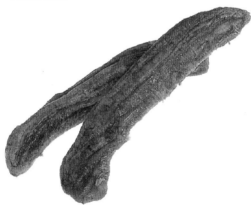

Dried Banana

NUTRITIONAL INFORMATION No detailed analysis is available. Drying reduces the vitamin C content by half and increases the kilojoule content fivefold (e.g., 30 g of raw banana provides 100 kJ, whereas 30 g of the dried equivalent provides 500 kJ).

DESCRIPTION Sometimes available whole, usually in rounds.

ORIGIN AND HISTORY Drying the banana is an Australian development which is also practised in South-East Asia. The banana is sliced and dried as chips or flakes, which may then be powdered as a flour. It has value as a nourishing food supply in Third World countries. Dried banana is produced in Queensland, Australia.

BUYING AND STORAGE The dried banana keeps for up to 1 year.

PREPARATION AND USE Soak the banana chips and flakes in hot water for 30 minutes, then drain and use in cakes and batter mixtures. Banana flour may be used in baked products or in a porridgelike pudding.

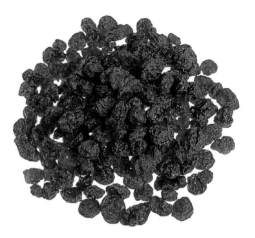

Dried Currant

MAJOR NUTRIENTS		SERVE SIZE 10 G	
Energy	100 kJ	Cholesterol	0
Protein	0	Sodium	0
Fat	0	Dietary Fibre	5 g
Carbohydrate	6 g	Magnesium	30 mg

NUTRITIONAL INFORMATION The energy comes from carbohydrate; excellent source of dietary fibre (1 teaspoon provides one-fifth of the daily needs); good source of magnesium. Drying destroys the vitamin C in the fruit.

DESCRIPTION The currant is a dried grape, processed from the tiny, purple, seedless Corinth grape, native to Greece.

ORIGIN AND HISTORY The currant came originally from Greece and was an important export commodity from Crete, along with the sultana, during the Aegean era. It was probably one of the dried fruits found in the Egyptian tombs. The early white settlers introduced currants, sultanas and raisins, and other dried fruits, into North America and Australia. Today California and the Murray Irrigation Area of Australia, as well as Greece, produce currants commercially. The currant grape varieties of Zante and Corinth are so small that they dry quickly and are usually dried naturally in the sun.

BUYING AND STORAGE The currant will store for up to 1 year. Also may be frozen.

PREPARATION AND USE Wash the fruit carefully, drain, then dry well in a clean, dry tea towel. Spread currants on baking trays and dry off in a low oven, or toss lightly in plain flour if used for baking.

Use fruit in cakes, yeast mixtures, biscuits and pastries; use in stuffings for vine leaves, game or fish; add to savoury rice and sauces.

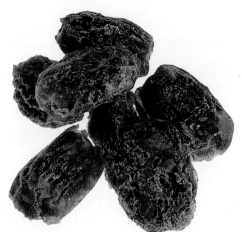

Dried Date

MAJOR NUTRIENTS			SERVE SIZE 33 G
Energy	350 kJ	Sodium	0
Protein	1 g	Dietary Fibre	3 g
Fat	0	Magnesium	19 mg
Carbohydrate	21 g	Iron	0.5 mg
Cholesterol	0	Niacin Equiv.	0.7 mg

NUTRITIONAL INFORMATION The energy comes from carbohydrate; good source of fibre; moderate source of iron, magnesium and vitamin B6. The date is very nutritious, as it contains a wide variety of nutrients. What makes the date slightly unusual is that it contains folate, niacin, and magnesium.

DESCRIPTION The dried date retains the shiny skin of the raw fruit, but is less plump.

ORIGIN AND HISTORY The date, along with the fig, is amongst the oldest known cultivated fruits. The date palm tree is native to the fertile country between the Euphrates and Tigris rivers in Asia. It has been cultivated for more than 7000 years and is a staple food in the Arab world. The date was traded with the Romans and was enjoyed at Roman banquets. It was probably introduced to other European countries by the Crusaders returning from the Holy Land.

The date palm tree can live for 100 years and can produce up to 45 kg of fruit every year. The date is grown commercially in Iraq and North Africa and was introduced into California at the beginning of the 20th century.

BUYING AND STORAGE Choose clean, firm, dry dates, preferably a reliable brand which is well packaged.

Store in a cool dry place, in a glass storage jar if loose or once package is opened. Dates store for up to 6 months.

PREPARATION AND USE The better quality fruit is packed whole in long boxes. Eat in the hand as a sweetmeat or use as a decoration; stuff with marzipan or dip in chocolate as confectionery; or stuff with cream cheese

as a savoury. Poorer quality dates are stoned and compressed into blocks for marketing. These may be chopped and used in baked products such as cakes, biscuits, slices and puddings. The fruit may also be chopped and served with a fruit dessert.

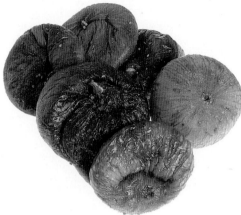

Dried Fig

MAJOR NUTRIENTS			SERVE SIZE 30 G
Energy	340 kJ	Sodium	0
Protein	0	Dietary Fibre	10 g
Fat	0	Calcium	90 mg
Carbohydrate	20.9 g	Magnesium	30 mg
Cholesterol	0	Iron	0.5 mg

NUTRITIONAL INFORMATION High in carbohydrate, and even richer in fibre than the prune. The fig is unusual in that it provides magnesium, calcium, and iron. As drying concentrates nutrients, dried figs are higher in kilojoules by weight than their raw counterparts, so weight-watchers should beware of overindulging.

DESCRIPTION The plump fig compresses easily when dried.

ORIGIN AND HISTORY The fig tree originated in western Asia, probably in Syria. The Phoenicians took it by trade caravan along the silk route to India and China. The Romans probably introduced it to Europe. The fresh fig does not travel well owing to its thin skin, but there are no problems when it has been dried, so the dried fig has been much more available than the fresh fig in most of the world. It is now grown in many hot countries.

BUYING AND STORAGE Dried figs will keep fresh in an airtight container for up to 1 year.

PREPARATION AND USE Peel the figs carefully, if desired, then stew gently for 10–15 minutes or until tender. Serve stewed figs for breakfast or dessert, or drain well, macerate in port and serve with ricotta cheese as a sweetmeat.

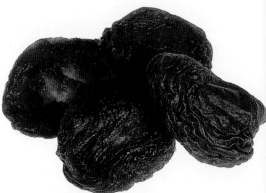

Dried Nectarine

NUTRITIONAL INFORMATION No data are available.

DESCRIPTION It may be bought whole, like the dried peach.

ORIGIN AND HISTORY The nectarine originated in China and followed the peach into Europe much later. From there it was introduced to North America and Australia, by the early white settlers. The nectarine is picked fully ripe for drying and is dried in a similar way to the peach. It is produced in California and in the Riverland district of the Murray Irrigation Area of Australia.

BUYING AND STORAGE As for the dried peach.

PREPARATION AND USE As for the dried peach.

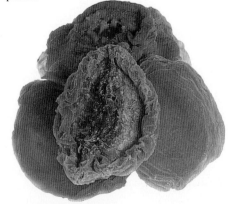

Dried Peach

MAJOR NUTRIENTS			SERVE SIZE 25 G
Energy	225 kJ	Sodium	0
Protein	0	Dietary Fibre	4 g
Fat	0	Vitamin A	83 µg
Carbohydrate	13 g	Niacin Equiv.	1.5 mg
Cholesterol	0	Iron	1.7 mg

NUTRITIONAL INFORMATION The energy source is carbohydrate; good vitamin A; moderate niacin. Drying reduces the vitamin C content to an insignificant amount, but other nutrients, and kilojoules, are concentrated. The dried peach has twice the iron content of the raw equivalent and consequently can be a valuable source of this mineral, particularly in vegetarian diets.

DESCRIPTION The dried peach is purchased whole.

ORIGIN AND HISTORY The peach was probably first dried in California along with the apricot, although the peach tree is native to China. The peach is dried by a similar process to the apricot, but, after being in the sulphur houses for 8–12 hours, it is placed in direct sunlight for about a week in order to complete the drying process naturally. The fruit is produced in the Riverland district of the Murray Irrigation Area in Australia and also in California. The dried peach had the honour of being eaten and enjoyed by Neil Armstrong while he was on the moon.

BUYING AND STORAGE The dried peach stores well for up to 1 year. Also freezes successfully.

PREPARATION AND USE Soak for 8 hours in cold water or in boiling water for 30 minutes. Stew gently until tender, or drain and use according to recipe.

Serve stewed for breakfast or dessert, puree and use as a sauce or in homemade ice cream, add to curries, chicken and game casseroles, and savoury rice. Dried peach may also be eaten as a healthy snack.

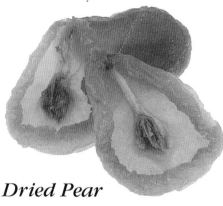

Dried Pear

MAJOR NUTRIENTS SERVE SIZE 87 G

Energy	961 kJ	Dietary Fibre	5 g
Protein	0	Potassium	466 mg
Fat	0	Iron	1.8 mg
Carbohydrate	60 g	Niacin Equiv.	2.5 mg
Cholesterol	0	Vitamin C	6 mg
Sodium	0		

NUTRITIONAL INFORMATION An excellent source of fibre, iron, vitamin C; good source of niacin; moderate source of phosphorus, potassium. High in carbohydrate. Dried pears contain a significant amount of potassium and individuals on low potassium diets should consult their dietitian regarding this.

DESCRIPTION Dried pear is usually bought halved.

ORIGIN AND HISTORY The process of drying the pear was probably developed in California along with the drying of stone fruits. Harvested when ripe but still firm, each pear is halved and the calyx and core are removed; the fruit is then dried in the sulphur houses on metal trays for 18–24 hours. After this the trays are stacked in tiers and dried off in natural sunshine for 2–3 weeks. Dried pear is produced in California and in the Murray Irrigation Area of Australia.

BUYING AND STORAGE Dried pear stores successfully for up to 6 months. Also freezes well.

PREPARATION AND USE Soak for 8 hours in cold water or in boiling water for 30 minutes, then stew gently until tender, or drain and use according to recipe.

Use in dried fruit salad, serve as a dessert, or with breakfast cereal or muesli. Chop drained, soaked pears and add to stuffing for roast pork and goose.

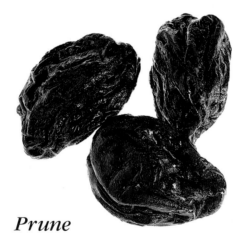

Prune

MAJOR NUTRIENTS SERVE SIZE 50 G

Energy	340 kJ	Sodium	0
Protein	0	Dietary Fibre	9 g
Fat	0	Phosphorus	42 mg
Carbohydrate	20 g	Iron	1.6 mg
Cholesterol	0	Vitamin A	115 µg

NUTRITIONAL INFORMATION The energy source is carbohydrate; excellent vitamin A. The prune is quite nutritious, being particularly high in fibre, and is traditionally used for its laxative effect. It contains a significant amount of iron and is therefore recommended for vegetarians. It also contributes a significant amount of phosphorus.

DESCRIPTION The prune is a whole dried plum with a dark, wrinkled appearance. The plum used is the d'Agen sugar plum, which is processed without removing the stone.

ORIGIN AND HISTORY Long ago, the prune is known to have travelled from Syria to ancient Rome. Later the Benedictine monks, returning from the Crusades, are reported to have taken the fruit from Persia and Turkey back to France. Today the USA is the major producer of prunes. In California they are dried by artificial heat. Prunes are also produced in the Murrumbidgee Irrigation Area in Australia. After mechanical harvesting, the plum is washed, then placed in a dehydrator to dry in a blast of hot air for 14–24 hours, resulting in the characteristic wrinkled appearance.

BUYING AND STORAGE Prunes are readily available in packets, and if kept sealed will last for up to 6 months. Canned prunes have a shelf life of up to 1 year.

PREPARATION AND USE Some prunes will require soaking in water overnight, others for only 1 hour, depending on how dry they are. Canned prunes have already been soaked. The soaked fruit may be drained and stoned, then stuffed and served as a savoury or in the classic Devils on Horseback. It may be chopped and used in stuffing for pork or game, added to hare or rabbit casseroles, stewed and served as a compote for dessert, added to breakfast cereal, chopped and added to cakes, or preserved in brandy.

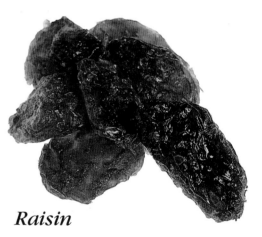

Raisin

MAJOR NUTRIENTS SERVE SIZE 20 G

Energy	210 kJ	Cholesterol	0
Protein	0	Sodium	0
Fat	0	Dietary Fibre	2 g
Carbohydrate	13 g		

NUTRITIONAL INFORMATION The energy source is carbohydrate; excellent fibre. The raisin, like most stone and dried fruit, has a significant amount of fibre.

DESCRIPTION A dried dark-skinned grape which has a shiny, wrinkled appearance. Muscat and Waltham Cross grapes are used.

ORIGIN AND HISTORY It is recorded that raisin cakes were festive fare among the Israelites when David became their king. The Romans enjoyed raisin wine and ate raisins as a snack at their banquets.

The grape is dipped in or sprayed with a safe alkaline solution to kill any insects before drying mechanically. A special machine is used to remove seeds from the raisin before packaging. Raisins are produced commercially today in Australia, South Africa, and the eastern Mediterranean.

BUYING AND STORAGE Raisins will store well for up to 1 year. May be frozen.

PREPARATION AND USE Rinse the fruit in warm water, drain well, then dry in a clean dry tea towel. If still damp, spread on a baking tray and dry off in a low oven or, if using for baking, coat lightly in a little plain flour. Some brands are sold washed and ready to use.

Use in homemade muesli, add to savoury rice and salads, use in cakes, biscuits, slices and puddings, or serve with cheese.

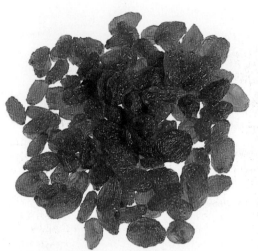

Sultana

MAJOR NUTRIENTS		SERVE SIZE 10 G	
Energy	100 kJ	Cholesterol	0
Protein	0	Sodium	0
Fat	0	Dietary Fibre	3 g
Carbohydrate	6 g	Vitamin E	1 mg

NUTRITIONAL INFORMATION The sultana contains excellent fibre, and moderate vitamin E, which is not normally found in fruit in any significant amount.

DESCRIPTION The sultana is a dried grape, with light-coloured skin.

ORIGIN AND HISTORY The products of the grapevine apparently played an important role in ancient Greece. The dried grape was an important export item from Crete during the Aegean era. The sultana was originally obtained by drying the juicy, sweet, seedless sultana grape in the sun, resulting in a dried fruit much softer and sweeter than its relations, the currant and raisin. Today the sultana grape is dipped or sprayed in a safe alkaline solution to kill insects and preserve its golden colour before drying. It is either sun-dried or mechanically dried. Produced commercially in Australia, South Africa and the eastern Mediterranean region; the best variety is said to come from Turkey.

BUYING AND STORAGE Sultanas can be stored successfully for up to 1 year. They also freeze well.

PREPARATION AND USE Rinse and drain, then dry well in a clean dry tea towel. If required for baking, spread on a baking tray and dry off in a low oven or toss in plain flour. Some brands of sultana are sold washed and ready to use.

Use in cakes, biscuits, slices, pastries and puddings. Add to muesli, breakfast cereal, salads, savoury rice, stuffings, curries and casseroles, or eat in the hand for a healthy snack.

FUNGI

There are hundreds of varieties of mushrooms, which fall into two types: cultivated and wild.

Cultivated varieties include the common mushroom, oyster mushroom, shiitake, straw mushroom, truffle and wood ear. Wild varieties include beefsteak fungus, blewit, boletus, cep, chanterelle, field mushroom, matsutake, morel, parasol mushroom and rubber brush.

Wild varieties of mushroom were used by the Sumerians 3500 years BC. The Greeks gathered them and exported them to the Romans who considered them food for the gods. The Egyptians served them only to the pharoahs, as they appeared magically overnight and were therefore too good for the ordinary people. In 1678 a Frenchman analysed how the edible fungi grew and crude cultivation of the mushroom was started. The methods were refined over the next 200 years and other international growers adopted the French method of cultivation in the late 19th century.

Today the cultivation of several types of fungi is a thriving industry, the common mushroom being the most popular.

Wild mushrooms are those that so far have defied cultivation. They grow in the country meadows and woodlands, in the ground and even on the tree trunks. Wild mushrooms are hand-picked and some varieties have a delicious flavour.

Wild mushrooms must be identified as being edible by a reputable source before they are cooked and eaten, as there are many varieties of inedible fungi which cause nausea and vomiting, and a few varieties which are extremely poisonous. Today, certain areas of various countries, known for their excellent wild mushrooms, are kept wild, so that the mushrooms may thrive. Such areas occur in France, Finland, Germany and Russia.

Mushrooming is a popular pastime in rural and semi-rural areas in Australasia, where field mushrooms appear as if by magic following rain. Most people, however, purchase mushrooms from the vegetable market or supermarket.

Mushroom cultivation is a successful industry and high quality graded mushrooms are available throughout the year. Although most mushrooms are still used in cooking, raw cultivated mushrooms are becoming popular in salads and hors d'oeuvre.

These foods are very light, and in the quantities eaten they are not nutritionally significant; but their delicious flavour enhances soups, meats, salads and other dishes and adds to the enjoyment of food, which is an important aspect of healthy eating.

Mushrooms provide dietary fibre and they contribute few kilojoules (or calories) to the diet. When prepared without the addition of fat they are a handy food for those wishing to reduce their fat intake and stay within the healthy weight range.

Nutritional information is not available for all entries in the Fungi chapter. It is included where possible.

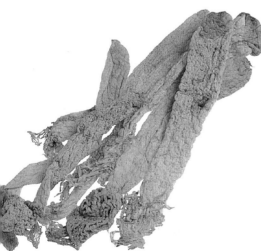

Bamboo Fungus

DESCRIPTION A lacy fungous growth which is gathered from bamboo plants in Szechuan and its neighbouring provinces in China. Before sale it is dried, which turns it a deep yellow-brown and gives it a musty, earthy flavour and crunchy texture.

ORIGIN AND HISTORY Bamboo fungus was one of the rare ingredients sought after by chefs of the Imperial households in the gourmandising Ming era, when exotica in menus was paramount.

BUYING AND STORAGE Sold in specialist shops and in some herbalists. It can be kept for many months provided it does not come into contact with moisture, which causes mould.

PREPARATION AND USE It is a rare and very expensive ingredient used only in Chinese vegetarian cooking, and occasionally in banquet dishes. It should be thoroughly rinsed after soaking, and simmered until tender — without overcooking, which can cause it to break up.

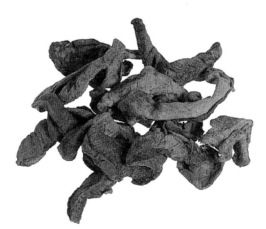

Boletus *Boletus granulatus*

also called Yellow mushroom

DESCRIPTION A mushroom with a yellow cap, popular in Europe.

ORIGIN AND HISTORY Found growing wild under conifer trees in woods in France,

Italy, Poland and Germany. Sometimes available, tinned or dried, in other countries.

BUYING AND STORAGE Pick wild in summer and autumn. Select boletus which have a fruity aroma. Store as for cultivated mushrooms.

PREPARATION AND USE Brush or wipe clean, trim ends off stalks. Wash only if very dirty. Fry, sauté or bake.

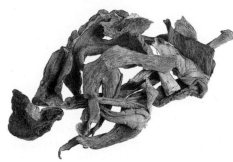

Cep *Boletus edulis*

also called **Cepe**

DESCRIPTION A round-capped mushroom with a thick stalk.

ORIGIN AND HISTORY Found growing wild in beech forests in France and under coniferous trees throughout Europe and in the Rocky Mountains, USA. Its botanical name comes from the word bolites, used by the Greeks and Romans to describe the best flavoured mushrooms. The cep continues to be much favoured in Europe today. It is sometimes available, tinned or dried, in other countries.

BUYING AND STORAGE Pick wild in summer and autumn. Select firm, dry, undamaged ceps. Store as for cultivated mushrooms but use as soon as possible.

PREPARATION AND USE Wipe clean with a damp cloth and trim off ends of stalks. Serve sautéed or use in soups, sauces and casseroles.

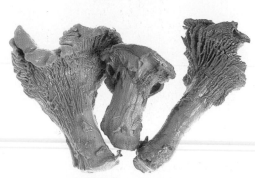

Chanterelle *Cantharellus cibarius*

also called **Egg mushroom, Girolle**

DESCRIPTION Shaped like a furled trumpet, with a firm-fleshed, apricot-yellow cap, rising out of a paler, ribbed stalk. Chanterelles vary in flavour according to their location.

ORIGIN AND HISTORY Found growing wild in beech woods in Europe, particularly France, Italy, Germany and Poland, and also in the USA. It is sometimes available, tinned or dried, in other countries.

BUYING AND STORAGE Pick wild from summer to midwinter. Select clean, firm, dry, spongy, undamaged chanterelles with an apricot aroma. Store as for shiitake.

PREPARATION AND USE Place in a colander and rinse under running cold water, then pat dry with a clean tea towel. Leave whole if small or cut into bite-size pieces if large. Need longer cooking than other mushrooms. Serve sautéed or in soups, sauces and with chicken.

If dried, soak well for an hour in warm water.

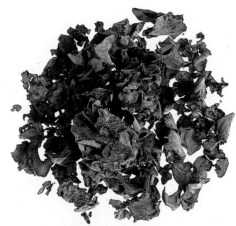

Cloud Ear Fungus
Auricularia polytricha

also called **Dried black fungus, Hed hunu, Jamar kuping, Kikurage, Kuping tikus, Mu erh, Tree ears, Wood ear fungus, You erh**

MAJOR NUTRIENTS			DRIED
			SERVE SIZE 1 G
Energy	12 kJ	Carbohydrate	1 g
Protein	0	Cholesterol	0
Fat	0	Iron	0.6 mg

NUTRITIONAL INFORMATION This is a good source of iron.

Since this food is used in very small amounts, it is nutritionally insignificant.

DESCRIPTION The black variety is a greyish-black, curled and crinkly dried fungus which has something of the appearance of clouds in a Chinese brush painting. When soaked, it expands to up to five times its dried size and resembles a type of curled seaweed. It has a bland mushroom flavour and an agreeable crisp texture. It grows on decaying logs

and has come to be known also as wood fungus. The albino form of this fungus is known as snow, white or silver fungus, and is listed separately.

ORIGIN AND HISTORY It first came into use in central and southern China. Mushrooms were obviously enjoyed during the T'ang dynasty (618–907). Wang Chen-po, a Buddhist sage, wrote of them being cooked in an ancient cauldron. A pharmacologist of the time mentioned the kind of 'black fungi that grows on the trunks of (various) trees to be very good'. In landlocked Laos, where the variety of ingredients is limited, all edible fungi are highly regarded.

BUYING AND STORAGE If fresh, store in the refrigerator. Usually sold by weight in small cellophane packs. A little goes a long way. Avoid damp which can cause it to grow mould. Stored in an airtight container, it can be kept indefinitely.

PREPARATION AND USE It is used extensively in Chinese cooking, particularly in vegetarian dishes, and increasingly in Malaysia and Singapore, Thailand and Indonesia. Soak in boiling water for about 20 minutes, until the fungus feels flexible and tender. Drain and chop. Add to stir-fried and braised dishes, soups and vegetables. This fungus accepts strong seasonings, so can be used in curries and pungent dishes using chilli, garlic and Chinese bean pastes.

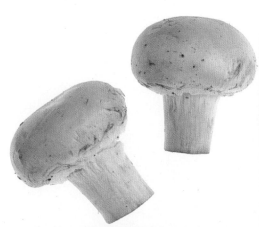

Cultivated Mushroom
Agaricus bisporus

also called **Champignon and Common mushroom**

MAJOR NUTRIENTS			SERVE SIZE 50 G
Energy	45 kJ	Sodium	0
Protein	1 g	Dietary Fibre	1 g
Fat	0	Phosphorus	84 mg
Carbohydrate	0	Riboflavin	0.2 mg
Cholesterol	0	Niacin Equiv.	2 mg

NUTRITIONAL INFORMATION An excellent source of pantothenic acid; good source of niacin, riboflavin, phosphorus (excellent if canned); moderate source of folate.

Mushrooms contain an appreciable amount of B group vitamins and iron — they are rather like a vegetable version of meat. Levels of B group vitamins are reduced by sautéeing or canning.

DESCRIPTION Cultivated common mushrooms are picked and sold in three sizes, since as they grow, they get larger and change their shape and name.

Buttons or babies are small unopened mushrooms with a delicate flavour. Cups or caps are slightly larger opened mushrooms with a stronger flavour. Flats or open mushrooms are large, soft, flat mushrooms with a rich, strong flavour. The brown type of *Agaricus bisporus* is becoming available and may be known as Swiss mushroom.

BUYING AND STORAGE Available all year round. Choose firm, dry, clean, undamaged mushrooms. Avoid withered ones. Store, unwashed, in a brown paper bag or a special cloth bag, in the refrigerator. Will keep for up to 7 days.

PREPARATION AND USE Brush or wipe mushrooms clean and trim off ends of stalks. Wash gently if very dirty. Do not peel. Use raw in salads or with dips. Slice, quarter, dice, chop or leave whole, then fry, grill, bake or microwave. Serve stuffed or use in stuffings, soups, sauces and casseroles.

PROCESSING Cultivated mushrooms may be canned, processed and frozen, and canned in soup.

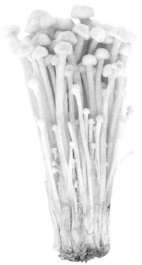

Enokitake Mushroom

DESCRIPTION A tiny mushroom with small round head on a slender stem which grows as long as 13 cm. The mushrooms grow in clumps on the stumps of the Chinese hackberry tree, which is called enoki in Japan. Cream-yellow in colour, they are mildly flavoured, with a crisp texture.

ORIGIN AND HISTORY Traditional Japanese cooking emphasises the use of seasonal ingredients, the arrival of each new season being heralded by the appropriate garnish and fresh ingredient. Enokitake mushrooms are winter food, and most usually find their way into donabe, Japanese one-pot dishes, or soups.

BUYING AND STORAGE Available in cans or jars, packed in water, they should be drained before use. Fresh ones are available in many Asian food stores. They can be kept, wrapped in plastic, in the vegetable compartment of the refrigerator for up to 1 week.

PREPARATION AND USE Their attractive appearance enhances any dish in which they are used. Trim and add in little clumps to soups, one-pot dishes and noodle dishes. Or serve lightly cooked as a salad with vinaigrette

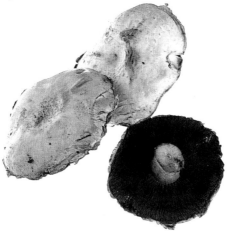

Field Mushroom   *Agaricus vaporarius*

DESCRIPTION Very similar in appearance to the cultivated common mushroom.

ORIGIN AND HISTORY Grows wild in fields, meadows and pastures.

BUYING AND STORAGE Collect wild in late summer and autumn. Store as for cultivated mushrooms.

PREPARATION AND USE Brush or wipe mushrooms clean and trim off ends of stalks. Wash only if very dirty. Peel only if very damaged. Use whole, quartered, sliced, diced, chopped. Fry, grill, bake or stuff, or use in soups, casseroles and savoury dishes.

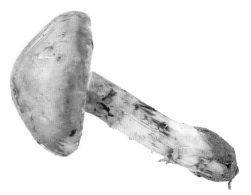

Matsutake Mushroom
Armillaria edodes

also called **Pine mushroom**

DESCRIPTION This mushroom is dark brown with a thick, meaty stem. It is usually eaten before the cap spreads open, and has a delicate flavour and the scent of the red pine woods in which it grows wild.

ORIGIN AND HISTORY Matsutake mushroom season in Japan has all the excitement of a truffle hunt in France. The season is short, a few weeks in mid autumn, and those who are lucky enough to find these earthy delicacies will immediately return to the kitchen to cook them by steam-grilling in a horaku, a 2-piece earthenware pot which is buried in hot coals.

BUYING AND STORAGE Matsutake are under very limited cultivation, so are expensive when available. They are never dried, but are sometimes canned, although the unique fresh flavour is lost in the process.

PREPARATION AND USE They are usually served by themselves, very lightly grilled or sautéed. To prepare them, do not wash, but wipe the cap with a damp cloth. Cut into thick slices after trimming just the base of the stem. Oyster mushrooms can be substituted in certain dishes.

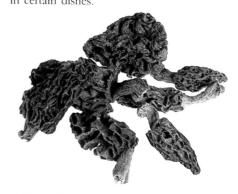

Morel   *Morchella esculenta*

also called **Morille, Sponge mushroom**

DESCRIPTION The morel grows on a thick stalk and has a brown, yellow or cream spongelike, pointed cap, pitted with hollows from which the spores fall. It can be as small as a strawberry or as large as an avocado.

ORIGIN AND HISTORY Grows wild on meadow clearings and pine heaths in the shade of the forests in Europe; thrives in France, Sweden and Finland, and on the west and east coasts of the USA.

BUYING AND STORAGE Collect wild in spring and early summer. Store in the refrigerator but use as soon as possible. It may be available canned or dried.

PREPARATION AND USE Brush clean and trim ends off stalks. Leave whole or slice lengthwise and rinse quickly in a colander, then dry with a clean tea towel. Chop and sauté the stalks, simmer the caps in cream and serve with chicken, rice or pasta. If dried, soak in warm water for 2 minutes or until they are soft enough to cut.

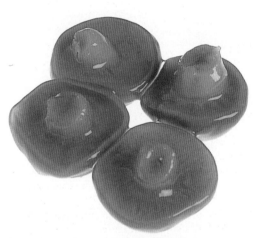

Nameko

DESCRIPTION This is a small, thick-capped Japanese mushroom with a dark yellow-amber colour. It has a pleasant woody flavour and agreeable, gelatinous coating.

ORIGIN AND HISTORY A fungus which has enjoyed continuous use in Japanese cooking since the earliest times. The rarity of these mushrooms in their fresh state has enhanced their reputation, so that even now that they are available in cans Japanese still consider them an impressive ingredient.

BUYING AND STORAGE Rarely available fresh as they spoil quickly, they are sold in cans and bottles packed in brine, which does not seem to detract too much from their flavour.

Chinese straw mushrooms are a good alternative to nameko in both appearance and flavour.

PREPARATION AND USE Drain the mushrooms and use whole in soups and Japanese one-pot dishes. They can also be served as a salad, with a mild vinegar dressing.

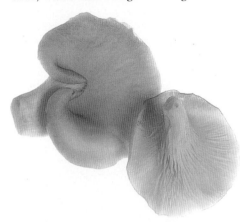

Oyster Mushroom

also called Abalone mushroom, Chinese mushroom, Hiratake, Hou goo, Shimeji

DESCRIPTION A pale grey-white mushroom which grows in close clusters, resulting in stems which are set off to the side, giving a lopsided appearance. It is more delicately textured than most other kinds of Asian mushroom and tastes quite distinctly like oysters.

ORIGIN AND HISTORY Until recent times, oyster mushrooms have not enjoyed the popularity of many of the related types of edible fungus outside Asia, but they have been available in China and Japan for centuries. Affectionately known as 'shellfish of the forest', they have been given the name oyster mushroom because of their distinct flavour. They are cultivated for sale in Asia, Europe, the USA and Australia.

BUYING AND STORAGE They are now readily available fresh in supermarkets and in Chinese food stores, and are also canned, although this impairs their flavour and texture. Store for a few days only.

PREPARATION AND USE Rinsed and sliced, they are used in Chinese stir-fried and vegetarian dishes, and added to soups and noodle dishes in place of black mushrooms.

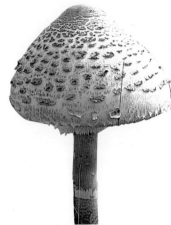

Parasol Mushroom
Lepiota procera

also called Umbrella mushroom

DESCRIPTION A large, tall mushroom with tiny scales on the cap.

ORIGIN AND HISTORY Grows wild on grassy hillsides, near trees in Europe, eastern North America and Australia. The botanical name derives from the Latin lepis (scale) and procerus (tall).

BUYING AND STORAGE Collect wild in late summer and autumn. Store in the refrigerator but use as soon as possible.

PREPARATION AND USE Remove and discard tough stalks. Brush or wipe caps clean. Use whole, sliced or chopped. Sauté or use in soups, sauces and savoury dishes.

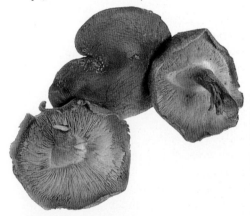

Shiitake Mushroom
Lentinus edodes

also called Chinese mushroom, Faa goo, Leong goo, Tung ku, Winter mushroom

MAJOR NUTRIENTS			BOILED
			SERVE SIZE 70 G
Energy	167 kJ	Cholesterol	0
Protein	0	Sodium	0
Fat	0	Dietary Fibre	0
Carbohydrate	10 g	Niacin Equiv.	1.2 mg

NUTRITIONAL INFORMATION A moderate source of niacin. Shiitake mushrooms are higher in kilojoules than cultivated mushrooms and do not have the extensive range of B vitamins and iron.

DESCRIPTION The mushrooms used in Chinese and Japanese cooking come in many sizes and grades. Japanese shiitake (*Cortinellus shiitake*) are cultivated by inserting the spore into prepared wood, which is usually the bark of *Pasania cuspidata*, a type of oak. In China a lighter coloured mushroom, with a thicker cap, is thought to have the best flavour. The large black mushrooms from the north, which may be known as winter mushrooms, also have good flavour.

ORIGIN AND HISTORY Mushrooms are also traditionally bought dried; these can be very expensive, some so much so that they are only enjoyed at very special banquets. The Chinese believe dried mushrooms to be very beneficial to the health. Workers involved in processing and packaging mushrooms are known to live long and healthy lives, particularly free from respiratory disorders.

Shiitake mushrooms were recorded in the Ming dynasty in China as generating stamina. In the 15th century they were important in the diet of warrior priests, to increase their energy. Shiitake grow in China and Japan on the wood of dead deciduous oak trees. They are called after the shii tree but also grow on oak and hornbeam trees. Cultivation is in an experimental stage in Australia.

BUYING AND STORAGE Available in spring and autumn. Select firm, dry mushrooms with a pungent smell. Store in a single layer in a brown paper bag or in a basket covered with damp muslin in the refrigerator. Will keep for at least a week.

Dried, they are sold by weight in small cellophane or plastic packs. Expect them to be expensive, for if not they will be of inferior quality. Stored in an airtight container away from damp, they can be kept indefinitely.

PREPARATION AND USE Shiitake have a distinctive flavour and aroma, which lends itself to many different styles of cooking. A plate of simmered top quality shiitake mushrooms, on poached lettuce, with a dressing of oyster sauce, is an unsurpassable treat. For fresh mushrooms, trim ends off the stalks and wipe caps clean with a damp cloth. Do not wash or peel. Slice and use in Japanese and Chinese dishes and stir-fries. Caps cook more quickly than stalks.

Dried mushrooms must be soaked to rehydrate. Twenty minutes in lukewarm water is sufficient for medium mushrooms; allow longer for larger, thicker ones. Some cooks prefer to soak them for several hours in cold water. Drain and squeeze out excess water. Remove stems by cutting close to the cap. Stems cannot be eaten, as they remain hard and woody. Use smaller or good quality mushrooms whole, others can be shredded. To serve as a vegetable, they should be simmered gently in well-flavoured stock.

Reserve liquid used for soaking or cooking to add to soups and braised dishes, as it adds an agreeable flavour.

Chinese oyster sauce provides a complementary flavour.

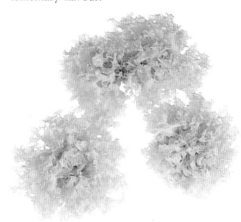

Snow Fungus

*also called **Seet gnee, Shirokikurage, Silver fungus, White fungus***

DESCRIPTION A fine, cream, crinkly dry fungus which is used in many ways in Chinese cooking. It dramatically increases in size when soaked in water, and although it has little taste, is prized for its crunchy texture.

ORIGIN AND HISTORY The Chinese believe that it is a beneficial food for toning the system. It is expensive, and the better qualities are reserved for serving at special Chinese banquets where it may be served in a vegetable dish, or as a dessert in sugar syrup. Chinese women take dishes containing white fungus to beautify their complexion.

BUYING AND STORAGE Sold in small packs by weight in dry form, it is also available canned in water or syrup. The canning process removes much of the delicate flavour and softens its crisp texture.

Dry snow fungus can be kept in an airtight container in a dry cupboard for many months.

PREPARATION AND USE Rinse, then soak in cold clean water until the fungus softens and increases in size. For vegetarian dishes, cut it into small pieces and simmer in stock until tender. The hard 'eye' in the centre can be cut away with kitchen scissors. As a dessert, simmer in sugar syrup until tender, drain, and serve in clear sugar syrup, or in fruit juice with fresh fruit.

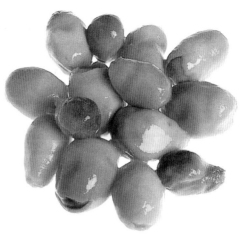

Straw Mushroom
Volvariella volvacea

*also called **Grass mushroom, Jelly mushroom, Paddy-straw mushroom***

MAJOR NUTRIENTS		CANNED, DRAINED SERVE SIZE 50 G	
Energy	60 kJ	Cholesterol	0
Protein	1 g	Sodium	130 mg
Fat	0	Iron	0.6 mg
Carbohydrate	2 g		

NUTRITIONAL INFORMATION A moderate source of iron. Contains a moderate amount of sodium.

DESCRIPTION A cultivated Chinese mushroom about the size and shape of a quail's egg, resembling a truffle, cream at the base and grey-black on top. The flavour is earthy and distinct. Straw mushrooms, as the name implies, grow naturally or are cultivated by their spore being implanted on paddy-straw, the residual straw of the rice crop after harvest. They spoil quickly, becoming acrid in taste and gelatinous in texture.

ORIGIN AND HISTORY The Chinese have been harvesting wild straw mushrooms from discarded paddy-straw for centuries. Straw mushrooms are enjoyed for their delicate flavour, but are also often included in banquet dishes as a fun item — the ultimate test of one's agility with chopsticks.

Cultivation is in an experimental stage in Australia.

BUYING AND STORAGE Sold fresh, as they cannot be successfully dried, they are also sold canned in water. They may be cream in the can, having the outer dark skin removed. Store opened cans of straw mushrooms in the refrigerator for several days, changing the water daily.

PREPARATION AND USE They are an attractive addition to stir-fried, braised and steamed dishes and are delicious in soups. Small ones may be left whole, large ones cut in halves or sliced.

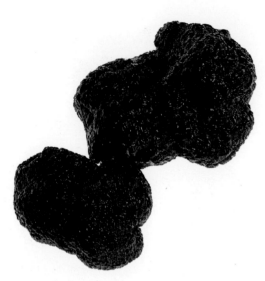

Truffle   *Tuber* spp.

DESCRIPTION Truffles are woody-looking tubers which grow underground, near the roots of oak or beech trees.

ORIGIN AND HISTORY Oak and beech groves are planted in France and Italy to encourage them to grow. The black Perigord truffle grows in France, the white Piedmontese in northern Italy, the red-grained in England and the violet truffle throughout Europe. Pigs and dogs are used to scent them out, and they form a much prized flavouring in European cuisine. The French writer Colette used to delight her friends by cooking a whole dish of truffles alone, but usually they are added in small quantities to flavour other foods, especially meat.

BUYING AND STORAGE Available during autumn, fresh truffles are usually marketed in the regions in which they are found.

Choose firm, undamaged, medium-sized, aromatic truffles; store in the refrigerator, but use as soon as possible. They are also available canned.

PREPARATION AND USE Wash thoroughly in cold water, then drain and dry with a clean tea towel. Slice thinly, or grate or chop, and use in classical pâté de foie gras, in sauces, soups, egg dishes, with meat, pasta and rice, and for garnishing.

PROCESSING Truffles are canned.

VARIETIES
Black Perigord truffle (*Tuber melanosporum*); white Piedmontese truffle (*T. magnatum*); red-grained black truffle (*T. aestivum*); violet truffle (*T. brumale*).

MEATS

Meat has played a vital part in the human diet since tens of thousands of years before recorded history, and man's earliest art records the great significance of animals hunted for food by prehistoric families and communities. An interesting example is Australia, where the Aboriginal people remained hunters and gatherers until the incursions by the Europeans which began in the 18th century. These settlers brought with them the food sources and styles of their homelands, not all of which adapted easily to the new environment. The First Fleet arrived carrying 2 bulls, 6 cows, 44 fat-tailed sheep, pigs, goats and poultry as well as salted beef and pork. Imported salted meat was vital to the survival of the colony when the local production of crops and meat failed in the early years.

Meat remained an important part of the diet in the new colony, where farming techniques were developed to suit the climate and soils, and a growing population ensured continued requirement of meat and meat products.

Consumption of meat in societies like those of Australia has, however, declined steadily since the 1930s. Many factors have contributed to the drop in meat consumption. Amongst these are the less formal eating patterns with 'lighter' and more varied meals and snacks, the desire for convenience and quickly prepared meals, the increased use of chicken in the home and its wide use as a takeaway food.

Today more people are turning to a vegetarian diet, for ecological reasons, and in a desire to avoid killing animals. Others have decided to eat less meat for 'health' reasons. They have been concerned about reducing fat and cholesterol, but they have often ignored the valuable contribution of other nutrients which meat makes in the diet.

Doctors and other health workers have reinforced this 'healthy' message and have often given the simplistic and poor advice to avoid red meat and dairy products, as part of the attempt to reduce fat consumption in order to lower the prevalence of heart disease. The advice should be: use moderate amounts of lean meats and reduced fat and low fat dairy products. This is not to say that a vegetarian diet cannot be a nutritious diet, it can be highly nutritious, but it needs careful planning, not just the removal of meat from a mixed diet.

Beef and sheep in former colonies like New Zealand and Australia are pasture-fed, and they are slaughtered at a younger age than the cattle and sheep in America and Europe. This makes the meat leaner than in northern hemisphere countries. The selvage of subcutaneous fat is narrower and there is less marbling of the lean muscle tissue with fat.

The meat industries in many countries have recognised the need to produce lean meat and have made changes in both farm production and processing to achieve this. A grading system is being introduced to assist the consumer in meat selection. Lean cuts of beef, veal, lamb and pork make it easy for the consumer to select lean meat. It is then important to avoid the addition of large amounts of fat to the meat in preparation.

Meats are major contributors of protein, iron, zinc and niacin equivalents. The iron and zinc are well absorbed from meat, and a small amount of meat in a meal improves the absorption of the iron from vegetables and cereals. Nutritional anaemia is common amongst women of child-bearing age and the iron requirements of these women are higher than those of men. Women, however, eat considerably less meat than men and thus miss out on a good source of iron.

Meat is the most important source of vitamin B12 and it does contribute small amounts of folate. The average cut of meat contains about equal amounts of saturated and monounsaturated fats with only small amounts of polyunsaturated fat. As the fat level falls, the proportion of monounsaturated and polyunsaturated fats increases.

Liver and kidneys deserve a special comment. It is true that they contain two to three times the amount of cholesterol as muscle meats. However they are a much richer source of iron, zinc and niacin equivalents and they are the only meats containing significant amounts of vitamin A. When fresh, they also contain vitamin C. These meats are a very rich source of vitamin B12 and folate. Their percentage of fat is similar to that of lean meat, but they contain more polyunsaturated fats.

Beef

DESCRIPTION   Beef is the meat of the many types of cattle which have been domesticated for human consumption through the centuries of history, ever since people developed settled agricultural communities.

ORIGIN AND HISTORY Beef has always been a favoured meat in Europe, where its use is recorded in antiquity. The primary producers raised and butchered their own beef cattle throughout early history, and by the Middle Ages there were powerful butchers' guilds which controlled the cuts of meat and to a certain extent the popular taste in beef consumption in towns and cities.

In England in the late 16th century the systematic planting of clover, hay crops and turnips made it possible to feed cattle over the winter months and provide fresh meat year round. There remained difficulties in providing fresh meat to a growing urban population, since meat had to be sold quickly or salted — there was no refrigeration until 1880. But despite these difficulties the 19th century was the century for great English beef.

Only in the last 200 years have cattle been systematically selected for either milk or beef, once it was discovered that cattle thrived on the natural grasslands of the New World. Great advances were made in cattle-feeding methods and breeding techniques in the USA, which has become the world's leading producer of beef today.

BUYING AND STORAGE Quality and tenderness will vary not only with the cut of beef but also with sex, age, condition of the beast, and the handling practices of the processer. In Australia, branding criteria have been introduced by the authorities to identify young, tender, quality beef. A gold strip brand is rolled onto the external fat selvages of grass-fed beef that meets the criteria and a purple brand is used to identify the lot-fed beef, that is, beef that has been fed on grain for 90 days.

Beef should be stored in the meat keeper or the coldest part of the refrigerator, on a plate or a rack with loose plastic wrap or foil, allowing the air to circulate around the beef.

When freezing, place beef in freezer bags (high density plastic) in meal-size portions — interleave steaks with plastic, extract air from the bag, seal, label, date and freeze as quickly as possible.

Small cuts of meat and steaks can be cooked frozen. Larger cuts should be removed from bags and thawed in the refrigerator or thawed in the microwave according to distributors' instructions.

PREPARATION AND USE   It is important to select the correct cooking methods for the cut of beef used. Meat is muscle. Those muscles less frequently used have less connective tissue, will be more tender and will therefore require less cooking. Forequarter cuts are generally less tender, and therefore are best cooked using a moist method. Hindquarter cuts are more tender and can generally be cooked by a quick, dry method.

HINDQUARTER CUTS

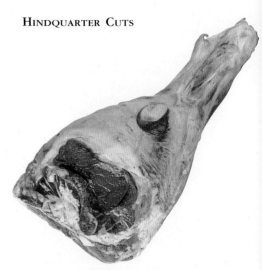

Butt   This contains shin, round, topside and silverside.

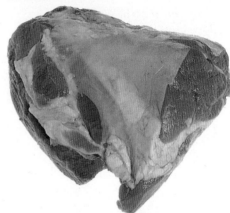

Fillet   Lies under the rump and the sirloin and is the most tender cut of beef. The whole or long fillet is the entire fillet and the butt fillet is that section under the rump. In a piece the fillet can be roasted (wrapped in pastry and roasted — Beef Wellington) or cut into steaks and grilled or pan fried.

MAJOR NUTRIENTS		**TRIMMED, GRILLED** SERVE SIZE 120 G	
Energy	1030 kJ	Phosphorus	260 mg
Protein	36 g	Magnesium	26 mg
Fat	12 g	Iron	4.7 mg
Cholesterol	100 mg	Zinc	5 mg
Carbohydrate	0	Thiamin	0.15 mg
Total Sugars	0	Riboflavin	0.4 mg
Sodium	70 mg	Niacin Equiv.	12.7 mg
Potassium	450 mg		

NUTRITIONAL INFORMATION An excellent source of protein with moderate levels of fat, which contribute 44% of energy. Is one of the best sources in the diet for phosphorus, iron, zinc, niacin and vitamin B. Contains cholesterol which should not affect blood cholesterol levels if remainder of diet is fat-controlled. Further trimming may reduce fat content further.

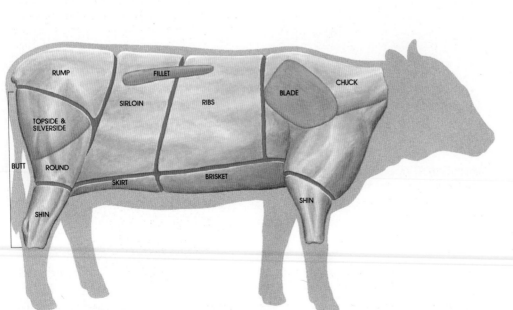

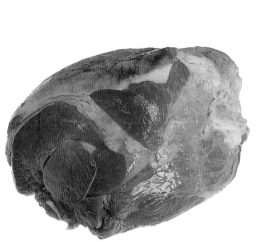

Round The boneless piece of meat taken from the front of the butt, off the femur bone. In one piece it can be roasted, as steak it can be braised, and is best marinated to tenderise prior to grilling, pan frying or barbecuing.

MAJOR NUTRIENTS		ROASTED SERVE SIZE 120 G	
Energy	1060 kJ	Phosphorus	260 mg
Protein	35 g	Magnesium	46 mg
Fat	13 g	Iron	2.4 mg
Cholesterol	85 mg	Zinc	7.2 mg
Carbohydrate	0	Thiamin	0.1 mg
Total Sugars	0	Riboflavin	0.2 mg
Sodium	80 mg	Niacin Equiv.	10.6 mg
Potassium	410 mg		

NUTRITIONAL INFORMATION An important source of vital iron and zinc which are well absorbed from this food source; especially good source of niacin and B12. Fats contain cholesterol but in a low fat diet this amount is not thought to elevate blood cholesterol levels. Extra trimming may further reduce fat content.

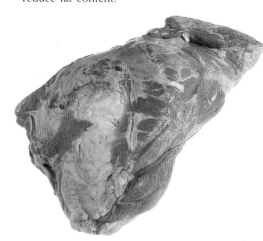

Rump The boneless piece of meat that covers the hip bone. It can be roasted in a piece or used as steaks for grilling, pan frying, or barbecuing.

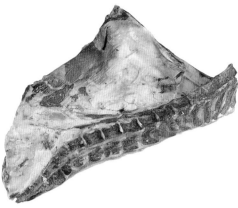

Rump and Loin The rump and the loin is the remainder of the hindquarter after the removal of the butt. It produces the most tender meat.

MAJOR NUTRIENTS		GRILLED SERVE SIZE 120 G	
Energy	1070 kJ	Phosphorus	265 mg
Protein	11 g	Magnesium	22 mg
Fat	11 g	Iron	4.3 mg
Cholesterol	100 mg	Zinc	5.8 mg
Carbohydrate	0	Thiamin	0.15 mg
Total Sugars	0	Riboflavin	0.45 mg
Sodium	65 mg	Niacin Equiv.	9.4 mg
Potassium	425 mg		

NUTRITIONAL INFORMATION An excellent source of protein with moderate levels of fat, which contribute 38% of energy; one of the best sources in the diet for phosphorus, iron, zinc, niacin and vitamin B.

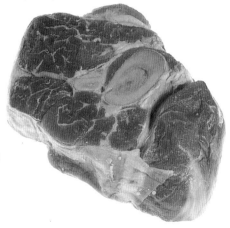

Shin Beef From both the fore and hindquarter, contains the shank bone. It is lean and most commonly used with the bone in for soups and stocks.

MAJOR NUTRIENTS		BRAISED SERVE SIZE 120 G	
Energy	990 kJ	Potassium	310 mg
Protein	42 g	Phosphorus	230 mg
Fat	8 g	Magnesium	24 mg
Cholesterol	70 mg	Iron	3.2 mg
Carbohydrate	0	Zinc	5.6 mg
Total Sugars	0	Riboflavin	0.45 mg
Sodium	75 mg	Niacin Equiv.	14.7 mg

NUTRITIONAL INFORMATION With less than 30% of energy coming from fat this cut of meat is an exceptionally useful source of protein, minerals and vitamins. The iron and zinc in meat are exceptionally well absorbed by the body.

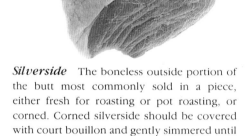

Silverside The boneless outside portion of the butt most commonly sold in a piece, either fresh for roasting or pot roasting, or corned. Corned silverside should be covered with court bouillon and gently simmered until tender (approximately 30 minutes per 500 g).

MAJOR NUTRIENTS		CORNED, BOILED SERVE SIZE 60 G	
Energy	380 kJ	Potassium	120 mg
Protein	14 g	Phosphorus	90 mg
Fat	4 g	Iron	1.4 mg
Cholesterol	45 mg	Zinc	2.1 mg
Carbohydrate	0	Riboflavin	0.15 mg
Total Sugars	0	Niacin Equiv.	4.2 mg
Sodium	830 mg		

NUTRITIONAL INFORMATION A moderately lean cut of meat with fats contributing about 38% of total energy. Contains excellent amounts of minerals and vitamins especially iron, zinc and vitamin B12. Because of the method of preparation may have a high sodium content and so should be used with discretion in a sodium-controlled diet. If silverside is soaked and washed with water, the sodium level can be reduced substantially.

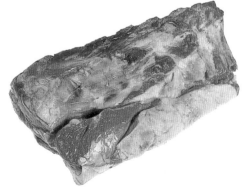

Sirloin The piece of meat between the rump and the ribs. The section of the sirloin nearest the rump contains some fillet. In a piece with the bone in or boneless it can be roasted. Sirloin steak with bone in or T-bone with bone in and fillet attached, or boneless, is for grilling, pan frying or barbecuing.

MAJOR NUTRIENTS ROLLED, ROASTED, TRIMMED
SERVE SIZE 60 G

Energy	530 kJ	Potassium	225 mg
Protein	16 g	Phosphorus	105 mg
Fat	7 g	Magnesium	15 mg
Cholesterol	35 mg	Iron	2.1 mg
Carbohydrate	0	Zinc	3.6 mg
Total Sugars	0	Riboflavin	0.05 mg
Sodium	50 mg	Niacin Equiv.	6.6 mg

NUTRITIONAL INFORMATION An excellent source of protein with moderate levels of fat, which contribute 44% of energy. One of the best sources in the diet for phosphorus, iron, zinc, niacin and vitamin B. Contains cholesterol which should not affect blood cholesterol levels if remainder of diet is fat controlled.

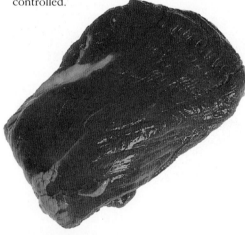

Skirt Steak The flank cut from mid to hindquarter from the underside of the rump and loin. Cut into pieces and stewed, or stuffed, rolled and braised. Also sold as flank steak.

MAJOR NUTRIENTS STEWED, TRIMMED
SERVE SIZE 120 G

Energy	1000 kJ	Potassium	315 mg
Protein	42 g	Phosphorus	195 mg
Fat	8 g	Magnesium	24 mg
Cholesterol	100 mg	Iron	3.5 mg
Carbohydrate	0	Zinc	12 mg
Total Sugars	0	Riboflavin	0.5 mg
Sodium	75 mg	Niacin Equiv.	14.5 mg

NUTRITIONAL INFORMATION An excellent beef cut with fat content providing less than 30% total fat. Can be considered an extremely useful source of all nutrients noted especially iron, zinc and vitamin B12 which are well absorbed from this source.

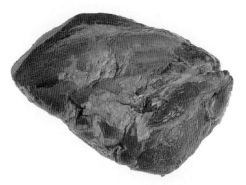

Topside The boneless inside portion of the butt, off the femur bone. In a piece it can be roasted or pot roasted, for steaks it can be braised, and is best if marinated to tenderise before grilling, pan frying or barbecuing.

MAJOR NUTRIENTS ROASTED, TRIMMED
SERVE SIZE 60 G

Energy	420 kJ	Phosphorus	120 mg
Protein	17 g	Magnesium	20 mg
Fat	4 g	Iron	1.7 mg
Cholesterol	75 mg	Zinc	2.5 mg
Carbohydrate	0	Thiamin	0.05 mg
Total Sugars	0	Riboflavin	0.1 mg
Sodium	35 mg	Niacin Equiv.	6.7 mg
Potassium	185 mg		

NUTRITIONAL INFORMATION A moderate source of fat contributing 33% of total energy. Contains important amounts of minerals and vitamins, especially iron, zinc, niacin and vitamin B12. Cholesterol content is only significant if remainder of diet is high in fat.

FOREQUARTER CUTS

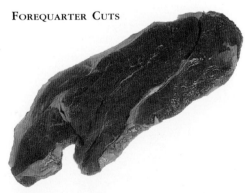

Blade That piece of meat that surrounds the shoulder blade outside and underneath. Available in a piece with bone in or boneless for roasting or pot roast, or as steaks for braising.

MAJOR NUTRIENTS TRIMMED, GRILLED
SERVE SIZE 120 G

Energy	970 kJ	Phosphorus	265 mg
Protein	34 g	Magnesium	26 mg
Fat	11 g	Iron	3.1 mg
Cholesterol	80 mg	Zinc	7.8 mg
Carbohydrate	0	Thiamin	0.1 mg
Total Sugars	0	Riboflavin	0.25 mg
Sodium	90 mg	Niacin Equiv.	10.4 mg
Potassium	445 mg		

NUTRITIONAL INFORMATION Contains fat which provides over 40% of total energy. Excellent levels of phosphorus, iron, zinc, niacin and vitamin B12. These nutrients are known to be especially well absorbed from beef sources. Extra trimming may reduce fat content further and so reduce energy and cholesterol levels.

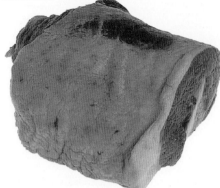

Brisket The undersection of the forequarter and ribs. Available in a piece with bone in, boned and rolled for roasting, or corned for boiling.

MAJOR NUTRIENTS CORNED, BOILED
SERVE SIZE 60 G

Energy	610 kJ	Potassium	105 mg
Protein	17 g	Phosphorus	90 mg
Fat	8 g	Iron	1.5 mg
Cholesterol	45 mg	Zinc	3.5 mg
Carbohydrate	0	Riboflavin	0.2 mg
Total Sugars	0	Niacin Equiv.	4.7 mg
Sodium	500 mg		

NUTRITIONAL INFORMATION This cut of meat is relatively high in fat with 48% of total energy coming from fat sources. Cholesterol level is about 15% of recommended daily intake but in an otherwise fat controlled diet this level is not excessive. Still an excellent source of phosphorus, iron and zinc.

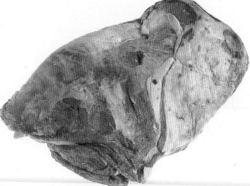

Chuck That section above the ribs and onto the neck with the blade removed. In a piece with bone in, boneless for roasting or pot roasting, or boneless steak for braising or stewing. The chuck is a flavoursome piece of meat suitable for curries, steak and kidney pudding, and pies.

MAJOR NUTRIENTS		TRIMMED, STEWED SERVE SIZE 120 G	
Energy	1100 kJ	Phosphorus	195 mg
Protein	43 g	Magnesium	23 mg
Fat	10 g	Iron	4.5 mg
Cholesterol	100 mg	Zinc	14 mg
Carbohydrate	0	Thiamin	0.05 mg
Total Sugars	0	Riboflavin	0.4 mg
Sodium	60 mg	Niacin Equiv.	15.8 mg
Potassium	280 mg		

NUTRITIONAL INFORMATION A leaner cut of beef with 33% of energy coming from fats. Excellent source of protein, phosphorus, iron, zinc, niacin and vitamin B12.

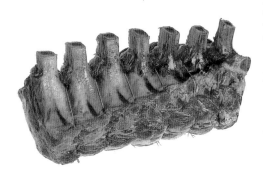

Ribs As the name implies, these are the ribs of the forequarter. Rib steak has the bone in. Rib eye — sometimes referred to as Scotch fillet — has the bone and the spare ribs removed. Both are suitable for grilling, pan frying or barbecuing. Ribs with the bone in, boneless and rolled, and rib eye, are all excellent pieces for roasting.

MAJOR NUTRIENTS	RIB EYE, TRIMMED, GRILLED SERVE SIZE 120 G		
Energy	1070 kJ	Phosphorus	265 mg
Protein	37 g	Magnesium	30 mg
Fat	12 g	Iron	4.2 mg
Cholesterol	100 mg	Zinc	6.1 mg
Carbohydrate	0	Thiamin	0.1 mg
Total Sugars	0	Riboflavin	0.4 mg
Sodium	55 mg	Niacin Equiv.	12.9 mg
Potassium	435 mg		

NUTRITIONAL INFORMATION This cut of meat provides 41% of total energy from fat. An excellent source of protein and especially iron, zinc, niacin and vitamin B12. Useful easy-to-prepare cut which does not require additional fats for tenderness.

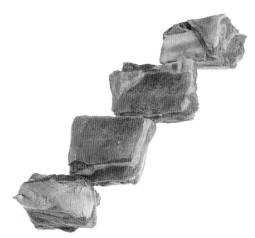

Spare Ribs These are cut from the tail of the ribs above the brisket. Spare ribs are removed when rib steaks or rib eye are prepared and have gained popularity because of the sweet meat that clings to the bone. They are usually marinated and grilled or barbecued.

MAJOR NUTRIENTS		BARBECUED SERVE SIZE 90 G	
Energy	1130 kJ	Potassium	340 mg
Protein	23 g	Phosphorus	100 mg
Fat	20 g	Iron	2 mg
Cholesterol	80 mg	Zinc	4.5 mg
Carbohydrate	0	Riboflavin	0.25 mg
Total Sugars	0	Niacin Equiv.	7.7 mg
Sodium	55 mg		

NUTRITIONAL INFORMATION A tasty but high fat cut of beef, with over 65% of energy coming from fats which also contain significant quantities of cholesterol. Good source of usual nutrients found in beef but not in such concentrated quantities as leaner cuts. Fat levels can be reduced by painstaking defatting process. Better to include only occasionally in diet, being aware of high fat content.

Bones

NUTRITIONAL INFORMATION No detailed analysis of bones is available.

ORIGIN AND HISTORY The Latin poet Horace (65BC–AD8) mentioned dried marrow and liver were popular aphrodisiacs in his time. Bones have been used extensively in most cuisines through the ages for the flavour and substance (gelatine) that they produce.

BUYING AND STORAGE Bones can be purchased fresh or are available in a processed form as gelatine. Fresh bones should be stored as fresh meat.

PREPARATION AND USE Bones require long, slow, moist cooking to extract the maximum flavour for stock, soup and stews. Bone marrow is highly regarded for its flavour and texture — veal shin or shank is used for osso buco, a famous Italian dish prized for the bone marrow. To gain maximum flavour and softening of the marrow, have bones cut transversely into sections approximately 50 mm long. Lamb shin or shanks can be braised or casseroled. Ham and bacon bones are used because of their distinctive flavour. Traditionally ham bones are used with dried peas or lentils as a thickener for soup.

DESCRIPTION The skeleton of any beast.

VARIETIES
May be of beef, lamb, pork or veal.

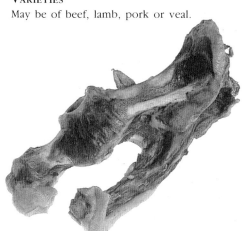

Bacon Bones

Brains

MAJOR NUTRIENTS		LAMB'S BRAINS, BOILED SERVE SIZE 45 G	
Energy	230 kJ	Potassium	125 mg
Protein	6 g	Phosphorus	145 mg
Fat	4 g	Iron	0.6 mg
Cholesterol	850 mg	Zinc	0.6 mg
Carbohydrate	0	Thiamin	0.05 mg
Total Sugars	0	Riboflavin	0.15 mg
Sodium	50 mg	Niacin Equiv.	2 mg

NUTRITIONAL INFORMATION A relatively high fat product with almost 65% of energy coming from the fat, and this fat contains high levels of cholesterol — about three times the recommended daily intake. They should therefore be used as an occasional meal and prepared without the addition of extra fats.

DESCRIPTION The brain provides a very soft, pale meat which is formed into convoluted patterns to provide the maximum of surface area inside the head of the animal.

ORIGIN AND HISTORY Brains have always been a popular offal.

BUYING AND STORAGE Choose brains that are pink, moist and plump. Lamb's brains are widely available, however calf's and pig's brains will need to be ordered from the butcher. See Offal for storage instructions.

PREPARATION AND USE The fine membrane which covers the brain can be removed to improve the appearance, by soaking in cold water for 30 minutes and carefully pulling the membrane from the brain. Soak for 1 hour to whiten.

Brains can be sautéed or poached and then deep-fried or grilled.

SEE ALSO Offal.

VARIETIES

Sheep, lamb, pig, calf, ox.

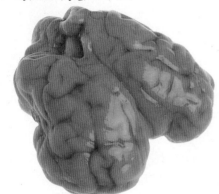

Lamb's Brains

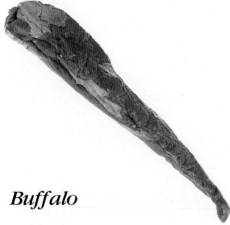

Buffalo

MAJOR NUTRIENTS			BOILED SERVE SIZE 100 G
Energy	646 kJ	Carbohydrate	0
Protein	21 g	Total Sugars	0
Fat	40 g	Sodium	0
Cholesterol	N/A		

NUTRITIONAL INFORMATION No analysis has been done for cholesterol, B vitamins and fat-soluble vitamins. An excellent source of protein and iron. Low in fat.

DESCRIPTION The buffalo is a member of the ox family. The meat of young animals is sinewy, and that of older ones is tough.

ORIGIN AND HISTORY An important food animal for prehistoric Europeans, the buffalo was frequently depicted in Stone Age cave paintings. It is found in many hot countries around the world and has long been domesticated in the Orient.

The milk is often drunk and can be made into cheeses, such as the famous mozzarella. In India the butter is clarified and called ghee. In northern parts of Australia, buffalo have been domesticated and are slaughtered for meat.

BUYING AND STORAGE Available in some specialist butcher shops, buffalo fillets are a special item on some restaurant menus. The meat must be kept refrigerated and can be frozen.

PREPARATION AND USE Buffalo is marinated in wine and herbs and roasted, or cut into steaks and pan-fried. The fillet is considered to be the best cut and even in the Northern Territory of Australia, where the animal is bred, it needs to be specially ordered.

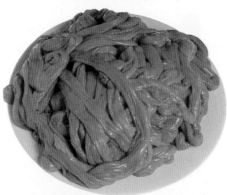

Chitterlings

also known as Chitlins

MAJOR NUTRIENTS			SERVE SIZE 100 G
Energy	350 kJ	Sodium	70 mg
Protein	14 g	Potassium	15 mg
Fat	3 g	Phosphorus	140 mg
Cholesterol	110 mg	Zinc	1.4 mg
Carbohydrate	0	Niacin Equiv.	2.7 mg
Total Sugars	0		

NUTRITIONAL INFORMATION These are a good source of protein and contain high levels of zinc and folate. If cooked in milk total fat and energy levels will increase and dish will become a significant source of calcium riboflavin.

DESCRIPTION Chitterlings are the small intestines of the pig.

ORIGIN AND HISTORY In the southern states of America they are considered to be a great delicacy. Formerly, however, they used to be given to the slaves to eat, along with other offal. Chitterlings are also normally the main ingredient in the famous French andouille sausage.

BUYING AND STORAGE Not easily obtained, chitterlings may be specially ordered from some butchers. In North America they are also available frozen. Use the fresh chitterlings within 24 hours of purchase.

PREPARATION AND USE The favoured method of preparation is to clean the intestines well and cook in boiling water with a few spices until tender. Cut into pieces about the size of an oyster, dip in cornmeal and fry in deep hot lard until golden brown. They may also be baked or stewed in milk or stock with onions and vegetables.

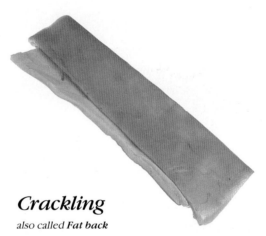

Crackling

also called Fat back

MAJOR NUTRIENTS			SERVE SIZE 15 G
Energy	380 kJ	Carbohydrate	0
Protein	2 g	Total Sugars	0
Fat	9 g	Sodium	10 mg
Cholesterol	16 mg	Potassium	30 mg

NUTRITIONAL INFORMATION Contains large amounts of fat contributing 89% total energy. Fat sources more than 50% saturated.

DESCRIPTION The long strip of fat that goes from the shoulder butt to the leg and protects the loin is called fat back in North America. It is usually rendered down for lard or may be fried to make pork crackling. It is also used in sausage making, especially the famous Spanish chorizo.

ORIGIN AND HISTORY The leftovers from the pig were given to the slaves who worked on the plantations in the southern states of the USA. Nothing was wasted: the fat was saved to be rendered down into lard and the bits of skin that floated to the top were crisply fried to make crackling. In Central America, pork crackling is a great favourite and is called chicharrones.

BUYING AND STORAGE Your friendly butcher may save the fat back for you if you want to make your own crackling. Store in the refrigerator and use as soon as possible. Now commercially made in Australia, pork crackling should be stored in an airtight container once the packet is opened.

PREPARATION AND USE Served with and in salads and as a crisp appetiser or snack food. In the south, crisp fried crackling is added to cornbread batter to make a flavoursome treat known as cracklin' bread.

To make crackling cut the fat back into thin squares. Fry in deep fat until they are curled and golden brown. Drain on absorbent paper and serve warm or cold, or use for crackling bread.

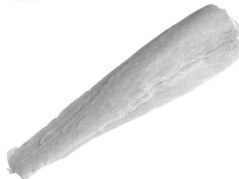

Crocodile

NUTRITIONAL INFORMATION No nutritional data are available for crocodile flesh.

DESCRIPTION The crocodile has a long snout that tapers to a point, a strong body and powerful tail. It is an agile and aggressive reptile which lives on small aquatic and shore animals and has been known to attack large animals, including dogs, cattle, and people.

ORIGIN AND HISTORY The eating of crocodile in Australia has had great importance for Aborigines throughout history.

Crocodiles are a protected species and their slaughter is illegal in the wild, unless carried out under the special dispensations for people of Aboriginal descent, which apply in some states.

Permits have been issued for the farming of crocodiles, and crocodile meat is available in some areas, particularly on restaurant menus, although the demand remains very much higher than the supply.

In general, because of food standards regulations, crocodile flesh is classed on its own and may not be sold with other meats in retail shops.

BUYING AND STORAGE If crocodile meat is acquired from a specialist supplier, it should be stored in the refrigerator.

PREPARATION AND USE Because the musk glands of the neck give the meat a musky flavour, they must be removed. It has been recommended that the meat be cut into thin steaks, grilled and served in a red wine sauce flavoured with sugar and ginger.

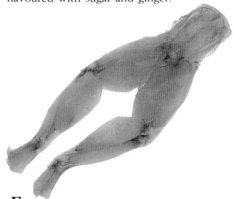

Frog

MAJOR NUTRIENTS			SERVE SIZE 100 G
Energy	310 kJ	Sodium	N/A
Protein	16 g	Phosphorus	145 mg
Fat	0	Iron	1.5 mg
Cholesterol	N/A	Thiamin	0.15 mg
Carbohydrate	0	Riboflavin	0.3 mg
Total Sugars	0	Niacin Equiv.	1 mg

NUTRITIONAL INFORMATION Frogs' legs are an excellent protein source and contain more iron and riboflavin than fish fillets.

DESCRIPTION A web-footed amphibian, the frog varies in colour (brown to green) and in size. In the USA and Asia some species are more than twice the size of those indigenous to Europe. Frogs eaten in France are very muscular and plump. The meat is light and easily digestible, rather like chicken in flavour.

ORIGIN AND HISTORY Frogs' legs have long been a French delicacy. The French chef Escoffier is credited with making them acceptable to the English. In China they are served at banquets and are known as fried chickens. Keen frog eaters still go frogging in streams and lakes.

BUYING AND STORAGE Available canned and frozen. Once opened or thawed keep in refrigerator 3 days. Wrap in plastic wrap and place in airtight container.

SEASON All year.

PREPARATION AND USE Not all frogs are edible. The ones that are purchased either frozen or canned come from special frog farms. The best preparation is to blanch and skin, then sauté gently in oil/butter until cooked. They can also be poached in white wine or 'southern fried' like chicken legs. They require only a short cooking time.

PROCESSING Frozen or canned.

VARIETIES

There are over 20 species of edible frogs.

Game

Game meats are the flesh of animals which have been traditionally hunted for food. Some of these creatures are now fully protected by law, while others are available under restricted conditions. Others again are raised in captivity and their flesh can be bought in specialist stores.

Those listed in this chapter are buffalo, crocodile, frog, goanna, goat, hare, kangaroo, possum, rabbit, snake, venison, wild boar and, by way of special interest, witchetty grub.

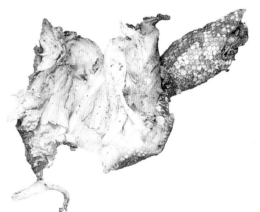

Goanna   *Varanus* spp.

MAJOR NUTRIENTS			SERVE SIZE 100 G
Energy	765 kJ	Cholesterol	0
Protein	34 g	Sodium	60 mg
Fat	5 g	Iron	3 mg
Carbohydrate	0	Zinc	4.5 mg

NUTRITIONAL INFORMATION Like most wild meat, goanna is low in fat.

DESCRIPTION A plump reptile that yields succulent flesh.

ORIGIN AND HISTORY The goanna is a relative of the iguana, which in ancient Peru and Mexico was a great delicacy, relished by the kings. The Aborigines of Australia judge the goanna by the amount of fat in the body, which determines its value as a food and delicacy.

BUYING AND STORAGE Goannas are a fully protected species in Australia and the laws relating to killing and eating them are similar to the ones which apply to snakes. Goanna flesh is not available commercially.

PREPARATION AND USE According to traditional cooking methods, if the goanna has plenty of fat it must not be held up too long by the neck, or the thin membrane holding the fat will break. It is placed on the fire and turned over until all scales become crisp. It may also be cooked lengthwise in a ground oven.

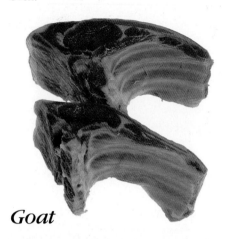

Goat

MAJOR NUTRIENTS   SERVE SIZE 100 G

Energy	540 kJ	Sodium	0
Protein	13 g	Phosphorus	150 mg
Fat	9 g	Iron	1.5 mg
Carbohydrate	0	Thiamin	1.5 mg
Cholesterol	N/A	Niacin Equiv.	7.6 mg

NUTRITIONAL INFORMATION Goat meat is very similar in nutritional value to beef. It is an excellent source of niacin and thiamin; a good source of phosphorus and iron; and it contains moderate amounts of fat.

DESCRIPTION The meat of young kid goats is mild and succulent.

ORIGIN AND HISTORY In Mediterranean countries and parts of the Middle East, chevreau or kid is eaten as a delicacy. Aged between six weeks to four months, it is cooked whole and, at festivities on certain Mediterranean islands, is wrapped in myrtle leaves and slowly baked in an underground oven. There are many varieties of wild goats to be found. The chamois and Rocky Mountain goat meats are valued in North America for their mild, gamy character. Wild goats in Australia should be treated in the same way as venison.

BUYING AND STORAGE Only the domestic varieties are available commercially and may be purchased from specialist butcher shops that cater for ethnic groups. The meat must be refrigerated and may be frozen.

PREPARATION AND USE Kid may be roasted whole, either on a spit or in the oven, and the meat is popular in curries. Treat more mature meat as venison.

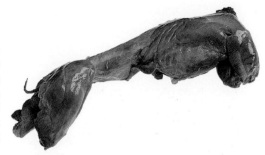

Hare

MAJOR NUTRIENTS   STEWED
               SERVE SIZE 100 G

Energy	804 kJ	Total Sugars	0
Protein	30 g	Sodium	0
Fat	8 g	Phosphorus	250 mg
Cholesterol	71 mg	Iron	10.8 mg
Carbohydrate	0		

NUTRITIONAL INFORMATION No data are available for vitamin content. Excellent source of protein, iron and phosphorus; moderate in fat and cholesterol.

DESCRIPTION The long-eared, swift-running hare lives above ground and, unlike the rabbit, sleeps in a 'form' among grass. It has been hunted through the centuries both for the speed and excitement of the chase and for the distinctive flavour of its flesh.

ORIGIN AND HISTORY Originally from Europe, hares belong to the same family as the rabbit, but are a larger, longer-legged species, with reddish-brown flesh and a rich, gamy flavour. A young hare, up to the age of six months, is known as a leveret. It has soft ears, white teeth, and smooth fur.

BUYING AND STORAGE Can be purchased skinned and cleaned, ready to cook, from a number of butchers, specialty poultry and game stores, and delicatessens. Keep refrigerated and use as soon as possible.

PREPARATION AND USE Young hares do not need hanging and can be fresh roasted. Older animals are usually hung for a few days to improve the flavour, then gutted and skinned. The traditional British method is to 'jug' the hare by gently casseroling the joints in a well-flavoured red wine sauce to which the hare's blood is added just before serving.

Heads

NUTRITIONAL INFORMATION There are no detailed analyses available for whole heads.

DESCRIPTION Heads can be purchased whole or in separate parts, that is, skin (lamb's heads are sold shorn, pig's and calf's heads have hair removed), snout, cheek, ears, tongue, and brains. Ox heads are large and are not usually available.

ORIGIN AND HISTORY Boar's head made its appearance as a gala dish in England in the 14th century. At medieval feasts it was preceded by trumpets and followed by a train of ladies and gentlemen. The tradition of serving boar's head at Christmas to the accompaniment of carols has been carried over to the 20th century at Queen's College in Oxford. Head cheese is a kind of sausage consisting of meat from calf's and pig's head, seasoned and moulded in its own natural jelly. Head cheese (called brawn in England) is traditional in English and northern European cuisine.

BUYING AND STORAGE See Offal for purchasing and storage instructions. Fresh heads can be cleaned and prepared for cooking and then successfully frozen, but ensure they have not been frozen before purchase.

PREPARATION AND USE Also see section on Brains and Tongue. Pigs' heads are used mainly for brawn and sausages. Calf and lamb may be boned or left whole but they are usually divided into pieces — tongue, cheeks and so on. Soak head in salted water to draw out the blood — add vinegar to the water for calf's or pig's head to lighten the skin and keep covered with acidulated water until required for cooking.

Blanch the head by covering it with cold water, bring to the boil and simmer for 5 minutes, drain, refresh.

Poach the head in court bouillon for 2–3 hours until tender.

After precooking the head can be braised, sautéed or grilled. Lamb's head can be roasted without precooking. Heads are used to make brawn or head cheese, which is discussed in the chapter on sausages and preserved meats.

VARIETIES
Pig, calf, lamb.

SEE ALSO Brains, Brawn, Offal, Tongue.

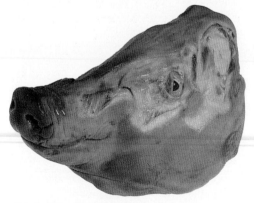

Pig's Head

Hearts

MAJOR NUTRIENTS		HEART OF LAMB OR CALF, ROASTED SERVE SIZE 120 G	
Energy	1190 kJ	Phosphorus	470 mg
Protein	136 g	Magnesium	26 mg
Fat	9 g	Iron	9.2 mg
Cholesterol	225 mg	Zinc	4.5 mg
Carbohydrate	0	Thiamin	0.4 mg
Total Sugars	0	Riboflavin	1.7 mg
Sodium	90 mg	Niacin Equiv.	12.7 mg
Potassium	320 mg	Vitamin C	13 mg

NUTRITIONAL INFORMATION Although only 28% of the total energy comes from fat, the fat in this product contains significant amounts of cholesterol, almost 100% of total recommended daily intake. Provides almost total daily requirements of phosphorus, iron, zinc, niacin and vitamin B12, so has a useful role in a varied low total fat diet.

DESCRIPTION The heart of a beast is its most hard-working muscle and has dark red meat surrounded by fatty tissue.

ORIGIN AND HISTORY Eating the heart of an animal has always had strong symbolic meaning for people, but present-day cuisine does not give it a special place.

BUYING AND STORAGE Lamb and calf hearts have a flavour not unlike the normal meat of these animals. Ox hearts have a strong beefy flavour. Heart is a popular pet food, therefore should be ordered to ensure the freshest and the best quality available.

See Offal for storage instructions.

PREPARATION AND USE Remove any fat from around the heart. Rinse well and remove flaps, lobes and membrane dividing the cavities. Soak ox heart in cold water with 1 tablespoon of vinegar added. Drain, rinse and dry. Leave whole, stuff and roast, or cut as required and braise, sauté, grill or use in casseroles or stews.

Heart has a dense muscular structure and care should be taken not to overcook it as it will dry and toughen. If grilling or roasting is the selected method be sure to serve the heart while still pink.

VARIETIES
Calf, lamb, ox, pig.

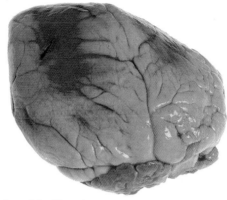

Lamb's Heart

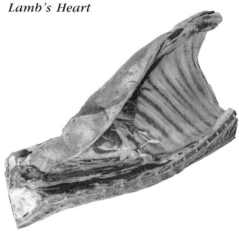

Hogget

also called Two-tooth

NUTRITIONAL INFORMATION The nutritional value of cuts of hogget is similar to that of lamb cuts.

DESCRIPTION Hogget is the name given to sheep meat that is older than lamb but not as old as mutton. A hogget is judged by dentition and has no more than one pair of permanent incisors, which usually means it is between 15 and 30 months old. Hogget is an underrated meat which, though not as sweet or tender as lamb, produces dishes that are tasty and flavoursome.

ORIGIN AND HISTORY Like young lamb, hogget has come to be more appreciated in Europe in this century. Previously, more mature sheep meat was preferred.

BUYING AND STORAGE Hogget can be identified at point of purchase by an official brown HGT strip brand applied to the external fat selvage by meat inspectors. If the meat does not have a brand it has to be considered mutton. Hogget is a darker red in colour than lamb and has firm, white fat. It should be stored in the same way as lamb.

PREPARATION AND USE See Lamb for cuts.

Depending upon the season and the condition of the animal, the loin and chump may not be suitable for grilling or pan frying. These cuts may be better braised or roasted.

SEE ALSO Lamb.

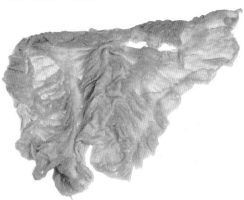

Hog Maw

MAJOR NUTRIENTS		SERVE SIZE 100 G	
Energy	250 kJ	Sodium	45 mg
Protein	9 g	Potassium	10 mg
Fat	2 g	Iron	0.5 mg
Cholesterol	110 mg	Zinc	1.5 mg
Carbohydrate	0	Niacin Equiv.	1.5 mg
Total Sugars	0		

NUTRITIONAL INFORMATION An excellent source of protein with low amounts of accompanying fats although the fat does contain significant amounts of dietary cholesterol.

DESCRIPTION Hog maw is a term meaning the stomach of a pig.

ORIGIN AND HISTORY In the USA, the Pennsylvania Dutch are well known for their thriftiness in the kitchen and make use of everything edible, including hog maw. It is stuffed and made into a large sausage which is called stuffed goose. In southern USA soul cooking, it is boiled for hours until tender, chopped finely and mixed with salad and mayonnaise.

BUYING AND STORAGE Your friendly butcher will have to order this in specially and there is no guarantee you will get it. Keep refrigerated and use as soon as possible.

PREPARATION AND USE To make stuffed hog maw, thoroughly clean the stomach and remove excess fat from the lining. Dry and stuff loosely with combined stuffing ingredients of well-flavoured minced pork, vegetables and herbs, then seal and braise with cider and beef stock for 3 hours.

Serve sliced, hot or cold.

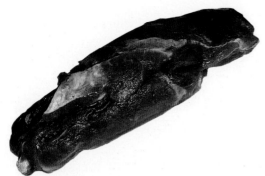

Kangaroo *Macropus* spp.

MAJOR NUTRIENTS		SERVE SIZE 100 G	
Energy	660 kJ	Cholesterol	56 mg
Protein	25 g	Sodium	25 mg
Fat	4 g	Iron	7 mg
Carbohydrate	0	Zinc	3.5 mg

NUTRITIONAL INFORMATION Like other wild meat, kangaroo is low in fat, and its balance of fatty acids is better than that found in the meat of domesticated animals. A rich source of iron and zinc.

DESCRIPTION The kangaroo is a marsupial native to Australia, and has always been one of the principal animals hunted by the people of the land.

ORIGIN AND HISTORY Early settlers from Europe shot kangaroo as a pest rather than for food, but all of the meat is good to eat. It has been described as more tender than beef and more nourishing than mutton, and the flavour has been compared to that of wild rabbit. There are many recipes for both kangaroo and wallaby in early Australian cookery books and the meat has been grilled, curried, jugged, larded, braised, potted, roasted, and made into pies, soup and stews.

BUYING AND STORAGE The kangaroo is a protected species throughout Australia, and it is illegal to slaughter the animal in the wild, except under special government permit.

Kangaroos have been raised in captivity for many years, for the export meat trade. Regulations within Australia are changing with relation to domestic consumption, and kangaroo meat is becoming steadily more available to the consumer, depending on the food standards regulations in the various states.

PREPARATION AND USE The head of a kangaroo, split open and thoroughly washed, makes an excellent stew along with the tail. The tail can be used as a basis for stews or made into soup. The leg can be cooked by a long, slow method in well-seasoned stock. Simmer fillets in kangaroo stock for an hour with bouquet garni, redcurrant jelly, lemon zest and raisins.

Kidney

MAJOR NUTRIENTS		LAMB, OX AND CALF SERVE SIZE 90 G	
Energy	510 kJ	Phosphorus	320 mg
Protein	24 g	Iron	8 mg
Fat	4 g	Zinc	2.8 mg
Cholesterol	460 mg	Thiamin	0.3 mg
Carbohydrate	0	Riboflavin	2.3 mg
Total Sugars	0	Niacin Equiv.	8.8 mg
Sodium	160 mg	Vitamin C	6 mg
Potassium	240 mg		

NUTRITIONAL INFORMATION A low total fat containing product with 29% of energy coming from fats. The fats present contain significant quantities of cholesterol, more than is recommended as the ideal daily intake. Especially good source of protein, iron and vitamin B12, although pig's kidney has a lower B12 level than other sources.

DESCRIPTION Lamb's kidneys have only one lobe, while calf and ox kidneys have numerous lobes. Kidneys are encased in suet fat which is usually removed before sale.

ORIGIN AND HISTORY Early Europeans believed that kidneys bestowed courage and strength on those who ate them. Since the beginning of this century kidneys have not enjoyed the same popularity, although they are still featured in classic French cuisine. In parts of the Middle East where whole animals are roasted, the kidney is considered the choicest part. Throughout Africa, kidneys are still singled out as a treat.

BUYING AND STORAGE Choose round, plump kidneys. The colour will vary from light to dark browny-red, depending upon the age of the animal. For storage, see Offal.

PREPARATION AND USE Make a split in the surface membrane and peel off with the fingers. Halve the kidney and remove the fatty core. The flavour can be reduced by soaking in cold water for 30 minutes. Drain, rinse and dry well before using.

Kidneys can be grilled, sautéed and braised. Ox kidneys are traditionally used in steak and kidney pudding.

VARIETIES
Calf, lamb, ox, pig.

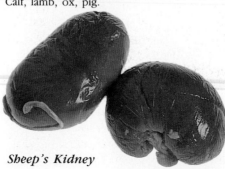

Sheep's Kidney

Lamb

DESCRIPTION There are three types of sheep meat: lamb, hogget and mutton. Lamb is sweet, tender meat which is deep pink in colour with fine, white fat, while the older meats are darker, with a more pronounced flavour.

ORIGIN AND HISTORY Sheep have been domesticated for many thousands of years. In early times sheep and goats were kept to provide milk.

In Victorian times mutton was favoured over young lamb. Mutton under two years old was considered by the epicure of the day to be 'flabby, pale and savourless' and to suit this discerning palate the sheep would never be killed earlier than 3 years or later than 5 years. Opinions about the merits of mutton and lamb changed at the beginning of the century when the popularity of the sweet, succulent flavour of lamb grew.

Modern breeding techniques have produced lambs which gain weight rapidly so it is possible to produce a leaner, meaty product younger.

Sheep meats have featured in the cuisine of many nations. In the cuisines of the British Isles, Europe, North Africa, the Middle East, and Muslim India sheep meat is the dominant meat. Archaeological evidence in Iraq shows that the preference for sheep meat was already established in 9000 BC, so it is understandable that the Middle Eastern countries have a whole gamut of mutton and lamb recipes.

BUYING AND STORAGE Lamb is at its very best during spring.

In Australia sheep meats are branded according to their age, judged by the dentition of the beast. The red lamb brand is applied to sheep without any permanent teeth (usually younger than 12 months), a brown HGT brand is applied to sheep with one pair of permanent incisors (usually between 15–30 months and called hogget or two-tooth) and any sheep meat that is not branded must be sold as mutton.

Store lamb in the meat keeper or in the coldest part of the refrigerator, on a plate or rack loosely covered with plastic film or foil, allowing a little air to circulate around the meat.

To freeze, pack lamb in meal-size portions into freezer bags (high density plastic bags). Interleave small cuts with plastic. Remove all the air from the bag, seal, label and date. Freeze as quickly as possible.

To thaw loosen the packaging and thaw in

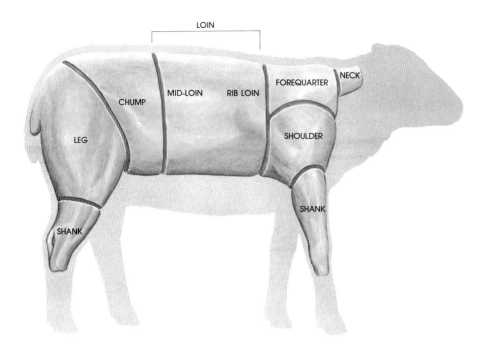

LOIN

CHUMP | MID-LOIN | RIB LOIN | FOREQUARTER | NECK

LEG

SHOULDER

SHANK

SHANK

MAJOR NUTRIENTS		LAMB LEG, TRIMMED, ROASTED
		SERVE SIZE 60 G
Energy	690 kJ	Potassium	175 mg
Protein	18 g	Phosphorus	120 mg
Fat	7 g	Iron	1.4 mg
Cholesterol	65 mg	Zinc	2.7 mg
Carbohydrate	0	Riboflavin	0.15 mg
Total Sugars	0	Niacin Equiv.	5.7 mg
Sodium	40 mg		

NUTRITIONAL INFORMATION Has moderate levels of fat which contribute 37% of total energy. Excellent source of protein, phosphorus, iron, zinc, niacin and vitamin B12. Extra trimming before cooking may reduce fat levels.

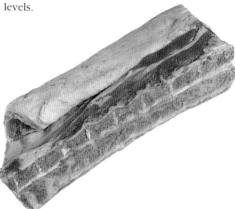

Loin Contains the eight ribs and the mid-loin which is the most tender cut of the lamb.

the refrigerator, or in the microwave in accordance with distributors' instructions. Small cuts are best cooked frozen.

HINDQUARTER CUTS

excellent, their value to the total diet is compromised by the high fat (predominantly saturated fat) and also cholesterol levels. Fat levels may be reduced by trimming before cooking.

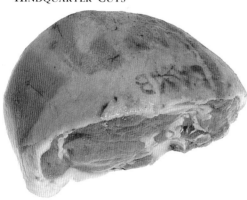

Chump Cut between the legs and the loin: available in a piece for roasting, or cut into chops and grilled, pan fried or barbecued.

MAJOR NUTRIENTS	LAMB CHUMP CHOPS, GRILLED
	SERVE SIZE 120 G
Energy	1410 kJ	Phosphorus	250 mg
Protein	35 g	Magnesium	31 mg
Fat	22 g	Iron	3.7 mg
Cholesterol	130 mg	Zinc	5 mg
Carbohydrate	0	Thiamin	5.65 mg
Total Sugars	0	Riboflavin	0.3 mg
Sodium	85 mg	Niacin Equiv.	9.6 mg
Potassium	310 mg		

NUTRITIONAL INFORMATION Fat can contribute over 57% of total energy of this cut of lamb. If eaten in the untrimmed form, although levels of protein, phosphorus, iron, zinc, riboflavin, niacin and vitamin B12 are

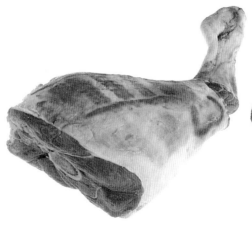

Leg Most commonly roasted on the bone. The bone can be removed either by cutting through the meat down to the bone and then cutting along the length of the bone to remove it, or by tunnel boning, that is, tunnelling down the side of the bone from the top of the leg, loosening, turning and removing the bone, leaving the leg whole. The boned leg is usually filled with a stuffing before roasting. A butterfly leg is boned and laid flat. It can be marinaded and then roasted or barbecued.

Legs are also available corned for boiling. Hoggett and mutton leg are most commonly used for corning. Leg steaks are cut from the top of the leg for grilling or braising.

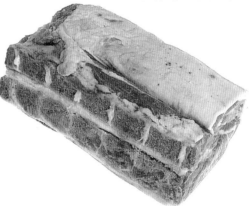

Mid-loin or Short loin Available in a piece with the bone in, boned for roasting, or cut into chops for grilling or dry frying.

Lamb fillets should be cut from the underside of the mid-loin but it is a very small piece of meat in a lamb and the rib eye is better for a recipe asking for this cut.

MAJOR NUTRIENTS		MID-LOIN CHOPS, GRILLED
		SERVE SIZE 70 G
Energy	1060 kJ	Potassium	175 mg
Protein	15 g	Phosphorus	150 mg
Fat	22 g	Iron	1.4 mg
Cholesterol	80 mg	Zinc	2.1 mg
Carbohydrate	0	Riboflavin	0.1 mg
Total Sugars	0	Niacin Equiv.	4.8 mg
Sodium	60 mg		

NUTRITIONAL INFORMATION Fat can contribute over 77% of total energy of this cut of lamb. If eaten in the untrimmed form, although levels of protein, phosphorus, iron, zinc, riboflavin, niacin and vitamin B12 are excellent, their value to the total diet is compromised by the high fat and cholesterol levels. Fat levels may be reduced markedly by trimming before cooking.

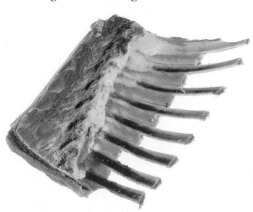

Ribs In a piece for roasting, racks of lamb, guard of honour and crown roasts are all made from the ribs.

Rib Chops Trimmed for cutlets; can be grilled. Cutlets are popular coated with egg and breadcrumbs, then pan fried.

MAJOR NUTRIENTS		LAMB RIB-LOIN CUTLETS/ RIB CHOPS SERVE SIZE 70 G	
Energy	990 kJ	Sodium	60 mg
Protein	16 g	Potassium	195 mg
Fat	19 g	Phosphorus	140 mg
Cholesterol	75 mg	Iron	1.3 mg
Carbohydrate	0	Zinc	1.9 mg
Total Sugars	0	Niacin Equiv.	5.6 mg

NUTRITIONAL INFORMATION Fat can contribute over 77% of total energy of this cut of lamb. If eaten in the untrimmed form, although levels of protein, phosphorus, iron, zinc, riboflavin, niacin and vitamin B12 are excellent, their value to the total diet is compromised by the high fat and cholesterol levels.

Rib Eye The piece of meat that runs through the ribs with the fat and bone removed. Suitable for pan frying or roasting.

MAJOR NUTRIENTS		LAMB RIB EYE, ROASTED SERVE SIZE 60 G SLICES	
Energy	475 kJ	Potassium	170 mg
Protein	18 g	Phosphorus	240 mg
Fat	4 g	Iron	1.5 mg
Cholesterol	65 mg	Zinc	2.8 mg
Carbohydrate	0	Riboflavin	0.17 mg
Total Sugars	0	Niacin Equiv.	5.8 mg
Sodium	40 mg		

NUTRITIONAL INFORMATION Moderate to low levels of fat in this lamb cut, with about 30% of total energy coming from fat sources and less than 20% of daily recommended cholesterol intake quantities. Therefore an excellent dietary source of protein, phosphorus, iron, zinc, niacin and vitamin B12.

FOREQUARTER CUTS

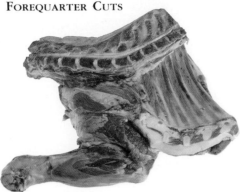

Whole Forequarter Can be roasted with bone in but it is much easier to carve if the bones are removed. A square cut forequarter has the shank, neck and breast removed — the boned forequarter can be stuffed and rolled before roasting.

MAJOR NUTRIENTS		STUFFED, ROASTED SERVE SIZE 60 G	
Energy	720 kJ	Potassium	145 mg
Protein	11 g	Phosphorus	90 mg
Fat	13 g	Iron	1.1 mg
Cholesterol	70 mg	Zinc	1.7 mg
Carbohydrate	0	Riboflavin	0.15 mg
Total Sugars	0	Niacin Equiv.	3.7 mg
Sodium	130 mg		

NUTRITIONAL INFORMATION High fat with over 65% of energy coming from fats. If roasted with polyunsaturated fats, however, the total cholesterol level is only about 20% of recommended daily intake. Contains excellent amounts of protein, phosphorus, iron, zinc, niacin and vitamin B12. Useful if consumed in an overall low fat diet.

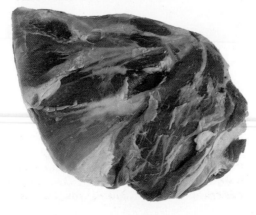

Shoulder Includes the shank clod, bone in, or boned for easy carving, or cut into pieces for kebabs or casseroles.

MAJOR NUTRIENTS		ROASTED SERVE SIZE 60 G	
Energy	790 kJ	Potassium	155 mg
Protein	15 g	Phosphorus	90 mg
Fat	12 g	Iron	1.1 mg
Cholesterol	70 mg	Zinc	3.1 mg
Carbohydrate	0	Riboflavin	0.15 mg
Total Sugars	0	Niacin Equiv.	2.4 mg
Sodium	50 mg		

NUTRITIONAL INFORMATION High fat cut with over 65% of energy coming from fats, although if roasted with polyunsaturated fats the total cholesterol level is only about 20% of recommended daily intake. Contains excellent amounts of protein, phosphorus, iron, zinc, niacin and vitamin B12. Useful if consumed in an overall low fat diet. Trimming fat before cooking could reduce total fat intake.

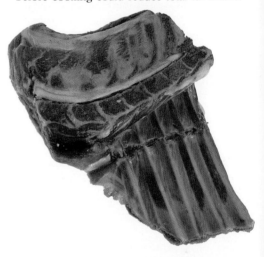

Neck Chops Those referred to as best neck chops are cut from the section where the neck joins the forequarter. The small rosettes are cut from higher on the neck. Neck chops are usually braised or used in stews.

MAJOR NUTRIENTS		STEWED SERVE SIZE 110 G	
Energy	1630 kJ	Potassium	230 mg
Protein	30 g	Phosphorus	190 mg
Fat	30 g	Magnesium	22 mg
Cholesterol	120 mg	Iron	2.6 mg
Carbohydrate	0	Zinc	8.5 mg
Total Sugars	0	Riboflavin	0.25 mg
Sodium	60 mg	Niacin Equiv.	7.8 mg

NUTRITIONAL INFORMATION High levels of fat in this cut with over 68% of energy and up to 40% of recommended daily cholesterol intake coming from fat. This serving provides major amounts of zinc and vitamin B12 as well as being an important source of iron and niacin. The fat level may be reduced by trimming before cooking.

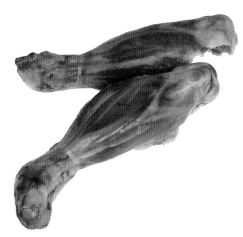

Shank Forequarter shanks are used in casseroles and stews.

MAJOR NUTRIENTS			STEWED SERVE SIZE 250 G
Energy	1400 kJ	Potassium	360 mg
Protein	46 g	Phosphorus	285 mg
Fat	16 g	Magnesium	34 mg
Cholesterol	110 mg	Iron	4.8 mg
Carbohydrate	0	Zinc	13 mg
Total Sugars	0	Riboflavin	0.3 mg
Sodium	120 mg	Niacin Equiv.	10.3 mg

NUTRITIONAL INFORMATION Moderate fat levels in this tasty cut, with up to 42% of energy being supplied by fats, which contain over one-third of recommended daily cholesterol intake. Excellent protein, iron, zinc, riboflavin, niacin and vitamin B12 make this a useful, relatively inexpensive source of these nutrients in an otherwise low fat diet.

SEE ALSO Hogget, Mutton.

Lights

also called **Lungs**

NUTRITIONAL INFORMATION No nutritional analysis available. Not widely or regularly used in quantities to make a significant contribution to nutrition.

DESCRIPTION Lights is the name used for the lungs, which provide lean meat for stuffing and sausages. In Australia, lights are only available fresh in NSW and are not used in manufactured meats.

ORIGIN AND HISTORY A less widely used form of offal.

BUYING AND STORAGE Lungs should be bright red in colour and spongy in texture. They will need to be ordered, purchased fresh and used within 24 hours. For storage, see notes under Offal.

PREPARATION AND USE Remove loose pieces of fat, gristle and the windpipe. Cut as required. Lungs can be braised or grilled, used in stuffing or homemade sausages.

VARIETIES
Calf, pig.

SEE ALSO Offal, Pluck.

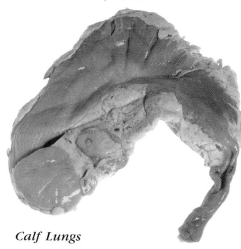

Calf Lungs

Liver

MAJOR NUTRIENTS	LIVER OF LAMB, CALF OR OX, BRAISED SERVE SIZE 90 G		
Energy	830 kJ	Phosphorus	420 mg
Protein	23 g	Magnesium	22 mg
Fat	10 g	Iron	6 mg
Cholesterol	370 mg	Zinc	5 mg
Carbohydrate	0	Vitamin A	1755 µg
Total Sugars	0	Thiamin	0.1 mg
Sodium	65 mg	Riboflavin	4.4 mg
Potassium	260 mg	Niacin Equiv.	10.6 mg

NUTRITIONAL INFORMATION Although it is moderately high in fats, with 42% of energy coming from fat, these are very concentrated sources of cholesterol. A serving provides more than the recommended daily intake. Very high levels of vitamin A, folate and vitamin B12 mean that these products can have a useful role as a small part of a varied diet.

DESCRIPTION The liver is the organ which purifies the blood of an animal. The meat is dark brown and glistening, with a strong, distinctive flavour. It is easily cut or minced when raw, and stiffens on contact with heat.

ORIGIN AND HISTORY Liver was considered to be the repository of the manly virtues such as courage and virility. The Latin poet Horace (65BC–AD8) mentioned liver as a popular aphrodisiac of his time. Perhaps this is the reason why liver has featured in many cuisines of many different nations. Liver is considered a valuable supplement for those who suffer from anaemia, and for athletes in training.

BUYING AND STORAGE The colour of the liver will vary from light red-brown (calf liver) through to dark red (ox or pig liver).

Calf liver is generally considered the best and is highly prized for its tenderness and flavour. It should be purchased in one piece and sliced just before use.

See Offal for storage instructions.

PREPARATION AND USE Rinse liver; carefully remove the membrane that covers the liver by making a small incision, loosen and gently (with the fingers) pull the membrane away. Hold liver down to prevent tearing. If the membrane is difficult to remove soak in cold water for 10 minutes.

Ox and pig livers are best if sliced and soaked in milk for 1–2 hours to reduce the strong flavour before roasting or braising the pig's liver or braising or stewing the ox liver. Lamb, calf and chicken livers can be grilled, fried or roasted.

PROCESSING Livers can be processed and baked in a terrine or cooked and processed for pâtés.

SEE ALSO Offal.

VARIETIES
Lamb (usually called lamb's fry), pig, calf.

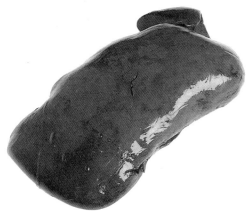

Calf's Liver

Mutton

NUTRITIONAL INFORMATION The major nutrients of mutton are detailed under the different cuts of lamb. Cuts may have greater visible fat covering than equivalent lamb cuts and this should be well trimmed or removed before cooking.

DESCRIPTION Mutton is mature sheep meat.

ORIGIN AND HISTORY See Lamb.

BUYING AND STORAGE Mutton should be dark red in colour with hard, white fat. It should be well trimmed of visible fat before using to produce a strong-flavoured dish. See Lamb for storage.

PREPARATION AND USE Mutton is best suited to moist cooking methods such as stewing or braising, as these help to tenderise the meat. It is ideal for curries.

The legs can be roasted and are often sold corned for boiling.

SEE ALSO Hogget, Lamb.

Offal

also called *Variety meats, Fancy meats*

NUTRITIONAL INFORMATION The major nutrients of offal are listed under brains, hearts, hog maw, kidneys, lights, liver, oxtail, pig's trotters, sweetbreads, tongue and tripe.

DESCRIPTION Offal are the edible off-cuts taken from a carcass when it is dressed. Head, brains, eyeballs, ears, tongue, liver, kidneys, tripe, sweetbreads, heart, spleen, lungs, bones, tail and feet are all offal.

ORIGIN AND HISTORY Throughout history controversy has surrounded the eating of offal. It has been alternately condemned on religious, social or economic grounds or prized for its cultural, nutritional or culinary benefits. Most countries have traditional offal recipes that reflect the cuisine of the region, and offal supplies a rich variety of nutritious meats that have delighted epicures through the ages.

STORAGE AND BUYING Most offal will need to be ordered from a meat supplier to ensure the freshest and best quality is available. Offal deteriorates faster than carcass meat and is best eaten within 24 hours of purchase. Fresh offal should be unwrapped, placed on a dish, covered loosely with plastic wrap or foil, as a little air must be allowed to circulate around the meat, and stored in the coldest part of the refrigerator.

Freezing should be avoided (except for bones, tails or feet), as it adversely affects the flavour, texture and appearance of most offal. If needed offal can be packed in meal-size portions into freezer bags; extract air with a freezer pump, seal, label and store in freezer for up to 2 months. If the offal has been frozen DO NOT REFREEZE. Defrost in the refrigerator 24 hours before required. Most offal with the exception of liver or oxtail can be thawed in cold water.

PREPARATION AND USE Method of cookery will vary with the type of offal. Many offal require gentle poaching or precooking to tenderise, skin or firm the meat for ease of handling. Moist methods of cookery are used to extract flavour from bones, oxtail and so on, and to tenderise tongues, tripe, or trotters. Delicately structured offal — like liver, kidney and brains — need only be quickly sautéed or grilled and simply garnished.

SEE ALSO Bones, Brains, Heads, Heart, Hog Maw, Kidney, Lights, Livers, Oxtail, Pig's Trotters, Sweetbreads, Tongue and Tripe.

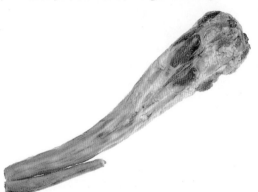

Oxtail

MAJOR NUTRIENTS			STEWED
			SERVE SIZE 300 G
Energy	1700 kJ	Potassium	135 mg
Protein	26 g	Calcium	20 mg
Fat	35 g	Phosphorus	170 mg
Cholesterol	70 mg	Iron	3 mg
Carbohydrate	0	Zinc	5.5 mg
Total Sugars	0	Riboflavin	0.4 mg
Sodium	65 mg	Niacin Equiv.	6.1 mg

NUTRITIONAL INFORMATION Generally a very high fat product, if cooked as purchased. Over 75% of energy comes from fat sources. Otherwise excellent source of protein, phosphorus, iron, zinc, riboflavin and vitamin B12. Careful trimming before cooking can remove much of the fat and as these are best eaten stewed, more fat can be removed if oxtails are cooked the day before eating and excess fat skimmed off.

DESCRIPTION Oxtail is the skinned tail of an ox, used to make soup and stew. It is regarded as an off-cut and is therefore considered an offal or variety meat.

ORIGIN AND HISTORY The oxtail has been a valued flavouring meat for soups and stews over the centuries.

BUYING AND STORAGE Ask the butcher to joint the oxtail. This will produce pieces approximately 5 cm long when cut at the cartilage between the vertebrae. See Offal for notes on storage instructions.

PREPARATION AND USE Oxtail is particularly valued for the rich beef gravy it produces. Rinse in cold water and dry before using in braises, stews, casseroles and soups. Oxtail will require three hours' gentle, moist cooking and is best if cooked the day before serving. Refrigerate to facilitate the removal of fat, which will set on top of the dish. Standing will improve the flavour.

SEE ALSO Offal.

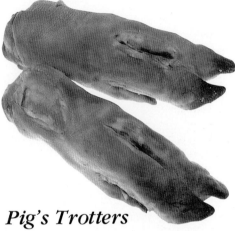

Pig's Trotters

NUTRITIONAL INFORMATION An excellent source of gelatinous protein essential for growth and repair. If eaten with skin, will contain large amounts of fat.

DESCRIPTION Trotters are the feet of the pig.

ORIGIN AND HISTORY Pig's trotters are considered a delicacy by many peoples, and are popular in Europe today, particularly in France.

BUYING AND STORAGE See Offal. Trotters are suitable for freezing but care should be taken to ensure they have not been frozen before purchase.

PREPARATION AND USE Trotters are rich in gelatine and are used to add flavour and body to stocks. They require long, slow simmering to soften the flesh. The trotters can then be grilled or baked.

Pluck

Pluck is the name given to the combination of the heart, lungs and liver of a lamb, goat or pig. For information, see the entries for these meats.

Pork

DESCRIPTION Pork is the white, succulent meat of the domestic pig, prized for its richness and flavour.

ORIGIN AND HISTORY China is perhaps the leading pork-eating nation in the world, though it is also the principal meat of the Pacific and Indonesian islands and of South-East Asia. In ancient Greece and Rome, pigs roamed freely in the streets, and, even in medieval times, wandered around the thoroughfares of London and Paris, where they lived on the refuse. For centuries pork was virtually the only meat eaten by European peasants and the pig has aptly been described as nothing but an immense dish which walks while waiting to be served.

BUYING AND STORAGE Because of consumer demand, pork meat has become leaner and new cuts have recently been developed to allow consumers a wider choice. These should be readily available at most butcher shops. Keep refrigerated, on a plate and lightly covered, and use as soon as possible. May be frozen. The lean of pork should be pale pink, smooth and finely grained and the fat white and firm. It should have no smell.

PREPARATION AND USE Pork should not be undercooked.

HINDQUARTER CUTS

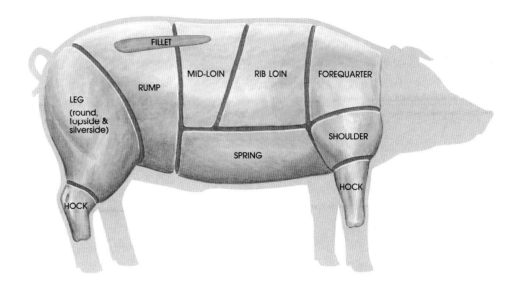

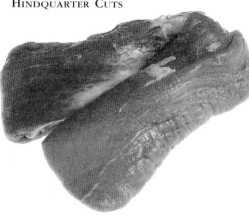

Fillet Medallions, noisettes, escalopes — pan fry or grill. Mignon strips prepared from the tail end of the fillet — quick pan fry dishes such as goulash, stroganoff, curries and Chinese or Malay-style stir-fry dishes.

MAJOR NUTRIENTS		GRILLED SERVE SIZE 100 G	
Energy	780 kJ	Phosphorus	250 mg
Protein	32 g	Magnesium	30 mg
Fat	6 g	Iron	1.2 mg
Cholesterol	85 mg	Zinc	2.9 mg
Carbohydrate	0	Thiamin	0.55 mg
Total Sugars	0	Riboflavin	0.2 mg
Sodium	70 mg	Niacin Equiv.	16.5 mg
Potassium	430 mg		

NUTRITIONAL INFORMATION A leaner cut of pork but still 43% of energy coming from fat. Excellent source of many nutrients if prepared without additional fat.

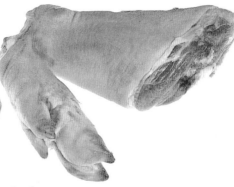

Hock Trussed with bone in — roast, spit roast, pot roast, braise or smoke. Cubed — stew and ragout.

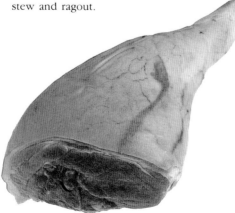

Leg Roast. Skin is scored for a crisp crackling.

MAJOR NUTRIENTS		ROAST, TRIMMED SERVE SIZE 60 G	
Energy	545 kJ	Potassium	170 mg
Protein	19 g	Phosphorus	135 mg
Fat	7 g	Iron	1 mg
Cholesterol	55 mg	Zinc	2 mg
Carbohydrate	0	Thiamin	0.4 mg
Total Sugars	0	Riboflavin	0.15 mg
Sodium	30 mg	Niacin Equiv.	3.5 mg

NUTRITIONAL INFORMATION A moderately lean source of animal protein with fat contributing 47% total energy. Contains important amounts of zinc, phosphorus and niacin as well as other nutrients. Final fat level depends on amount added in cooking and degree of trimming: fats are predominantly monounsaturated.

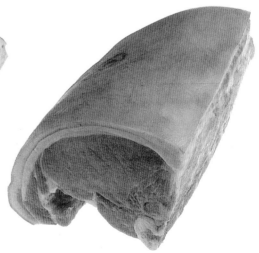

Mid-loin Boned — roast. Rosette, steak, chop — pan fry or grill.

101

MAJOR NUTRIENTS

TRIMMED
SERVE SIZE 150 G

Energy	1730 kJ	Phosphorus	400 mg
Protein	46 g	Magnesium	20 mg
Fat	22 g	Iron	1.5 mg
Cholesterol	150 mg	Zinc	3 mg
Carbohydrate	0	Thiamin	1.3 mg
Total Sugars	0	Riboflavin	0.4 mg
Sodium	100 mg	Niacin Equiv.	9.2 mg
Potassium	460 mg		

NUTRITIONAL INFORMATION Although an excellent source of protein, this cut contains about 47% of total energy in the form of fat with significant amounts of cholesterol. As such a concentrated source of iron, zinc, thiamin, riboflavin and niacin, it can be included regularly in the diet. Fat content (predominantly monounsaturated) may be reduced by more careful trimming.

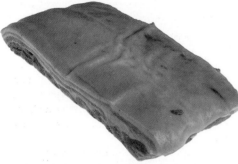

Pork Spring (rib section) Roast, smoke, grill or pan fry. Spare ribs can be presented in either Chinese or USA style. Boned and rolled with its lean meat surface on the outside, and a pocket filled with minced pork and fresh herbs, pork spring is presented in stretch netting for roasting.

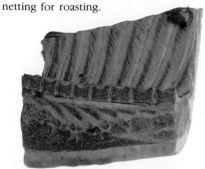

Rib Loin Crown roast, guard of honour, or rack roast. Cutlet, steak, USA-style spare ribs — grill or barbecue.

MAJOR NUTRIENTS

PORK SPRING, SPARE RIBS, BRAISED
SERVE SIZE 90 G

Energy	1240 kJ	Phosphorus	150 mg
Protein	13 g	Magnesium	25 mg
Fat	26 g	Iron	2.1 mg
Cholesterol	90 mg	Zinc	2.2 mg
Carbohydrate	0	Thiamin	0.4 mg
Total Sugars	0	Riboflavin	0.2 mg
Sodium	50 mg	Niacin Equiv.	7.1 mg
Potassium	350 mg		

NUTRITIONAL INFORMATION A very tasty cut of pork but extremely high in fat with over 77% of energy coming from fat. Excellent source of many nutrients but because of the high fat content (predominantly monounsaturated), it should not be included on a regular basis in a diet. Sodium level will increase if cooked with soya sauce. With perseverance excess fat can be removed in the kitchen before cooking. It is not possible to turn this into a lean cut.

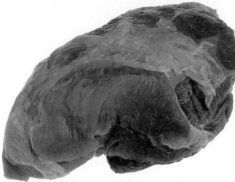

Round Roast, pot roast, braise, smoke or pickle.

MAJOR NUTRIENTS

TRIMMED
SERVE SIZE 150 G

Energy	1005 kJ	Phosphorus	375 mg
Protein	45 g	Magnesium	45 mg
Fat	6 g	Iron	2.4 mg
Cholesterol	126 mg	Zinc	4.5 mg
Carbohydrate	0	Thiamin	1.2 mg
Total Sugars	0	Riboflavin	0.5 mg
Sodium	90 mg	Niacin Equiv.	17 mg
Potassium	645 mg		

NUTRITIONAL INFORMATION A very lean source of protein with fat contributing only 22% of total energy, but the fat still contains significant amounts of cholesterol. Especially useful source of iron, zinc, thiamin and niacin. If conventional cuts used, fat content will be higher.

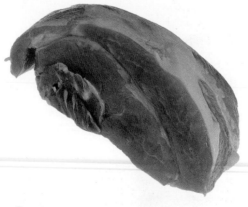

Rump In the piece — roast, pot roast, braise. Steak/escalope — pan fry or grill. Cubed — braise, stew or shashlik.

MAJOR NUTRIENTS

TRIMMED
SERVE SIZE 150 G

Energy	1005 kJ	Phosphorus	375 mg
Protein	45 g	Magnesium	45 mg
Fat	6 g	Iron	2.3 mg
Cholesterol	126 mg	Zinc	4.5 mg
Carbohydrate	0	Thiamin	1.2 mg
Total Sugars	0	Riboflavin	0.55 mg
Sodium	90 mg	Niacin Equiv.	17 mg
Potassium	645 mg		

NUTRITIONAL INFORMATION A very lean source of protein with fat contributing only 22% of total energy, but the fat still contains significant amounts of cholesterol. Especially useful source of iron, zinc, thiamin and niacin. If conventional cuts used, fat content will be higher.

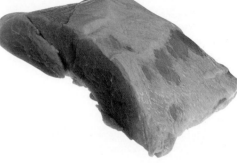

Silverside Roast, smoke or pickle. Main silverside muscle — paupiette or roulade. Slice for medallion — pan fry or grill.

MAJOR NUTRIENTS

TRIMMED
SERVE SIZE 150 G

Energy	1005 kJ	Phosphorus	375 mg
Protein	45 g	Magnesium	45 mg
Fat	6 g	Iron	2.3 mg
Cholesterol	126 mg	Zinc	4.5 mg
Carbohydrate	0	Thiamin	1.2 mg
Total Sugars	0	Riboflavin	0.5 mg
Sodium	90 mg	Niacin Equiv.	18 mg
Potassium	645 mg		

NUTRITIONAL INFORMATION A very lean source of protein with fat contributing only 22% of total energy, but the fat still contains significant amounts of cholesterol. Especially useful source of iron, zinc, thiamin and niacin. If conventional cuts used, fat content will be higher.

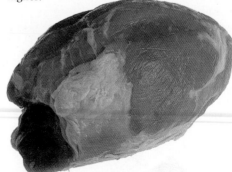

Topside Rolled and trussed — braise or pot

roast. Cubed — stew or ragout. Some of the meat is also suitable for shashlik and escalope.

MAJOR NUTRIENTS

		TRIMMED SERVE SIZE 150 G	
Energy	1005 kJ	Potassium	645 mg
Protein	45 g	Phosphorus	375 mg
Fat	6 g	Magnesium	45 mg
Cholesterol	126 mg	Iron	2.2 mg
Carbohydrate	0	Zinc	4.4 mg
Total Sugars	0	Thiamin	1.2 mg
Dietary Fibre	0	Riboflavin	0.5 mg
Sodium	90 mg	Niacin Equiv.	17.2 mg

NUTRITIONAL INFORMATION A very lean source of protein with fat contributing only 22% of total energy, but the fat still contains significant amounts of cholesterol. Especially useful source of iron, zinc, thiamin and niacin. If conventional cuts used, fat content will be higher.

FOREQUARTER CUTS

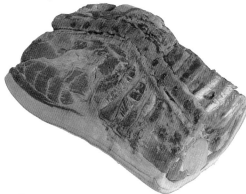

Forequarter Foreloin, chops and neck muscle. Roast, grill, pan fry, ragout, fricassee, shashlik, satay.

MAJOR NUTRIENTS

		FOREQUARTER CHOP, GRILLED SERVE SIZE 190 G	
Energy	1860 kJ	Calcium	57 mg
Protein	49 g	Phosphorus	320 mg
Fat	27 g	Magnesium	30 mg
Cholesterol	175 mg	Iron	3 mg
Carbohydrate	0	Zinc	8 mg
Total Sugars	0	Thiamin	0.9 mg
Sodium	150 mg	Riboflavin	0.55 mg
Potassium	656 mg	Niacin Equiv.	15.7 mg

NUTRITIONAL INFORMATION A moderately high fat cut of pork, 50% of energy coming from fat sources. Excellent source of phosphorus, iron, zinc, thiamin, riboflavin and niacin and so should be considered as a regular food in a varied diet. There is a predominance of monounsaturated fats. Can be further de-fatted.

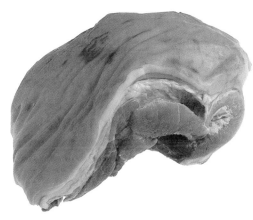

Shoulder Boned. Tempura, Mongolian barbecue meat, tandoori-style, barbecue, Chinese stir-fry dishes, teriyaki style dishes, ragout or fricassee.

MAJOR NUTRIENTS

		BONED, DE-FATTED SERVE SIZE 120 G	
Energy	1240 kJ	Phosphorus	280 mg
Protein	32 g	Magnesium	32 mg
Fat	18 g	Iron	1.5 mg
Cholesterol	105 mg	Zinc	4.2 mg
Carbohydrate	0	Thiamin	2.5 mg
Total Sugars	0	Riboflavin	2.3 mg
Sodium	70 mg	Niacin Equiv.	13.1 mg
Potassium	450 mg		

NUTRITIONAL INFORMATION A moderately high fat cut of pork, 55% of energy coming from fat sources. Excellent source of phosphorus, iron, zinc, thiamin, riboflavin and niacin and so should be considered as a regular food in a varied diet. Moderate source of magnesium.

SEE ALSO Chitterlings, Crackling, Hog maw, Pig's trotters.

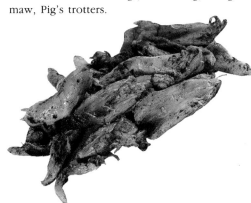

Possum Trichosurus spp.

also called Opossum

MAJOR NUTRIENTS

		SERVE SIZE 100 G	
Energy	700 kJ	Cholesterol	0
Protein	34 g	Sodium	200 mg
Fat	4 g	Iron	10 mg
Carbohydrate	0	Zinc	4 mg

NUTRITIONAL INFORMATION Like most wild meat, possum flesh is low in fat.

DESCRIPTION The possum is a furred marsupial which forages at night and has plump, white flesh.

ORIGIN AND HISTORY Australian possums were part of the Aboriginal meat diet and, judging by the number of recipes in early Australian cookery books, were also enjoyed by the early settlers. Because gum leaves are the natural diet of the possum, the flesh has a delicate eucalyptus flavour which is an acquired taste.

BUYING AND STORAGE Possums are a fully protected species throughout Australia, and only one variety, the common brushtail possum, may be hunted — and only in Tasmania, during an open season which lasts for several months of the year. Possum flesh is not legally classed as meat and may not be retailed to the consumer as such.

PREPARATION AND USE In the early days, the possum was cleaned, jointed and put into a hollowed-out pumpkin which was then roasted until the meat was cooked. The Aboriginal way was to simply toss the whole possum on the fire. When it was cooked, the burnt skin and shrunken entrails were removed.

The animal has four musk sacs which must be removed, otherwise the meat will taste 'strong'.

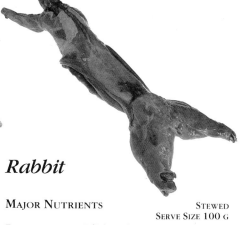

Rabbit

MAJOR NUTRIENTS

		STEWED SERVE SIZE 100 G	
Energy	749 kJ	Phosphorus	200 mg
Protein	27 g	Magnesium	22 mg
Fat	8 g	Iron	2 mg
Cholesterol	71 mg	Thiamin	0.10 mg
Carbohydrate	0	Riboflavin	0.28 mg
Total Sugars	0	Niacin Equiv.	12 mg
Sodium	0		

NUTRITIONAL INFORMATION No data are available for fat-soluble vitamins. Excellent source of protein, phosphorus, iron, riboflavin, niacin, vitamin B12 and vitamin B6; moderate source of magnesium.

DESCRIPTION The rabbit is a furred, burrowing animal which has long been both hunted and raised in captivity for its lean, appetising flesh.

ORIGIN AND HISTORY Originally from Africa, the rabbit migrated across the Mediterranean and then to many other parts of the world. The wild rabbit and hutch rabbit belong to the same species, though their flavour and colour are dissimilar because of the differences in habitat and diet. The wild rabbit is more sinewy, has darker flesh and a gamy taste, whilst the flesh of the hutch rabbit has tender, fine-grained, pale flesh with a slightly nutty flavour.

BUYING AND STORAGE Young rabbits are best to eat and can be identified by their soft ears, white teeth, and smooth fur. Rabbits can be purchased skinned and cleaned, ready to cook, from a number of butchers and delicatessens. Keep refrigerated and use as soon as possible.

PREPARATION AND USE Before cooking, rabbit should be washed and soaked in cold salted water for several hours. Rinse and pat dry, then cook. Young rabbits are usually roasted or sautéed, while older animals are best braised, casseroled or stewed gently with small pieces of salt pork, vegetables and wine, in traditional European fashion.

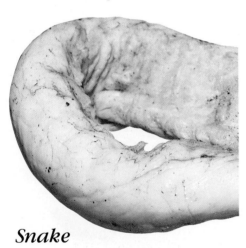

Snake

MAJOR NUTRIENTS   SERVE SIZE 100 G

Energy	490 kJ	Cholesterol	0
Protein	16 g	Sodium	210 mg
Fat	6 g	Iron	10 mg
Carbohydrate	0	Zinc	3 mg

NUTRITIONAL INFORMATION Snake meat is relatively low in fat.

DESCRIPTION Snake meat is firm, appetising, and a favourite with many peoples of the world, including the Australian Aborigines, who have appreciated it for tens of thousands of years.

ORIGIN AND HISTORY The snake has commanded people's respect and admiration since the beginning of time — for its graceful shape, lithe swiftness of movement and the dazzling patterns and colours of its skin. Snakes, both venomous and harmless, have been eaten and relished by native peoples wherever they are found. Rattlesnake meat was served as a ritual food in North American Indian tribal ceremonies and the meat has been compared in flavour to eel, chicken, and rabbit. In Africa, recipes recommend that a python be curried. In Australia, the Aborigines consider the firm, white flesh of snake to be much better than fowl.

BUYING AND STORAGE In most states of Australia, snakes are protected. It is only legal to kill them in self-defence, unless under the special dispensations applying to Aboriginal people living a traditional way of life.

Snake flesh may not be sold commercially and is not legally classed as meat.

PREPARATION AND USE In traditional Australian cooking, over a fire, two cooks are required: one to hold the head, and one the tail. This is to prevent the snake from curling up into disconcerting shapes over the heat. When the snake's body has completely ceased to wriggle and twist, it is laid lengthwise on the ground and cuts are made right along both sides close to the backbone. It is then rolled up like a pinwheel, tied together with reeds or a piece of string, slipped under hot coals, covered with ashes and left to cook. The gut is removed before serving.

Sweetbreads

MAJOR NUTRIENTS   BOILED
                              SERVE SIZE 60 G

Energy	500 kJ	Calcium	22 mg
Protein	12 g	Phosphorus	240 mg
Fat	6 g	Iron	1.1 mg
Cholesterol	190 mg	Zinc	1.3 mg
Carbohydrate	0	Riboflavin	0.15 mg
Total Sugars	0	Niacin Equiv.	3.4 mg
Sodium	135 mg	Vitamin C	11 mg
Potassium	160 mg		

NUTRITIONAL INFORMATION A moderate source of fat with about 45% of energy coming from fat, which contains about one-third of recommended daily cholesterol intake. Contains significant amounts of vitamin C which other flesh products do not.

DESCRIPTION Sweetbread is the thymus gland of calves and lambs. The thymus is made up of the rounded centre lobe, suspended close to the heart, called the heartbread, and two elongated side lobes called throatbreads. Collectively these are known as sweetbreads.

ORIGIN AND HISTORY A popular form of offal.

BUYING AND STORAGE Calf sweetbreads are generally considered better than lamb. They should be pale pink in colour. See Offal for storage. Poached sweetbreads may be refrigerated for 2–3 days. Frozen sweetbread will be a little darker in colour and should be used immediately after thawing.

PREPARATION AND USE Cover the sweetbreads with cold, lightly salted water and soak for 2–3 hours, changing the water several times. Sweetbreads are easier to handle if poached.

To poach, cover sweetbreads with cold water, bring to the boil and simmer — calf 7–10 minutes, lamb 2–3 minutes. Refresh and remove outer membranes and tubes. Press sweetbreads between two plates with a 1 kg weight on top. Refrigerate 2 hours before cutting and cooking as required. They can then be poached, deep-fried, sautéed, braised or grilled.

VARIETIES
Calf, Lamb.

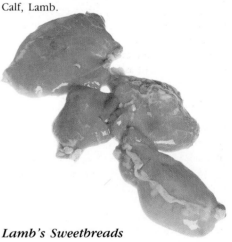

Lamb's Sweetbreads

Tongue

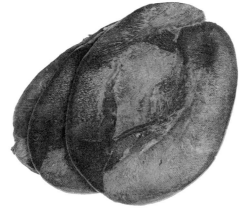

Ox Tongue

MAJOR NUTRIENTS		TONGUE OF OX OR LAMB, STEWED SERVE SIZE 60 G SLICE	
Energy	720 kJ	Potassium	140 mg
Protein	13 g	Phosphorus	120 mg
Fat	14 g	Iron	1.9 mg
Cholesterol	75 mg	Zinc	2.3 mg
Carbohydrate	0	Riboflavin	0.3 mg
Total Sugars	0	Niacin Equiv.	5.3 mg
Sodium	50 mg		

NUTRITIONAL INFORMATION A high fat animal product with 72% of energy coming from fat. This cannot be reduced, as little visible fat on product. Good levels of protein, phosphorus, iron, zinc and vitamin B12 make small serves a useful source of these in a varied diet. Pickling or salting will add at least 500 mg of sodium.

ORIGIN AND HISTORY This has always been a popular form of offal.

BUYING AND STORAGE Fresh or corned tongues are available. Ox tongues are also available smoked. See Offal for storage instructions.

PREPARATION AND USE Tongues require moist methods of cookery to tenderise. Scrub tongue if necessary, using a stiff brush. Soak fresh tongues in salted water for 1 hour, corned tongue should be soaked for 10–12 hours. Rinse well after soaking. Tongues will need to be poached gently to remove the skin. Ox tongues can be partially cooked, skinned and used as a substitute for beef in casseroles and stews. (Remove any bone and gristle after poaching if necessary. The bone and gristle is often removed by the butcher prior to purchase.) Tongue can be completely cooked by poaching, then skinned, pressed and sliced for salads and sandwiches, or sliced, egg breadcrumbed and pan fried. Or it can be partly cooked for 1 hour before skinning, then braised.

To poach, cover with fresh water and add onion, carrot and celery. Herbs can also be added. Add salt to fresh tongue and simmer gently. To completely cook, poach lamb and pig tongues for 2 hours, calf tongues 3 hours, ox tongues 4 hours — test with a skewer for tenderness.

To skin, allow to become completely cold in the water. Remove any fat, bones or gristle — split the skin and gently peel off.

VARIETIES
Lamb, Calf, Ox, Pig.

Tripe

MAJOR NUTRIENTS		STEWED IN MILK SERVE SIZE 90 G	
Energy	370 kJ	Potassium	90 mg
Protein	13 g	Calcium	135 mg
Fat	4 g	Phosphorus	80 mg
Cholesterol	145 mg	Iron	0.6 mg
Carbohydrate	0	Zinc	2 mg
Total Sugars	0	Niacin Equiv.	2.1 mg
Sodium	65 mg	Vitamin C	2.5 mg

NUTRITIONAL INFORMATION A moderate source of fat with up to 40% of energy coming from fat and significant amounts (almost 50%) of recommended daily intake of cholesterol in this size of serve. Contains some useful vitamin C. Excellent source of calcium because of the method of cooking, so useful to include in diets where calcium intake may be low. Use of new modified low fat high calcium milks for cooking could reduce the total fat content of the product and increase useful calcium levels.

DESCRIPTION Tripe is the name given to the four stomachs of ruminant animals. Tripe proper is available from beef, while sheep's stomach is known as paunch and pig's as hog maw.

ORIGIN AND HISTORY Tripe is a popular form of offal for which there are many traditional recipes.

BUYING AND STORAGE Colour can vary from white to a creamy-yellow depending upon the sex of the animal from which it is obtained but the colour does not affect the quality. There is very little difference in flavour between the tripes, but blanket and seam tripes are better for slow cooking recipes as they are less likely to disintegrate than honeycomb tripe.

See Offal for storage.

PREPARATION AND USE In Australia tripe is purchased ready for the pot and it is best blanched before further cooking. Rinse tripe, cover with cold water, bring to the boil. Drain, rinse, dry and cut into pieces as required.

Tripe can be boiled in a flavoured mixture of water and milk for 1½ hours or until tender, and served with a sauce made from the cooking liquid. It can also be sautéed, grilled, deep-fried or braised.

VARIETIES

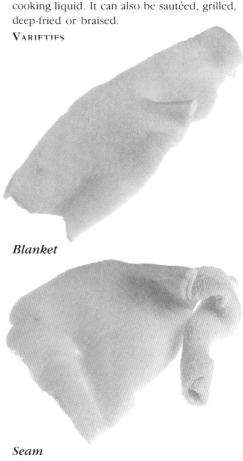

Blanket

Seam

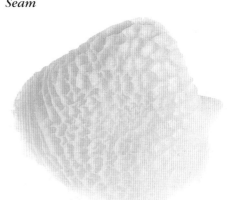

Honeycomb

SEE ALSO Hog Maw.

Veal

DESCRIPTION Veal is derived from young cattle with no physiological signs of maturity. The very best veal comes from calf that has just been weaned.

ORIGIN AND HISTORY Veal was popular in the time of the Romans and has maintained its reputation with modern Italians. Although it is impossible to verify, some say the very name of the country Italy comes from the Italian word for veal, 'vitello' Alpine countries like Austria and Italy made great use of veal in the past because calves born to ensure the necessary lactation of the cow over the winter months could not be fattened on snow-covered mountain pastures. It is in Italian cuisine that the now internationally famous dishes like vitello tonnato (veal with tuna fish sauce) and veal parmigiana (with parmesan cheese) have their origins.

BUYING AND STORAGE Veal should be pale pink, with very little or no visible selvage fat. See Beef for storage instructions.

PREPARATION AND USE Veal is very lean, tender meat and because of its immaturity has very little connective tissue or strong flavour of its own. Therefore it lends itself well to dishes that have a strong-flavoured sauce or accompaniment.

HINDQUARTER CUTS

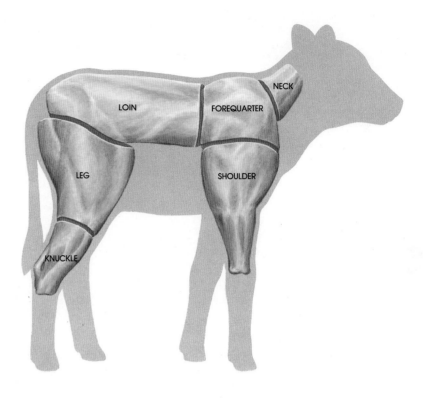

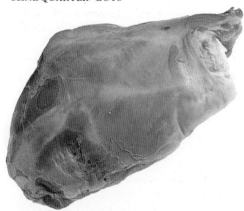

Leg Cuts from the leg include silverside, topside, round (nut of veal), knuckle and, from the top of the leg, rump and butt tenderloin or fillet.

The leg can be divided into these parts and sliced for steaks and schnitzels. Steaks can be pan fried or braised. The braising process is employed to combine the flavours of the sauce rather than to tenderise the veal, for example veal scallopine, veal parmigiana.

Legs can be roasted with the bone in or boned, stuffed, rolled and roasted. Care should be taken not to dry the veal and French roasting — that is, adding 1 cup water,

stock or wine to the roasting pan — is recommended. Allow approximately 35–40 minutes per 500 g.

MAJOR NUTRIENTS		**BONED, ROASTED** **SERVE SIZE 60 G**	
Energy	400 kJ	Sodium	50 mg
Protein	17 g	Potassium	295 mg
Fat	3 g	Phosphorus	215 mg
Cholesterol	65 mg	Iron	1.2 mg
Carbohydrate	0	Zinc	2 mg
Total Sugars	0	Niacin Equiv.	4.6 mg

NUTRITIONAL INFORMATION A low fat source of animal protein, with over 15% of daily phosphorus, iron, zinc and vitamin B12 recommended intakes.

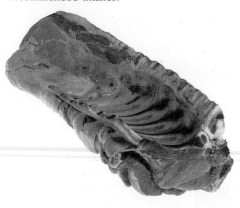

Loin Cut between the hip bone and the 5th rib with the flank and breast removed.

Divided into the short loin and ribs.

Cut into short loin chops and rib chops or cutlets, veal can be grilled, pan fried, crumbed and fried, or barbecued.

In the piece the short loin can be roasted with the bone in or boned and rolled. The ribs can be made into racks and roasted. (With the tail of the rib bone trimmed of meat it is called a French rack. The veal is usually tied to maintain a good shape.)

The tenderloin or fillet which comes from under the loin and the rump is trimmed of the side straps and silver skin and either left in the piece, cut into medallions, or laid flat, that is, butterflied. It can be roasted or pan fried and requires very little cooking as it is the most tender cut of veal.

MAJOR NUTRIENTS		**LOIN CHOP, GRILLED** **SERVE SIZE 75 G**	
Energy	370 kJ	Sodium	55 mg
Protein	16 g	Potassium	200 mg
Fat	3 g	Phosphorus	325 mg
Cholesterol	60 mg	Iron	1.1 mg
Carbohydrate	0	Zinc	2.1 mg
Total Sugars	0	Niacin Equiv.	4.4 mg

NUTRITIONAL INFORMATION De-fatted chops contain only small amounts of fat, with only 30% of total energy coming from fat. Excellent source of protein and accompanying phosphorus as well as iron, zinc and vitamin B12.

FOREQUARTER CUTS

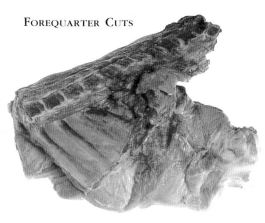

Forequarter Cuts from the forequarter include the shoulder, forequarter chops, neck and the shank or the shin.

MAJOR NUTRIENTS		FOREQUARTER, STEWED SERVE SIZE 100 G	
Energy	550 kJ	Sodium	35 mg
Protein	17 g	Potassium	120 mg
Fat	5 g	Phosphorus	260 mg
Cholesterol	60 mg	Iron	1.4 mg
Carbohydrate	0	Zinc	2.4 mg
Total Sugars	0	Niacin Equiv.	3.5 mg

NUTRITIONAL INFORMATION A low fat source of animal protein, with over 15% of daily phosphorus, iron, zinc and vitamin B12 recommended intakes.

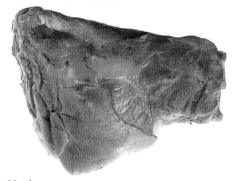

Neck Can be cut into steak or chops, and depending on the size of the carcass can be used for braising.

NUTRITIONAL INFORMATION Similar to the nutrients listed for forequarter.

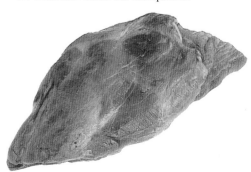

Shoulder The shoulder can be roasted with

the bone in, or boned, stuffed and rolled. It can be cut into steaks or cubed for braising or casseroling.

MAJOR NUTRIENTS		SHOULDER STEAK, GRILLED SERVE SIZE 120 G	
Energy	810 kJ	Phosphorus	310 mg
Protein	34 g	Magnesium	24 mg
Fat	6 g	Iron	2.1 mg
Cholesterol	110 mg	Zinc	3.8 mg
Carbohydrate	0	Thiamin	0.5 mg
Total Sugars	0	Riboflavin	0.2 mg
Sodium	150 mg	Niacin Equiv.	9.2 mg
Potassium	500 mg		

NUTRITIONAL INFORMATION A low fat high protein meat. Contains excellent amounts of phosphorus, iron, zinc, thiamin, niacin and vitamin B12, all of which are known to be well absorbed from this type of animal product.

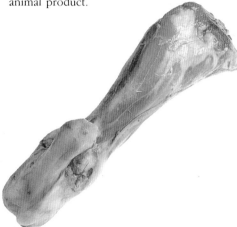

Veal Knuckle Renowned for its use in the famous Italian dish osso buco. The hind or forequarter shank or knuckle is cut through into medallions and gently simmered to allow the prized bone marrow to tenderise. The knuckle can also be trimmed of meat at the thin end (hoof end). This is called Frenched Knuckle (jarret de veau); it is cooked by gently simmering.

MAJOR NUTRIENTS		SERVE SIZE 110 G	
Energy	240 kJ	Potassium	70 mg
Protein	9 g	Phosphorus	250 mg
Fat	2 g	Iron	1 mg
Cholesterol	40 mg	Zinc	2 mg
Carbohydrate	0	Riboflavin	0.1 mg
Total Sugars	0	Niacin Equiv.	2.4 mg
Sodium	30 mg		

NUTRITIONAL INFORMATION A tasty low fat, high protein, cheaper meat cut. Provides excellent amounts of phosphorus and vitamin B12 with good quantities of iron, zinc, riboflavin and niacin being present.

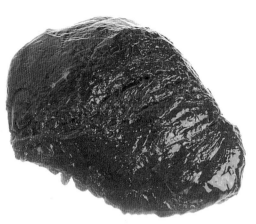

Venison

MAJOR NUTRIENTS		ROASTED SERVE SIZE 100 G	
Energy	832 kJ	Sodium	0
Protein	35 g	Phosphorus	290 mg
Fat	6 g	Iron	8 mg
Cholesterol	N/A	Magnesium	33 mg
Carbohydrate	0	Thiamin	0.20 mg
Total Sugars	0	Niacin Equiv.	12 mg

NUTRITIONAL INFORMATION No data for other water-soluble or fat-soluble vitamins. Excellent source of protein, iron, phosphorus, thiamin, niacin.

DESCRIPTION Though the name 'venison' used to apply to the flesh of any sort of game or wild beast, it now usually means the flesh of the roe deer, fallow deer, red deer, moose or reindeer.

ORIGIN AND HISTORY People have been eating deer since prehistoric times and there have been periods when they were the principal food of some societies. Deer are now bred for the table and there are several farms in Australia and New Zealand supplying the domestic and export markets.

BUYING AND STORAGE Good deer meat should be dark red with a fine grain and firm, white fat. Best parts are the haunch, fillet, loin and chops. The meat of the buck is tastier than that of the doe, but it should be eaten when the animal is young, or not older than three years old. Available from specialty game shops, venison must be kept refrigerated.

PREPARATION AND USE Venison is dry and a little tough, so it should be larded before roasting in an oven. It is also delicious when roasted on a spit. It may be marinated before cooking and served with redcurrant jelly and a port wine sauce, according to the traditional English recipes for venison which date back to times when the sport of hunting deer in the forests of Europe was reserved only for royalty.

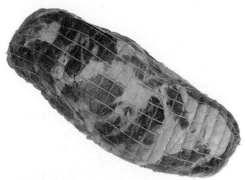

Wild Boar

DESCRIPTION The wild relative of the domestic pig has a longer snout and tougher hair in a variety of colours. Its behaviour can be considerably more aggressive, being particularly dangerous in a mature boar, which is equipped with a pair of sharp, curved tusks.

ORIGIN AND HISTORY The wild boar is still hunted in Europe and in many parts of Asia, though it has long been extinct in Britain. Stuffed boar was the main attraction at Roman banquets; the head also was splendidly stuffed, boiled or roasted, placed on a large platter, decorated with laurel leaves and borne in procession and triumph to the dining hall. It has been a popular food in New Zealand ever since Captain Cook released pigs there in the 18th century.

BUYING AND STORAGE While not available commercially in Australia, it may be bought from specialist butchers in New Zealand.

PREPARATION AND USE Young animals aged 6 to 12 months provide the most tender flesh, especially delicious when cooked in a Maori hangi, or earth oven, which is the traditional New Zealand method. Because of its gamy flavour, boar flesh of any age responds well to marinating and braising.

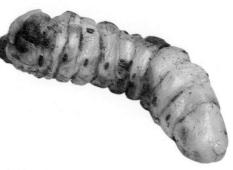

Witchetty Grubs

MAJOR NUTRIENTS		SERVE SIZE 50 G	
Energy	1370 kJ	Sodium	25 mg
Protein	14 g	Calcium	130 mg
Fat	26 g	Iron	15 mg
Carbohydrate	11 g	Zinc	1.5 mg
Cholesterol	0		

NUTRITIONAL INFORMATION Witchetty grubs and other grubs of the same type are very rich sources of protein, fat and energy. A large proportion of the fatty acids are monounsaturated.

DESCRIPTION These are the long, fat grubs, up to 10 cm in length, which are found on the superficial roots of the 'witchetty bush', around Alice Springs and throughout Central Australia.

ORIGIN AND HISTORY These have been one of the staple foods of the Australian desert dwellers for countless thousands of years. In Aboriginal tradition, they are gathered by the women, who locate and then dig up the affected roots and harvest the grubs, which are often eaten on the way back to camp.

BUYING AND STORAGE Witchetty grubs must be found and eaten fresh.

PREPARATION AND USE The traditional method is to cook the grubs quickly in the ashes of a fire, when they swell and the skin stiffens. Inside the crisp skin, the flesh is solid and a bright yellow, with a taste which has often been compared to almonds.

SAUSAGES & PRESERVED MEATS

The word sausage is derived from the Latin word salsus meaning salted or preserved. Historical records reveal that about 3500 years ago the Babylonians and the Chinese were making and eating sausages. It is recorded that in about 1300 BC the ruling Chinese Emperor decided to take advantage of the popularity of salting meat by imposing a tax on salt.

In the Odyssey, Homer referred to sausage as the favourite food of the Greeks, and the Romans liked sausages so much that no festive occasion was complete without them. In fact, sausages became so popular during the wild festivals of Rome, that, as the Christian era began, they were banned. Strong public protest eventually forced a repeal of the ban.

The exact nature of these early sausages is not clear. Indications are that they were composed of fat and blood in a natural casing which was roasted. Perhaps they resembled the modern black pudding.

Climate influenced the development of sausages. The Germans, because of their cool climate, became adept at the manufacture of a moist sausage. Further south in the dry Mediterranean area it was necessary to dry and/or highly season meat to prolong its usefulness. The Italians in particular became famous for their range of salamis, most of which bear the name of the locality of origin.

Today's sausage industry began when home-makers decided to duplicate their recipes for commercial purposes to meet the demand of a growing population. The current process is a unique combination of old and new methods and has steadily grown into a highly scientific industry that still represents the old art of sausage making with all its wonderful variety and flavour.

The Preserved Meats section of this chapter includes meats which have been cured, smoked or otherwise preserved so that they can be used later as joints, slices or spreads.

Like the sausages, they can also be heated for selected dishes, but they are listed here separately since in the main they correspond to what are known as cold cuts. They include various types of preserved poultry.

Many ways of preserving meats go back very far in time. Salting meat was a favoured way of preserving meat for long journeys or voyages in the past, and for keeping meat edible when no freshly slaughtered meat was available for the table.

Preserving in fat, the method used when making pâtés and terrines, was another popular method. Cooked liver, for instance, is the ingredient of the liverwursts listed here. Although wurst means sausage in German, these are not used as a sausage but as a spread, and are really more akin to the pâtés.

Another form of curing is with sugar, as the bacon and ham entries show.

These meats are popular and convenient. They became part of traditional diets in the days before most houses had a refrigerator, when their good keeping qualities were important. They are a favourite for sandwiches and snacks because of their ready availability and ease of handling.

They differ from fresh meat in three major respects. They contain high levels of fat; they have high levels of sodium salts, including common salt (sodium chloride); they contain significant amounts of food additives, which according to the different varieties may include nitrites and nitrates, sulphur dioxide, ascorbic acid, phosphates, smoke flavour and other flavourings.

It would be difficult to implement the dietary guidelines 'eat less fat' and 'eat less salt' while consuming a lot of sausage and preserved meats.

Manufacturers are working to reduce the use of salt and preservative and reduce the level of fat in such foods. But there is a limit to the reductions which can be made, because the salt and other preservatives are essential if the products are to be safely stored, and fat is important to the texture and flavour.

It is only possible for manufacturers to use additives which are approved by food law, but sulphur dioxide and the nitrates and nitrites are additives which health authorities are anxious to restrict. Many asthmatics have an intolerance to sulphur dioxide and they need to avoid foods containing it.

The higher incidence of cancer of the oesophagus and stomach, in countries such as China and Japan where salt-cured meats are frequently consumed, have caused official experts in other countries such as the USA and Australia to advise that the consumption of foods preserved by salt-curing or smoking be minimised.

Salami and related products are processed by fermentation which means that they can be safely kept without refrigeration for prolonged periods.

Since most of the important nutrients in meat are contained in the lean tissues the relative amounts of protein, minerals and vitamins in sausages and preserved meats are lower than in fresh lean meat, but the same range of nutrients occurs in both, as a study of the individual nutritional information shows.

SAUSAGES

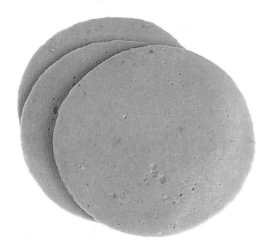

Berliner Fleischwurst

MAJOR NUTRIENTS		SERVE SIZE 100 G	
Energy	1320 kJ	Sodium	820 mg
Protein	13 g	Potassium	199 mg
Fat	27 g	Phosphorus	130 mg
Cholesterol	80 mg	Iron	1.9 mg
Carbohydrate	0	Zinc	1.8 mg
Total Sugars	0	Riboflavin	0.1 mg
Dietary Fibre	0	Niacin Equiv.	4.1 mg

NUTRITIONAL INFORMATION Over 75% of energy coming from fats. Contains excellent amounts of phosphorus, iron and vitamin B12 and good amounts of zinc, riboflavin and niacin. Use in moderation, not as a daily animal protein source. Preboiling may reduce fat content.

DESCRIPTION A smoked and water-cooked sausage made from a very fine mixture of pork and veal with no garlic. Similar to Pariser. Berliner Fleischwurst is popular in Australia, however the Berliner available in the USA is a coarser product.

ORIGIN AND HISTORY A German sausage from Berlin, from which it takes its name.

BUYING AND STORAGE Sold sliced/kg. Berliner should be wrapped in plastic and stored in the refrigerator. Best used within 3–5 days of purchase.

PREPARATION AND USE Finely sliced, this is an excellent cold meat to accompany salads or as a sandwich filling. In true German style serve on fresh rye bread with a glass of German beer.

VARIETIES
Pariser includes a touch of garlic and natural herbs. There is also chicken pariser.

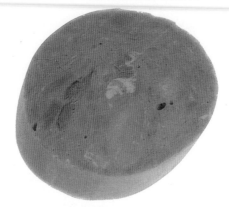

Bierschinken

MAJOR NUTRIENTS		SERVE SIZE 30 G	
Energy	1300 kJ	Dietary Fibre	0
Protein	4 g	Sodium	200 mg
Fat	5 g	Potassium	30 mg
Cholesterol	15 mg	Phosphorus	50 mg
Carbohydrate	0	Iron	1 mg
Total Sugars	0	Zinc	1 mg

NUTRITIONAL INFORMATION Over 60% of energy coming from fats which are predominantly unsaturated. A serving contains good amounts of phosphorus, iron, zinc and niacin. Use in moderation to add flavour rather than as a major source of these vitamins.

DESCRIPTION A cooked and lightly smoked sausage made from beef and pork which is distinguishable by small chunks of ham/ham fat and pistachio nuts.

ORIGIN AND HISTORY West German.

BUYING AND STORAGE Usually bought already sliced/kg. Seal in plastic to prevent drying and keep refrigerated. Best used within 2–3 days of purchase.

PREPARATION AND USE Ideal as a cold platter meat to be served with salads or as a sandwich fill.

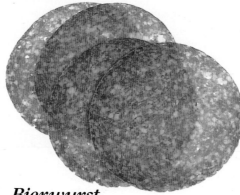

Bierwurst

MAJOR NUTRIENTS		SERVE SIZE 20 G	
Energy	200 kJ	Dietary Fibre	0
Protein	3 g	Sodium	145 mg
Fat	4 g	Potassium	20 mg
Cholesterol	11 mg	Phosphorus	35 mg
Carbohydrate	0	Iron	0.5 mg
Total Sugars	0		

NUTRITIONAL INFORMATION Over 75% of energy coming from fats, which are predominantly unsaturated. A serving contains good amounts of phosphorus and iron.

DESCRIPTION A cooked, spicy, lightly smoked pork or pork/beef large diameter sausage. Soft in texture it is sometimes flavoured with garlic.

ORIGIN AND HISTORY German.

BUYING AND STORAGE Usually bought sliced/kg. Keep refrigerated in plastic wrap. Best used within 2–3 days of purchase.

PREPARATION AND USE For sandwiches or with beer and bread.

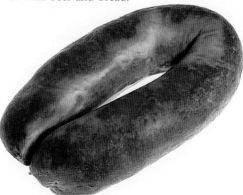

Black Pudding

MAJOR NUTRIENTS		SERVE SIZE 90 G	
Energy	1140 kJ	Potassium	70 mg
Protein	15 g	Calcium	35 mg
Fat	17 g	Phosphorus	210 mg
Cholesterol	65 mg	Magnesium	28 mg
Carbohydrate	6 g	Iron	10 mg
Total Sugars		Zinc	3 mg
less than 1 g		Thiamin	0.1 mg
Dietary Fibre	0.5 g	Riboflavin	0.6 mg
Sodium	870 mg	Niacin Equiv.	3.8 mg

NUTRITIONAL INFORMATION High fat and carbohydrate containing sausage which uses blood as a binder and so has particularly high levels of useful iron. In addition it contains excellent levels of phosphorus, zinc, riboflavin and vitamin B12. The high levels of cholesterol and fat mean that this product should be eaten in moderation. The fats are predominantly monounsaturated.

DESCRIPTION Traditionally black pudding is a large black sausage made of pig's blood, suet and seasonings enclosed in an intestine. The essential ingredient for all varieties is fresh pig's blood.

ORIGIN AND HISTORY Black pudding is reported to be one of the few dishes made by the Assyrians which survive today, even if prepared in a vastly superior way. Perhaps it was a type of black pudding referred to in Homer's *Odyssey* translated as follows: 'in the same way as a man, having filled the stomach with fat and blood, stands in front of a great fire and turns it this way and that, in his eagerness to get it roasted'.

The black pudding was brought to England by the Romans, whose recipes were highly spiced as recorded by Apicius, a gourmet of AD100.

Traditionally black pudding is from the Midlands and north of England, though it is made under different names in most regions.

BUYING AND STORAGE Purchase by the ring and keep refrigerated.

PREPARATION AND USE Black puddings are usually sliced and fried, however, they can be heated through in boiling water. In Wales black pudding is served with rashers of thick salty bacon.

VARIETIES

There are many local versions of black pudding in England, notably in north Staffordshire, Stretford, and Yorkshire. Other varieties include: Black Pudding, Caribbean, West Indies; Black Pudding, Scotland; Blood Pudding, 'Pwdin Gwaed' Wales; Drisheen, Ireland; Karvariza, Bulgaria; Packet, Limerick, Southern Ireland.

SEE ALSO Boudin Noir.

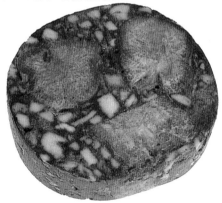

Blood Sausage

MAJOR NUTRIENTS		SERVE SIZE 90 G	
Energy	1140 kJ	Potassium	70 mg
Protein	15 g	Calcium	35 mg
Fat	17 g	Phosphorus	210 mg
Cholesterol	65 mg	Magnesium	28 mg
Carbohydrate	6 g	Iron	10 mg
Total Sugars		Zinc	3 mg
	less than 1 g	Thiamin	0.1 mg
Dietary Fibre	0.5 g	Riboflavin	0.65 mg
Sodium	870 mg	Niacin Equiv.	2.8 mg

NUTRITIONAL INFORMATION A high fat, carbohydrate containing sausage which uses blood as a binder and so has particularly high levels of useful iron. In addition it contains excellent levels of phosphorus, zinc, riboflavin and vitamin B12 and good quantities of magnesium and thiamin. The high levels of cholesterol and fat mean that this product should be eaten in moderation. The fats are predominantly monounsaturated. The manufacture requires the addition of salt resulting in a final high sodium content.

DESCRIPTION Pork or pork fat is diced and mixed with beef blood and mildly spiced, then cooked. Very dark in appearance. Similar to black pudding.

ORIGIN AND HISTORY In Germany the general term for a blood sausage is blutwurst.

BUYING AND STORAGE Available in both sections and rings in the USA. Purchase by the unit. Keep refrigerated.

PREPARATION AND USE Slice and brown lightly in butter. Serve with mashed potatoes or sauerkraut. These go very well with all kinds of pastry, so place thick slices in baked puff or short pastry shells and top with some warm, unsweetened apple sauce and a few raisins.

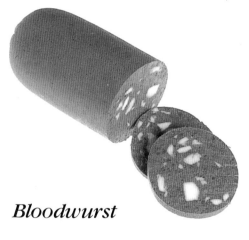

Bloodwurst

MAJOR NUTRIENTS		SERVE SIZE 90 G	
Energy	1140 kJ	Potassium	70 mg
Protein	15 g	Calcium	35 mg
Fat	17 g	Phosphorus	210 mg
Cholesterol	65 mg	Magnesium	28 mg
Carbohydrate	6 g	Iron	9.8 mg
Total Sugars		Zinc	2.8 mg
	less than 1 g	Thiamin	0.1 mg
Dietary Fibre	0.5 g	Riboflavin	0.6 mg
Sodium	870 mg		

NUTRITIONAL INFORMATION Moderately high fat, carbohydrate containing sausage which uses blood as a binder and so has particularly high levels of useful iron. In addition it contains excellent levels of phosphorus, zinc, riboflavin and vitamin B12 and good quantities of calcium and magnesium. The high levels of cholesterol and fat mean that this product should be eaten in moderation.

DESCRIPTION A blood sausage made from pig's blood, onions, diced pieces of speck and aspic jelly. Fully cooked.

ORIGIN AND HISTORY The Australian equivalent of the blood sausage (blutwurst in Germany).

BUYING AND STORAGE Usually sold per slice/kg. Seal in plastic wrap and refrigerate for up to 7 days.

PREPARATION AND USE Serve as a cold platter food.

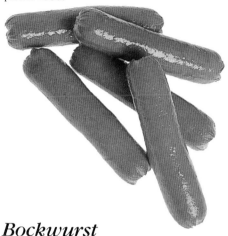

Bockwurst

MAJOR NUTRIENTS		SERVE SIZE 90 G	
Energy	1110 kJ	Sodium	630 mg
Protein	11 g	Potassium	120 mg
Fat	22 g	Phosphorus	60 mg
Cholesterol	50 mg	Iron	1.1 mg
Carbohydrate	0	Zinc	1.2 mg
Total Sugars	0	Niacin Equiv.	5.1 mg
Dietary Fibre	0		

NUTRITIONAL INFORMATION Over 80% of energy coming from fats. A serving contains good amounts of phosphorus, iron, zinc, niacin and vitamin B12. Use to add flavour rather than as a major source of these vitamins.

DESCRIPTION A sausage made from veal and pork with a taste and bite similar to that of a frankfurter, but white in colour and generally thicker in diameter.

ORIGIN AND HISTORY Originally a delicate fresh German veal sausage made in spring at a special festival for which bock beer was made. It contained onion and/or chives, parsley and nutmeg. Traditionally bockwurst was pan fried and served with bock beer.

BUYING AND STORAGE Sold by the unit/kg. Refrigerate for 3–5 days.

PREPARATION AND USE Steam or heat in boiling water, then serve.

VARIETIES

Regional varieties available in the USA include farmer-style bockwurst, coarsely ground; Swiss-style, very mildly seasoned; Thuringer bockwurst, coarsely textured with a speckled appearance.

Bologna

Major Nutrients · Serve Size 30 g

Energy	410 kJ	Sodium	230 mg
Protein	4 g	Potassium	36 mg
Fat	8 g	Phosphorus	70 mg
Cholesterol	20 mg	Iron	0.7 mg
Carbohydrate	Trace	Zinc	1.1 mg
Total Sugars	Trace	Thiamin	0.05 mg
Dietary Fibre	0	Niacin Equiv.	1 mg

Nutritional Information A high fat content with over 72% of energy coming from fats, which are predominantly monounsaturated. A serving contains good amounts of phosphorus, iron, zinc, niacin and thiamin. Use to add flavour rather than as a major source of vitamins.

Description Bologna is a fully cooked, mildly seasoned sausage made from beef and/or pork.

Origin and History Mortadella was the original Bolognese sausage, but bologna is one of the most famous. It is the second most popular sausage sold in the USA, accounting for around 20% of all sausages sold.

Buying and Storage Generally made in a large skin; some varieties, like Berliner, are produced in sections and sticks. If purchased sliced, wrap and keep refrigerated. Best used within 3–5 days.

Preparation and Use Snack item, ideal as a sandwich fill. Particularly popular with children.

Varieties

Balleron A mildly seasoned sausage which includes pieces of smoked beef tongue and pistachio nuts.

Berliner/New England (USA) Sausage Bologna with pieces of ham or chopped beef.

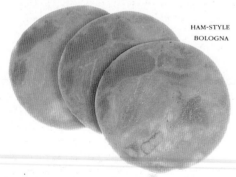

HAM-STYLE
BOLOGNA

Ham-Style/Ham Bologna Contains cured ham pieces.

German Medium texture, no garlic, in a large skin.

Turkey Bologna Contains turkey meat.

See Also Schinkenwurst.

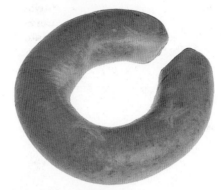

Boudin Blanc

Nutritional Information There are no detailed data available on the nutritional composition of this sausage.

Description A very delicate, expensive, fresh white sausage made from white meat, which can include pork, cream, eggs, onions and fine breadcrumbs.

Origin and History French.

Buying and Storage Purchased by kg. Must be refrigerated. Use within 2–3 days of purchase.

Preparation and Use Always eaten hot, the boudin blanc can be poached or brushed with melted butter and grilled. Preferred method is to sauté gently in butter and serve with mashed potatoes.

Varieties

Morcilla blanca from Spain made from chicken and hard boiled eggs.

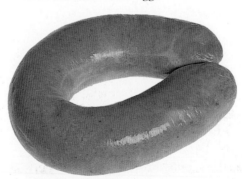

Boudin Noir

Major Nutrients · Serve Size 90 g

Energy	1140 kJ	Potassium	70 mg
Protein	15 g	Calcium	35 mg
Fat	17 g	Phosphorus	210 mg
Cholesterol	65 mg	Magnesium	28 mg
Carbohydrate	6 g	Iron	10.2 mg
Total Sugars		Zinc	3.4 mg
	less than 1 g	Thiamin	0.1 mg
Dietary Fibre	0.5 g	Riboflavin	0.6 mg
Sodium	870 mg		

Nutritional Information A high fat, carbohydrate containing sausage which uses blood as a binder and so has particularly high levels of useful iron. In addition it contains excellent levels of phosphorus, zinc, riboflavin and vitamin B12 and significant amounts of calcium, magnesium and thiamin. The high levels of cholesterol and fat mean that this product should be eaten in moderation.

Description The French equivalent of the English black pudding. The principal ingredient is pig's blood.

Origin and History Boudin noir has a long history and is still popular today. In some regions of France this sausage is traditionally served on returning from midnight mass on Christmas Eve. The village of Manziat holds a competition each year to see who can eat the most boudin noir. Montagne-au-Perche, west of Paris, organises an annual competition for the best black pudding from each country and attracts some 600 entries.

Buying and Storage Purchase by the ring and keep refrigerated.

Preparation and Use Slice and fry as black pudding. Morcilla is used as an ingredient in the famous Spanish dish fabada, a stew of butter beans, pork, tomato puree, garlic and sliced chorizo and morcilla.

Varieties

Morcilla, Spain; biroldo, Italy; blood sausage, Sweden; staburpoelse, Norway.

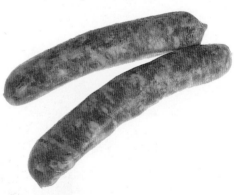

Bratwurst

Major Nutrients · Serve Size 100 g

Energy	1520 kJ	Potassium	200 mg
Protein	13 g	Calcium	50 mg
Fat	32 g	Phosphorus	190 mg
Cholesterol	65 mg	Iron	1.6 mg
Carbohydrate	0	Zinc	1.4 mg
Total Sugars	0	Riboflavin	0.2 mg
Dietary Fibre	0	Niacin Equiv.	6.1 mg
Sodium	520 mg		

Nutritional Information A high fat content with over 78% of energy coming from fats. A serving contains good amounts of calcium, phosphorus, iron, zinc, riboflavin, niacin and vitamin B12. Use in moderation to add flavour rather than as a major source of these vitamins. Fat content may be reduced if cooked slowly and fats released are discarded.

DESCRIPTION A fresh, uncooked sausage made from pork and veal, chopped onion and fairly heavily seasoned. Finely textured, pale in colour, it is produced in longish links. Bratwurst produced in Australia is coarser in texture and has a redder, more meaty colour than the traditional bratwurst.

In the USA, bratwurst are being produced cooked as well as fresh. The cooked variety are known as 'white hots' and are similar to a frankfurter without the Nitrites 250 (which give frankfurters the pink colour).

ORIGIN AND HISTORY Bratwurst is the German word for a frying sausage.

BUYING AND STORAGE Purchased by the unit/kg. Must be refrigerated and consumed/cooked within 2–3 days of purchase.

PREPARATION AND USE Usually grilled or fried. A traditional German dish is bratwurst cooked in beer, Berlin style. Scald approximately 500 g bratwurst. Sauté onion and when soft add sausage. Add bay leaves, peppercorns to taste and 150 ml beer. Reduce for a few minutes, then add another 150 ml beer and simmer gently for 15 mins. Thicken with potato flour.

Also excellent when barbecued and served with horseradish, mustard, warm German potato salad, sauerkraut, and a glass of German Riesling.

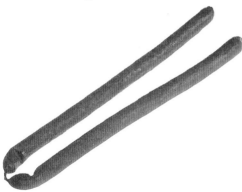

Cabanossi

also called **Kabanos**

MAJOR NUTRIENTS		SERVE SIZE 30 G	
Energy	460 kJ	Sodium	240 mg
Protein	5 g	Potassium	35 mg
Fat	9 g	Phosphorus	40 mg
Cholesterol	21 mg	Iron	1.1 mg
Carbohydrate	1 g	Zinc	0.9 mg
Total Sugars	0	Thiamin	0.05 mg
Dietary Fibre	0	Niacin Equiv.	1.6 mg

NUTRITIONAL INFORMATION A high fat content with over 70% of energy coming from fats, which are predominantly monounsaturated. A serving contains good amounts of phosphorus, iron, zinc, niacin and vitamin B12. Use to add flavour rather than as a major source of these vitamins and minerals. Also, the preservation process requires the addition of sodium, so intake should be moderated in sodium-controlled diets.

DESCRIPTION A coarsely textured sausage made from pork and/or beef, seasoned and smoked. The casings are red and twisted to form thin links about 30 cm or more in length.

ORIGIN AND HISTORY A sausage made only from pork in Russia and as kabanos found all over Poland, where it was originally taken on hunting expeditions.

BUYING AND STORAGE Buy by the link. Refrigerate.

PREPARATION AND USE Already cooked, cabanossi is ready to eat and is an ideal snack item, or cut into bite-size pieces and serve with your favourite drink. Often used in an antipasto.

VARIETIES
Kabana, a wider diameter cabanossi developed in Australia.

Cervelat

also called **Cervelas**

MAJOR NUTRIENTS		SERVE SIZE 30 G	
Energy	510 kJ	Sodium	380 mg
Protein	5 g	Potassium	90 mg
Fat	13 g	Phosphorus	50 mg
Cholesterol	33 mg	Iron	0.5 mg
Carbohydrate	0	Zinc	0.9 mg
Total Sugars	0	Thiamin	0.05 mg
Dietary Fibre	0	Niacin Equiv.	1.6 mg

NUTRITIONAL INFORMATION A high fat content with over 90% of energy coming from fats. A serving contains significant amounts of phosphorus, iron, zinc, niacin and vitamin B12. Use to add flavour rather than as a major source of these vitamins and minerals. Also, the preservation process requires the addition of sodium, so intake should be moderated in sodium-controlled diets.

DESCRIPTION In general, a cervelat is a lightly cooked, semi-dry, finely minced mixture of pork/beef. Mildly seasoned and smoked to a golden brown.

ORIGIN AND HISTORY Name originated from the Latin word for brains, however, brains are not now found amongst the ingredients of cervelat. The cervelat family is an example of the moist cooked-type sausage developed in Germany's cooler climate, where heavy salting and seasoning was not necessary for good keeping quality.

BUYING AND STORAGE Purchase sliced/kg. Refrigerate for up to 1 week.

PREPARATION AND USE Use as a cold cut, in fine/medium slices.

VARIETIES

Farm-Style/Summer Sausage USA. A soft cervelat.

Goettinger A distinctively flavoured hard cervelat from Germany.

Goteborg A salty, heavily smoked and coarsely textured product from Sweden.

Gothaer A German variety made from very lean pork.

Holsteinerwurst German, produced in rings.

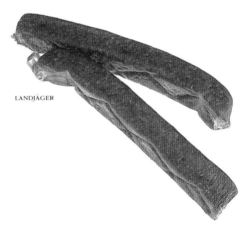

LANDJÄGER

Landjäger A black, wrinkly, flat cervelat from Switzerland which is heavily smoked.

Thuringer

NUTRITIONAL INFORMATION Information on the major nutrients of this product is unavailable. May contain Nitrites 250.

DESCRIPTION Some thuringers are fresh sausages made from finely ground pork and/or veal for frying or grilling. The German variety, containing pork, liver and seasoning, is boiled, dyed red and cold smoked over sawdust and juniper berries. In the USA the term thuringer is a little confused as there are many varieties. In some parts the name is interchangeable with summer sausage. The most popular interpretation in the USA is that a cooked thuringer is mostly pork with a similar flavour to fresh pork breakfast links.

ORIGIN AND HISTORY German. As with other sausages this sausage was sold fresh, but now many processers are offering thuringer in cooked form for better shelf life.

BUYING AND STORAGE Buy by the link/ kg. If fresh, keep refrigerated and use within 2–3 days. If purchased precooked, refrigerate and use within 7 days.

PREPARATION AND USE Excellent in a cassoulet or with potatoes or dried beans. A cassoulet is a haricot bean stew which is a specialty of the Languedoc region (a former province of southern France). Traditionally it contains preserved goose/duck, sausages, ribs of pork and loin of mutton with haricot beans, tomatoes, and onions.

SEE ALSO Saveloy.

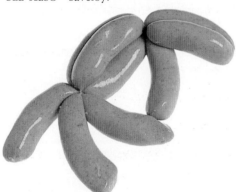

Chipolata

MAJOR NUTRIENTS
GRILLED
SERVE SIZE 50 G

Energy	760 kJ	Sodium	500 mg
Protein	7 g	Potassium	100 mg
Fat	12 g	Phosphorus	110 mg
Cholesterol	25 mg	Iron	0.8 mg
Carbohydrate	5 g	Zinc	0.8 mg
Total Sugars	0	Niacin Equiv.	3.1 mg
Dietary Fibre	0		

NUTRITIONAL INFORMATION About 58% of energy comes from fats. A serving contains good amounts of phosphorus, iron, zinc, niacin and vitamin B12. Use to add flavour rather than as a major source of these vitamins and minerals. Also, the preservation process requires the addition of sodium, so intake should be moderated in sodium-controlled diets.

DESCRIPTION A small fresh pork or pork/ beef sausage with special flavourings, around half the size of a standard pork sausage.

ORIGIN AND HISTORY The chipolata was originally an Italian ragout/stew with onion but the word was adopted by the French to mean a small sausage.

BUYING AND STORAGE Purchase by kg. Refrigerate. Best used or cooked within 2–3 days of purchase.

PREPARATION AND USE Pan-fry, use as a garnish for meat and poultry dishes, or eat as a cocktail snack. Antony and Araminta Hippisley Coxe give an English recipe for chipolata with tomatoes. Brown the chipolatas, then fry onion and garlic, and add a can of tomatoes, white wine, and bouquet garni. Simmer. Cook noodles of choice, mix in some butter and grated cheese. Arrange chipolatas, pour sauce over, then noodle mixture. Add more cheese on top and place under grill.

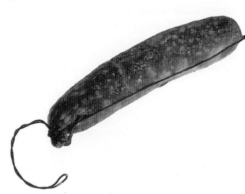

Chorizo

also called **Chaurice**

MAJOR NUTRIENTS
SERVE SIZE 60 G

Energy	950 kJ	Potassium	70 mg
Protein	10 g	Phosphorus	80 mg
Fat	18 g	Iron	1.4 mg
Cholesterol	45 mg	Zinc	1.9 mg
Carbohydrate	0	Thiamin	0.15 mg
Total Sugars	0	Riboflavin	0.1 mg
Dietary Fibre	0	Niacin Equiv.	3.6 mg
Sodium	280 mg		

NUTRITIONAL INFORMATION Over 70% of energy comes from predominantly mono-unsaturated fats. A serving contains good amounts of phosphorus, iron, zinc, niacin and vitamin B12. Use to add flavour rather than as a major source of these vitamins and minerals. Also, the preservation process requires the addition of sodium, so intake should be moderated in sodium-controlled diets.

DESCRIPTION A coarsely textured fairly dry spicy sausage made from pork and red pepper which are the essential ingredients common to all varieties. Other ingredients can include a little beef, cayenne pepper, chilli, paprika, salt and pepper. They may be smoked or unsmoked.

ORIGIN AND HISTORY A spicy sausage originating in Spain, regional variances are owing to the proportion of red pepper used. In Somerset Maugham's novel *Catalina*, a 16th

century wedding breakfast menu consisted of bread, cheese, cold chicken, chorizo sausage and a bulging skin of wine. 'Who could want anything better?' the hero asked.

BUYING AND STORAGE Chorizo is sold as a sausage approximately 10 cm in length by unit/kg. Can be hung in a cool draughty area for up to 1 week. After this time the sausage matures and assumes a wrinkled appearance and becomes spicier. Alternatively, refrigerate.

PREPARATION AND USE Chorizo may be eaten in the same way as any sausage: fried, grilled, in a stew, soup, or as an ingredient in traditional Spanish dishes. The length of cooking depends on the heat used. Larousse recommends cooking with garbanzos (chickpeas) stewed Spanish style, or as an ingredient in a thick French soup, made in an earthenware pot. It is also good sliced and eaten on bread garnished with pickled vegetables; for a drink have a glass of dry sherry. Fabada is a famous Spanish stew of vegetables, sliced chorizo and morcilla.

VARIETIES
A typical country sausage with each region having its own particular recipe. Most varieties are from Spain, but chorizo piquante is Mexican and chorizo from the River Plate (Uruguay) is Argentinean. Best varieties are reputed to come from Estramadura, near the Portuguese border, and Pamplona, not far from the French frontier, where the pigs are fed on acorns. Chaurice is a Creole version from New Orleans, USA.

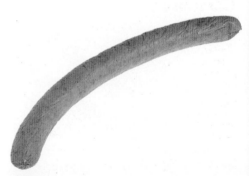

Clobassy

MAJOR NUTRIENTS
SERVE SIZE 30 G

Energy	420 kJ	Dietary Fibre	0
Protein	5 g	Sodium	255 mg
Fat	9 g	Potassium	35 mg
Cholesterol	25 mg	Phosphorus	50 mg
Carbohydrate		Iron	0.8 mg
less than 1 g		Zinc	1 mg
Total Sugars	0	Thiamin	0.05 mg

NUTRITIONAL INFORMATION A high fat content with over 79% of energy coming from predominantly monounsaturated fats. A serving contains good amounts of phosphorus, iron, zinc, thiamin and vitamin B12. Use to add flavour rather than as a major source of these vitamins and minerals. Also, the preservation process requires the addition of sodium, so intake should be moderated in sodium-controlled diets. Slow cooking may reduce fat content marginally.

DESCRIPTION A long, round sausage made from pork and beef, finely seasoned and often with a touch of garlic. Smoked.

ORIGIN AND HISTORY Clobassy is the term for smallgoods in Poland.

BUYING AND STORAGE Sold by the unit. Hang in a cool place for up to 3 months to enhance flavour. To prevent maturation clobassy can be refrigerated.

PREPARATION AND USE Can be served hot or cold, grilled, barbecued, or used as a bacon substitute. Excellent as a snack with drinks.

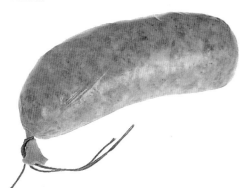

Cotechino

also called *Italian-style pork sausage*

MAJOR NUTRIENTS		SERVE SIZE 100 G	
Energy	1520 kJ	Potassium	200 mg
Protein	13 g	Calcium	50 mg
Fat	32 g	Phosphorus	190 mg
Cholesterol	85 mg	Iron	1.5 mg
Carbohydrate	0	Zinc	2.5 mg
Total Sugars	0	Riboflavin	0.2 mg
Dietary Fibre	0	Niacin Equiv.	5.8 mg
Sodium	520 mg		

NUTRITIONAL INFORMATION A high fat content with over 79% of energy coming from fats. A serving contains good amounts of phosphorus, iron, zinc, riboflavin, niacin and vitamin B12. Use to add flavour rather than as a major source of these vitamins and minerals. Also, the preservation process requires the addition of sodium, so intake should be moderated in sodium-controlled diets. Slow cooking may reduce fat content marginally.

DESCRIPTION A large fresh lean and fat pork sausage, lightly salted.

ORIGIN AND HISTORY Italian. The New

Year's Eve in modern Rome would be incomplete without boiled cotechino with lentils which dates back to ancient Rome.

BUYING AND STORAGE In Italy, cotechino are made fresh and are not meant for keeping, however, a part-cured and cooked type is now commercially available.

PREPARATION AND USE Pan fry or braise the cooked variety. If fresh, wrap in a cloth and simmer for 2 hours. Serve with beans, lentils or mashed potatoes. Cotechino is also one of the ingredients in a bollito misto, a glamorous Italian dish consisting of various cooked meats in hot stock, cotechino, and served with pickled Italian vegetables and green sauce (salsa verde). Robert Carrier recommends cotechino with cooked spinach.

VARIETIES
Pizza Sausage (USA).

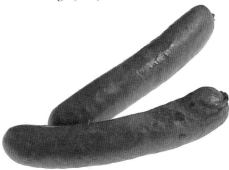

Frankfurter

also called *Wiener*

MAJOR NUTRIENTS		SERVE SIZE 100 G	
Energy	1040 kJ	Potassium	90 mg
Protein	14 g	Phosphorus	130 mg
Fat	20 g	Iron	2.2 mg
Cholesterol	60 mg	Zinc	2.2 mg
Carbohydrate	3 g	Thiamin	0.2 mg
Total Sugars	0	Riboflavin	0.13 mg
Dietary Fibre	0	Niacin Equiv.	3.2 mg
Sodium	770 mg		

NUTRITIONAL INFORMATION Even though these sausages may not appear to be as fatty as some others, they contain 70% of energy from fats. A serving contains good amounts of phosphorus, iron, zinc, thiamin and vitamin B12. Use sparingly, not as a daily source of these vitamins and minerals. Also, the preservation process requires the addition of sodium, so intake should be moderated in sodium-controlled diets.

DESCRIPTION In general a frankfurter is a blend of beef, pork and/or poultry meat, mildly seasoned with spices and smoked. May be contained in a casing, however, 95% of frankfurters sold in the USA are skinless.

ORIGIN AND HISTORY Frankfurter originated near Frankfurt, Germany; Wiener from

Vienna, Austria. Today they are known to millions of North Americans as hot dogs.

BUYING AND STORAGE Sold as units/kg. Also available in vacuum packs. Keep refrigerated and can be stored for up to 1 week. If purchased in a vacuum pack observe the use-by date recommended by the processer.

PREPARATION AND USE Already cooked frankfurter can be eaten cold, but is more commonly simmered in water for 3–5 minutes. Serve as a hot dog in a bread roll with fried onion and sweet mustard. Cocktail frankfurter is usually heated and served with a tomato-based sauce as a party snack.

VARIETIES

Australian Frankfurter Formulated to appeal to Anglo-Saxon tastes.

Cocktail Frankfurter/Cheerio Half the size of a regular frankfurter.

Continental Frankfurter Finely textured, mildly spiced.

Foot-long Frankfurter

Red Hots

Smoked Frankfurter/Smoked Link/ Smoky

Vienna-Style / Vienna / Wiener Short links and canned.

Fresh Sausage

DESCRIPTION Fresh sausages are made from chopped, minced or blended meats that are neither cured nor smoked. They are seasoned and usually stuffed into casings (skins) and must be fully cooked before serving. Today there are many exotic types of sausages being produced with entire shops specialising in sausages like turkey and sage, satay, tomato and onion, lamb and mint to name a few.

ORIGIN AND HISTORY The word sausage comes from the Latin salsus, meaning salted. However, the French are credited with developing the modern sausage. The Greeks and Romans encouraged sausage making, and it is believed that the Germans, who claim to have invented the sausage, learned their skill from the Romans, but it was left to the French to develop the idea so imaginatively. After those, the most varied contributions to sausage making came from Germany and Italy.

BUYING AND STORAGE Purchase by the unit/kg. Fresh sausages should be placed promptly in the coolest part of the refrigerator, and cooked within 2–3 days of purchase. Most fresh sausages can be sealed in plastic wrap and frozen. If purchased in a vacuum-sealed pack observe the use-by date.

PREPARATION AND USE All fresh sausages should be thoroughly cooked at a low to moderate temperature. Fresh sausage is fully cooked and ready to eat when the colour turns from pink to grey. Different methods of cooking include pan frying, braising, baking, grilling, barbecuing and microwaving. Mustard as an accompaniment to sausages has a history which goes back to the Greeks and Romans. Ketchups and sauces, including the English Worcestershire sauce, pickles and chutneys complement a sausage. A favourite English meal is bangers and mash, simply fried sausages and mashed potatoes.

VARIETIES

Banger The English breakfast sausage made from pork, with cereal. Plump and around 10 cm in length.

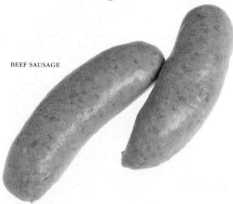

BEEF SAUSAGE

Beef Sausage A standard sausage made from beef which may be thick or thin in diameter but usually around 10 cm in length.

MAJOR NUTRIENTS		GRILLED	
		SERVE SIZE 100 G	
Energy	1100 kJ	Sodium	1100 mg
Protein	13 g	Potassium	190 mg
Fat	17 g	Calcium	75 mg
Cholesterol	50 mg	Phosphorus	210 mg
Carbohydrate	15 g	Iron	1.5 mg
Total Sugars	0	Zinc	1.5 mg
Dietary Fibre	0.5 g	Niacin Equiv.	7.1 mg

NUTRITIONAL INFORMATION Over 57% of energy comes from fats. A serving contains excellent amounts of protein, phosphorus,

iron, niacin and vitamin B12 and good amounts of calcium and zinc. It should not be used as a daily source of animal protein despite its economic price. Also, the preservation process requires the addition of sodium, so intake should be moderated in sodium-controlled diets. Slow cooking or preboiling may enable total fat content to be reduced slightly. Addition of spices will not affect nutrient analysis.

Breakfast Sausage Small and finely textured, usually a pork sausage which may contain a variety of spices. Mild in flavour.

Country-Style Pork Sausage A pork sausage with a coarser texture than a regular pork sausage.

Cambridge Sausage A very popular English sausage made from pork, rice and sausage meal. Its distinctive flavour comes from the seasoning of sage, cayenne, mace, nutmeg, pepper and salt.

English Country Pork Sausage A coarsely textured pork sausage produced in England.

Link Sausages A general term covering fresh sausages which may contain pork, or pork/beef or other meats with seasonings.

Oxford Sausage An English sausage containing veal, pork, beef suet, herbs and spices.

Paprika Sausage A fresh, dark, fairly coarsely textured sausage made from lamb and beef, paprika, coriander, fennel and seasonings.

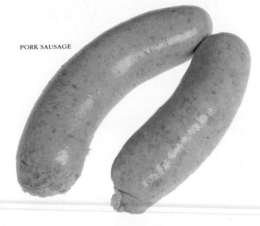

PORK SAUSAGE

Pork Sausage A general term for a sausage made from pork. Seasonings will vary according to the processer. In the USA a pork sausage is often seasoned with pepper and sage.

MAJOR NUTRIENTS		GRILLED	
		SERVE SIZE 100 G	
Energy	1320 kJ	Potassium	200 mg
Protein	13 g	Calcium	55 mg
Fat	25 g	Phosphorus	220 mg
Cholesterol	55 mg	Iron	1.5 mg
Carbohydrate	12 g	Zinc	1.5 mg
Total Sugars		Riboflavin	0.15 mg
	less than 1 g	Niacin Equiv.	5.8 mg
Dietary Fibre	0.5 g		
Sodium	1000 mg		

NUTRITIONAL INFORMATION Over 79% of energy coming from fats. A serving contains excellent amounts of protein, phosphorus, iron, niacin and vitamin B12 and good amounts of zinc and riboflavin. However, it should not be used as a daily source of animal protein despite its economical price. Also, the preservation process requires the addition of sodium, so intake should be moderated in sodium-controlled diets. Slow cooking or preboiling may enable total fat content to be reduced slightly.

Skinless Sausages Sausage meat sold without casings. Sometimes shaped into patties.

Spiced English Sausage A pale pink sausage that incorporates pork and spices. Smooth in texture.

Spiced French Sausage A fairly coarsely textured sausage, highly spiced and well seasoned with garlic.

SEE ALSO Bratwurst, Chipolata, Cotechino, Loukanika, Merguez, Salsiccie, Saucisson, Toulouse Sausage.

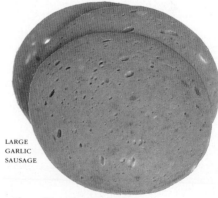

LARGE GARLIC SAUSAGE

Garlic Sausage

MAJOR NUTRIENTS		SERVE SIZE 100 G	
Energy	1040 kJ	Potassium	90 mg
Protein	14 g	Phosphorus	130 mg
Fat	20 g	Iron	2 mg
Cholesterol	60 mg	Zinc	2 mg
Carbohydrate	3 g	Thiamin	0.2 mg
Total Sugars	0	Riboflavin	0.1 mg
Dietary Fibre	0	Niacin Equiv.	3.2 mg
Sodium	770 mg		

NUTRITIONAL INFORMATION Over 71% of energy coming from fats. A serving provides an excellent source of iron and good amounts of phosphorus, zinc, thiamin, riboflavin, niacin and vitamin B12. Use to add flavour rather than as a major source of these vitamins and minerals. Also, the preservation process requires the addition of sodium, so intake should be moderated in sodium-controlled diets. Slow cooking may reduce fat content marginally.

DESCRIPTION Similar to the frankfurter, except that garlic is a prime spice ingredient. The shape is also distinctive, very short and squat, about 12 cm in length and 5 cm thick. Usually smoked with a reddish-brown skin.

'Garlic sausage' in Australia usually means a soft, devon-like product. Devon is listed in the second half of this chapter.

ORIGIN AND HISTORY German.

BUYING AND STORAGE These should be bought and kept in the same way as frankfurters.

PREPARATION AND USE Heat through and serve with a sauce.

VARIETIES
Cervela, Knoblauchwurst, German.

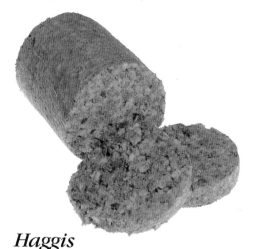

Haggis

MAJOR NUTRIENTS		SERVE SIZE 100 G
Energy	1120 kJ	Calcium	55 mg
Protein	11 g	Phosphorus	120 mg
Fat	19 g	Iron	8 mg
Cholesterol	70 mg	Zinc	2 mg
Carbohydrate	15 g	Vitamin A	1500 µg
Total Sugars	0	Thiamin	0.15 mg
Dietary Fibre	0	Riboflavin	0.5 mg
Sodium	820 mg	Niacin Equiv.	4 mg
Potassium	170 mg		

NUTRITIONAL INFORMATION Over 79% of energy comes from predominantly unsaturated fats. A serving contains an excellent amount of vitamin A, iron, zinc, riboflavin, niacin and vitamin B12 and good amounts of

thiamin. Use in moderation. Also, the preservation process requires the addition of sodium, so intake should be moderated in sodium-controlled diets.

DESCRIPTION A large spherical sausage made from the liver, heart and lungs of a sheep, all mixed with beef or mutton, suet and oatmeal, seasoned with onion and cayenne pepper.

ORIGIN AND HISTORY The concept of chopping pork meat and meal and stuffing it into an animal's gut was promoted by the Romans. When introduced into Scotland, the Scots preferred mutton and the idea was adapted to suit local tastes. Haggis is the national dish of Scotland, served on Burns's night, 25 January, and Scotland's New Year celebration, Hogmanay. The derivation of the word is unknown.

BUYING AND STORAGE Precooked haggis is now commercially available.

PREPARATION AND USE Traditionally prepared haggis requires long cooking. Simmer in all-but boiling water, long enough to be thoroughly hot and steaming when a slit is made in the paunch for a large tablespoon to be inserted and the haggis scooped out. Traditional accompaniments are neeps (turnips), potatoes, and, of course, whisky.

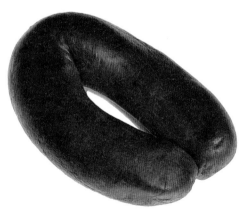

Hog's Pudding

MAJOR NUTRIENTS		BLACK HOG'S PUDDING SERVE SIZE 100 G
Energy	1120 kJ	Calcium	55 mg
Protein	11 g	Phosphorus	120 mg
Fat	19 g	Iron	8 mg
Cholesterol	70 mg	Zinc	2 mg
Carbohydrate	15 g	Vitamin A	1500 µg
Total Sugars	0	Thiamin	0.15 mg
Dietary Fibre	0	Riboflavin	0.5 mg
Sodium	820 mg	Niacin Equiv.	4 mg
Potassium	170 mg		

NUTRITIONAL INFORMATION Over 63% of energy comes from fats with significant amounts of cholesterol, a very rich source of

vitamin A and iron. Contains excellent amounts of phosphorus, zinc, riboflavin, niacin and vitamin B12. As it used to be a relatively inexpensive product it was considered a very nutritious budget food, but now, because of labour costs it is quite expensive. Also, the preservation process requires the addition of sodium, so intake should be moderated in sodium-controlled diets. White hog's pudding will have a reduced iron and zinc content.

DESCRIPTION An English West Country dish, similar to haggis, which contains the pig's pluck (liver, heart and lungs). Devon and Cornwall also have their varieties of hog's pudding, the difference being in the seasoning.

ORIGIN AND HISTORY English. Recorded recipes date back to 1689.

BUYING AND STORAGE Commercially available.

PREPARATION AND USE As for haggis.

VARIETIES
Black hog's pudding, contains blood; white hog's pudding, no blood, with cream and eggs.

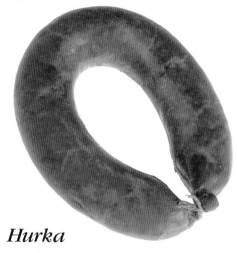

Hurka

NUTRITIONAL INFORMATION No detailed analysis is available, but normally at least 40% by weight will be carbohydrate; protein, phosphorus, iron and zinc levels will be lower than 100% meat-filled sausage.

DESCRIPTION A ring sausage made from cooked pork and beef with cooked rice, onion and seasonings. Black hurka contains pig's blood while white hurka does not.

ORIGIN AND HISTORY Polish.

BUYING AND STORAGE Purchased by the unit/ring. Refrigerate and use within 1 week of purchase.

PREPARATION AND USE Slice and use as cold cut or an interesting snack.

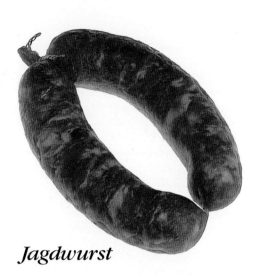

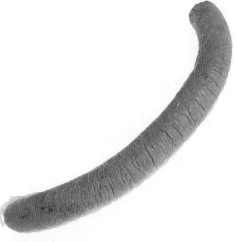

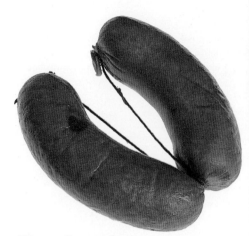

Jagdwurst

MAJOR NUTRIENTS		SERVE SIZE 30 G	
Energy	460 kJ	Sodium	250 mg
Protein	4 g	Potassium	80 mg
Fat	10 g	Phosphorus	45 mg
Cholesterol	40 mg	Iron	1.1 mg
Carbohydrate	0	Zinc	2 mg
Total Sugars	0	Niacin Equiv.	1.6 mg
Dietary Fibre	0		

NUTRITIONAL INFORMATION Over 79% of energy comes from fats. A serving contains excellent amounts of phosphorus, iron, zinc, niacin and vitamin B12. Use to add flavour rather than as a major source of these vitamins and minerals. Also, the preservation process requires the addition of sodium, so intake should be moderated in sodium-controlled diets.

DESCRIPTION There are various types of this 'hunter's sausage'. Generally it is a large smoked sausage made from finely minced pork and pork fat. In the USA jagdwurst denotes a bologna-style product in a stick form.

ORIGIN AND HISTORY German. Huntsmen often carried this sausage in their pockets to nibble on when out for several days hunting.

BUYING AND STORAGE Usually bought by slice/kg; in the USA per unit. Store in refrigerator, wrapped, and use within 3–5 days.

PREPARATION AND USE The jagdwurst is usually sliced and eaten cold. A traditional German dish is Brunswick salad where strips of jagdwurst are mixed with finely chopped pickled cucumber, tomato, grated apple and cooked French beans. This is dressed with olive oil mixed with the juice of the pickled cucumber.

VARIETIES

Schinken jagdwurst, contains pieces of ham.

Kielbasa

*also called **Polish sausage***

MAJOR NUTRIENTS		SERVE SIZE 30 G	
Energy	560 kJ	Sodium	665 mg
Protein	7 g	Potassium	50 mg
Fat	11 g	Phosphorus	50 mg
Cholesterol	30 mg	Iron	1 mg
Carbohydrate	0	Zinc	0.9 mg
Total Sugars	0	Thiamin	0.5 mg
Dietary Fibre	0	Niacin Equiv.	2.1 mg

NUTRITIONAL INFORMATION A high fat content with over 72% of energy coming from predominantly monounsaturated fats. A serving contains good amounts of phosphorus, iron, zinc, niacin and vitamin B12. Use to add interesting flavour rather than as a major source of these vitamins and minerals. Also, the preservation process requires the addition of sodium, so intake should be moderated in sodium-controlled diets. Slow cooking may reduce fat content marginally.

DESCRIPTION A Polish smoked sausage made from ground beef and pork, highly spiced with garlic. In the USA kielbasa is used to describe Polish or Polish-style sausages.

ORIGIN AND HISTORY 'Kielbasa' is the Polish word for 'sausage'.

BUYING AND STORAGE Around 10 cm in length and 4 cm in diameter, kielbasa are purchased by unit/kg. Refrigerate.

PREPARATION AND USE Fry and serve with potatoes or steam and accompany with lentils.

A kielbasa salad consists of the diced sausage mixed with cold cooked kidney beans, spring onions, diced beetroot, capers and a French dressing. Another version uses green lentils, shredded green pepper and hard boiled egg.

Knackwurst

MAJOR NUTRIENTS		SERVE SIZE 100 G	
Energy	1560 kJ	Potassium	195 mg
Protein	12 g	Phosphorus	150 mg
Fat	33 g	Iron	1.5 mg
Cholesterol	100 mg	Zinc	2.2 mg
Carbohydrate	0	Thiamin	0.1 mg
Total Sugars	0	Riboflavin	0.15 mg
Dietary Fibre	0	Niacin Equiv.	3.9 mg
Sodium	1190 mg		

NUTRITIONAL INFORMATION Over 79% of energy comes from fats. A serving contains good amounts of phosphorus, iron, zinc, thiamin and vitamin B12. Use to add flavour rather than as a major source of these vitamins and minerals. Also, the preservation process requires the addition of sodium, so intake should be moderated in sodium-controlled diets. Slow cooking may reduce fat content marginally.

DESCRIPTION A coarsely ground beef, pork and veal sausage smoked to a reddish-brown. Highly seasoned with garlic.

ORIGIN AND HISTORY German.

BUYING AND STORAGE A short chunky sausage which is purchased by the unit/kg. Refrigerate for up to 1 week.

PREPARATION AND USE Simmer or steam to warm, or cook with sauerkraut. Can be substituted for frankfurters.

VARIETIES

Schueblig, Switzerland.

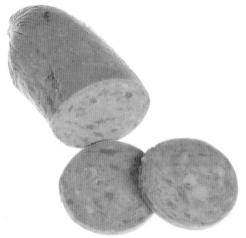

Kolbasa

MAJOR NUTRIENTS — SERVE SIZE 30 G

Energy	560 kJ	Sodium	665 mg
Protein	7 g	Potassium	50 mg
Fat	11 g	Phosphorus	50 mg
Cholesterol	30 mg	Iron	1 mg
Carbohydrate	0	Zinc	1.1 mg
Total Sugars	0	Thiamin	0.5 mg
Dietary Fibre	0	Niacin Equiv.	2.1 mg

NUTRITIONAL INFORMATION Over 73% of energy comes from predominantly unsaturated fats. A serving contains excellent amounts of thiamin and good amounts of phosphorus, iron, zinc, niacin and vitamin B12. Use to add flavour rather than as a major source of these vitamins and minerals. Also, the preservation process requires the addition of sodium, so intake should be moderated in sodium-controlled diets. May contain Nitrites 250.

DESCRIPTION A type of spicy sausage made from beef and pork, either fresh or smoked.

ORIGIN AND HISTORY Russian. There is a Hungarian version, known as Kolbasz.

BUYING AND STORAGE Keep in refrigerator.

PREPARATION AND USE As for kielbasa.

Kransky

MAJOR NUTRIENTS — SERVE SIZE 100 G

Energy	1560 kJ	Potassium	195 mg
Protein	12 g	Phosphorus	150 mg
Fat	33 g	Iron	1.5 mg
Cholesterol	45 mg	Zinc	2.2 mg
Carbohydrate	0	Thiamin	0.1 mg
Total Sugars	0	Riboflavin	0.10 mg
Dietary Fibre	0	Niacin Equiv.	3.9 mg
Sodium	1190 mg		

NUTRITIONAL INFORMATION Over 79% of energy comes from fats. A serving contains excellent amounts of protein, phosphorus, iron and vitamin B12 and good amounts of zinc, thiamin, riboflavin and niacin. Use to add flavour rather than as a major source of these vitamins and minerals. Also, the preservation process requires the addition of sodium, so intake should be moderated in sodium-controlled diets. Slow cooking may reduce fat content marginally.

DESCRIPTION A coarsely textured sausage made from pork or pork/beef, seasoned and smoked, and including pepper.

ORIGIN AND HISTORY Kranj is a town north of Ljubljana, Yugoslavia which gives this sausage its name.

BUYING AND STORAGE Purchase in links of 7–10 cm or by the kg. Store in the refrigerator for up to 1 week.

PREPARATION AND USE Eat cold or simmer for 3–5 minutes and serve with sauerkraut.

VARIETIES
Kranjska kobasica, Yugoslavia.

Lap Cheong

*also called **Chinese sausage, Cantonese sausage***

MAJOR NUTRIENTS — SERVE SIZE 30 G

Energy	540 kJ	Dietary Fibre	0
Protein	7 g	Sodium	440 mg
Fat	11 g	Potassium	35 mg
Cholesterol	25 mg	Phosphorus	50 mg
Carbohydrate	1 g	Iron	1 mg
Total Sugars		Zinc	1 mg
less than 1 g		Niacin Equiv.	1 mg

NUTRITIONAL INFORMATION Over 75% of energy comes from fats. A serving contains good amounts of protein, phosphorus, iron, zinc, niacin and vitamin B12. Use to add flavour rather than as a major source of these vitamins and minerals. Also, the preservation process requires the addition of sodium, so intake should be moderated in sodium-controlled diets. Slow cooking may reduce fat content marginally.

DESCRIPTION Thin, hard, linked sausages each about 15 cm long, with a sweet, smoky taste and smell, similar in appearance to a small pepperoni sausage. These are made with highly seasoned pork and pork fat in a natural casing, smoked and dried.

ORIGIN AND HISTORY The Chinese learned even before Han times (206 BC–AD220) that meats could be hung to dry, and thus began what is the world's longest history of the preservation of foods by air-drying. Encased within an intestinal skin, the meat was further protected and dried into a firm shape which was easy to use and transport. The techniques applied in those early times are little changed today. Chou, the last king of Shang, kept so much meat drying on racks that it was described as 'jou lin', a 'meat forest'.

BUYING AND STORAGE Sold in packs of 8–10 sausages, weighing 500 g, and in some Chinese delicatessens these can be bought singly. They will keep refrigerated for many months.

PREPARATION AND USE These sausages should be steamed or blanched in simmering water before use to soften. Used primarily to add their unique flavour to certain Chinese stir-fried dishes, and a prime ingredient in 'sticky' rice and certain stuffings. They can be steamed on top of rice as a simple snack.

A stronger tasting similar Chinese sausage contains duck and pork liver with pork meat. It is used with discretion in stir-fried dishes and may be served as an accompaniment to rice 'congee', a soup-like bland rice dish eaten in the morning.

VARIETIES
Pork and pork fat, duck liver.

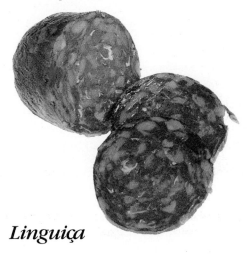

Linguiça

*also called **Longaniza***

MAJOR NUTRIENTS			SERVE SIZE 100 G
Energy	1560 kJ	Potassium	195 mg
Protein	12 g	Phosphorus	150 mg
Fat	33 g	Iron	1.5 mg
Cholesterol	100 mg	Zinc	2 mg
Carbohydrate	0	Thiamin	0.1 mg
Total Sugars	0	Riboflavin	0.1 mg
Dietary Fibre	0	Niacin Equiv.	3.9 mg
Sodium	1190 mg		

NUTRITIONAL INFORMATION Over 79% of energy comes from fats. A serving contains excellent amounts of protein, phosphorus, iron and vitamin B12 and good amounts of zinc, thiamin, riboflavin and niacin. Use to add flavour rather than as a major source of these vitamins and minerals. Also, the preservation process requires the addition of sodium, so intake should be moderated in sodium-controlled diets. Slow cooking may reduce fat content marginally.

DESCRIPTION Linguiça is a small slim Portuguese sausage with lots of garlic and paprika. It is often smoked. The Spanish longaniza is usually fresh.

ORIGIN AND HISTORY Portuguese.

BUYING AND STORAGE Wherever it is obtained, it should be kept refrigerated.

PREPARATION AND USE A favourite ingredient in Portuguese and Brazilian soups, stews and casseroles but can be grilled over charcoal. Tripe dishes, baked eggs and Portuguese gazpacho also include linguiça. A popular choice is a mixed pork grill including linguiça, an open-topped sausage pie, sautéed morcilla slices served with pickled onions, and a wonderful-tasting combination of sausage and clams called cataplana.

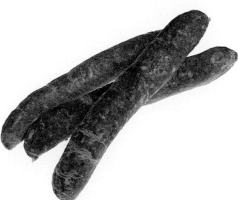

Loukanika

MAJOR NUTRIENTS			SERVE SIZE 30 G
Energy	560 kJ	Sodium	665 mg
Protein	7 g	Potassium	50 mg
Fat	11 g	Phosphorus	50 mg
Cholesterol	30 mg	Iron	1 mg
Carbohydrate	0	Zinc	1 mg
Total Sugars	0	Thiamin	0.5 mg
Dietary Fibre	0	Niacin Equiv.	2.1 mg

NUTRITIONAL INFORMATION Over 72% of energy comes from predominantly mono-unsaturated fats. A serving contains good amounts of protein, phosphorus, iron and vitamin B12 and significant amounts of zinc, thiamin and niacin. Use to add flavour rather than as a major source of these vitamins and minerals. Also, the preservation process requires the addition of sodium, so intake should be moderated in sodium-controlled diets.

DESCRIPTION A lamb and pork fresh sausage which has been marinated in red wine or port. Sometimes the sausage is hung for up to 2 weeks.

ORIGIN AND HISTORY From Greece and Cyprus.

BUYING AND STORAGE Purchased by the link/kg. Refrigerate and use within 2–3 days.

PREPARATION AND USE In Greece the loukanika is often cut into 4 cm chunks, grilled and served as an hors d'oeuvre. A traditional Greek stew, spetsofagi, consists of loukanika cooked with green peppers. Often fried and served with eggs or accompanied by a baked rice pilaf.

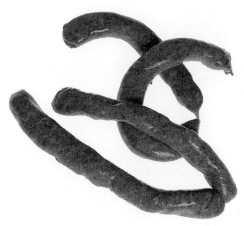

Merguez

NUTRITIONAL INFORMATION No detailed nutritional analysis available on this product, as ingredients can vary owing to traditional recipes.

DESCRIPTION A highly spiced sausage which is made from goat or mutton and flavoured with harissa (a mixture of hot pepper and cumin).

ORIGIN AND HISTORY From Algeria.

BUYING AND STORAGE Available at certain delicatessens. Keep refrigerated.

PREPARATION AND USE Grill. It is often served with couscous, a traditional North African dish.

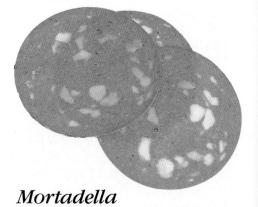

Mortadella

MAJOR NUTRIENTS			SERVE SIZE: 30 G
Energy	410 kJ	Sodium	231 mg
Protein	4 g	Potassium	40 mg
Fat	9 g	Phosphorus	50 mg
Cholesterol	20 mg	Iron	1 mg
Carbohydrate		Zinc	1 mg
	less than 1 g	Niacin Equiv.	1.1 mg
Total Sugars	0		
Dietary Fibre	0		

NUTRITIONAL INFORMATION A popular cold meat often not recognised for its very high fat content. Over 80% of energy comes from fats. A serving contains good amounts of protein, phosphorus, iron, zinc and vitamin B12. Use to add flavour in a sandwich rather than as a major source of these vitamins and minerals. Also, the preservation process requires the addition of sodium, so intake should be moderated in sodium-controlled diets.

DESCRIPTION Mortadella is an Italian-style cooked sausage composed of finely chopped cured pork and beef with added cubes of pork back fat. Delicately spiced and smoked.

ORIGIN AND HISTORY This is the original bolognese sausage, produced before 1376, the year in which the Guild of Sausage-makers was formed. In monastery kitchens pork was broken down with a pestle and mortar. It is said that the mortar was known as a 'mortaio della carne di maiale' which became 'mortadella'.

BUYING AND STORAGE A large diameter sausage, mortadella is usually purchased finely sliced. Keep refrigerated and use within 2–3 days of purchase.

PREPARATION AND USE To be enjoyed as a cold cut, as a sandwich slice, or as part of an antipasto. The Bolognese use it in many different ways, as a pasta stuffing, added to sauces and vegetable gratinée, pies and the famous Genoa torta.

VARIETIES
Mortadella with pistachio nuts.

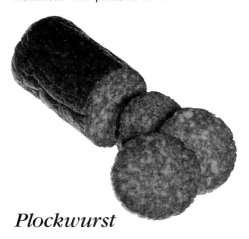

Plockwurst

MAJOR NUTRIENTS		SERVE SIZE 100 G	
Energy	1320 kJ	Sodium	830 mg
Protein	19 g	Potassium	200 mg
Fat	27 g	Phosphorus	130 mg
Cholesterol	70 mg	Iron	1.5 mg
Carbohydrate	0	Zinc	2.1 mg
Total Sugars	0	Niacin Equiv.	5.9 mg
Dietary Fibre	0		

NUTRITIONAL INFORMATION Over 80% of energy comes from fats. A serving contains good amounts of protein, phosphorus, iron, zinc, thiamin and vitamin B12 and significant quantities of zinc, thiamin and niacin. Use to add flavour rather than as a major source of

these vitamins and minerals. Also, the preservation process requires the addition of sodium, so intake should be moderated in sodium-controlled diets.

DESCRIPTION Beef or beef/pork sausage, which has been smoked. Dark in colour owing to the high proportion of beef. A similar sausage is known in the USA as polka sausage.

ORIGIN AND HISTORY German.

BUYING AND STORAGE Keeps well in the refrigerator.

PREPARATION AND USE Use as a snack, like other smoked sausages.

VARIETIES
Pfeffer plockwurst, with peppercorns.

Salami

MAJOR NUTRIENTS		SERVE SIZE 30 G	
Energy	610 kJ	Potassium	51 mg
Protein	6 g	Phosphorus	50 mg
Fat	11 g	Iron	0.9 mg
Cholesterol	35 mg	Zinc	0.8 mg
Carbohydrate		Thiamin	0.05 mg
	less than 1 g	Riboflavin	0.15 mg
Total Sugars	0	Niacin Equiv.	1.9 mg
Dietary Fibre	0		
Sodium	440 mg		

NUTRITIONAL INFORMATION Over 67% of energy comes from predominantly mono-unsaturated fats. A serving contains good amounts of iron, zinc and vitamin B12 and significant amounts of thiamin, riboflavin and niacin. It should be used in moderation. Also, the preservation process requires the addition of sodium, so intake should be moderated in sodium-controlled diets.

DESCRIPTION Most salamis are made from fresh pork and have a coarsely ground texture with garlic as the main spice. They are generally cured during processing and may or may not be smoked.

ORIGIN AND HISTORY Salami appears to have originated in the ancient Grecian town of Salamis, on the Cypriot East Coast. It was under the Romans that Salamis enjoyed great prosperity as the principal town of Cyprus. Salami is one of the original sausages developed when salting, drying and smoking were the only ways to preserve meat. By the Middle Ages sausage making had become a commercial art. Climate was an important factor in the development of the regional varieties. Dry and semi-dry sausages originated in the warm

Mediterranean climates of Italy, Spain, and southern France while the cooler climates of Germany and Austria resulted in the making of fresh and cooked sausages. Dry salamis are the true salami, being made from fresh uncooked meat. Semi-dry salamis are made from cooked meat.

BUYING AND STORAGE Most salamis are available as single units or sliced. Dry salamis when purchased as a single unit may be stored in a cool dry place for up to 3 months. During this time they will mature and the flavour will intensify with the slow drying out process. Occasionally wipe with a lightly oiled or damp cloth. If purchased sliced, refrigerate and use within 3–5 days.

PREPARATION AND USE Salamis are generally ready to eat, with salad, as a sandwich filling, as a snack. Excellent as an ingredient in an antipasto, pizza topping, in hotpots or as a garnish in salads. Add julienne strips of salami to your favourite pasta dish for added flavour.

VARIETIES

Arles A tangy French provincial salami, coarsely ground.

Alpina Salami/Alessandria Italian-style salamis of USA origin.

Beer From Bavaria, Germany. Made from pork and veal, coarsely textured and so named because in its country of origin it is considered the ideal sausage to serve with beer.

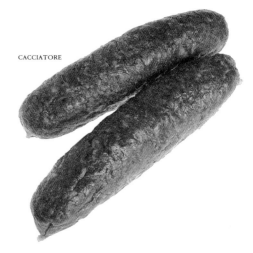

CACCIATORE

Cacciatore An Italian salami which can be either mild or hot. Made from pork and beef, spices and a touch of garlic. Small in size, they are said to have originated near Como, Italy. Cacciatore means hunter and implies that these salamis were made to be suitable for a sportsman's pocket, when out hunting.

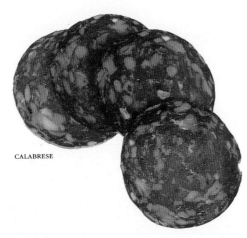

CALABRESE

Calabrese A hot spicy salami which includes chilli, red peppers, red wine and other spices. It originates from Calabria, southern Italy, and it is reported that the further south one travels the stronger the seasoning. It can contain quite large pieces of white fat.

Cappicola Of Italian origin. Made from boneless pork butt seasoned with red hot and sweet peppers, mild cured and air-dried.

Casalingo Cacciatore Cacciatore-style, 'casalingo' simply means homemade in Italian.

Cervelatwurst Quite different from the Cervelat family of products. It is a pork-based mild dry salami of German origin. No garlic.

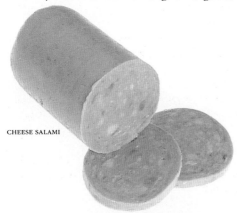

CHEESE SALAMI

Cheese Salami A mild flavoured Austrian pork/veal salami with cubes of Emmentaler cheese.

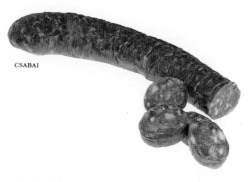

CSABAI

Csabai A mild Hungarian-style salami seasoned with cracked peppercorns and paprika.

Culatello (culatello di Zibello) Zibello is a village near Parma which became famous several hundred years ago, when the Lords of Lower Parma found the local salami so delicious that they sent it as a 'rare and precious offering' to the Sforzas, the ruling family. The secret of their recipe has been lost.

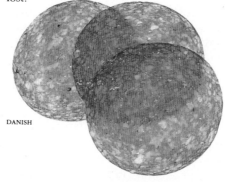

DANISH

Danish Salami/Spegelpoelse A bright red, coarsely textured salami seasoned with black pepper and garlic. The Danes have been making their own style of salami since before the 15th century.

Felinetti/Salame de Felino From the village of Felino, southwest of Parma, Italy. It is a delicate salami containing white peppercorns and a little garlic. 'Expensive but succulent.'

Frizzes Italian-style salamis found in the USA. Sweet and peppery types are made, both scented with aniseed. The sweet is corded with blue string, the hot with red.

French Pepper/French Herb Small diameter salami made from pork and beef with coarse fat and coated with peppercorns or herbs.

Genoa Salami A good quality, quite fat Italian salami studded with whole peppercorns.

German Generally the German varieties of salami are made of finely ground beef and pork, and tend to be more heavily smoked than their Italian counterparts.

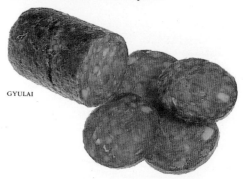

GYULAI

Gyulai Mildly smoked salami with sweet pepper. This salami takes its name from its place of origin in Hungary, Gyula, near the Romanian border.

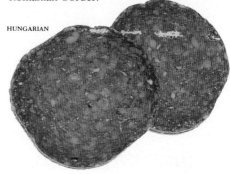

HUNGARIAN

Hungarian and White Hungarian Salami A mild semi-coarse salami made from pork and beef and a blend of spices. It is reported that the Hungarians were making salami over a century ago, and it was first made in 1859 in Szeged. Hungarian salami keeps well and its flavour grows sharper with age. White Hungarian is so named because of its white-coloured casing.

Italian Salami A mild, delicately flavoured salami that should be thinly sliced.

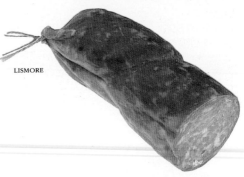

LISMORE

Lismore Salami A natural soft salami, coarsely minced, with a very sweet flavour. Slice thickly and fry with eggs for breakfast.

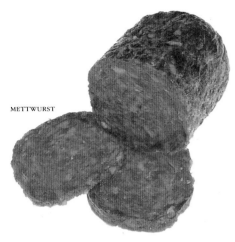

METTWURST

Mettwurst A medium-textured German-style salami made from fresh pork, mildly seasoned and usually without garlic.

Milano Salami A regional Italian salami, of finely textured pork/beef with garlic, pepper and white wine. A classic antipasto ingredient.

Napoli Salami A long thin salami made with pork and beef, seasoned with both black and red pepper to make it quite hot.

Paprika Salami A Hungarian-style salami of fine texture, spiced with Hungarian paprika.

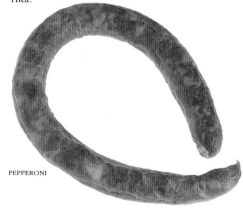

PEPPERONI

Pepperoni Italian in origin, pepperoni (sometimes spelt pepperone) is made from ground pork and beef with added fat. Ground red pepper is the major flavour ingredient. The popularity of pizza has added greatly to the consumption of pepperoni — this is its most common use.

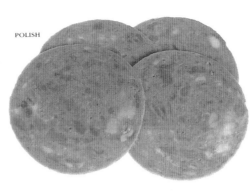

POLISH

Polish Salami

MAJOR NUTRIENTS		SERVE SIZE 30 G	
Energy	560 kJ	Sodium	665 mg
Protein	7 g	Potassium	50 mg
Fat	11 g	Phosphorus	50 mg
Cholesterol	30 mg	Iron	1 mg
Carbohydrate	0	Zinc	1 mg
Total Sugars	0	Thiamin	0.5 mg
Dietary Fibre	0	Niacin Equiv.	2.1 mg

NUTRITIONAL INFORMATION Over 79% of energy comes from predominantly mono-unsaturated fats. A serving contains excellent amounts of thiamin, good amounts of protein, phosphorus, iron and vitamin B12 and significant quantities of zinc and niacin. Use in moderation to add flavour rather than as a major source of these vitamins and minerals. Also, the preservation process requires the addition of sodium, so intake should be moderated in sodium-controlled diets.

DESCRIPTION A fine/medium texture semi-dry, cooked salami made from pork/beef, seasonings and some garlic.

ORIGIN AND HISTORY Polish.

BUYING AND STORAGE Usually bought in medium/thick slices. Must be refrigerated and best used within 3–5 days of purchase.

PREPARATION AND USE A tasty snack and cold cut with salad. Also excellent when fried with eggs.

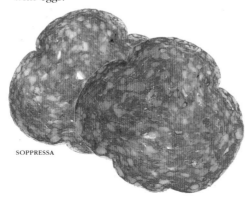

SOPPRESSA

Soppressa Salami An Italian salami made of pork and beef found around Verona, Padua and the surrounding Italian countryside.

Spegelpoelse See Danish Salami.

Toscana Salami This recipe is centuries old. A slightly sweet flavour contrasts with the diced fat pieces.

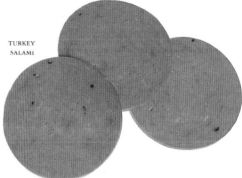

TURKEY SALAMI

Turkey Salami

MAJOR NUTRIENTS		SERVE SIZE 30 G	
Energy	135 kJ	Total Sugars	0
Protein	6 g	Dietary Fibre	0
Fat	1 g	Sodium	70 mg
Cholesterol	50 mg	Potassium	90 mg
Carbohydrate	0	Phosphorus	70 mg

NUTRITIONAL INFORMATION A lean animal protein source with only 27% of energy coming from fats. Forms a good basic meat for a cold platter to which small amounts of the higher fat, tasty cuts can be added.

DESCRIPTION A moist cooked salami made from the turkey thigh with seasonings. Can contain peppercorns. Low fat and salt varieties are available.

ORIGIN AND HISTORY Popular in the USA and England, and now available in Australia.

BUYING AND STORAGE Bought sliced/kg or in a vacuum sealed portion/knob. Keep refrigerated and use within 3–5 days if purchased sliced or observe the use-by date recommended by the processer.

PREPARATION AND USE Use as a cold meat, for platters, as a sandwich filling and as a snack.

Veneto Salami A mild slightly sour-sweet flavoured salami with coarse pepper berries and Venetian seasoning.

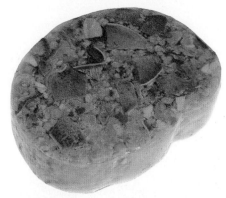

Salsiccie

also called **Salsiccie casalinga**

MAJOR NUTRIENTS		SERVE SIZE 100 G	
Energy	1560 kJ	Potassium	195 mg
Protein	12 g	Phosphorus	150 mg
Fat	33 g	Iron	1 mg
Cholesterol	100 mg	Zinc	2.1 mg
Carbohydrate	0	Thiamin	0.10 mg
Total Sugars	0	Riboflavin	0.15 mg
Dietary Fibre	0	Niacin Equiv.	3.9 mg
Sodium	1190 mg		

NUTRITIONAL INFORMATION Over 79% of energy comes from fats. A serving contains good amounts of iron, zinc, niacin and vitamin B12 and a significant amount of thiamin. Use in moderation. Also, the preservation process requires the addition of sodium, so intake should be moderated in sodium-controlled diets.

DESCRIPTION An Italian pork sausage usually flavoured with garlic and peppercorns.

ORIGIN AND HISTORY Salsiccie is the Italian word for pork sausage and casalinga means homemade.

BUYING AND STORAGE Buy by the unit/kg. Store as a fresh sausage, in a refrigerator and cook within 2–3 days of purchase.

PREPARATION AND USE Poach, grill or fry. Robert Carrier recommends pricking the sausages with a needle, then poaching for a few minutes before drying them and sautéeing in a mixture of butter and oil.

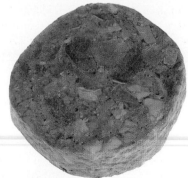

Saucisson

also called **Saucisson fumé, Saucisson fumé aux herbes**

MAJOR NUTRIENTS		SERVE SIZE 30 G	
Energy	510 kJ	Sodium	380 mg
Protein	5 g	Potassium	90 mg
Fat	13 g	Phosphorus	50 mg
Cholesterol	33 mg	Iron	0.5 mg
Carbohydrate	0	Zinc	1.1 mg
Total Sugars	0	Thiamin	0.05 mg
Dietary Fibre	0	Niacin Equiv.	1.8 mg

NUTRITIONAL INFORMATION One of the highest fat content smallgoods available. Over 90% of energy comes from fats. A serving contains an excellent amount of vitamin B12 and significant amounts of iron, zinc, thiamin and niacin. Use to flavour rather than as a major animal protein food. Also, the preservation process requires the addition of sodium, so intake should be moderated in sodium-controlled diets.

DESCRIPTION There are three types of saucissons; all large, one kind is boiled before eating while the other two, saucisson sec and saucisson fumé, are eaten raw. The boiling sausage is usually referred to by the place of origin, and sometimes is called saucisse.

Saucisson fumé aux herbes is made from a basic sausage mixture into which garlic has been blended, then dried and/or smoked. Sometimes a generous coating of herbs is added.

ORIGIN AND HISTORY Varieties of this sausage abound all over France, the most well known being the saucisson de Lyon. These sausages have even inspired a number of poems and are recorded in A. & A. Hippisley Coxe's *Book of Sausages*.

BUYING AND STORAGE Keep refrigerated.

PREPARATION AND USE The fresh sausages can be cooked by boiling. Treat the others like other smoked sausages.

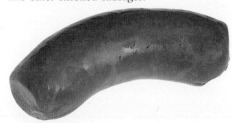

Saveloy

MAJOR NUTRIENTS		SERVE SIZE 100 G	
Energy	1090 kJ	Potassium	160 mg
Protein	10 g	Phosphorus	210 mg
Fat	21 g	Iron	1.5 mg
Cholesterol	120 mg	Zinc	1.5 mg
Carbohydrate	10 g	Thiamin	0.15 mg
Total Sugars		Riboflavin	0.1 mg
	less than 1 g	Niacin Equiv.	3.6 mg
Dietary Fibre	0.5 g		
Sodium	890 mg		

NUTRITIONAL INFORMATION A popular sausage not often considered to be high in fat, it contains over 71% energy from fats. A serving contains excellent amounts of protein, phosphorus, iron and vitamin B12 and good amounts of zinc, riboflavin and niacin. Do not use as a daily source of animal protein despite its relatively cheaper price. Also, the preservation process requires the addition of sodium, so intake should be moderated in sodium-controlled diets. Slow cooking or preboiling may enable total fat content to be reduced slightly.

DESCRIPTION The modern commercial saveloy may contain any part of a pig or beef cut which has been dried, smoked and cooked.

ORIGIN AND HISTORY An English version from the cervelat family. After the 'banger', Britain's most famous sausage.

BUYING AND STORAGE Sold by the unit/kg. Also available in vacuum packs. Keep refrigerated and can be stored for up to 1 week. If purchased in a vacuum pack observe the use-by date recommended by the processer.

PREPARATION AND USE Already cooked saveloys can be eaten cold, however, usually they are simmered for 3–5 minutes, and served with mustard or tomato sauce in a bread roll. Traditionally served with pease pudding.

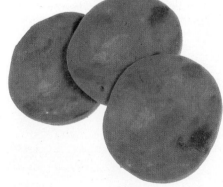

Schinkenwurst

also called **Ham bologna, Hamwurst**

MAJOR NUTRIENTS		SERVE SIZE 30 G	
Energy	645 kJ	Sodium	665 mg
Protein	6 g	Potassium	50 mg
Fat	14 g	Phosphorus	50 mg
Cholesterol	40 mg	Iron	1 mg
Carbohydrate	0	Zinc	1.1 mg
Total Sugars	0	Thiamin	0.5 mg
Dietary Fibre	0	Niacin Equiv.	1.9 mg

NUTRITIONAL INFORMATION Over 80% of energy comes from fats. They are a relatively cheap item and although a serving contains excellent amounts of thiamin and vitamin B12, good amounts of iron and zinc and significant niacin, they should be used in moderation. Also, the preservation process requires the addition of sodium, so intake should be moderated in sodium-controlled diets.

DESCRIPTION An old-world sausage closely related to bologna. Ham pieces and diced pistachios are set in a finely textured mixture of pork and veal. No garlic.

ORIGIN AND HISTORY A specialty from Westphalia, Germany.

BUYING AND STORAGE Purchase by the slice/kg. Seal in plastic wrap and refrigerate, and best used within 2–3 days of purchase.

PREPARATION AND USE A cold cut suitable for platters, or with salads, as a sandwich filling, snacks.

VARIETIES
Schinken kalbfleischwurst, sometimes flavoured with peppercorns and caraway seeds; Schinken plockwurst, firm texture, containing large pieces of fat; Gekochte schinkenwurst, contains beer and coarsely chopped lean pork; Lyoner, a German version of what was originally the French sausage from Lyon.

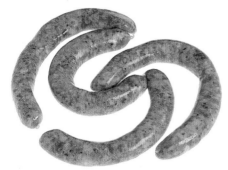

Toulouse Sausage

MAJOR NUTRIENTS		SERVE SIZE 100 G	
Energy	1520 kJ	Potassium	160 mg
Protein	10 g	Calcium	40 mg
Fat	32 g	Phosphorus	160 mg
Cholesterol	70 mg	Iron	1 mg
Carbohydrate	0	Zinc	1 mg
Total Sugars	0	Riboflavin	0.1 mg
Dietary Fibre	0	Niacin Equiv.	4.6 mg
Sodium	760 mg		

NUTRITIONAL INFORMATION Over 78% of energy comes from fats. A serving contains excellent amounts of phosphorus, niacin and vitamin B12, good amounts of iron, and significant amounts of zinc and riboflavin. Use sparingly as an additional flavour rather than main protein source. Also, the preservation process requires the addition of sodium, so intake should be moderated in sodium-controlled diets.

DESCRIPTION A long, fresh coarsely textured pork and pork fat sausage, flavoured with pepper. Some varieties include garlic and white wine.

ORIGIN AND HISTORY This sausage takes its name from the city of Toulouse in France. It is considered to be one of the best and most versatile sausages in France.

BUYING AND STORAGE Purchased by the unit/kg. Refrigerate and use within 2–3 days of purchase.

PREPARATION AND USE Toulouse sausages are usually skewered into a coil and grilled or included in soups or stews. These sausages feature in many French recipes, the most famous being the cassoulet of Toulouse, a haricot bean stew which originated in the former Languedoc region of France.

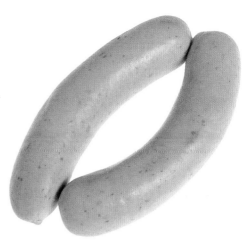

Weisswurst

MAJOR NUTRIENTS		SERVE SIZE 100 G	
Energy	1280 kJ	Sodium	620 mg
Protein	11 g	Potassium	125 mg
Fat	27 g	Phosphorus	230 mg
Cholesterol	80 mg	Iron	1.2 mg
Carbohydrate	0	Zinc	2 mg
Total Sugars	0	Riboflavin	0.1 mg
Dietary Fibre	0	Niacin Equiv.	3.5 mg

NUTRITIONAL INFORMATION Over 78% of energy comes from fats. A serving contains excellent amounts of phosphorus and vitamin B12, good amounts of iron, zinc and niacin and significant amounts of riboflavin. Use as a flavour rather than the main source of animal protein. Also, the preservation process requires the addition of sodium, so intake should be moderated in sodium-controlled diets.

DESCRIPTION A delicate small white German sausage made from veal, cream and eggs.

ORIGIN AND HISTORY German.

BUYING AND STORAGE Keep in the refrigerator.

PREPARATION AND USE Traditionally it is served after midnight at Oktoberfest with rye bread and sweet German mustard.

VARIETIES
Münchner weisswurst, a Bavarian specialty which should be eaten the day it is made.

PRESERVED MEATS

Bacon

MAJOR NUTRIENTS BREAKFAST RASHERS, GRILLED			SERVE SIZE 70 G
Energy	670 kJ	Phosphorus	180 mg
Protein	21 g	Magnesium	21 mg
Fat	8 g	Iron	1 mg
Cholesterol	52 mg	Zinc	2 mg
Carbohydrate	0	Thiamin	0.6 mg
Sodium	1500 mg	Riboflavin	0.15 mg
Potassium	280 mg	Niacin Equiv.	5.7 mg

NUTRITIONAL INFORMATION Bacon is an excellent source of phosphorus, thiamin, niacin and vitamin B12, as well as a good source of iron, zinc and riboflavin. Contains cholesterol and sodium. Contains up to 44% fat which can be reduced by trimming visible fat before cooking. Intake should be limited, especially if on a controlled sodium diet.

DESCRIPTION Bacon is the fat and lean rib section of a pig carcass which is preserved by curing and usually smoked. Smoking gives bacon its distinctive flavour, golden brown rind and deep pink flesh.

ORIGIN AND HISTORY Bacon has long been a favourite meat because of its comparative ease of smoke-curing and its keeping qualities. One story relates that Genghis Khan and his Mongol hordes were frustrated in their conquering progress as they could move only as fast as the herds of sheep and goats, needed to feed the hordes. One day some meat was left lying on the seashore. The following day it was noticed that the side of meat lying on the salty sand was a pink colour and remained unspoiled over the next few days. From then on meat was laid on salt on both sides and carried over the backs of horses. The men were then able to proceed at full tilt pillaging the herds of the victims.

Considered a 'poor man's meat' in medieval Europe, it was the subject of a famous saying used by Rabelais, writing in Paris in the 1540s, 'Let us flee and save our bacon.'

BUYING AND STORAGE Fresh bacon has a smooth rind, white fat and deep red flesh. Wrap in waxed or greaseproof paper, then foil or plastic wrap to prevent loss of moisture. Refrigerate for up to 7 days.

If purchased in a vacuum pack observe the use-by date recommended by the processer. Keep refrigerated.

PREPARATION AND USE Grilled or fried, bacon is the traditional accompaniment to eggs and served for breakfast. Also popular as an ingredient in a number of cooked dishes, salads, entrées and as a garnish.

VARIETIES

Beef Bacon Made from boneless beef short plates which are cured and processed similarly to regular bacon. Available in the USA.

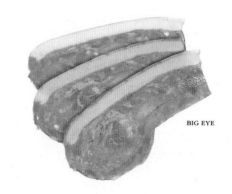

BIG EYE

Big Eye

MAJOR NUTRIENTS			SERVE SIZE 70 G
Energy	670 kJ	Potassium	280 mg
Protein	21 g	Phosphorus	180 mg
Fat	8 g	Magnesium	21 mg
Cholesterol	52 mg	Iron	1 mg
Carbohydrate	0	Zinc	2 mg
Total Sugars	0	Thiamin	0.6 mg
Dietary Fibre	0	Riboflavin	0.15 mg
Sodium	1500 mg	Niacin Equiv.	4 mg

NUTRITIONAL INFORMATION Contains up to 44% fat which can be reduced by trimming visible fat before cooking. Then bacon is an excellent source of phosphorus, thiamin and niacin, as well as a good source of iron, zinc and riboflavin. Processing results in a high salt content so intake should be limited, especially if on a sodium-controlled diet.

DESCRIPTION These bacon rashers are made with trimmings from old pigs, and are also called breakfast rashers and picnic rashers.

ORIGIN AND HISTORY A traditional type of bacon.

BUYING AND STORAGE A lesser quality bacon which is usually sold in vacuum packs and shaped to the processer's design.

PREPARATION AND USE Use and cook as ordinary bacon.

Canadian Bacon

MAJOR NUTRIENTS			SERVE SIZE 100 G
Energy	1680 kJ	Potassium	290 mg
Protein	25 g	Phosphorus	160 mg
Fat	34 g	Iron	1.5 mg
Cholesterol	80 mg	Zinc	3 mg
Carbohydrate	0	Thiamin	0.4 mg
Total Sugars	0	Riboflavin	0.2 mg
Dietary Fibre	0	Niacin Equiv.	4.5 mg
Sodium	2020 mg		

NUTRITIONAL INFORMATION Contains up to 74% fat which can be reduced by trimming visible fat before cooking. This bacon is an excellent source of phosphorus, thiamin and niacin, as well as a good source of iron, zinc and riboflavin. Processing results in a high salt content so intake should be limited, especially if on a sodium-controlled diet.

DESCRIPTION This bacon is sugar-cured loin of pork and can be known as smoked pork loin. As it is produced from one large muscle, there is very little intermuscular and external fat present, making leanness one of its predominant characteristics.

ORIGIN AND HISTORY The name comes from Canada but this product is also known in Britain under the name of back bacon.

BUYING AND STORAGE Purchased sliced or as a slab.

PREPARATION AND USE Cut thickly, the Canadian-style bacon can be used as a 'bacon steak'.

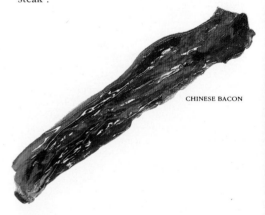

CHINESE BACON

Chinese Bacon

MAJOR NUTRIENTS			SERVE SIZE 50 G
Energy	610 kJ	Potassium	160 mg
Protein	8 g	Iron	0.5 mg
Fat	12 g	Zinc	0.9 mg
Carbohydrate	2 g	Thiamin	0.35 mg
Cholesterol	N/A	Riboflavin	0.1 mg
Dietary Fibre	0	Niacin Equiv.	4 mg
Sodium	700 mg		

NUTRITIONAL INFORMATION This bacon is an excellent source of thiamin, niacin and vitamin B12. It is a moderate source of potassium, iron, zinc and riboflavin. It also contains a large amount of sodium. It is an excellent source of protein but it has a high fat content which is predominantly monounsaturated.

DESCRIPTION Strips of red-brown, smoked belly pork which have been hung until they turn hard and dry. Each strip is around 20 cm long and 2 cm thick, and has a flavour like any well-smoked bacon.

ORIGIN AND HISTORY Dried meats are the earliest form of preserved food in the history of Chinese cooking. Even in the Han era, strips of meat suspended on bamboo racks to dry were an everyday part of domestic Chinese life.

BUYING AND STORAGE Sold fresh or packed in plastic vacuum-sealed packs, it is available in Chinese delicatessens and can be kept for many weeks, tightly wrapped in plastic, in the refrigerator, or it may be frozen.

PREPARATION AND USE The bacon is sliced or cubed and used to add a rich smoky flavour to braised, simmered and steamed dishes and to soups and stuffings.

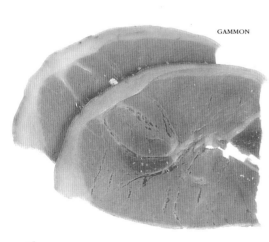

GAMMON

Gammon

MAJOR NUTRIENTS		BOILED, TRIMMED SERVE SIZE 60 G	
Energy	420 kJ	Phosphorus	110 mg
Protein	17 g	Iron	1 mg
Fat	3 g	Zinc	2 mg
Cholesterol	50 mg	Thiamin	0.6 mg
Carbohydrate	0	Riboflavin	0.2 mg
Sodium	660 mg	Niacin Equiv.	6.7 mg
Potassium	150 mg		

NUTRITIONAL INFORMATION This is a lean source of protein with about 26% of energy coming from fats. Excellent source of phosphorus, thiamin and niacin; good source of iron and zinc. Contains significant amounts of cholesterol, but as total fat content is low this should not be of serious consequence in a low fat diet. Although sodium levels are high they are lower than some other bacon prod-

ucts. Sodium levels could be further reduced by soaking before boiling.

DESCRIPTION Gammon is the cured whole leg of a pig. It is called gammon when eaten hot, but it is known as ham when served cold.

ORIGIN AND HISTORY English.

BUYING AND STORAGE Gammon is particularly popular in Britain, where it is often sold in smaller pieces and called English bacon. Gammon steaks are lean and should have the rind removed before cooking. They are best fried slowly in a little oil or lard, and turned often during cooking.

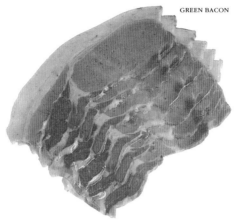

GREEN BACON

Green Bacon

MAJOR NUTRIENTS		SERVE SIZE 100 G	
Energy	1680 kJ	Potassium	290 mg
Protein	25 g	Phosphorus	160 mg
Fat	34 g	Iron	1.5 mg
Cholesterol	80 mg	Zinc	2.8 mg
Carbohydrate	0	Thiamin	0.4 mg
Total Sugars	0	Riboflavin	0.2 mg
Dietary Fibre	0	Niacin Equiv.	8.5 mg
Sodium	2020 mg		

NUTRITIONAL INFORMATION Contains up to 74% fat which can be reduced by trimming visible fat before cooking. Then bacon is an excellent source of phosphorus, thiamin and niacin, as well as a good source of iron, zinc and riboflavin. Processing results in a high salt content so intake should be limited, especially if on a sodium controlled diet.

DESCRIPTION This bacon has been cured but not smoked.

ORIGIN AND HISTORY Green bacon is known in all countries where bacon is popular.

BUYING AND STORAGE The rind should be pale and the flesh a deep pink.

PREPARATION AND USE Use when a mild bacon flavour is desired.

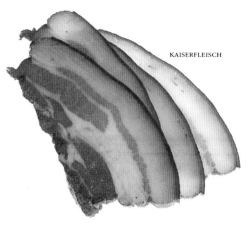

KAISERFLEISCH

Kaiserfleisch

MAJOR NUTRIENTS		SERVE SIZE 20 G	
Energy	550 kJ	Total Sugars	0
Protein	2 g	Dietary Fibre	0
Fat	13 g	Sodium	355 mg
Cholesterol	90 mg	Potassium	45 mg
Carbohydrate	0	Thiamin	0.1 mg

NUTRITIONAL INFORMATION Over 80% of energy comes from fats. A serving contains good amounts of phosphorus, iron, zinc and niacin. Use to add flavour rather than as a major source of these vitamins.

Moderate source of thiamin allows correct carbohydrate usage and nerve function.

Contains large amounts of fat (the most concentrated source of kilojoules), cholesterol (non-essential in diet since it is produced by the body), and sodium, which plays a central role in maintaining fluid balance and muscle function.

DESCRIPTION Smoked stomach pork.

ORIGIN AND HISTORY Kaiserfleisch originated in Austria and is known as belly bacon. It is popular in North America and Europe.

BUYING AND STORAGE Available cooked or smoked and ready to eat.

PREPARATION AND USE As for ordinary bacon.

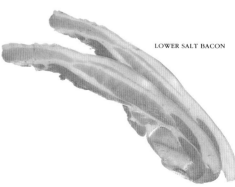

LOWER SALT BACON

Lower Salt Bacon

NUTRITIONAL INFORMATION Has a similar nutritional content to big eye/breakfast rashers/picnic rashers except for markedly reduced sodium levels. Product would still contribute significant levels of sodium to diet.

DESCRIPTION This product looks like ordinary breakfast bacon.

ORIGIN AND HISTORY It was developed to provide a bacon for people wanting to reduce the salt in their diet.

BUYING AND STORAGE Quite readily available. Store like breakfast bacon.

PREPARATION AND USE As for other bacons.

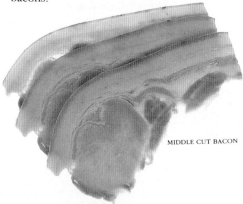

MIDDLE CUT BACON

Middle Cut Bacon

MAJOR NUTRIENTS		SERVE SIZE 100 G	
Energy	1720 kJ	Potassium	290 mg
Protein	25 g	Phosphorus	160 mg
Fat	35 g	Iron	1.5 mg
Cholesterol	80 mg	Zinc	3 mg
Carbohydrate	0	Thiamin	0.4 mg
Total Sugars	0	Riboflavin	0.2 mg
Dietary Fibre	0	Niacin Equiv.	7.9 mg
Sodium	2000 mg		

NUTRITIONAL INFORMATION Contains up to 74% fat which can be reduced by trimming visible fat before cooking. Then bacon is an excellent source of phosphorus, thiamin and niacin, as well as a good source of iron, zinc and riboflavin. Processing results in a high salt content so intake should be limited, especially if on a sodium-controlled diet.

DESCRIPTION Can contain a large 'eye' of lean meat.

ORIGIN AND HISTORY A traditional cut of bacon.

BUYING AND STORAGE Middle cut bacon is cut from the middle rib area and is graded as premium or regular according to the shape of the eye and amount of visible fat. Usually available sliced, thin, regular, thick, or as a slab.

PREPARATION AND USE The ideal choice for bacon and eggs.

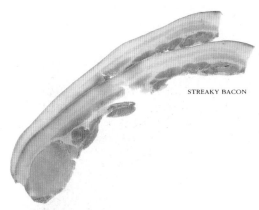

STREAKY BACON

Streaky Bacon

MAJOR NUTRIENTS		GRILLED SERVE SIZE 100 G	
Energy	1750 kJ	Potassium	290 mg
Protein	24 g	Phosphorus	160 mg
Fat	36 g	Iron	1.5 mg
Cholesterol	75 mg	Zinc	2.8 mg
Carbohydrate	0	Thiamin	0.4 mg
Total Sugars	0	Riboflavin	0.15 mg
Dietary Fibre	0	Niacin Equiv.	7.8 mg
Sodium	1990 mg		

NUTRITIONAL INFORMATION Contains up to 76% fat which can be reduced by trimming visible fat before cooking. Then bacon is an excellent source of phosphorus, thiamin and niacin, as well as a good source of iron, zinc and riboflavin. Processing results in a high salt content so intake should be limited, especially if on a sodium-controlled diet.

DESCRIPTION This is bacon from the tail end of the loin, with alternate streaks of lean and fat.

ORIGIN AND HISTORY A traditional cut of bacon.

BUYING AND STORAGE Sold in narrow strips.

PREPARATION AND USE This bacon is often used to lard other meats when oven-roasting.

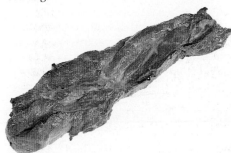

Barbecue Pork, Chinese

MAJOR NUTRIENTS		SERVE SIZE 100 G	
Energy	790 kJ	Potassium	380 mg
Protein	21 g	Magnesium	22 mg
Fat	7 g	Iron	1 mg
Carbohydrate	10 g	Zinc	2.4 mg
Cholesterol	60 mg	Thiamin	0.9 mg
Dietary Fibre	0	Riboflavin	0.25 mg
Sodium	1050 mg	Niacin Equiv.	10 mg

NUTRITIONAL INFORMATION Barbecue pork is an excellent source of protein, iron, vitamin B12, thiamin, niacin and zinc. It is also a good source of riboflavin and potassium and a moderate source of magnesium. It contains a large amount of sodium and a moderate amount of fat, which is predominantly monounsaturated. It also contains high amounts of cholesterol.

DESCRIPTION Strips of roasted, marinated pork fillet called cha siew, which have the flavour of Chinese five spice and soy sauce, and a rich sweet red-brown glaze. The meat inside is moist and tender.

ORIGIN AND HISTORY This is a Chinese specialty served all over the country, but particularly popular in south China where pork is the most commonly used meat. Grill-roasting of meat — which in ancient times meant beef, mutton and pork — on old rectangular-shaped, four-legged iron stoves, the earliest form of meat cooking known in China, is not all that different from a barbecue today. Around the 10th century Cheng's restaurant in Kaifeng was noted to have upwards of 50 ovens turning out cakes, buns and pastries, many with a filling of roast pork.

BUYING AND STORAGE Sold by the portion in Chinese delicatessens; it can be bought sliced if requested. Refrigerate in a plastic container or wrapped loosely in paper for several days only.

PREPARATION AND USE The marinated pork is barbecued over charcoal, or roasted by suspending it from hooks in special upright ovens, over high temperature, to keep the meat rare while crisping the surface. Used cold or warm in Chinese stir-fried and noodle dishes and in soups. As an appetiser it is usually served with roasted peanuts or sweet pickled vegetables. Diced, it is used as a filling in buns — particularly the sweet steamed bun known as cha siew pow — pastries and in rolls of steamed riceflour dough as dim sum foods.

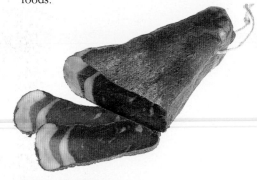

Basderma

also called **Pastourma**

MAJOR NUTRIENTS			SERVE SIZE 30 G
Energy	330 kJ	Sodium	830 mg
Protein	7 g	Phosphorus	60 mg
Fat	4 g	Iron	4.7 mg
Cholesterol	N/A	Magnesium	17 mg
Carbohydrate	4 g	Thiamin	0.05 mg
Dietary Fibre	0	Niacin Equiv.	200 mg

NUTRITIONAL INFORMATION An excellent source of iron; a good source of protein and niacin; a moderate source of magnesium, thiamin and phosphorus. Basderma has a high sodium content and the high fat content can vary up to twice as much, depending on the type of meat used and the extent of processing.

DESCRIPTION Air-dried beef, highly spiced and flavoured, with a spicy coating on the outside, and a dark colour when cut, similar in appearance to prosciutto. Pieces are long and slender, about 8 cm in diameter. It bears a similarity to the pastrami popular in the USA and Australia. However, pastrami is cooked during its preparation.

ORIGIN AND HISTORY Armenian in origin, basderma is regarded as the bacon of the Armenians, Greeks, and Turks. It has been prepared for many centuries as a means of preserving beef during the summer months, and preparation methods have changed little over the centuries.

Lean pieces of beef from the butt are cut into long strips about 10 cm in diameter, processed with a brine solution and weighted to extract moisture over a period of 10 days, then air-dried for 1–2 weeks. When sufficiently dried, a paste of fenugreek, paprika, cumin, allspice, chilli powder, garlic, salt and pepper is spread over the meat, left for a week or two in a bowl, then air-dried for a further week. With today's technology, short cuts are possible, but purists maintain the homemade product is the best.

BUYING AND STORAGE It is more readily available from Greek food stores under the name of pastourma. Purchase by weight, wrap in thick greaseproof paper, overwrap with foil and store in the refrigerator. It keeps for several months, providing it is not allowed to 'sweat' in plastic wrap or containers.

PREPARATION AND USE Cut in paper-thin slices and serve on bread as a light meal, or on crackers as an appetiser. Slice about the thickness of bacon, fry in butter and serve with fried eggs.

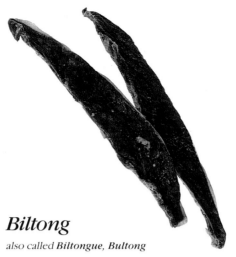

Biltong

*also called **Biltongue, Bultong***

MAJOR NUTRIENTS			SERVE SIZE 50 G
Energy	510 kJ	Potassium	200 mg
Protein	20 g	Phosphorus	150 mg
Fat	5 g	Magnesium	30 mg
Cholesterol	30 mg	Iron	3.1 mg
Carbohydrate	0	Zinc	3.8 mg
Total Sugars	0	Thiamin	0.8 mg
Dietary Fibre	0	Riboflavin	0.35 mg
Sodium	1050 mg	Niacin Equiv.	8.2 mg

NUTRITIONAL INFORMATION A fairly lean dried meat with only 36% of energy coming from fats. A readily transportable high protein source which contains excellent levels of phosphorus, iron, zinc, thiamin, riboflavin, niacin and vitamin B12. In addition it contains good amounts of magnesium.

DESCRIPTION Strips of meat dried by a method developed in South Africa which enables it to keep for years, while retaining its nutriment and flavour.

ORIGIN AND HISTORY The name comes from Afrikaans, bil meaning buttock (its source) and tong meaning tongue, from its appearance. The old ladies of the veldt claim that biltong has medicinal properties and is often fed finely grated to the sick.

BUYING AND STORAGE Buy by the strip. Store/hang in a cool dry place. Biltong will keep indefinitely.

PREPARATION AND USE The strips can be grated or sliced and eaten raw.

VARIETIES
Bunderfleisch, Swiss air-dried beef; jerked beef; jerky, the name being a corruption of a Spanish word used in South America.

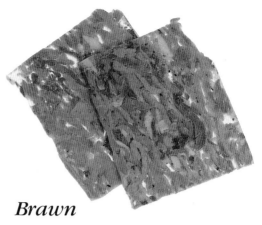

Brawn

*also called **Head cheese***

MAJOR NUTRIENTS			SERVE SIZE 60 G
Energy	380 kJ	Sodium	450 mg
Protein	7 g	Potassium	50 mg
Fat	7 g	Phosphorus	35 mg
Cholesterol	30 mg	Iron	0.5 mg
Carbohydrate	0	Zinc	1.2 mg
Total Sugars	0	Niacin Equiv.	1.5 mg
Dietary Fibre	0		

NUTRITIONAL INFORMATION Over 68% of energy comes from fats. The cholesterol level is not as high as one would expect with this level of fat. A serving contains good amounts of phosphorus, iron, zinc and niacin. Use to add flavour rather than as a major source of these vitamins.

DESCRIPTION Brawn is a preparation of boned meat, traditionally from the pig's head, however, other meats are now used. Set in a thick gelatine with seasoning, brawn is usually square with no casing.

Known as head cheese in the USA, it is available in two styles, French and German (sulze). The French variety consists of cured pork pieces suspended in vinegar flavoured gelatine with pickles and pimentos. The German sulze is composed of cured pork pieces with some beef and the gelatine is soft, so requires a casing.

ORIGIN AND HISTORY It is recorded that 'brawn' figured on most 'meat' days in the accounts of the Lords of the Star Chamber, from 1534 to 1590, either as 'collars' or 'rounds' of brawn, or simply 'in brawn'. According to Wynkyn de Worde's *Boke of Kervynge*, brawn used to be served at the very beginning of the meal; 'Fryste sette ye forthe mustarde and brawne' (*Furnivall's Early English Meals and Manners*, 1868).

BUYING AND STORAGE Purchased by the slice/kg. Keep refrigerated. Consume as soon as possible after slicing as the edges tend to dry out.

PREPARATION AND USE Use as a cold cut with salads.

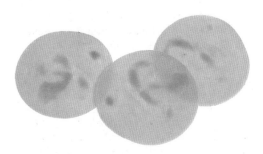

Chicken Roll

*also called **Chicken loaf***

MAJOR NUTRIENTS			SERVE SIZE 30 G
Energy	190 kJ	Dietary Fibre	0
Protein	4 g	Sodium	201 mg
Fat	2 g	Potassium	30 mg
Cholesterol	14 mg	Phosphorus	35 mg
Carbohydrate	2 g	Zinc	1 mg
Total Sugars	0	Thiamin	0.05 mg

NUTRITIONAL INFORMATION A moderate source of protein, phosphorus, zinc, thiamin and niacin.

Contains large amounts of fat, the most concentrated source of kilojoules. Significant amounts of cholesterol and sodium.

DESCRIPTION Processed chicken meat with flavourings, styled into a roll or loaf shape.

ORIGIN AND HISTORY A late 20th century product which was developed in line with increased production and consumption of chicken/poultry meat worldwide.

BUYING AND STORAGE Purchased as a set weight unit/knob or by the slice/kg. Seal in plastic wrap and refrigerate. Best used within 3–5 days of purchase.

PREPARATION AND USE This is a cold cut/sandwich meat. Popular with children and as an economical cold platter food.

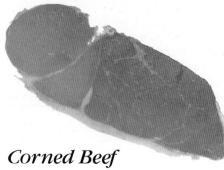

Corned Beef

*also called **Corned silverside***

MAJOR NUTRIENTS			SERVE SIZE 60 G
Energy	380 kJ	Sodium	830 mg
Protein	14 g	Potassium	120 mg
Fat	4 g	Phosphorus	90 mg
Cholesterol	45 mg	Iron	1.5 mg
Carbohydrate	0	Zinc	2.2 mg
Total Sugars	0	Riboflavin	0.15 mg
Dietary Fibre	0	Niacin Equiv.	4.2 mg

NUTRITIONAL INFORMATION This is a moderately lean protein source which contains excellent quantities of phosphorus, iron and vitamin B12 as well as good amounts of zinc, riboflavin and folate. Processing has resulted in increased sodium levels. Home-prepared products can be soaked before cooking and so sodium level is reduced.

DESCRIPTION Corned beef is a cut of beef, brisket, which has been cured. Brisket has alternating layers of fat and lean and is often rolled and tied. Corned silverside is solid meat with a layer of fat on one side. Both corned beef and corned silverside have a strong rosy red colour.

ORIGIN AND HISTORY English. In the 16th century the word corn was synonymous with grain and meat rubbed with grains of salt was thus 'corned'.

BUYING AND STORAGE Both cuts are available raw, ready to cook. As a cold cut, corned silverside is the most common. Available as small pieces for home carving or purchased by the slice/kg.

PREPARATION AND USE The traditional accompaniments when served hot are carrots and cabbage. If purchased cooked it is an ideal salad meat and sandwich filling.

VARIETIES

Bresaola, a cured smoked plate (underside) of beef from Italy; bully beef, a canned beef which was used as part of army rations during the war; salt beef, a cut of beef, usually brisket.

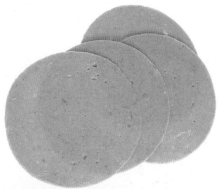

Devon

MAJOR NUTRIENTS			SERVE SIZE 30 G
Energy	290 kJ	Sodium	230 mg
Protein	4 g	Potassium	15 mg
Fat	5 g	Phosphorus	50 mg
Cholesterol	14 mg	Iron	0.5 mg
Carbohydrate	2 g	Zinc	1 mg
Total Sugars	0	Thiamin	0.05 mg
Dietary Fibre	0		

NUTRITIONAL INFORMATION Over 63% of energy comes from fats. A serving contains good amounts of phosphorus, iron, zinc, thiamin and vitamin B12. Use to add flavour rather than as a major source of these vitamins and minerals. Also, the preservation process requires the addition of sodium, so intake should be moderated in sodium-controlled diets. Slow cooking may reduce fat content marginally.

DESCRIPTION A finely textured cooked sausage made from pork/beef trimmings. Mildly seasoned.

ORIGIN AND HISTORY Devon was developed in Australia as fritz but renamed devon after the British county as a show of patriotism after World War I. In the UK there is a similar canned product made of minced pork, called Spam.

BUYING AND STORAGE Buy by the slice/kg. Often available as a portion/knob. Refrigerate in foil or plastic wrap for 3–5 days. If in a vacuum pack, observe the use-by date while keeping refrigerated.

PREPARATION AND USE Use as an economical cold meat. A particular favourite with Australian children as a snack and sandwich filling.

VARIETIES

Beef German, garlic sausage, ham and chicken, ham sausage, luncheon, Spam.

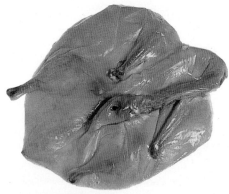

Dried Duck

*also called **Pressed duck***

MAJOR NUTRIENTS			SKIN AND FAT SERVE SIZE 50 G
Energy	1170 kJ	Dietary Fibre	0
Protein	11 g	Sodium	1050 mg
Fat	43 g	Potassium	210 mg
Carbohydrate	3 g	Iron	2.4 mg
Cholesterol	110 mg	Zinc	1.3 mg

NUTRITIONAL INFORMATION Dried duck is an excellent source of iron and a moderate source of zinc. It also contains a moderate amount of potassium. No nutritional data are available for vitamin A, vitamin D, thiamin, riboflavin, niacin, vitamin C, vitamin B12 and folate. It contains large amounts of fat, which is predominantly monounsaturated. It is an excellent source of protein. Cholesterol and sodium content are high.

DESCRIPTION Chinese duck which has been deboned leaving only wing and leg bones, seasoned with salt and spices and pressed flat, then hung until dry.

ORIGIN AND HISTORY The Chinese have been drying meat for over 2000 years as a method of preservation. Dried poultry not only keeps well, but like so many other dried foods, actually intensifies in flavour. Many old Chinese drawings of village and domestic life depict bamboo racks of flattened whole ducks, suspended by their long necks, drying in the sun.

BUYING AND STORAGE They are sold whole in stores where processed Chinese meats are sold, or are cut into portions, packaged in airsealed plastic and sold by weight in Asian supermarkets. The duck should keep, in cool, dry conditions, for many months.

PREPARATION AND USE Wipe it with a clean cloth and steam, or add to a braising or simmering dish. Cook until tender. Used primarily to add an intense flavour to stocks and braised dishes.

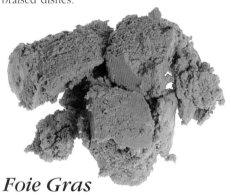

Foie Gras

MAJOR NUTRIENTS		SERVE SIZE 30 G	
Energy	370 kJ	Potassium	30 mg
Protein	5 g	Phosphorus	70 mg
Fat	7 g	Iron	2.8 mg
Cholesterol	50 mg	Zinc	1.1 mg
Carbohydrate	0	Vitamin A	2500 µg
Total Sugars	0	Riboflavin	0.5 mg
Dietary Fibre	0	Niacin Equiv.	2.2 mg
Sodium	290 mg		

NUTRITIONAL INFORMATION Over 79% of energy comes from fats. A serving contains excellent amounts of iron and vitamin A and good amounts of phosphorus, zinc, niacin and vitamin B12. Use to add flavour rather than as a major source of these vitamins and minerals. The price may ensure that this dietary moderation is enforced. Intake should be moderated in sodium-controlled diets.

DESCRIPTION A rich smooth preparation made from the livers of specially fattened geese and ducks, normally studded with truffles. The quality of foie gras is judged by its colour and texture, which is creamy-white, tinged with pink and very firm.

ORIGIN AND HISTORY Foie gras, literally translated from the French, means fat liver. Recipes date back to 1762, although goose liver has been consumed for many centuries. Pliny speaks of the exquisite taste of the fattened goose liver. Horace, before him, mentioned it in his *Satires*, Martial (AD43) in his *Epigrams*. Modern-day popularity is attributed to the Marechal de Contades, Military Governor of the French province of Alsace, who resided in Strasbourg, 1762–1788. Other French towns with the reputation for fine foie gras include Toulouse, Périgueux, and Nancy.

BUYING AND STORAGE Foie gras is presented in various shapes and sizes and in different types of containers, including tins. Refrigerate.

PREPARATION AND USE Usually served cold, and eaten at the beginning of a meal in order to savour its great delicacy. Can be garnished with jelly. Best presented on the plate in the shape of shells, scooped out of the terrine with a spoon, or in slices. A slice of foie gras is an essential ingredient in the famous French dish tournedos rossini. A slice of foie gras is placed on the tournedos, topped with sliced truffles then served with a Madeira demi glace.

VARIETIES

Bloc tunnel de foie gras truffé, a tunnel-shaped length of foie gras specially prepared for slicing; pâté de foie gras truffé en croûte, a long cylindrical pie filled with foie gras, coated with jelly and covered with an edible crust; suprême de foie gras truffé, a block of foie gras in aspic jelly. The jelly is usually flavoured with madeira. There are also terrines de foie gras truffé, foie gras packed in decorated terrines of various sizes.

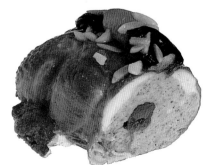

Galantine

NUTRITIONAL INFORMATION No detailed nutrient analysis is available, owing to varying recipes, but a galantine is usually a good source of protein; a moderate source of phosphorus, iron and zinc. May contain Nitrites 250.

DESCRIPTION A prepared dish made from boned poultry or other meat with a forcemeat stuffing pressed into a symmetrical shape and set in gelatine. A galantine is usually an individually prepared masterpiece and is not readily available commercially.

ORIGIN AND HISTORY The origin of the word is not clear, however the Gothic word gal meaning jelly would appear to have relevance as would the words geline or galine which in Old French mean chicken. Originally this dish was made from chicken but towards the end of the 17th century other birds or meats were used.

BUYING AND STORAGE Available from specialty shops, if at all. More commonly seen on a restaurant menu.

PREPARATION AND USE This is served in medium slices, cold.

Ham

MAJOR NUTRIENTS		COOKED, OFF THE BONE SERVE SIZE 60 G	
Energy	300 kJ	Potassium	145 mg
Protein	10 g	Phosphorus	165 mg
Fat	4 g	Iron	1 mg
Cholesterol	30 mg	Zinc	1 mg
Carbohydrate	0	Thiamin	0.2 mg
Total Sugars	0	Riboflavin	0.13 mg
Dietary Fibre	0	Niacin Equiv.	3.6 mg
Sodium	832 mg		

NUTRITIONAL INFORMATION Fat content can be up to 49% but this will vary depending on the amount of visible fat incorporated on the slice. Excellent source of protein, phosphorus and thiamin. Contains good quantities of iron, zinc, riboflavin and niacin. Should be eaten in moderation if a sodium-restricted regime is being adhered to.

DESCRIPTION Ham is the cured meat from the hind leg or shoulder of a pig. Generally smoked and cooked. There are many varieties and styles.

ORIGIN AND HISTORY Curing of pork to produce ham began thousands of years ago when it was discovered that drying and salting meats prevents spoilage. As early as the 5th century BC covering pork with salt was used as a method of dry cure. Later it was discovered that immersing the pork in a salt solution (brine) produced even better results. The smoking of meat dates back to ancient Egyptian times when meat was smoked by simply hanging it over a fire. However it was the Gauls, great devotees of pig meat, who first became renowned for the salting, smoking and curing of the various cuts of pork. At that period France was forest-covered, with herds of pigs feeding on the vegetation, without cost to the Gauls for whom they were a valuable asset. Such was the skill of the Gauls in the curing of hams that they became suppliers of ham to Rome and to the whole of Italy.

BUYING AND STORAGE Hams purchased in vacuum-sealed bags may be stored in the refrigerator up to the processer's recommended use-by date. Pack must be tight, not punctured. When opened the packet should be discarded and product wrapped in a damp cheese (muslin) cloth which should be rinsed daily in a mild vinegar solution. Leg ham on the bone will keep for 3–4 weeks in the refrigerator. Sliced ham is best consumed within 3–5 days of purchase. Ham wrapped in foil can be frozen for up to 3 months, however, there is some loss of quality and sliceability.

PREPARATION AND USE Raw ham like coppa, Parma/prosciutto, Bayonne, Westphalian is often served at the beginning of a meal as a dish by itself, sometimes with a slice of melon. It is always cut wafer-thin and is extremely delicate in taste.

Cooked hams can be baked (leg ham on the bone) or served cold. Ideal with salads, as a sandwich filling, snacks, or combined with other ingredients to make croquettes, rissoles, added to vol-au-vent fillings, soups.

VARIETIES

Ardennes A boneless, quality ham from Belgium.

Baked Virginia The whole leg is trimmed of surplus fat and skin, then sugar-cured, and smoked. Long maturing period.

Bayonne A salted, smoked boneless ham from the Basque region of France. This is a raw ham type (a jambon cru).

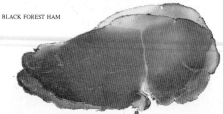

BLACK FOREST HAM

Black Forest Ham This fine quality ham

takes its name from the Black Forest area in Germany.

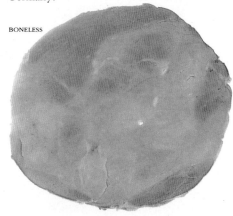

BONELESS

Boneless Leg Ham A whole, half or portion of the leg with the bone removed and trimmed of most of the external fat. This lean meat is rolled or formed into various shapes.

Bradenham A black-skinned ham on the bone from England. The ham is dry-cured then treated with spices and molasses to give its black colour.

Canned Hams These may include meat from the hindquarter, shoulder or trimmings pressed into a mould. Product names include leg ham, shoulder ham, pork shoulder picnic, flakes of ham and deli ham.

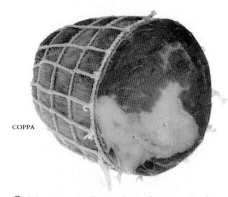

COPPA

Coppa A small raw ham from Italy, boneless, which has been air-dried for a long period. Similar in taste to Parma ham.

Danish Ham Boneless, mild, honey-cured ham of firm texture.

Easy-Cut or Semi-Boneless Leg Ham The shank and the aitch bone have been removed leaving only the round leg bone, thereby achieving a traditional ham-on-the-bone presentation that is easy to carve.

Epicam Ham An English ham cured to a very old and famous recipe.

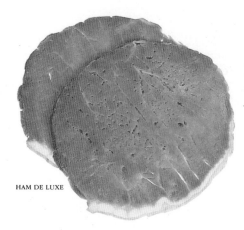

HAM DE LUXE

Ham de Luxe Also known as lachsschinken in Germany. A luxury cut made from the cured loin of lean tender pork, which is smoked.

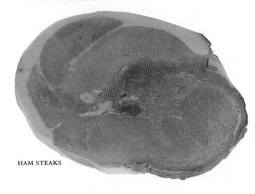

HAM STEAKS

Ham Steaks Thick slices of ham cut from the shoulder, forequarter, or formed from trimmings. Available fresh or in vacuum packs. Best grilled, fried or barbecued.

Irish Ham As a general rule these hams are dry-salt cured and are smoked, often peat-smoked.

Karlsbader A leg ham which has been cured and cooked but not smoked, then boned and pressed into a round shape.

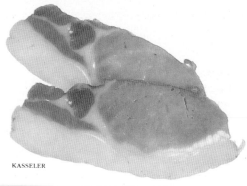

KASSELER

Kasseler A famous German ham.

Kentucky Ham A USA ham produced from Hampshire hogs. It is dry-salted and smoked over hickory and apple wood and has a long maturing period.

Leg Ham on the Bone (or Bone-In Leg Ham) Leg ham from the leg of a young porker which has been cured, smoked and cooked.

Prager Ham Moist quality boneless leg ham which takes its name from Prague, Czechoslovakia.

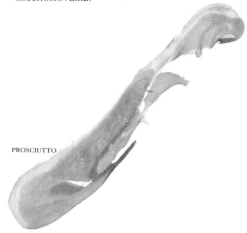

PROSCIUTTO

Prosciutto or Parma Ham A fine quality raw ham which originated in Parma, Italy. Hams are rubbed with a special mixture, then rested for some days before the process is repeated. After maturing the hams are pressed, steamed and rubbed with pepper.

Smithfield This leg ham on the bone takes its name from a USA town in Virginia where the particular curing process was first developed. The hams are dry-salted (hand-rubbed with salt), then heavily smoked and dried.

Soccerball Leg Ham An Australian specialty produced from a boned leg of pork which has been formed into a soccerball shape, then smoked and cooked.

Suffolk An expensive English ham, like the Bradenham ham, which has been treated with molasses.

Turkey Ham/Hamwich A boneless ham made from thigh and leg meat of a turkey.

Westphalian One of the most famous of the German raw hams. This rich dark ham is dry-cured, rested, cured and smoked with juniper twigs and berries over a beechwood fire.

York A fine English ham which is firm and tender and is famous for its delicate taste. It is cured with dry salt instead of brine, then lightly smoked.

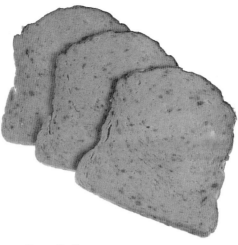

Leberkäse

also called Liver cheese

MAJOR NUTRIENTS		SERVE SIZE 60 G	
Energy	420 kJ	Potassium	50 mg
Protein	10 g	Phosphorus	60 mg
Fat	7 g	Iron	1.1 mg
Cholesterol	31 mg	Zinc	1.2 mg
Carbohydrate	0	Thiamin	0.05 mg
Total Sugars	0	Riboflavin	0.15 mg
Dietary Fibre	0	Niacin Equiv.	2.6 mg
Sodium	450 mg		

NUTRITIONAL INFORMATION Over 60% of energy comes from fats. A serving contains good amounts of protein, phosphorus, iron and vitamin B12 and significant quantities of riboflavin and niacin. Use to add flavour rather than as a major source of these vitamins and minerals. Intake should be moderated in sodium-controlled diets. Liver-containing varieties will have increased levels of iron, zinc and vitamin A.

DESCRIPTION A baked meat loaf, finely seasoned. May contain liver.

ORIGIN AND HISTORY A specialty of southern Germany.

BUYING AND STORAGE Various styles of meat loaf containing liver can be found at delicatessens.

PREPARATION AND USE It is served with salads or as a sandwich filling. Can also be grilled/fried and served hot.

Liverwurst

MAJOR NUTRIENTS		PORK LIVERWURST SERVE SIZE 30 G	
Energy	380 kJ	Potassium	25 mg
Protein	5 g	Phosphorus	70 mg
Fat	8 g	Iron	1.5 mg
Cholesterol	45 mg	Zinc	1.2 mg
Carbohydrate	0	Vitamin A	2500 µg
Total Sugars	0	Thiamin	0.05 mg
Dietary Fibre	0	Riboflavin	0.5 mg
Sodium	230 mg	Niacin Equiv.	2.8 mg

NUTRITIONAL INFORMATION Over 79% of energy comes from fats, which are predominantly monounsaturated. A serving contains excellent amounts of protein, phosphorus, iron, riboflavin, vitamin A and vitamin B12, and good amounts of zinc, thiamin and niacin. Use to add flavour rather than as a major source of these vitamins and minerals. Intake should be moderated in sodium-controlled diets.

DESCRIPTION There are many varieties: in general, liverwurst is a smooth spreadable mixture of ground pork, liver, onions and seasonings.

ORIGIN AND HISTORY Liverwurst developed in many different regions in Europe, each with its particular style and flavourings. Liverwurst provided piquancy to the continental feast and was used as an embellishment to roasted and grilled meats, game and fowl. It was set conveniently on the table to be scooped up by the feaster to complement the flavour of the freshly baked bread and prepared the palate to savour more of the finest local beer or wine.

BUYING AND STORAGE Sold as a piece/kg or in a prepackaged knob/portion. Keep refrigerated and use within 3–5 days of purchase, or observe the use-by date recommended by the processer.

PREPARATION AND USE Use as a savoury spread on freshly baked bread or savoury biscuits. An old Polish recipe suggests that the liverwurst be opened, stuffed with whole boiled eggs and chopped onions, and then served on toast with a garnish of orange slices and parsley.

VARIETIES

Chicken Liverwurst Made from chicken livers, highly seasoned.

CONTINENTAL LIVER SAUSAGE

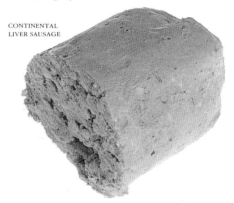

Continental Liver Sausage Smooth and creamy, no garlic.

English Liver Sausage Smooth but firm.

Ganselandleberwurst German country-style liverwurst made from goose livers.

Ganseleberwurst A German liverwurst, made from goose livers.

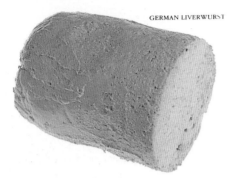

GERMAN LIVERWURST

German Liverwurst A mild product which can include cooked beef livers.

Gutsleberwurst German-style liverwurst.

Gasleverkorv A Swedish liverwurst.

Hausmacher Leberwurst A German homemade liverwurst made from pork livers.

Kalbs/Kalbsleberwurst A German liverwurst made from pig and calf's livers, finely minced and seasoned, with a creamy consistency.

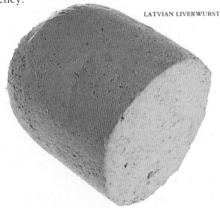

LATVIAN LIVERWURST

Latvian Liverwurst A Latvian variety which originated in the city of Riga. Superfine pork liver paste with cubes of pork fat.

Leberwurst A general term for liverwurst made in Germany, and most other countries.

Leberstreichwurst An Austrian variety. A small, fairly coarsely textured liver sausage.

Leverkorv A Swedish variety.

Onion and Liver Sausage England. A liver sausage made from liver, pork and pork fat with seasonings including onion.

Onionwurst/Zwiebelwurst German. Similar to kalbs but includes fresh onion.

Pfälzer A strong German liverwurst.

Saucisson au Foie de Porc A French variety.

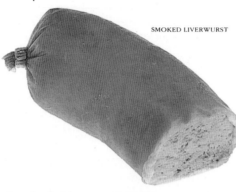

SMOKED LIVERWURST

Smoked Liverwurst German liverwurst made from specially selected calf's liver finely smoked.

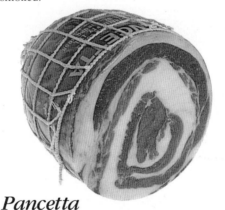

Pancetta

MAJOR NUTRIENTS		SERVE SIZE 20 G	
Energy	550 kJ	Total Sugars	0
Protein	2 g	Dietary Fibre	0
Fat	13 g	Sodium	355 mg
Cholesterol	90 mg	Potassium	45 mg
Carbohydrate	0	Thiamin	0.1 mg

NUTRITIONAL INFORMATION Most energy comes from predominantly unsaturated fats. A serving contains good amounts of protein and thiamin. Use to add flavour rather than as a major source of these vitamins and minerals. Also, the preservation process requires the addition of sodium, so intake should be moderated in sodium-controlled diets. May contain Nitrites 250.

DESCRIPTION Cured pork belly.

ORIGIN AND HISTORY Italian.

BUYING AND STORAGE Available at delicatessens.

PREPARATION AND USE Best if served thinly sliced, and can be substituted for bacon.

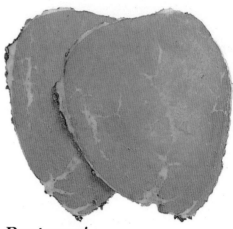

Pastrami

MAJOR NUTRIENTS		SERVE SIZE 20 G	
Energy	550 kJ	Carbohydrate	0
Protein	2 g	Sodium	355 mg
Fat	13 g	Potassium	45 mg
Cholesterol	90 mg		

NUTRITIONAL INFORMATION A little fat may be removed by cutting off the visible fat round the red meat. Preservation process requires the addition of sodium, so intake should be moderated in sodium-controlled diets. Over 87% of energy comes from fats. It should be used in moderation to give interesting flavour rather than as a major source of nutrients.

DESCRIPTION Made from the eye of silverside, cured and spiced. It is dry-cooked, then rubbed in dried chilli and black peppercorns. Always lean.

ORIGIN AND HISTORY This began as a Rumanian treat made of brisket.

BUYING AND STORAGE A deep red in colour, the flavour of pastrami is enhanced when sliced wafer-thin. Keep refrigerated. Best used as soon as possible following purchase as it dries out fairly quickly.

PREPARATION AND USE Pastrami is used as a sandwich filler, or served as part of a cold meat platter or smorgasbord.

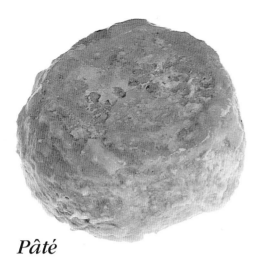

Pâté

*also called **Terrine***

MAJOR NUTRIENTS		SERVE SIZE 30 G	
Energy	370 kJ	Potassium	30 mg
Protein	5 g	Phosphorus	70 mg
Fat	7 g	Iron	3.2 mg
Cholesterol	50 mg	Zinc	1.1 mg
Carbohydrate	0	Vitamin A	2500 µg
Total Sugars	0	Riboflavin	0.5 mg
Dietary Fibre	0	Niacin Equiv.	1.7 mg
Sodium	290 mg		

NUTRITIONAL INFORMATION Over 70% of energy comes from fats and, because of liver content, has significant amounts of cholesterol. A serving contains excellent amounts of protein, iron, vitamin A, riboflavin and vitamin B12, and good amounts of zinc and niacin. Use to add flavour rather than as a major animal protein source. Sodium level will vary greatly according to the place of manufacture, so intake may have to be moderated in sodium-controlled diets.

DESCRIPTION In general, a pâté is a fine paste/spread which can be made from a variety of meats, poultry or fish, and can be flavoured with vegetables, fruits, herbs, spices, nuts, wines, spirits and liqueurs. A terrine can be either smooth or coarser in texture than a pâté, and takes its name from the earthenware dish in which it is cooked.

ORIGIN AND HISTORY Pâté comes from the French term pâté en croûte meaning savoury pie. Pâté was originally enclosed in a pastry case and baked in an oven. Then the words pâté and terrine came to be used to describe a preparation put into a dish (terrine), lined with strips of bacon and baked.

BUYING AND STORAGE If purchased by the slice (from bulk), refrigerate and use within 1–2 days. Commonly available in vacuum sealed portions, which should be kept refrigerated and served before the expiry of the use-by date. If prepared from fresh ingredients at home, keep refrigerated and use within 3–5 days.

PREPARATION AND USE A pâté and/or terrine is often served as an entrée with melba toast or freshly toasted wedges of bread. With the different flavours and textures available now, it is common to serve a variety of pâtés/terrines when entertaining.

Pâté is used when making Beef Wellington, a fillet of beef browned, then topped with pâté and mushrooms, enclosed in pastry, then baked until golden brown.

VARIETIES There are many types of terrine, including confit, made from minced pork, goose or duck. The flavourings used in pâtés are varied. Favourites are herbs (especially parsley and thyme), liqueurs such as Grand Marnier, fruits such as orange, and spices, like the many types of pepper.

SEE ALSO Foie Gras.

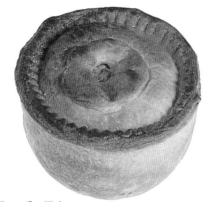

Pork Pie

MAJOR NUTRIENTS		SERVE SIZE 150 G	
Energy	2080 kJ	Calcium	90 mg
Protein	15 g	Phosphorus	180 mg
Fat	40 g	Magnesium	27 mg
Cholesterol	60 mg	Iron	2 mg
Carbohydrate	37 g	Zinc	1.5 mg
Total Sugars	4 g	Thiamin	0.25 mg
Dietary Fibre	1 g	Riboflavin	0.15 mg
Sodium	1080 mg	Niacin Equiv.	5.4 mg
Potassium	285 mg		

NUTRITIONAL INFORMATION Over 71% of energy comes from fats and significant amounts of cholesterol. A serving contains excellent amounts of protein, phosphorus, iron, thiamin, niacin and vitamin B12, and good amounts of calcium and zinc with significant quantities of riboflavin. Use in moderation, not as a daily snack or main meal item. Intake should be moderated in sodium-controlled diets.

DESCRIPTION A traditional English raised pie made with hot-water crust pastry, filled with seasoned pork and jellied stock.

ORIGIN AND HISTORY English.

BUYING AND STORAGE Purchased by the unit. Usually a small pork pie is an individual serve, larger sizes to serve 4–6 are available.

PREPARATION AND USE Eaten when cold. Can be accompanied with salads or selection of breads.

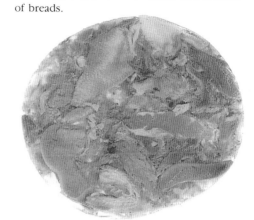

Presswurst

MAJOR NUTRIENTS		SERVE SIZE 60 G	
Energy	380 kJ	Sodium	450 mg
Protein	7 g	Potassium	50 mg
Fat	7 g	Phosphorus	35 mg
Cholesterol	60 mg	Iron	0.5 mg
Carbohydrate	0	Zinc	1 mg
Total Sugars	0	Niacin Equiv.	1.3 mg
Dietary Fibre	0		

NUTRITIONAL INFORMATION Over 68% of energy comes from fats. A serving contains significant amounts of protein, phosphorus, iron, zinc and vitamin B12. Use to add flavour rather than as a major source of these vitamins and minerals. Intake should be moderated in sodium-controlled diets.

DESCRIPTION Presswurst looks like a large sausage-shaped brawn. Produced from pork cheek, pig/ox tongue, trimmings and seasonings including paprika, set in aspic.

ORIGIN AND HISTORY Unknown. Presswurst is a German word which when translated means a pressed sausage.

BUYING AND STORAGE Sold per slice/kg. Keep refrigerated. Best used within 2–3 days of purchase.

PREPARATION AND USE Serve as a cold cut.

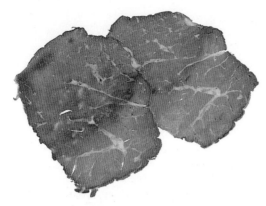

Roast Beef

MAJOR NUTRIENTS		SERVE SIZE 60 G	
Energy	420 kJ	Potassium	185 mg
Protein	17 g	Phosphorus	120 mg
Fat	4 g	Magnesium	20 mg
Cholesterol	75 mg	Iron	1.5 mg
Carbohydrate	0	Zinc	2.5 mg
Total Sugars	0	Thiamin	0.05 mg
Dietary Fibre	0	Riboflavin	0.1 mg
Sodium	35 mg	Niacin Equiv.	7.2 mg

NUTRITIONAL INFORMATION Provides excellent amounts of protein, phosphorus, iron, zinc, niacin and vitamin B12; also a moderate source of magnesium, thiamin, riboflavin and folate. Contains significant amounts of cholesterol, good source of lean protein.

DESCRIPTION Premium beef which has been tenderised, then cooked.

ORIGIN AND HISTORY Wide commercial sale of cooked joints of this kind has only been possible since refrigeration.

BUYING AND STORAGE When cooked it is vacuum packed and usually sold sliced and used as a cold cut. Keep refrigerated.

PREPARATION AND USE Best used within 3–5 days of purchase.

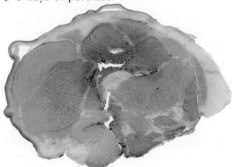

Roast Pork

MAJOR NUTRIENTS		SERVE SIZE 60 G	
Energy	545 kJ	Potassium	170 mg
Protein	19 g	Phosphorus	135 mg
Fat	7 g	Iron	1 mg
Cholesterol	55 mg	Zinc	2 mg
Carbohydrate	0	Thiamin	0.4 mg
Total Sugars	0	Riboflavin	0.15 mg
Dietary Fibre	0	Niacin Equiv.	6.1 mg
Sodium	30 mg		

NUTRITIONAL INFORMATION A moderately lean source of animal protein especially if all visible fat is removed before consumption. Provides excellent amounts of protein, phosphorus, thiamin, niacin and vitamin B12 and good amounts of iron and zinc; also a moderate source of magnesium and riboflavin. Contains significant amounts of cholesterol. Good source of lean protein.

DESCRIPTION Pork leg, tenderised and cooked.

ORIGIN AND HISTORY Widespread commercial sale of such cooked joints of meat has only been possible since refrigeration.

BUYING AND STORAGE Purchase sliced and use as a cold cut for a meat platter or as a sandwich meat. Refrigerate.

PREPARATION AND USE Use within 3–5 days of purchase.

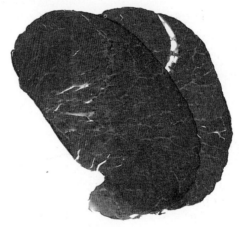

Smoked Beef

MAJOR NUTRIENTS		SERVE SIZE 60 G	
Energy	380 kJ	Sodium	800 mg
Protein	14 g	Potassium	120 mg
Fat	4 g	Phosphorus	90 mg
Cholesterol	45 mg	Iron	1.5 mg
Carbohydrate	0	Zinc	2.1 mg
Total Sugars	0	Riboflavin	0.15 mg
Dietary Fibre	0	Niacin Equiv.	4.2 mg

NUTRITIONAL INFORMATION The fat content is over 38% of total energy. This tasty cold cut provides excellent quantities of phosphorus, iron and vitamin B12. In addition it is a good source of zinc, riboflavin, niacin and folate. A useful cold cut meat. Fat level may be reduced by careful removal of all visible fats.

DESCRIPTION Selected silverside which is cured and cold smoked.

ORIGIN AND HISTORY Reportedly it is of Dutch origin.

BUYING AND STORAGE Smoked beef should be dark in colour when bought.

PREPARATION AND USE Its flavour is enhanced if sliced wafer-thin. Serve as part of a cold meat platter.

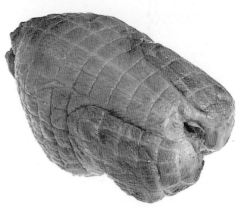

Smoked Chicken

MAJOR NUTRIENTS		SERVE SIZE 60 G	
Energy	400 kJ	Sodium	40 mg
Protein	17 g	Potassium	160 mg
Fat	3 g	Phosphorus	130 mg
Cholesterol	55 mg	Iron	0.5 mg
Carbohydrate	0	Riboflavin	0.1 mg
Total Sugars	0	Niacin Equiv.	7.7 mg
Dietary Fibre	0		

NUTRITIONAL INFORMATION A moderate fat content with fats providing about 17% of total energy. Excellent source of protein, phosphorus and niacin, but also contains significant quantities of iron and riboflavin.

DESCRIPTION Whole chicken which has been cured and smoked. Delicate in flavour and pale pink in colour.

ORIGIN AND HISTORY A recent development in line with the increasing popularity of poultry-based products.

BUYING AND STORAGE Purchased usually as the whole chicken. Keep refrigerated. Observe the use-by date stamped on the packaging. When opened, cover and use within 1 week.

PREPARATION AND USE A tasty cold cut. Carve and serve on a cold meat platter, or with a salad, or as a sandwich filling.

Dice or chop to add to other favourite recipes, pasta, vol-au-vents.

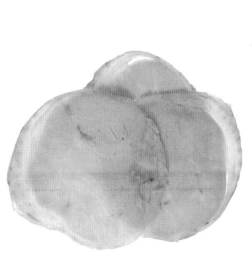

Smoked Turkey

MAJOR NUTRIENTS — SERVE SIZE 60 G

Energy	330 kJ	Sodium	30 mg
Protein	17 g	Potassium	170 mg
Fat	less than 1 g	Phosphorus	120 mg
Cholesterol	47 mg	Iron	0.5 mg
Carbohydrate	0	Zinc	1 mg
Total Sugars	0	Riboflavin	0.1 mg
Dietary Fibre	0	Niacin Equiv.	7.7 mg

NUTRITIONAL INFORMATION A very lean source of protein and is an excellent source of phosphorus, niacin and vitamin B12, as well as containing significant quantities of iron, zinc and riboflavin. A very useful cold cut to use in conjunction with higher fat items.

DESCRIPTION Breast of turkey cured and delicately smoked. Finely textured and pale pink in colour.

ORIGIN AND HISTORY A recent innovation and addition to the many turkey products being produced worldwide.

BUYING AND STORAGE Purchase by the unit/slice. Observe the use-by date recommended or, if purchased sliced, keep refrigerated and use within 3–5 days of purchase.

PREPARATION AND USE Serve as a cold cut, on a party platter. Best sliced thinly, and particularly enjoyable piled into a sandwich.

VARIETIES Smoked turkey breast (buffe), full breast of turkey on the bone; smoked turkey half breast, boneless breast; smoked turkey breast roll, natural breast of turkey, boned and rolled.

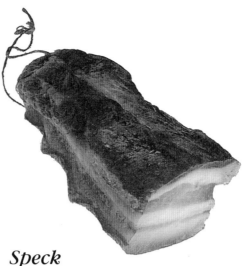

Speck

also called **Spec, Ham spec, Smoked ham spec**

MAJOR NUTRIENTS — SERVE SIZE 20 G

Energy	550 kJ	Total Sugars	0
Protein	2 g	Dietary Fibre	0
Fat	13 g	Sodium	355 mg
Cholesterol	90 mg	Potassium	45 mg
Carbohydrate	0	Thiamin	0.1 mg

NUTRITIONAL INFORMATION Over 87% of energy comes from predominantly unsaturated fats. Use to give interesting flavour rather than as a major source of nutrients. Preservation process requires the addition of sodium, so intake should be moderated in sodium-controlled diets. Some fat may be removed by cutting off the visible fat round the red meat. May contain Nitrites 250.

DESCRIPTION The topside of leg of a mature pig, cut to shape and smoked.

ORIGIN AND HISTORY Austrian.

BUYING AND STORAGE Buy as a piece or sliced. Refrigerate. The piece will keep for up to 2 weeks, if sliced 1 week.

PREPARATION AND USE Serve as a cold slice, a tasty snack with drinks.

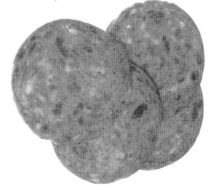

Strassburg

MAJOR NUTRIENTS — SERVE SIZE 30 G

Energy	310 kJ	Sodium	260 mg
Protein	4 g	Potassium	25 mg
Fat	6 g	Phosphorus	40 mg
Cholesterol	15 mg	Iron	1 mg
Carbohydrate	1 g	Zinc	1 mg
Total Sugars	0	Niacin Equiv.	1.6 mg
Dietary Fibre	0		

NUTRITIONAL INFORMATION Over 71% of energy comes from fats. A serving contains good amounts of iron, zinc and vitamin B12, and significant amounts of phosphorus and niacin. Use as an addition rather than a major protein source. Intake should be moderated in sodium-controlled diets.

DESCRIPTION A cooked sausage made from a blend of pork and beef, coarsely cut specks of fat, seasonings and mildly smoked.

ORIGIN AND HISTORY From Strasbourg, France.

BUYING AND STORAGE Usually it is purchased pre-sliced. Store, wrapped, in the refrigerator. Best used within 2–3 days of purchase.

PREPARATION AND USE A year-round sandwich filling, snack or cold cut.

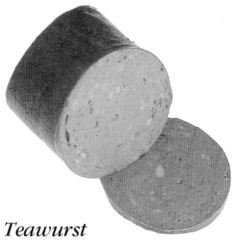

Teawurst

also called **Teewurst**

MAJOR NUTRIENTS — SERVE SIZE 20 G

Energy	160 kJ	Dietary Fibre	0
Protein	2 g	Sodium	160 mg
Fat	3 g	Potassium	60 mg
Cholesterol	15 mg	Phosphorus	55 mg
Carbohydrate	1 g	Iron	1 mg
Total Sugars	0	Niacin Equiv.	1.2 mg

NUTRITIONAL INFORMATION Over 69% of energy comes from fats. A serving contains good amounts of iron and vitamin B12, and significant amounts of phosphorus and niacin. Use to add flavour rather than as a major protein source. Intake should be moderated in sodium-controlled diets.

DESCRIPTION A very fine mixture of pork, beef and seasonings with garlic and small cubes of white lard. Fully cooked. Some varieties are smooth and pastelike and therefore suitable for spreading.

ORIGIN AND HISTORY Originally it was German, but many countries have their own variety of this popular sausage. Translated literally, teawurst means tea-sausage and it can be assumed that it was served at times when tea was consumed.

BUYING AND STORAGE Sold sliced. Seal in plastic wrap and refrigerate. Best used within 2–3 days of purchase.

PREPARATION AND USE A tasty cold meat for sandwiches, party platters, or added as a garnish to salads or scrambled eggs. Mix with cheese, onion and sour cream for a savoury dip.

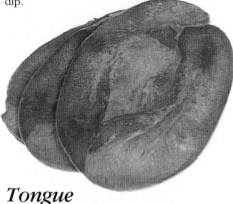

Tongue

MAJOR NUTRIENTS		PICKLED TONGUE SERVE SIZE 60 G	
Energy	530 kJ	Sodium	510 mg
Protein	9 g	Potassium	125 mg
Fat	9 g	Phosphorus	85 mg
Cholesterol	80 mg	Iron	1.5 mg
Carbohydrate	0	Riboflavin	0.2 mg
Total Sugars	0	Niacin Equiv.	3.4 mg
Dietary Fibre	0		

NUTRITIONAL INFORMATION Over 63% of energy comes from fats with a significant level of cholesterol. A serving contains excellent amounts of iron and vitamin B12, good amounts of phosphorus, riboflavin and niacin. Use with some discretion. Intake should be moderated in sodium-controlled diets.

DESCRIPTION Usually beef or ox tongue, smoked, corned or pickled.

ORIGIN AND HISTORY Tongue is a popular form of offal in many countries.

BUYING AND STORAGE Normally purchased by the slice/kg. Refrigerate and use within 3–5 days of purchase.

PREPARATION AND USE Serve as a cold cut.

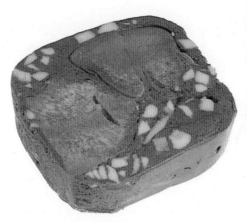

Zungenwurst

NUTRITIONAL INFORMATION No detailed nutritional information is available on this product.

DESCRIPTION A cooked and lightly smoked sausage made from pork fat and large pieces of tongue, and sometimes including liver and blood.

ORIGIN AND HISTORY German.

BUYING AND STORAGE This is purchased sliced/kg. Keep refrigerated in plastic wrap. Use within 3–5 days of purchase.

PREPARATION AND USE Serve as a cold cut.

VARIETIES
Tonguewurst, tongue sausage.

POULTRY AND EGGS

'An egg,' as Oscar Wilde once remarked, 'is always an adventure.' It is impossible to imagine a human diet without eggs, which must have been one of the first foods gathered by man. And it is equally hard to envisage what the world's tables would be like without the sight of poultry, which from the early days, when it was spitted over a fire, has become one of the most spectacularly served creatures in the culinary repertoire. The traditional Russian royal banquet tables groaned under the weight of whole, decorated swans, and those of Europe, especially in the Middle Ages, saw fantastic centrepieces made from pheasants and other ornamental fowl, surrounded by enormous aureoles made from their own feathers. Birds today are still chosen by many societies as the focal point for ceremonial feasts, the Thanksgiving turkey of the USA being only one example.

The popularity of chicken means that the ingenuity of cooks and food experts is constantly exercised by the need to invent new and interesting recipes, and this white meat, which lends itself to a very wide range of flavours, is continually being served in a rich variety of ways.

Chicken has become an almost everyday food in the diets of the Western world. The use of turkey and duck is also increasing, but not to the same extent as chicken over the last three or four decades; geese, guinea fowls and pigeons remain specialty foods.

Chicken is widely used in the home, the hospitality industry, in institutional and industrial catering and as a takeaway food.

In a national dietary survey of adults in Australia in 1983, men consumed an average of 29 grams and women 21 grams of poultry and game daily. Ninety-five percent of this was chicken. Industry statistics clearly confirm the change. In 1950 the industry processed 3 million chickens, by the mid-1980s the annual production had almost reached 270 million, a ninety-fold increase. Initially this came in the form of frozen chicken, but these have largely been replaced by chilled and fresh chickens and a variety of ready-to-cook chicken pieces and fillets. The growth in takeaway food has made a significant contribution to the increase.

Selective breeding and automated production have brought down the relative price of poultry and improved the general quality. Poultry often offers a cheaper alternative to the more expensive meat cuts, and specialty retail poultry outlets have made marketing attractive and purchasing simple. The poultry industry, like the meat industry, has responded to consumer demand for convenient, quickly prepared cuts. These have been promoted along with recipe suggestions which reflect modern food habits.

The interest in health and nutrition and the emphasis on reducing fat intake have resulted in a fall in the consumption of red meat and an increase in consumption of white meat such as poultry. There has been a lot of misunderstanding about the relative nutritional value of red meat and chicken: the facts show that each is a very nutritious food. When lean cuts of meat are selected and the meat is trimmed of fat before cooking, and when the skin and fat are trimmed from poultry and these foods are prepared with the minimum of fat, both foods are very suitable for healthy diets.

In contrast to the growth in the popularity of poultry, the consumption of eggs has dropped in the last fifty years. There are a number of reasons for the decline, including the concern about cholesterol, the replacement of the cooked breakfast by a cereal breakfast and fewer home-cooked desserts, cakes and biscuits. Australians, for instance, consume less than half an egg daily.

It should be remembered that there is not a direct correlation between dietary cholesterol and blood cholesterol. The amount of saturated fat in the diet is more important than the amount of dietary cholesterol in affecting the blood cholesterol level.

Eggs are a convenient food for people of all ages, being particularly useful in the diets of children and the elderly. People who are at risk of coronary heart disease should restrict their intake of egg yolks to three or less weekly, but the rest of the population can include an average of five eggs weekly in a healthy diet.

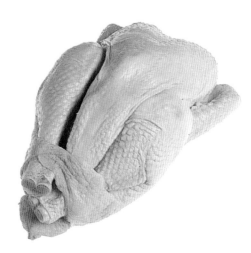

Chicken

MAJOR NUTRIENTS		ROASTED MEAT AND SKIN SERVE SIZE 100 G	
Energy	963 kJ	Phosphorus	170 mg
Protein	26 g	Magnesium	22 mg
Fat	14 g	Iron	1 mg
Carbohydrate	0	Zinc	1.6 mg
Cholesterol	128 mg	Riboflavin	0.2 mg
Sodium	0	Niacin Equiv.	10 mg

NUTRITIONAL INFORMATION An excellent source of protein, phosphorus and niacin; good source of iron, zinc, riboflavin; moderate source of magnesium. High in fat and cholesterol. The white meat alone contains less fat, and any chicken meat without the skin contains moderate fat.

DESCRIPTION Chicken is one of the world's most popular meats. In every country where chicken is eaten, cooks using local ingredients and traditional cooking techniques have learned to prepare it in ways that suit their culture and lifestyle. Cooks can roast, fry, boil, grill, barbecue, poach, steam or casserole the versatile chicken.

ORIGIN AND HISTORY All the domestic

breeds of chicken are descended from the wild red jungle fowl of India. Originally regarded as a sacred bird, the fowls were used in religious ceremonies where entrails were examined in a search for omens and the meaning of life.

Historians believe that from India chickens were taken to China and the Pacific Islands. Their arrival in the Mediterranean regions has been dated by the 1350 BC paintings in Tutankhamen's tomb. The Hebrews of the Old Testament do not appear to have known chicken, as it is not listed in the dietary prescriptions of Deuteronomy and Leviticus. In 720 BC the Greeks were issuing ordinances banning crowing cocks from city streets; chickens were thought to be too scrawny for good eating and were kept for the eggs. The Romans in the 5th century BC apparently felt the same way, and it was not until the Romans discovered that hand-fed chickens were tenderer, tastier and meatier than ones that scratched for their own food, that fattened chicken started to be featured at Roman banquets. Many recipes for chicken are to be found in the cookbooks of Apicus, one of the earliest food writers. By the Middle Ages, most of Europe was eating chicken. An Italian medieval cookbook of the 13th century gives recipes for stuffed chicken, while a German cookbook of the same period provides instructions for chicken stew.

These days chicken appears in such differing national dishes as Indian murgh biriani; Indonesian ayam panggang; Malaysian rendang ayam; Chinese shui ng heung gai; Japanese tori teriyaki; Thai kai yang; Scottish cock-a-leekie; Italian pollo al vino bianco; French poule au pot; Russian cotletki pojarski; English roast chicken; and another culinary development of this century, American Kentucky Fried chicken.

BUYING AND STORAGE 'Poussin', 'spring chicken', 'roaster' and 'boiler' are used to identify sizes and styles of chicken. Poussin and spatchcock are much the same thing — birds about 6 weeks old — and a spring chicken is one about 8 weeks old. A roaster can be any age under 6 months, whilst boilers are hens that are well past their laying prime and can be 18 months old or more.

To simplify matters, in many countries a numerical system has been adopted: it is used to show weight and indicates age as well.

In Australia, for instance, a number 5 chicken could be called a spatchcock or a poussin. It weighs about 500 g and as with all chickens up to number 9 (900 g and 8 weeks old) the flesh is very tender but with very little flavour. These birds need to have flavour added in the way of marinades and can be grilled, barbecued or roasted whole for a single serve. Numbers 10 to 14, that is chickens weighing 1–1.4 kg, still have tender flesh but possess more flavour and roast, sauté and deep-fry well. A number 14 chicken is about 3 months old. With numbers 15 to 27 (1.5–2.7 kg), the birds have tender flesh and much more flavour and can be roasted in the oven or cooked whole in a pot on the stove top. The number 27 is about 6 months old.

Free-range chickens are birds that have been allowed to roam freely in fenced runs instead of being raised in cages above the ground. The free-range birds are always more expensive than other chickens but the flavour is said to be better. They are cooked and treated in the same ways as other chickens.

Boilers are old hens that have stopped laying and are always very tough, and need moist heat in cooking to tenderise the flesh.

Capons are male birds that have been neutered. They are always more expensive than other chickens and can be found in chicken specialty shops. They have a greater proportion of white breast meat to darker meat than other chickens and are very tender.

The quantity of chicken to buy will vary according to individuals, but the following gives a rough guideline.

For roasted chicken allow 375 g per serving; for barbecued, grilled or fried chicken about 500 g per serve; for chicken casserole or stew between 250–500 g depending on the other ingredients.

Whole chickens are readily available both fresh and frozen. In a young chicken, the breast bone is soft and pliable. In an old bird, the bone is rigid and hard. Generally speaking, a large bird is better value than a smaller one as the proportion of meat to bone is higher. Chicken is also available cut up into individual portions: breast, breast fillet, thigh, thigh fillet, drumstick, maryland, halves, quarters and wings.

Fresh, uncooked chicken should be stored in the coolest part of the refrigerator and used within 2 or 3 days of purchase. Fresh giblets deteriorate quickly and need to be used within 24 hours. Frozen chicken can be stored for 3 months in a freezer section of a refrigerator or for up to 6 months in a separate freezer. Do not buy frozen chickens with pinkish ice in the pack — this indicates the chicken may have been defrosted and then refrozen. Also avoid chickens with brown marks. This is 'freezer burn', caused by incorrect storage. When thawing frozen chicken, leave it in its wrapper and thaw quickly to prevent loss of flavour and proliferation of harmful micro-organisms. Thaw chicken overnight in the refrigerator or in a sinkful of cold water or in the microwave oven.

Cooked chicken needs to be cooled rapidly, wrapped loosely and stored in the refrigerator. It will keep 2 to 3 days. It can be frozen for up to a month. Chicken in sauce can be refrigerated for 3 days, or kept frozen for 3 months.

PREPARATION AND USE There are many ways of varying the taste of chicken, and cooks all over the world have their own unique national ways. The English like the taste of bread stuffings, with thyme and onions. The French use red wine to create classic coq au vin. Mexicans add chocolate and chilli to sauces for dishes called moles. The Japanese blend soya sauce, rice wine and grated ginger to make chicken teriyaki. The Burmese add coconut milk and spices to their chicken curries. The Chinese cook slivered, marinated chicken for their stir-fry dishes. The Russians stuff flattened breasts with cold butter for chicken Kiev. With all recipes it needs to be remembered that the flesh of young chickens is very delicate and will shrink, dry out and become stringy if too high a heat is used during cooking. These chickens can be fried, grilled, roasted, barbecued or poached. Older birds always need the slower ways of cooking such as stewing, casseroling and steaming.

THE CUTS

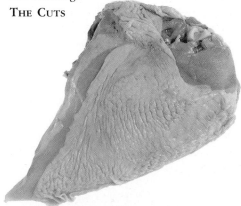

Breast The tenderest meat, which can be poached, baked, sautéed or grilled. Chicken breasts are called supremes when they are boned, skinned and halved. The thin strip of meat lying next to the breastbone is called the fillet.

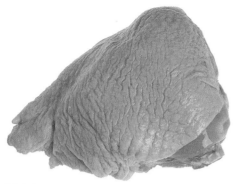

Thighs These can be fatty and may need to be trimmed and skinned. Thighs can be fried, baked, casseroled and barbecued. Boned thighs can be stuffed or the flesh used as a cheaper substitute for expensive breast meat.

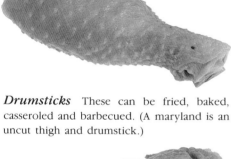

Drumsticks These can be fried, baked, casseroled and barbecued. (A maryland is an uncut thigh and drumstick.)

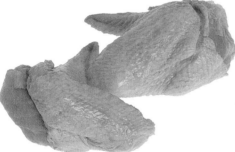

Wings These are often used in soups and can also be fried, baked, casseroled and barbecued.

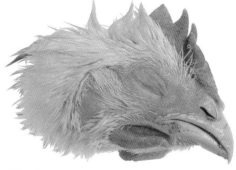

Giblets The edible parts of the entrails of the bird. They consist of the gizzard, heart, neck and liver. The livers can be sautéed or made into pâté and the other giblets can be used for soups and stocks.

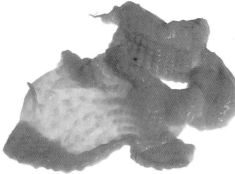

Skin This can be crisped in an oven for a snack, but it must be remembered that skin has a high fat content.

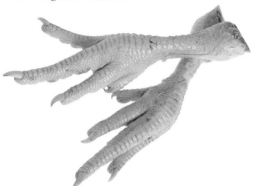

Feet These can be added to the stock pot, and the Chinese serve them hot or cold as snacks.

Head This can be used for stocks, and some people regard it as a delicacy.

VARIETIES

There are more than 100 breeds of chicken and they can be divided into five classes — Asiatic, Continental European, Mediterranean, English and Continental — but the number kept for meat or egg production is very limited.

The major breeds are the Australorp, an Australian bird bred for egg production and eating; the Cornish, an English breed, popular in the USA and bred for the table; the Leghorn, found in Europe, North America and the southern hemisphere and regarded as the most prolific egg producer; the American New Hampshire which provides both eggs and meat; the English-originated Orpington, mainly an egg producer but in the USA raised

for its meat; the famous white-fleshed Bresse chicken of France and the heavy Jersey White Giant of America, both raised for their meat; the American Plymouth Rocks largely bred for the table; and the Rhode Island Red used extensively for egg production. On a smaller scale, tiny Bantams, once fighting birds from Indonesia, are largely kept for their beauty and not for their flesh or eggs.

SEE ALSO Barbecue Chicken, Fried Chicken, Smoked Chicken.

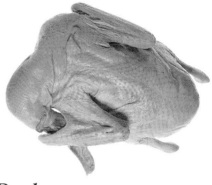

Duck

MAJOR NUTRIENTS		ROASTED MEAT AND SKIN SERVE SIZE 100 G	
Energy	1410 kJ	Phosphorus	150 mg
Protein	20 g	Iron	2.7 mg
Fat	29 g	Zinc	1.8 mg
Carbohydrate	0	Thiamin	0.2 mg
Cholesterol	160 mg	Riboflavin	0.3 mg
Sodium	80 mg	Niacin Equiv.	8 mg

NUTRITIONAL INFORMATION An excellent source of protein, phosphorus, iron, thiamin, riboflavin, niacin, vitamins B6, B12, pantothenic acid; good source of zinc. Very high in fat and cholesterol.

Duck contains approximately the same level of nutrients as chicken except that duck contains twice the amount of fat.

DESCRIPTION Ducks are web-footed waterbirds, of which there are many different species, all with differing characteristics and appearance, though all have a long body and attractive plumage. The ducks most commonly bred for the table are the ones with a natural habitat of fresh water.

ORIGIN AND HISTORY Wild ducks have been eaten in all parts of the world for thousands of years. The Egyptians and Greeks ate wild duck, while the Romans thought only the breast and brains of the bird were worth eating. The Chinese claim to be the first to domesticate the wild bird and the duck in China came to symbolise fidelity. Others believe credit for domesticating the duck could be given to either the American Indians or the Aztecs. The Chinese influence, however, is to be found in the ducks from Beijing, which have been used in breeding worldwide.

The hunting season for ducks differs for each country. In Australia, some states have totally banned the shooting of wild ducks. In New South Wales and Victoria, however, the duck and pheasant shooting season runs from March to May, while in South Australia shooting is only permitted in years when the duck breeding season has resulted in a great number of birds. In New Zealand the shooting season for ducks and pheasants starts in May and ends in June.

BUYING AND STORAGE Ducks are not as meaty as chicken, so allow 750 g duck per person. Ducks are available both fresh and frozen and should have creamy white skin and plump breasts. The webbing between the toes should be soft and pliable and so should the end of the beak. The term 'duck' applies to birds between two and three months and weighing between 2 kg and 3 kg. A 'duckling' is between six weeks and two months and weighs from 1½–2 kg. A 'drake' is a male bird and is a little larger than the female. Male and female birds are usually sold without detailing the differences but a female has a more meaty breast.

PREPARATION AND USE The French and Chinese cuisines are noted for their duck dishes. From the French have come such classic favourites as caneton à l'orange from a domestic bird, and a pressed duck recipe, canard sauvage à la presse, from a wild one. Traditional Chinese buck ging ngap (Peking duck) takes hours to prepare and eat. Chinese cooking also uses duck in braises, stir-fries and roasts. Duck can be casseroled, roasted or fried. Always rinse and dry ducks before use and remove all visible fat. The fat sac at the base of the tail needs to be cut out. For roasting, prick the duck all over with a fine skewer and place on a rack in the baking dish.

VARIETIES

There are over 80 varieties of freshwater ducks eaten in the world, with different countries favouring different breeds. The ducks most eaten in Australia are a cross between the English Aylesbury and the Chinese Peking. In France the most highly regarded ducks for the table are the Nantais and Rouennais, while in England the Aylesbury, Gadwell and Garganey (called Teal in other parts of the world) are prized. Other popular international breeds are Long Island, Barbary, Mallard and Pintail. The Muscovy duck's tail glands give its flesh a musky taste that some people dislike, but the French

crossbreed it with a Rouennais or a Nantais for a bird with the meaty flesh of the Muscovy but without the strong taste.

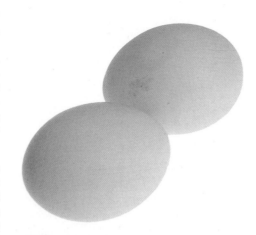

Egg

MAJOR NUTRIENTS		DOMESTIC HEN SERVE SIZE 50 G	
Energy	334 kJ	Sodium	0
Protein	6 g	Phosphorus	109 mg
Fat	5 g	Iron	1.2 mg
Carbohydrate	0	Vitamin A	80 µg
Cholesterol	230 mg	Riboflavin	0.15 mg

NUTRITIONAL INFORMATION An excellent source of phosphorus, iron, vitamin B12, pantothenic acid; good source of vitamin A, folate; moderate source of protein, riboflavin, vitamin D. Eggs are high in cholesterol and contain moderate fat. Cooking does not significantly affect their nutrient content.

DESCRIPTION An egg is the roundish reproductive body laid by a bird. There are many varieties that are eaten — goose, quail, pheasant, duck, guinea fowl, gull, ostrich, emu — but most eggs eaten are from the domestic hen. No one has ever attempted to count the many, many ways in which eggs can be used in cooking. Apart from eating them whole, in or out of the shell, every country has its own ways of using them, from the simplest of peasant food to the French haute cuisine.

ORIGIN AND HISTORY Eggs have been a staple food since prehistoric times when nests of wild birds were raided for their eggs. Many cultures believed that eggs had magical powers of renewal and rebirth, and this belief is remembered in the eggs of Easter time. For centuries there were arguments and discussions on philosophical, metaphysical or biological levels about which came first — the chicken or the egg. Ancient philosophers saw the egg as a perfect symbol of the world: the shell was the earth, the white was water, the

yolk was fire, and the air was in the round end of the shell.

BUYING AND STORAGE Eggs are graded and sold according to the minimum weight of each egg and are available in five sizes: 65 g, 60 g, 55 g, 50 g and 45 g. The grade size is always marked on the carton. A high quality egg will have a smooth, well-shaped shell free of blemishes and cracks. It will have a small air cell at the round end and will be infertile and without a blood spot. Blood spots in eggs do not always indicate a fertilised egg, as they can occur if the hen is upset during the formation of the egg. Faults in eggs are generally detected during candling, a process that throws light into eggs to check the quality. As eggs age, changes take place. Moisture seeps through the porous shell and is replaced by air so that the air cell found at the round end of the egg becomes larger. The yolk enlarges and is easily broken. The thick white becomes runny. The use-by date on cartons is an indication of the freshness of eggs, but eggs are still usable past this date if they have been stored properly. Very fresh eggs have a rough shell and will sink to the bottom of a bowl of water, as the air cell is very small. Another way to determine freshness is to break an egg onto a flat plate. A fresh egg will have a well-rounded yolk and a thick gelatinous white, while in an older egg, the white is less gelatinous and the yolk is no longer rounded, but flattened. In bad eggs, yolk and white run together and the smell is very unpleasant. Eggs begin to lose quality as soon as they are laid, and need to be stored correctly. They are best kept stored in their cartons in the refrigerator with the pointed end down. If they are left out of the refrigerator they can lose as much quality in one day at room temperature as they do in 5 days in the refrigerator. The carton provides protection for the fragile shells, slows down moisture loss and helps prevent the eggs from absorbing strong odours from such foods as cheese, sausages or smoked fish. Unbroken egg yolks can be stored for 3 days in the refrigerator, covered with a little water. If yolks are broken, press plastic wrap onto the surface to exclude air. Egg whites can be stored in an airtight container in the refrigerator for at least a week or frozen for 9 months. Eggs in the shells should never be frozen but beaten eggs or separated yolks and whites can be. To freeze yolks, always add 1 teaspoon of salt or 1 tablespoon of sugar for every 6 yolks. Do not add anything to the whites and for convenient use, freeze egg whites in ice cube trays, one white for every space.

Many people believe that brown eggs are

better nutritionally and in flavour than white ones. Shell colour, however, usually depends on the breed of hen. The yolk colour also can vary, and will be determined by the feed of the hen. A corn-fed chicken, for instance, lays an egg with a bright orangy yolk, while a wheat-fed chicken's egg yolk is much paler.

PREPARATION AND USE Eggs can be boiled, poached, baked, fried, scrambled and pickled. They can be cooked in the shell or out of it, simply or elaborately, on their own or with something sweet or savoury. They make cakes and soufflés rise, they enrich and thicken sauces, bind croquettes together, combine with oil for mayonnaise and with butter for hollandaise and other sauces. They provide the base for coating foods with crumbs or batter and give a golden glow as a glaze for baking.

Eggs need to be at room temperature before using, and whites will not whip successfully if they are too fresh, too cold, or have the tiniest speck of yolk or oil in them. The size of eggs can affect the result of some recipes, particularly cake recipes. Most recipes are based on a medium-sized egg.

VARIETIES

Balut

NUTRITIONAL INFORMATION No reliable data are available.

DESCRIPTION Fertilised eggs in which the embryo has formed into a chick.

ORIGIN AND HISTORY Eating such eggs is a custom adopted in the Philippines. Some say eating balut symbolises strength and purity. There is a suggestion that the eggs may be considered aphrodisiac.

BUYING AND STORAGE Rarely available in the West. Eggs can be matured at home.

PREPARATION AND USE Eggs at just the right stage of development are broken open and the entire contents eaten raw. A potent local wine usually accompanies this activity, no doubt to mask the taste.

Bantam Egg
This is half the size of a hen egg and the main appeal is in the pretty shell colours. The charm of their size makes bantam eggs favourites with small children. The eggs are not usually found in poultry shops, but may be available from breeders.

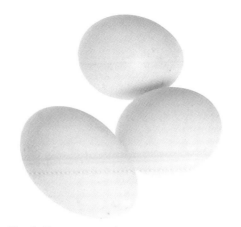

Duck Egg
This is larger than a hen egg and has an oilier, stronger taste. Duck eggs can be found in some poultry shops and a few specialist delicatessens. The eggs are often laid in dirty places and can pick up harmful bacteria, so they need at least 15 minutes of cooking time before they are eaten. This time makes them unsuitable for boiling, scrambling or poaching, but they are good for cakes. They should not be preserved in any way, and the whites must not be used for meringues.

Duck Egg, Salted

DESCRIPTION In China duck eggs are preserved in a coating of finely ground charcoal and brine until the egg has changed consistency, due to osmosis of the salt entering the shell. The yolks become quite hard, resembling dried apricots. The whites take on a pleasant salty flavour. The result is called haam daan.

ORIGIN AND HISTORY The Chinese moon cakes made for the mid-autumn festival contain salted duck egg surrounded by a sweet lotus seed paste and wrapped in layers of flaky lard-based pastry, which is stamped with coloured dyes.

BUYING AND STORAGE Unopened, salted eggs can be kept indefinitely. Separated yolks should be wrapped in plastic and will keep under refrigeration for several days.

PREPARATION AND USE The yolks should be mashed and sweetened to include in fillings for cakes and pastries. They are sometimes crumbled over dishes as a colourful garnish. Whole eggs are scraped clean of their charcoal coating, thoroughly washed and then boiled to serve with congee (rice gruel) or used in fillings or soup.

Emu Egg
This is ten times the size of a hen egg. The dark green shell is hard to crack and the egg has a strong flavour. All native birds in Australia are protected and it is against the law to collect, sell and eat them or their eggs unless under special dispensation applying to

Aboriginal people. The eggs can be scrambled but are best used in baking or in savoury dishes.

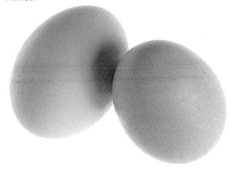

Free-Range Egg
It is possible to obtain eggs laid by chickens that have been allowed to roam freely in wired runs. Most supermarket eggs come from hens laying in confined cages above the ground. The space needed for free-range chickens makes their eggs much more expensive, but the flavour is said to be better. Generally speaking, free-range chickens are fed the same diet as other hens but their laying cycles are not speeded up like those of battery hens.

Goose Egg
Twice the size of a hen egg, and with a slightly oily taste. The shell is hard to crack. The eggs are not freely available in poultry shops but may be obtained from breeders. They should be used when very fresh; their strong flavour makes them more suitable for cakes. Like ducks, geese often lay their eggs in dirty, wet places and the eggs need long cooking to kill harmful bacteria.

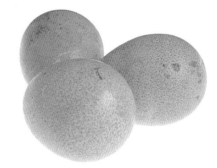

Guinea Fowl Egg
This is smaller than a hen egg and has a more delicate taste. The shell is usually brown with dark speckles. The eggs are rarely found in poultry shops but may be available from breeders. The eggs are eaten hard boiled with salad.

Ostrich Egg
This may be 8 to 10 times the size of a hen egg. It has a strong flavour and the pale shell is very hard to crack. The eggs are not freely available in Australia but may be obtainable from breeders of the birds. They are best used in baking.

Pheasant Egg This is smaller than a hen egg and the shell colour can vary from white, buff, olive or speckled. The eggs are not freely available from poultry shops but may be obtainable from breeders. They can be served hard boiled in salads, in aspics, or pickled in brine.

Pullet Egg This is the small egg laid by a young hen. These eggs weigh about 35 g and their charm lies in their tiny size and their delicate flavour. They are usually only to be found at egg farms.

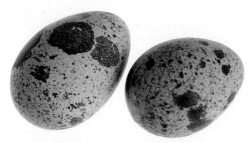

Quail Egg This is one-third the size of a hen egg. The shell is greenish-beige with dark spots. Usually available in poultry shops, and can be served hard boiled in salads, in aspics, or pickled.

Seagull Egg The colour varies depending on the species of gull, but the shells are always mottled with dark spots as camouflage. The eggs have a slightly fishy taste. In Australia, gulls are protected species and it is prohibited by law to collect, eat or sell the eggs except under the special dispensations applying to Aboriginal people. In England there is no restriction on collection and eggs are available in specialist poultry shops. One way of serving the eggs is to hard boil for 5 minutes, cool and serve with celery salt.

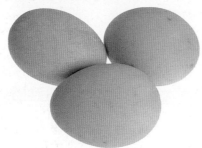

Thousand-Year Egg

MAJOR NUTRIENTS		BOILED SERVE SIZE 20 G	
Energy	160 kJ	Potassium	160 mg
Protein	3 g	Iron	0.7 mg
Fat	3 g	Zinc	0.7 mg
Carbohydrate	N/A	Riboflavin	0.1 mg
Cholesterol	105 mg	Vitamin A	N/A
Sodium	340 mg	Vitamin C	N/A

NUTRITIONAL INFORMATION It is an excellent source of vitamin B12; a good source of iron; a moderate source of riboflavin, potassium, zinc and protein. It contains a large amount of cholesterol and sodium. The fat is predominantly monounsaturated.

DESCRIPTION Duck eggs which have been coated with a mixture of lime, ash, salt and tea leaves or rice husks, then packed in tubs to cure for 2–4 months. They are also known as ancient eggs and 100-day eggs. The chemicals osmose through the eggshell and preserve and flavour the egg. The yolk turns a dark grey-green and the white becomes firm and pale amber in colour. Chicken eggs are also preserved in this way, but duck eggs have a better texture and taste. The flavour of the white is slightly sulphurous, its texture firmly gelatinous; the yolk is somewhat like a mild blue cheese, its texture creamy. The Chinese name is pay dun.

ORIGIN AND HISTORY A Chinese discovery of ancient times, this food was originally an attempt to preserve eggs using juice extracted from the bark of a native tree resembling the chestnut. Later eggs were to be stacked between layers of ash and earth, as a means of preservation. They are packed for maturation and transport, into large glazed jars similar to those used for pickled mustard greens. Ancient eggs symbolise the connection with the past and longevity, and are served accompanied by sliced vinegar-pickled ginger at banquets.

BUYING AND STORAGE Sold by the piece in Chinese food stores. They should be wrapped in paper and can be kept for up to 1 month in the refrigerator or at least 1 week unrefrigerated.

PREPARATION AND USE Scrape the shells, then peel and rinse. Dry and cut into wedges. Serve with sweet pickled ginger as an appetiser.

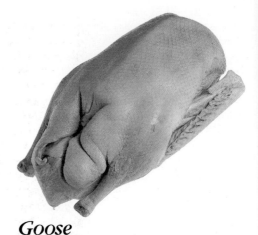

Goose

MAJOR NUTRIENTS		ROASTED DARK MEAT SERVE SIZE 100 G	
Energy	1330 kJ	Sodium	150 g
Protein	29 g	Magnesium	31 mg
Fat	22 g	Phosphorus	270 mg
Carbohydrate	0	Iron	4.6 mg
Cholesterol	N/A		

NUTRITIONAL INFORMATION No analysis has yet been performed for B group vitamins or cholesterol. An excellent source of protein, phosphorus, iron; moderate source of magnesium; very high in fat. Although goose has a higher iron content than chicken, it contains twice as much fat and therefore twice as many kilojoules.

DESCRIPTION Goose is a web-footed waterbird widely bred for the table in Europe, while it is less popular in the southern hemisphere. Geese are mainly natives of the northern hemisphere, and each country has its own favourite breed.

ORIGIN AND HISTORY Domestic geese are descended from the Greylag goose. Archaeologists believe that geese were probably domesticated in Neolithic times when fledglings of wild birds were caught and fattened. The Greeks raised geese, feeding them on soft grain. Geese were part of Roman religious rituals and were associated with the goddess Juno, guarding her temples. Legend says that in 390 BC their loud calls saved Rome from capture by the invading Gauls. The Romans did not eat geese, as the flesh was thought to be not palatable. The Gauls, however, were fattening geese and supplied Rome with birds after the Roman invasion of their country. By the Middle Ages goose was the most popular meat, next to pork, and large flocks of geese were common. In Elizabethan England, the queen celebrated a victory by declaring 29 September as St Michael's Day, with roast goose to be always a feature of the day. In Europe goose is always associated with celebrations and holidays.

BUYING AND STORAGE In Australia and New Zealand, geese usually need to be ordered from specialist poultry shops. They are generally sold frozen, but can sometimes be purchased fresh. They are eaten at 3 months, when they weigh between 3 kg and 5 kg. Allow 500 g per person. The male bird is called a gander and is slightly larger than the female.

PREPARATION AND USE Rinse and dry goose, remove all visible fat and prick all over with a fine skewer. Young goose is best when it is roasted on a rack. Older geese are often poached before baking. The liver of the goose is used to make pâté de foie gras, and a classic dish of France is confit d'oie, where goose flesh is preserved in its own fat as a traditional accompaniment for cassoulet.

VARIETIES

The domestic geese of Europe are the Emden, the Toulouse, the Strasburg, the Roman and the Brecon, while in Asia they eat the Chinese goose, the largest of all geese.

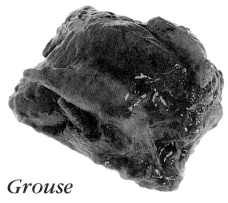

Grouse

also called Moor fowl

MAJOR NUTRIENTS			ROAST MEAT SERVE SIZE 100 G
Energy	730 kJ	Magnesium	41 mg
Protein	31 g	Phosphorus	340 mg
Fat	5 g	Iron	7.6 mg
Carbohydrate	0	Thiamin	0.3 mg
Cholesterol	N/A	Riboflavin	0.5 mg
Sodium	100 mg	Niacin Equiv.	14 mg
Potassium	470 mg		

NUTRITIONAL INFORMATION Has yet to be analysed for vitamins B6, B12, pantothenic acid and cholesterol. An excellent source of protein, phosphorus, iron, thiamin, riboflavin, niacin; good source of magnesium; moderate in fat and potassium. As grouse is a game bird, it is higher in protein and iron than domestic chicken.

DESCRIPTION Grouse is the common name given to a number of ground-scratching game birds in the northern hemisphere. Grouse is not freely available in the southern hemisphere.

ORIGIN AND HISTORY Grouse is hunted as a game bird. The English have named the day the shooting season starts in that country — 12 August — as the Glorious Twelfth. The season ends on 10 December.

BUYING AND STORAGE Freshly killed grouse are generally hung for 3 days before plucking and cleaning, to tenderise them and improve the gamy flavour. Allow one grouse per person. Weight of the birds ranges from 750 g–1.5 kg. Canned grouse, shown above, is available in Australasia.

PREPARATION AND USE After hanging and cleaning, grouse can be grilled or roasted. Older birds are casseroled.

VARIETIES

Birds include the red grouse of Britain, the ruffled grouse of North America, the black grouse of Germany. Others are the European wood and hazel grouse, the Canadian spruce grouse, and the American Franklin's, blue and Sierra grouse.

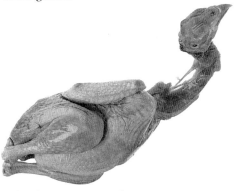

Guinea Fowl

NUTRITIONAL INFORMATION Not available, but likely to resemble that of pheasant.

DESCRIPTION Guinea fowl is a domestic and game bird very like pheasant.

ORIGIN AND HISTORY Guinea fowl come from the Guinea coast of Africa. They were being eaten in Greece in 500 BC and the Romans called them Carthaginian hens. After the collapse of the Roman Empire, Guinea fowl disappeared from Europe and only came back when the Portuguese colonised Guinea. The birds are difficult to domesticate as they will not lay in confinement and are extremely noisy. The shooting season in England lasts all year round.

BUYING AND STORAGE Guinea fowl are available from specialist poultry shops. Allow one per person and use within 2–3 days of purchase.

PREPARATION AND USE Guinea fowl is often hung undressed after killing, to tenderise the flesh and improve the flavour.

Any recipe for chicken or pheasant can be used, but care must be taken during cooking as the flesh can dry out and become stringy. Guinea fowl can be roasted or braised. The liver is highly regarded by gourmets.

VARIETIES

There are over 20 different species of Guinea fowl but the one most commonly eaten has the scientific name of *Numida melagris* and has white-spotted grey plumage.

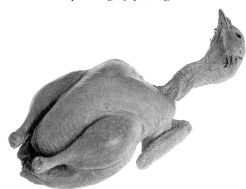

Partridge

MAJOR NUTRIENTS			ROAST MEAT SERVE SIZE 100 G
Energy	890 kJ	Sodium	100 mg
Protein	38 g	Calcium	46 mg
Fat	7 g	Magnesium	36 mg
Carbohydrate	0	Phosphorus	310 mg
Cholesterol	N/A	Iron	7.7 mg

NUTRITIONAL INFORMATION Has yet to be analysed for vitamins A, D, C, E, folate, all B group vitamins and cholesterol. An excellent source of protein, phosphorus, iron; good source of magnesium; moderate source of calcium; moderate in fat.

DESCRIPTION The partridge is a small game bird.

ORIGIN AND HISTORY The partridge is a native of the northern hemisphere and gourmets have been praising its flesh since Roman times. It was introduced into England in the late 19th century for the shooting season, which starts on 1 September and ends on 1 February. An interesting feature of the hen partridge is the way the scent that the bird gives off is suppressed while she is hatching eggs. The American 'partridge' is not a true partridge, but one of the grouse family. It is thought that the partridge in a pear tree in the well-known Christmas song was not a live bird, but a dead one, hung from a branch.

BUYING AND STORAGE Freshly killed partridge are generally hung for 3 days before plucking and cleaning to tenderise them and improve the flavour. Allow one per person. Weight of the birds ranges from 750 g–1.5 kg.

PREPARATION AND USE After hanging and cleaning, partridge can be grilled or roasted. Older birds are casseroled.

VARIETIES

There are several different varieties but the two main birds eaten are the European grey and the French red-legged partridge. Others include the rock and snow partridges.

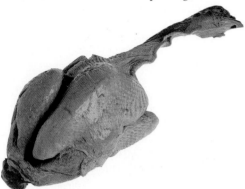

Pheasant

MAJOR NUTRIENTS

		ROASTED MEAT SERVE SIZE 100 G	
Energy	890 kJ	Calcium	49 mg
Protein	32 g	Magnesium	35 mg
Fat	9 g	Phosphorus	310 mg
Carbohydrate	0	Iron	8.4 mg
Cholesterol	N/A	Riboflavin	0.15 mg
Sodium	100 mg	Niacin Equiv.	16 mg

NUTRITIONAL INFORMATION As yet no analysis performed for vitamins A, D, E, B6, B12, folate, pantothenic acid and cholesterol. An excellent source of protein, phosphorus, iron, niacin; good source of magnesium and riboflavin; moderate source of calcium; moderate in fat.

DESCRIPTION Pheasant is regarded by many as having the best-flavoured flesh of all game birds. Cock pheasants have beautifully coloured feathers, and often have long tails. They are slightly larger than the duller hen birds.

ORIGIN AND HISTORY Legend says that Jason of the Argonauts brought the birds back to Greece along with the Golden Fleece, and historians believe the birds originated in Asia. From Roman times the birds have been served cooked and re-feathered at exotic and ceremonial banquets. In England the shooting season for pheasants starts on 1 October and ends on 1 February.

BUYING AND STORAGE Pheasant is available from specialist poultry shops and weighs approximately 1.5 kg. Allow 500 g per person. Store in the refrigerator and use within 2–3 days.

PREPARATION AND USE Pheasant was always hung uncleaned to tenderise the flesh and improve the flavour. These days some people prefer it unhung if the birds are young. After plucking and cleaning, the young birds can be roasted and the older birds casseroled. Care needs to be taken to prevent the tender flesh from drying out and larding with strips of fat and basting during the cooking keeps the flesh moist.

VARIETIES

There are many varieties of pheasant in the world — Reeves, Lady Amherst, golden, silver, peacock, Impeyan, crested fireback, Chinese ring-necked. The ring-necked pheasant is the bird raised commercially in Australia.

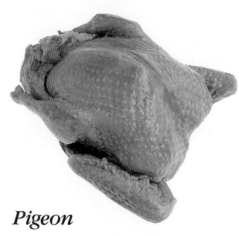

Pigeon

MAJOR NUTRIENTS

		ROASTED MEAT SERVE SIZE 100 G	
Energy	960 kJ	Sodium	100 mg
Protein	28 g	Magnesium	3.4 mg
Fat	13 g	Phosphorus	400 mg
Carbohydrate	0	Iron	19 mg
Cholesterol	100 mg	Niacin Equiv.	13 mg

NUTRITIONAL INFORMATION As yet no analysis for vitamins A, D, E and B group vitamins. An excellent source of protein, iron, phosphorus, niacin; good source of magnesium; high in fat and cholesterol. Higher in fat and consequently in kilojoules than roast chicken, and extremely high in iron compared to other birds.

DESCRIPTION The pigeon is a small game bird with attractive plumage, often in greys and greens.

ORIGIN AND HISTORY Once trapped in the wild, pigeons are now bred in captivity for the table. Pigeons mate for life, and if one dies the remaining bird takes a long time to find a new mate.

BUYING AND STORAGE In Australia and New Zealand, the word 'squab' is used to describe pigeons bred for the table. In the USA on the other hand, a squab is a very small young chicken. Pigeons are available in specialist poultry shops and weigh approximately 500 g. Allow one per person. Store in the refrigerator and use within 2–3 days of purchase.

PREPARATION AND USE Wild pigeons are hung uncleaned for 2 days in a cool room to tenderise the flesh and improve the flavour. Domestic pigeons are starved for 24 hours before killing. Young birds are usually roasted or grilled and the older tougher birds are casseroled. Pigeon pie is a traditional English dish and the French like to leave the liver inside the bird when it is cooking, as it contains no bitter gall.

VARIETIES

There are over 290 species of pigeons in the world, all with different plumage. The wood pigeon or ring-dove is the species that is most eaten.

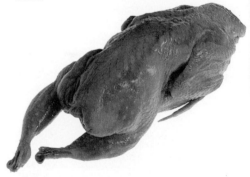

Quail

NUTRITIONAL INFORMATION No reliable data are available.

DESCRIPTION The quail is a small game bird found in Europe, Asia, Africa and Australia. It has mottled or dark plumage, and some varieties have an erect head feather.

ORIGIN AND HISTORY True quail are migratory birds and immense numbers are netted in the Mediterranean region during their flights north in summer, and south during the winter months. As quail prefer to run from danger rather than fly, they are easily caught. They are a protected species in England, as shooting almost exterminated them. These days in the United Kingdom quail are raised on farms.

BUYING AND STORAGE Quail is available both fresh and frozen in specialist poultry shops. A bird weighs approximately 150 g. Allow 1 or 2 per person. Store in the refrigerator and use within 2 days of purchase.

PREPARATION AND USE Quail can be roasted, braised, sautéed or made into pies and pâtés. The flesh is very delicate and care needs to be taken to prevent it drying out, by wrapping the bird in bacon or fat and basting during roasting. The French like to present the quail boned in a variety of ways, while the English simply roast it.

VARIETIES

As well as the common quail of Europe, there are the rain quail, African and Australian stubble quail. The American Californian and bobwhite quail are not true quail and belong to a branch of the family which includes grouse.

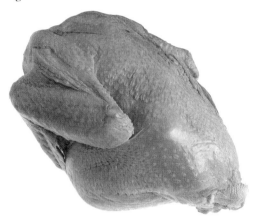

Turkey

MAJOR NUTRIENTS		ROASTED MEAT AND SKIN SERVE SIZE 100 G	
Energy	720 kJ	Sodium	50 mg
Protein	28 g	Magnesium	24 mg
Fat	7 g	Phosphorus	200 mg
Carbohydrate	0	Iron	0.9 mg
Cholesterol	79 mg	Zinc	2.1 mg

NUTRITIONAL INFORMATION No analysis available for vitamins A, D, E, folate and B group vitamins. An excellent source of protein, phosphorus; good source of iron and zinc; moderate in fat.

Roast turkey has half the fat content and a third less cholesterol when compared to domestic chicken. Without the skin, 100 g of turkey meat contains 1 g of fat, and 62 mg of cholesterol.

DESCRIPTION The turkey is a large domestic fowl originally from the Americas but now bred in all countries. The colour of the feathers varies, but all birds have the distinctive red wattles and make the 'gobble gobble' cry.

ORIGIN AND HISTORY Spanish explorers of the 16th century are given the credit for taking the turkey from the Americas to Europe but there is some dispute over this. The pictorial Norman Bayeux Tapestry of 1087 shows a turkey in the marginal decorations and it is believed that the Norsemen could have had settlements in North America from 985 to 1121 and some turkeys came to Europe with them. The Spaniards, however, did re-introduce turkeys and by the end of the 16th century turkey was being eaten all over Europe. A German cookbook of that period gives 20 different ways of cooking the bird.

For North Americans, the turkey has long been associated with Thanksgiving, when the Pilgrims celebrated their landfall with a turkey dinner after crossing the Atlantic. The French sympathies were with the Americans during the American Revolution and turkey eating was a practical way of showing their support for the American cause. Turkey is always associated with holidays and festivals.

BUYING AND STORAGE Turkeys are available both fresh and frozen. The hen is considered more tender than the male bird. The numerical system is used to show the weight of the turkey and indicates its age. For example, a number 35 weighs 3.5 kg and is 8 weeks old. Number 55 weighs 5.5 kg and is 12 weeks old. As turkeys age, they become very tough, and birds over 12 months old can be inedible except for the breast meat. Frozen turkeys should be thawed in the refrigerator or in a microwave oven. Store fresh turkeys in the refrigerator and use within 2–3 days of purchase. Store cooked meat loosely wrapped in paper in the refrigerator. If the cooked turkey has been stuffed, the stuffing needs to be removed from the bird before refrigerating as meat stuffings can deteriorate and cause food poisoning.

Turkey is also available as turkey buffe, which is breast meat with the bone intact. The breast is also available in halves, rolled for roasting or as fillets. Turkey hindquarters are also sold.

PREPARATION AND USE Young whole turkey can be roasted and barbecued while older ones can be casseroled. Birds for roasting are usually stuffed in the body cavity and the crop. Fashions in stuffing change continually but traditionalists like sage and onion, forcemeat, or chestnut.

Turkey breast pieces can be roasted, fried or sautéed, and hindquarters roasted or casseroled. Leftover cooked turkey can be used in sandwiches, salads, soups, and casseroles.

VARIETIES

These include the traditional English Norfolk Black, But 5 and But 6. The Holland White is a new turkey with a high percentage of the most popular white breast meat.

FISH AND SHELLFISH

Food from the sea, lakes and rivers has been important in human diets since prehistoric times. Archaeologists have identified shellfish middens amongst the remains of primitive societies in many locations around the world, providing good evidence that these foods were eaten before the dawn of agriculture.

Today, fish remains a staple food in the diets of a minority of people such as the Inuit and other North American Indians, and groups living in fishing communities. In most industrialised societies, however, the average consumption is low.

In some regions, such as Australasia, there has been a recent increase brought about by improvements in the harvesting, promotion and marketing of seafoods and freshwater fish and by the heightened public interest in the nutritional and health significance of fish. There have also been developments in fish farming which are resulting in improvements in the supply and quality of fish such as rainbow trout and Atlantic salmon, although these are beyond the budget of most households as a regular item of the family diet.

Fish and other foods from the oceans and rivers have long been recognised as nutritious foods, but observations in the last decade, noting the correlation between the consumption of two or more fish meals per week and a lower prevalence of coronary heart disease, have highlighted the possibility of additional health benefits associated with eating fish. These benefits have been linked to the long-chain, highly polyunsaturated omega-3 fatty acids, eicosapentaenoic acid and docosahexaenoic acid, which are found in fish.

These fatty acids are converted to hormonelike compounds called prostaglandins, which affect metabolic processes in body tissues. They have been shown to lower the level of triglycerides in the blood, to reduce the risk of blood clotting, and, possibly, to reduce inflammation in conditions such as rheumatoid arthritis and to improve the immune system.

Fish and seafoods are an excellent source of protein. Most fish caught in tropical and subtropical waters have a very low fat content (0.5–2 per cent), but the cold water fish such as salmon, trout, tuna, sardines, herrings, pilchards, mackerel and eels have a much higher fat content (10–20 per cent). The fats are rich in polyunsaturated fatty acids.

Fish is often prepared with fat or oil and a low-fat fish, when fried, will thus contain 10 per cent or more fat.

In some societies, fish is eaten raw, sometimes with the accompaniment of sauces: the Japanese sashimi is an example, and raw fish is a frequent ingredient of the small delicacies, sushi.

Like most animal products, seafoods contain cholesterol: fish and molluscs contain only 40–100 mg per 100 g and crustaceans have 100–200 mg per 100 g. Roe and caviar are very high in cholesterol.

Seafoods are the best food source of iodine: freshwater fish contain about half the iodine found in saltwater varieties. They also provide an excellent source of selenium and fluoride. Other minerals which are provided in moderate amounts are iron, zinc and magnesium. The level of iron is approximately a third to a half that in red meat.

Crustaceans and molluscs are good sources of calcium, and fish with edible bones, such as canned sardines, whitebait and salmon, are excellent sources of calcium. Sardines and whitebait are excellent sources of magnesium. Sardines, crabs and oysters are excellent sources of zinc.

Seafood in general is an excellent source of niacin and vitamin B12, and a moderate source of thiamin, riboflavin and vitamin B6. Eel, roe and salmon are good sources of vitamin A.

The health hazards associated with the consumption of fish contaminated with heavy metals such as mercury have received worldwide publicity since the reports of severe cases of poisoning amongst Japanese fishermen and their families, who ate large amounts of fish caught in Minimata Bay, where waters were polluted with factory effluent. Large carnivorous fish such as tuna, swordfish and shark eat smaller plant-eating fish and as we move up the food chain these heavy metals become more concentrated in the flesh of the fish. Problems have only arisen when individuals eat large amounts of fish which have fed in contaminated waters.

There has also been concern about the safety of oysters, and these are now carefully monitored by the growers and health authorities.

The fish listed have been chosen according to availability and palatability. The naming of fish in the marketplace can be confusing (the term 'ocean trout', for instance, has been used to describe several different types of fish, including salmon) and care has been taken to list common names where relevant.

Shellfish fall into two groups — crustaceans and molluscs. Crustaceans have an external skeleton which forms a sometimes fragile jointed shell. This group includes prawns, crabs, lobsters, crayfish, yabbies, and scampi. Molluscs are invertebrates, usually protected by a strong shell, and are estuary and shore dwelling creatures. This group includes oysters, mussels, pipis, scallops, abalone, cockles, clams, whelks, periwinkles, cuttlefish, squid and octopus.

They are similar in food value to fish, but crustaceans contain about twice as much cholesterol as other seafoods. Molluscs used to be classified as foods high in cholesterol, but it is now known that most of the sterols in these foods are compounds other than cholesterol.

The last section of this chapter deals with preserved seafood. The drying, salting and smoking of fish were methods of preservation used long before commercial processing was introduced. In most preservation, including canning, a lot of salt is introduced, but 'no added salt' canned sardines, salmon and tuna are now readily available and are excellent foods in a healthy diet.

Smoking is perhaps one of the oldest forms of food preparation. As well as having a preserving effect, it also yields a beautiful appearance, smell and flavour. Moist, oily and firm-fleshed fish are the best to use. The moister the fish, the faster the smoke flows over the surface, and the quicker the smoke vapour is absorbed into the flesh.

Cold smoking involves light brining of fish and smoke temperatures do not normally rise above 29°C. The source of the smoke is usually placed outside the smokehouse, allowing it to cool down before reaching the fish. All cold-smoked products require cooking. Examples of cold-smoked products are smoked gemfish, tailor, cod and haddock. With hot smoking, fish are generally smoked and cooked at temperatures between 80°C and 90°C. Smoke reaches the fish directly, while still hot. Examples of hot-smoked products are smoked trout, salmon and eel.

In general, the nutrients in preserved fish are similar to those in fresh fish, but there would be some loss of vitamins. The retention of nutrients in the canned products is excellent.

There is every reason to encourage the consumption of fish and to promote low fat methods of preparation.

These foods are nutritious and, when eaten as a regular part of the diet, they may be protective against heart disease and possibly other diseases.

In general, to benefit from maximum flavour and nutritional value, fish should be bought and eaten when it is as fresh as possible. The usual signs of freshness in whole fish are bright, bulging eyes; flesh that is firm and resilient to the touch; and a smell that is pleasantly reminiscent of the sea. Filleted fish should be white

(or tinged with the natural creaminess or pinkness common to some types of fish). Do not buy any fish that has traces of discoloration, such as brown blotches.

To store fish, it is best to scale, gill and gut it, and fins can be trimmed. If it is not to be eaten immediately, it should be wrapped in plastic film and stored in an airtight container in the refrigerator for a maximum of 3 days. Do not keep deep frozen for longer than 6 months.

When buying smoked fish, beware of a sweaty appearance and rancid smell. To store, wrap in paper or foil or keep in an airtight container. Do not use plastic wrap, as this will cause the fish to sweat. Keep up to 7 or 10 days in the refrigerator. Smoked fish can be successfully frozen, but may display an extra saltiness when eaten.

When buying frozen fish, always look out for 'freezer burn'. This is caused when the fish has been incorrectly wrapped for freezing and has dehydrated. Freezer burn is obvious when there are white or brown blotches and 'dry' markings on the flesh. Never refreeze fish that has already been frozen.

FISH

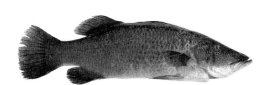

Barramundi *Lates calcarifer*

MAJOR NUTRIENTS		SERVE SIZE 100 G	
Energy	390 kJ	Sodium	120 mg
Protein	18 g	Calcium	51 mg
Fat	2 g	Phosphorus	180 mg
Carbohydrate	0	Magnesium	20 mg
Cholesterol	60 mg	Thiamin	0.3 mg

NUTRITIONAL INFORMATION Very little analysis is available on the nutrients of some of the fish found in Australian waters, but the figures above are supplied as a general guide to this variety.

DESCRIPTION Dark bluish-grey on the upper body and silver below, with a yellow tinge on the caudal fin. The eyes are bright pinkish-red and glow at night. A deep-bodied fish with a large mouth and powerful tail, its flesh is white, tender and firm with a large flake. The taste is distinctive, yet mild.

ORIGIN AND HISTORY The word barramundi was used by Australian Aboriginal people for certain river fish with large scales.

At night, people would wade into the water holding a spear and a bundle of lighted sticks. The fish were attracted to the light and then speared with great precision. If the hunters were in a canoe they would make a small fire in the bow on sand or stone and attract the fish in this way. Alternatively, a fire could be lit on the shore. As the fish made towards the bank, they were speared. Aboriginal people often wrapped barramundi in the wild ginger plant and baked it in hot ashes.

Barramundi ranges from the Mary River in Queensland, where it is not very plentiful, and along the northern Australian coast as far as Western Australia. It is very plentiful in Princess Charlotte Bay on the eastern shores of Cape York Peninsula and in rivers flowing into the Gulf of Carpentaria. The barramundi in Australia grows to a weight of upwards of 54 kg and fish of 27–45 kg are by no means rare. There is, however, a record of one caught in the Bay of Bengal that weighed 267 kg.

BUYING AND STORAGE Although available fresh in certain areas it is mainly sold in frozen fillets. When purchasing whole barramundi, look for firm flesh, bright bulging eyes and a pleasant sea smell. Fillets should be white with no brown markings, firm and not spongy.

Season: October to March (southern hemisphere).

PREPARATION AND USE If using whole fish, scale and clean first. Before cooking either whole fish or fillets, scoring is essential.

Barramundi fillets can be skinned. This versatile fish suits all methods of cooking.

PROCESSING Barramundi is filleted and frozen.

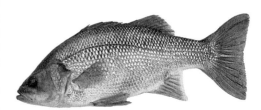

Bass, Australian *Macquaria novemaculeata*

also called **Freshwater perch**

MAJOR NUTRIENTS		SERVE SIZE 100 G	
Energy	390 kJ	Carbohydrate	0
Protein	19 g	Cholesterol	80 mg
Fat	1 g	Sodium	70 mg

NUTRITIONAL INFORMATION No data are available on vitamin and mineral content.

DESCRIPTION Bass flesh is white, tender but firm with a low fat content. It has very good eating qualities.

ORIGIN AND HISTORY The name bass is derived from the Old English word byrst meaning to bristle, which accurately describes the attitude displayed by the dorsal fins of the bass. Bass are members of a large, ravenous family of fishes. Australian bass are found on the east coast, from Queensland to New South Wales.

BUYING AND STORAGE Available whole, or as fillets, cutlets, and steaks. The bass is also a popular game fish.

PREPARATION AND USE Can be filleted or served whole. Suits most methods of cooking but because of its low fat content it is more suited to moist methods of cooking.

VARIETIES

There are hundreds of varieties of bass. Bass is usually described by a qualifying word, such as small-mouthed, spotted etc., and many local names. To add to the confusion, there are also some saltwater fish called bass.

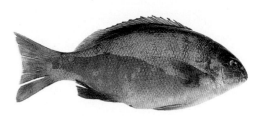

Blackfish *Girella tricuspidata, G. elevatus*

MAJOR NUTRIENTS		SERVE SIZE 100 G	
Energy	390 kJ	Sodium	120 mg
Protein	18 g	Calcium	51 mg
Fat	2 g	Phosphorus	180 mg
Carbohydrate	0	Magnesium	20 mg
Cholesterol	60 mg	Thiamin	0.3 mg

NUTRITIONAL INFORMATION Very little analysis is available on the nutrients contained in some of the fish found in Australian waters, but the figures above are supplied as a general guide to this variety.

DESCRIPTION A deep-bodied fish, medium in size. Colourings vary from silver to brown. The flesh is white, moist, soft and with a distinctive flavour, and is good eating if the fish is bled as soon as it is caught.

ORIGIN AND HISTORY Blackfish are estuarine fish. Family members are found worldwide. In Australia the greatest number are found in southern Queensland, New South Wales and Victoria, and the family includes the drummer also. The blackfish lives in shallow flats with abundant weeds, and although it is mainly vegetarian it is not averse to some meat. It is one of the gamest fighters in Australian waters and has an enthusiastic following of anglers.

BUYING AND STORAGE Available whole or in fillets.

Season: all year.

PREPARATION AND USE When caught, should be bled as soon as possible. Best used in fillet form but can be cooked whole. Suits all methods of cooking. If using fillets, skin. Strong flavourings suit blackfish because of its distinctive flavour.

VARIETIES

Luderick, rock blackfish.

SEE ALSO Drummer.

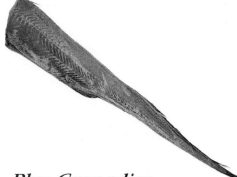

Blue Grenadier *Macruronus novaezelandiae*

MAJOR NUTRIENTS		SERVE SIZE 100 G	
Energy	390 kJ	Sodium	120 mg
Protein	18 g	Calcium	51 mg
Fat	2 g	Phosphorus	180 mg
Carbohydrate	0	Magnesium	20 mg
Cholesterol	60 mg	Thiamin	0.3 mg

NUTRITIONAL INFORMATION Very little analysis is available on the nutrients contained in some of the fish found in Australian waters, but the figures above are supplied as a general guide to this variety.

DESCRIPTION Blue grenadier is a long silver fish with no scales, similar in appearance to gemfish. Its flesh is cream-pink in colour, very moist and soft. It has a medium to large flake and a mild taste.

ORIGIN AND HISTORY It is a deep-sea fish, mainly caught on the south coast of New South Wales and in Victoria. Family members are worldwide.

BUYING AND STORAGE Available in fillets or cutlets.

Season: winter (southern hemisphere).

PREPARATION AND USE When using thick fillets, score first. Skin can either be left on or removed. Lends itself to most methods of cooking, and most flavourings. Be careful with the soft flesh.

PROCESSING Occasionally frozen commercially.

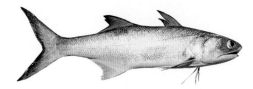

Blue Threadfin *Eleutheronema tetradactylum*

also called Cooktown salmon

MAJOR NUTRIENTS		SERVE SIZE 100 G	
Energy	390 kJ	Sodium	120 mg
Protein	18 g	Calcium	51 mg
Fat	2 g	Phosphorus	180 mg
Carbohydrate	0	Magnesium	20 mg
Cholesterol	60 mg	Thiamin	0.3 mg

NUTRITIONAL INFORMATION Very little analysis is available on the nutrients contained in some of the fish found in Australian waters, but the figures above are supplied as a general guide to this variety.

DESCRIPTION The blue threadfin can reach a weight of 18.5 kg. It is dull blue-green above and clean white to silvery over the stomach; the pectoral fins are yellow, the forked tail dusky.

ORIGIN AND HISTORY Seen in southern Asian waters as well as Western Australian coastal warm waters, it also ranges from the Northern Territory into the Gulf of Carpentaria and along the tropical Queensland coastline. It is an important commercial and sport fish. It is attracted to a trolled lure or plug, especially towards dusk.

BUYING AND STORAGE It is mainly available in fillet form. The flesh is large-flaked and white. Look out for already frozen fillets — they can be spongy and are not good for refreezing.

Season: all year.

PREPARATION AND USE With age, this fish can develop great bony nodules along the backbone, making filleting difficult. If fillets are very thick, score them to allow even heat penetration. If using whole fish, trim fins before serving. This fish suits most methods of cooking.

VARIETIES

It is often associated with the king threadfin, from which it is readily distinguishable by the number and length of trailing 'fingers' to the pectoral fin. They are short in the blue threadfin and are only 3 or 4 in number, whereas the king threadfin has 5.

PROCESSING Fillets can be frozen commercially.

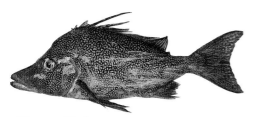

Boarfish *Zanclistius elevatus*

MAJOR NUTRIENTS			SERVE SIZE 100 G
Energy	390 kJ	Sodium	120 mg
Protein	18 g	Calcium	51 mg
Fat	2 g	Phosphorus	180 mg
Carbohydrate	0	Magnesium	20 mg
Cholesterol	60 mg	Thiamin	0.3 mg

NUTRITIONAL INFORMATION Very little analysis is available on the nutrients contained in some of the fish found in Australian waters, but the figures above are supplied as a general guide to this variety.

DESCRIPTION Boarfish are short, deep-bodied fish with large eyes and protruding snouts. Some are brightly coloured, but the majority are brown in colour. The flesh is white, firm and moist with a medium flake and is very good eating.

ORIGIN AND HISTORY Fishermen often give appropriate names to their catch and boarfish is no exception. The boarfish actually looks like a boar! It is found in the Atlantic Ocean and in parts of the Pacific. In Australia it is found along the southern half of the continent including Tasmania.

BUYING AND STORAGE Usually available in fillet form. There are few bones in boarfish fillets.

Season: all year.

PREPARATION AND USE Because of its appearance boarfish should not be served whole. Filleted, it lends itself to baking, shallow frying, poaching, barbecuing and grilling. Most flavourings are compatible with boarfish. The fillets are meaty and can be used for hearty meals.

VARIETIES
Giant boarfish, *Paristiopterus labiosus*; long-snouted boarfish, *Pentaceropsis recurvirostris*.

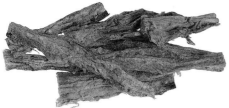

Bombay Duck *Harpodon nehereus*

also called **Bomeloe, Boomla, Bummalow**

MAJOR NUTRIENTS			SERVE SIZE 20 G
Energy	280 kJ	Cholesterol	N/A
Protein	12 g	Sodium	N/A
Fat	2 g	Calcium	340 mg
Carbohydrate	0	Iron	0.5 mg

NUTRITIONAL INFORMATION An excellent source of protein, it contains high amounts of sodium in the salted, dried form.

DESCRIPTION The Bombay duck is a predatory fish which hunts in shoals, particularly in the Arabian Sea around the port of Bombay. The body is long and tapering, growing up to 40 cm in length, pale in colour and almost translucent. It has a large head with hard, needle-like teeth, and feeds on small crustaceans on the seabed.

ORIGIN AND HISTORY Fished off the west coast of India during the monsoon season, it probably acquired the appellation 'duck' because it swims close to the surface at this time of year. Better known in the West in its dried form, it is also eaten fresh as it has soft, delicately flavoured flesh.

BUYING AND STORAGE Dried, it is sold whole or cut into pieces of about 2.5 cm, and should be stored in an airtight container in a cool, dry cupboard. Fresh, it should be eaten soon, as it decomposes quickly.

PREPARATION AND USE Bombay duck is served as an accompaniment to Indian meals. It should be deep fried or grilled until crisp, when its pungent smell will dissipate.

PROCESSING Air or sun-dried and salted.

Bream Family Sparidae

MAJOR NUTRIENTS			SERVE SIZE 100 G
Energy	420 kJ	Sodium	65 mg
Protein	21 g	Calcium	55 mg
Fat	2 g	Phosphorus	250 mg
Carbohydrate	0	Iron	0.8 mg
Cholesterol	70 mg		

NUTRITIONAL INFORMATION No data are available on vitamin content. Fat content can vary from low fat to moderate fat (1%–5%).

DESCRIPTION Bream are a most attractive fish, varying in colour from silvery yellow to silvery black depending upon their habitat. The flesh is white, soft and sweet, making bream a most popular table fish.

There are both saltwater and freshwater bream. It must be noted here that the name bream has been used incorrectly for many other species of fish.

ORIGIN AND HISTORY A popular angling fish, mainly found in tidal rivers, estuaries and coastal lagoons. Fish caught in rivers and estuaries tend to be dark in colour, and are often called black bream. Those caught in clear ocean waters are much lighter in colour, and are thus called silver bream. One type of sea bream is called porgy in North America.

BUYING AND STORAGE Bream is nearly always sold whole, but can be purchased in fillets. To store: scale, gill, clean (gut) and trim fins.

Season: all year, particularly March to May.

PREPARATION AND USE Suits all methods of cooking. Scale, gut, clean, trim fins and score whole fish before cooking.

VARIETIES
There are many varieties of bream. The main ones are listed below.

Pikey Bream

Southern Bream

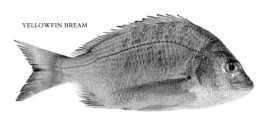

YELLOWFIN BREAM

Yellowfin Bream also called Silver bream, Surf bream and Black bream.

Tarwhine

MAJOR NUTRIENTS			SERVE SIZE 100 G
Energy	390 kJ	Sodium	120 mg
Protein	18 g	Calcium	51 mg
Fat	2 g	Phosphorus	180 mg
Carbohydrate	0	Magnesium	20 mg
Cholesterol	60 mg	Thiamin	0.3 mg

NUTRITIONAL INFORMATION Very little analysis is available on the nutrients contained in some of the fish found in Australian waters, but the figures above are supplied as a general guide to this variety.

DESCRIPTION The tarwhine, *Rhabdosargus sarba*, is a small to medium-sized silver fish. The flesh is white, fine-flaked, sweet, and can be bony. Tarwhine is similar to yellowfin bream but can be distinguished by the shape of the head and by the presence of narrow golden stripes along the back and sides. Tarwhine is smaller than the average black bream.

ORIGIN AND HISTORY Found mainly in Australian coastal waters, from southern Queensland to Victoria.

BUYING AND STORAGE It is always sold whole. To store: scale, gill, clean (gut) and trim fins from whole fish.

Season: all year.

PREPARATION AND USE Depending upon the size of the fish it is acceptable to serve a plate-size per person. Suits all methods of cooking. Scale, gut, clean, trim fins and score whole fish before cooking.

SEE ALSO Porgy.

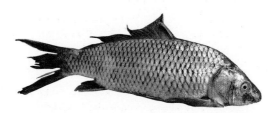

Carp Cyprinus carpio

also called **Black carp, Crucian carp, Grass carp, Silver carp**

MAJOR NUTRIENTS		SERVE SIZE 100 G	
Energy	480 kJ	Sodium	50 mg
Protein	18 g	Calcium	50 mg
Fat	4 g	Phosphorus	255 mg
Carbohydrate	0	Iron	0.9 mg
Cholesterol	70 mg	Niacin Equiv.	1.5 mg

NUTRITIONAL INFORMATION Fat content can vary from moderate to high.

DESCRIPTION Freshwater fish enjoyed in Asia, particularly China and Japan, as both an ornamental and table fish. There are several main types used in cooking.

Rock carp have small heads, thick rounded bodies and many small bones; they are considered the most delicious.

Grass carp have rounder, longer bodies similar to mullet.

Crucian carp are similar to bream and are silver-coloured. The very large *black* and *silver carp* are meaty and can weigh up to 70 kg.

European carp, shown above, also occurs in Australian waters.

ORIGIN AND HISTORY Native to China, and brought from there to Japan, and to most European countries, where they inhabit slow-moving rivers. Carp arrived in England in the reign of Henry VIII and in Australia in 1876. Chinese consider the carp a special food, not only for its delicate texture and flavour, but also its shiny golden scales, which are equated — like all things golden in colour — with wealth and prosperity. The carp family (Cyprinidae) embraces other freshwater fish: tench, bream, roach, dace and the ornamental goldfish. They have a habit of burrowing into mud on the bottom of a river, which can give

the meat a muddy taste, and which is one of the reasons — the other being an excess of bones — why carp are not eaten in many countries. They can live to a great age and grow to enormous size. Carp for the table are mostly bred in special ponds or tanks.

BUYING AND STORAGE Buy fresh carp in preference to frozen.

PREPARATION AND USE Muddiness can be eliminated by soaking well-washed carp in a mild vinegar-water solution for 2–3 hours. Score whole fish before cooking. Because carp have a dry flesh it is best to use moist methods of cooking. Braise, steam or poach in flavoured stock. In central China, various types of carp are cooked with strong sauces containing chilli, garlic and preserved black soya beans.

VARIETIES

Rock carp, grass carp, crucian carp and European carp.

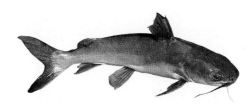

Catfish Families Atiidae, Ictaluridae, Siluridae

MAJOR NUTRIENTS		SERVE SIZE 100 G	
Energy	430 kJ	Sodium	60 mg
Protein	17 g	Phosphorus	330 mg
Fat	3 g	Iron	0.4 mg
Carbohydrate	0	Niacin Equiv.	1.5 mg
Cholesterol	60 mg		

NUTRITIONAL INFORMATION Fat content can vary from low fat to high fat (0.5%–11%).

DESCRIPTION The majority of catfish are scaleless; however, some have heavy scales. They vary in size from tiny specimens to ones weighing many kg. The flesh is white with a very good flavour.

ORIGIN AND HISTORY The name catfish derives from the arrangement of long whiskers about the mouth. Catfish constitute a large group of mainly freshwater fishes distributed around the world. South America is especially rich in quantity and species of catfish. Most prefer sluggish conditions of lakes and rivers. They are important commercially and are considered a fine sport fish.

BUYING AND STORAGE Available whole and in fillet form. Sometimes available in cutlets and steaks if catfish are large.

Season: all year.

PREPARATION AND USE If cooking catfish whole, scoring is essential. Suits most methods of cooking and most flavourings.

PROCESSING Can be smoked.

VARIETIES

Bullhead, including brown, black and yellow varieties; Eurasian catfish (family Siluridae) of which a well-known type is the blue catfish, with forked tail, which can weigh up to 45 kg; the North American freshwater catfish belonging to the family Ictaluridae; and sea catfish, Atiidae.

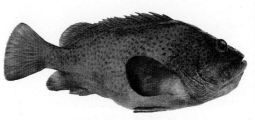

Cod Family Gadidae

also called **Codfish**

MAJOR NUTRIENTS		SERVE SIZE 100 G	
Energy	320 kJ	Sodium	75 mg
Protein	17 g	Phosphorus	170 mg
Fat	1 g	Magnesium	25 mg
Carbohydrate	0	Thiamin	0.05 mg
Cholesterol	40 mg	Niacin Equiv.	1.5 mg

NUTRITIONAL INFORMATION See the introduction to this section for general comments.

DESCRIPTION Members of the cod family are medium to large in size. Therefore their flesh has medium to large flakes. The flesh is white and moist with a mild to distinct flavour.

ORIGIN AND HISTORY Members of the cod family live in the cold waters of both the Atlantic and Pacific Oceans. History relates that English ships travelled to Iceland early in the 15th century to obtain codfish. Later that century, codfish was discovered in abundance as explorers combed North American waters, and for about 300 years thereafter it remained an important trade commodity. Drying and salting were the first processing methods used and, within a few years of pioneer settlers going to the New England area of America, a profitable export business to Europe had been established. Cod is still very valuable commercially, and today most is frozen.

It must be noted that in Australia the names perch and cod are used with little discrimination: most so-called cod in Australia are, in fact, members of the perch family.

BUYING AND STORAGE Most cod is available in fillet, steak and cutlet form. However some smaller cod are sold whole.

Season: all year.

PREPARATION AND USE If using small whole fish or thick fillets, scoring is essential. Cod is a very versatile fish: its thick moist flesh suits all methods of cooking, and its distinctive flavour combines well with most flavourings.

PROCESSING Frozen, salted and dried. A variety known as stockfish is dried and widely sold in the northern hemisphere.

VARIETIES
The many varieties of cod are too numerous to list.

SEE ALSO Cod, Smoked.

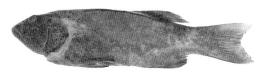

Coral Trout *Plectropoma maculatum*

also called Coral cod, Leopard cod

MAJOR NUTRIENTS		SERVE SIZE 100 G	
Energy	390 kJ	Sodium	120 mg
Protein	18 g	Calcium	51 mg
Fat	2 g	Phosphorus	180 mg
Carbohydrate	0	Magnesium	20 mg
Cholesterol	60 mg	Thiamin	0.3 mg

NUTRITIONAL INFORMATION Very little analysis is available on the nutrients contained in some of the fish found in Australian waters, but the figures above are supplied as a general guide to this variety.

DESCRIPTION Medium-sized fish — average weight 1.8–4.5 kg. The skin is pink to reddish-brown with small blue spots over the head and body. Moist, white, firm, sweet flesh makes this an excellent eating fish.

ORIGIN AND HISTORY These fish are generally found around coral reefs off Queensland, the Northern Territory and Western Australia.

BUYING AND STORAGE Mainly available whole. Look for bright and bulging eyes, firm but resilient flesh and a pleasant sea smell. One of the few fish that can be frozen whole and successfully filleted upon thawing.

Season: all year, most common in winter.

PREPARATION AND USE Coral trout can be cooked whole or in fillet form. It is a sweet delicate fish, and therefore strong flavourings should be avoided. It deserves simple cooking: shallow frying, grilling or poaching. Accompany with a mild cream sauce or light

mayonnaise. Whole fish may be poached and served chilled.

PROCESSING Whole fish and fillets can be frozen commercially.

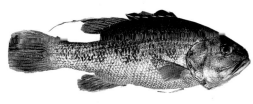

Dhu-fish, Western Australia *Glaucosoma hebraicum*

MAJOR NUTRIENTS		SERVE SIZE 100 G	
Energy	390 kJ	Sodium	120 mg
Protein	18 g	Calcium	51 mg
Fat	2 g	Phosphorus	180 mg
Carbohydrate	0	Magnesium	20 mg
Cholesterol	60 mg	Thiamin	0.3 mg

NUTRITIONAL INFORMATION Very little analysis is available on the nutrients contained in some of the fish found in Australian waters, but the figures above are supplied as a general guide to this variety.

DESCRIPTION These fish are silver-blue with a large mouth and an enormous blue eye. There is a pearly lustre from a prominent bone above the pectoral fin. The flesh is white, moist, sweet and medium-flaked and is considered one of the finest eating fish in Australia. The name seems to be an alternative spelling of 'Jewfish'. This species is not, however, related to the other fish known by that name, listed in this chapter.

ORIGIN AND HISTORY This fish is caught around offshore reefs on the western side of the continent and is almost identical to the silver perch, caught on the east coast. Their colouring is similar, but the dhu-fish has browner marble tonings.

BUYING AND STORAGE Nearly always sold whole.

Season: mainly autumn–winter.

PREPARATION AND USE Scale, gill and gut whole fish. Trim fins. Score whole fish to allow even heat penetration. Because of the delicate flavour of the fish use mild flavourings and cook gently. Pan fry, grill lightly or poach.

SEE ALSO Perch.

Dory *Zeus faber, Zenopsis ocellata, Zenopsis nebulosus, Cyttus australis*

MAJOR NUTRIENTS		SERVE SIZE 100 G	
Energy	350 kJ	Calcium	40 mg
Protein	18 g	Phosphorus	180 mg
Fat	1 g	Magnesium	20 mg
Carbohydrate	0	Iron	1 mg
Cholesterol	70 mg		

NUTRITIONAL INFORMATION No data are available on vitamin content.

DESCRIPTION Dory is a deep-bodied, silver-smooth fish with a large mouth and a turned-up snout. The ventral fins are very long. The flesh is fine, white, moist and tender. An excellent table fish, John Dory is the best of the species, known for the black spot on its side which distinguishes it from the silver and mirror dory.

ORIGIN AND HISTORY The dories live in the middle depths of the sea. They are caught in the Atlantic off the coast of North America, from the British Isles southward to Africa, and in the Mediterranean and the Pacific Ocean, particularly around southern Australia. John Dory is known as St Peter Fish, a name given to it on account of the dark blotches on the sides, which are supposed to represent the imprint of St Peter's thumb, made as he took a piece of money from the fish's mouth. The fish was caught in the Sea of Galilee but, contrary to the legend, the John Dory does not occur there.

BUYING AND STORAGE Available whole or in fillets. Whole fish: eyes should be bright and bulging, flesh firm and resilient with a pleasant sea smell. Fillets: look for pinkish-white, firm flesh and a pleasant sea smell. There should be no discoloration.

Season: all year.

PREPARATION AND USE Scale, gill and gut whole fish. Fillet if desired. With the John Dory all bones are removable when filleting correctly. Small fish yield better quality flesh. Use gentle methods of cooking and delicate flavourings.

PROCESSING Some dory are filleted and frozen commercially.

VARIETIES

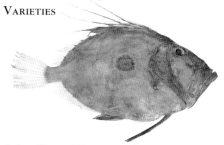

John Dory (European) Zeus faber.

John Dory (American) Zenopsis ocellata.

Mirror Dory Zenopsis nebulosus.

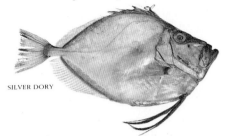

SILVER DORY

Silver Dory Cyttus australis.

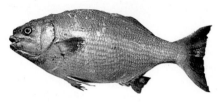

Drummer *Kyphosus sydneyanus*

also called *Silver drummer*

MAJOR NUTRIENTS   SERVE SIZE 100 G

Energy	390 kJ	Sodium	120 mg
Protein	18 g	Calcium	51 mg
Fat	2 g	Phosphorus	180 mg
Carbohydrate	0	Magnesium	20 mg
Cholesterol	60 mg	Thiamin	0.3 mg

NUTRITIONAL INFORMATION Very little analysis is available on the nutrients contained in some of the fish found in Australian waters, but the figures above are supplied as a general guide to this variety.

DESCRIPTION A deep-bodied, medium-sized fish. Colourings vary from silver to brown with markings. The flesh is good eating if fish are bled as soon as they are caught. The flesh is white, moist, soft and with a distinct flavour.

ORIGIN AND HISTORY Drummer is an estuarine fish whose family members (including the blackfish) are found worldwide. In Australia the greatest numbers are found in southern Queensland, New South Wales and Victoria. The drummer lives in shallow flats with abundant weeds. Although mainly vegetarian, it is not averse to some meat. It is one of the most game fighters in Australian waters and has an enthusiastic following of anglers.

BUYING AND STORAGE Available whole or as fillets.

Season: all year.

PREPARATION AND USE These fish should be bled as soon as possible after being caught. They may be cooked whole, but are best in fillet form. Fillets should be skinned. All methods of cooking and strong flavourings

are suited to the distinctive flavour of this fish.

SEE ALSO Blackfish.

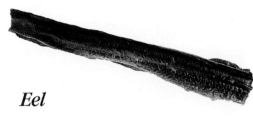

Eel

MAJOR NUTRIENTS   SERVE SIZE 100 G

Energy	700 kJ	Magnesium	20 mg
Protein	17 g	Iron	0.7 mg
Fat	13 g	Thiamin	0.15 mg
Carbohydrate	11 g	Riboflavin	0.35 mg
Cholesterol	140 mg	Niacin Equiv.	3 mg
Sodium	85 mg	Vitamin A	1900 μg
Phosphorus	230 mg		

NUTRITIONAL INFORMATION Limited data are available: the high fat content is variable, tending to increase together with the vitamin A level as the fish matures.

DESCRIPTION Eels have slim snakelike bodies that lack pelvic fins. In most species, the dorsal, caudal and anal fins are joined to form one continuous fin over the rear of the body. The pinky-white flesh is rich and fatty. Most species make good eating.

ORIGIN AND HISTORY Much has been written about eels over the centuries. Aristotle stated that there were neither males nor females and the eels did not seem to possess reproductive organs! In Ancient Greece eels were esteemed as a delicacy. To the Ancient Romans, however, they had no such appeal. Indeed, they were referred to as the 'cousin' of the snake. The customary method of correcting children in Rome was to use straps made of eel skins. Perhaps that is why the Romans did not fancy them on their dinner plates.

Known as tuna by New Zealand Maoris, eel is a traditional food caught by a variety of ingenious methods, one of which was to establish permanent weirs on rivers where eels are plentiful. Eel is still appreciated in New Zealand today.

BUYING AND STORAGE Sold whole or in cutlets, smoked or fresh. Fresh eel should be skinned and cut into cutlets, then wrapped in plastic or placed in an airtight container, and stored in the fridge for up to 2 days.

Season: all year.

PREPARATION AND USE Remove the skin before cooking. The skin is extremely tough. To remove, make an encircling cut behind the gills and use pliers to loosen skin from the

flesh, working downwards towards tail with a sharp knife. Discard head and skin and cut body into desired lengths. Or cut eel into cutlets and boil in stock or water for a minute or two. This softens the skin which is then easily removed. Eel may be marinated before cooking.

PROCESSING Smoked, dried.

VARIETIES There are both freshwater (family Anguillidae) and saltwater varieties of eel. Freshwater: American eel, European eel, Japanese eel, Australian eel. Saltwater: Moray eel, conger eel, snake eel, swallower eel, gulper eel.

SEE ALSO Eel, Smoked.

Emperor *Lutjanus sebae,* *Lethrinus chrysostomus, L. nebulosus*

MAJOR NUTRIENTS   SERVE SIZE 100 G

Energy	390 kJ	Sodium	120 mg
Protein	18 g	Calcium	51 mg
Fat	2 g	Phosphorus	180 mg
Carbohydrate	0	Magnesium	20 mg
Cholesterol	60 mg	Thiamin	0.3 mg

NUTRITIONAL INFORMATION Very little analysis is available on the nutrients contained in some of the fish found in Australian waters, but the figures above are supplied as a general guide to this variety.

DESCRIPTION Emperors are medium-sized fish. The red emperor is a spectacular fish: its body is salmon-pink and its fins are narrowly edged with white. The sweetlip emperor is olive-green above and silver below. The spangled emperor is also olive-green with blue streaks along the flanks. The flesh of emperors is white, moist and sweet: excellent eating.

ORIGIN AND HISTORY Found in Australian tropical waters, emperors are bottom dwelling, inhabiting reefs, rocky outcrops and gravel beds in deep and shallow waters. They are abundant along the Great Barrier Reef on the east coast of Australia. The red emperor is a good sporting fish — actually a sea perch, it has been known as the red emperor for decades, and the red emperor it remains.

BUYING AND STORAGE Emperor is sold whole and in fillets.

Season: all year.

PREPARATION AND USE If using whole fish or very thick fillets, score. Emperor is characterised by a moist flesh that lends itself to most methods of cooking. Suits most flavourings, although be careful about strong herbs and spices. Especially suits cream sauces, tropical fruit, coconut. Can be served hot or cold.

VARIETIES

Red emperor (*Lutjanus sebae*), sweetlip emperor (*Lethrinus chrysostomus*), spangled emperor (*L. nebulosus*).

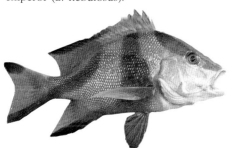

Red Emperor

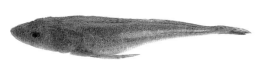

Flathead Family Platycephalidae

MAJOR NUTRIENTS		SERVE SIZE 100 G	
Energy	390 kJ	Sodium	120 mg
Protein	18 g	Calcium	51 mg
Fat	2 g	Phosphorus	180 mg
Carbohydrate	0	Magnesium	20 mg
Cholesterol	60 mg	Thiamin	0.3 mg

NUTRITIONAL INFORMATION The figures above are supplied as a general guide to this variety.

DESCRIPTION The flathead is a bottom-dwelling fish, recognised by its extremely depressed or flattened head and slender body. Its eyes are set on top of the head. The flesh is white with a fine to medium flake. It can be dry, but is generally a very good table fish.

ORIGIN AND HISTORY The family of flatheads is most widely represented in Australian waters: around the coast of Australia there are over 30 species, several of which are of commercial importance. None of these species are found in European or American waters, but this family has its greatest concentration from Australia through the East Indies to India and Japan.

BUYING AND STORAGE Sold whole and in fillets. Check that flesh is firm and that there are no brown markings or open flesh on stomach.

Season: all year, mainly autumn.

PREPARATION AND USE Scale, gill and gut, but keep the skin on as it is very fine. Some people even keep the scales on as they can actually 'cook'. Whole fish: trim all fins including the back fin. The 'wing' part of the fillet can also be trimmed. The whole fish may be stuffed and baked or poached, casseroled, or dipped in a thin batter, deep fried and served with a sauce.

VARIETIES

The main ones are sand flathead, dusky flathead, bartailed flathead, marbled flathead, rock flathead, tiger flathead.

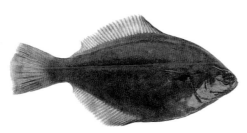

Flounder Family Pleuronectidae

MAJOR NUTRIENTS		SERVE SIZE 100 G	
Energy	280 kJ	Calcium	61 mg
Protein	15 g	Phosphorus	195 mg
Fat	1 g	Magnesium	30 mg
Carbohydrate	0	Iron	0.8 mg
Cholesterol	50 mg	Thiamin	0.05 mg
Sodium	55 mg	Niacin Equiv.	1.5 mg

NUTRITIONAL INFORMATION As for fish in general.

DESCRIPTION Flounder are flat fish with small scales and a white stomach. They have a fine bone structure and white soft flesh with a fine flake and mild taste.

ORIGIN AND HISTORY Although a flat fish, the flounder does not start life as such. The newly hatched fish are as symmetrical as any other fish, with one eye on each side of the head. When they are little more than a centimetre long, one eye begins to move towards the top of the head and then crosses the other side to lie adjacent to the other eye. Flounder (and also sole) always swim on their sides.

BUYING AND STORAGE If fish is small allow one whole fish per person. Allow 2 to 3 fillets per person.

Season: all year.

PREPARATION AND USE Scale, gill and gut. Fillet, if fish is too large. Grill, bake, poach, or pan fry gently.

PROCESSING Filleted and frozen.

VARIETIES

Flounder is often used as a generic term applying to hundreds of different kinds of flat fishes around the world. Major species of flounder are winter flounder, summer flounder, large-toothed flounder, small-toothed flounder, long-snouted flounder, greenback flounder. Plaice is a member of the flounder family.

SEE ALSO Sole.

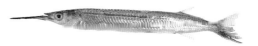

Garfish

also called Needlefish

MAJOR NUTRIENTS		SERVE SIZE 100 G	
Energy	390 kJ	Sodium	120 mg
Protein	18 g	Calcium	51 mg
Fat	2 g	Phosphorus	180 mg
Carbohydrate	0	Magnesium	20 mg
Cholesterol	60 mg	Thiamin	0.3 mg

NUTRITIONAL INFORMATION Very little analysis is available on the nutrients contained in some of the fish found in Australian waters, but the figures above are supplied as a general guide to this variety.

DESCRIPTION The garfish has a prolongation of the lower jaw into a 'beak' which is usually tipped with bright orange or scarlet. The body is bluish-green to silver in colour, depending upon the species. The meat is white, fine and sweet. Very good eating, but bony.

ORIGIN AND HISTORY These fish are found in most warm seas and are herbivorous, feeding upon minute scraps of vegetable matter, seaweeds etc. Swimming in big shoals at the surface, they are usually captured by net fishermen. They may leap from the water or skip along the surface at a great pace, especially when surrounded by nets.

BUYING AND STORAGE Sold whole but occasionally available in fillet form. Body should be firm and not 'sagging' and should have a pleasant sea smell. Best to clean (gut) and scale the garfish; the head may be removed. This fish keeps extremely well and may be refrigerated for up to 4 days.

Season: all year (southern hemisphere); all year, except July to August (northern hemisphere).

PREPARATION AND USE Remove scales before cooking. To butterfly: cut off head, run a sharp knife down either side of rib cage and break the backbone at the base of the tail, using a rolling pin or milk bottle. Lift the base of the backbone with your fingers and remove by pulling it towards the head. Use the blunt side of the knife to free the flesh as you pull the bone.

PROCESSING Occasionally deboned or filleted.

Varieties

There are more than fifty species. The main ones are eastern garfish, also known as sea garfish (*Hyporhampus australis*); northern garfish, also known as snub-nose garfish (*Arrhampus sclerolepis*); river garfish (*Hymorhampus ardelio*); long-beaked or long-finned garfish (*Euleptorhampus viridis*).

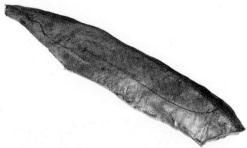

Gemfish *Rexea solandri*

Major Nutrients		Serve Size 100 g	
Energy	390 kJ	Sodium	120 mg
Protein	18 g	Calcium	51 mg
Fat	2 g	Phosphorus	180 mg
Carbohydrate	0	Magnesium	20 mg
Cholesterol	60 mg	Thiamin	0.3 mg

Nutritional Information Very little analysis is available on the nutrients contained in some of the fish found in Australian waters, but the figures above are supplied as a general guide to this variety.

Description A long, silver fish with minute scales. The flesh is large-flaked, white, with a mild flavour.

Origin and History Gemfish is a deep-sea fish and the most important species in the trawling industry of the waters of south-eastern Australia. Originally gemfish were known as hake. However, because of the confusion with the true hake which is imported into Australia, the name gemfish (derived from the family name Gempylidae, which includes the barracouta) was adopted.

Buying and Storage Because of its size and unattractive appearance, gemfish is sold in fillet or cutlet form. It is also available either hot- or cold-smoked.

Season: winter (southern hemisphere).

Preparation and Use Very thick fillets can be scored by a sharp knife to allow even heat penetration. The skin may be left on or removed. The middle bone may be removed from cutlets and filling placed in the cavity.

Processing Filleted and frozen, smoked.

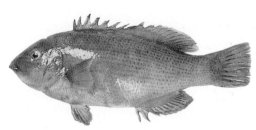

Groper *Achoerodus viridus*

also called **Grouper**

Major Nutrients		Serve Size 100 g	
Energy	360 kJ	Sodium	60 mg
Protein	19 g	Phosphorus	195 mg
Fat	1 g	Magnesium	25 mg
Carbohydrate	0	Iron	0.8 mg
Cholesterol	50 mg	Niacin Equiv.	3 mg

Nutritional Information No data are available on other vitamins and minerals.

Description Gropers vary in size. Generally medium to large. They are good eating with firm white flesh that can be fatty, and a medium to large flake.

Origin and History These fish are members of the sea bass family and are widely distributed in the Atlantic and Pacific waters. Some gropers have the ability to change their colour: the Nassau groper is capable of eight different colourings. Their habitat is rocky caves and crevices.

Buying and Storage Mostly available in fillets, cutlets or steaks. Sometimes available whole.

Season: all year.

Preparation and Use Groper fillets, cutlets and steaks tend to be thick — therefore score before cooking. Use dry methods of cooking due to the fat content. Also use in soups and casserole cooking.

Varieties

Red groper (*Epinephelus morio*), black groper (*Mycteroperca bonaci*), Nassau groper (*E. striatus*), Warsaw groper (*E. nigritus*).

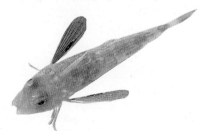

Gurnard Family **Triglidae**

Major Nutrients		Serve Size 100 g	
Energy	390 kJ	Sodium	120 mg
Protein	18 g	Calcium	51 mg
Fat	2 g	Phosphorus	180 mg
Carbohydrate	0	Magnesium	20 mg
Cholesterol	60 mg	Thiamin	0.3 mg

Nutritional Information Very little analysis is available on the nutrients contained in some of the fish found in Australian waters, but the figures above are supplied as a general guide to this variety.

Description Gurnards have a bony head structure with beautiful pectoral fins that open out like a fan. The flesh is dry and firm with a fine flake. The fillet resembles the flathead fillet in shape.

Origin and History The gurnard takes its name from the French words for growling (*gronder*) and for grunting (*grogner*). The gurnard has the ability to emit short, sharp noises, made by a vibrating muscle in the air bladder wall which acts as a resonating chamber.

Buying and Storage Sold whole and in fillet form.

Season: all year (southern hemisphere); all year except July, August, September (northern hemisphere).

Preparation and Use Gurnard should be filleted, with or without skin. The dry flesh requires moist methods of cooking: poach, pan fry or deep fry.

Varieties

Grey gurnard, yellow gurnard, red gurnard, sharp-beaked gurnard (also known as latchet), spotted gurnard.

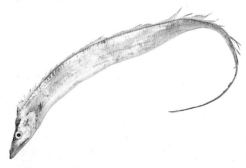

Hairtail *Trichiurus coxii*

also called **Ribbon-fish**

Description A brilliant silver fish with no scales, a tapered body and long, hairlike tail. It has ferocious jaws. Flesh is soft and white, with delicate flavour. Fair eating.

Origin and History This fish is coastal and may enter estuaries in winter. It is usually caught by anglers, and is plentiful off the coast of Queensland. It is not often marketed.

Buying and Storage Available in cutlet form.

Season: autumn–winter (southern hemisphere).

Preparation and Use If in whole form, cut off head, gut and cut crosswise into cutlets of desired thickness. Suits shallow frying, grilling and casseroling. Because of the mild taste use only mild flavourings.

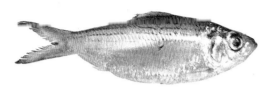

Herring *Elops australis, Harengula konigsbergeri*

MAJOR NUTRIENTS		SERVE SIZE 100 G	
Energy	970 kJ	Phosphorus	210 mg
Protein	17 g	Magnesium	30 mg
Fat	18 g	Iron	0.8 mg
Carbohydrate	0	Riboflavin	0.2 mg
Cholesterol	70 mg	Niacin Equiv.	4 mg
Sodium	65 mg	Vitamin A	45 µg

NUTRITIONAL INFORMATION The high fat content is variable.

DESCRIPTION In Australasian waters are the giant herring, which is not good eating, and the spotted herring (*Harengula konigsbergeri*), pictured above Flesh is soft with a fine flake and a strong taste.

ORIGIN AND HISTORY The Atlantic herring is a most abundant pelagic fish in the cool waters of the North Atlantic. The Pacific herring occurs throughout the north Pacific southward to San Diego, along the north American coast and also off the coasts of Japan and Northern Asia. Australasian varieties are mentioned above.

BUYING AND STORAGE Sold whole. Be careful not to buy herrings with broken stomachs — this is a sign they are deteriorating.

Season: April to November (northern hemisphere); all year (southern hemisphere).

PREPARATION AND USE The flesh is soft so gentle cooking is advised. Scale, clean and wash stomach cavity well. The cavity can be filled with a stuffing and either fried, baked, grilled or barbecued. Because of the oil content dry methods of cooking are ideal.

PROCESSING Smoked, canned, pickled, salted, cured and frozen.

VARIETIES

Atlantic herring (*C. harengus harengus*), Pacific herring (*C. harengus pallasi*), Giant herring (*Elops australis*), Spotted herring (*Harengula konigsbergeri*).

Soft Herring Roe

MAJOR NUTRIENTS		SERVE SIZE 100 G	
Energy	340 kJ	Sodium	90 mg
Protein	13 g	Thiamin	0.2 mg
Fat	3 g	Riboflavin	0.5 mg
Carbohydrate	0	Niacin Equiv.	2 mg
Cholesterol	700 mg	Vitamin C	5 mg

NUTRITIONAL INFORMATION Roe is a rich source of dietary cholesterol and should be avoided on cholesterol lowering diets. As it contains all the nutrition required for growth in the young fish, it is an excellent source of protein and vitamin B including thiamin, niacin and vitamin B12. Unlike fish it is an excellent source of riboflavin and vitamin C. Although no data are available for other vitamins and minerals, it does also contain vitamins D and E.

DESCRIPTION Soft roe is the milt or sperm of the male fish. It has a creamy texture and is very rich in flavour. When cooked it becomes firmer.

ORIGIN AND HISTORY Herring roe (soft) is available mostly in the northern hemisphere.

BUYING AND STORAGE Available fresh from fish retailers. Store in plastic wrap or airtight container in refrigerator for 2–3 days.

PREPARATION AND USE The flesh should be washed in cold water and stripped of any blood vessels. Can be cooked and added to omelettes, sauces, or used as a soft roe paste. Pairs can be gently cooked in butter and served with bread and butter with plenty of lemon squeezed over them.

PROCESSING Soft herring roe paste.

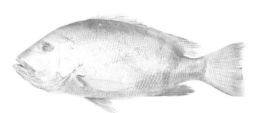

Hussar *Lutjanus amabilis*

MAJOR NUTRIENTS		SERVE SIZE 100 G	
Energy	390 kJ	Sodium	120 mg
Protein	18 g	Calcium	51 mg
Fat	2 g	Phosphorus	180 mg
Carbohydrate	0	Magnesium	20 mg
Cholesterol	60 mg	Thiamin	0.3 mg

NUTRITIONAL INFORMATION Very little analysis is available on the nutrients contained in some of the fish found in Australian waters, but the figures above are supplied as a general guide to this variety.

DESCRIPTION A small pink fish no more than 46 cm long. A fair table fish. Good bait for the red emperor.

ORIGIN AND HISTORY Found in tropical waters in reef localities. In Australia it is found in southern Queensland, but is rarely seen north of Townsville.

BUYING AND STORAGE Available whole and sometimes filleted.

Season: all year.

PREPARATION AND USE Whole hussar should be scored. Fillets can be bony. Suits all methods of cooking.

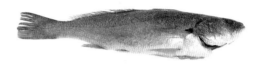

Jewfish *Argyrosomus hololepidotus*

also called **Butterfish, Jewie, Mulloway, Silver Jew**

MAJOR NUTRIENTS		SERVE SIZE 100 G	
Energy	390 kJ	Sodium	120 mg
Protein	18 g	Calcium	51 mg
Fat	2 g	Phosphorus	180 mg
Carbohydrate	0	Magnesium	20 mg
Cholesterol	60 mg	Thiamin	0.3 mg

NUTRITIONAL INFORMATION The figures above are supplied as a general guide to this variety. Limited data indicate that jewfish has a moderate fat content.

DESCRIPTION A medium to large silver fish with a convex tail. The flesh is pale pink with a large flake and firm texture. Mild flavoured, it can sometimes be a little dry. An excellent table fish.

ORIGIN AND HISTORY Jewfish is found mainly in Australian waters. The name jewfish is apparently a corruption of 'dewfish' — which was given on account of the beautiful silvery-grey colour. Found in locations varying from deep offshore reefs to coastal beaches and mouths of estuaries.

BUYING AND STORAGE Sold whole and in cutlet form.

Season: all year, mainly late spring–summer.

PREPARATION AND USE Score whole fish unless wrapping in foil for baking. Bone may be removed from cutlet if desired. As jewfish can be a little dry, moist methods of cooking are recommended.

VARIETIES

The spotted jewfish (*Epinephelus itajara*) is much larger than most commercial jewfish. It is found in the Caribbean and northward to the coast of Florida and also in the Pacific from Panama to the Gulf of Carpentaria.

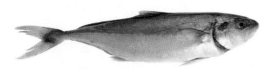

Kingfish *Seriola lalandi*

MAJOR NUTRIENTS		SERVE SIZE 100 G	
Energy	440 kJ	Carbohydrate	0
Protein	18 g	Cholesterol	70 mg
Fat	3 g	Sodium	80 mg

NUTRITIONAL INFORMATION No data are available on mineral and vitamin content. Fat content can vary from low fat to high fat.

DESCRIPTION The kingfish is purple-blue above the lateral line to the snout, with a green lateral band separating the silver undersides and a yellow tail. Varies in size, but fairly large, average 2–8 kg. The flesh is pink, soft and dry with a mild taste and makes very good eating.

ORIGIN AND HISTORY Members of the kingfish family are found worldwide. They are popular gamefish because of their fighting capabilities and eating qualities. They are both oceanic and estuarine fish.

BUYING AND STORAGE Sold whole and in cutlet form. Occasionally small kingfish fillets are available. Look for firm pink flesh but remember that kingfish flesh is soft.

Season: all year, mainly autumn.

PREPARATION AND USE Cut whole fish into cutlets or use whole if small. Use moist methods of cooking as kingfish can dry out. It is a very popular fish eaten raw (sashimi etc.). Most flavourings go well with kingfish.

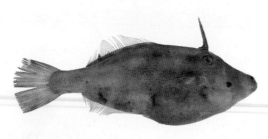

Leatherjacket Family Monacanthidae

also called File fish

MAJOR NUTRIENTS		SERVE SIZE 100 G	
Energy	390 kJ	Sodium	120 mg
Protein	18 g	Calcium	51 mg
Fat	2 g	Phosphorus	180 mg
Carbohydrate	0	Magnesium	20 mg
Cholesterol	60 mg	Thiamin	0.3 mg

NUTRITIONAL INFORMATION Very little analysis is available on the nutrients contained in some of the fish found in Australian waters, but the figures above are supplied as a general guide to this variety.

DESCRIPTION Small to medium-sized fish, with a strong and prominent dorsal spine, and spines covering the skin. Leatherjackets have a tough skin — hence the name. Usually they are drab in colour. The flesh is white, soft and has a very mild flavour, although leatherjackets found in tropical waters may have a bitter taste.

ORIGIN AND HISTORY These fish occur worldwide in both offshore and estuarine waters. Some species can grow to a length of 60 cm.

BUYING AND STORAGE Leatherjacket is always sold whole and headless. The tough leather skin is usually removed by the retailer.

Season: all year.

PREPARATION AND USE Skin should be removed and fins may be trimmed. Allow one to two fish per person, depending upon size. Leatherjacket can be a little dry, so use moist methods of cooking, or grill, basting with lemon juice, wine or melted butter. Suits mild flavourings.

VARIETIES There are about 50 species in Australian waters.

Ling *Gerypterus blacodes, G. tigerinus*

MAJOR NUTRIENTS		SERVE SIZE 100 G	
Energy	390 kJ	Sodium	120 mg
Protein	18 g	Calcium	51 mg
Fat	2 g	Phosphorus	180 mg
Carbohydrate	0	Magnesium	20 mg
Cholesterol	60 mg	Thiamin	0.3 mg

NUTRITIONAL INFORMATION Very little analysis is available on the nutrients contained in some of the fish found in Australian waters, but the figures above are supplied as a general guide to this variety.

DESCRIPTION Pink ling, as its name implies, is pink-orange in colour with irregular brown marks. It grows to about 1.5 metres in length and 20 kg in weight. Fillets are nearly boneless, flesh is white, firm, moist with a large flake. Excellent eating. Rock ling grows to about 1 metre and 9 kg in weight. Its flesh is soft and white. Also very good eating.

ORIGIN AND HISTORY The name ling comes from 'long'. Two species of ling, a member of the cod family, are found in Australian waters. They are not to be confused with lingcod (*Ophiodon elongatus*), which is found in North American and Alaskan waters. Lingcod is a member of the greenling family and not strictly a ling or a cod.

Pink ling is a deep-water fish whereas rock ling is a shallow-water species. Rock ling is less abundant than pink ling.

BUYING AND STORAGE Mostly sold in fillet form. Look for skinless white fillets with no brown markings and a very firm flesh.

Season: winter.

PREPARATION AND USE If fillets are very thick, score to allow even heat penetration. Always make sure the fillets are skinless. Because ling is so moist, it suits dry methods of cooking very well. A great fish for the dieter because it grills well, it may also be poached, pan fried, baked, steamed and barbecued.

VARIETIES Pink ling (*G. blacodes*), rock ling (*G. tigerinus*).

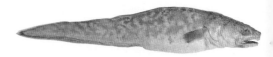

Rock Ling

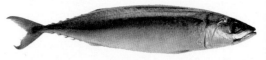

Mackerel Family Scombridae

MAJOR NUTRIENTS		SERVE SIZE 100 G	
Energy	930 kJ	Magnesium	30 mg
Protein	19 g	Iron	1 mg
Fat	16 g	Vitamin A	45 µg
Carbohydrate	0	Thiamin	0.1 mg
Cholesterol	80 mg	Riboflavin	0.35 mg
Sodium	130 mg	Niacin Equiv.	8 mg
Phosphorus	240 mg		

NUTRITIONAL INFORMATION The high fat and Vitamin D content vary.

DESCRIPTION Mackerel vary in size. They have a streamlined body with a pointed head and a tapered tail. The flesh texture and flavour varies depending upon species. However, most have a strong flavour. A good eating fish.

ORIGIN AND HISTORY Mackerel are schooling fish of the open sea. They are speedy fish which feed on herrings, sardines and other school fish. Many species are important commercially.

BUYING AND STORAGE Mainly sold in cutlets and steaks. Smaller mackerel sometimes sold whole.

Season: summer (southern hemisphere); December to July (northern hemisphere).

PREPARATION AND USE Mackerel vary — some are dry, while others are oily. Little preparation is required for fillets, cutlets or steaks. Just be aware that if the mackerel is dry it lends itself to moist methods of cooking. If the mackerel is oily it suits drier methods. Mackerel suits most flavourings.

PROCESSING Smoked.

VARIETIES

Spanish mackerel, chub mackerel, Atlantic mackerel, king mackerel, frigate mackerel, wahoo.

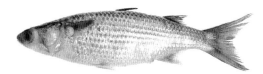

Mullet Family Mugilidae

MAJOR NUTRIENTS		SERVE SIZE 100 G	
Energy	610 kJ	Phosphorus	220 mg
Protein	20 g	Magnesium	30 mg
Fat	7 g	Iron	1.8 mg
Carbohydrate	0	Thiamin	0.1 mg
Cholesterol	50 mg	Niacin Equiv.	5 mg
Sodium	80 mg		

NUTRITIONAL INFORMATION The fat content can vary from low fat to high fat (0.5%–15%).

DESCRIPTION Mullet is blunt-nosed and small-mouthed, small to medium in size and silver to black in colour. The flesh is fatty with a distinctive flavour, but good eating.

ORIGIN AND HISTORY Mullet was one of the favourite foods of the Ancient Romans who were reputed to have paid high prices for it. The mullet family ranges throughout the world and is one of the most uniform fish families, with a great similarity between the many species of fish. All are valuable food fishes.

BUYING AND STORAGE Sold whole and in fillet form. Some species of mullet are prone to a condition known as earthiness, identified by picking a scale off the fish and smelling the flesh. If the flesh smells earthy then chances are the fish will taste earthy, but this should not be considered a bad sign. Mullet can become earthy swimming at the bottom of the river amongst the mud. Fillets of mullet are moist and pink with a medium flake.

Mullet should be stored according to usual guidelines for fish. Note, however, that oily species of mullet freeze only up to 3 months. Red mullet, one of the exceptions to this rule, can be frozen up to 6 months.

Season: mainly autumn, early winter (southern hemisphere); all year (northern hemisphere).

PREPARATION AND USE Use the fish whole, filleted or butterflied. Scale, gill and clean (gut). Most species of mullet have a rich oil content so should be baked, barbecued, shallow fried or grilled. Good smoked. When cooked and flaked, particularly good as a filling for crepes, pastry cases, and bread loaves. Mullet has a distinct flavour and so stronger herbs can be used.

VARIETIES

Striped mullet (also called black mullet), white mullet, fantail mullet, grey mullet, sea mullet, sand mullet, red mullet.

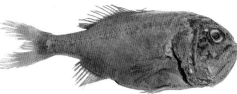

Orange Roughy Hoplostethus atlanticus

also called **Orange roughie, Sea perch**

MAJOR NUTRIENTS		SERVE SIZE 100 G	
Energy	390 kJ	Sodium	120 mg
Protein	18 g	Calcium	51 mg
Fat	2 g	Phosphorus	180 mg
Carbohydrate	0	Magnesium	20 mg
Cholesterol	60 mg	Thiamin	0.3 mg

NUTRITIONAL INFORMATION Very little analysis is available on the nutrients contained in some of the fish found in Australian waters, but the figures above are supplied as a general guide to this variety.

DESCRIPTION An orange thick-skinned fish. Medium-sized with a medium flake. White, moist flesh with a delicate flavour.

ORIGIN AND HISTORY This is a deep-sea fish, a member of the perch family, mainly caught in New Zealand and exported. It is also sold as sea perch. The fat underneath the skin can be rancid and must be removed by skinning the fillet. A popular fish that is important commercially.

BUYING AND STORAGE Always sold in fillet form.

Season: mainly in the winter (southern hemisphere).

PREPARATION AND USE Fillets *must* be skinned. They are a thin fillet so cook quickly. They suit most methods of cooking, but be careful when grilling as they can break easily. Suit delicate flavourings.

PROCESSING Filleted and frozen.

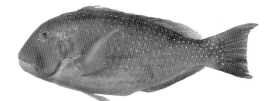

Parrot Fish Scarus rivulatus, S. sordidus, S. ghobban

MAJOR NUTRIENTS		SERVE SIZE 100 G	
Energy	390 kJ	Sodium	120 mg
Protein	18 g	Calcium	51 mg
Fat	2 g	Phosphorus	180 mg
Carbohydrate	0	Magnesium	20 mg
Cholesterol	60 mg	Thiamin	0.3 mg

NUTRITIONAL INFORMATION Very little analysis is available on the nutrients contained in some of the fish found in Australian waters, but the figures above are supplied as a general guide to this variety.

DESCRIPTION A brightly coloured, small to medium-sized fish. The flesh is white, moist, sweet and soft with excellent eating qualities.

ORIGIN AND HISTORY The parrot fish is related to the tusk fish, and is found in reef areas along the Queensland coastline. At night some parrot fish cover themselves in a protective mucus, enabling them to rest for the night.

BUYING AND STORAGE Nearly always sold in whole form. Look for a brightly coloured skin, with no hint of dullness.

Season: all year, mainly winter.

PREPARATION AND USE Scale, gill and gut. Fillet if desired, but because these fish are so beautiful, they are most attractive cooked whole. Score whole fish to allow even heat penetration. Use mild flavourings due to the delicate flavour of the fish. Suits most methods of cooking.

Surf parrot fish (*Scarus rivulatus*) shown above, green-finned parrot fish (*S. sordidus*) and blue-barred orange parrot fish (*S. ghobban*).

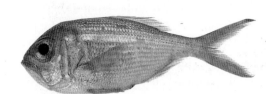

Ocean Perch

Perch Family Percidae

MAJOR NUTRIENTS		SERVE SIZE 100 G	
Energy	360 kJ	Phosphorus	190 mg
Protein	19 g	Iron	1 mg
Fat	1 g	Zinc	1 mg
Carbohydrate	0	Thiamin	0.2 mg
Cholesterol	40 mg	Niacin Equiv.	2 mg
Sodium	60 mg		

NUTRITIONAL INFORMATION For general information see introduction to this section.

DESCRIPTION Perch vary in colour and size. However, generally the flesh is white, moist and with a sweet delicate flavour.

ORIGIN AND HISTORY Mainly freshwater, although there are some saltwater species. Perch is found throughout the world. The Chinese have, for centuries, marinated perch fillets in wine and soy sauce before steaming and serving with herb-toasted rice. The French prepare medium-sized perch for frying and stuff and bake the larger-sized fish. Some species are cultivated throughout Europe, Asia and North America. Most are to be found in rivers, lakes and reservoirs. Australia is renowned for its beautiful Murray perch.

BUYING AND STORAGE Perch is sold whole or in fillets.

Season: June to December (northern hemisphere); autumn–winter (southern hemisphere).

PREPARATION AND USE Smaller perch may be cooked whole. Scale, clean and trim fins and score. Thick perch fillets should also be scored before cooking. Because of the mild flavour it is important that no strong herbs or spices be used; most fruits go well. All methods of cooking are suitable.

PROCESSING Some species are filleted and frozen and provide a good export commodity for some countries.

VARIETIES

Ocean perch, sea perch, silver perch, yellow perch, European perch, walleye perch, English redfin perch, golden perch, Macquarie perch, Murray perch, pearl perch (*Glaucosoma scapulare*, which is almost identical to the dhu-fish of Western Australia).

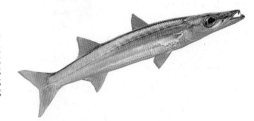

Pike Family Esocidae

MAJOR NUTRIENTS		SERVE SIZE 100 G	
Energy	370 kJ	Sodium	50 mg
Protein	19 g	Magnesium	175 mg
Fat	1 g	Iron	0.7 mg
Carbohydrate	0	Zinc	1.3 mg
Cholesterol	80 mg		

NUTRITIONAL INFORMATION No data are available on vitamin content.

DESCRIPTION The pike is a sharp-nosed fish. The meat is firm and white with a medium to large flake and can be dry. The size varies.

ORIGIN AND HISTORY Nearly all species are freshwater. However, some pike, found mainly in Australia, are saltwater. Pike is very popular in Europe and North America. Medieval records indicate that pike was used in aspics, puddings and other dishes.

BUYING AND STORAGE Pike is mainly sold whole.

Season: all year (southern hemisphere); August to February (northern hemisphere).

PREPARATION AND USE Scale and clean. Can be stuffed with breadcrumbs, rice, shellfish, fruits or vegetables. Suits poaching, grilling, frying, barbecuing or baking. Pike has soft flesh so gentle cooking is desirable.

VARIETIES

Blackspotted pike, blue pike, grass pike, great northern pike, jackpike, waterwolf, silver pike.

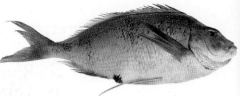

Porgy Family Sparidae

NUTRITIONAL INFORMATION No reliable figures are available.

DESCRIPTION The porgy is small to medium in size. The skin is tough, but the flesh is tender with a delicate flavour.

ORIGIN AND HISTORY As a group porgies have worldwide distribution. They live mainly in warm seas, although a few live in cooler waters. Most are prevalent around reefs, but some are found only over sandy bottoms. Most species can change their colouring from solid to blotched, and from dark to light, thus providing a camouflage. The porgy is a sea bream, with many varieties.

BUYING AND STORAGE Porgy is usually sold whole.

Season: all year.

PREPARATION AND USE When cooking whole, score first. Whole fish can be stuffed with either breadcrumbs, cooked rice, shellfish, fruit or vegetables. Bake, shallow fry, grill or barbecue.

VARIETIES

More than 100 species.

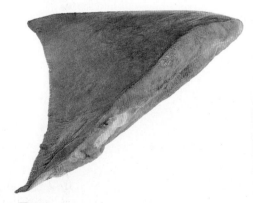

Ray Family Rayidae

also called Skate, Roker

MAJOR NUTRIENTS		SERVE SIZE 100 G	
Energy	410 kJ	Sodium	100 mg
Protein	21 g	Calcium	65 mg
Fat	1 g	Phosphorus	200 mg
Carbohydrate	0	Magnesium	30 mg
Cholesterol	70 mg	Iron	1.2 mg

NUTRITIONAL INFORMATION No data are available on vitamin content.

DESCRIPTION The dorsal and anal fins are small, and the pelvic fins are deeply notched so that they appear as four fins rather than two. The pectoral fins are large and winglike, joined at the front of the head. The tail is slender. The meat from the flaps is pink, sweet and moist.

ORIGIN AND HISTORY Rays are found worldwide. Most live in shallow water, but there are some deepwater species. Rays are bottom dwellers. They are brown or grey in colour and can be mottled. When resting they usually fan the sand or soft sediment over themselves as camouflage. By forming a suction with their body, they can cling to the bottom so tightly that they are difficult to dislodge.

BUYING AND STORAGE The flesh available in markets or shops is usually the flaps of a stingray, with skin on. Look for moist, pink flesh with a pleasant sea smell, often sold as 'flake'.

Season: August to April (northern hemisphere); all year (southern hemisphere).

PREPARATION AND USE Skin must be removed before using. Frying and poaching are optimum methods of cooking. Ray suits most flavourings.

VARIETIES

More than 100 species, including Banks's shovelnose skate, blue skate, stingray or stingaree.

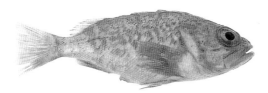

Redfish *Centroberyx affinis*

also called *Nannygai*

MAJOR NUTRIENTS		SERVE SIZE 100 G	
Energy	390 kJ	Sodium	120 mg
Protein	18 g	Calcium	51 mg
Fat	2 g	Phosphorus	180 mg
Carbohydrate	0	Magnesium	20 mg
Cholesterol	60 mg	Thiamin	0.3 mg

NUTRITIONAL INFORMATION Very little analysis is available on the nutrients contained in some of the fish found in Australian waters, but the figures above are supplied as a general guide to this variety.

DESCRIPTION A small red-orange fish with heavy scales. It has a fine to medium flake and a delicate flavour. Flesh is pale pink.

ORIGIN AND HISTORY Redfish are mainly distributed along the east coast of Australia from southern Queensland to Tasmania in depths of 10–400 metres.

BUYING AND STORAGE Available whole and in fillets.

Season: spring (southern hemisphere).

PREPARATION AND USE The scales are so tightly knit that it is best to fillet and skin. (Should be cooked in fillet form only.) Suits shallow or deep frying, and mincing. Because of the delicate taste of the fish use mild flavourings.

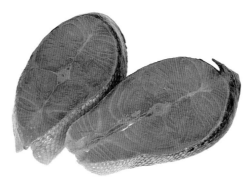

Salmon *Arripis trutta, Salmo salar,* genus *Onchorhynchus*

MAJOR NUTRIENTS		SERVE SIZE 100 G	
Energy	760 kJ	Magnesium	25 mg
Protein	18 g	Iron	0.7 mg
Fat	12 g	Zinc	0.8 mg
Carbohydrate	0	Thiamin	0.2 mg
Cholesterol	70 mg	Riboflavin	0.15 mg
Sodium	100 mg	Niacin Equiv.	7 mg
Phosphorus	280 mg		

NUTRITIONAL INFORMATION Fat content can vary from low fat to high fat.

DESCRIPTION In maturity, the salmon is a large, strong fish, varying in skin colour, markings and flesh colour according to the species. There are both Pacific and Atlantic salmon, both having firm flesh with a medium to large flake and a rich flavour. Salmon is an excellent, highly valued fish for the table.

The Atlantic salmon, *Salmo salar,* is also fished in New South Wales, Australia, and in New Zealand.

In the genus *Onchorhynchus,* the Pacific salmon, there are five species. One is the quinnat salmon, which is fished successfully in lakes in Victoria, Australia, and in rivers and streams in the USA and New Zealand. Another is red salmon: this is the Alaskan sockeye, also known as the Columbia river blueback. Australian salmon, *Arripis trutta,* is a highly popular sportfish with beach anglers in New South Wales and Victoria.

ORIGIN AND HISTORY This fine fish spends most of its life in the sea but returns to rivers to spawn. The tiny salmon are called fingerlings and, as they grow, are known as parr until they leave the river. Young salmon

at sea are known as smolt. Thereafter they live in the ocean until their return the next season to the river where they were spawned. Salmon have been recorded to have made the journey from one side of the Atlantic to the other during their time in the ocean.

They have been fished by anglers from time immemorial, and are taken by the fishing industries of many countries, in very great numbers. They are also raised on fish farms, which supply a growing proportion of the market.

BUYING AND STORAGE Available whole, or as cutlets, steaks and fillets.

Season: March to October (northern hemisphere); winter (southern hemisphere).

PREPARATION AND USE The optimum ways to cook salmon are to poach and bake. Can be served hot or cold. Use mild flavourings. Cream sauces go well.

PROCESSING Canned, smoked, frozen.

VARIETIES

Atlantic Salmon *Salmo salar.*

Australian Salmon *Arripis trutta,* called Kahawai in New Zealand.

Pacific Salmon Five species.

Silver Salmon

MAJOR NUTRIENTS		SERVE SIZE 100 G	
Energy	640 kJ	Calcium	175 mg
Protein	19 g	Phosphorus	230 mg
Fat	8 g	Potassium	420 mg
Carbohydrate	0	Magnesium	30 mg
Cholesterol	70 mg	Iron	0.5 mg
Sodium	50 mg	Thiamin	0.1 mg

NUTRITIONAL INFORMATION Fat content can vary from moderate fat to high fat.

DESCRIPTION The silver salmon is a Pacific salmon (*Onchorhynchus kisutch*) which is also known as coho. Most silver salmon weigh between 2.25 and 4.5 kg. The body is greenish on top and pink underneath, with black spots on the upper portion of the tail. Flesh has a mild flavour with a medium to large flake.

ORIGIN AND HISTORY Silver salmon are a favourite of sport fishermen in the USA and are found from California to Alaska. When caught they generally fight near the surface and make spectacular leaps into the air. Silver salmon has been introduced into the Great Lakes of North America and has become a successful replacement for lake trout.

BUYING AND STORAGE Available whole, and in cutlets, steaks and fillets.

Season: March to November (northern hemisphere).

PREPARATION AND USE The optimum ways to cook silver salmon are to poach and bake. Can be served hot or cold. Use mild flavourings. Cream sauces go well.

PROCESSING Canned, smoked, frozen.

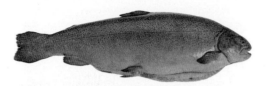

Salmon Trout   *Salmo trutta*

NUTRITIONAL INFORMATION No reliable figures are available.

DESCRIPTION Salmon trout is similar in shape to salmon, but narrower and smaller. It has a pale pink flesh, which is soft and has a delicate flavour.

ORIGIN AND HISTORY Salmon trout is found in the North Atlantic, Baltic and North Sea. It is often confused with salmon as it returns from the sea to spawn in coastal rivers.

BUYING AND STORAGE Available whole.

PREPARATION AND USE The salmon trout may be used in similar ways to salmon, but the flesh is too delicate for smoking. Stuff the fish with breadcrumbs flavoured with herbs or shellfish and bake or steam.

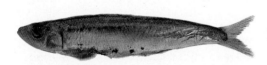

Sardine   *Sardinops sagax, Sardina pilchardus, Sardinella anchovia*

also called **Pilchard**

MAJOR NUTRIENTS		**SERVE SIZE 100 G**	
Energy	670 kJ	Cholesterol	80 mg
Protein	19 g	Phosphorus	215 mg
Fat	9 g	Magnesium	25 mg
Carbohydrate	0	Iron	1.8 mg

NUTRITIONAL INFORMATION No data are available for vitamin content. The fat content can vary from low fat to high fat.

DESCRIPTION A small, slim, bluish-black fish with silver sides. Flesh is soft and oily with very fine pink flakes.

ORIGIN AND HISTORY The sardine is a member of the herring family and a very important commercial fishery. Most live in ocean waters; however a few are found in fresh water. Some confusion reigns as to the relationship between the pilchard and the sardine: originally the term 'sardine' was applied only to young pilchards. Sardine shoals can usually be distinguished by the luminescence they cause on very dark nights, or by the breaking of surface waters in a manner that gives the impression of heavy rain falling.

BUYING AND STORAGE Available whole.

Season: autumn, winter, spring (southern hemisphere); April to November (northern hemisphere).

PREPARATION AND USE Sardines should be cooked whole. Suitable for baking, frying, grilling and barbecuing. Can be butterflied (opened out with the backbone removed). Suits strong flavourings.

PROCESSING Canning, freezing.

VARIETIES

Pacific sardine, European sardine, Spanish sardine, whose scientific names are given in order above.

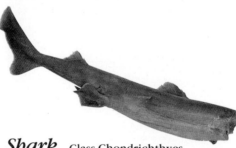

Shark   Class Chondrichthyes

MAJOR NUTRIENTS		**SERVE SIZE 100 G**	
Energy	420 kJ	Cholesterol	50 mg
Protein	21 g	Phosphorus	160 mg
Fat	1 g	Iron	1.5 mg
Carbohydrate	0	Niacin Equiv.	4.5 mg

NUTRITIONAL INFORMATION See general introduction to this section.

DESCRIPTION Some sharks are handsomely streamlined, others are so flattened and expanded laterally that they resemble rays. Sharks are usually drab, grey-brown creatures but there are some spectacular exceptions, like the tiger and zebra sharks. The flesh varies in colour from white and cream to pink. It is moist and chunky and in many cases good eating. The only fault is that in some flesh the taste of ammonia is present. The ammonia is not harmful.

ORIGIN AND HISTORY Sharks are an extremely interesting group. They are living representatives of groups that have survived almost unchanged from remote geological times, and could almost be called living fossils. They are essentially scavengers, tending to swim over the bottom picking up food here and there; however, when they come to the surface, they are usually attracted by shoals of fish. Sharks hunt their food by smell: their eyesight is not good. Some species are very important commercially.

BUYING AND STORAGE Available in fillet form.

Season: all year.

PREPARATION AND USE If fillets are very thick, score before cooking. Shark is an excellent food for children as it is boneless, having only cartilage. All methods of cooking and most flavourings are suitable.

PROCESSING Filleted and frozen.

VARIETIES

There are about 225–250 species of sharks.

SEE ALSO Shark's fin.

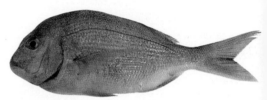

Snapper   Family Sparidae

MAJOR NUTRIENTS		**SERVE SIZE 100 G**	
Energy	390 kJ	Phosphorus	215 mg
Protein	20 g	Magnesium	30 mg
Fat	1 g	Iron	1 mg
Carbohydrate	0	Thiamin	0.15 mg
Sodium	70 mg	Niacin Equiv.	3.5 mg

NUTRITIONAL INFORMATION See the general introduction to this section.

DESCRIPTION Many fish are classified under the name of snapper. In USA and Europe, snappers come under the family Lutjanidae. Australian snappers belong to the family Sparidae.

A medium to large fish. Colour varies according to species. Some species are a beautiful orange-red and others even have all the colours of the rainbow in a muted pattern. The flesh is white, moist, firm, with a medium to large flake. A most delicious fish with a mild, yet distinct flavour.

ORIGIN AND HISTORY Snapper has a number of names which vary according to stage of growth, age, and where it is caught: cockney bream, under 700 g; red bream, between 700–850 g; squire, between 850 g–1.5 kg; snapper, over 1.5 kg. The name of the fish is often incorrectly spelt schnapper.

BUYING AND STORAGE Available whole

and in cutlets, fillets and steaks.

Season: all year, mainly spring.

PREPARATION AND USE If using whole fish, score first. Whole fish can be stuffed with shellfish, breadcrumbs, rice, fruits or vegetables. If fillets are thick they may also be scored. Cutlet bone may be removed and a stuffing put in its place. All methods of cooking suit this versatile fish. The heads and bones of snapper make excellent stock. Suits all flavourings.

PROCESSING Is sometimes frozen whole or in fillets.

VARIETIES
Over 250 species worldwide.

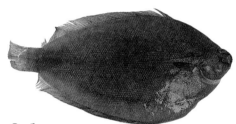

Sole Family Soleidae

MAJOR NUTRIENTS		SERVE SIZE 100 G	
Energy	340 kJ	Sodium	95 mg
Protein	17 g	Phosphorus	200 mg
Fat	1 g	Iron	0.5 mg
Carbohydrate	0	Thiamin	0.1 mg
Cholesterol	50 mg	Niacin Equiv.	3.5 mg

NUTRITIONAL INFORMATION See the introduction to this section.

DESCRIPTION Sole is a flat fish, small to medium in size, with a fine, white flesh and a mild flavour; a very good table fish. Sole is frequently confused with flounder. The main difference lies in the prominence of the lower jaw and cheekbone, those of the sole being less conspicuous.

ORIGIN AND HISTORY Large numbers of sole occur worldwide. In Australia they live in estuaries and the ocean and some in fresh water, but few reach the market in profitable numbers. The lemon sole is found in northern European waters and also off the coast of New Zealand, which exports it.

BUYING AND STORAGE Available whole and in fillets.

Season: all year.

PREPARATION AND USE Because of the fine flesh use gentle methods of cooking, i.e. shallow frying, poaching, a light grilling. The whole fish may be stuffed with shellfish or breadcrumbs flavoured with mild herbs; fillets can be filled with breadcrumbs, rolled and poached. White wine sauces go especially well with sole.

PROCESSING Filleted and frozen.

VARIETIES

Black Sole

Dover Sole

NUTRITIONAL INFORMATION As for sole in general.

DESCRIPTION A flat fish, small to medium in size. White fine flesh with a mild flavour. Also called the common sole.

ORIGIN AND HISTORY Like other flat fish, the left eye moves up and over to the right side as the sole matures. Soles lie on the bed of the sea, dark side up: they are bottom dwelling fish rarely going near the surface of the water. They are found worldwide.

BUYING AND STORAGE Available whole and in fillets.

Season: all year.

PREPARATION AND USE Do not overcook the fine flesh. Use gentle methods, i.e. poaching, shallow frying. Fillets can be filled with a stuffing and rolled and poached. Delicate flavourings are ideal for use with Dover sole.

PROCESSING Frozen — whole and filleted.

European Sole A major variety, *Solea solea*.

Lemon Sole

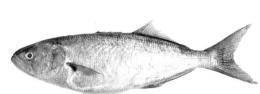

Tailor Pomatomus saltatrix
also known as **Bluefish**

MAJOR NUTRIENTS		SERVE SIZE 100 G	
Energy	490 kJ	Sodium	5 mg
Protein	20 g	Phosphorus	240 mg
Fat	4 g	Iron	0.6 mg
Carbohydrate	0	Thiamin	0.1 mg
Cholesterol	60 mg	Niacin Equiv.	1.9 mg

NUTRITIONAL INFORMATION Fat content can vary from low fat to high fat depending on location and season.

DESCRIPTION The body is elongated and covered with very small scales, blue-green above fading to a silver below. The tail fin is forked. The flesh is pink to red in colour, soft and slightly oily.

ORIGIN AND HISTORY Often described as a small marine game fish, tailor is surf-fished in the USA and Australia. A cannibal, it travels in schools and will attack and feed on other fish time and time again to the point of vomiting up the prey and attacking again with an empty stomach. The larger fish are tremendous fighters. It is an important commercial species. Ideally all fish should be bled and chilled immediately upon capture. The flesh is then very good eating; if not bled, however, it becomes soft and loses flavour.

BUYING AND STORAGE Sold whole, but occasionally filleted. Flesh should be firm but note that this fish is soft fleshed. Do not freeze for more than 3 months.

Season: summer–autumn (southern hemisphere).

PREPARATION AND USE Scale, gill and gut whole fish. Be careful to wash the stomach cavity thoroughly. When cooking whole fish, score to allow even heat penetration. Because of its oil content tailor is good for grilling, baking and barbecuing.

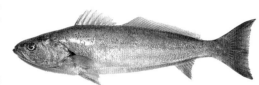

Teraglin Atractoscion aequidens
also called **Trag**

MAJOR NUTRIENTS		SERVE SIZE 100 G	
Energy	390 kJ	Sodium	120 mg
Protein	18 g	Calcium	51 mg
Fat	2 g	Phosphorus	180 mg
Carbohydrate	0	Magnesium	20 mg
Cholesterol	60 mg	Thiamin	0.3 mg

NUTRITIONAL INFORMATION Very little analysis is available on the nutrients contained in some of the fish found in Australian waters, but the figures above are supplied as a general guide to this variety.

DESCRIPTION Similar in shape and colour to the jewfish, but much smaller in size. The scales are finer than on the jewfish and its tail fin is slightly concave whereas the jewfish has a convex tail. The inside of the mouth is reddish-grey in colour. The flesh is pale pink and a little softer than jewfish, with a medium flake and a mild flavour. Very good eating fish.

ORIGIN AND HISTORY Teraglin comes from the same family as the jewfish. It is found off the east coast of Australia (New South Wales and southern Queensland).

BUYING AND STORAGE Available whole and in fillet form.

Season: mainly spring–summer.

PREPARATION AND USE Teraglin can be cooked whole if small enough. Score fish first. Fillets may need scoring if thick. Suits all methods of cooking and most flavourings.

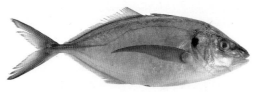

Trevally

MAJOR NUTRIENTS		SERVE SIZE 100 G	
Energy	440 kJ	Carbohydrate	0
Protein	18 g	Cholesterol	70 mg
Fat	3 g	Sodium	80 mg

NUTRITIONAL INFORMATION No data are available for mineral and vitamin content. Fat content can vary from low to high.

DESCRIPTION Trevally are deep-bodied, generally greenish on the upper half and silver on the lower. The fins of many species are yellow. The flesh tends to be pink and, in the larger fish, dry. However, they are good eating.

ORIGIN AND HISTORY The trevally is a member of a large family of fishes which have worldwide distribution. This family includes the yellowtail kingfish, yellowtail, and jack mackerel or cowanyoung. Trevally are fast swimming fish, usually inhabiting the mid and near surface waters where they hunt in schools. Trevally occur mainly in tropical waters.

BUYING AND STORAGE A budget-priced fish. Buy whole or in fillets.

Season: all year.

PREPARATION AND USE Trevally are far better cooked in fillet form. However, if whole fish is to be cooked, wash cavity of fish thoroughly. The cavity can be filled with a stuffing of breadcrumbs, shellfish etc. If fillets are to be cooked, it is best to remove the skin which can be tough. Trevally is a dry fish so use a moist method of cooking such as frying, poaching or casseroling.

VARIETIES

Silver trevally (*Pseudocaranx dentex*), blue trevally (*Caranx bucculentus*), cale cale trevally (*Ulua mentalis*), golden trevally (*Gnathanodon speciosus*), great trevally (*Caranx sexfasciatus*), lowly trevally (*Caranx ignobilis*), herring trevally (*Alepes kallas*).

Trout   Family Salmonidae

MAJOR NUTRIENTS		SERVE SIZE 100 G	
Energy	570 kJ	Phosphorus	270 mg
Protein	24 g	Magnesium	30 mg
Fat	5 g	Iron	1 mg
Carbohydrate	0	Riboflavin	0.15 mg
Cholesterol	60 mg	Niacin Equiv.	5 mg
Sodium	90 mg		

NUTRITIONAL INFORMATION Fat content can vary from low to high.

DESCRIPTION A small to medium-sized fish, colours vary according to species. The flesh is pinkish-white, soft and can be bony. It has a delicate flavour but can occasionally taste 'muddy'.

ORIGIN AND HISTORY The name 'trout' comes from a Greek word for 'gnawer', suggested by the sharp teeth that help identify the different species. Trout are a very popular sport and commercial food fish. They are a coldwater fish and a member of the same family as salmon. The rainbow trout is perhaps one of the most popular worldwide species. The various names and colour markings change with the area in which they are found. Rainbow trout in particular change their colour to adapt to local habitats.

BUYING AND STORAGE These fish are available unsmoked and smoked, whole and filleted. When buying fresh, look for firm, cream-pink fillets.

Season: all year (southern hemisphere); March to September (northern hemisphere).

PREPARATION AND USE Scale (very fine scales), gill and gut. Whole fresh trout and fillets can be poached or baked. Most cream sauces and herbs and spices suit trout. Smoked trout can be eaten cold.

PROCESSING Filleted, frozen and smoked.

VARIETIES

Brook trout, brown trout, cutthroat trout, golden trout, lake trout, rainbow trout.

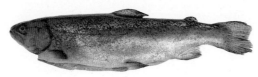

Rainbow Trout

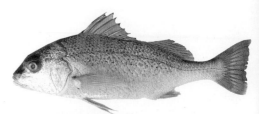

Trumpeter   *Latris lineata*

also called **Blue moki, Striped trumpeter, Tasmanian trumpeter**

MAJOR NUTRIENTS		SERVE SIZE 100 G	
Energy	390 kJ	Sodium	120 mg
Protein	18 g	Calcium	51 mg
Fat	2 g	Phosphorus	180 mg
Carbohydrate	0	Magnesium	20 mg
Cholesterol	60 mg	Thiamin	0.3 mg

NUTRITIONAL INFORMATION Very little analysis is available on the nutrients contained in some of the fish found in Australian waters, but the figures above are supplied as a general guide to this variety. Limited data indicate that trumpeter has a high fat (5%) content.

DESCRIPTION The Tasmanian trumpeter is a deep bronze with white lines running along the body. The mouth is large with thick lips. The flesh is whitish-pink and moist. A good eating fish.

ORIGIN AND HISTORY Trumpeter is both a sport and food fish. It is caught in New Zealand waters and off the southeast coast of Australia. The silver trumpeter is found abundantly in Tasmania and is often referred to as the Tasmanian trumpeter. Trumpeter can grow up to 1 metre in length and weigh up to 25 kg, but smaller ones up to 3 kg are usually regarded as best for eating.

BUYING AND STORAGE Can be sold whole or in fillets.

Season: spring–summer.

PREPARATION AND USE Best served in fillet form. Fillets may or may not be skinned. Use as a main course, in casseroles, in salads, soups. Nearly all flavourings suit the trumpeter, but use stronger ones in moderation. Ideal cooking methods are grilling, shallow frying, poaching, baking or barbecuing.

PROCESSING Sometimes smoked.

Tuna

MAJOR NUTRIENTS		SERVE SIZE 100 G	
Energy	560 kJ	Phosphorus	350 mg
Protein	25 g	Magnesium	50 mg
Fat	3 g	Iron	2.5 mg
Carbohydrate	0	Thiamin	0.1 mg
Cholesterol	45 mg	Riboflavin	0.15 mg
Sodium	35 mg	Niacin Equiv.	9.5 mg

NUTRITIONAL INFORMATION Fat content can vary from low to high (1%–10%) depending on location, season, the variety of the tuna and in particular the part of fish selected.

DESCRIPTION A streamlined body with a pointed head and tapered tail. Most tuna are ocean blue or greenish on the back with silvery sides and belly. The flesh is pink to crimson in colour, has a large flake and the flavour is rich and gamy.

ORIGIN AND HISTORY Tuna are mainly schooling fish of the open sea, closely related to the mackerel family. They are amongst the finest sporting fishes of the world. They are also extremely important commercially; most of the catch is canned.

BUYING AND STORAGE Sold in cutlets, steaks and fillets. Look for firm, moist flesh. Ideally, white lines of fat permeating the meat should be seen — this 'marbling' is highly prized for sashimi. The colour is a good indication of freshness. A freshly cut surface is very dull. To store, wrap in plastic or put in airtight container in refrigerator up to 6 days. Freeze for no longer than 3 months.

Season: all year, mainly autumn–winter.

PREPARATION AND USE Tuna cutlets can be grilled, shallow fried or barbecued. Large tuna pieces can be wrapped in foil and baked. Tuna can also be sliced thinly and served raw as sashimi. A variety of marinades and accompanying sauces suit tuna, e.g. soya sauce, honey and ginger marinade, garlic and sherry marinade.

VARIETIES

Albacore *Thunnus alalunga*

MAJOR NUTRIENTS		SERVE SIZE 100 G
Energy	606 kJ	Carbohydrate	0
Protein	24 g	Cholesterol	70 mg
Fat	5 g		

NUTRITIONAL INFORMATION No data available. Vitamin and mineral content would be similar to tuna. Fat content can vary from low to high (0.5%–18%).

DESCRIPTION This is a small variety of tuna, characterised by its spindle-shaped body which enables it to be extremely fast moving. Most weigh around 5 kg. The flesh is soft and oily, but tends to cook dry. The greater part of the meat is white.

ORIGIN AND HISTORY Albacore is only one of many species of tuna but, in many countries, it has become a generic term for tuna.

Albacore is a speedy and voracious fish, often referred to as 'chicken or pork of the sea' because of its white flesh. The sashimi (raw fish) market uses albacore thinly sliced.

BUYING AND STORAGE Available sometimes whole, but mostly in cutlet (steak) or fillet form. Look for firm, moist flesh with marbling, as for tuna.

Season: all year, but mainly autumn–winter.

PREPARATION AND USE Skin can be left on. Thickness of cutlets and fillets should depend on use. Albacore is soft so careful cooking is required. It suits most methods of cooking, but is a bit soft for poaching. Whole pieces can be wrapped in foil and baked or barbecued. Or why not save cooking time and serve raw with a soya sauce?

PROCESSING In some countries it is canned.

Bluefin Tuna *Kishinoella tonggoi*

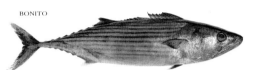

BONITO

Bonito Family Scombrinae

MAJOR NUTRIENTS		SERVE SIZE 100 G
Energy	700 kJ	Carbohydrate	0
Protein	24 g	Cholesterol	70 mg
Fat	7 g		

NUTRITIONAL INFORMATION The vitamin and mineral content would be similar to mackerel with a variable fat content.

DESCRIPTION There are many names given to the bonito, some common ones being Atlantic bonito, California bonito, Pacific bonito.

Basically the bonito is a bluish-green fish with a pattern of stripes that run along the side. The flesh is pink-red in colour with a beautiful coarse grain and a rich flavour.

ORIGIN AND HISTORY Bonito are found from the Black Sea to Normandy, as well as in the Atlantic and Pacific Oceans. Closely related to the mackerel family, they are free-ranging, speedy and voracious with a spindle body specially adapted for fast movement. They are a hardfighting fish. Members of the family include the leaping bonito and Australian bonito.

BUYING AND STORAGE Sold in cutlets, steaks and fillets. Look for firm, moist flesh and 'marbling' if the fish is to be eaten as sashimi. The nature of the colour is a good indication of freshness. A freshly cut surface is very dull. Will keep for 6 days in refrigerator, but only 3 months in freezer.

Season: all year, but mainly autumn–winter.

PREPARATION AND USE Bonito has a soft flesh so quick and careful cooking is required. Bonito cutlets can be grilled, shallow fried or barbecued. Large bonito pieces can be wrapped in foil and baked. Bonito can also be sliced thinly and served raw as sashimi.

PROCESSING In some countries this species of tuna is canned. Can also be smoked.

Yellowfin Tuna *Thunnus albacares*.

SEE ALSO Bonito Flakes; Tuna, Canned.

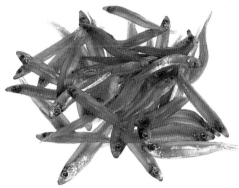

Whitebait *Galaxias attenuatus, G. maculatus*

also called **Inanga, Jollytails, Minnows**

MAJOR NUTRIENTS		SERVE SIZE 100 G
Energy	390 kJ	Sodium	120 mg
Protein	18 g	Calcium	51 mg
Fat	2 g	Phosphorus	180 mg
Carbohydrate	0	Magnesium	20 mg
Cholesterol	60 mg	Thiamin	0.3 mg

NUTRITIONAL INFORMATION Very little analysis is available on the nutrients contained in some of the fish in Australian waters, but the figures above are supplied as a general guide to this variety. Whitebait are eaten whole and so are an excellent source of calcium.

DESCRIPTION Silver fish. Matchstick in size, although the size of the fish varies depending on where caught.

ORIGIN AND HISTORY Whitebait used to be a rich man's pleasure, and fashionable summer whitebait parties were popular during the Victorian era. Traditionally a gourmet's delight, considered a great delicacy in the United Kingdom, New Zealand, and Mediterranean countries.

BUYING AND STORAGE Sold whole, fresh and frozen. Place fish in a colander and wash thoroughly. Store in a container (such as a colander) that allows liquid to drain from fish. Some people use a clean canvas bag. *Do not* put in a plastic bag as they sweat. When whitebait are drained properly they will remain firm to the touch and can be kept, covered, in the refrigerator for 3 days.

Season: January to September (northern hemisphere); all year (southern hemisphere), except New Zealand's North Island (1 August–30 November) and South Island (1 September–15 November).

PREPARATION AND USE Wash fish well. Whether you remove the head and gut depends upon the size of the fish and your personal preference, but it is not really necessary. The best and most popular way of cooking whitebait is to coat them in flour and deep fry. Alternatively, make fritters: make a batter, add the whitebait and ladle spoonfuls of the mixture into hot oil. Remove when golden. Good with pre-dinner drinks or on a mixed seafood platter. They have a beautiful crunchy texture.

PROCESSING Frozen.

VARIETIES
Over time, the juveniles of many kinds of fish have been known as whitebait. In the southern oceans, the most prevalent fish caught in whitebait nets or traps is *Galaxias*, but juvenile anchovies and other species are often sold as whitebait in some areas.

Whiting *Sillago ciliato, S. bassensis, S. maculata, Sillaginodes punctatus*

MAJOR NUTRIENTS		SERVE SIZE 100 G	
Energy	390 kJ	Sodium	130 mg
Protein	21 g	Calcium	42 mg
Fat	1 g	Phosphorus	190 mg
Carbohydrate	0	Magnesium	30 mg
Cholesterol	30 mg	Iron	1 mg

NUTRITIONAL INFORMATION The nutrients are typical of fish in general.

DESCRIPTION Small to medium fish with elongated bodies and small mouths, varying in colour, but mainly silver-white with different markings.

ORIGIN AND HISTORY These fish are caught worldwide. Their popularity varies from country to country. Southern and northern hemisphere whiting are not related and as the southern hemisphere fish is a better eating fish it will be more appropriate to concentrate on it. The Australian whiting is relatively small and has at least 6 species. It spends its life in sandy situations, in shallow coastal waters, bays and estuary mouths. Whiting is very important commercially.

BUYING AND STORAGE Available whole and in fillets.

Season: all year.

PREPARATION AND USE Whole fish (if a good size) can be stuffed with breadcrumbs, rice, shellfish, fruits or vegetables and baked, poached or shallow fried. Perhaps one of the most delightful ways to prepare whiting is to lay fillets flat and place a delicately flavoured stuffing on top, roll up and secure with a skewer. Poach in white wine and serve with a mild flavoured sauce. Use strong flavourings sparingly.

PROCESSING Filleted and frozen.

VARIETIES
Sand or silver whiting; school whiting; trumpeter whiting, and King George or spotted whiting, whose scientific names are given in order above.

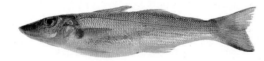

Sand Whiting

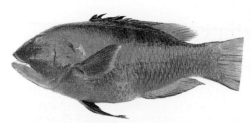

Wrasse *Cheilinus chlororus, C. trilobatus, C. undulatus*

MAJOR NUTRIENTS		SERVE SIZE 100 G	
Energy	390 kJ	Sodium	120 mg
Protein	18 g	Calcium	51 mg
Fat	2 g	Phosphorus	180 mg
Carbohydrate	0	Magnesium	20 mg
Cholesterol	60 mg	Thiamin	0.3 mg

NUTRITIONAL INFORMATION Very little analysis is available on the nutrients contained in some of the fish found in Australian waters, but the figures above are supplied as a general guide to this variety.

DESCRIPTION A small to medium-sized fish. Mainly reef-dwelling fish, inhabiting tropical waters, with colourful and intricate markings. Some species are better eating than others. The flesh is white and moist with a mild flavour. Most are very good food fishes.

ORIGIN AND HISTORY Wrasse are not only characterised by their beautiful colours, but by the variation of colour displayed during the course of their growth. These reef dwelling fish have an interesting habit of wrenching pieces of living coral off and grinding it with their teeth.

BUYING AND STORAGE Mostly available whole, although occasionally in fillets.

Season: all year.

PREPARATION AND USE Can be cooked whole or in fillets. If whole, scale, clean, score and stuff with breadcrumbs, rice or tropical fruits. Both whole fish and fillets suit baking, barbecuing, shallow frying, steaming and poaching.

VARIETIES
Main varieties are yellow-dotted Maori wrasse; tripletail Maori wrasse and hump-headed Maori wrasse, whose scientific names are given in order above.

SHELLFISH

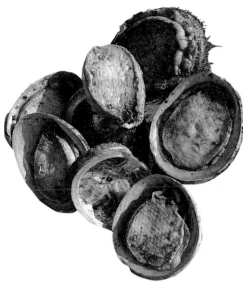

Abalone *Haliotis ruber,* *H. laevigata*

also called Awabi, Bau yeu, Ear shell, Mutton fish, Ormer, Paua, Sea ear

MAJOR NUTRIENTS		SERVE SIZE 100 G	
Energy	580 kJ	Phosphorus	180 mg
Protein	25 g	Magnesium	35 mg
Fat	2 g	Iron	8.8 mg
Carbohydrate	5 g	Zinc	2.1 mg
Cholesterol	70 mg	Niacin Equiv.	2.5 mg
Sodium	990 mg	Vitamin A	110 µg

NUTRITIONAL INFORMATION See the introduction to this chapter.

DESCRIPTION A mollusc which lives in subtidal zones, attaching itself strongly to rocks and ledges by its muscular foot which is the edible part. The epipodium, a part of the foot, can be of different colours and the various types are identified by this. The abalone foot, which is greyish-brown in colour, nestles in a roughly oval–shaped shell with a grey exterior and a vari-coloured opalescent lining.
Blacklip: the shell is basically red and roughly corrugated. The interior is lined with mother-of-pearl, and there is a spiral row of holes around one edge of the shell. Once opened, the muscle (foot) is very meaty. The name comes from the black mantle (epipodium).
Greenlip: the shell is red, streaked with pale green and is roughly corrugated. The common name comes from the green mantle.

ORIGIN AND HISTORY Commonly found along American, Asian, Australian and New Zealand shores of the Pacific Ocean. Less commonly found on the Atlantic coasts of France, Spain and Portugal. In Britain they are unlikely to be found north of the Channel Islands. Abalone is an important food to the Aboriginal people of Australia and the Maoris of New Zealand. The pearly lining of the abalone shell is used for jewellery, and the so called marine opal is cut from the New Zealand paua shell.

Only limited reference is made to abalone in the history of Chinese food. Harvesting is dangerous as their habitat often coincides with that of man-eating sharks. Because of its comparative rarity and expense, fresh abalone is usually only served on very important occasions, but dried abalone became the source of vigorous trade some centuries ago in coastal China.

No other shellfish quite matches the unique flavour and chewy-tender texture of abalone, though many in Western countries wonder what all the fuss is about. The Japanese love abalone, a dish that heralds summer, but prefer it young and tender. Many of their favourite harvesting grounds have been overfished, and they have had to resort to importing abalone from Australia and New Zealand.

BUYING AND STORAGE Occasionally sold fresh, the best coming from the south-coastal waters of Australia. More commonly sold canned in water, or dried. Canned and dried abalone will keep indefinitely. If buying fresh abalone, touch the meat: it should still move if very fresh. If fresh, abalone should be kept in clean salt water for 2 days, changing the water several times, until the contents of the stomach have been expelled. Shuck (remove meat from shell) when needed. If bought dead, shuck as soon as possible and refrigerate. Store in airtight container for 2–3 days. Freeze up to 3 months.

Season: all year.

PREPARATION AND USE To remove shell use a domestic paint scraper or the tip of a tyre iron. Forcing blade tip in at thin end of shell underneath the flesh, move blade until muscle becomes free. Remove meat and wash well, discarding intestine.

Some Asian countries cook abalone whole in their shells, without first removing the intestine. The mantle may be removed, although some say there is more flavour in the mantle than in the heel (meat). Trim off tough dark portions. Heel may be left whole or cut into very thin slices. Pound each slice between plastic wrap or greaseproof paper, until limp, using light strokes. It may be chopped and minced instead of sliced.

Dried abalone should be soaked overnight to soften, then simmered in clean water for up to 4 hours to tenderise. Slice thinly and stir-fry quickly, coat with batter and deep fry, or simmer in rich stock. Oyster sauce is the traditional Chinese accompaniment to abalone.

PROCESSING Can be smoked — very tasty, although a bit leathery. Large amounts are frozen.

VARIETIES
The main species of abalone are blacklip and greenlip, whose scientific names are listed above, and tiger (rare).

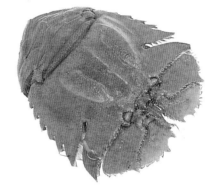

Balmain Bug *Ibacus incisus*

NUTRITIONAL INFORMATION Major nutrients similar to lobster.

DESCRIPTION This is a species of sand lobster (crayfish). It is a member of the crustacean group of shellfish, characterised by an orange-red shell, white medium-flaked flesh and a rich sea taste. Excellent eating qualities. The eyes of Balmain bugs are in the centre of the head whereas those of Moreton Bay bugs are on the outer edge of the head.

ORIGIN AND HISTORY Often called the shovel-nosed lobster because the shape of its head resembles a shovel. Found along the southeastern coast of Australia.

BUYING AND STORAGE When uncooked (green): whole. Cooked (red): whole. Avoid buying bugs with a garlicky smell, a sure sign of deterioration. Keep live bugs in a damp hessian bag which allows them more oxygen than if placed in a bucket of water.

If cooked, wrap in plastic or foil and then place in an airtight container and store in the refrigerator up to 3 days. Freeze up to 3 months.

Season: all year.

PREPARATION AND USE Before cooking, drown bugs in fresh water or freeze them. Then place in cold water and bring slowly to the boil. Bugs should be split lengthwise to get the maximum amount of meat, although cutting across the top of the tail is a more attractive way of serving — break tail carefully away from body to extract the meat.

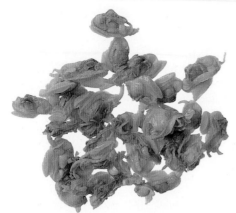

Clam *Mya arenaria, Pinna dolobiata, Venus mercenaria*

MAJOR NUTRIENTS		SERVE SIZE 100 G	
Energy	340 kJ	Cholesterol	190 mg
Protein	14 g	Sodium	35 mg
Fat	2 g	Phosphorus	185 mg
Carbohydrate	1 g	Iron	3.5 mg

NUTRITIONAL INFORMATION No data are available for vitamins.

DESCRIPTION Clams are generally described as either hard-shell or soft-shell bivalves. The clam has a tapering shell formed from two valves hinged along one side, pointed at one end and widely curved at the other. Has a rich flavour, and can occasionally be tough.

ORIGIN AND HISTORY America's supply of and fondness for clams surpasses most other nations. However, efforts were made to introduce them into France in the second half of the 19th century and they have now acclimatised along the Atlantic coast of France. The New England area of America is famous for its summer clambakes. Clam chowder is also famous: there are many recipes for it, with variations according to the resources of the different towns down the east coast of America.

BUYING AND STORAGE Can be purchased in shell or meat form. Shells and meat should have a pleasant sea smell. Store shells in a damp hessian bag or a bucket of water. Store meat in plastic or airtight container in fridge. Unopened shells can last 4 days, meat 2 to 3 days. Can be frozen up to 3 months.

Season: June to September (northern hemisphere).

PREPARATION AND USE To open shell: insert strong knife between halves and slide from one end to the other; sever the muscles that hold the meat to the shell. Wash well. Suits most methods of cooking but beware of overcooking. Suits most flavourings, especially rich sauces.

PROCESSING Canned, smoked.

VARIETIES

Bar clam, bean clam, butter clam, Californian

jackknife, cherrystone soft or long-necked (*Mya arenaria*), chowder clam, hard or little-necked (*Venus mercenaria*), razor clam (*Pinna dolobiata*), also known as razor fish (found in Australian waters).

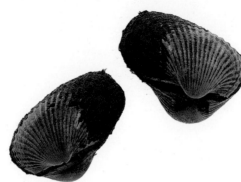

Cockle *Katylesia* spp.

MAJOR NUTRIENTS		SERVE SIZE 100 G	
Energy	200 kJ	Calcium	130 mg
Protein	11 g	Magnesium	50 mg
Fat	0	Phosphorus	200 mg
Carbohydrate	0	Iron	26 mg
Sodium	3520 mg	Zinc	1.2 mg

NUTRITIONAL INFORMATION No data are available for vitamins.

DESCRIPTION The cockle is a mollusc with two ridged oval shells hinged by a ligament near the pointed end. The outside of the shell is light sandy brown with deep markings of light purple while the inside is yellow and purple. Has a rich sea taste, but can be tough and gritty.

ORIGIN AND HISTORY Found throughout most of the world, cockles are not considered very good eating. Sometimes referred to as the 'poor man's oyster'.

BUYING AND STORAGE Always sold in the shell; do not buy if open. Should have a pleasant sea smell. Store in a damp hessian bag or in a bucket of water. Do not keep more than 24 hours.

Season: early summer.

PREPARATION AND USE Soak in fresh water for a few hours before cooking to remove the sediment. Salt can be added to draw out sediment. Cockles may be knifed open but it is better to cook them in their shell so that flavour and moisture will be retained.

Crab

MAJOR NUTRIENTS		SERVE SIZE 100 G	
Energy	530 kJ	Magnesium	50 mg
Protein	20 g	Iron	1.3 mg
Fat	5 g	Zinc	5.5 mg
Carbohydrate	0	Thiamin	0.1 mg
Cholesterol	100 mg	Riboflavin	0.15 mg
Sodium	370 mg	Niacin Equiv.	2.5 mg
Phosphorus	350 mg		

NUTRITIONAL INFORMATION The nutrients are typical of crustaceans.

DESCRIPTION This crustacean has a short, broad, flattened body with the abdomen, or so-called tail, small and folded under the thorax. Species vary in colour when alive but, once cooked, turn orange-red. The flesh is white and moist with a delicate, sweet flavour. The claw meat is usually the choicest.

ORIGIN AND HISTORY The most common edible crab in the world is the agile, fast-swimming blue swimmer. It is mostly caught in baited traps and is very valuable commercially. The mangrove crab is one of the most delicious of all crabs and is widely distributed in the tropical Pacific and Indian Oceans. Most crab species have a broad carapace, providing a large area for meat production.

BUYING AND STORAGE Sold whole, cooked and uncooked. Cooked crabs: limbs should be intact and heavy in proportion to size with no discoloration of joints. Lift a crab and shake before buying; there should be no sound of water.

Green (raw): Blue swimmer crabs are acceptable dead; however most other uncooked crabs must be alive until point of cooking, as once dead, the flesh goes bad very quickly.

To store alive: keep in damp hessian bag to provide more oxygen. To store cooked: wrap in foil or store in airtight container in refrigerator up to 3 days. Freeze up to 3 months.

Season: January to September (northern hemisphere); all year, mainly summer (southern hemisphere).

PREPARATION AND USE Cooked crabs: insert knife at 'seam' area at back, using a lever action to lift off shell. Wash inside thoroughly and remove meat. Break off claws and snap with a shellfish cracker to remove meat. Use as desired.

For some Asian dishes, the live crab must be cracked and cleaned before cooking:

1. Place a board near the sink.
2. Grasp live crab from the rear with a good hold on the back and place with back on board.
3. Put point of knife into shell between eyes.

Hit the back of the knife with a hard, quick blow which kills the crab instantly.

4. Firmly grasping hold of a front claw, twist off where it joins the body, repeat with the other claw and legs. Scrub and rinse well.

5. Pull off top shell with knife, if necessary. Remove gills and spongy parts under shell. Wash body and leg pieces thoroughly.

6. Crack each claw with a mallet to open each section and lift out all meat. Also remove meat from body cavity.

To cook live crabs: never, never put into boiling water as this toughens the meat and the claws can fall off. It is generally thought to be more painful for the crab. Put the crab into cold water (after first drowning or freezing). Cover pan and bring to boil, simmer 5–20 minutes depending upon size (about 8 minutes per 500 g once the water is simmering).

PROCESSING   Frozen, canned.

VARIETIES

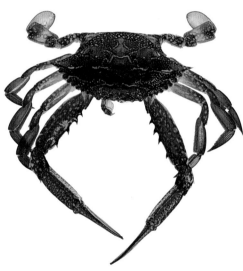

Blue Swimmer Crab   Also known as blue manna, sand crab, Atlantic blue crab, *Portunus pelagicus.*

Coral Crab   Also known as crucifix crab, *Charybdis cruciata.*

Giant King Crab   Also known as Japanese spider crab, *Macrochira kaempferi.*

Giant Tasmanian Crab   *Pseudocarcinus gigas.*

Green Shore Crab   *Carcinus maenas.*

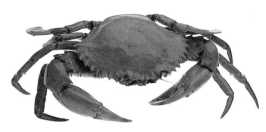

Mud Crab   Also known as mangrove crab, *Scylla serrata.*

Red Spot Crab   *Portunus sanguinolentus.*

Spanner Crab   Also known as frog crab, *Ranina ranina.*

Crayfish

*also called **Cray, Marron, Murray cray, Yabbie, Yabby***

MAJOR NUTRIENTS		SERVE SIZE 100 G	
Energy	300 kJ	Calcium	77 mg
Protein	15 g	Phosphorus	200 mg
Fat	1 g	Iron	1.5 mg
Carbohydrate	1 g	Niacin Equiv.	2 mg
Cholesterol	160 mg		

NUTRITIONAL INFORMATION   The nutrients are typical of crustaceans.

DESCRIPTION   Size varies. Most species found in the northern hemisphere are small–medium. In Australia some species are larger.

Marron — May grow to a maximum of 2 kg. Meat is mild tasting and moist.

Murray Crayfish — The claws and underside are white, while the top of the body and head are blue; the shell is spiny. The meat is mild and moist. Can grow up to 2 kg.

Yabbie — A freshwater crayfish, usually brown, but can be green-blue or purple. It can reach a size of up to 30 cm in length and 300 g in weight. The meat is in the tail and claws and is mild and moist. Shell is smooth.

ORIGIN AND HISTORY   The three largest species of freshwater crayfish in the world are found in Australia, occurring in creeks, rivers and billabongs. The yabbie, marron and Murray crayfish have increased in popularity and are now being cultivated commercially.

BUYING AND STORAGE   Available live and cooked. If cooked look for intact claws, firm shell and a pleasant sea smell. Green species should be alive and intact. Live species should be stored in a damp hessian bag for approximately 2 days. Cooked species may be wrapped in foil or stored in an airtight container in refrigerator up to 2 days. Freeze up to 3 months.

Season: January to February, May to August (northern hemisphere); all year (southern hemisphere).

PREPARATION AND USE   To cook live crayfish — place in cold water, bring to the boil and simmer until pink-red in colour. Alternatively, kill by putting a knife between the eyes, and then grill, bake or barbecue. The smaller species are best served whole, but the larger species should be halved before serving. Small freshwater crays are ideal for entrées, seafood platters and garnishes for seafood dishes. Mild flavourings go best with these delicate shellfish.

VARIETIES

Marron   *Cherax tenuimanus.*

Murray Crayfish   *Euastacus armatus.*

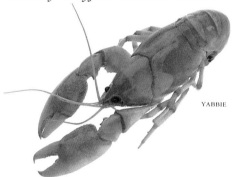

YABBIE

Yabbie   *Cherax destructor.*

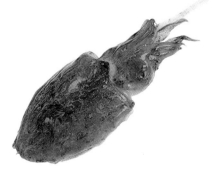

Cuttlefish   *Sepia* spp.

MAJOR NUTRIENTS		SERVE SIZE 100 G	
Energy	340 kJ	Iron	0.8 mg
Protein	16 g	Thiamin	0.05 mg
Fat	1 g	Niacin Equiv.	6 mg
Carbohydrate	1 g	Vitamin B12	1 µg

NUTRITIONAL INFORMATION   The nutrients are typical of molluscs.

DESCRIPTION   The cuttlefish is a mollusc. It

is generally smaller than a squid with a thicker mantle (body). Inside the mantle is a hard cuttlebone and an ink sac. Cuttlefish have 10 tentacles, two of which are much longer than the others. The cream flesh is covered by a brown-grey, sometimes mottled, skin; it has delicate flavour, but can be tough if incorrectly prepared or cooked.

ORIGIN AND HISTORY Cuttlefish are found worldwide. Their popularity is increasing: in fact, to some gourmets, they have more flavour than squid. In Japanese cuisine they are highly prized. The hard cuttlebone of the cuttlefish is given to caged birds to peck at as it is a source of lime. Ground, it was once used as tooth powder, jewel polish and face powder by Roman ladies.

BUYING AND STORAGE Available whole. Look for firm flesh and undamaged bodies with a pleasant sea smell. Don't be put off by a broken ink sac: sacs are often broken when cuttlefish are caught. Prepare before storing: remove gut and wash thoroughly. Wrap in plastic wrap and place in airtight container. Keeps 3 days in the refrigerator. Freezes 3 months.

Season: all year.

PREPARATION AND USE Place bone side down on a board and slit mantle with a sharp knife. Open gently, and remove and discard gut. The ink sac and tentacles can be used in cooking. Cut mantle in two. You will then be left with two flaps. Remove skin, then either cut flaps into thin strips or score diagonally on both sides of the flap. Suited to frying, stir-frying and barbecuing, but cook very quickly as cuttlefish can toughen. Grill, basting with wine, marinades, lemon juice, soya sauce. Delicious as a snack with pre-dinner drinks and entrées, or in sauces for pastas or rice. The ink sac is often used in the Italian black rice dish *risotto nero*.

PROCESSING Canned.

VARIETIES
The many species of cuttlefish are similar in outward appearance, but are distinguished from one another by the sculptured shape of the internal cuttlebone.

Lobster

also called Crawfish, Lobby

MAJOR NUTRIENTS			SERVE SIZE 100 G
Energy	500 kJ	Phosphorus	280 mg
Protein	22 g	Magnesium	35 mg
Fat	3 g	Iron	0.8 mg
Carbohydrate	0	Zinc	1.8 mg
Cholesterol	150 mg	Thiamin	0.1 mg
Sodium	330 mg	Niacin Equiv.	1.5 mg
Calcium	62 mg		

NUTRITIONAL INFORMATION The nutrients are typical of crustaceans.

DESCRIPTION A large, sea-dwelling crustacean. The colour varies from pink to red-brown to deep maroon, from creamy-yellow to orange to purple, depending on the species. Lobsters have a pair of stalked compound eyes, two pairs of antennae and five pairs of legs, of which the first pair is modified into enormous pincers, one being heavier than the other. There are also swimming legs, but the chief swimming organ is the tail, by means of which they can make sudden backward movements. Lobsters feed on animals, both living and dead, and are usually caught in traps.

Norway lobsters (Dublin Bay prawns) are not treated as lobsters, although they do have the eight walking legs and two claws of a true lobster. Norway lobsters are about 25 cm long. They are often marketed as shrimps (prawns).

ORIGIN AND HISTORY For centuries arguments have existed about whether all lobster-like crustaceans are entitled to be called lobsters. The original scientific name, *Astacus verus*, meaning 'true lobster', was abandoned after 17th century explorers discovered that the New World contained new lobsters. Since 1910, two species of crustaceans have been recognised as true lobsters. They are *Homarus vulgaris* (European lobster) and *Homarus americanus* (American lobster). Rock lobsters, spiny lobsters and Norway lobsters are considered to be crayfish.

BUYING AND STORAGE When uncooked (green): whole (alive or frozen) or in lobster tails and lobster meat. Cooked: whole, or in lobster tails.

Uncooked (green) lobsters should have limbs intact and be active. Do not buy a dead green lobster as the flesh will go off quickly. Cooked whole lobsters should have limbs intact, with no discoloration at joints. The tail should be curled and should spring back when raised; the eyes should be bright. Lobsters should be heavy in weight in proportion to their size. The smaller the species, the more tender the flesh.

Keep live lobsters in a damp hessian bag which allows them more oxygen than if placed in a bucket of water. If cooked, wrap in plastic or foil and place in an airtight container in the refrigerator up to 3 days. Freeze up to 3 months.

Season: March to October (northern hemisphere); all year (southern hemisphere).

PREPARATION AND USE Never, never, put a live lobster into a pot of boiling water. Boiling water not only toughens the flesh, but makes legs fall off and is supposed to be more painful for the lobster. For maximum flavour and texture drown the lobster in fresh water or freeze it, and then place in cold water and bring slowly to the boil. Once boiling, allow 8 minutes per 500 g.

For serving on the half shell: Place cooked lobster on its back. Cut along the mid-line with a sharp knife, starting at mid-tail: ease knife down to the end, then work back to the head. Split open and wash thoroughly. Save the coral-coloured roe, if any, and the green or yellow liver, which is considered a delicacy, to add to sauces. (The liver should be cooked before adding to cold sauces, such as mayonnaise, etc.)

In recipes where live lobster are not boiled first but grilled green, place the point of a strong sharp knife on the shell between the eyes, then plunge the blade in strongly and quickly, at the same time pulling it down through the body and tail. Finally, turn lobster around and cut through the head.

To grill green lobster tails: with a sharp knife slit underside of tail a couple of times to allow heat penetration. Place under grill, brush with butter, grill 20 cm from heat for about 5–8 minutes each side.

PROCESSING Frozen — either whole in shell or as meat only.

VARIETIES

American Lobster Can be sold as Maine lobster, *Homarus americanus*.

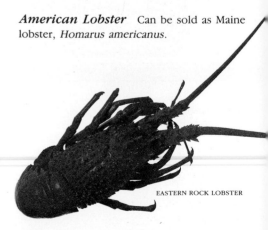

EASTERN ROCK LOBSTER

Eastern Rock Lobster Also known as

spiny rock lobster, and green or packhorse lobster, *Jasus verreauxii*.

European Lobster *Homarus vulgaris*.

Flapjack A lobster without antennae, found in Queensland, *Scyllarides squamosus*.

Norway Lobster Also called Dublin Bay prawn.

SOUTHERN ROCK LOBSTER

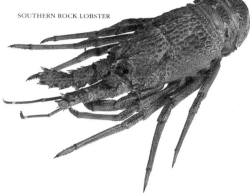

Southern Rock Lobster *Jasus novae-hollandiae*.

Spiny Lobster Found mainly in New Zealand, *Jasus edwardsii*.

Tropical Rock Lobster Also called painted lobster, *Panulirus ornatus*.

Western Rock Lobster *Panulirus cygnus*.

SEE ALSO Balmain Bug, Moreton Bay Bug.

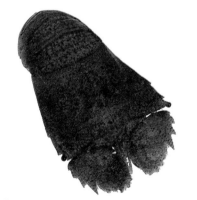

Moreton Bay Bug *Thenus orientalis*

also called **Bay lobster**

NUTRITIONAL INFORMATION Since this is a variety of lobster, the nutrients are similar to those found under Lobster.

DESCRIPTION This is really a species of lobster, yellow-brown in colour with brown spots all over, except the tail, which is golden.

The eyes of the Moreton Bay bug are on the outer edge of the head, whereas those of the Balmain bug are in the centre of the head. It has white, medium-flaked flesh with a rich sea taste. Excellent eating qualities.

ORIGIN AND HISTORY Found off the northern coast of Australia from Moreton Bay in Queensland to Exmouth Gulf in Western Australia.

BUYING AND STORAGE When uncooked (green): whole. Cooked (red): whole.

Avoid specimens with a garlicky smell, a sure sign of deterioration. Keep live bugs in a damp hessian bag to allow them oxygen.

Wrap cooked species in plastic or foil and then place in an airtight container and store in the refrigerator up to 3 days. Freeze up to 3 months.

Season: all year (southern hemisphere).

PREPARATION AND USE To make the most of their flavour and texture drown bugs in fresh water or freeze them. Then place in cold water and bring slowly to the boil. Bugs should be split lengthwise to get maximum amount of meat, although cutting across the top of the tail is a more attractive way of serving — in this case, break tail carefully away from body to extract meat.

SEE ALSO Lobster.

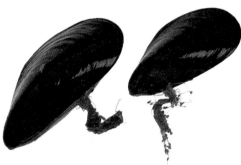

Mussel *Mytilus edulis planulatus, Mytilus edulis canaliculus*

MAJOR NUTRIENTS		SERVE SIZE 100 G	
Energy	366 kJ	Phosphorus	330 mg
Protein	17 g	Magnesium	25 mg
Fat	2 g	Iron	7.7 mg
Carbohydrate	0	Zinc	2.1 mg
Cholesterol	100 mg	Vitamin A	70 µg
Sodium	210 mg	Riboflavin	0.4 mg
Calcium	60 mg	Niacin Equiv.	2 mg

NUTRITIONAL INFORMATION Nutrients typical of molluscs.

DESCRIPTION The shell is smooth, thin and crescent-shaped, brown to purple-black (blacklip) or emerald green (greenlip). All the meat is edible, with a distinct sea flavour, but it can be chewy. The greenlip is larger than the blacklip.

ORIGIN AND HISTORY Mussels are available worldwide. They usually grow on rocks and in beds on coarse sandy bottoms of shallow ocean waters. They are also cultivated on long rope-like poles. In years gone by the mussel shell has been used for making buttons.

BUYING AND STORAGE Approximately 25 to a kilo. Sold fresh in the shell (tightly closed — do not buy open mussels as they are dead) or pickled in jars.

To store: never store live mussels in the refrigerator for a long time as the cold temperature will kill them. Store in a damp hessian bag or in a bucket of water (salt or fresh) in a cool place. If soaking in water, add some oatmeal. The mussels eat the oatmeal and get plump. They have a life of 1–3 days. Discard any that open.

Season: September to April (northern hemisphere); all year (southern hemisphere).

PREPARATION AND USE Scrub mussels thoroughly under running water and remove the beard (fibrous hair-like threads) attached. Do not overcook as they can easily toughen. Steam, boil, grill, microwave, bake or barbecue in the shell. Mussels are very good for hors d'oeuvres, entrées, sauces and stuffings. The shell is ovenproof.

PROCESSING Smoked, canned.

VARIETIES
Blacklip, New Zealand greenlip, whose scientific names are given above. The latter is also marketed as Kiwiclam.

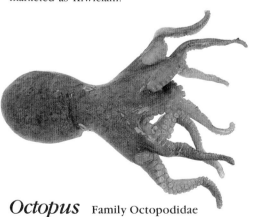

Octopus Family Octopodidae

MAJOR NUTRIENTS		SERVE SIZE 100 G	
Energy	290 kJ	Carbohydrate	0
Protein	14 g	Niacin Equiv.	2 mg
Fat	1 g		

NUTRITIONAL INFORMATION The nutrients are typical of molluscs.

DESCRIPTION The octopus has eight tentacles and no internal backbone. The colour varies from grey-brown to pink. It has a large head armed with a strong beak and a small oval sac-like body. The eight tentacles are united at the base by a membrane and are usually provided with two rows of suckers to cling to prey or to other objects. Upon cooking the meat goes white and the skin pink. It has a delicate flavour.

ORIGIN AND HISTORY The octopus is a cephalopod. Found worldwide, they live on the bottom of the ocean, among the rocks, and are caught in traps, nets and by spearing.

In Greece octopus is eaten readily. However, in many other European countries, America and Australia, although its popularity is on the increase, people are still hesitant.

BUYING AND STORAGE Available whole in varying sizes. Small octopus are the best for cooking. Look for firm flesh and a pleasant sea smell. Clean before storing. Wrap in plastic wrap or store in an airtight container. Keep in refrigerator for 3 days. Freeze up to 3 months.

Season: all year.

PREPARATION AND USE Remove gut from octopus either by cutting off the head entirely or by slitting open the head and removing gut and beak only. Skin can be left on, as it is difficult to remove and does not interfere with the delicate flavour of octopus. Octopus needs tenderising. Fishermen often bash octopus on rocks to tenderise it. Another method is to beat it with a kitchen mallet. Long slow cooking is perhaps the best way. Simmer in red wine or its own juices until fork-tender (1–1½ hours). Eat as is or stir-fry, grill, or barbecue quickly.

VARIETIES

There are a number of species of octopus in various genera. Some small species are highly venomous.

Oyster

MAJOR NUTRIENTS		SERVE SIZE 100 G	
Energy	220 kJ	Magnesium	40 mg
Protein	11 g	Iron	6 mg
Fat	1 g	Zinc	45 mg
Carbohydrate	0	Thiamin	0.1 mg
Cholesterol	50 mg	Riboflavin	0.2 mg
Sodium	510 mg	Niacin Equiv.	1.5 mg
Calcium	190 mg	Vitamin A	75 µg
Phosphorus	270 mg		

NUTRITIONAL INFORMATION The nutrients are typical of molluscs.

DESCRIPTION Oysters are bivalve molluscs

usually eaten raw. The shells are mostly grey-black in colour, the flesh creamy-grey and moist with an evocative smell of the sea and a rich flavour.

ORIGIN AND HISTORY Oysters date from antiquity. Shells have been found in ancient ruins and in excavated shell heaps of North American Indians and Australian Aboriginal people. The Romans fattened oysters in tanks and also cultivated them to provide a continuous supply. The Celts gathered oysters and ate them abundantly. The Greeks prized oysters highly and knew how to prepare them in a number of ways. (Incidentally, they also used oyster shells for casting their votes, a voter inscribing his choice with a sharp point on the white mother-of-pearl shell.) From the Middle Ages to the 19th century oysters were a great bargain. Enormous quantities were sold and, by the middle of the 19th century, oysters were so abundant that anyone could afford them.

BUYING AND STORAGE Most oysters are sold raw, whether intact in their shell, opened and in half shells, or bottled. Some are processed and canned. In New Zealand, bluff oysters are sometimes dipped in batter, fried and sold over the counter. Fresh oysters should be plump, a natural creamy-grey colour, shiny and fresh-smelling with clear liquid, free of shell particles. If bought in shell, they should be alive.

Unopened oysters should be stored in a bucket and covered with a wet bag or placed in a wet hessian bag. Oysters in half shells should be placed on crushed ice in the refrigerator and covered with plastic wrap. If removed from the shell, place in a container, cover with water and store in refrigerator. Oysters will remain fresh for a week to 10 days. If bottled, store in refrigerator.

Season: all year (southern hemisphere); September to April (northern hemisphere).

PREPARATION AND USE Rinse the oysters well in water. To open, place oyster on board flat side up and hold it with one hand; with the other, force an oyster knife (or a very sharp pointed small knife) between the shells at the thin end. Lever the top shell off. The best way to eat oysters is *au naturel*, with lemon, pepper, bread and butter, but they are delicious grilled, poached or fried with accompanying sauces. The distinct flavour of the bluff oyster makes it a favourite for oyster soups and seafood casseroles. The Pacific oyster can be a bit chewy so try cutting in half and incorporating in soups, casseroles or even steak and kidney pudding.

PROCESSING Canned, smoked.

VARIETIES

Black-lip Oyster *Saccostrea echinata.*

Bluff Oyster From New Zealand, *Ostrea lutaria.*

Coral Rock Oyster *Saccostrea cuccullata.*

Pacific Oyster Also called Japanese oyster, *Crassostrea gigas.*

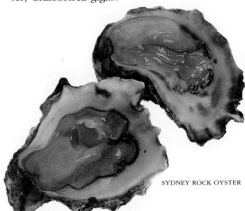

SYDNEY ROCK OYSTER

Sydney Rock Oyster *Saccostrea commercialis.*

Prawn

also called **Shrimp**

MAJOR NUTRIENTS		COOKED SERVE SIZE 100 G	
Energy	450 kJ	Calcium	116 mg
Protein	23 g	Phosphorus	350 mg
Fat	2 g	Magnesium	50 mg
Carbohydrate	0	Iron	1.1 mg
Cholesterol	200 mg	Zinc	1.6 mg
Sodium	400 mg	Niacin Equiv.	1.5 mg

NUTRITIONAL INFORMATION The nutrients are typical of crustaceans.

It must be noted here that prawn and shrimp tend to be interchangeable. In Australia larger species of this crustacean tend to be called prawns. However, in some countries it can be the opposite.

DESCRIPTION Prawns are crustaceans with slender legs, long antennae, a large strong compressed abdomen and a prominent, serrated rostrum. They vary in size and colour according to species. Colours range through cream, yellow, green, blue and light brown, when uncooked. Cooked prawns turn an orange-red colour. The flesh is firm, sweet and succulent. Excellent eating.

ORIGIN AND HISTORY Prawns are abundant in all tropical and temperate regions, and most Australian tidal lakes, estuaries and tidal rivers carry prawns. The prawn industry is very important in Australia.

BUYING AND STORAGE If uncooked, look for firm bodies and a pleasant sea smell. Should not be sweaty or have any discoloration.

Cooked prawns: Look for firm flesh and a tight shell; avoid black, loose heads and black legs. Leave in shell until ready to eat because the shell keeps in the moisture and flavour. Store in refrigerator in an airtight container or in a plastic bag. However, the best way is to place prawns in water in the refrigerator until ready to use. This prevents oxidation. Keep in refrigerator for 3 days depending upon freshness when purchased. Freeze up to 3 months.

Season: all year.

PREPARATION AND USE The preparation depends upon use. To peel: break or cut off the head, remove the tail and shell. (Tail may be left on — depends on cooking.) Devein by slitting the centre back with a very fine bladed knife or using a slender sharp skewer. Suit all methods of cooking — but remove once prawns turn orange/red. Particularly suit grilling, barbecuing, pan/stir-frying. Suitable for stuffing whole fish.

PROCESSING Frozen, canned.

VARIETIES

Banana Prawn Penaeus merguiensis.

Brown Tiger Prawn P. esculentus.

Eastern King Prawn P. plebejus.

Greasyback Prawn Also called greentail prawn, Metapenaeus macleayi.

Royal Red Prawn Haliporoides sibogae.

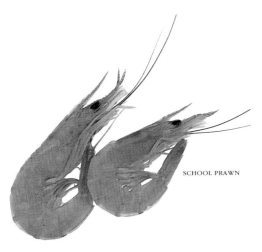

School Prawn M. bennettae.

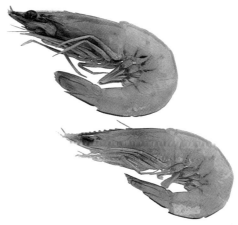

Western King Prawn Also called blue leg prawn, P. latisulcatus.

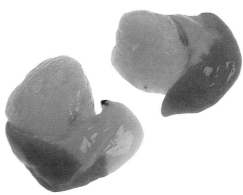

Scallop Family Pectinidae

MAJOR NUTRIENTS			COOKED SERVE SIZE 100 G
Energy	450 kJ	Potassium	480 mg
Protein	23 g	Calcium	120 mg
Fat	1 g	Phosphorus	340 mg
Carbohydrate	0	Magnesium	40 mg
Cholesterol	50 mg	Iron	3 mg
Sodium	270 mg		

NUTRITIONAL INFORMATION No data are available for zinc and vitamin B group except folate, which is 15 µg.

DESCRIPTION The scallop is a bivalve mollusc. The shell is radially ribbed, and the edge undulated. The shell is cream–pink in colour. The meat is white–cream with an orange roe. Excellent rich sea flavour.

ORIGIN AND HISTORY The French name for scallop is *coquille Saint Jacques*. Saint James is the patron saint of both shellfish and the gatherers of shellfish; during the Middle Ages pilgrims would wear a scallop-shell badge. Scallops generally do not attach themselves on the seabed but propel themselves by opening and closing the valves. Scallop shells are ovenproof and are often used as baking dishes.

BUYING AND STORAGE Available in shell and meat form. Also available pickled. Look for white-cream meat, without brown markings and with roe intact (if roe still remains). Should be firm with a pleasant sea smell. If buying meat, don't buy out of containers of water, as scallops absorb water which is then weighed with the scallop. If buying scallops in shell make sure the shells are firmly closed. To store: place meat in airtight container in the refrigerator up to 3 days. Freeze up to 3 months.

Season: September to April (northern hemisphere); all year (southern hemisphere).

PREPARATION AND USE Wash thoroughly and remove meat from shell either by levering the point of a knife between the valves or by placing scallops in a very slow oven and removing as shells open. Wash meat and remove brown vein. Leave the roe on. In some countries roe is removed during shucking. Large scallops may be cut in half, depending upon the recipe. Cook quickly, i.e. if deep frying, 30 seconds to 1 minute. If poaching, about 3 minutes. Scallops can toughen very easily.

PROCESSING Shucked and frozen; pickled.

VARIETIES

Commercial Scallop, *Pecten fumata*; Saucer Scallop, *Amusium balloti*.

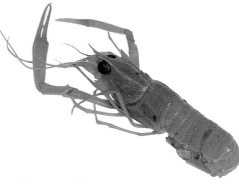

Scampi

*also called **Langoustine***

NUTRITIONAL INFORMATION The nutrients are similar to those of the prawn.

DESCRIPTION Scampi are marine prawns with long thin claws. When raw they are pale pink in colour. When cooked they are orange-red with white, delicately flavoured flesh.

ORIGIN AND HISTORY Scampi is technically a nocturnal creature with some physical traits of both lobsters and prawns. It inhabits the deep water of the Atlantic coast from Scandinavia to North Africa. It occurs off northwestern Australia also.

BUYING AND STORAGE Available whole. Wrap in plastic wrap or store in airtight con-

SCHOOL PRAWN

tainer. Keeps 3 days in refrigerator. Freezes 3 months.

Season: all year (northern hemisphere).

PREPARATION AND USE Wash and cook as desired. The head and body are really quite beautiful and are often served as garnishes. Suitable for grilling, barbecues, stir/pan frying, and in Japan scampi are eaten raw. Suits most flavourings.

PROCESSING Sometimes frozen.

VARIETIES

European Scampi, *Nephrops norvegicus*; Australian Scampi, *N. australis*.

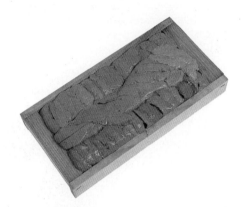

Sea Urchin *Heliocidaris* spp.

also called Sea egg, Kina

NUTRITIONAL INFORMATION No reliable data available.

DESCRIPTION Most of the sea urchins are sharp-spined and have a patterned shell.

ORIGIN AND HISTORY Sea urchin is a gourmet's delight, plentiful in many parts of the world. Most are rock-clinging, living from just below low tide level into deep water; however, some graze on sea grass.

BUYING AND STORAGE While sea urchin can be sold in the shell, the roe is more commonly available on its own. It is often packed in small wooden boxes. If bought in the shell, the crusty mouthparts should be removed before storing. Put in airtight container and store in refrigerator up to 24 hours.

Season: all year.

PREPARATION AND USE Remove the 'eye' (crusty mouthparts) with a small pair of scissors. Discard the watery viscera, then with a spoon scrape out the edible ovaries (containing the roe) which cling in five rows to the inside of the lower part of the shell. When pureed and mixed with butter or mayonnaise, the roe makes an unusual seafood dip or sauce. It is used as a topping for sushi.

VARIETIES

Green sea urchin, black sea urchin.

Squid

MAJOR NUTRIENTS		SERVE SIZE 100 G	
Energy	350 kJ	Cholesterol	190 mg
Protein	16 g	Phosphorus	120 mg
Fat	1 g	Iron	0.5 mg
Carbohydrate	2 g		

NUTRITIONAL INFORMATION In fact a mollusc, the squid provides similar nutrients to those of fish.

DESCRIPTION Squid has a long cylindrical body or mantle with fins on the sides, usually towards the tail, well-developed eyes and ten tentacles encircling the parrot-like beak. It has a delicate internal backbone or 'quill'. The meat is white and mild in flavour. Can be tough in large species or if overcooked.

ORIGIN AND HISTORY Squid is caught worldwide. Mediterranean countries understand how to prepare and cook squid perhaps better than most other countries. Squid is also used in Asian countries, and is becoming more and more popular in Australia.

BUYING AND STORAGE Sold whole, in tube or ring form. Some rings are already breadcrumbed ready for use. Whole squid: look for firm flesh and make sure that head and tentacles are intact. Skin which is difficult to remove is a sign of staleness. Fresh tubes or rings should be white without any brown markings. Clean before storing. Freeze only up to 3 months.

Season: all year.

PREPARATION AND USE Remove the head and tentacles from hood. Slide clear 'quill-like' membrane from hood and discard. Then remove skin from hood and flaps by pulling firmly, starting underneath flap. Remove flaps if desired. Use hood whole or cut into rings. Use tentacles and flaps as required. (If skin is hard to remove use salt on fingers for a firm grip.) May be cooked whole, or cut into rings. Requires very little cooking — DO NOT OVERCOOK. Pan fry, deep fry, bake, steam or barbecue. The ink may be used in a sauce to accompany the squid flesh.

PROCESSING Hoods (bodies, tubes) may be frozen whole, cut into rings and frozen or cut into rings and crumbed and frozen.

VARIETIES

Etheridge's Squid *Loligo etheridgi.*

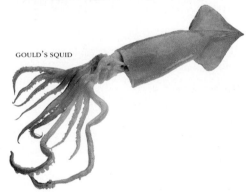

GOULD'S SQUID

Gould's Squid *Nototodarus gouldi.*

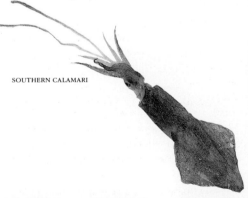

SOUTHERN CALAMARI

Southern Calamari *Sepioteuthis australis.*

PRESERVED SEAFOOD

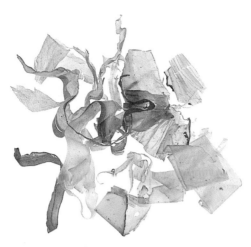

Bonito Flakes *Scomber japonicus*

*also called **Hana-katsuo, Katsuo-bushi, Kezuri-bushi***

NUTRITIONAL INFORMATION Adds flavour mainly because of high sodium content. Contains significant amounts of naturally occurring monosodium glutamate and amines.

DESCRIPTION A member of the mackerel family, bonito is not eaten fresh but is dried by a unique method for use as an essential ingredient in Japanese cooking. Katsuo-bushi, the Japanese name for dried bonito, looks like pieces of petrified wood, shaved into shreds or tissue-thin flakes. Bonito flakes are sold by weight. They have a mild seafood aroma and an intense flavour.

ORIGIN AND HISTORY *Katsuo-bushi* has been an important ingredient in Japanese cooking for many centuries, and bonito, in its dried form, has been used since the 15th century. It is interesting that such dark, unappealing meat, virtually impossible to eat fresh, should have achieved such importance in Japanese cuisine. For without the distinctive flavour of dried bonito, Japanese food would resemble much more that of its major neighbour, China.

ORIGIN AND HISTORY The coffee-coloured flakes are scraped from the rock-hard dried bonito fillets. The bonito is a variety of tuna. It is commonly found in the Mediterranean or on the Atlantic coast where French fishermen know it as *germon*.

BUYING AND STORAGE Packaged dried bonito flakes are known as *hana-katsuo* (literally 'flower bonito'), or *kezuri-bushi* ('shaved bonito fillets'). They should be firm and dry to the touch and a pale rose-pink to ochre colour. Also sold prepacked in infusion bags with seasoning for use as instant stock, under the name dashi no moto. Hon dashi, granules of katsuo-bushi and seasonings, is sold in small jars. It is an instantly dissolving stock which should be mixed with water in the ratio of 3–4 cups hot water to 1 teaspoon hon dashi.

Stocked by Japanese and some Asian food stores. Store in an airtight container in the freezer.

PREPARATION AND USE Dried and flaked bonito is a popular ingredient in oriental cooking, especially in Japan where the amount of bonito required for flavouring is simply scraped off and added to the dish.

Dashi stock is the base of many Japanese dishes, giving them the unique 'of the sea' flavour characteristic of Japanese cooking. Chicken or fish stock (broth) may be substituted, but at the loss of this special taste.

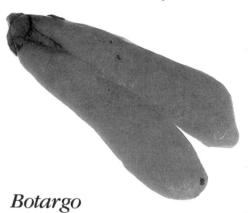

Botargo

*also called **Dried mullet roe, Bottarga, Avgotaraho***

NUTRITIONAL INFORMATION No reliable figures are available.

DESCRIPTION The salted and dried roe of the grey mullet. The roe come in pairs, as when taken from the fish. They are pale to deep amber in colour and elongated in shape. Flavour is pleasantly fishy but not salty; texture is slightly grainy. It tends to stick to the teeth, particularly if very dry.

ORIGIN AND HISTORY Prized for centuries in countries to the north of the Mediterranean, especially Sardinia and Greece. Also known in England in Samuel Pepys's day: his diary entry for 6 June 1661 states: 'We sat talking and singing and drinking great draughts of claret, and eating botargo and bread and butter until twelve at night.'

BUYING AND STORAGE Fishmongers and some delicatessens stock the dried roe. Look for roe with a medium to rich amber colour — a dark amber indicates 'drier' roe, preferred by connoisseurs. If vacuum-packed or wax-coated, leave intact and store in refrigerator; once cut, wrap in plastic and return to refrigerator. Will keep for several weeks.

PREPARATION AND USE Remove packag-

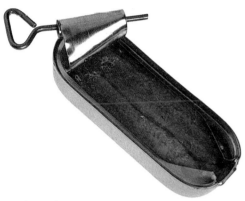

Anchovy, Canned

MAJOR NUTRIENTS		SERVE SIZE 12 G	
Energy	110 kJ	Cholesterol	10 mg
Protein	3 g	Sodium	660 mg
Fat	2 g	Phosphorus	60 mg
Carbohydrate	0		

NUTRITIONAL INFORMATION As these fish are normally eaten in very small amounts, they provide few nutrients. Large amounts of salt (sodium) and oil are added to the fillets in processing.

DESCRIPTION Anchovies are very small fish of the herring family, usually about 3 cm long for canning. They have a strong flavour, but if used sparingly are delicious. They are slightly oily.

ORIGIN AND HISTORY Anchovies are usually salted before being canned in oil. They can also be canned in brine or pickled.

BUYING AND STORAGE Canned anchovies are available worldwide. Shelf life of 12 months.

PREPARATION AND USE Anchovies can give a lift to many dishes without imparting a strong fishy taste. They can be added to meat as well as seafood, or used in vegetable, egg and pasta dishes. They can be used in canapés, in sauces, and rolled and stuffed on pizzas. When using anchovy paste or essence use sparingly.

ing and pull fine skin from portion to be sliced. If wax-coated, remove wax and skin from portion required. Slice thinly and serve with bread and butter or cracker biscuits as a snack or appetiser. Botargo may be used for making taramosalata.

PROCESSING At spawning time, the mullet are trapped and the roe removed intact. The pairs of roe are heavily salted, rinsed lightly, weighed, then air-dried for several days. Before refrigeration, drying had to be thorough so that the roe could keep for many months. When dry, they are coated with beeswax, but today vacuum packaging has replaced this method for most of the botargo prepared for retail sale.

SEE ALSO Tarama.

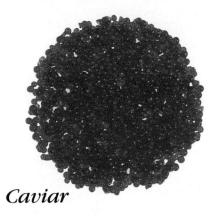

Caviar

MAJOR NUTRIENTS		SERVE SIZE 10 G	
Energy	50 kJ	Cholesterol	30 mg
Protein	2 g	Sodium	200 mg
Fat	1 g	Phosphorus	90 mg
Carbohydrate	0		

NUTRITIONAL INFORMATION As caviar is normally eaten in small amounts it provides few nutrients other than a large amount of sodium. When any fish roe is eaten in larger portions it will provide similar nutrients to soft herring roe.

DESCRIPTION Caviars come in a variety of sizes and colours. Sevruga is small grained and green-black. Osetra is larger grained and golden brown, bottle green or slate grey in colour. It can also be pale, almost bluish-white. Beluga is the largest and the best caviar and is grey in colour. It may be fresh, pasteurised or pressed.

ORIGIN AND HISTORY The most prolific source of caviar is Russia, mainly the Caspian Sea — and caviar seems to have remained a Russian delicacy until the Middle Ages, when it first appeared in Europe. It has remained highly favoured (and very expensive) ever since.

BUYING AND STORAGE Available in specialty shops around the world. Caviar can be kept 10–14 days in an airtight container in refrigerator.

PREPARATION AND USE By rights caviar should be eaten with small caviar spoons. Of course not everyone has these! Serve accompanied with sour cream and black bread, on canapés, as a garnish on seafood or simply as it is with a squeeze of lemon and a sprinkling of black pepper.

PROCESSING Caviar is processed by pouring it into cheesecloth bags and draining it of some of its liquid. The eggs are pressed in the process. A solid mass results, quite salty. 1 kg caviar will reduce to make 500 g when pressed.

VARIETIES

Fish that are used for commercial caviar production are the sevruga, osetra and the beluga. These are from the sturgeon family.

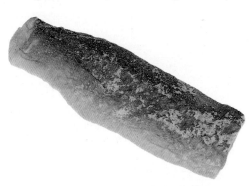

Cod, Dried and Salted

also called ***Bacalao, Bacalhau, Bakaliaros, Morue***

MAJOR NUTRIENTS		SOAKED, BOILED SERVE SIZE 100 G	
Energy	590 kJ	Sodium	400 mg
Protein	32 g	Phosphorus	160 mg
Fat	1 g	Magnesium	35 mg
Carbohydrate	0	Iron	1.8 mg
Cholesterol	40 mg	Niacin Equiv.	6 mg

NUTRITIONAL INFORMATION Note the very high sodium content.

DESCRIPTION Salted, dried fillets of the North Atlantic cod. Skin is left on, and the filleted side is creamy-yellow. It has a strong, somewhat fetid odour, but when properly prepared and cooked, it has a pleasant flavour and flaky texture. Much used in the cooking of Spain, Portugal, Greece and southern France, the alternative names above are of these languages respectively; as salt cod is more often to be found in these cuisines, the alternative names are more relevant.

ORIGIN AND HISTORY From the discovery of Newfoundland in 1497 by English navigator John Cabot, fishermen from England and France, followed by those from Spain and Portugal, used Newfoundland as a station for the rich fishing grounds in the region. The Basques of Spain and the Portuguese still head for these waters, spending six months of the year fishing for the prized cod, using mother ships as their bases. Once the fleets return, the fish are filleted, salted and dried on racks ready for local use and export.

Greece, France, and to a lesser extent Italy, depend on imports for salt cod, which was established in their traditional diet through the need for foods which could keep without refrigeration. Besides, it was a handy food to have for the fast days and 'fish' days of religious significance. The English also used salt cod a great deal for the same reasons, but eat it to a much lesser extent today.

BUYING AND STORAGE Purchase from stores stocking Hispanic, Greek and Italian foods. As the fillets are large, purchase by weight. Seal well in a plastic bag and store in the refrigerator or a cool place and use within 2 days of purchase, if only to eliminate its odour from the kitchen.

PREPARATION AND USE Cut fillet in pieces, rinse off excess salt and place in a bowl of cold water. Leave for 12–24 hours, changing water frequently. Drain and rinse pieces, then simmer in fresh water or milk for 15–20 minutes until flesh flakes easily. Remove skin and bones before completing dish.

Use for fish pies mixed with white sauce, for rich fish casseroles, stews and soups of Portuguese, Basque, French or Greek origin. Partially boiled, boned and skinned pieces of salt cod can be dipped in batter, fried and served with garlic sauce, or flaked and made into fritters.

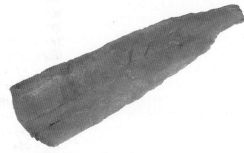

Cod, Smoked

MAJOR NUTRIENTS		SERVE SIZE 100 G	
Energy	330 kJ	Magnesium	25 mg
Protein	18 g	Phosphorus	190 mg
Fat	1 g	Iron	0.4 mg
Carbohydrate	0	Thiamin	0.1 mg
Cholesterol	40 mg	Niacin Equiv.	1.5 mg
Sodium	1170 mg		

NUTRITIONAL INFORMATION High salt content.

DESCRIPTION Smoked cod is a cold-smoked fish, readily available.

ORIGIN AND HISTORY See Cod, Dried and Salted.

BUYING AND STORAGE Keep in an airtight container (but not plastic wrap) in the refrigerator.

PREPARATION AND USE As it is cold-smoked, smoked cod must be cooked. It goes well with a white sauce or in fish pie.

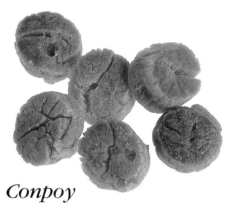

Conpoy

NUTRITIONAL INFORMATION No detailed analysis is available, but the data for the sea scallop suggest that conpoy is an excellent source of phosphorus, iron and niacin, and a good source of potassium and protein.

DESCRIPTION Amber discs of about 3 cm diameter and 1.5 cm thickness, conpoy are among the most expensive of Chinese ingredients, highly prized for their intense sea flavour. Conpoy comes from the long, cylindrical flesh of a sea scallop which the Chinese call ganbei. Never eaten fresh, as it is quite tough, it is cut into slices and sun-dried.

ORIGIN AND HISTORY Marco Polo noted during his stay in Hangchow, one of the great cities on the southeastern China coast, that among the proliferation of sea life served on the table were many kinds of shelled creatures, including a type of sea scallop. Its expense made conpoy a prized ingredient, to be featured in festive banquets and offered to the gods. During the Ch'ing dynasty which commenced in 1644, sea scallops on the menu heralded the coming of summer.

BUYING AND STORAGE Conpoy is always sold in dried form, and because it is costly, makes an impressive gift, ready packed in attractive gift wrapping. Dried conpoy can be kept for many months in a covered jar.

PREPARATION AND USE Conpoy must be soaked for up to 8 hours before using. It is steamed or simmered in a rich broth to be served alone at banquets, or added to braised and simmered dishes to enhance the flavour. A popular way of using conpoy is to deep-fry until crisp, crumble into shreds and scatter over braised or crisply fried green vegetables. It can be kept indefinitely in an airtight container in a cool dry cupboard.

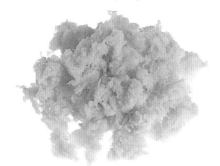

Crab, Canned

MAJOR NUTRIENTS		SERVE SIZE 100 G	
Energy	340 kJ	Calcium	120 mg
Protein	18 g	Phosphorus	140 mg
Fat	1 g	Magnesium	30 mg
Carbohydrate	0	Iron	2.8 mg
Cholesterol	100 mg	Zinc	5 mg
Sodium	550 mg	Niacin Equiv.	1 mg

NUTRITIONAL INFORMATION The canned crab is similar in nutritional value to fresh crab except for high level of salt (sodium) added in the processing.

DESCRIPTION Meat is fine to medium-flaked, white with tones of pink-red. Sweet flavour, although sometimes bland if quality is inferior.

ORIGIN AND HISTORY Most of the canned crabmeat comes from Asia.

BUYING AND STORAGE Canned crab is available worldwide. Shelf life of 12 months. Once opened store in refrigerator up to 24 hours.

PREPARATION AND USE Although canned crabmeat may be expensive it can be worthwhile in some recipes. There is no wastage and the meat needs no preparation. Add to salads, sauces, bread cases, vol-au-vent cases or dips. It can be a good extender for fresh seafood.

SEE ALSO Crab.

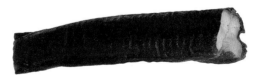

Eel, Smoked

NUTRITIONAL INFORMATION Major nutrients similar to eel except contains large amounts of sodium. For nutritional information see Eel.

DESCRIPTION The eel is a long, thin, dark fish. The pale flesh is densely textured and very oily and rich.

ORIGIN AND HISTORY Eel are smoked worldwide. Some consider smoked eel more delicious than smoked salmon.

BUYING AND STORAGE Look for firm skin and a pleasant smoky smell. Available in cutlet form, or whole. Wrap in foil or store in airtight container. Do not wrap in plastic wrap as it sweats. Keep in refrigerator for 7–10 days.

PREPARATION AND USE Skin eel cutlets. Serve as a starter or entrée. Accompany with sour cream, horseradish sauce or mayonnaise, and mild, fresh herbs.

SEE ALSO Eel, and other smoked fish.

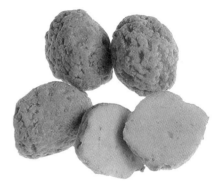

Fish Ball, Chinese

MAJOR NUTRIENTS		STEAMED SERVE SIZE 100 G	
Energy	220 kJ	Sodium	745 mg
Protein	12 g	Potassium	110 mg
Fat	1 g	Niacin Equiv.	3 mg
Carbohydrate	0	Vitamin A	N/A
Cholesterol	0	Vitamin C	N/A
Dietary Fibre	0		

NUTRITIONAL INFORMATION Fish balls are an excellent source of vitamin B12 and a good source of niacin. They also contain copper, and a large amount of sodium. The fat is predominantly polyunsaturated, and a high proportion of this is omega-3 fatty acids.

DESCRIPTION A small, round ball made from finely pulverised fish, or other seafood such as crab, prawns or scallops.

ORIGIN AND HISTORY Coastal southern China is the region where fish ball making was perfected. It required a technique whereby the flesh remained tender but the ball was sufficiently firmly packed to retain its shape when cooked. The pulverised meat is squeezed through furled index finger and thumb, and then scooped in a perfect ball into simmering liquid to cook. Chiu Chou Chinese in Fukien province particularly favour crab fish balls served with a sauce peculiar to this region (which is famed for its soya sauce factories) — a thick sweet rice soy flavoured with molasses or maltose.

BUYING AND STORAGE Sold singly in some Chinese delicatessens, or in plastic packs or tubs. Can be kept in the refrigerator for several days, or may be frozen.

PREPARATION AND USE Used in Chinese cooking, in particular soups. Precooked, they need only to be reheated, or may be fried or grilled, and are usually scored with a cross on the surface before cooking in this way to prevent cracking.

PROCESSING Finely minced fish meat with seasonings and, perhaps, a binder of cornflour or egg white, kneaded and pulverised until formed into a homogeneous mass. They are formed into balls and are simmered in lightly salted water, drained and cooled, then packed into plastic bags and sold fresh or frozen.

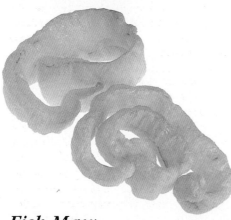

Fish Maw

NUTRITIONAL INFORMATION No detailed data are available.

DESCRIPTION A gelatinous white membrane removed from the stomach of certain very large fish. When dried, it resembles a cream-coloured polyurethane foam sheet. It is actually the air bladder, usually of the conger pike, which is a balloon-like organ used by the fish as a pressure regulator.

ORIGIN AND HISTORY Maw is prized in Chinese cooking for its subtle seafood flavour and its soft and slightly chewy texture. It has virtually no flavour — although it readily absorbs accompanying flavours — and has a texture that is spongy by contrast with the agreeable crunch of, say, dried jellyfish skin.

BUYING AND STORAGE Sold by the piece in Chinese delicatessens, maw is usually on

display hanging on racks above the counter as it is too large to store elsewhere. Store in very dry conditions.

PREPARATION AND USE The dried sheets should be soaked in warm water until softened, then drained and rinsed in clean water. Scrape any apparent impurities from the surface, and then cut into pieces. Maw requires only a few minutes' cooking in water slightly acidulated with white vinegar, and is usually cooked separately. It should be drained and the cooking liquid squeezed out before adding to the dish in the final stages of cooking. Do not overcook or it will become chewy, and then break up into a gelatinous mass.

PROCESSING Fish maw is rinsed thoroughly, air dried and then deep fried, which causes it to blow up into its bulky state.

VARIETIES
Pike maw, fried conger pike maw.

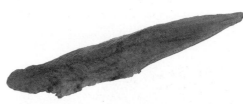

Haddock, Smoked

MAJOR NUTRIENTS		SERVE SIZE 100 G	
Energy	430 kJ	Phosphorus	250 mg
Protein	23 g	Magnesium	25 mg
Fat	1 g	Iron	1 mg
Carbohydrate	0	Thiamin B1	0.1 mg
Cholesterol	60 mg	Riboflavin B2	0.1 mg
Sodium	1220 mg	Niacin Equiv.	1.5 mg
Calcium	60 mg		

NUTRITIONAL INFORMATION For general comments, see the introduction to this section.

DESCRIPTION The flesh is white and has a mild smoky flavour. The skin is a beautiful orange colour.

ORIGIN AND HISTORY A great deal of haddock is smoked. It is available worldwide.

BUYING AND STORAGE Look for firm flesh, with a pleasant smoky smell. Wrap in foil or store in airtight container and keep in refrigerator for 7–10 days. Do not wrap in plastic wrap as the fish sweats.

PREPARATION AND USE Wash fillets thoroughly. Poach, steam, bake, gently fry or barbecue. Use mild flavourings to complement this fish.

PROCESSING The fish is salted, hung and then smoked for 24 hours.

SEE ALSO Other smoked fish.

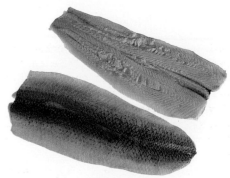

Herring, Matjes

NUTRITIONAL INFORMATION Similar to fresh herring, but with a high sodium content.

DESCRIPTION Matjes are salted herrings. They have pink, translucent, slippery flesh and an excellent flavour.

ORIGIN AND HISTORY Matjes are the best salted herrings. Fat female fish are used and are only slightly salted.

BUYING AND STORAGE Available from good fish retailers and delicatessens in Europe and America. To store, wrap in foil or put in airtight container. Keep in refrigerator for 7–10 days.

PREPARATION AND USE Matjes herrings do not need to be soaked like some strongly salted smoked fish. Poach, grill or gently steam, and serve with delicate flavourings.

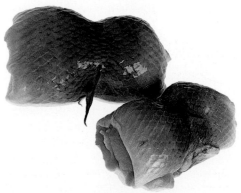

Herring, Rollmop

NUTRITIONAL INFORMATION Major nutrients similar to raw herring except contains large amounts of sodium. For nutritional information see Herring, Fresh.

DESCRIPTION Rollmop herrings are herrings that are boned lengthways, halved, rolled tightly around peppercorns and slices of onion and fastened with a wooden skewer before being put into jars to which is added hot spiced white vinegar. They may be wrapped around a gherkin or pickled cucumber.

ORIGIN AND HISTORY Rollmops originated in Europe and are particularly popular in Scandinavian countries. They can be easily made in Europe, where the appropriate herring is available. In Australia the best substitute is the garfish, although the flesh is a little softer than the European herring.

BUYING AND STORAGE Rollmops pickled in jars are readily available in most countries. Once opened store in refrigerator. Keep 2–3 months.

PREPARATION AND USE If using ready prepared rollmops, eat as they are. If making your own, clean and fillet the herrings and flatten, skin side down. Cover each fillet with a mixture of chopped gherkins, shallots and capers. Roll up from the tail, skewer with a toothpick and place in a glass jar. Pour over a spiced vinegar and leave in the refrigerator for 4 days before using.

SEE ALSO Herring.

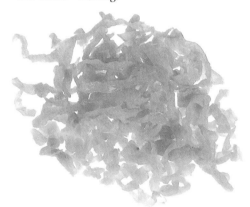

Jellyfish, Dried *Callinema ornata, Rhopilema eculenta*

NUTRITIONAL INFORMATION No specific data are available, but this food is high in salt.

DESCRIPTION Found worldwide, the jellyfish has a transparent, saucer-shaped body (umbrella), on the lower side of which is its mouth. It swims by relaxation and contraction of the umbrella. In spite of its bulk the tissues are composed mostly of water so that, when it is dried, very little solid matter is left. It has a distinctive flavour and texture — it remains soft on the outside and quite crunchy on the inside.

The salted and sundried skin of the marine jellyfish is a popular ingredient of Chinese cooking. In its dry state the thin golden top skin resembles a large disc of semi-transparent plastic. Although it has virtually no taste, it is enjoyed for its crunchy texture.

ORIGIN AND HISTORY There are very few creatures for which the Chinese have not devised a culinary use. The jellyfish, bane of swimmers and fishermen, is a delicacy to Chinese gourmets, who are addicted to foods with an interesting 'crunch'. The Chinese also

find it beneficial in lowering the blood pressure and keeping the bones supple.

BUYING AND STORAGE Jellyfish is available dried and salted, in sheets or precut into thin shreds. It can be kept indefinitely, but as with all dried Asian products, moisture is the enemy. Store in a dark cool place for up to 6 months.

PREPARATION AND USE Jellyfish must be soaked in several changes of cold water for several hours. Sometimes it can be bought already presoaked. Jellyfish does not have to be cooked; after soaking, it should be marinated for a short while in warm water or stock, with ginger, onion and Chinese rice wine. Do not use boiling water as the jellyfish will shrink and toughen.

Usually served cold in the form of a salad served as an appetiser, or as a snack with Chinese wine. Sesame oil is the preferred dressing for jellyfish salad. Alternatively, cut into slivers and either stir-fry, barbecue or grill. These methods produce curls which have a crunchy texture.

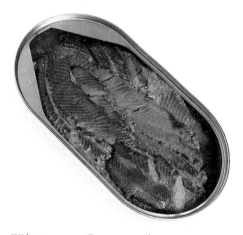

Kipper, Canned

NUTRITIONAL INFORMATION The major nutrients are similar to those of herring.

DESCRIPTION Soft, moist, filleted flesh with a strong flavour.

ORIGIN AND HISTORY Kippers are in fact herrings: 'kippering' is the name given to the process by which some herrings are smoked.

BUYING AND STORAGE Available canned, mostly in Europe and America. Available in some specialty shops in Australia. Store in a cool dark place. Recommended storage life 12 months.

PREPARATION AND USE The flesh is soft so grill carefully. Otherwise eat as they are. Accompany with lemon wedges, bread and butter.

SEE ALSO Other smoked seafood; Herring.

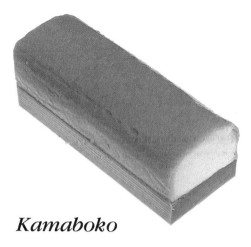

Kamaboko

MAJOR NUTRIENTS		STEAMED SERVE SIZE 100 G	
Energy	220 kJ	Sodium	745 mg
Protein	12 g	Potassium	110 mg
Fat	1 g	Niacin Equiv.	3 mg
Carbohydrate	0	Vitamin A	N/A
Cholesterol	0	Vitamin C	N/A
Dietary Fibre	0		

NUTRITIONAL INFORMATION Kamaboko is an excellent source of vitamin B12 and a good source of niacin. It also contains copper and a large amount of sodium. The data for carbohydrate depend on the amount of flour, corn starch or potato starch and the Japanese kuzu starch that is used in the preparation. Kamaboko is a high protein food. The fat is predominantly polyunsaturated and a high proportion of this is omega-3 fatty acids.

DESCRIPTION An important Japanese cooking ingredient, kamaboko is a processed fish cake with a smooth, firm, slightly rubbery texture similar to that of processed sausage.

ORIGIN AND HISTORY The Japanese first made chikuwa, a type of kamaboko, in the 14th century: the name kamaboko is in fact the medieval word for 'cat tail'. Ita-kamaboko is kamaboko moulded onto a slip of cypress wood before steaming, giving it a distinctive woody aroma.

ORIGIN AND HISTORY A fish paste made in Japan. The most familiar type of kamaboko is moulded into a Nissen-hut shape, tinted pink or light green, and placed in a small piece of cypress wood. It is an important part of oden (fish hot pot), a dish served at New Year celebrations.

BUYING AND STORAGE Sold in specialist Japanese food stores which stock perishable items, packed in vacuum-sealed plastic wrap. Will keep in the refrigerator for several weeks, before opening, and up to a week afterwards.

PREPARATION AND USE Slice and serve hot or cold, with or without a dipping sauce. Served in soups and sometimes with wasabi.

PROCESSING Made from pounded fish meat

(cod or shark) bound with potato starch or the Japanese kuzu, a starch derived from a wild native vine. The fish paste is formed into various shapes — most common being a flat loaf of about 15 cm length — and steamed. Variations in processing include painting the surface with food colourings, usually crab-shell pink-red, or grilling the surface so that it turns a rich golden brown.

VARIETIES
Ita-kamaboko, chikawa kamaboko.

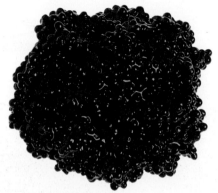

Lumpfish Roe

NUTRITIONAL INFORMATION Major nutrients similar to caviar.

DESCRIPTION Red or black eggs of the Arctic lumpfish. Has a pleasant fishy flavour and an appealing appearance, since the normally pale eggs are dyed red or black for commercial sale.

ORIGIN AND HISTORY Lumpfish roe has long been a favoured substitute for the more expensive caviar.

BUYING AND STORAGE Available in jars or cans worldwide. Once opened, store in refrigerator and use within 2 months.

PREPARATION AND USE Because of the colourings in lumpfish roe it is best to drain the roe on a slice of bread to prevent the colour running across canapés, other seafood, etc. Use lumpfish roe as is as a garnish, or mash with sour cream and grated onion and serve with black bread.

PROCESSING The roe is salted, coloured and pressed.

VARIETIES
Sold as German or Danish caviar.

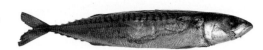

Mackerel, Smoked

NUTRITIONAL INFORMATION Major nutrients similar to mackerel except contains large amount of sodium.

DESCRIPTION Silver on top of the fish and gold on the bottom. A firm, slightly fatty, smoked fish with a strong flavour. This fish is usually hot-smoked so can therefore be eaten without cooking.

ORIGIN AND HISTORY These fish are smoked worldwide.

BUYING AND STORAGE Look for firm flesh, not sweaty and with a pleasant smoky smell. Wrap in foil or place in an airtight container. Keeps in refrigerator for 7–10 days.

PREPARATION AND USE Skin fish and eat as is. Suits mild flavourings and accompaniments such as sour cream, mayonnaise.

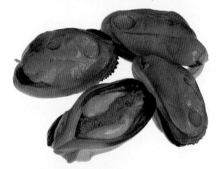

Mussel, Canned

NUTRITIONAL INFORMATION Similar in nutritional value to fresh mussel except may be higher in oil and sodium, depending on canning liquid. For nutritional information see Mussel.

DESCRIPTION Mussels are usually canned in oil. Their shape is retained, although their texture becomes softer. They have a distinctive flavour.

ORIGIN AND HISTORY Most mussels are canned in Asia.

BUYING AND STORAGE Canned mussels are sold throughout the world and come in a variety of forms, smoked, in oil, in barbecue sauce, in tomato sauce, etc. Store can in cool, dark place. Recommended storage life 12 months. Once opened eat within 24 hours.

PREPARATION AND USE Mussels are mainly used straight from the can for hors d'oeuvres; however, they can be gently grilled on kebab sticks with fresh seafood or added to sauces (for example, a rich tomato sauce for pasta).

SEE ALSO Mussels, Fresh.

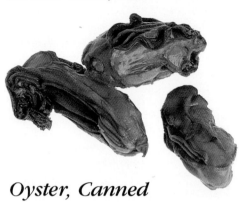

Oyster, Canned

NUTRITIONAL INFORMATION Fat content varies depending on liquid used in canning. Canned oysters are similar in nutritional value to fresh oysters except for high levels of salt (sodium) added during processing.

DESCRIPTION Once canned, oysters retain their shape but take on a distinct fishy flavour.

ORIGIN AND HISTORY Canned oysters come mainly from Asia.

BUYING AND STORAGE Sold throughout the world, canned oysters come in a variety of forms — smoked, in oil, in barbecue or in tomato sauce, etc. Store in cool, dark place. Recommended storage life 12 months.

PREPARATION AND USE Used straight from can. Suitable for savouries, vol-au-vent cases, bread cases, etc. They can be used in sauces, pies or stuffings.

SEE ALSO Oysters, Fresh.

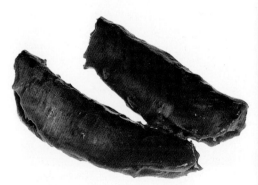

Pilchard, Canned

MAJOR NUTRIENTS			SERVE SIZE 100 G
Energy	530 kJ	Calcium	300 mg
Protein	19 g	Phosphorus	350 mg
Fat	5 g	Magnesium	40 mg
Carbohydrate	1 g	Iron	2.7 mg
Cholesterol	70 mg	Zinc	1.6 mg
Sodium	370 mg	Riboflavin	0.3 mg
Potassium	420 mg	Niacin Equiv.	7.6 mg

NUTRITIONAL INFORMATION Canned pilchards contain high levels of salt (sodium) added in processing.

DESCRIPTION Pilchards are canned in fillet form. The flesh is soft with a strong flavour. Usually available in a sauce.

ORIGIN AND HISTORY These fish are canned in Asian countries and some European countries.

BUYING AND STORAGE Canned pilchards are available worldwide. The cans should be stored in a cool, dark place. Shelf life of 12 months.

PREPARATION AND USE Pilchards are a little bigger than sardines but are less flavoursome. They can be eaten straight from the can, either hot or cold. Their flavour is enhanced by the accompanying sauce.

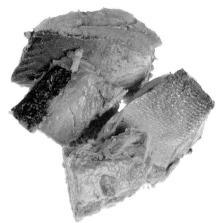

Salmon, Canned

MAJOR NUTRIENTS			SERVE SIZE 100 G
Energy	650 kJ	Phosphorus	240 mg
Protein	20 g	Magnesium	30 mg
Fat	8 g	Iron	1.4 mg
Carbohydrate	0	Zinc	0.9 mg
Cholesterol	90 mg	Vitamin A	90 µg
Sodium	570 mg	Riboflavin	0.2 mg
Calcium	93 mg	Niacin Equiv.	7 mg

NUTRITIONAL INFORMATION Salt free (no added sodium) varieties are available.

DESCRIPTION Salmon is the most popular fish for canning, giving a salty, pink flesh and edible bones.

ORIGIN AND HISTORY Canning factories on the coasts of the USA supply a high proportion of the world's market for canned salmon.

BUYING AND STORAGE Readily available and will store for long periods.

PREPARATION AND USE Salmon from a can is usually eaten cold, often with or in salad. The flesh may be mashed and added to soups and soufflés.

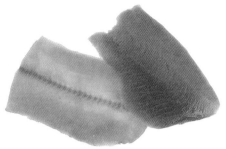

Salmon, Smoked

MAJOR NUTRIENTS			SERVE SIZE 100 G
Energy	600 kJ	Phosphorus	250 mg
Protein	25 g	Magnesium	30 mg
Fat	4 g	Iron	0.6 mg
Carbohydrate	0	Thiamin	0.15 mg
Cholesterol	70 mg	Riboflavin	0.15 mg
Sodium	1880 mg	Niacin Equiv.	9 mg
Potassium	420 mg		

NUTRITIONAL INFORMATION Has nutrients similar to those of the fresh fish, except for sodium.

DESCRIPTION Smoked salmon when purchased by the side or in slices is a beautiful pink–orange, with moist flesh, a mild smoky smell and a delicate flavour.

ORIGIN AND HISTORY There is much debate where the best smoked salmon comes from — Scotland, Norway or Canada. Who knows? It's all delicious. The traditional Scottish way of kippering salmon involves brining of boned slices of salmon, wiping, drying, oiling and then covering them in brown sugar. Other methods are soaking in whisky or olive oil and then smoking over a fire of peat and oak chips.

BUYING AND STORAGE Available in sides or sliced. Mostly smoked salmon is vacuum packed. Store in refrigerator up to 10 days once opened.

PREPARATION AND USE Smoked salmon can be eaten as purchased. It requires no preparation. Can be used for hors d'oeuvres, entrées, sandwiches. Serve with lemon wedges, bread and butter. Accompany with sour cream with mild herbs, such as dill, or mayonnaise. The Jewish people serve smoked salmon with bagels and cream cheese.

SEE ALSO Other smoked fish; Salmon.

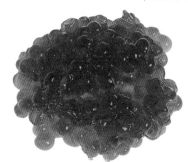

Salmon Roe

*also called **Keta-red caviar***

NUTRITIONAL INFORMATION For major nutrients and nutritional information refer to Caviar.

DESCRIPTION Bright orange in colour and large-grained.

ORIGIN AND HISTORY Not as expensive as other caviars, it has a very pleasant fresh flavour that is slightly bitter compared to other varieties.

BUYING AND STORAGE Available in cans or vacuum packed. Keeps for 10–14 days once opened.

PREPARATION AND USE Salmon roe can be eaten as it is or used on canapés, served with sour cream and black bread, or as a garnish on other seafood.

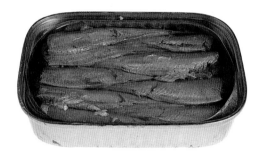

Sardine, Canned

MAJOR NUTRIENTS			SERVE SIZE 100 G
Energy	910 kJ	Calcium	550 mg
Protein	24 g	Phosphorus	520 mg
Fat	14 g	Magnesium	50 mg
Carbohydrate	0	Iron	3 mg
Cholesterol	100 mg	Zinc	3 mg
Sodium	650 mg	Riboflavin	0.35 mg
Potassium	430 mg	Niacin Equiv.	8 mg

NUTRITIONAL INFORMATION Salt-free (no added sodium) varieties are available.

DESCRIPTION Sardines are small silver fish belonging to the herring family. When canned they have a strong fishy flavour and are soft but good to eat. They are generally canned in olive oil, peanut oil, cottonseed oil or tomato sauce.

ORIGIN AND HISTORY The sardine canning industry developed in France in the 19th century as a result of two circumstances. First, the fishermen of southern Brittany evolved, for their own consumption, a method of preserving their sardines which produced something more delicate than the primitive dried cod. They cooked sardines in butter or olive oil, then packed them in clay jars sealed with more oil or butter. The delicacy became known to wealthy shipbuilders and merchants who saw the possibilities of applying this local method to the canning process which was then being developed. By 1824 a sardine canning factory had been established in Nantes, France. Olive oil soon proved to be a better preserving agent than butter. For over 50 years sardine canning remained a French monopoly. It was not until the 1880s that competition came from Spanish, Portuguese and American canners, using cheaper processing and inferior grades of fish (often not even sardines). By 1912 the French were taking action to protect the industry from misrepresentation, but the only concession they obtained was that the place of origin of the canned fish be stated on labels.

BUYING AND STORAGE Canned sardines are available worldwide. They come either in oil or in a sauce such as tomato. Shelf life 12 months.

PREPARATION AND USE Sardines can be used straight from the can. They can be spread (mashed) on toast and served as a snack or used in sandwiches and savouries. Sardines can be eaten whole, bones and all. Accompany with lemon or vinegar and bread and butter.

PROCESSING It is worth mentioning the process for canning: Sardines are gently brined, then dried and lightly cooked in olive oil (or other), and stored for about a year, so that the flavour of fish and oil are mingled.

VARIETIES

French, Portuguese, Spanish, English, American.

SEE ALSO Sardine.

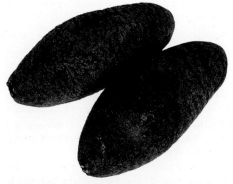

Sea Cucumber Class Holothuroidea

*also called **Bêche-de-mer, Hoy sum***

MAJOR NUTRIENTS		DRIED, SOAKED SERVE SIZE 100 G	
Energy	370 kJ	Sodium	N/A
Protein	19 g	Calcium	70 mg
Fat	0	Iron	9.2 mg
Carbohydrate	1 g	Vitamin A	100 μg
Cholesterol	N/A		

NUTRITIONAL INFORMATION Sea cucumbers provide an excellent source of protein and iron and a good source of calcium and vitamin A.

DESCRIPTION A marine animal without a shell. It is highly regarded in China for its delicate taste and interesting, crunchy-soft texture, and for its reputed qualities as an aphrodisiac. It is grey-black in colour, about 17 cm long and tapering towards both ends. It is called the sea cucumber because of its resemblance to a type of spiny wild cucumber.

ORIGIN AND HISTORY Its unaesthetic appearance has not prevented it from becoming a much sought after ingredient in Chinese cooking. Medicinally it is 'warm and restorative' and has a high protein content. Its phallic shape and the fact that the live animal swells when touched have earned it its reputation for improving a male's sexual vigour. It is not a common ingredient in other parts of Asia, and Chinese fishermen have been known to usurp foreign fishing rights as far away as the Pacific Islands in search of this prize. Like many of the expensive dried Chinese products — particularly mushrooms and birds' nests — sea cucumbers have over the centuries been the merchandise of thieves and black marketeers.

BUYING AND STORAGE Sea cucumbers are occasionally available fresh, but more usually sold in dried form. They must be soaked for several hours until softened. If dried whole, the stomach and its surrounding yellow membrane must be removed before cooking. They are cooked by steaming, simmering in a rich stock, or braising. Because they have little flavour of their own, sea cucumbers readily absorb seasonings, and are usually cooked with strong seasonings such as garlic, chilli, ginger and bean sauces.

PROCESSING The fresh animals are thoroughly cleaned, then sun dried.

Seaweed

MAJOR NUTRIENTS		SERVE SIZE 10 G	
Energy	130 kJ	Cholesterol	0
Protein	0	Sodium	N/A
Fat	0	Calcium	75 mg
Carbohydrate	8 g	Iron	0.8 mg

NUTRITIONAL INFORMATION The value of seaweed in an Asian-style diet is as a rich source of many minerals including calcium and iron. Seaweed is an excellent source of iodine and a good source of a wide variety of minerals — zinc, manganese, nickel, molybdenum, selenium, copper, cobalt and chromium. The mineral content of seaweed can vary with location, and it may contain excessive quantities of the poison arsenic. The amount of iodine present in 1 teaspoon of typical seaweed is 15 times the recommended daily intake. Large amounts of iodine taken regularly may cause goitre.

The chief carbohydrates in seaweeds are mannitol and polyssaccharides alginic acid and laminarin. Agar and alginic acid derived from the seaweeds are used to alter the texture and consistency of foods, especially in jelly making. Seaweeds are known to contain less than 1% fat.

DESCRIPTION There are a number of edible seaweeds used worldwide.

ORIGIN AND HISTORY These vary widely according to the type of seaweed. See the varieties below.

BUYING AND STORAGE Dried seaweed keeps indefinitely.

PREPARATION AND USE See the varieties below.

VARIETIES

Carrageen

NUTRITIONAL INFORMATION See above.

DESCRIPTION Also called Irish moss, Iberian moss, pear or sea moss and ling-bye, carrageen (*Chondrus crispus*) is a gelatinous seaweed, purplish-brown or reddish-green in colour.

ORIGIN AND HISTORY Carrageen is found along the coasts of Europe and North America. It derives its name from the village of Carragheen in Ireland.

BUYING AND STORAGE Carrageen is found in health food shops. Keeps indefinitely.

PREPARATION AND USE Needs to be softened in water or milk for at least 2 hours before use. Used as a substitute for isinglass (itself made from fish bladders) and gelatine to make jellies, blancmanges, moulds and aspics.

PROCESSING Dried.

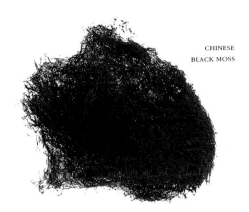

CHINESE
BLACK MOSS

Chinese Black Moss

NUTRITIONAL INFORMATION See above.

DESCRIPTION *Gracilaria verrucosa*, also called Fa ts'ai or hair vegetable, is a dried, edible seaweed used in Chinese cooking. It resembles a bundle of black hair, hence the common name 'hair vegetable'. The thin black strands have no distinct taste or texture.

ORIGIN AND HISTORY Commonly used at Chinese New Year because its Chinese name of fa ts'ai (fat choy in Cantonese) has auspicious connotations. It translates as 'prosperity' and is part of the Chinese New Year greeting, 'Kung hei fat choy'. It is considered cooling and cleansing to the system.

BUYING AND STORAGE Sold in small cellophane packs. It keeps well in dry conditions.

PREPARATION AND USE It should be soaked in several changes of cold water. Black moss is cooked with a butt of pork in a rich tasting Chinese New Year specialty dish.

It may be deep fried, and is occasionally used to make edible baskets for stir-fried ingredients, being cooked in a special double layered frying basket which forms it into its bowl-like shape.

Dulse

NUTRITIONAL INFORMATION Dulse is a typical seaweed.

DESCRIPTION *Rhodymenia palmata*, also known as dillisk, algue rouge, rodsallat, sol and soluum, is a coarse, red seaweed with broad leaves, which grow to about 30 cm in length. There is also a species, *Laurencia pinnatifida*, known as pepper dulse.

ORIGIN AND HISTORY Principally eaten by people of northern countries, in particular Scotland, Ireland and Iceland. Gathered on both sides of the North Atlantic and harvested commercially in the USA and Canada.

BUYING AND STORAGE Usually sold in dry form, either in sheets or shredded. Available at specialty shops. Keeps indefinitely.

PREPARATION AND USE Used as a vegetable, raw in salads and added to flavour

soups. In Ireland it is chewed as one would chew tobacco.

PROCESSING Dried.

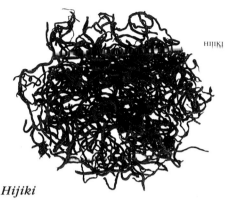

HIJIKI

Hijiki

NUTRITIONAL INFORMATION No specific data are available.

DESCRIPTION *Cystophyllum fusiforme*, also called bladder leaf seaweed, becomes short thin sticks of black seaweed when dried, resembling coarse black tea.

BUYING AND STORAGE Sold in small cellophane or plastic packs and can be kept unopened for many weeks in dry conditions. Once opened, transfer unused portion to a tightly sealed glass container.

PREPARATION AND USE This should be soaked for at least 15 minutes before use, and will expand to about three times its size. Cooked by simmering in stock or water and used in Japanese boiled dishes, and in combination with vegetables, seafood and chicken as a simple appetiser. Makes an interesting garnish for warm salads.

Kelp

NUTRITIONAL INFORMATION Kelp is a good source of iodine.

DESCRIPTION Any of the large brown seaweeds with thick leaves, sometimes ribbonlike.

ORIGIN AND HISTORY Kelp is possibly the oldest crop known. The Romans, Greeks and Chinese used it as a food, medicine and fertiliser, and Pliny the Elder praised its virtues in his book *Natural History* in the first century AD.

In the Pacific Northwest, Americans prepare kelp in a special way. The hollow middle ribs are peeled, cut into slices and pickled in a sweet-and-sour liquid containing vinegar, sugar and various spices.

In Japan, kelp is processed by a complicated series of dryings, boilings and compressions, to make kombu.

In Ireland, it is boiled for a long time until

it has been reduced to a sort of thick green gruel, which is then served with mutton.

BUYING AND STORAGE Available in tablet, granular and powder form, kelp will keep for some time if stored in a dry cool place.

PREPARATION AND USE Powdered kelp may be added in very small quantities to stews and casseroles and sprinkled on salads in place of salt. Commercially, kelp is added to ice cream, prepared desserts and salad dressings.

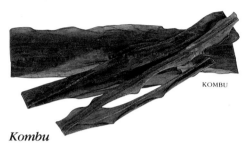

KOMBU

Kombu

MAJOR NUTRIENTS		SERVE SIZE 100 G	
Energy	N/A	Dietary Fibre	7 g
Protein	N/A	Sodium	3010 mg
Fat	1 g	Potassium	5275 mg
Carbohydrate	N/A	Calcium	1095 mg
Cholesterol	0	Phosphorus	240 mg

NUTRITIONAL INFORMATION Kombu is an excellent source of calcium and phosphorus. It contains a large amount of sodium and potassium and is a rich source of iodine.

DESCRIPTION *Laminaria japonica* is a wide-leafed, ribbon-like kelp, found mainly in Japan. It is deep olive brown to grey-black in colour, ranges from 6–30 cm in width and is very long.

ORIGIN AND HISTORY A vital ingredient in Japanese cooking, kombu or konbu is mainly harvested off the northernmost Japanese island of Hokkaido. Some of the oldest paintings and writing surviving today illustrate seaweed gathering as an ancient occupation. From early times, it was known that seaweed was a natural source of many valuable dietary minerals.

Tororo and oboro konbu are other varieties of kombu used in cooking. The former is shaved along the length of the kelp and is sold in shred form, the latter is shaved across and comes in thin sheets. What remains is known as shiraita kombu, beige coloured and as fine as silk. It is folded into small squares and packed in cellophane.

BUYING AND STORAGE Sold in bundles of folded sheets, or narrow strips. They should be stored in very dry conditions and will keep for many months. In moist climates, transfer the kelp to an airtight glass jar and keep in a cool, dry cupboard away from light.

PREPARATION AND USE Dried kombu develops a fine speckling of salt over the surface. This should be removed before use by wiping with a clean damp cloth. Do not wash. It can be lightly scored with a sharp knife to release its flavour. One piece of kombu can be used several times to make stock, the intensity of its flavour diminishing with each use.

Kombu is one of the most important ingredients in Japanese cooking. In combination with shaved dried bonito (katsuo-bushi) it gives a characteristic 'of the sea' flavour to many dishes, is used to flavour stock for soup and sauces, or may be crumbled over hot rice. It can also be deep fried or sautéed as a vegetable. To make dashi stock use a piece of kombu of about 25 g with 4–5 cups water. Bring to the boil and simmer gently for a few minutes. Add a handful of katsuo-bushi. Cool. The kelp can then be removed, dried and kept for a further use.

Kombu is used extensively in Korean cooking, particularly in full flavoured soups, often fiercely hot from chilli.

PROCESSING It is sun-dried, then the leaves are cut into usable sizes which are generally about 30 cm long and 6 to 10 cm in width. They are folded and packed in cellophane or plastic bags.

SEE ALSO Bonito Flakes, Kelp.

Mekabu

NUTRITIONAL INFORMATION A typical seaweed in its nutrient value.

DESCRIPTION Mekabu is a lobe-leaf seaweed, usually dried in curled strands.

ORIGIN AND HISTORY Used mainly in Japanese cooking.

BUYING AND STORAGE Available dried in specialty shops. Keeps indefinitely.

PREPARATION AND USE Mainly used in soups and salads, and as a garnish.

PROCESSING Dried.

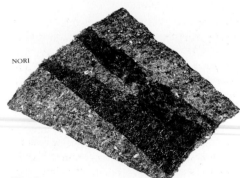

NORI

Nori

NUTRITIONAL INFORMATION Nutritionally, nori is a typical seaweed.

DESCRIPTION A species of the *Porphyra* genus of red algae, it ranges from bright deep green to a dull purple in colour. Nori is gathered from the ocean in cooler parts of Europe and in Japan, where it is cultivated by means of bamboo stakes placed in the sheltered waters off Tokyo Bay, the seaweed attaching itself to the stakes from which it can be easily harvested. Called tsu ts'ai in Chinese, it is gathered off the coasts of northern China, where it is usually a deep purple in colour, and around Korea. It is generally agreed that the brightest green nori has the best flavour. Known in Japan as asakusa nori, or commonly as nori, it is called keem in Korea.

ORIGIN AND HISTORY An ingredient used since ancient times, nori must be kept absolutely dry or it will mildew, spoiling its delicate flavour. Beautifully formed wooden boxes and intricately painted metal and lacquered wood boxes used for storing nori are delightful acquisitions, the better ones being collectors' items.

BUYING AND STORAGE Sold in packs of flat square sheets or discs, usually about eight to a pack. Store away from moisture in an airtight container.

PREPARATION AND USE Nori can be used fresh in stewed dishes and soups, but in Asia it is most commonly used in its dried compressed sheet form. In Japan nori is used as an edible wrapper for several types of sushi, or rice cakes. In Japan and in Korea and northern China, it is cut into fine shreds to scatter as a garnish over soups, rice dishes and noodles. It lends a refreshing flavour of the ocean and an interesting crisp texture. Sheet nori should be crisped by holding briefly over a flame before use. Nori cut into fine shreds is an important ingredient in many Japanese condiment mixtures.

PROCESSING The frothy alga is laid on bamboo trays to sun dry, then is compressed into thin sheets or discs by rolling. Sheets are cut into squares of about 23 cm and packed in cellophane.

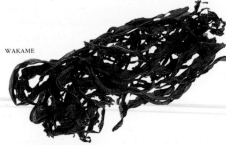

WAKAME

Wakame

NUTRITIONAL INFORMATION Wakame is a typical seaweed in its nutrient value.

DESCRIPTION *Undaria pinnatifida* is a deep green, curly-leafed seaweed of the brown algae group, known also as lobe-leaf seaweed or salad seaweed. It has a fresh taste of the sea. When dry, the seaweed strands are almost black in colour, resembling Chinese black fungus. After soaking, it expands dramatically and becomes green.

ORIGIN AND HISTORY A typical seaweed, wakame is low in kilojoules — the perfect dieters' food. It is therefore always popular with Japanese women, being excellent for both the complexion and the figure.

BUYING AND STORAGE Sold at oriental food stores in small packs, a little goes a long way. Store in an airtight jar. Dry, it will keep indefinitely.

PREPARATION AND USE Used extensively in Japanese cooking, often as a salad ingredient, and also in Korean and northern Chinese cooking in soups and simmered dishes. The hard central spine should be cut away as it will not soften during cooking. Wakame should be cooked only briefly so as to retain both its flavour and its valuable minerals. Soften wakame in cold water, drain and then simmer for no more than a few minutes in boiling water or dashi stock. Drain. Serve as a salad with a vinegar dressing, or add to soups or other dishes in the final few minutes of cooking.

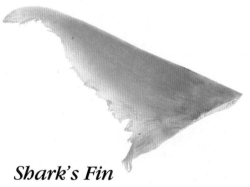

Shark's Fin

also called **Yu chee**

MAJOR NUTRIENTS		SERVE SIZE 20 G	
Energy	305 kJ	Carbohydrate	0
Protein	17 g	Iron	2 g
Fat	0		

NUTRITIONAL INFORMATION An excellent source of protein and iron.

DESCRIPTION The cartilage from the fin of the shark. When purchased it is dried, cream-coloured and quite matted in appearance.

ORIGIN AND HISTORY Highly prized as an ingredient in Chinese cooking, and priced to match, it is served at banquets and special occasions when the intention is to impress.

When shark's fin is fresh there is very little flavour, so therefore it must be cured or dried in the sun to develop the flavour. Believed to be highly beneficial to health and virility, shark meat has been eaten by Chinese for well over 2000 years, either fresh or in the form of a salty pickle. The refinement of braising the jelly-like strands contained within the fin came in the Sung era (AD960–1279). Marco Polo was one of the first Europeans to enjoy the benefits of this delicacy. The most famous recipe is of course shark's fin soup.

BUYING AND STORAGE In some countries it can be purchased in ready prepared form; however, in most it is only available canned or in cakes of compressed 'needles' which require a preliminary soaking and simmering. The top of the range cleaned 'needles' have been precleaned and softened and have the best flavour.

PREPARATION AND USE The basic form is a whole fin still covered with dark grey skin. This must be soaked until the skin is soft enough to scrape away, then simmered gently in lightly salted water to soften the thread-like cartilages. Refined shark's fin also requires soaking overnight or even longer in many changes of water, until it becomes like firm jelly. It should then be simmered to obtain the perfect softened, gelatinous product. Mainly used in soup.

PREPARATION AND USE Shark's fin soup relies on a richly flavoured stock of chicken and pork. Similarly, when shark's fin is braised to serve as a main meal, it is cooked in an intensely flavoured stock which is usually supplemented with oyster sauce or dried Chinese scallops. Chinese red rice, vinegar, white pepper, finely shredded lemon leaves, crisp pretzels and chrysanthemum petals are traditional accompaniments to shark's fin soup and braised shark's fin. Also available canned, either as chunks or as soup. Canned shark's fin is ideal for use in stuffings.

PROCESSING Cured, sun-dried or canned.

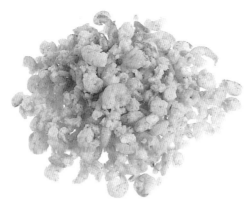

Shrimp, Canned

MAJOR NUTRIENTS		SERVE SIZE 100 G	
Energy	490 kJ	Calcium	320 mg
Protein	24 g	Phosphorus	270 mg
Fat	2 g	Magnesium	110 mg
Carbohydrate	0	Iron	1.8 mg
Cholesterol	180 mg	Zinc	5.3 mg
Sodium	3840 mg	Niacin Equiv.	3 mg

NUTRITIONAL INFORMATION Typical nutrients for crustaceans.

DESCRIPTION Small varieties of shrimp are canned whole, packed in a brine solution.

ORIGIN AND HISTORY As with salmon, shrimp are a popular canned food.

BUYING AND STORAGE Readily available, and being canned will store for long periods.

PREPARATION AND USE Widely used in easily prepared entrées such as shrimp cocktail, or as part of a snack, often with mayonnaise.

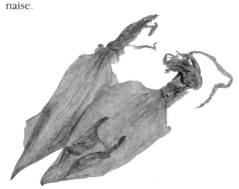

Squid, Dried

MAJOR NUTRIENTS		SERVE SIZE 25 G	
Energy	340 kJ	Potassium	150 mg
Protein	16 g	Magnesium	N/A
Fat	1 g	Iron	1 g
Carbohydrate	1 g	Niacin Equiv.	45 mg
Cholesterol	N/A	Copper	N/A
Dietary Fibre	0	Zinc	N/A
Sodium	235 mg	Vitamin A	N/A

NUTRITIONAL INFORMATION Dried squid is an excellent source of iron and niacin and it is only a moderate source of potassium. It contains a large amount of sodium. No data

are available for nutrients followed by N/A.

DESCRIPTION Sun-dried and salted squid.

ORIGIN AND HISTORY Used in Asian (mainly Chinese) cooking.

BUYING AND STORAGE Whole dried squid are sold by the piece, rolled in cellophane packs, from Chinese stores. Can be kept indefinitely in an airtight container in dry conditions.

PREPARATION AND USE Used to add an intense seafood flavour to stir-fried and braised dishes and soups, and are popular in regions where fresh seafoods are unobtainable. In central China, shredded dried squid is deep fried until crisp and puffy, resembling thick crisp noodles.

Whole dried squid should be soaked for several hours in warm water to reconstitute, then simmered in cold water with a pinch of bicarbonate of soda, to soften. They should be rinsed thoroughly before adding to a dish.

Rolled, dried squid roasted over charcoal and cut into strips is served as a chewy snack food, 'Chinese chewing gum'.

PROCESSING Whole dried squid are flattened and dried on racks or bamboo trays, are packed whole or may be further flattened by passing through a series of rollers to compress them into thin rectangular sheets.

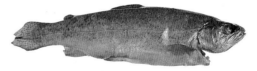

Trout, Smoked

NUTRITIONAL INFORMATION Similar to trout except for large amount of sodium.

DESCRIPTION Trout is usually smoked whole. The skin becomes a rich golden colour and slightly crinkled. It is easily peeled away to reveal beautiful pink, moist flesh with a delicate smoky flavour.

ORIGIN AND HISTORY Smoked trout is readily available in Europe, America and Australia. Smoking is a method of preserving the fish as well as yielding a unique odour, flavour, texture and appearance. The odour is mainly caused by deposited smoke particles and the flavour is a combination of smoke, salt and the trout itself.

BUYING AND STORAGE This is available in whole or fillet form. Trout should have a pleasant smoky odour, not at all rancid, and with a firm, not sweaty, flesh. Wrap in foil or store in airtight container. Keep in refrigerator 7–10 days. Freezing not recommended.

PREPARATION AND USE Peel skin gently away and serve either whole (head on or off) or as fillets — two fillets each side. Serve simply, with bread and butter and lemon. However, it can be made into pâtés, sliced thinly and folded through pasta or incorporated in salads.

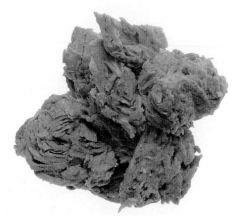

Tuna, Canned

MAJOR NUTRIENTS		SERVE SIZE 100 G	
Energy	460 kJ	Phosphorus	190 mg
Protein	22 g	Magnesium	30 mg
Fat	2 g	Iron	1.1 mg
Carbohydrate	0	Zinc	0.8 mg
Cholesterol	45 mg	Niacin Equiv.	7.5 mg
Sodium	390 mg		

NUTRITIONAL INFORMATION The fat content of canned tuna is low unless the tuna is canned in oil. Salt-free (no added sodium) varieties are available. For more nutritional information see Fish.

DESCRIPTION Tuna meat can be canned either in oil or brine. The meat varies in colour and flavour, depending upon the species. Albacore and southern bluefin tuna are the best. The meat has a medium flake and a rich fish taste. Varying shades of pink in colour.

ORIGIN AND HISTORY Most tuna is caught in the Pacific Ocean. Tuna spend a great deal of their life in cold, temperate waters but favour warm waters for spawning. Summer–autumn is the best time for commercial fishing. For canning, tuna should be aged between 3–8 years and weigh 7–50 kg.

BUYING AND STORAGE Canned tuna is available worldwide. Store in a cool, dark place. Shelf life of 12 months. Once opened should be refrigerated and eaten within 24 hours.

PREPARATION AND USE The canned tuna needs no preparation. Can be eaten hot or cold. Useful for mornays, sauces, sandwiches, canapés, fish cakes or salads.

PROCESSING Canned, in brine or oil.

SEE ALSO Tuna, fresh.

BREADS

Bread was first made from grains harvested from wild plants, ground into a coarse meal, mixed with water and formed into cakes which were dried in the sun or baked on hot stones.

Nine thousand years ago, when wheat and barley were first being cultivated in the Middle East, flat bread was made from crude flour milled from these grains. The ancient Egyptians are credited with first finding a way to leaven bread: tomb paintings from four thousand years ago clearly show leavened breads being prepared and baked.

Wheat contains the proteins gliadin and glutenin which, when mixed with water, form the elastic gluten which makes it possible for dough to 'stretch' and rise, as the yeast ferments the sugars and releases carbon dioxide. This process produces a lighter loaf. Rye, oats and barley also contain the proteins which produce gluten, but the concentrations are lower and the bread heavier.

Bread today is usually made from wheat flour, salt, yeast, water and optional other ingredients, mixed together to form an elastic dough, which is fermented, shaped as desired and baked.

Bread is a constant, daily element in the diet of most people. The most common variety of bread worldwide is white bread, but different styles of brown bread are also part of strong popular tradition. As nutritional analysis of foods has become of more interest to the consumer, especially in Western countries, consciousness about the flours used in the various breads has been heightened, and wholemeal breads — also known as wheatmeal and wholegrain breads — are now more sought after.

Bread is usually purchased fresh as required. It should be stored at room temperature for immediate use, or in the refrigerator in hot, humid weather. For longer storage, it can be frozen for up to four months, depending on the variety. Crusty breads are best eaten on the day of baking, as they dry out quickly.

Since bread is rich in complex carbohydrates (starch and dietary fibre), it is possible to use it to replace some of the high fat foods in the diet.

There is a lot of misunderstanding about the nutritional quality of bread: two popular misconceptions are that bread is 'fattening', and that white bread is a poor quality food.

Bread is a low fat food and it is not 'energy dense'; the spreads and fillings served with bread often provide more kilojoules than the bread itself.

One important measure of the nutritional value of a food is the balance between the energy provided and the other nutrients it contains, such as protein, vitamins, minerals and dietary fibre. Bread has an excellent balance of energy and nutrients.

White bread is a food of good nutritional quality. Brown, mixed grain and wholemeal breads provide more dietary fibre, minerals and vitamins, but it is a mistake to condemn white bread or the people who prefer to eat the more highly refined loaf. Children, in particular, often prefer white bread, and many of them will come to appreciate the more flavoursome wholemeal loaves later in life.

One advantage of white bread is the higher availability of the minerals. In wholemeal bread, some of the minerals, such as iron, are bound to phytates, making it more difficult for them to be absorbed from the digestive tract. The iron in bread is not as well absorbed as the haem-iron from flesh foods, but the absorption is improved by taking foods rich in vitamin C with the bread. This higher availability of iron from white bread compensates, in part, for its lower iron content.

Brown and mixed grain breads provide almost twice as much dietary fibre as white bread, and wholemeal bread provides about two and a half times the amount as white bread. Nevertheless, white bread is a valuable source of dietary fibre.

All breads contain about 9% protein and they are an excellent source of the complex carbohydrates, starch and dietary fibre.

The individual food entries show that bread contributes significant amounts of several nutrients. In addition to the nutrients listed it also contributes folate, with the highest levels in wholemeal bread.

One nutritional disadvantage of bread is its high sodium content. Most breads contain about 140 mg sodium per slice, which is equivalent to approximately 350 mg salt (sodium chloride). Salt-reduced breads contain approximately two-thirds this level of sodium, and low salt bread must contain no more than 36 mg per 30 g slice. Salt-free or 'no added salt' bread contains insignificant amounts of sodium.

Most breads carry nutritional labelling, providing information about sodium as well as other nutrients.

Although bread is a low fat food, some foods which may be substituted for bread (for example, croissants), are high fat foods. When such substitutions are made on a regular basis, it is important to be aware of the nutritional consequences. The individual entries on the following pages are a valuable guide.

The breads included in the entries in this chapter relate to the two main categories of bread, which, are discussed.

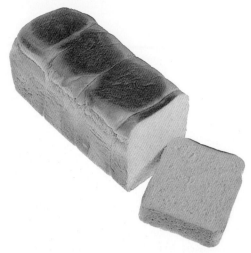

White Bread Made from white bread flour milled from wheat, and other permitted ingredients, white breads come in many different shapes, sizes and textures. Sometimes up to 10% of another cereal — or a vegetable flour, seeds, herbs, or a mixture of these — is added for variety. For a full description of white flour, see the chapter on Grains and Cereals.

MAJOR NUTRIENTS		SERVE SIZE 60 G	
Energy	620 kJ	Potassium	70 mg
Protein	6 g	Iron	0.7 mg
Fat	2 g	Magnesium	16 mg
Carbohydrate	27 g	Zinc	0.4 mg
Cholesterol	0	Thiamin	0.1 mg
Dietary Fibre	2 g	Niacin Equiv.	1.5 mg
Sodium	260 mg	Riboflavin	0.05 mg

NUTRITIONAL INFORMATION 60 g represents 2 slices of bread. These are a good source of thiamin and iron; a moderate source of protein, fibre, niacin, sodium and magnesium. Commercial white bread contains enough thiamin to ensure the body can use the carbohydrate present in the bread, as well as augmenting the body pool of thiamin.

White bread is an often undervalued food. Some people believe that bread is too fattening and has no nutritional value. These beliefs are unfounded.

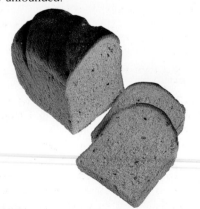

Wholemeal, Wheatmeal, Wholegrain Bread Bread made 100% from flour milled from the whole grain (usually wheat) — or it may legally contain 90% wholemeal and 10% white flour.

MAJOR NUTRIENTS		SERVE SIZE 60 G	
Energy	540 kJ	Potassium	160 mg
Protein	6 g	Iron	1.4 mg
Fat	2 g	Magnesium	32 mg
Carbohydrate	23 g	Zinc	0.8 mg
Cholesterol	0	Thiamin	0.15 mg
Dietary Fibre	4 g	Niacin Equiv.	2.5 mg
Sodium	280 mg	Riboflavin	0.05 mg

NUTRITIONAL INFORMATION 60 g represents 2 slices. These are a good source of fibre, thiamin, niacin, iron and magnesium; a moderate source of protein, sodium and zinc. Wholemeal bread has three times the amount of niacin and twice the amount of fibre in white bread. For those who are interested in reducing their sodium intake, salt-reduced and salt-free wholemeal breads are available.

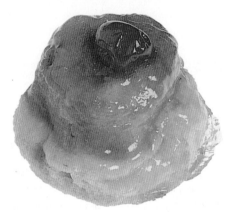

Baba

*also called **Baba au rhum, Savarin***

NUTRITIONAL INFORMATION No nutritional analysis available. The nutrient content will depend upon the recipe used.

DESCRIPTION A light yeast-leavened cake studded with raisins, resembling a gugelhupf with a honeycomb texture. The baked cake is soaked in a rum- or kirsch-flavoured syrup and often glazed with apricot jam.

Babas may be made as small or large cakes. The ring-shaped version is called a savarin. In France a baba is sometimes presented in a fish shape at Easter.

ORIGIN AND HISTORY Originally a Polish Easter cake baked only by women, baba resembled the Russian kulich in shape. Baba traditionally contained raisins, vanilla, ground almonds and saffron soaked in vodka. Some sources say King Stanislaus Leczinski took the familiar gugelhupf, sprinkled it with rum, set it alight and named it after Ali Baba, one of the heroes from *The Thousand and One Nights*. This practice was taken to Paris at the beginning of the 19th century where babas became a specialty of the establishment operated by the pastry cook Sthorer, who brushed them with syrup to soften the crust before sale.

BUYING AND STORAGE Available from most French patisseries and better pastry cooks. Refrigerate 1–2 days or freeze for up to 4 months.

PREPARATION AND USE Serve slightly warmed with whipped cream as an accompaniment to coffee, or as a dessert.

PROCESSING A dough rich with eggs and butter is allowed to ferment, then placed into deep round pans and allowed to prove before baking. The cooled babas are sprinkled heavily with rum or kirsch.

SEE ALSO Gugelhupf.

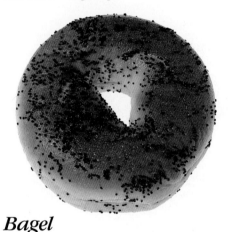

Bagel

MAJOR NUTRIENTS		PLAIN SERVE SIZE 60 G	
Energy	570 kJ	Cholesterol	n/a
Protein	5 g	Dietary Fibre	n/a
Fat	1 g	Sodium	370 mg
Carbohydrate	28 g	Potassium	40 mg

NUTRITIONAL INFORMATION 60 g represents 1 bagel. A moderate source of protein. There is no analysis available for vitamin content but it will be similar to that of white bread rolls.

DESCRIPTION A ring of baked yeast dough with a chewy centre and a crusty outside. Known as 'the roll with a hole', it is typically 8–10 cm in diameter and weighs 60–100 g.

ORIGIN AND HISTORY Originating in Eastern Europe, the bagel is thought to have been first made 300–400 years ago in Vienna to honour Jan Sobieski, the king of Poland, a famous horseman who helped drive the Turks out of Austria. The roll was shaped to resemble a stirrup and boiled before baking to preserve the shape (Bügel in German). The Jewish community in Vienna started making them commercially and using the name bagel.

BUYING AND STORAGE Made by specialist bakers and available from some specialty delicatessens, freezer cabinets in supermarkets and food stores in areas with concentrated Eastern European populations. Becoming better known as distribution improves. Bagels will store at room temperature in their original packaging for up to 3 days, or in the freezer for months.

PREPARATION AND USE Serve warm with cream cheese and savoury or sweet toppings at breakfast or lunch or for a snack.

PROCESSING Bagels are shaped from proved yeast dough, boiled briefly to preserve their shape, then baked.

VARIETIES

Plain and egg are the most common types, often sprinkled with caraway seeds, poppy seeds or coarse salt. Wholemeal, rye and onion-flavoured bagels are also available.

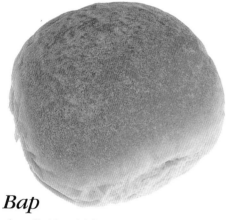

Bap

also called **Scottish bap**

NUTRITIONAL INFORMATION No nutritional analysis available. Baps have a similar nutrient value to white bread rolls.

DESCRIPTION A small, very light yeast roll, oval in shape with a soft floury crust and soft inner crumb.

ORIGIN AND HISTORY The origin remains obscure but there are references to baps in 16th century Scottish history books, where it is reported that they sold at 'nine for twelve pence'.

BUYING AND STORAGE Buy individually or in bags of 8 or 10 from most small bakeries. Baps keep well in a polythene bag for up to 4 days. Freeze for up to 4 months; thaw at room temperature.

PREPARATION AND USE Serve warm for breakfast with preserves, or filled for lunches.

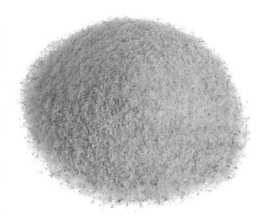

Breadcrumbs

MAJOR NUTRIENTS		DRIED SERVE SIZE 20 G	
Energy	300 kJ	Potassium	30 mg
Protein	2 g	Iron	0.3 mg
Fat	0	Magnesium	7 mg
Carbohydrate	16 g	Zinc	0.2 mg
Cholesterol	0	Thiamin	0.05 mg
Dietary Fibre	1 g	Niacin Equiv.	0.5 mg
Sodium	150 mg	Riboflavin	0

NUTRITIONAL INFORMATION A good source of thiamin and iron. A moderate source of protein, fibre, niacin, sodium and magnesium. The nutrient content of dried breadcrumbs is similar to that of white bread, the major difference being the moisture content, which is lower in dried breadcrumbs.

Soft breadcrumbs will have the same nutrient value as the bread they are made from.

DESCRIPTION Crumbs from the soft inner portion of a loaf of bread, or crisp crumbs crushed from bread which has been dried out.

ORIGIN AND HISTORY See introduction: the history is that of bread.

BUYING AND STORAGE Buy crisp or toasted crumbs in packets from supermarkets. They will keep almost indefinitely in an airtight container. A bay leaf buried in the crumbs seems to keep weevils and other insects away. Make soft fresh breadcrumbs and buttered crumbs at home. Store in the freezer for up to 6 months.

PREPARATION AND USE Soft crumbs: Either crumb the inner part of a 2 or 3 day-old-loaf in a blender or food processor or grate on the coarse part of a grater. Dried or toasted crumbs: Dry thin slices of soft bread in a slow oven until very crisp and pale straw in colour. Cool, then break into pieces and either roll with rolling pin or crumb in a blender or food processor. Use for stuffings, for toppings, as extenders for more expensive foods, to thicken sauces, and for coating foods to be fried.

Buttered crumbs are made by cooking soft breadcrumbs in a little butter until crisp. They may be combined with chopped herbs or grated cheese and sprinkled onto foods before baking.

VARIETIES

Dried, soft (fresh).

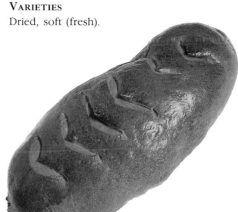

Brioche

NUTRITIONAL INFORMATION No nutritional analysis available.

DESCRIPTION A light and delicate yeast-leavened cake-type loaf or small roll richly flavoured with butter and eggs. Small brioches often have a topknot and are called brioche à tête.

ORIGIN AND HISTORY Brioche, sometimes known as apostle or prophet cake, is generally considered to be of French origin but also has a long history in Poland and Austria. The first brioche was a loaf made with fine white flour and smaller quantities of butter and eggs; it was not until later that the very rich, buttery fluted bread we now call brioche became popular. One possible derivation of the name is that the 'bri' part comes from the name of brie cheese (used for making early brioches) and the 'oche' part comes from occhi, which were large, very popular Hyrcanian figs similar in shape to the brioche head. Baker's yeast replaced brewer's yeast for leavening these breads in the mid-18th century.

BUYING AND STORAGE Available from good French patisseries and pastry cooks. Store brioche dough at room temperature for up to 1 week or freeze for up to 4 months; thaw at room temperature.

PREPARATION AND USE Traditionally it is served warm with jam for breakfast. Small brioches may be hollowed out and filled with hot savoury mixtures to serve at luncheon. Brioche dough is often used to encase meat or sausage for protection during baking. Stale brioche makes particularly fine bread and butter custard.

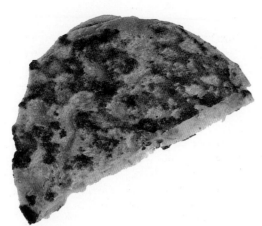

Chapatti

also called Chappati

MAJOR NUTRIENTS		MADE WITHOUT FAT SERVE SIZE 100 G	
Energy	860 kJ	Iron	1 mg
Protein	7 g	Calcium	40 mg
Fat	1 g	Magnesium	37 mg
Carbohydrate	44 g	Zinc	0.5 mg
Cholesterol	0	Thiamin	0.1 mg
Dietary Fibre	3 g	Niacin Equiv.	2.5 mg
Sodium	120 mg	Riboflavin	0.05 mg
Potassium	150 mg		

NUTRITIONAL INFORMATION A good source of protein, fibre, thiamin and the minerals iron and magnesium; moderate source of niacin and calcium. If this serve size of chapattis is made with oil the fat content may be as high as 13 g.

The nutrient content of chapattis will differ depending on the flour used in preparation. In India chapattis are usually high in vitamins and minerals owing to the low extraction of fibre and bran from the flour.

DESCRIPTION A flat disc of bread which may be unleavened or slightly leavened, wholemeal or white or a combination of both, made from milled wheat flour called atta.

ORIGIN AND HISTORY Chapatti, along with other types of roti (bread), originated in India, where history stretches back into the mists of time. Chapatti is one example of a number of primitive breads indigenous to different continents, such as the Ethiopian injera and Mexican tortillas, that are made from unleavened or very slightly leavened doughs rolled into discs and baked over a fire on metal or pottery griddles.

In India, chapattis are either homemade or bought fresh from street hawkers or from the bazaars for every meal, as they become stale quickly. They have long been the food of the people, particularly in northern India where they are also used like a plate to hold other food. Pieces of torn chapatti are still curved to form a primitive but efficient replacement for a spoon for eating curries and other foods.

BUYING AND STORAGE Buy fresh from Indian takeaway restaurants. Use within a few hours. Chapattis do not freeze well.

PREPARATION AND USE A stiff dough made from atta, water and salt is divided into pieces weighing from 30 g to 100 g. These are rolled into circles about 3–5 mm thick and cooked on a hotplate lightly greased with ghee. Constant pressure is applied to the chapatti during cooking to prevent large air pockets from forming. After cooking for 1 minute, the chapatti is turned and cooked for another minute on the second side.

Chapattis are eaten warm with vegetables and rice.

SEE ALSO Paratha, Puri (Indian).

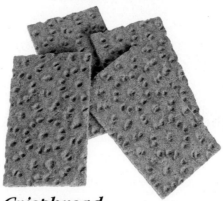

Crispbread

NUTRITIONAL INFORMATION The ingredients of crispbread vary with the maker: commercially available crispbreads often carry a nutritional breakdown on the packet.

DESCRIPTION A thin flat square or disc of dry bread made from rye, barley, wheat or combinations of these grains.

ORIGIN AND HISTORY Crispbreads originated in Scandinavia and other parts of northern Europe where, because of the short seasons, grain often had to be harvested before it was fully ripe. Green (unripened) grain does not store well, so it was ground by the farmer and afterwards baked into bread, often by the visiting craftsman baker, who would bake sufficient bread to last the household until the next harvest before moving on to the next farm.

For baking the dough was shaped, either into large discs with a hole through the centre that could be threaded onto a rod and hung from the rafters to continue drying out, or into squares or rectangles that were stored, after baking, in a chest or cupboard set aside for the purpose.

In times of famine similar bread was made from the inner bark of trees or from ground acorns.

BUYING AND STORAGE Packaged crispbreads are available from supermarkets. Unwrapped round rye bread discs are available from some specialty Scandinavian bakeries. They are softer, but may be hung in the same way as the original breads; they will dry gradually.

PREPARATION AND USE In Scandinavia these crispbreads were traditionally broken into pieces and soaked in sour milk overnight ready for eating at breakfast.

PROCESSING A rye sourdough ferment is added to rye flour, rye meal and various other ingredients depending on the flavour and nature of the final crispbread. The dough is mixed and fermented, then rolled out into a large sheet, cut into desired shapes and docked (pricked) thoroughly to prevent large bubbles from forming during baking. After slow baking the bread is strung up to dry out slowly. Some breads are baked twice.

SEE ALSO Sourdough Bread.

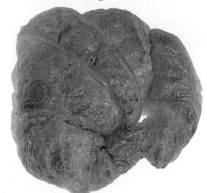

Croissant

MAJOR NUTRIENTS		SERVE SIZE 80 G	
Energy	1314 kJ	Cholesterol	14 mg
Protein	89 g	Dietary Fibre	1 g
Fat	19 g	Sodium	50 mg
Carbohydrate	28 g	Potassium	100 mg

NUTRITIONAL INFORMATION High in carbohydrate and fat. There is no analysis available for vitamin content, but it is likely to be similar to that of white bread.

DESCRIPTION A rich, flaky Danish pastry roll shaped into a crescent.

ORIGIN AND HISTORY First created in 1686 in Budapest where the Turks were besieging the city. Bakers, who worked at night, heard the noise made by the Turks as they tunnelled under the city to reach the centre of town. The alarm was raised, the Turks were repulsed, and as a reward the bakers were granted the privilege of baking a pastry in the shape of the crescent on the Ottoman flag. The rolls did not become known as croissants until after Marie Antoinette introduced them to the French court when she married Louis XVI. In the early days the croissant was a rich crescent-shaped roll; it only became the flaky pastry we know today in the 1920s.

BUYING AND STORAGE Readily available prepacked from supermarkets or loose from bakers and pastry cooks. Keep at room temperature for 3–4 days. Freeze for up to 6 months; thaw at room temperature.

PREPARATION AND USE Serve warm with butter and preserves for breakfast or brunch. Split and fill with savoury or sweet mixtures for a light snack or dessert.

SEE ALSO Danish Pastry.

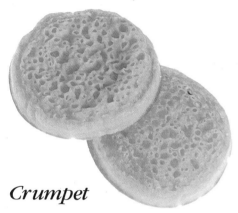

Crumpet

MAJOR NUTRIENTS			PLAIN SERVE SIZE 55 G
Energy	450 kJ	Potassium	55 mg
Protein	3 g	Iron	0.7 mg
Fat	1 g	Magnesium	13 mg
Carbohydrate	24 g	Zinc	0.4 mg
Cholesterol	0	Thiamin	0.05 mg
Dietary Fibre	1.5 g	Niacin Equiv.	1 mg
Sodium	165 mg		

NUTRITIONAL INFORMATION A good source of iron; a moderate source of fibre, thiamin and niacin. Bran and wholemeal crumpets will have more fibre, thiamin, niacin and riboflavin than plain crumpets. The nutrient content of bran and wholemeal crumpets will be similar to that of wholemeal bread.

DESCRIPTION Traditional yeasted flour-based product 8–10 cm in diameter and 1 cm thick. It is baked on one side only and has an open honeycomb structure which appears on the top surface.

ORIGIN AND HISTORY Well known in Britain where their origin has been lost in time, crumpets were very popular at the turn of the century, when they were sold in the streets along with muffins. In some areas crumpets were called muffins and vice versa, making it difficult to trace the history of either food.

BUYING AND STORAGE Available from supermarkets, crumpets are essentially a winter product. They may be refrigerated for up to 2 weeks or frozen for up to 4 months. They can be toasted when frozen.

PREPARATION AND USE Serve hot, toasted and liberally spread with butter.

VARIETIES
Bran, wholemeal.

SEE ALSO Muffin (English).

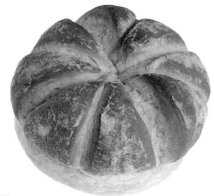

Damper

*also called **Bush damper***

MAJOR NUTRIENTS			SERVE SIZE 60 G
Energy	810 kJ	Potassium	60 mg
Protein	5 g	Iron	0.5 mg
Fat	6 g	Magnesium	16.5 mg
Carbohydrate	33 g	Zinc	0.1 mg
Cholesterol	0	Thiamin	0.1 mg
Dietary Fibre	1 g	Niacin Equiv.	1.5 mg
Sodium	710 mg	Riboflavin	0.05 mg

NUTRITIONAL INFORMATION A good source of thiamin; moderate source of protein, niacin, iron and magnesium. The nutrient content of damper is very similar to white bread except that damper contains more than twice the amount of sodium, as it is made with self-raising flour. The yeast-leavened 'dampers' will have a similar nutrient content to white bread.

DESCRIPTION Round, chemically leavened bread with a thick rough crust and soft inner crumb.

ORIGIN AND HISTORY Originally made by the settlers in the Australian bush, damper became the staple food in the early days, when four, salt and water were the only ingredients. It was baked in the hot ashes of the fire. Camp ovens came into use later. Baking powder and powdered milk were added when they became available. Johnny cakes were made by winding strips of the dough around green sticks and cooking these over the fire.

BUYING AND STORAGE Yeast-leavened 'dampers' are available from some bakeries.

They have a texture, flavour and shelf life similar to conventional white bread.

PREPARATION AND USE Make a dough with self-raising flour, milk powder, butter and water. Knead lightly and form into a ball. Flatten slightly to fit into a well-greased camp oven or ovenproof casserole with a lid. Bake the camp oven in the hot ashes of a fire or the casserole in a hot oven for 40–50 minutes.

VARIETIES
Johnny Cakes Named after the somewhat similar American product (see under Origin and History).

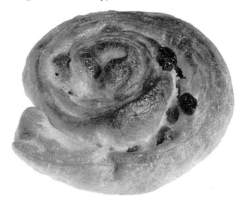

Danish Pastry

MAJOR NUTRIENTS			SERVE SIZE 80 G
Energy	1030 kJ	Cholesterol	28 mg
Protein	6 g	Dietary Fibre	1 g
Fat	12 g	Sodium	30 mg
Carbohydrate	30 g	Potassium	120 mg

NUTRITIONAL INFORMATION High in carbohydrate and fat. There is no vitamin content analysis available.

DESCRIPTION Yeast-leavened flaky pastry, very light and buttery with many tissue-thin layers, also known as apple Danish, apricot Danish, depending on the ingredients used.

ORIGIN AND HISTORY The Danish pastry originated when the bakers of Copenhagen went on strike just over 100 years ago. Their employers refused to give in to their demands for cash wages instead of room and board, which was the traditional form of payment up to that time. Instead they fired the local Danish bakers and brought in Austrian and German bakers in their place. The Viennese method of making pastry was by rolling and folding butter into yeast dough, a method enthusiastically accepted by the Danish populace. When the Danish bakers finally returned to work they continued to make the new Danish pastries and went on to improve them by the addition of jam, custard, fruit and other fillings. The Danes to this day call Danish pastry Wienerbrod — Vienna bread.

BUYING AND STORAGE Buy from specialist pastry cooks and store at room temperature for 2–3 days or in the freezer for up to 2 months. Danish pastries are best eaten on the day they are made.

PREPARATION AND USE A yeast dough enriched with eggs and milk is mixed and then chilled in the refrigerator. Butter is then interleaved into the mixture, which is rolled and folded several times to produce a layered dough. To maintain a low temperature, which will prevent the butter from melting during handling, the dough is chilled and rested between rollings. The resulting pastry may be formed into a variety of shapes, filled with fruit, custard, crème pâtissière, nuts or jam. After baking, glazes or icing are applied. They may be decorated with nuts. Serve slightly warmed or cold with coffee.

VARIETIES
Made in traditional shapes — e.g. envelopes, snails, cockscombs — with a variety of fillings.

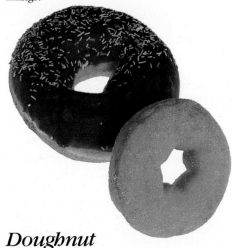

Doughnut

MAJOR NUTRIENTS			PLAIN
			SERVE SIZE 40 G
Energy	590 kJ	Sodium	25 mg
Protein	2 g	Potassium	45 mg
Fat	6 g	Iron	0.8 mg
Carbohydrate	20 g	Magnesium	6.5 mg
Cholesterol	0	Zinc	0.2 mg
Dietary Fibre	0.5 g	Niacin Equiv.	0.5 mg

NUTRITIONAL INFORMATION Doughnuts are high in fat and have limited nutrient value.

DESCRIPTION A small deep-fried cake made from yeast dough or baking powder raised batter. Doughnuts may be in the form of rings, twists, or round balls with jam in the centre. They are tossed in spiced sugar or coated with icing.

ORIGIN AND HISTORY Fried cakes and doughnuts of varying kinds can be found in a number of cuisines, but the best-known is the American version. Historians are divided on how the doughnut with a hole came into being. One story, no doubt apocryphal, which has been handed down for generations tells of the Indian brave who shot an arrow into the bread dough his spouse was shaping. She was so startled she dropped the cake into a pan of hot bear fat and the result was the first doughnut. A bronze plaque in Rockport, Massachusetts, commemorates the birthplace of one Captain Henson Gregory, crediting him with the invention of the doughnut in 1847. Fed up with the soggy centres in his mother's fried cakes, he simply cut the centres out and fried the rings (no mention is made of the fate of the centres). However, the *official* invention is attributed to a man named John Blondel who patented a doughnut cutter with a hole in the 1870s.

BUYING AND STORAGE Available from specialty doughnut shops or takeaway outlets, they are sold as required. They keep well at room temperature for a few days, or up to 2 months in the freezer.

PREPARATION AND USE Serve at room temperature, or warmed slightly; doughnuts are always 'ready to eat'.

VARIETIES
Cake doughnuts, yeast doughnuts.

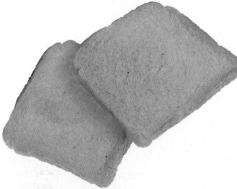

Fibre-increased Bread

NUTRITIONAL INFORMATION This bread will be similar to one of the breads analysed in the introduction, depending on whether it is white or wholemeal: the amount of increased fibre is generally shown on the package when the bread is bought.

DESCRIPTION Bread made with the addition of extra fibre to provide higher levels than usual. Fibre-increased meal breads provide at least 50% more fibre than wholemeal breads and white varieties have sufficient extra fibre added to make them comparable with normal wholemeal breads.

Both varieties usually have added gluten and are generally labelled protein-increased.

The fibre source is usually wheat or rice bran, but soya hulls are also permitted. Purified cellulose, used in some countries overseas, is not a permitted additive in Australia.

ORIGIN AND HISTORY These breads have been developed to accompany the increased consciousness of the importance of dietary fibre in foods.

BUYING AND STORAGE Readily available in most supermarkets and groceries.

PREPARATION AND USE As for other breads.

VARIETIES
White, wholemeal.

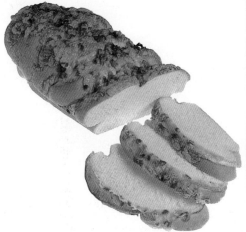

Flavoured Breads

NUTRITIONAL INFORMATION For type 1 below, the analysis will not differ greatly from those given in the introduction. For type 2, added butter will considerably increase the fat content.

DESCRIPTION These breads may be:
1. Plain white, wholemeal or rye doughs with various flavourings added to the dough or sprinkled on top of the dough before baking as loaves or rolls.
2. Baked loaves — usually rolls or French sticks — cut into slices, spread with flavoured butter, reassembled and reheated as a loaf.

ORIGIN AND HISTORY These are varieties of bread which are probably almost as old as bread itself, especially those sprinkled with seeds.

BUYING AND STORAGE Available fresh at bakeries and at supermarkets, wrapped in clear packaging. Garlic breads may be bought refrigerated, wrapped in foil. These breads freeze better when preprepared.

PREPARATION AND USE As for other breads. Filled breads such as garlic loaf are heated in an oven before serving.

VARIETIES

Loaves covered with cheese, cheese and bacon or other mixtures; herbs, garlic or other breads served hot.

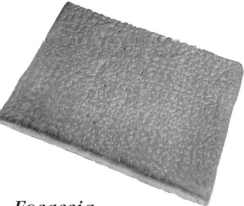

Focaccia

also called **Pinze, Sardenaira, Schiacciata**

NUTRITIONAL INFORMATION The nutrient value will depend on the local recipe used: in the main, focaccia resembles pizza dough, and the topping is usually a thin paste of tomato and/or cheese.

DESCRIPTION A flat disc or rectangle of peasant bread, savoury or sweet and variously flavoured according to the district where it is made.

ORIGIN AND HISTORY Focaccia and similar types of bread are known in the villages of both France and the Italian Riviera. Originally thought to have come from Genoa, the breads were taken much further afield by the Romans and during their travels the name and character changed many times. Thus focaccia may be called by any of a number of names and may be crisp or soft, thin or thick, weighed down with toppings or almost plain. Flavours will also vary according to what is available.

BUYING AND STORAGE Buy fresh from Italian bakeries, and eat while still fresh.

PREPARATION AND USE These breads are usually eaten as a snack or light meal.

PROCESSING Made from a fairly plain yeasted dough which has been proved at least once. The dough is rolled or patted out to fit a well-oiled pan about 25 cm in diameter. Indentations are made with the fingertips all over the surface of the dough, which is then topped with a sprinkling of coarse salt or herbs, onions sautéed in olive oil, tomatoes, garlic, olives or some combination of these, and baked in a hot oven. The best focaccia is baked on the sole of the oven, and a fine spray of water across the surface during the first few minutes of baking also improves the finished bread.

Some bakers shape the dough into a rectangle, while others add ricotta cheese mixed with prosciutto, parmesan and nutmeg, or bake a sweet brioche-type dough topped with crystallised sugar, sandwiching it with ice cream when it is cold.

VARIETIES

Savoury, sweet.

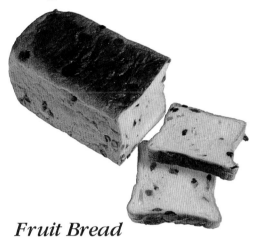

Fruit Bread

MAJOR NUTRIENTS		SERVE SIZE 60 G	
Energy	670 kJ	Potassium	150 mg
Protein	5 g	Iron	1.2 mg
Fat	2 g	Magnesium	16 mg
Carbohydrate	32 g	Zinc	0.5 mg
Cholesterol	0	Thiamin	0.05 mg
Dietary Fibre	2 g	Niacin Equiv.	1.5 mg
Sodium	115 mg	Riboflavin	0.1 mg

NUTRITIONAL INFORMATION A good source of iron; a moderate source of protein, fibre, thiamin, niacin, riboflavin and magnesium. The nutrient content is similar to that of white bread, but fruit bread has almost double the amount of iron and less thiamin than white bread.

DESCRIPTION Many styles of bread include dried fruit and/or fruit peel. The table above gives representative figures for these breads.

ORIGIN AND HISTORY Preserving fruits by drying is an age-old method, so it is safe to assume that fruit breads have a long history.

BUYING AND STORAGE Bought sliced or whole, fruit breads tend to be moister than the ordinary loaf, and will keep up to 4 days at room temperature.

PREPARATION AND USE Usually served hot with butter.

SEE ALSO Hot Cross Bun.

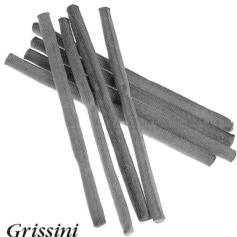

Grissini

also called **Grissine**

NUTRITIONAL INFORMATION No nutritional analysis available.

DESCRIPTION These are pencil-shaped, thin crispbread sticks which may be as long as an arm. Traditional handmade grissini are irregular and knobbly in shape.

ORIGIN AND HISTORY Turin seems to have been the home of grissini; they were first made there in the mid-17th century. They were thought to be good for the digestion and some say they were so successful they became well known all over Italy within a short time. When Napoleon met with 'les petits batons de Turin', so the story goes, he started a fast postal service to ensure they were delivered to the court daily.

BUYING AND STORAGE Both the locally made grissini and those imported from Italy are available from supermarkets, Italian food stores and most delicatessens in boxes containing various weights. Stored in the original box or in a closed container, they will keep for months.

PREPARATION AND USE Usually found on the tables in Italian restaurants. Grissini are eaten plain as a snack, although some non-Italians break them into pieces and spread them with butter.

PROCESSING Made from a lean yeasted dough, small pieces of which are rolled into pencillike sticks 25–30 cm long. They are then rolled in salt or seeds and baked until crisp, dry and golden brown.

VARIETIES

Plain, salt-crusted or seeded; made from wholemeal or white flour.

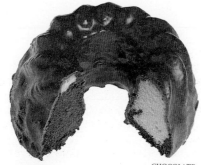

Gugelhupf

also called Gugelhopf, Kugelhoff, Kugelhopf, Kugelhupf

NUTRITIONAL INFORMATION No nutritional analysis available. The nutrient content will depend upon the recipe used.

DESCRIPTION A light yeast or sponge cake containing rum-soaked raisins or currants baked in a deep, distinctively sculptured fluted ring mould called a gugelhupf pan.

ORIGIN AND HISTORY Said to have originated in Austria, Poland and Germany. In the mid-17th century it was leavened with brewer's yeast (barm). Gugelhupf was taken to Paris by the chef to the Austrian Ambassador, who gave the recipe to Carême, the great French cook of the early 19th century. At this time, Carême had set up shop in Paris as a pastry cook.

BUYING AND STORAGE Available from most good French patisseries and pastry cooks. Store in the refrigerator 2–3 days or in the freezer in a rigid container for up to 4 months.

PREPARATION AND USE Warm slightly, dust top with icing sugar and serve with coffee.

SEE ALSO Baba.

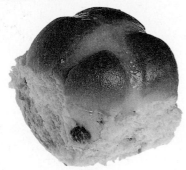

Hot Cross Bun

also called Easter bun

MAJOR NUTRIENTS		SERVE SIZE 40 G	
Energy	450 kJ	Potassium	100 mg
Protein	3 g	Iron	0.7 mg
Fat	3 g	Magnesium	7.5 mg
Carbohydrate	19 g	Zinc	0.3 mg
Cholesterol	0	Thiamin	0.05 mg
Dietary Fibre	1 g	Niacin Equiv.	1 mg
Sodium	70 mg	Riboflavin	0.05 mg

NUTRITIONAL INFORMATION A good source of iron; moderate source of thiamin and niacin.

DESCRIPTION A small bun made from sweet dough flavoured with dried fruits and spices, finished with a cross on the top made by slashing the bun, or by piping choux pastry or icing. Glazed with sugar syrup.

ORIGIN AND HISTORY Dates back to sacrificial breads that were part of pagan worship in many countries including Egypt, Greece and Saxon England where the practices were adopted by the early Christian church. Originally baked to honour the Anglo-Saxon goddess of spring, Easter. The round shape was seen to represent the moon and the cross the four seasons of the year.

BUYING AND STORAGE Available pre-packed in trays of 6 or 8 buns from supermarkets and bakeries from the beginning of Lent. They will keep for up to 4 days at room temperature and up to 6 months in the freezer. Thaw at room temperature.

PREPARATION AND USE Warm in microwave oven, electric frypan or oven, or toast under the griller. Serve with butter or cream cheese.

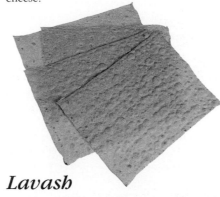

Lavash

MAJOR NUTRIENTS		SERVE SIZE 60 G	
Energy	700 kJ	Sodium	340 mg
Protein	6 g	Potassium	80 mg
Fat	1 g	Iron	3.3 mg
Carbohydrate	31 g	Thiamin	0.20 mg
Cholesterol	0	Niacin	1.5 mg

NUTRITIONAL INFORMATION An excellent source of thiamin and niacin; a good source of protein and iron.

DESCRIPTION Oval sheets of bread approximately 0.5 cm thick, very pliable and with a chewy texture. Made from white wheaten flour, yeast, salt and water. It is oven-baked on a heated metal plate.

ORIGIN AND HISTORY Dates back 3000 years to biblical times. Originally made by the Babylonians and Assyrians, this bread of the people has spread to many areas of the Middle East, and is especially well known in Armenia and Iran.

BUYING AND STORAGE Available from some supermarkets in packets containing 8 sheets approximately 28 cm by 23 cm. Stored at room temperature they will become dry and crisp and will keep indefinitely.

PREPARATION AND USE Sprinkle lightly with tepid water, wrap in a clean towel and allow to soften. Roll around fillings and serve hot or cold.

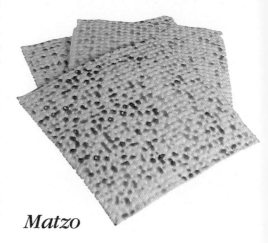

Matzo

MAJOR NUTRIENTS		SERVE SIZE 30 G	
Energy	490 kJ	Potassium	45 mg
Protein	3 g	Iron	0.5 mg
Fat	1 g	Magnesium	6 mg
Carbohydrate	26 g	Zinc	0.2 mg
Cholesterol	0	Thiamin	0.05 mg
Dietary Fibre	1 g	Niacin Equiv.	1 mg
Sodium	5 mg		

NUTRITIONAL INFORMATION A moderate source of thiamin, niacin and iron.

DESCRIPTION A thin sheet of unleavened bread made with wheaten flour and water and, sometimes, salt.

ORIGIN AND HISTORY This is the original unleavened bread, mentioned in the Bible, which is baked for the Jewish community, under supervision, to commemorate the flight of the Israelites from ancient Egypt. They fled in such haste they did not take their leaven with them. Always eaten at Passover to remind them of that flight from bondage.

BUYING AND STORAGE Buy from kosher stores in bags of various weights. Matzos will keep indefinitely in a dry cupboard.

PREPARATION AND USE Served as a cracker or as a substitute for leavened bread, particularly during Passover.

PROCESSING Matzos must be baked under the supervision of a rabbi to ensure the product meets the requirements of the Jewish faith.

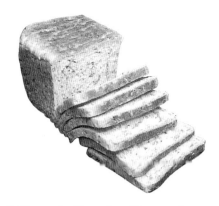

Mixed Grain Bread

MAJOR NUTRIENTS		SERVE SIZE 60 G	
Energy	590 kJ	Potassium	130 mg
Protein	6 g	Iron	1.2 mg
Fat	1 g	Magnesium	27.5 mg
Carbohydrate	27 g	Zinc	0.8 mg
Cholesterol	0	Thiamin	0.1 mg
Dietary Fibre	3 g	Niacin Equiv.	2 mg
Sodium	280 mg	Riboflavin	0.05 mg

NUTRITIONAL INFORMATION 60 g represents 2 slices. A good source of thiamin and niacin; moderate source of protein, fibre and the minerals sodium, iron, magnesium and zinc. The nutrient content of different mixed grain breads will differ slightly depending on the ratio of white flour to wholemeal flour.

DESCRIPTION Bread made from white and/or wholemeal flour with kibbled grains added to the mix.

ORIGIN AND HISTORY Dr K. C. Alfred Vogel, a Swiss biochemist and naturopath, was the first person to manufacture white bread with mixed grains added. After experimenting for a number of years he finally won a gold medal for his loaf in the mid-1950s. Vogel's mixed grain bread has been made under licence in Australia since the late 1950s. At first it was sold only in health food stores, but it gradually became available in supermarkets across the country. Other brands and varieties of mixed grain bread soon followed and it has now replaced brown bread in most areas. 'Brown bread' was the general term used for a type of bread which was usually made from roughly half white flour and half wholemeal flour. As interest has grown in the precise ingredients contained in bread, the terms manufacturers and customers use to describe the different breads have become more specific. Mixed grain bread is sold in Britain and is just becoming available in the United States. It is popular for its nutty taste and crunchy texture.

BUYING AND STORAGE Buy from supermarkets, health food stores, delicatessens, in fact anywhere bread is sold. Store in its wrapper at room temperature, or in the refrigerator during hot humid weather. Freeze for longer storage. Always pack the loaf (in its original wrapper) in a good quality freezer bag. Remove as much air as possible without distorting the bread. Seal and label and store for up to 4 months.

PREPARATION AND USE Mixed grain bread may be made at home. Choose a favourite basic recipe, and use a mixture of wholemeal and white flours, replacing up to 30% of the flour with kibbled (cracked) grains of your choice. Measure some of the water from the recipe, bring to the boil and pour over the grain, allow to stand so the grain will soften, then add to the dry ingredients. Follow recipe directions as usual.

Use mixed grain bread for sandwiches, toast, savouries, as a base for spreads, or crumbed in meat loaves and hamburgers, desserts and puddings, and as an extender for more expensive foods.

PROCESSING Most commercial mixed grain breads are a mixture of flour and kibbled rye and/or wheat, with added gluten and bran, yeast, emulsifier, salt and water. Milk, fat and vinegar may be present. The label on the wrapper lists the ingredients.

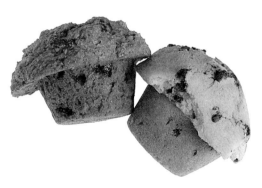

Muffin (American)

MAJOR NUTRIENTS		PLAIN SERVE SIZE 40 G	
Energy	470 kJ	Dietary Fibre	n/a
Protein	10 g	Sodium	70 mg
Fat	2 g	Potassium	20 mg
Carbohydrate	7 g	Iron	0.1 mg
Cholesterol	0	Niacin Equiv.	1.6 mg

NUTRITIONAL INFORMATION A good source of protein; moderate source of niacin. American muffins contain insignificant amounts of thiamin and riboflavin. The nutrient content will alter if the muffins contain extra ingredients like corn, chocolate chips and pumpkin.

DESCRIPTION A small, chemically leavened cake 6–8 cm in diameter weighing about 60 g, with light fluffy inside crumb and a rounded top with a pebbly texture.

ORIGIN AND HISTORY Early American settlers lived isolated lives, especially as they moved west. Food supplies were uncertain and the resourceful women, who excelled at baking, developed many recipes for quickly made products collectively known as quick breads. They were quick because they were made with baking powder instead of yeast or sourdough which took hours to rise. In this way, hospitality could be offered to passing travellers who unexpectedly dropped in with frontier news.

Australians have home-baked these muffins for generations. They were probably brought to this country by the goldminers and in early recipe books.

BUYING AND STORAGE Many varieties are readily available, either fresh from pastry cooks and takeaway counters or frozen from supermarkets.

Fresh muffins keep well for up to 2 days in summer, 1 week during cool weather. Frozen muffins will keep for 6 months.

PREPARATION AND USE Warm in the microwave oven or a moderate oven. Serve plain, spread with butter or cream cheese for breakfast or as a snack.

PROCESSING Often homemade from recipes readily available in good cookbooks.

VARIETIES
Bran, corn, fruit, nut, chocolate chip, carrot, pumpkin or combinations of these flavours.

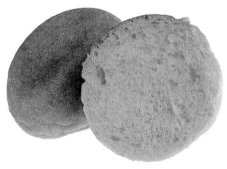

Muffin (English)

MAJOR NUTRIENTS		PLAIN SERVE SIZE 70 G	
Energy	640 kJ	Potassium	65 mg
Protein	6 g	Iron	1 mg
Fat	1 g	Magnesium	17 mg
Carbohydrate	31 g	Zinc	0.5 mg
Cholesterol	0	Thiamin	0.1 mg
Dietary Fibre	2 g	Niacin Equiv.	1.5 mg
Sodium	210 mg	Riboflavin	0.05 mg

NUTRITIONAL INFORMATION A good source of thiamin and iron; a moderate source of protein, fibre, niacin and magnesium.

Plain muffins have a similar nutrient content to white bread. The nutrient content will differ if the muffins contain bran, corn, fruit or muesli.

DESCRIPTION A round yeasted teacake, baked on both sides, 8–10 cm in diameter and 2 cm thick. It has a moist inner crumb with mildly acid flavour and a slightly tough crust.

ORIGIN AND HISTORY Muffins were popular in 18th century England. Early recipes were published in the 1754 edition of *The Art of Cookery Made Plain and Easy.* Muffin men sold their wares in the streets of Victorian England. Muffins are sometimes confused with crumpets, and the interchangeability of the two names makes the history of these foods difficult to trace.

BUYING AND STORAGE Readily available from bakeries and supermarkets in packs of 6 or 8. They will keep well at room temperature in their original wrapping for up to 10 days. Freeze for up to 2 months.

PREPARATION AND USE Thaw frozen muffins at room temperature or toast from the frozen state. Top with desired sweet or savoury filling. Serve for breakfast, as a quick snack or as a replacement for toast.

VARIETIES

Bran, corn, fruit, muesli.

SEE ALSO Crumpet.

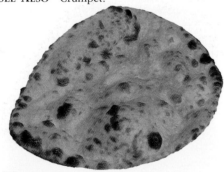

Naan

MAJOR NUTRIENTS		SERVE SIZE 60 G	
Energy	850 kJ	Iron	2 mg
Protein	59 g	Calcium	95 mg
Fat	79 g	Thiamin	0.10 mg
Carbohydrate	309 g	Phosphorus	80 mg
Cholesterol	0	Niacin Equiv.	3 mg
Sodium	220 mg		

NUTRITIONAL INFORMATION An excellent source of thiamin and niacin; a good source of protein.

DESCRIPTION Flat bread shaped like a teardrop, slightly leavened with yeast.

ORIGIN AND HISTORY A traditional Indian bread.

BUYING AND STORAGE Buy fresh from Indian takeaway restaurants. Will stay fresh for up to 3 hours, but best eaten while still

warm. Naan does not freeze successfully.

PREPARATION AND USE The dough (leavened slightly with yeast or baking powder) is mixed to a firm consistency, then divided into pieces weighing 150–200 g which are rolled or flattened to form a teardrop shape about 15 mm thick. The flattened dough piece is then plastered onto the hot side of a tandoori oven, where it is baked for approximately 3 minutes.

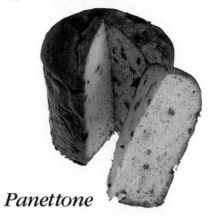

Panettone

NUTRITIONAL INFORMATION No nutritional analysis available.

DESCRIPTION A tall, light, cylindrical yeast cake with sultanas and candied peel.

ORIGIN AND HISTORY The history of panettone, which originated in Milan, is buried in legend. Some sources say it was originally called pan de Tonio, 'Tony's bread', after a 15th century Milanese baker.

BUYING AND STORAGE Available from most Italian or continental delicatessens and Italian bakeries. At Christmas panettone is exported from Milan to all corners of the globe. Store homemade panettone 1–2 days at room temperature. Follow manufacturer's instructions on the packet for imported panettone.

PREPARATION AND USE Serve with coffee for breakfast.

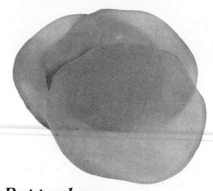

Pappadum

also called Pappadam

MAJOR NUTRIENTS		FRIED	
		SERVE SIZE 10 G	
Energy	155 kJ	Cholesterol	0
Protein	2 g	Sodium	240 g
Fat	2 g	Iron	1 g
Carbohydrate	4 g		

NUTRITIONAL INFORMATION Frying makes pappadums high in energy.

DESCRIPTION A thin, crackly wafer of lentil, potato or rice flour, eaten with Indian foods.

ORIGIN AND HISTORY Not known.

BUYING AND STORAGE Buy in packets from supermarkets and Asian food stores. Stored in the original wrapping in a cool dry place, pappadums will keep for months. If they become damp, pappadums should be dried out in the sun or a warm oven before they are cooked.

PREPARATION AND USE Fry pappadums in 1–2 cm of hot vegetable oil. During frying they will expand and bubble. Turn over to the other side as soon as they start to become straw-coloured. Drain thoroughly on absorbent paper and stand upright in a deep dish lined with more paper. They may be served warm or cold. Pappadums are served as an accompaniment to drinks or as a crisp addition to savoury dishes. They are best when cooked just before serving, but if they are cooked ahead, drained well and cooled, they may be stored in an airtight container for 2–3 hours before use.

VARIETIES

Pappadums are available plain, and flavoured with chilli, cumin seeds or cracked black pepper.

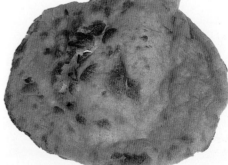

Paratha

also called Parata, Paratta

MAJOR NUTRIENTS		SERVE SIZE 30 G	
Energy	400 kJ	Dietary Fibre	1 g
Protein	2 g	Sodium	40 mg
Fat	4 g	Iron	0.5 mg
Carbohydrate	13 g	Vitamin A	40 µg
Cholesterol	11 mg	Thiamin	0.05 mg

NUTRITIONAL INFORMATION Frying makes paratha high in energy.

DESCRIPTION Unleavened, flaky, layered whole wheat bread.

ORIGIN AND HISTORY This Indian bread is usually reserved for special occasions.

BUYING AND STORAGE Parathas are usually homemade as they become stale quickly, although they may be available from takeaway sections of Indian restaurants.

PREPARATION AND USE Parathas are made from a combination of wholemeal and white flours (or wholemeal alone), salt and ghee, mixed to a dough with water. Pieces of dough are rolled into a disc shape, spread with cooled melted ghee and folded, then rolled again to a round, fairly thin pancake shape, and fried or cooked on a very well-greased griddle until golden brown. They may also be stuffed with vegetable mixtures. Place a spoonful of filling in the centre of a thin disc of dough, gather the edges together and crimp to seal into a ball shape. Flatten gently between the palms of the hands, then fry until golden.

Parathas, plain or filled, are served hot. The plain ones are usually served with kebabs and sambals.

SEE ALSO Chapatti, Puri (Indian).

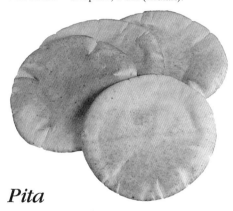

Pita

also called **Khoubiz, Pide, Pitta, Pocket Bread**

MAJOR NUTRIENTS		SERVE SIZE 60 G	
Energy	670 kJ	Sodium	310 mg
Protein	6 g	Calcium	55 mg
Fat	1 g	Iron	1 mg
Carbohydrate	35 g	Thiamin	0.15 mg
Cholesterol	0	Niacin Equiv.	2 mg
Dietary Fibre	2.5 mg		

NUTRITIONAL INFORMATION A good source of protein, iron, thiamin, and niacin; a moderate source of dietary fibre and calcium; this bread has a high sodium content. Wholemeal varieties could contain twice as much thiamin and three times as much dietary fibre.

DESCRIPTION Pita is a two-layered flat bread with a small amount of crumb adhering to both crusts.

Pitta is a Greek flat bread, 0.5 cm thick, with a pronounced yellow colour. Both breads may be from 12 cm to 20 cm in diameter.

Pide is the Arab term for a similar bread.

Khoubiz, or khoubiz sorj, is the bread sheet of Lebanon and Syria, cooked on an iron dome (sorj) over an open fire.

ORIGIN AND HISTORY Indicative of the breads of prehistoric and ancient times when grain pastes were shaped into flat cakes and cooked on hot stones. When the Egyptians discovered leavening, a secret they zealously guarded for many years, bread became lighter and easier to eat — a big improvement on the tough, chewy primitive breads.

BUYING AND STORAGE The various flat pocket breads are widely available from supermarkets, delicatessens and specialty food shops. Store in a sealed plastic bag at room temperature for 1–2 days, or in the freezer for up to 2 months.

PREPARATION AND USE If breads are required warm, heat briefly in oven or under griller. To open pocket breads, slit halfway around edge with a sharp knife and open gently. Large pocket breads can be halved and opened. All flat breads may be cut or broken into serving sized pieces.

Fill pocket breads with desired hot or cold ingredients, or roll any flat bread around fillings. Round flat breads can be used as a quick base for pizzas. All the breads can accompany meals or be used to scoop up dips and purees.

PROCESSING Whole or split flat breads can be brushed with butter or oil and sprinkled with spicy mixtures such as za'tar, sesame or poppy seeds, and heated in the oven; seed-topped breads can be left until crisp. Cut into serving portions before or after heating.

SEE ALSO Lavash, Naan.

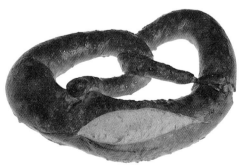

Pretzel

NUTRITIONAL INFORMATION No detailed analysis available.

DESCRIPTION A crunchy, loosely knotted rope of savoury bread.

ORIGIN AND HISTORY Pretzels, which originated in Germany and neighbouring Alsace, are traditionally made in the shape of a loose knot that may be an ancient symbol of the solar cycle. Pretzels were held in special reverence and authorities decreed that they must all be baked of fine white flour. Failure to do so resulted in severe punishment.

BUYING AND STORAGE The pretzels available in packets from supermarkets are usually either shaped in the traditional knot or in the form of thin sticks up to 10 cm long. This variety has been well baked to extend the shelf life to some months. The traditional crusty pretzels with soft centres are not available in Australia.

PREPARATION AND USE Traditionally, a yeast-leavened dough is made from fine white flour, which is shaped and boiled in water before baking, in much the same way as bagels are prepared. The water for boiling contains sodium bicarbonate and ammonium carbonate. After boiling they are drained well, brushed with egg and sprinkled with coarse salt or cumin seeds and sometimes poppy or sesame seeds, then oven-baked until crisp.

Pumpernickel

NUTRITIONAL INFORMATION See Dark Rye variety under Rye Bread.

DESCRIPTION A heavy, dark bread made from a mixture of rye flour, rye meal and kibbled or cracked rye grains.

ORIGIN AND HISTORY Pumpernickel is a regional rye bread which originated in Westphalia, Central Germany. It is an unusual bread as it is steamed and baked in the oven for many hours, resulting in a dense dark bread with a strong but mellow flavour.

BUYING AND STORAGE Buy from most stores where bread is sold. Imported and local varieties are usually vacuum packed for long shelf life and, if left unopened, will keep for many months. Once opened, pumpernickel should be kept in a sealed container in the refrigerator, particularly during hot weather.

PREPARATION AND USE The strong flavour of pumpernickel goes very well with strongly flavoured foods, particularly cheese, spicy sausage and cured or pickled fish. It is also used to make desserts and stuffings.

SEE ALSO Rye Bread.

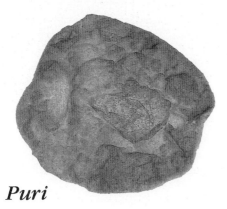

Puri

MAJOR NUTRIENTS   SERVE SIZE 30 G

Energy	415 kJ	Sodium	40 mg
Protein	2 g	Iron	0.7 mg
Fat	49 g	Thiamin	0.05 mg
Carbohydrate	14 g	Niacin Equiv.	2 mg
Cholesterol	12 mg		

NUTRITIONAL INFORMATION Frying increases the energy content. Puri are a moderate source of iron, thiamin and niacin.

DESCRIPTION The Georgian puri is a long, thin flat loaf of peasant bread, also called Dada's puri or mother's bread. The Indian puri is a flat disc of unleavened or slightly leavened deep-fried wholemeal bread which has puffed during cooking to form a pocket.

ORIGIN AND HISTORY Puri is the traditional peasant bread of Georgia, the area between the Black Sea and the Caspian Sea. It is usually made in the home and baked in an outside oven called the tone, which very closely resembles the tandoori oven of northern India. The sourdough starter used to leaven the dough was handed down from generation to generation. Each starter imparted a different flavour, so it was possible to identify each family's bread. In India, puris were probably originally the food of the wealthy, as they are deep-fried, requiring a pan suitable for frying and the oil for cooking — both expensive commodities.

BUYING AND STORAGE Georgian puri is not readily available. Indian puri is not available in stores, but some Indian restaurants may sell takeaway puri.

PREPARATION AND USE The Georgian bread is made from stone-ground wholemeal flour mixed with salt, water and sourdough starter. After shaping and proofing, the dough is slapped against the hot bricks lining the oven where it hangs until baked. For Indian puri, prepare a chapatti dough, roll out into circles 0.5 cm thick and deep-fry in hot oil until golden and puffy. Drain well and serve hot. They are usually served with curries.

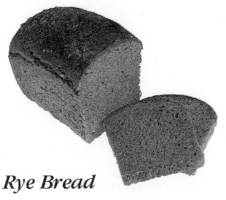

Rye Bread

NUTRITIONAL INFORMATION   See Varieties.

DESCRIPTION Bread made from rye flour, or including a large proportion of rye flour. Loaves are usually either baton-shaped or square. For further information see Varieties.

ORIGIN AND HISTORY Rye bread has been a staple food of Germany, Russia and northern Europe for thousands of years. In the very early days the rye flour was often mixed with barley to produce a heavy flat bread that could be baked on hot stones.

Today the big round dark rye loaves, small rectangular light loaves and small oval rolls of northern Europe are much the same as those of medieval Germany. These everyday breads are depicted in a 15th century portrait of a Nuremberg monastery baker.

The famous Gebild Brote, or picture breads, were baked for festive occasions. Many were embossed with animals, birds, flowers or a sheaf of grain, while others were sculpted to resemble people. Others bore Christian symbols such as the loaves and fishes, which may have derived from symbolic offerings to the gods of long ago in Egypt, Rome and northern Europe, where bread took the place of the sacrificial beasts and other offerings the poor could not afford. For example: Zopf, a plaited loaf, represented hair; Kipfel, a crescent roll, represented the moon. Originally, these breads were probably made from rye or a mixture of rye and wheat, if wheat was available. These breads are still made today for special occasions, by craftsmen bakers in many countries.

Rye breads are still important in the Scandinavian countries and Russia, where they are the basic food of the people.

BUYING AND STORAGE Choose a variety with the flavour which will best suit the foods to be served with the bread. Generally, dark ryes are served with strongly flavoured foods — herring, smoked ham, sharp cheddar cheeses — while the milder light ryes are served with cold meats, corned beef, pickles and milder-flavoured cheeses.

Store at room temperature for up to 4 days. Freeze wrapped for up to 6 months. Some varieties are vacuum packed in 250 g sealed packets and have a shelf life of 6 months.

PREPARATION AND USE Pure food regulations state that rye breads must contain at least 30% rye flour. Many varieties have much more rye flour and/or meal.

PROCESSING The black ryes are usually naturally fermented and baked slowly at lower temperatures, resulting in products which have a long shelf life and mellow flavours. Some varieties are based on sourdough.

VARIETIES

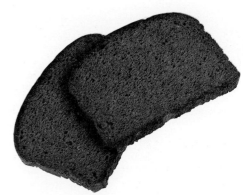

Dark or Black Rye (including Schinkenbrot)

MAJOR NUTRIENTS   SERVE SIZE 45 G

Energy	450 kJ	Potassium	100 mg
Protein	4 g	Iron	1.2 mg
Fat	1 g	Magnesium	25 mg
Carbohydrate	18 g	Zinc	0.5 mg
Cholesterol	0	Thiamin	0.05 mg
Dietary Fibre	3.5 g	Niacin Equiv.	1.5 mg
Sodium	230 mg	Riboflavin	0.1 mg

NUTRITIONAL INFORMATION 45 g represents 1 slice. A good source of fibre and iron; moderate source of protein, thiamin, niacin, riboflavin and magnesium. One slice of dark rye bread has more than twice as much fibre, riboflavin, iron and magnesium as 1 slice of light rye bread.

DESCRIPTION A dense, heavy, strongly flavoured bread with dark colour, usually made with 100% rye flour.

Light Rye

MAJOR NUTRIENTS		SERVE SIZE 60 G	
Energy	610 kJ	Potassium	90 mg
Protein	6 g	Iron	0.8 mg
Fat	1 g	Magnesium	21.5 mg
Carbohydrate	27 g	Zinc	0.6 mg
Cholesterol	0	Thiamin	0.1 mg
Dietary Fibre	3.5 g	Niacin Equiv.	1.5 mg
Sodium	310 mg	Riboflavin	0.05 mg

NUTRITIONAL INFORMATION 60 g represents two slices. A good source of thiamin and iron; moderate source of protein, fibre, niacin, sodium and magnesium. Light rye bread has similar nutrient content to white bread.

DESCRIPTION A light, softer, milder-flavoured bread with a paler fawn crumb. The varieties include sweet and sour breads, which often contain caraway seeds.

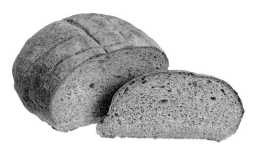

Sourdough Bread

NUTRITIONAL INFORMATION No nutritional analysis available, but nutrient content would be similar to those of other breads made from similar ingredients.

DESCRIPTION Crisp, crackly crusted bread with soft springy inner crumb and distinctive, sour aroma and flavour. Sourdough bread is, ideally, baked on the solid oven floor.

ORIGIN AND HISTORY Six thousand years ago the Egyptians discovered that if a flour and water dough was exposed to airborne yeast spores it would ferment and produce light, leavened bread. This method of leavening bread has long been employed in Europe where it has become a fine art, with starters being handed down through generations.

Using a piece of dough from the previous batch was a simple if slow way to ferment home-baked bread, and European settlers took the tradition with them to the New World. In the Californian goldfields sourdough starter was the only form of yeast available for bread making. Californian goldminers brought the habit to the Australian goldfields in the mid-19th century.

BUYING AND STORAGE Available from specialist bakers.

Store at room temperature for up to 2 days. Freezer storage will spoil the crisp crust.

PREPARATION AND USE The characteristic flavour of sourdough bread depends entirely on the quality and flavour of the yeast ferment or starter used to leaven the bread. Many home bakers make their own starter by leaving a batter of flour, a little yeast and water, milk or yoghurt to stand at room temperature for several days until wild yeasts in the air settle on it and help yeast already present to begin to ferment the mixture. Part of this starter is added to bread ingredients to provide the leavening which will cause the dough to rise. The remaining batter is fed with more flour and water or milk at regular intervals until required for the next batch of bread. Country cooks sometimes just save a piece of dough from a batch of bread to add to the mixture next time they bake. Care must be taken when making a starter, as it is not always successful, particularly in crowded cities where pollution in the air can provide undesirable yeasts which impart unpleasant flavours.

Manufacturers of sourdough breads guard their starters very carefully, taking great care to ensure no off flavours occur. They may also buy specially stabilised starters for commercial use. Dried starters for domestic use are available in the United States, particularly on the West Coast where the famed San Francisco sourdough bread is popular. Home bakers there also use it for hotcakes, muffins and 'biscuits' (scones).

VARIETIES
Wholemeal, white, rye.

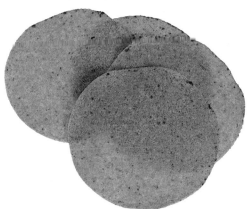

Tortilla

NUTRITIONAL INFORMATION No detailed analysis available.

DESCRIPTION Flat cornbread baked in discs by the people of Mexico and the Latin American countries.

ORIGIN AND HISTORY Central and Latin American. Basic tortillas are known to have been served at the court of Montezuma.

BUYING AND STORAGE Available at stores specialising in Mexican food and in dried form at groceries and supermarkets.

PREPARATION AND USE Tortillas are eaten alone as a bread or fried to make tacos and rolled around fillings or served with toppings as nachos, tortedos enchiladas, and tacquitos burritos tamales. The dough is also baked as corn chips for snacks.

PROCESSING Corn or maize is steeped overnight in water containing a very small quantity of lime. It is then passed between heated rollers, partially gelatinising the starch, then dried and ground into a meal (coarse flour) called nixtamal. A dough is mixed from the meal and water and cooked as flat discs 10–15 cm in diameter and 2–3 cm thick on a heated flat plate.

GRAINS AND CEREALS

Cereals are the edible grains or seeds of the grasses, named after Ceres the ancient Roman goddess of tillage and corn. Cereals are unique amongst foods because of their small bulk and excellent keeping qualities. This made them a very important survival food in early human history.

A hybrid wheat appeared in the Middle East and in other places after the Ice Age. The cultivation of cereals marked the transition of humans from hunter gatherers to agriculturalists. There is evidence that wheat was being cultivated sometime between 15 000 and 10 000 years BC. In other areas, different grasses grew, which were the forerunners of other major cereal crops.

There are important cereal crops in most geographic zones. Wheat and barley spread from Egypt and the Middle East to Greece and Rome, then throughout southern Europe to Britain, and then to India and parts of Asia and the colonies of the imperial powers. Rice was the staple in Asia and it too has spread in tropical and temperate zones. Corn or maize was the staple cereal in the Americas, and millet in Africa and Asia. In northern Europe, where the climate was too cold for wheat, oats and rye became the staple cereals. Older strains such as amaranth are being revived in the USA, while newer ones such as quinoa are also being developed.

Cereal crops have given rise to a wealth of foods in the various food cultures, such as breads, pastas, noodles, tortillas, breakfast cereals, semolina and couscous, cornmeal, polenta, cornstarch, flour and the innumerable products based on flour.

Cereals are the main food for the majority of humans. In some developing countries, they supply most of the energy and up to 90% of the protein. In Western countries they provide approximately 25% of the energy and protein. They vary in the amount of protein and the vitamins and minerals they contain, as the individual entries illustrate. In general, wholegrain cereals are an excellent source of thiamin, but in the milling process some of the thiamin is lost. White flour is still a valuable source of thiamin, but white rice does not contain sufficient thiamin to metabolise the carbohydrate in the cooked grain. Parboiled rice and brown rice are good sources of thiamin. Most cereals contribute some riboflavin and niacin to the diet, and wholegrain cereals provide folate.

The quality of the protein from grains is not as good as the quality of animal protein. Most cereals lack the amino acids leucine, lysine, threonine, tryptophan and methionine. When cereals are used in a mixed diet, other foods can provide these amino acids. When small amounts of pulses (dried peas, beans, lentils), nuts, other seeds, milk, cheese or flesh foods are combined with cereals, a good source of protein is provided.

From the individual entries it will also be seen that the amount of dietary fibre in cereals varies, with wholegrain cereals being the most valuable source. Oats and barley provide the soluble dietary fibres which assist in lowering blood cholesterol levels, the other cereals contain the insoluble fibres which assist in preventing constipation. Agricultural research into the improvement of cereal crops for yield and nutritive value, and the development of crops to grow under different climatic conditions, is important in the international effort to feed the populations in developing countries. A great deal has already been achieved. Much is also being done to encourage people in developing countries to maintain their own food customs and to build on these to improve their nutrition and health. This is often achieved by developing plant crops to supplement the staple cereals.

Increased affluence usually leads to a decline of the use of cereal products, and an increase in the use of animal products such as meat, dairy products and eggs. It is sensible to eat more bread and cereals, particularly the wholemeal and wholegrain varieties, and to use these to replace some of the high fat foods being consumed at present.

At the end of this chapter is a section on flour, where flours other than cereal flours are also included, for ease of reference.

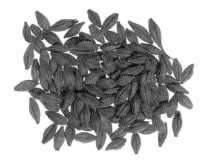

Barley *Hordeum distichon, H vulgare*

also called **Barleycorn**

MAJOR NUTRIENTS			SERVE SIZE 40 G
Energy	550 kJ	Iron	2.4 mg
Protein	4 g	Magnesium	36 mg
Fat	1 g	Zinc	0.9 mg
Carbohydrate	28 g	Thiamin	0.1 mg
Dietary Fibre	4 g	Niacin Equiv.	3 mg
Sodium	0	Cholesterol	0
Potassium	225 mg		

NUTRITIONAL INFORMATION An excellent source of fibre and niacin; good source of thiamin, folate, iron and magnesium; moderate source of protein and zinc. As with other cereals, the nutritive value of barley is influenced by milling or other processing. Usually the fibre, vitamin and mineral content is decreased with increased milling and processing.

ORIGIN AND HISTORY One of the first grains to be cultivated, barley was grown by the ancient Egyptians. It was used as a bread grain by the ancient Romans and Greeks who incorporated either grains or ears of barley into the design of their early coins. The ancient Greeks also looked on barley as a symbol of fertility while the Jews used it as a form of payment for the workers whose job it was to cut down the cedars of Lebanon. Barley was the general food of the Roman gladiators and calcined remains of stone-age coarse barley cakes have been found in Switzerland. Barleycorn was another name for a grain of barley. John Barleycorn was a name for whisky or spirits.

BUYING AND STORAGE Barley grains are sold in health food and stock feed stores. Keep in a cool dry place. Many farmers grow barley as a cash crop.

PREPARATION AND USE Use of barley for human food (other than beer) is fairly small in Western countries. Asia, North Africa and the Middle East eat it mainly as flour baked into flat breads or ground grain cooked as porridge. In developed countries barley is mainly used for stock feed and for malting for the baking, brewing and distilling industries. Small quantities are milled for other barley products.

PROCESSING It is important to remove the completely indigestible husk or hull from the grain before processing. The grains are cleaned, graded according to size, then steeped in water and allowed to germinate under strictly controlled conditions. After drying, the sprouted grains are ground and dried again to make malt flour. Barley grains may also be popped, rather like popcorn. Boil the whole grains in water for 30 minutes (they will triple in volume). Drain well, then rinse and remove as much excess water as possible and allow to dry for some hours. Deep-fry small amounts of prepared grain in hot oil for a minute or until it pops, then drain on absorbent paper. Season with parmesan cheese, seasoned salt or cayenne pepper.

VARIETIES

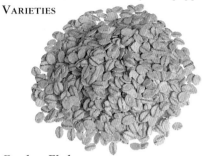

Barley Flakes

DESCRIPTION Flattened grains similar in appearance to rolled oats.

ORIGIN AND HISTORY See Barley.

BUYING AND STORAGE Buy from health food stores and store in a cool dry place. Refrigerate during hot weather.

PREPARATION AND USE Barley flakes may need soaking for a short while to soften the flakes before adding them to baked products. They are also used to make porridge or gruel, milk puddings and breakfast cereals such as muesli.

PROCESSING The outer husks are removed, then the whole grains are passed through rollers which press and flatten the grain, producing flakes which are slightly thicker and chewier than rolled oats.

Barley Grits

DESCRIPTION Hulled barley, broken into small particles. Also known as barley groats.

ORIGIN AND HISTORY See Barley.

BUYING AND STORAGE Barley grits or groats are sold in health food stores. Store in a cool dry place in a sealed container. Refrigerate in very hot weather.

PREPARATION AND USE Soak parboiled grits in water, squeeze out excess and use in salads and baked goods. Use groats (not boiled) in casseroles, meat loaves, hamburgers, soups, stews and as an ingredient in breakfast cereals.

PROCESSING Outer hulls are removed and the inner grain is broken into small particles. Sometimes the particles are steamed or parboiled, then dried.

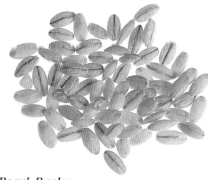

Pearl Barley

DESCRIPTION Dehulled small round polished barley grains with a shiny appearance. Also called pearled barley.

ORIGIN AND HISTORY Pearl barley was well known to the ancients and a very early recipe instructs the cook to pound pearl barley in a mortar and mix the flour with the very finest oil (amount determined by experience). The mixture was cooked gently while being enriched at regular intervals with gravy from a fat chicken or succulent lamb until this was absorbed. This was perhaps the forerunner of pilaf. Barley water, known as a diet drink (ptisana) called barley broth, was much favoured by Hippocrates. To make barley broth, barley was soaked in water until it swelled, then sun-dried, the husk removed, and the grain ground, boiled again for a longer period and dried once more. A small quantity of this flour was boiled, the water strained off and a little vinegar added to the liquid before drinking.

BUYING AND STORAGE Buy pearl barley from supermarkets in packets, either by itself or as an ingredient in a soup mix — a mixture of pulses and cereals suitable for enriching homemade soups. Store in a cool dry place. Buy barley water as a drink base (see below).

PREPARATION AND USE Pearl barley is used to make a refreshing drink base made from the water in which barley has been boiled, sweetened and flavoured with lemon, lime or orange or a combination of these fruits. Dilute with water to taste. Commonly known as lemon barley water, it is available in both powder and liquid form.

The grains are also used to thicken soups, stews, casseroles and desserts. Served as kasha in some areas in place of buckwheat.

PROCESSING The husk and pellicle are removed, then the grain is completely rounded by grinding and polishing.

Bran

NUTRITIONAL INFORMATION See the variety Wheat Bran.

DESCRIPTION The coarse outer layers of most cereal grains which are removed from the grains during the early stages of milling. In some countries the word refers to wheat bran. Bran particles may be large (flakes) or fine.

ORIGIN AND HISTORY Being a part of the cereal grain, bran has been in use since cereals were first cultivated. It is best known today as a source of dietary fibre, and its importance is much emphasised in the marketplace.

BUYING AND STORAGE Buy from supermarkets and health food stores.

PREPARATION AND USE Used in baked goods, breakfast cereals and health bars, and as a coating for foods to be fried. Also added to flour to increase the fibre content of biscuits, cakes and bread.

VARIETIES

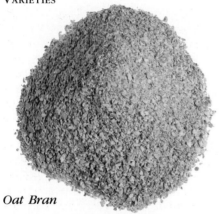

Oat Bran

MAJOR NUTRIENTS			SERVE SIZE 10 G
Energy	145 kJ	Sodium	0
Protein	1 g	Iron	1 mg
Fat	1 g	Zinc	0.5 mg
Carbohydrate	6 g	Thiamin	1 mg
Dietary Fibre	2 g	Niacin	2 mg

NUTRITIONAL INFORMATION This is an excellent source of fibre, particularly the soluble fibre. It is also a good source of iron, thiamin and niacin.

DESCRIPTION Oats and barley have a very rough outer hull which must be removed and discarded. Oat bran is in reality a fibre-rich layer of cells located under the husk. Fine pale brown particles of fibre with creamy specks form the centre of the groat distributed throughout the mixture.

ORIGIN AND HISTORY See Oats.

BUYING AND STORAGE Sold as oat bran, although the correct name is oat fibre. Always look for white flecks as they indicate the presence of the portions of the groat with the

potential health benefit. Buy in small quantities from some supermarkets and from health food stores. Store in a cool dry place.

PREPARATION AND USE Oat fibre is added to commercial breads, muffins and porridge as a fibre source for the health conscious. It is also used as a filler or extender in meat loaves, sausages and similar foods. For home baking, add to breads, quick breads, muffins, biscuits, meat loaves, rissoles or hamburgers and similar recipes.

PROCESSING The groats are dehusked, then the fairly thin underlying layer of fibre-rich cells is removed by milling. As it is impossible to remove the layer cleanly, small flakes of the white starch containing the centre part of the grains will also be present.

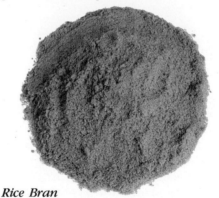

Rice Bran

MAJOR NUTRIENTS			SERVE SIZE 15 G
Energy	270 kJ	Magnesium	105 mg
Protein	2 g	Iron	0.8 mg
Fat	3 g	Zinc	0.8 mg
Carbohydrate	7 g	Phosphorus	110 mg
Dietary Fibre	3.8 g	Thiamin	0.45 mg
Sodium	1 mg	Niacin	6.3 mg

NUTRITIONAL INFORMATION Rice bran contains more fat than any other cereal bran. It is an excellent source of magnesium, phosphorus, thiamin and niacin, but due to the large amounts of fibre and other chemicals present, these nutrients may not be readily absorbed.

DESCRIPTION The fine outer bran layers are separated from the rice grain after the hull has been removed during processing of white rice.

BUYING AND STORAGE Buy fairly small amounts of coarsely or finely milled rice bran from health food stores. 'Unprocessed' bran has a short shelf life due to the presence of oil which quickly becomes rancid. Store in the refrigerator and use as soon as possible. Heat stabilised (defatted) rice bran has been treated to reduce rancidity and prolong shelf life. Stored in a cool dry place, it will keep for some months.

Defatted rice bran has good foaming capacity and stability — important properties in the manufacture of whipped toppings and meringues.

PREPARATION AND USE Rice bran is a permitted fibre additive for bread.

Add with wheat flour to such baked products as multigrain breads, doughnut and pancake mixes. As an extender, bran increases the fibre in fish and meat dishes and is used as an additive to soups and stews. Rice bran syrups are used as sugar substitutes in special diets. Raw rice bran is used as stock food.

PROCESSING During polishing the outer fibrous bran layers are separated from the grains and milled to make a light-textured, slightly sweetish powder which may be coarse or fine depending on the intended use. Rice oil is extracted from stabilised bran for use as a lubricator for drilling in the oil industry.

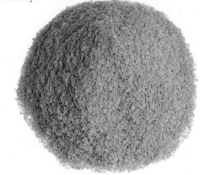

Wheat Bran

MAJOR NUTRIENTS			SERVE SIZE 10 G
Energy	80 kJ	Iron	1.2 mg
Protein	1 g	Magnesium	40 mg
Fat	1 g	Zinc	0.5 mg
Carbohydrate	2 g	Thiamin	0.1 mg
Dietary Fibre	4.5 g	Niacin Equiv.	2.5 mg
Sodium	0	Riboflavin	0.05 mg
Potassium	130 mg	Cholesterol	0

NUTRITIONAL INFORMATION An excellent source of fibre and iron; good source of thiamin and magnesium.

Despite the relatively high concentrations of vitamins and minerals in bran, to a varying extent they are biologically unavailable to humans. The presence of dietary fibre and phytic acid decreases the availability of the vitamins and minerals in the human gastrointestinal tract.

DESCRIPTION Outer layers of the wheat grain which are removed during the early stages of milling. May be coarsely or finely milled. It is often recommended for its excellent laxative properties.

ORIGIN AND HISTORY Emmer, the forerunner of modern wheat, had an outer husk which had to be removed by rubbing with sand. At the time of the Old Testament wheat was ground between millstones and sieved to remove the bran, sand and any chips from the grinding stones. By AD 50 sieving (bolting) of flour was widespread, being carried out by the Spanish, Egyptians and the Gauls. In Greece and Rome bran was probably mixed with bean flour, millet or barley to make it go further, and used to make a type of 'black' bread. Whether it was intended for human or animal consumption, even the poor endeavoured to sieve their flour. The laxative effects of bran were well tabulated at this time by the early medical writers who generally agreed that wholemeal bread increased faecal bulk and cleared the gut while white bread was more nutritious and recommended for people suffering from diarrhoea. Through the ages bran was eaten mostly by the poor until the 1830s when Sylvester Graham, an American evangelist who lectured on food up and down the east coast of America, urged people to put the bran back into wheat flour as a way of curing the indigestion so prevalent at the time. Graham teas were held over bran tea and Graham milk toast so that ladies could discuss intimate female problems. About this time the American Physiological Society was formed to broadcast Graham's teachings. Now, in the 20th century, bran has become a very popular food for people on healthy diets.

BUYING AND STORAGE Buy from supermarkets and health food stores. Store in a cool dry place in a covered container. Bran is also available in dry commercial breakfast cereals and some muesli.

PREPARATION AND USE Sprinkle on breakfast cereal or fruit, mix with fruit juices, add to biscuits, cakes, muffins, breads and quick breads. Finely ground bran can be added to casseroles and meat loaves, and used for coating foods for frying, although it does tend to soak up the fat or oil.

Commercial uses include prepared breakfast cereals and coatings for foods; also used in sausage and prepared meat products, and added to various packet mixes for cakes and puddings.

PROCESSING Bran is separated from other components of the wheat grain during milling. Because of the structure of the grain it is difficult to peel the bran cleanly from the grain, so small particles are still found in white flours of high extraction.

SEE ALSO Wholemeal Flour, Wholemeal and Fibre-increased Breads.

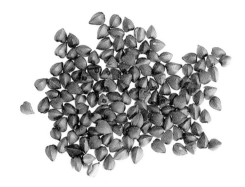

Buckwheat *Fagopyrum esculentum*

*also called **Buckweizen, Kasha, Piroshki***

MAJOR NUTRIENTS			SERVE SIZE 40 G
Energy	560 kJ	Potassium	130 mg
Protein	4 g	Sodium	15 mg
Fat	1 g	Iron	1.3 mg
Carbohydrate	29 g	Magnesium	34 mg
Dietary Fibre	4.5 mg	Thiamin	0.1 mg
Cholesterol	0	Niacin Equiv.	2 mg

NUTRITIONAL INFORMATION A good source of protein, thiamin, niacin, iron and magnesium; moderate source of fibre.

As with other cereals, nutritive value of buckwheat is influenced by milling and processing. Usually the fibre, vitamin and mineral content is decreased with increased processing.

DESCRIPTION An annual plant which produces triangular seeds which are said to resemble miniature beechnuts. The name is derived from the German word buckweizen. Buckwheat is not a cereal (grass), but the seeds can be used in much the same way as the cereal grains, so many people think of it as a cereal.

ORIGIN AND HISTORY A native of northern Europe and Asia, buckwheat has been a staple food in China for at least 1000 years. Migrating tribes from Manchuria and Siberia introduced buckwheat to eastern Europe and Mediterranean countries.

German and Dutch settlers took buckwheat to the New World where some people enjoy its strong distinctive taste when used alone, and others mix it with other flours for pancakes, dumplings and cakes.

Buckwheat is still a staple food in Russia and eastern Europe, where it is very popular in Jewish and in Polish cuisines.

BUYING AND STORAGE Buy buckwheat as rounded, plump, shiny seeds, toasted groats, or flour. The whole grain will keep for up to a year, and the flour, for many months, in a cool, dry area.

PREPARATION AND USE Untoasted groats are used for stuffings or kasha, a dish resembling pilaf. Cooked kasha is used as a stuffing for meatballs and vegetables such as cabbage or capsicums, and for piroshki. The flour is also used to make blini (pancakes) and, in China and Japan, for soba noodles.

SEE ALSO Soba, Piroshki.

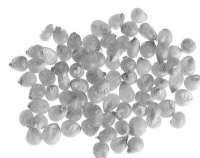

Maize *Zea mays*

*also called **Corn, Indian corn, Sweet corn***

MAJOR NUTRIENTS			SERVE SIZE 40 G
Energy	600 kJ	Sodium	0
Protein	4 g	Potassium	130 mg
Fat	0	Iron	2 mg
Carbohydrate	25 g	Thiamin	0.15 mg
Dietary Fibre	4 g	Niacin Equiv.	1 mg

NUTRITIONAL INFORMATION An excellent source of fibre; good source of thiamin and iron; moderate source of protein and niacin. The nutritive value of maize resembles that of other cereals, except that it contains some carotene which can be converted to vitamin A.

The niacin in maize is bound and does not become biologically available until the maize has been treated with heat and an alkaline solution. In Central America where maize is the principal source of energy, lime water has been used as the alkali. The lime water not only makes the niacin more available but also leaves a significant amount of calcium in the maize.

DESCRIPTION A kernel of grain made up of four basic parts: the outer hull; the soft endosperm which is made into cornflour; the hard endosperm milled for corn meal and grits; and the soft oily part of the grain called the germ which is much valued for the oil it yields.

ORIGIN AND HISTORY Corn is the only cereal native to the American continent where Indians began cultivating white, yellow, red and blue corn around 5000 BC. It was a particularly important crop for the Incas, the Aztecs and the Mayans of Mexico and Latin America who included it in their religious ceremonies. It has since become one of the most important food crops in North America where the whole plant is used both for human consumption and for stock feed. Explorers in the 16th century took corn to Europe where it is called maize. It has also become a staple food in many African countries. It is not an important food source in Australia.

BUYING AND STORAGE Buy fresh corn on the cob and cook as soon as possible as it loses flavour very quickly. Cobs should have firm, juicy kernels covered by fresh green husks with dark golden silk which feels damp to the touch. Avoid dried kernels which are a sure sign of age. Wrap cobs, still with husks, in damp paper towelling and store in the coldest part of the refrigerator for up to 24 hours if necessary. Freeze for longer storage.

PREPARATION AND USE To cook corn on the cob, remove most of the husk, all the silk and trim both ends of the cobs. Place in a large pan of water and add a pinch of sugar for each cob (do not add salt), bring to the boil and cook 3–5 minutes. Test to see if cooked. Serve hot with butter and freshly ground pepper. Cobs may also be roasted or barbecued. Soak husks in cold water for up to half an hour, drain and roast 20 to 25 minutes over a slow fire. Wrap de-husked cobs in aluminium foil with a little butter and cook as above. One cob yields approximately two-thirds of a cup of kernels.

PROCESSING Corn is milled to produce grits, meal and flour. Principal food uses are tortillas, cornbread, hominy, mealies, breakfast cereals, popcorn, snack foods, and as a vegetable. It is also used extensively as a filler in meat products, for manufacturing corn syrups, for glucose and for brewing and distilling. The oil extracted from the germ is used for cooking and as salad oil.

VARIETIES

Most common varieties are white and yellow, but other strains are available in Africa and blue corn is much favoured in Mexico.

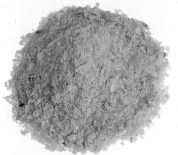

Corn Meal

MAJOR NUTRIENTS		SERVE SIZE 40 G	
Energy	620 kJ	Potassium	115 mg
Protein	4 g	Iron	1.7 mg
Fat	1 g	Thiamin	0.1 mg
Carbohydrate	30 g	Niacin Equiv.	1.2 mg
Dietary Fibre	n/a	Cholesterol	0
Sodium	0		

NUTRITIONAL INFORMATION A good

source of thiamin and iron; a moderate source of protein and niacin. The vitamins and minerals of corn meal are to a varying extent biologically unavailable. The protein is poor quality, even when compared to other grains.

Untreated corn is much less nutritious than treated corn.

DESCRIPTION Yellow-white coarse granular flour made from corn or maize. Also called polenta.

ORIGIN AND HISTORY Originally, polenta was a staple food made as a porridge from millet or spelt. Called puls or pulmentum, it was the field rations of the early Roman soldiers. Later, barley replaced millet and today polenta is made with corn meal.

BUYING AND STORAGE Available from supermarkets and specialist health food stores in packets weighing 375 g or 500 g. Store in a screw-topped jar in a cool place for up to 6 months, or refrigerate for longer storage. Sometimes an imported quick-cooking variety is available from specialist delicatessens.

PREPARATION AND USE Corn meal is used to make many foods of American origin, particularly from southern USA, Mexico and other Latin American countries. Cornbread, muffins, stuffings for turkey and fish, tamale pie, and innumerable recipes for quick breads are all popular. In northern Italy polenta is a staple food. Polenta is usually made from maize, mixed with water and a little salt and then cooked to a very thick porridge. It is traditionally served on a round wooden board, shaped into a large flat loaf and cut with a wooden knife. Sometimes it is cut into thick slices and served with stews or fried in oil or bacon fat and served with a rich tomato sauce.

Gnocchi are sometimes made from corn meal.

Romanians make mamaliga, a type of corn meal mush which is sometimes layered with goat cheese and baked, then served with sour cream. Cooked mealie, a corn meal mush, is a staple food for many African tribes.

Hominy

MAJOR NUTRIENTS		SERVE SIZE 40 G	
Energy	610 kJ	Potassium	30 mg
Protein	3 g	Iron	0.4 mg
Fat	0	Thiamin	0.05 mg
Carbohydrate	31 g	Niacin Equiv.	1 mg
Dietary Fibre	n/a	Cholesterol	0
Sodium	0		

NUTRITIONAL INFORMATION A moderate source of thiamin, niacin and iron. The niacin may be bound and not biologically available.

DESCRIPTION Whole dried kernels of corn

which have been treated to remove the germs and hulls; also called pozole.

ORIGIN AND HISTORY It became a staple food in the southern states of America where the Algonquin Indians taught the early colonists to soak the kernels in a weak solution of wood-lye to loosen the outer skins. The bran and germ were washed off with the outer skin and the inner kernel called tackhummin was cooked with water or milk to produce a type of porridge.

BUYING AND STORAGE Available only rarely in Australia, usually from delicatessens and food stores that specialise in imported foods. Store dry hominy in an airtight container in a dry place for months. Canned hominy should be used as soon as possible after opening, or frozen.

PREPARATION AND USE Dried hominy must be soaked before long cooking until it is soft. It may be served as a potato substitute or added to soups and stews. Layer cooked hominy with grated cheese and onions in a casserole, bake, and serve with sour cream or flavour with onions or capsicum.

PROCESSING Hominy is made by pearling (polishing) the grains mechanically or by treating them chemically with baking soda, slaked lime or lye for several hours to loosen the skins of the kernels. The inner part of the kernel is then dried and ground into a meal.

VARIETIES

Hominy grits are ground, whole hominy particles which may be coarse, medium or fine. They are cooked the same way as corn meal. Often used as porridge or baked or fried like polenta. They are the traditional accompaniment to many recipes from the southern USA.

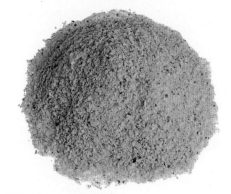

Matzo Meal

*also called **Matzah***

MAJOR NUTRIENTS		SERVE SIZE 50 G	
Energy	720 kJ	Sodium	5 g
Protein	5 g	Potassium	50 mg
Fat	less than 1 g	Phosphorus	45 mg
Carbohydrate	40 g	Thiamin	0.05 mg
Dietary Fibre	1 g		

NUTRITIONAL INFORMATION A moderate source of folate and thiamin. It is a carbohydrate flour with moderate protein content.

DESCRIPTION Coarse or fine meal ground from matzo.

ORIGIN AND HISTORY The history of matzo meal is very closely bound to matzo, the unleavened bread which is baked for Passover to commemorate the flight of the Israelites from Egypt. Before Passover all leaven and foods containing yeast are thrown out, the house is cleaned and only unleavened products are eaten during this religious festival. Matzo, the waferlike unleavened bread which is baked under supervision of the rabbi, is ground into a meal used to thicken dishes eaten at this time.

BUYING AND STORAGE Buy from delicatessens and supermarkets that specialise in kosher products. Store in a cool dry place and use as soon as possible.

PREPARATION AND USE Use in place of flour, in sweet or savoury baked dishes, particularly Pesach foods.

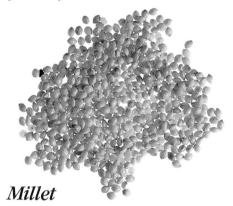

Millet

*also called **Bulrush millet, Finger millet, Ragi, Kaffir corn, Guinea corn, Teff, Adlay, Job's tears***

MAJOR NUTRIENTS		SERVE SIZE 40 G	
Energy	610 kJ	Cholesterol	0
Protein	2 g	Sodium	0
Fat	1 g	Iron	2.5 mg
Carbohydrate	30 g	Thiamin	0.15 mg
Dietary Fibre	4 g	Niacin Equiv.	2 mg

NUTRITIONAL INFORMATION An excellent source of fibre; good source of thiamin, niacin and iron; moderate source of protein.

Millet, like other cereals, is milled and processed before eating, which can decrease the vitamin and mineral content. Refined millet products are not widely available.

DESCRIPTION Millet is the name given to a group of cereal grasses, many of which are of the genus *Panicum*, and which are grown mainly in Asia, Africa, parts of India, Pakistan, USA, and USSR.

ORIGIN AND HISTORY Millets have been used for brewing and for food since prehistoric times in Asia, Africa and Europe. Sorghum, a member of the millet family, probably originated in North Africa.

The word millet is thought to have evolved from the Latin millesimum, meaning one-thousandth part — something extremely small, a good description of millet seeds. Evidence of early cultivation has been found on a carving discovered in an ancient Assyrian palace, although historians are certain it was first cultivated in Ethiopia, where it is still a staple crop. The Bantu tribes of Africa adopted millet, which was pulverised to make flour or meal and, in turn, made into porridge, bread and beer. From Ethiopia the cultivation of millets spread via Arabia and the Persian Gulf to India, where they have been grown since around 2000 BC, and to China, following the silk trade routes. Teff, although not strictly a millet, is usually grouped with them because it is the basic ingredient of injera, one of Ethiopia's finest breads.

BUYING AND STORAGE Buy from health food stores or from produce merchants. Millet is available as bird seed from supermarkets.

PREPARATION AND USE Millets are used principally for making porridge, for flat breads, and for brewing beer. Thick millet porridge is eaten throughout the USSR as kasha. In Australia very small quantities of millet are used for porridge and even smaller quantities are ground into flour to add texture and flavour to baked products. It is sometimes used for people on wheat-free diets. Sorghum is used mainly for brewing and for stock feed.

Oats

MAJOR NUTRIENTS		SERVE SIZE 40 G	
Energy	650 kJ	Cholesterol	0
Protein	6 g	Sodium	10 mg
Fat	3 g	Iron	1.5 mg
Carbohydrate	26 g	Thiamin	0.2 mg
Dietary Fibre	3 g	Niacin Equiv.	2.5 mg

NUTRITIONAL INFORMATION An excellent source of thiamin; good source of niacin and iron; moderate source of protein. Oatmeal contains more protein and more oil than other common cereals.

In milling of oats only the fibrous pericarp is usually removed and the germ is retained. Most forms of oatmeal are thus not highly refined and retain a high percentage of the vitamins and minerals present in the original grain.

ORIGIN AND HISTORY The oat was being cultivated by the Europeans at least 1000 BC in a wide sweep from Armenia to Spain. In classical times it was regarded as a weed and only used for medicinal purposes. It became an important crop in northern Europe and was grown in Denmark, Germany and Switzerland where it was used both as porridge and as a bread cereal.

In medieval England, the Isle of Man was known for growing fine crops. The monasteries mixed oats with beans to make a mixture known as 'Lenten gruelum'. In 18th century Britain oat bread was eaten by farmers and country villagers, particularly in northern England and Ireland. In Scotland, where oats were known as pilcorn, they became part of the daily fare and today are still much favoured as a staple crop where they retain traditional importance as a food.

BUYING AND STORAGE Buy in small quantities as required. The high fat content of oats means they will go rancid more quickly than other cereals. Store in the refrigerator in a sealed container.

PREPARATION AND USE Used to make groats, rolled oats, flakes, bran (fibre), oatmeal and flour. In Ireland a gruel called stirabout is made from oat groats.

PROCESSING Oats have a covered caryopsis, so the grains have to be de-husked before use.

VARIETIES

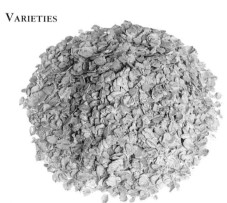

Oat Flakes

DESCRIPTION Large flattened flakes of oat grain.

ORIGIN AND HISTORY See Oats.

BUYING AND STORAGE Available from health food stores. Buy in small quantities and store in a cool dry place. They are sometimes sold as toasted flakes.

PREPARATION AND USE Use for breakfast cereals, in muesli, biscuits and breads and as an extender in meat loaves, and in all recipes calling for rolled oats. Oat flakes may be ground in a food processor to produce a fine flour which is used in breads and cakes.

PROCESSING The grains are cleaned, hulled, steamed, flattened and, if required, toasted until very fine.

Oatmeal

DESCRIPTION Tiny flakes of oat grain, sometimes milled until very fine.

ORIGIN AND HISTORY Oats were taken to the New World, where they grew well along the northeast coast of America. They were rolled and ground to make a meal which was cooked as porridge.

PREPARATION AND USE Primary use is for breakfast porridge, but it is also used in pancakes, muffins, bread, Scottish oatcakes, biscuits and quick breads. Oatmeal is the essential ingredient in the uniquely Scottish mixture called Athole Brose which is made from oatmeal, honey, whisky and water. Haggis, a national dish of Scotland, is a mixture of oatmeal, chopped sheep's offal and seasonings stuffed into a sheep's stomach and boiled.

PROCESSING Oats are cleaned to remove stones, poor grains and any other pieces of unwanted matter. After cleaning they are stabilised by steam treatment, inactivating enzymes in the grain which lead to oxidation. The process also seems to improve the development of the characteristic nutty flavour. After steaming, the oats are air-dried in a kiln to reduce the water content to a suitable level for milling. This makes the husk brittle so it becomes easier to remove. After drying the grains are graded, the husk removed and the inner groats are scoured. Before grinding into meal, the groats are cut into several pieces and are known as 'pinhead meal'. Any flour produced during cutting is sieved off to make pet food biscuits. Pinhead meal is ground to make medium or fine oatmeal containing nearly 100% of the oat groat.

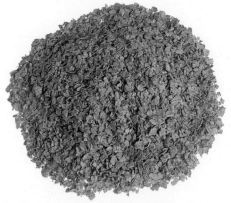

Quick Cooking Oats, Instant Oats

DESCRIPTION Flakes of oat grain, finer and thinner than rolled oats. Instant oats are precooked.

BUYING AND STORAGE Buy from health food stores and supermarkets. Store in a cool, dry place.

PREPARATION AND USE Instant oats cook more quickly, but either type may be used to make porridge, in cakes, pastries and breads, in hamburgers, in quick breads and muffins, and also in special diet foods for people with wheat allergies. Quick cooking and instant oats are also used in packaged breakfast cereals.

PROCESSING Oat groats are cut into pieces, then passed through rollers so they become very thin. For instant oats, the end groats are precooked before being rolled very thinly.

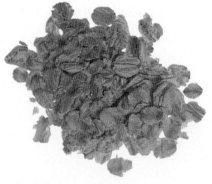

Rolled Oats

DESCRIPTION Flattened flakes of grain.

ORIGIN AND HISTORY Oat grains are much softer than wheat grains, so it was easy for them to be crushed by hand in a mortar and pestle. This flattening also made them much easier to cook.

BUYING AND STORAGE Buy from supermarkets. Store in a cool dry place or in the refrigerator, as they go rancid quickly owing to the high fat content.

PREPARATION AND USE Used to make porridge, for muesli, biscuits, shortbread, muffins and quick breads, and in meat loaves, rissoles and similar foods. Rolled oats may be ground in a food processor to make fine oat-

meal or oat flour for use in breads, cakes and muffins.

PROCESSING The grains are cleaned, hulled, steamed and flattened between rollers. Hulled oat grains (called groats) may be rolled by hand at home with a rolling pin.

Steel-cut Oats

DESCRIPTION Small pieces of oat groat.

ORIGIN AND HISTORY Originated in the USA where they were sold in grocery stores in the mid-1850s.

PREPARATION AND USE Used for porridge and oatcakes, breads, biscuits, muffins and quick breads.

PROCESSING The cleaned oat groats are cut into thin lengthways slices with sharp steel blades.

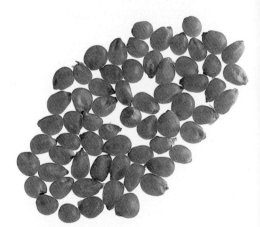

Popcorn   *Zea mays everta*

MAJOR NUTRIENTS		SERVE SIZE **15** G	
Energy	260 kJ	Dietary Fibre	2.5 g
Protein	2 g	Sodium	0
Fat	1 g	Cholesterol	0
Carbohydrate	12 g		

NUTRITIONAL INFORMATION A moderate source of fibre.

DESCRIPTION Popping corn is a type of corn having kernels which will pop open after drying and on the application of heat, exposing the light, puffy centre of the grain.

ORIGIN AND HISTORY Ancient corn poppers have been found in North, South and Central America. According to legend popcorn was introduced to the British colonists at the first Thanksgiving feast by the brother of one of the Indian chiefs. Sales of commercial popcorn in the US began around 1885.

BUYING AND STORAGE Popping corn is available at most supermarkets and specialty food stores. It will keep indefinitely in a cool dry place. Cooked popcorn is sold in sealed cellophane bags from sweet shops and in cardboard containers from popcorn machines located in stores, cinema foyers and at country fairs. A microwavable pop-in-the-bag product is also now available from supermarkets for home popping.

PREPARATION AND USE To prepare popcorn at home, a small amount of oil is heated in a large pan, the corn is added and the lid is immediately placed on the pan. The moisture inside the grain turns to steam and explodes the grains, the starch gelatinises and the corn is 'popped'. Flavours or salt may be added as desired.

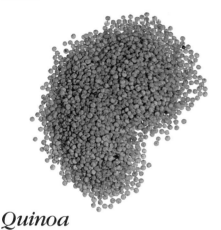

Quinoa

MAJOR NUTRIENTS — SERVE SIZE 100 G

Energy	1425 kJ	Fat	6 g
Protein	15 g	Dietary Fibre	8 g
Carbohydrate	60 g		

NUTRITIONAL INFORMATION Quinoa has a high protein content, compared with other grains. No data are available on vitamins and minerals.

DESCRIPTION Quinoa (pronounced keenwa) is a grain resembling millet.

ORIGIN AND HISTORY The Incas of South America grew it for thousands of years in the Andes, where it was known as 'the mother grain'. It is grown in and exported from Peru and the United States.

BUYING AND STORAGE Quinoa is becoming available in delicatessens and specialty food stores. Keep the packet sealed in a cool, dry place.

PREPARATION AND USE Easy to cook, the tiny pellets swell and become translucent, with the texture of caviar. They can be cooked in water or broth for 10–15 minutes, then served as for rice or cracked wheat.

Rice *Oriza sativa*

MAJOR NUTRIENTS

			BROWN RICE SERVE SIZE 50 G
Energy	780 kJ	Sodium	0
Protein	4 g	Iron	0.6 mg
Fat	1 g	Magnesium	55 mg
Carbohydrate	38 g	Zinc	0.8 mg
Dietary Fibre	2 g	Thiamin	0.2 mg
Cholesterol	0	Niacin Equiv.	3 mg

			WHITE RICE SERVE SIZE 50 G
Energy	770 kJ	Sodium	5 mg
Protein	4 g	Iron	0.4 mg
Fat	0	Magnesium	15 mg
Carbohydrate	39 g	Zinc	0.5 mg
Dietary Fibre	1 g	Thiamin	0.05 mg
Cholesterol	0	Niacin Equiv.	3 mg

NUTRITIONAL INFORMATION Brown rice is an excellent source of niacin and magnesium; good source of thiamin and iron; moderate source of protein, fibre and zinc. When brown rice is the major source of energy in the diet it provides valuable quantities of the above nutrients as well as riboflavin and calcium. The B group vitamins are all very soluble in water and heavy losses of these vitamins may occur if rice is boiled in excess water, fried at high temperatures or washed.

White rice is an excellent source of niacin; moderate source of protein, thiamin and iron. It has fewer vitamins and minerals than brown rice. The bran layer, which includes the embryo of the seed, is removed during the milling of white rice, giving brown rice a superior vitamin content.

White rice does not contain sufficient thiamin to enable the body to use the carbohydrate present in rice for energy.

DESCRIPTION Rice is a small, oval grain with an outer hull inside which is a brown kernel, whose outer layer is the rice bran. Underneath is the white inner kernel containing the rice germ.

ORIGIN AND HISTORY According to legend, rice was first eaten in China 5000 years ago. To mark the beginning of the planting season the Emperor Shen would plant the first (and best) rice seeds, followed by his sons who planted different varieties. Most Chinese people prefer to eat white rice, no doubt influenced by Confucius who always insisted it should be as white as possible. The early Chinese removed the outer husks from the grains and probably sold them for polishing precious gems.

Rice arrived in Egypt in the 4th century BC and around that time India was exporting it to Greece. Rice has been a staple crop in many countries and often the sole source of food. In a number of languages the word for rice is the same as the word for food. 'Have you had rice?' in some cultures means, 'Have you eaten?'

In Japan the importance of rice is emphasised by the many thousands of shrines to Inari the rice god which may be seen in the countryside. Freshly harvested rice was always thought to taste the best as it has a moist texture and needs less water for cooking. For centuries rice was a standard of wealth and often used in place of money. Samurai were paid in rice and when Japan invaded China the Chinese coolies in turn were also paid in rice. The growing of rice, and the success or failure of the crop, affected the history, art, literature, ceremonials and the very way of life of the people of India, China and Japan for centuries.

Spilling rice or upsetting a rice bowl is considered very bad luck.

Rice is the symbol of life and fertility and the tradition of throwing rice at weddings (nowadays symbolised by confetti) stems from this belief.

Although white rice has been popular throughout the millennia of human cultivation, brown rice has also been eaten, by the farmers and peasants of Asia, India and Africa. Rice husks are tough, adhering closely to the grain, and must be removed before the grain can be cooked. This was done by either crushing with a mortar or pounding with a large wooden hammer, both primitive methods which removed some of the bran layer and some of the germ and damaged many of the inner kernels.

BUYING AND STORAGE Brown rice can be bought from supermarkets and a quick-cooking variety is available.

Most of the world's rice is eaten as the white, polished whole grain. Stored in a cool, dry place away from vermin, sound rice will keep almost indefinitely.

PREPARATION AND USE Brown rice takes longer to boil or steam because the water has to penetrate the bran layers. 40–45 minutes is normal, but the quick-cooking variety will only take 18–20 minutes. See packet labels for directions. One cup of raw brown rice is equal to approximately 3 cups of cooked.

Brown rice can be used whenever white rice is suggested in dishes. In Japan natural fermentation occurs after the addition of koji (a rice culture) which reduces the starches in glutinous brown rice to sugars. This process results in the easily digested sweetener amazake.

The choice of short-, medium- or long-grain

rice for cooking depends on availability and personal preference. The different varieties tend to vary in stickiness and each one, whether brown, polished or parboiled, may be boiled, steamed, oven-cooked or fried. Steaming is the preferred method of cooking for many, as the flavour of the cooked rice is very full and the grains are soft without being mushy. For white rice, place clean, dry rice in a heavy-based saucepan and add water to cover to a depth of 2.5 cm. Bring to the boil, boil rapidly until small steam holes appear, then reduce heat, cover with a tight fitting lid and simmer 10 minutes. Remove from heat, allow to stand for 10 minutes. Remove lid and allow to stand 5 minutes more before serving. Also used for paella and pilau.

The basic method for pilau rice: Cook 1 measure rice in butter, ghee or oil with chopped vegetables, then add 1½ measures of liquid (water, stock, vegetable juice). Stir rice and simmer, covered, over low heat for 25 minutes (check to ensure rice is cooked as you like it), toss rice with a fork and allow to steam for a few minutes before serving. Pieces of meat, fish or chicken may be cooked with the rice to make a complete dish. The same method may be used to cook desserts, by adding fruit juice and fruit instead of vegetables and meat.

PROCESSING The grains are rubbed against abrasive discs to remove the outer hull and lightly polish the brown kernel (known as brown rice). The grains are further polished until the grain becomes white and glossy. Rice is also made into vinegar, Japanese sweet rice wine, mirin, and the stronger rice wine sake.

VARIETIES
Over two thousand varieties are grown worldwide.

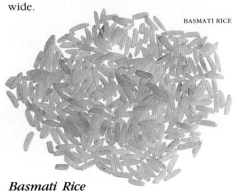
BASMATI RICE

Basmati Rice

MAJOR NUTRIENTS SERVE SIZE 50 G

Energy	750 kJ	Dietary Fibre	1 g
Protein	4 g	Cholesterol	0
Fat	0	Sodium	5 mg
Carbohydrate	40 g	Iron	0.5 mg

NUTRITIONAL INFORMATION There is no

analysis available of the vitamins and minerals (except iron) in basmati rice. This rice is likely to have a similar vitamin and mineral content to white rice.

There is little variation in the amount of protein, fat and carbohydrate between the different rices.

DESCRIPTION Aromatic, long, narrow-grained rice.

ORIGIN AND HISTORY Remains of cultivated rice dating back 7000 years have been found in eastern China and northern India where rice farmers are sometimes referred to as 'farmers of fifty centuries'. Basmati rice has been cultivated in the foothills of the Himalayas in areas stretching from northern India to Bangladesh, where the high altitudes and this particular variety combine to produce a rice so prized by the population for its firm texture and aromatic flavour that it commands premium prices.

BUYING AND STORAGE Buy from specialist Indian or Asian food suppliers or the supermarket. Stored in a covered container in a cool dry place, it will keep indefinitely.

PREPARATION AND USE Pick over the rice, discarding any stones, sticks and stray seeds. Soak in cold water for 15–20 minutes before cooking. Drain well and cook as directed in recipes for Indian dishes. It is particularly good in pilau, for fried rice or for biryani, as the grains stay firm and separate when cooked and the flavour enhances the other flavours in the dishes.

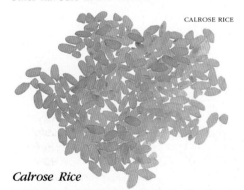
CALROSE RICE

Calrose Rice

MAJOR NUTRIENTS SERVE SIZE 50 G

Energy	760 kJ	Sodium	0
Protein	3 g	Potassium	30 mg
Fat	0	Iron	0.4 mg
Carbohydrate	39 g	Zinc	0.5 mg
Dietary Fibre	1 g	Thiamin	0.05 mg
Cholesterol	0	Niacin Equiv.	1.5 mg

NUTRITIONAL INFORMATION A moderate source of protein, thiamin, niacin, iron and magnesium. See White Rice.

DESCRIPTION Medium-grain white rice bred from the original American variety.

Calrose is accepted as an Australian rice variety.

PREPARATION AND USE Steam in a covered saucepan for maximum retention of nutrients. Serve as an accompaniment to cooked dishes.

Carolina Rice

NUTRITIONAL INFORMATION No nutritional analysis available. See white rice.

DESCRIPTION Variety of long-grain rice, also called patna rice. No longer grown in Australia — superseded by newer varieties e.g. Mahatma, Pelde.

ORIGIN AND HISTORY This long-grain, less starchy variety of rice was originally grown in India where it has been eaten as a staple food for thousands of years. By various means, it found its way to southern USA where the first crops were planted in the mid-17th century. Unfortunately the seeds died, probably due to the fact that they were sown in dry farmland, and no one bothered to try again until towards the end of the century when a ship bound for Liverpool docked at Charlestown. One of the city fathers obtained some of the unhulled rice grains which formed part of the cargo and planted them in swampy ground. This crop flourished to become the basis of rice growing in America. Much of the American rice imported into Britain is still called 'Carolina' although cultivation in that state ceased soon after the end of the American Civil War. Nowadays it is more likely to come from Arkansas, California, Argentina or Brazil or, until some years ago, Australia.

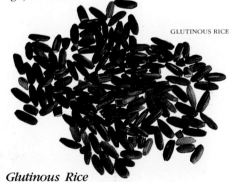
GLUTINOUS RICE

Glutinous Rice

MAJOR NUTRIENTS SERVE SIZE 50 G

Energy	750 kJ	Sodium	0
Protein	4 g	Iron	0.6 mg
Fat	1 g	Zinc	1 mg
Carbohydrate	37 g	Thiamin	1 mg
Dietary Fibre	1 g	Niacin Equiv.	1.5 mg
Cholesterol	0		

NUTRITIONAL INFORMATION A good source of thiamin and iron; moderate source of protein, niacin and zinc. See White Rice.

Of the cereal grains, rice protein is high quality protein.

DESCRIPTION Rice with fat opaque grains which become sweet and sticky on boiling, hence the alternative names, pudding rice and sticky rice. Black glutinous rice is normally aromatic. Long-grain deep red rice is used mainly for sweet dishes. Imported from Thailand, available at Asian supermarkets.

ORIGIN AND HISTORY Since before recorded history rice has been a staple crop in Japan. There are many thousands of varieties but glutinous or sticky rice has a special place in Japanese life. Sekihan (red rice) is made from glutinous rice and red beans steamed together, resulting in a dish which is specially prepared for ceremonial occasions, children's festivals, weddings and birthdays. It is also presented at the shrine as a gift to the gods. In China, glutinous rice has been traced back to archaeological excavations of the early Han period. At this time rice was considered to be a delicacy as millet was the staple cereal. One of the ancient festivals took place on the fifth day of the fifth month, when the people celebrated with a special mixture of glutinous rice and millet in a triangular package enclosed in bamboo leaves. It is also used for the special Eight Treasure rice puddings, particularly at Chinese New Year celebrations.

BUYING AND STORAGE Available from Asian food stores. The Vietnamese community imports black glutinous rice to make dishes for special occasions, while the red varieties are also popular for desserts.

PREPARATION AND USE Boil with sugar, water and spices to make desserts. Because it becomes sticky it is ideal for baking, for confectionery and for beer and wine. Glutinous rice is also used to make rice paper — transparent sheets which are used to wrap savoury Chinese foods (it may be used as a spring roll wrapper). Glutinous rice is used extensively in Asian cookery.

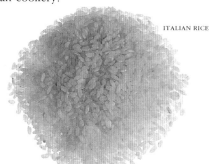

ITALIAN RICE

Italian Rice

NUTRITIONAL INFORMATION No nutritional analysis available.

DESCRIPTION Short round-grained pearly rice preferred for Italian cooking.

ORIGIN AND HISTORY Arborio, the name of a village in the Piedmont region of northern Italy, has become the generic name for the rice which is grown in this area. Italy is the largest European producer.

BUYING AND STORAGE Buy from Italian specialty shops and store in a cool dry place. Leftover cooked rice may be stored in the refrigerator for 2–3 days, or for up to 1 month in the freezer. Reheat over simmering water or in a microwave oven.

PREPARATION AND USE Cooked the same way as other rice, but it is especially suitable for risotto, a uniquely Italian technique for cooking rice, where the main objective is to enable it to gradually absorb hot liquid, a little at a time, until the grains become swollen and tender and the dish has a creamy velvet texture. Chopped onion is sautéed in butter, then the rice is added and sautéed for a minute or two before the liquid is added. Constant stirring is necessary to ensure the grains do not stick to the bottom of the pan. The temperature should be hot enough for the rice to cook evenly and absorb the liquid without being soggy. Risotto is always served with freshly grated parmesan cheese. Arborio is also used in soups, for baked cakes (budini di riso) and in desserts. Risotto alla Milanese is a famous risotto dish.

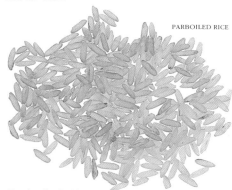

PARBOILED RICE

Parboiled Rice

MAJOR NUTRIENTS		SERVE SIZE 50 G	
Energy	780 kJ	Sodium	0
Protein	4 g	Iron	0.4 mg
Fat	1 g	Magnesium	32 mg
Carbohydrate	39 g	Zinc	0.6 mg
Dietary Fibre	1 g	Thiamin	0.1 mg
Cholesterol	0	Niacin Equiv.	3 mg

NUTRITIONAL INFORMATION An excellent source of niacin; good source of thiamin and magnesium; moderate source of protein, iron and zinc.

Parboiling drives the B group vitamins into the interior of the grain so that they are not removed with the bran when the grain is milled.

The levels of vitamins and minerals in parboiled rice are between white rice and brown rice.

DESCRIPTION 'Rough' or 'paddy' rice, known as siddha, ushna rice

ORIGIN AND HISTORY The practice of parboiling rough or paddy rice grains has been widely carried out for centuries by peasants in southern Asia (particularly on the Indian subcontinent) and in parts of Africa. However, it was not known outside this area until the beginning of the 19th century. The practice of parboiling received world attention when it was discovered that Chinese immigrants in Malaya who ate raw rice suffered from beri-beri while Indians who ate the parboiled product did not. Studies were then carried out to prove that the consumption of milled rice was associated with the disease.

BUYING AND STORAGE This rice is available in most Asian countries and in Australia. Store in a cool dry place as it is prone to oxidation and rancidity.

PROCESSING Rice is thoroughly saturated by soaking in water. The excess water is drained off and the grains are steamed or boiled to gelatinise the starch. After cooling they are dried either in the sun or by fanning hot air across the surface of the grains.

After treatment the grains become pale amber or light yellow.

PREPARATION AND USE Parboiled rice is very suitable for canning as the grains stay whole, and the loss of solids is significantly reduced during processing. It is preferred by the catering industry as it is less sticky when cooked, makes particularly good salads, and holds well when kept hot for serving large numbers of people. In Australia it is sold as 'the rice that cooks in the fridge'. Covered with hot tap water and left to stand for an hour, it rehydrates with very separate grains.

Parboiled waxy rice is used to make flaked rice in the Philippines.

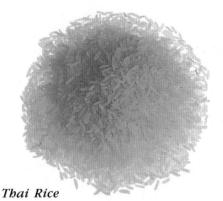

Thai Rice

NUTRITIONAL INFORMATION No nutritional analysis available.

DESCRIPTION A fragrant long-grained rice used in many South-East Asian recipes and also called jasmine rice.

ORIGIN AND HISTORY As for rice in general.

BUYING AND STORAGE As for rice in general.

PREPARATION AND USE Usually steamed or cooked, without salt, in a covered saucepan.

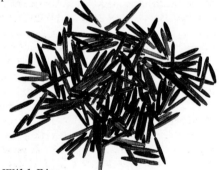

Wild Rice

NUTRITIONAL INFORMATION No nutritional analysis available.

DESCRIPTION Dark rice (*Zizania aquatica*) with black to brown grains, chewy texture and nutty flavour, also called tuscarora.

ORIGIN AND HISTORY Wild rice is not a close relative of rice. Rather, it is the grain of a water grass native to North America where it grows in the shallow lakes and marshy areas of the Great Lakes region. It was originally harvested by the Chippewa Indians who gathered it by hand. Nowadays it is grown in paddies and harvested by machine.

BUYING AND STORAGE Buy from stores that specialise in imported foods. Wild rice is very expensive and therefore usually sold in small quantities. Store in an airtight container in a cool dry place. Cooked leftover rice may be stored in the refrigerator for 2–3 days.

PREPARATION AND USE Wash thoroughly before cooking. Boil or steam with water, stock, wine or a combination of these liquids. Being such an expensive food, it is often extended by the addition of cooked white or brown rice, or burghul. Serve flavoured with sautéed onions, mushrooms or nuts. Use as an accompaniment to poultry or fish or as a stuffing for these foods. It is also used for soups and salads.

PROCESSING Wild rice is fermented for up to 2 weeks to make it easier to hull, then, after hulling, it is heated to partly gelatinise the starch. Fermenting the grain also helps to develop the characteristic nutty flavour.

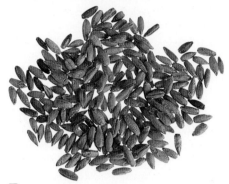

Rye *Secale cereale*

MAJOR NUTRIENTS		SERVE SIZE 40 G	
Energy	530 kJ	Sodium	15 mg
Protein	4 g	Potassium	205 mg
Fat	1 g	Iron	1.4 mg
Carbohydrate	26 g	Thiamin	0.1 mg
Dietary Fibre	5 g	Niacin Equiv.	0.5 mg
Cholesterol	0		

NUTRITIONAL INFORMATION An excellent source of fibre; good source of thiamin and iron; moderate source of protein. Also contains niacin and riboflavin.

Like other cereals, the nutritive value of rye is influenced by milling and other processing. Usually the fibre, vitamin and mineral content is decreased with increased milling and processing. See Rye Bread.

DESCRIPTION Long narrow cereal grain which is milled to meal and flour for baking.

ORIGIN AND HISTORY Early records suggest that rye originated in southern Asia, then moved to northern Europe where grains which were considered to be 'wild' were found in the Neolithic sites of Austria and Poland. It probably spread from there into Russia, Asia Minor and Germany. The Egyptians did not grow it, the Greeks considered it a weed, and it was not until the end of the Christian period that the Romans began harvesting wild rye seeds.

The present type of rye was taken to Britain by the Saxons. The basic bread of medieval Britain and probably Europe was made from a mixture of coarsely ground rye, pea and, sometimes, barley flours.

For several centuries rye was the major bread grain in Europe and, today, Eastern Europe and Russia are still the biggest users of the grain, where it has been able to tolerate severe climates and poor soils better than other grains. Here it is still made into a fermented slightly alcoholic drink, kvass.

The Scandinavians made aromatic light rye breads sweetened with honey and Dutch settlers took rye with them to the New World. There, Irish and Scottish settlers distilled it to make whiskey, one of the largest uses of rye in that country.

BUYING AND STORAGE Buy sound fresh rye grains from grain merchants and store in a cool dry place where they will keep indefinitely.

PREPARATION AND USE Cook cracked rye with milk or water to make a creamy porridge for breakfast. For variety, mix with cracked oats or other cereals. Rye grains are malted for whiskey in the USA and for beer (kvass) in the USSR.

PROCESSING Sound rye grains may be cracked or kibbled in a steel-bladed mill, food processor or blender, taking care not to grind the grains too finely.

SEE ALSO Pumpernickel, Rye Bread.

VARIETIES

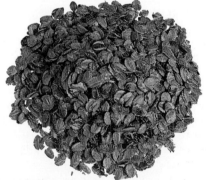

Rye Flakes

DESCRIPTION Flat flakes of crushed rye grain.

BUYING AND STORAGE Buy from health food stores and store in a cool dry place.

PREPARATION AND USE Rye flakes are cooked as a breakfast porridge or as a binder for hamburgers or meat loaves. Toasted rye flakes are often added to commercial breakfast cereals.

PROCESSING Sound rye grains are flattened between millstones or rollers in a roller mill. This process is fairly easy to carry out by hand with a mortar and pestle as the grain is rather soft.

Rye Meal

ORIGIN AND HISTORY See Rye Flour.

PREPARATION AND USE Used to make the traditional rye breads of northern and eastern Europe and for Scandinavian crispbreads.

BUYING AND STORAGE Buy rye meal from health food stores and bulk grocers and store in a cool dry place, preferably in the refrigerator, where it will keep indefinitely.

PROCESSING Sound rye grains are cleaned, conditioned and milled to make a coarse wholegrain flour.

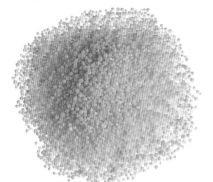

Sago *Metroxylon sagu*

MAJOR NUTRIENTS		SERVE SIZE 40 G	
Energy	610 kJ	Dietary Fibre	0
Protein	0	Sodium	0
Fat	0	Potassium	0
Carbohydrate	38 g	Cholesterol	0

NUTRITIONAL INFORMATION Very rich in starch, contains insignificant amounts of B vitamins.

DESCRIPTION Small balls of starch, prepared from the inner trunk of various kinds of palm trees. Sago resembles tapioca in appearance (the balls are smaller) and in its thickening ability.

ORIGIN AND HISTORY Sago comes from the starchy inner trunk of the sago palm which grows in the watery swamps of South-East Asia. The name sago originated in Malaysia and the East Indies where the trees were cut down just before flowering when the starch reserves had built up in the trunk.

BUYING AND STORAGE Sago is available in granules in 375 g packets from the supermarket. It may also be present in soup mixes. Stored in a cool dry place it will keep indefinitely.

PREPARATION AND USE Bark is peeled from the trunk and the inner part is cut into 1 m lengths. The logs are split, the pith scooped out and ground. After grinding, the mixture is washed and dried into flour which is usually consumed locally.

Pearl or granular sago is made by pushing the wet starchy paste through a sieve onto a hotplate where it dries quickly in small balls which are used in European cooking for puddings and sweet dishes. It is supposed to be beneficial for invalids as it has a soothing effect on the stomach. Stir into boiling soup to thicken or into boiling sweetened milk or flavoured water to make desserts. Lemon sago, a popular dessert many years ago, is still included in old recipe books but is virtually unknown today. Sago and tapioca may be used interchangeably.

PROCESSING Pearl sago may also be made from tapioca starch. The outer skin of the tapioca (cassava) tuber is peeled off, then the fibrous inner part is crushed finely in water. The starch slurry that forms is passed through a cloth screen to remove the cellular material and left in settling tanks until the water has drained off. The wet starch paste is pressed through a coarse screen into a hammock-shaped cloth which is then swung in a circle to spin out the water. If the water content is correct and the cloth is swung properly, this action causes the starch pellets to become roughly round in shape. After further sieving to remove any particularly large portions, the pearls are roasted to remove any remaining water and partially gelatinise the balls.

VARIETIES
The Indian Standards Institution established a standard for sago in 1956 stating that sago could be made from either sago or tapioca starch.

SEE ALSO Tapioca.

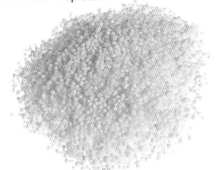

Tapioca *Manihot utilissima*

*also called **Cassava, Mandioca, Manioc, Yucca***

NUTRITIONAL INFORMATION No data are available.

DESCRIPTION Leafy shrub which grows up to 3 m. The leaves are often boiled as a vegetable and the starch extracted from the roots is an important food source.

ORIGIN AND HISTORY Tapioca was widely used as a food source in Brazil and neighbouring countries of South America before Columbus arrived. It was taken to the East Indies in the 19th century by Portuguese and Spanish explorers and from there it spread throughout Africa and Asia. It is an important food source in Papua New Guinea. Most of the world's flour production came from factories in Java until they were destroyed during World War II. Brazil was then the main source for some years but at present Thailand is the major producer and exporter. Tapioca root chips produced in Thailand and Malaysia are shipped to western Europe for animal feed.

BUYING AND STORAGE Sold in Western countries and parts of Asia as tapioca starch or flour or as pearled tapioca. Buy the starch in Asian food stores (although it is usually replaced by arrowroot or cornflour by Asians in Australia). Pearled tapioca is sold in grocery stores and in preprepared custard mixes. Stored in a cool dry place it will keep for years.

PREPARATION AND USE In many parts of the world the roots are baked or boiled as a vegetable. The starch is used to bake various kinds of breads and cakes. In Brazil and Latin America it is used to make farina de mandioca (tapioca meal), toasted and dried, and used as a basic food. Sometimes the meal is shaped into cakes and baked, then taken as a source of food during long journeys. Main commercial uses are for starch, or modified starches (pregelatinised) for manufactured food products. Good quality cooked starch produces a strong, almost tasteless gel. Granulated or pearled tapioca is used for thickening soups and stews and for puddings.

PROCESSING The starch is extracted by first washing and peeling the freshly dug roots, then grinding to a pulp. The pulp is sieved to remove fibres, then dried to a brilliant white powder. Granulated tapioca is processed by cooking, grinding and screening the starch which shortens the final cooking time. Pearled tapioca is a coarser form of the granulated.

VARIETIES
Over 2000 varieties of the plant are grown worldwide. They may be divided into 'bitter' and 'sweet'.

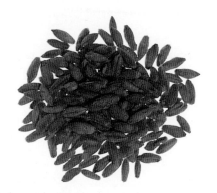

Triticale Triticosecale

MAJOR NUTRIENTS   SERVE SIZE 40 G

Energy	520 kJ	Fat	1 g
Protein	5 g	Carbohydrate	25 g

NUTRITIONAL INFORMATION No further nutritional analysis available.

DESCRIPTION Thin long kernels of grain resembling wheat in appearance.

ORIGIN AND HISTORY Triticale is a wheat–rye hybrid which first appeared at the turn of this century. Early examples, both naturally and artificially produced, were sterile but subsequent research more recently in Europe and especially in Canada and Mexico has overcome the problem. Many varieties have been bred during the past 15 years, including a durum–rye cross which is suitable for baking and a wheat–rye cross for stock feed.

BUYING AND STORAGE Buy flour or meal in small quantities from health food stores. Store in an airtight container in a cool dry place for up to 6 months.

PREPARATION AND USE Triticale can be milled to white flour but as it has only a small amount of endosperm in relation to the wholegrain, it is usually milled to wholegrain flour or meal. It is added to commercial breads and biscuits, usually in combination with wheat flour, and resembles rye products because of its weaker gluten compared to wheat. Home-baked biscuits, breads, cakes, muffins and pancakes made from triticale have a pleasant nutty flavour and are pale brown in appearance. It may be substituted for wheat flour in many domestic recipes, but adjustment to the liquid content may need to be made as finer particles of the flour absorb more liquid than the coarser particles. Triticale is also flaked and toasted for breakfast cereals and triticale macaroni is now available.

PROCESSING Although milled in the same way as wheat, triticale has a lower extraction rate as the presence of shrivelled grains prevents the effective separation into flour and bran.

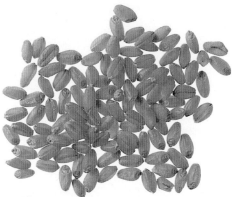

Wheat Triticum

MAJOR NUTRIENTS   SERVE SIZE 40 G

Energy	560 kJ	Sodium	5 mg
Protein	4 g	Potassium	200 mg
Fat	1 g	Iron	1.5 mg
Carbohydrate	25 g	Thiamin	0.15 mg
Dietary Fibre	4 g	Niacin Equiv.	2.7 mg
Cholesterol	0		

NUTRITIONAL INFORMATION An excellent source of fibre and niacin; good source of protein, thiamin and iron. Some of the vitamins and minerals may be biologically unavailable due to binding to phytic acid, a substance associated with fibre.

As with other cereals, the nutritive value of wheat is influenced by milling or other processing. Usually the fibre, vitamin and mineral content is decreased with increased processing.

DESCRIPTION Wheats can be divided into three distinct groups:
primitive, such as Einkorn and Emmer which were used for human food in very early times (still grown in some areas today);
durum for the production of pasta;
common bread wheats which are the source of flour for breads and other baked goods.

ORIGIN AND HISTORY First cultivated in the valley of the Tigris about 7000 BC. Wheat growing then spread through other parts of Asia Minor to Egypt and then Europe. Wheat is now grown throughout the world although it is more successful in the temperate regions.

VARIETIES

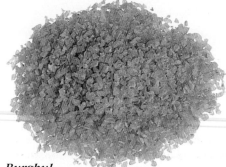

Burghul

DESCRIPTION Hulled wheat, steamed until partly cooked, then dried thoroughly and cracked or crushed in coarse or fine grades. It is also known as bulgur, pligouri and pourgouri.

ORIGIN AND HISTORY With wheat a staple grain of ancient civilisations of the Near and Middle East, the making of burghul could date back more than 4000 years, when wheat's principal use was as a porridge. Boiling softened the grain; after drying, it was more easily ground with primitive grindstones. Today it is an important food in Lebanon, Syria and Armenia, and also used in Turkish, Cypriot and Greek cooking.

BUYING AND STORAGE Middle Eastern and Greek food stores stock both fine and coarse grades. Packaged burghul, usually ungraded, is stocked in natural food stores and supermarkets. Store in an airtight container.

PREPARATION AND USE Burghul should be softened for dishes which do not require cooking; otherwise rinse, drain and squeeze out moisture, or use dry (with modern-day manufacture rinsing is unnecessary). To soften burghul, cover with water, drain and leave burghul in the bowl for 20 minutes to soften and swell.

Use for the popular Lebanese salad tabouli (coarse grade, softened); the ground lamb and burghul dish kibbeh (fine grade, rinsed only); burghul pilaus (coarse grade, dry or rinsed); and poultry stuffing (coarse grade, softened). Other uses may be found in the cuisines of the countries mentioned above.

PROCESSING A popular Middle Eastern cereal meal, kishk, is made with burghul mixed with thick yoghurt, allowed to ferment for several days, then dried in the sun and ground to a coarse powder. Kishk is used in soups and meat stews.

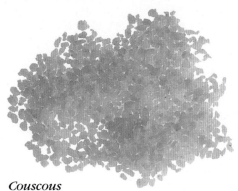

Couscous

MAJOR NUTRIENTS   SERVE SIZE 100 G

Energy	950 kJ	Sodium	0
Protein	6 g	Iron	5 mg
Fat	1 g	Thiamin	0.2 mg
Carbohydrate	51 g	Niacin Equiv.	2 mg
Cholesterol	0		

NUTRITIONAL INFORMATION An excellent source of thiamin and iron; good source of protein and niacin. The absorption of iron from grain products such as couscous can be improved by consuming a vitamin C-rich food at the same meal.

DESCRIPTION Tiny cream-coloured pellets, made from semolina moistened and coated with flour.

ORIGIN AND HISTORY The Berbers of North Africa devised this fascinating cereal product in ancient times. Originally made with millet; it is not known when wheat replaced the latter. Used widely in Algeria, Morocco and Tunisia, and to a lesser extent, Egypt, it is regarded as the national dish of Morocco. Couscous is still made by hand in North Africa; the semolina grains are sprinkled with lightly salted water and white flour and hand-rubbed into tiny pellets, steamed, and then dried. The French, through their North African links, developed a liking for couscous, and now use machinery to make it in France.

BUYING AND STORAGE Available loose or packaged from gourmet and Middle Eastern food stores. Store in a sealed container in a cool, dry place and use within 6 months.

PREPARATION AND USE There is a traditional vessel for cooking couscous called a *couscoussier* — a large, deep stew pot topped with a tight-fitting, lidded container with a perforated base. A muslin-lined steamer or colander can be used for the top container.

The traditional way to prepare couscous is to put it in a bowl, cover with water, then pour the excess off. Stand 15 minutes to allow pellets to swell, break up lumps, then place in the top container of the couscoussier, cover with a cloth and lid, and steam over water or a stew for 15 minutes. Turn into a bowl, break up lumps with a fork and sprinkle with a little water. Return to steamer and steam for 30 minutes more until tender. Turn into a bowl and toss with butter or oil to coat grains.

The couscous sold commercially is usually of the 'instant' variety. Soak the grains in water for 5 minutes, then warm and separate them in a steamer, or in a pan with a little butter.

Serve couscous with fruity, spicy meat stews. Traditionally it is eaten with mutton or chicken and sometimes fish. May be served with any meat or vegetable dish normally served with rice or pasta, or as a dessert tossed with sugar or honey, nuts and/or dried fruit.

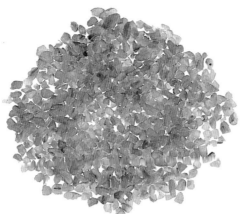

Cracked Wheat

NUTRITIONAL INFORMATION No nutrient analysis available. See Wheat.

DESCRIPTION Whole wheat grains which have been cracked or broken open during the early stages of milling for flour.

ORIGIN AND HISTORY Cracked wheat (also called kibbled wheat) probably dates from prehistoric times when the grains were crushed between two stones. The resulting coarse meal was mixed with water found in hollows of rocks and crudely cooked by dropping hot stones into the mixture. Later, when the Romans developed the quern, the grain was ground more finely.

BUYING AND STORAGE Buy in small quantities. Stored in the refrigerator, it will keep for up to 6 months.

PREPARATION AND USE Soak in water before use. Usually added to bread dough to provide texture and flavour.

Semolina

MAJOR NUTRIENTS		SERVE SIZE 40 G	
Energy	600 kJ	Sodium	5 mg
Protein	4 g	Potassium	68 mg
Fat	1 g	Iron	0.4 mg
Carbohydrate	31 g	Thiamin	0.05 mg
Cholesterol	0	Niacin Equiv.	1 mg
Dietary Fibre	0		

NUTRITIONAL INFORMATION A moderate source of protein, thiamin, niacin and iron.

DESCRIPTION The coarsely milled inner endosperm of wheat. It is granular in appearance and the colour may range from a clear yellow (durum) to a pale beige (hard wheat).

ORIGIN AND HISTORY Semolina has been a product of the milling of wheat ever since the process was first used.

PREPARATION AND USE Durum semolina is used for making extruded pasta products, e.g. spaghetti, hard wheat semolina is used to make puddings, cakes (especially those originating from the Middle East), the couscous of North Africa and breakfast cereals. Also sold as instant flour or gravy flour in 375 g shaker cartons, used for thickening sauces and stews. Shake straight into hot liquid and stir well for instant thickening.

VARIETIES
Durum, Hard wheat.

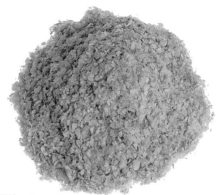

Wheatgerm

MAJOR NUTRIENTS		SERVE SIZE 10 G	
Energy	120 kJ	Potassium	105 mg
Protein	2 g	Iron	1 mg
Fat	1 g	Magnesium	30.5 mg
Carbohydrate	3 g	Zinc	0.8 mg
Dietary Fibre	2 g	Thiamin	0.15 mg
Sodium	0	Niacin Equiv.	1.3 mg
Cholesterol	0		

NUTRITIONAL INFORMATION A good source of thiamin and iron; moderate source of fibre, niacin, magnesium and zinc. Also contains riboflavin.

DESCRIPTION Small creamy flakes milled from the embryo or germ of the wheat grain.

ORIGIN AND HISTORY The wheatgerm is removed during the milling of white flour. Its nutritional significance has only seriously been considered in the present century.

BUYING AND STORAGE Available from supermarkets in 375 g and 500 g packets. Store in an airtight container in the refrigerator for up to 6 months. Because of its high fat content it goes rancid quickly.

PREPARATION AND USE Added to pastry, biscuits and cakes, breakfast cereals and breads. Sometimes used as a binder for meat loaves and similar products, and sprinkled onto savoury dishes, fruit or puddings.

FLOUR

Flour is the name given to any edible substance in powder form. Many cereals, roots and seeds are milled for flour worldwide, but, generally, wheat flour is accepted as flour in Western countries.

Prehistoric man first made a crude wheat flour by pulverising wheat grains between two stones. Later, the Romans developed the quern where the upper millstone was turned by men or beasts. Water-powered mills dated from the time of the birth of Christ. Windmills appeared in Europe at the beginning of the 14th century and were widely used until the invention of the steam engine in 1751. Later, the system of roller milling, still in use today, revolutionised the flour milling industry.

Buy from any supermarket and store in a cool dry place in a closed container. Do not put new supplies of flour on top of old.

Wheat flour is extremely important to the baking industry due to the presence of gluten (protein fractions of flour) which enables wheat flour mixtures to be leavened, producing light, airy, baked goods. The production of yeast breads, cakes, biscuits and pastries depends on this property to varying degrees. Wheat flour is also used as a thickening agent.

In Australia, domestic white flour retains 76–80% of the wheat grain (known as the extraction rate), a relatively high level in comparison with other Western countries.

SELF-RAISING FLOUR, SELF-RISING — American
Self-raising flour was first developed in the USA and the first successful product containing the new flour was marketed there as pancake flour in 1905. A similar flour was also produced in Britain and is still sold there, but it is not widely used in Europe as it is too limiting for serious cooks, particularly those who pride themselves on the quality of their cakes.

Self-raising flour is still sold in southern USA and may be found occasionally in the northern states but it has never really gained the general popularity it achieved in Australia after its introduction in the mid-1930s.

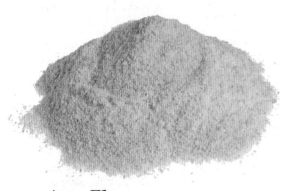

Atta Flour

MAJOR NUTRIENTS		WHITE PLAIN SERVE SIZE 40 G	
Energy	570 kJ	Cholesterol	0
Protein	4 g	Potassium	80 mg
Fat	0	Iron	1 mg
Carbohydrate	31 g	Zinc	0.5 mg
Dietary Fibre	2 g	Thiamin	0.15 mg
Sodium	5 mg	Niacin Equiv.	1 mg

NUTRITIONAL INFORMATION A good source of thiamin and iron; moderate source of protein, fibre and niacin.

DESCRIPTION Granular wheaten flour, made from the wheat grain.

ORIGIN AND HISTORY Atta is the name commonly given to a flour of about 85–95% extraction which is used to make chapattis in India, Tibet, China and other parts of Asia and the Pacific. It was originally made by pounding the wheat grains in a primitive form of mortar and pestle, then by stone grinding. Today it is roller milled.

BUYING AND STORAGE Buy from some supermarkets, health food stores and Asian food stores. Stored in a cool dry place, it will keep for up to a year.

PREPARATION AND USE Used mainly for chapattis, cakes and biscuits, also for some commercial prepackaged mixes.

VARIETIES

Brown Coarse The difference between white plain and brown coarse atta flour is related to the different extent of milling.

Brown coarse atta flour contains more protein and fibre and fewer carbohydrates, as well as higher levels of potassium and magnesium.

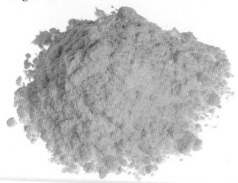

Baker's Flour

NUTRITIONAL INFORMATION No detailed nutritional analysis available. Baker's flour has a higher protein content than domestic flour.

DESCRIPTION Flour, preferably milled from blends of suitable wheats, usually with protein contents ranging from 12–16%.

BUYING AND STORAGE Buy from some health food stores in 1 kg packets, also in 10 kg or 25 kg bags directly from the flour mill.

PREPARATION AND USE Used for bread making, pre-mixes and packet mixes.

VARIETIES
White flour, Wholemeal flour.

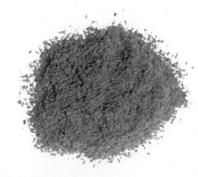

Barley Flour

NUTRITIONAL INFORMATION No data available, but see Barley.

DESCRIPTION Ground hulled barley.

ORIGIN AND HISTORY Coarsely ground barley flour was used as a bread ingredient in northern Europe.

BUYING AND STORAGE Barley flour is available from health food stores and many supermarkets. It is usually stone ground but may range from coarse meal to fine depending on the brand. Buy in small quantities and store in a cool place in a tightly sealed container.

PREPARATION AND USE Wholegrain barley flour has a nutty flavour. The colour is darker and it has a coarser texture than wheaten flour. Replace up to one-third of the wheat flour in baked products with barley flour and adjust the quantity of liquid accordingly as it absorbs more liquid than wheaten flour. Use barley flour in breads, pastries, muffins, pancakes and cakes, infant and invalid foods and special diet foods. Coarsely ground meal is used to make porridge and gruel.

PROCESSING Barley flour may be milled at home from the hulled grain or from pearl barley. Homemade flour will be wholegrain. Clean the grains and remove any loose hulls, weeds and other debris, then grind in a wheat mill, varying the degree of fineness depending on how you plan to use it. Pearl barley may be milled, half a cup at a time, in the blender or coffee grinder. Some experimentation may be necessary.

SEE ALSO Pearl Barley.

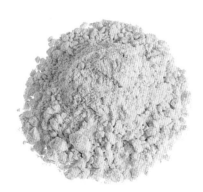

Besan

*also called **Gram flour***

MAJOR NUTRIENTS			SERVE SIZE 100 G
Energy	1380 kJ	Calcium	195 mg
Protein	22 g	Magnesium	134 mg
Fat	6 g	Iron	9.2 mg
Carbohydrate	50 g	Zinc	3.5 mg
Cholesterol	0	Thiamin	0.5 mg
Dietary Fibre	15 g	Riboflavin	0.15 mg
Sodium	40 mg	Niacin Equiv.	4 mg
Potassium	800 mg	Vitamin C	3 mg

NUTRITIONAL INFORMATION Besan is an excellent source of protein, calcium, magnesium, iron, zinc, thiamin, niacin and folic acid; a moderate source of riboflavin and vitamin C. It also contains copper, and provides a large amount of potassium.

DESCRIPTION This is a heavy textured, finely milled flour made from dried chickpeas (garbanzos) or channa Dal (Bengal gram/

pigeon peas). Pale yellow in colour, it is used extensively in Indian cooking.

ORIGIN AND HISTORY Two important factors have shaped the Indian cuisine: vegetarianism and the economy. These mean that a protein source has to be found in non-meat ingredients, and they must be within the financial reach of the average Indian. Chickpeas are an economical and easily grown crop and when milled into a flour have multiple applications.

BUYING AND STORAGE This flour should have a bright colour and not appear dry and lumpy. It has a leguminous aroma when fresh. Store in an airtight glass container for up to 3 months in dry conditions.

PREPARATION AND USE Use as a flour in batters, doughs and pastries. It is unleavened and produces a heavy texture, but has a pleasing flavour. It is also used occasionally as a thickener, and to make small dumplings as a meat substitute in vegetarian cooking. Finely ground lentils or mung beans could be substituted, although besan is now readily available in most good Asian food stores.

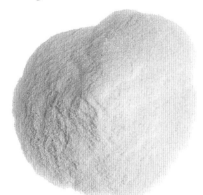

Continental Flour

NUTRITIONAL INFORMATION See Semolina.

DESCRIPTION Granular flour with a particle size between semolina and flour.

ORIGIN AND HISTORY Unknown, but this flour probably took the place of ground nuts which were commonly used in European cakes. Wheat flour was very expensive before the invention of the roller mill in the mid-19th century, but nut trees (particularly almond) grew in profusion and the nuts were ground into a type of flour used for baking.

BUYING AND STORAGE Buy from supermarkets and delicatessens. Store in a cool, dry place or in the refrigerator during summer.

PREPARATION AND USE Used for some continental European cakes and biscuits at the discretion of the individual cook.

PROCESSING Continental flour is usually sieved off during the milling of wheat into flour. Protein content is usually in the vicinity of 12%.

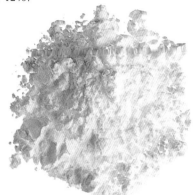

Cornflour

*also called **Maize starch, Corn starch, Wheat starch***

MAJOR NUTRIENTS			SERVE SIZE 10 G
Energy	150 kJ	Dietary Fibre	0
Protein	0	Sodium	5 mg
Fat	0	Potassium	5 mg
Carbohydrate	9 g	Cholesterol	0

NUTRITIONAL INFORMATION A source of carbohydrate. Unlike other flours cornflour contains no vitamins and insignificant amounts of minerals.

DESCRIPTION Fine white powder extracted from the starchy endosperm of maize (corn) or from wheat.

ORIGIN AND HISTORY The separation of starch from wheat was no doubt being carried out long before records were kept, although there are vague references to starch being used both as a food and as a strengthening agent by the classical writers of ancient times. The first really clear recording was by Cato (234–149 BC) when he described soaking wheat for 10 days, draining it and wrapping the soaked grains in a cloth before pressing or wringing out the starch which was used for stiffening clothes. It was also used to stiffen monks' habits. It is uncertain when starch was introduced to western Europe, although historians generally agree it was probably in the 14th century when we are told that weavers in Flanders used it for stiffening. In the mid–16th century coloured starches for ruffs and body linen were imported into England from Europe. The Puritans used blue starch but Queen Elizabeth I banned the use of starch in 1596, threatening offenders with imprisonment. The law was revoked later during the reign of James I and by the mid-1850s it was being used extensively in the perfume and confectionery industries. About this time it started to be used extensively as a thickener and an Englishman, John Polson, patented a complicated wet milling process for obtaining starch from maize. The two cereals were used side by side from that time but in America maize starch was being produced by a different method. John Polson's product was released on the domestic market as cornflour and it was exported to China, India, Europe and all the British colonies.

BUYING AND STORAGE Buy in 500 g packets from supermarkets. Both products are clearly labelled with the grain source. Stored in a cool dry place it will keep indefinitely.

PREPARATION AND USE Cornflour is used mainly as a thickening agent in domestic cookery, particularly for pie fillings and sauces, and for baking cakes. Wheaten cornflour may be used in recipes requiring maize cornflour, but the quantity used must be adjusted as their thickening powers are noticeably different. Maize cornflour produces a thicker, more viscous mixture than wheaten cornflour. Commercially, cornflour is used in packet mixes for instant puddings, sauces and gravies, pancake mixes, biscuits, wafers, baby foods, custard powder and canned and powdered soups, ice cream, baking powder, canned fruits and beverages, and as a carrier and filler for meat products.

VARIETIES
Wheaten cornflour, maize cornflour. The word 'cornflour' is confusing to many as it can refer to starch extracted from either wheat or from maize (corn).

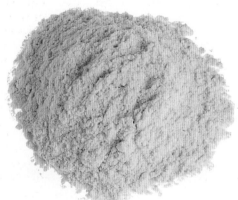

Gluten

MAJOR NUTRIENTS

	45% GLUTEN/55% PATENT FLOUR SERVE SIZE 100 G		
Energy	1580 kJ	Calcium	40 mg
Protein	40 g	Phosphorus	140 mg
Fat	2 g	Iron	n/a
Carbohydrate	47 g	Thiamin	n/a
Cholesterol	0	Riboflavin	n/a
Dietary Fibre	0.5 g	Niacin Equiv.	n/a
Sodium	5 mg		

NUTRITIONAL INFORMATION This flour is a high protein food. It is a good source of phosphorus and a moderate source of calcium. Gluten is a mixture of two proteins, gliadin and glutenin. It is present in wheat, rye, oats and barley but not in rice.

Coeliac disease occurs in individuals who are sensitive to gluten. Management of the disease requires a diet which does not contain gluten. This means that many common foods cannot be eaten.

DESCRIPTION Gluten is the complex protein product formed when wheat flour and water are mixed together, and gluten flour is a mixture of gluten and wheat flour.

ORIGIN AND HISTORY Origin unknown, although the means for separating starch from wheat were described by Marcus Porcius Cato (234–149 BC). The wheat was soaked for 10 days, then drained and wrapped in a cloth and the starchy liquid remaining was pressed or wrung out. The grains were used for animal fodder and the starch was retained. Gluten has also been used by vegetarians, particularly in Asia, as an important protein source, for hundreds of years. The method of separating gluten from wheat flour was first carried out in Australia in 1934 when the practice of adding it to commercial bread dough to produce Procera (protein increased) bread was introduced. Procera bread is no longer manufactured; it has been replaced by the familiar protein increased breads.

BUYING AND STORAGE Buy from health food stores and supermarkets. Buy only in small quantities as required and store in the refrigerator in an airtight container. Being a protein food, it is subject to insect infestation if not stored properly. Do not put fresh supplies on top of old.

PREPARATION AND USE Add gluten to flour when home-baking bread. One metric teaspoon of gluten added to 1 cup of wheat flour will increase the protein of the flour by 1%. Sift together at least twice to ensure even distribution through the flour. Gluten is also added to wheat and rye flours to increase protein content and strengthen soft flours for commercial bread making and, sometimes, in pasta and noodle manufacture. Gluten is an important protein source for vegetarians and is used as a binder to increase the protein level of sausages and other meat products, in breakfast foods, in special dietary foods, in textured vegetable protein (TVP) products and in pet foods. Textured or hydrolysed vegetable protein (TVP or HVP) products are used extensively in the commercial production of canned soups, sauces, bouillon cubes, and

some salad dressings, to name a few.

PROCESSING Gluten is separated from wheat flour by mixing a soft dough or batter, then washing out the starch. The elastic mass remaining is called wet gluten, which may be dried in much the same way that milk is powdered, then milled to even particle size.

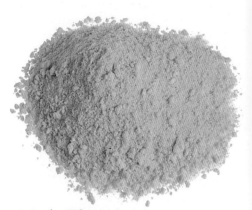

Malt Flour

also called Malt extract

NUTRITIONAL INFORMATION No nutrient analysis available.

DESCRIPTION Grains (particularly barley and wheat) are soaked to soften and allowed to germinate. During this time starch in the grains is converted to sugars by natural enzymes. After kiln drying, this product is called malt.

Malt is milled to break open the grain and release the sugar syrup which, in turn, is evaporated until a thick concentrated syrup remains. Further drying under vacuum produces dried malt extract. Malt flour is stone or roller-milled wheat or barley malt. Malted wheat is also flaked for breakfast cereals.

ORIGIN AND HISTORY During the Neolithic age wheat or barley was sprouted so that during the process of germination the largely indigestible starch in the grain was converted to digestible malt sugar. The grains were dried for storage and could be eaten dry, or mixed with water to make a paste. In Mesopotamia malting was carried out, but exactly how it was done is unknown. It seems likely that at that time the area now known as the Middle East was warmer and the rainfall heavier than it is today and that the malting happened by accident. It did not take long for the malted grain to be ground and mixed into a form of dough. Shaped into cakes and cooked slowly, it would dry out so that it could be stored as a ready source of food needing only to be crumbled and mixed with water to make a type of porridge. If left to ferment, which happened easily, it made a type of beer. The Saxons also knew how to malt barley, and ale, along with bread, cheese and meat, was a staple food and drunk at every meal. The Saxons often used drinking utensils made from hollowed out animal horns with pointed bases so they could not be put down until they were empty.

PREPARATION AND USE Malt products are important ingredients and colouring agents in the food industry. Malt flour is used as an improver in the baking industry.

Malt extract is sold in health food stores, supermarkets and Asian food stores (sometimes erroneously labelled as maltose).

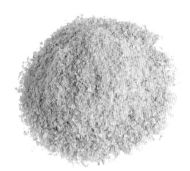

Oat Flour

NUTRITIONAL INFORMATION See Oats.

DESCRIPTION A fine flour made from milled oats.

ORIGIN AND HISTORY See Oats.

BUYING AND STORAGE Buy from health food stores.

PREPARATION AND USE For baby foods, ready-to-eat cereals and general baking. When baking bread, always use a mixture of oat flour and rye or wheat flour to produce a well-risen loaf.

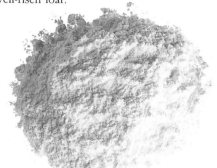

Rice Flour

MAJOR NUTRIENTS			SERVE SIZE 20 G
Energy	150 kJ	Dietary Fibre	0
Protein	0.64 g	Sodium	0
Fat	0	Potassium	25 mg
Carbohydrate	8 g	Cholesterol	0

NUTRITIONAL INFORMATION Very rich in starch; contains insignificant amounts of B vitamins.

DESCRIPTION Flour ground from broken pieces and the whole grains of medium-grained milled rice.

BUYING AND STORAGE Buy in 375 g and 500 g packets in supermarkets or in bulk from health food stores.

Stored in an airtight container in a cool place, it will keep indefinitely.

PREPARATION AND USE Used as a thickening agent, particularly in Asian countries. Mix with other flours for cakes, shortbread and biscuits. Also used to make rice noodles.

VARIETIES

Ground rice (slightly more granulated version).

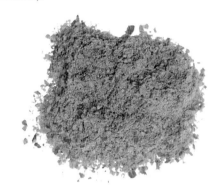

Rye Flour

NUTRITIONAL INFORMATION See Rye.

DESCRIPTION A flour made from milled rye.

ORIGIN AND HISTORY Rye flour has long been used to bake traditional breads, cakes and pastries in northern and eastern Europe and in Russia. Although rye grains were taken to medieval Britain and milled for flour for bread, rye was not popular for other baked goods.

BUYING AND STORAGE As for wheat flour.

PREPARATION AND USE Popular for bread making.

PROCESSING Sound rye grains of uniform size are cleaned, then conditioned by soaking in water to toughen the bran in much the same way as is done with wheat, after which they are ground and sifted to make flour. Rye wholemeal flour is usually milled from 100% of the grain while normal rye flour is less, the extraction rate varying from country to country. Lighter rye flours are sifted to remove some of the bran and sometimes bleached depending on the country of origin.

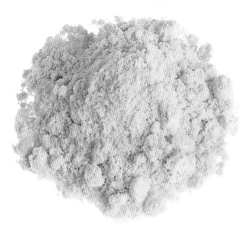

Soya Flour Glycine max; G. soja

also called *Soy flour, Kinako*

MAJOR NUTRIENTS			FULL FAT SERVE SIZE 20 G
Energy	370 kJ	Iron	1.5 mg
Protein	7 g	Magnesium	48 mg
Fat	5 g	Zinc	1 mg
Carbohydrate	5 g	Calcium	40 mg
Dietary Fibre	2.5 g	Thiamin	0.15 mg
Sodium	0	Niacin Equiv.	1.5 mg
Potassium	330 mg	Cholesterol	0

NUTRITIONAL INFORMATION An excellent source of magnesium; a richer source of protein, thiamin and iron than other flours; moderate source of fibre, niacin, calcium and zinc.

DESCRIPTION A creamy flour processed from soya beans. It has a strong flavour which limits its use in the kitchen, but is invaluable in food manufacturing industries because of its excellent binding properties and protein content.

ORIGIN AND HISTORY The soya bean was introduced into the United States in 1804, but it was not commercially exploited outside China until the 20th century. Soya flour was first produced in the United States in the 1930s, and began to be used commercially in the early 1940s. It is produced by a lengthy process: the soya beans are cleaned, cracked and hulled, broken into chips, then reduced to flakes. The oil is extracted with solvents, and the soluble carbohydrates are removed, ending up with soya grits (used in cereals). The grits are ground to produce soya flour.

BUYING AND STORAGE Soya flour is available at natural food stores. Store in a sealed container in a cool, dry place.

PREPARATION AND USE While it is attractive to those on gluten-free diets, its uses in the kitchen are limited. It may be used for batters in combination with cornflour (cornstarch), egg white and water. Use to increase protein content of muffins, quick breads and yeast breads, adding 1 part by volume of soya flour to each 3 parts by volume of wheat flour. Recipes may require the addition of more liquid. In Japan, soya flour is sweetened and used for confectionery.

PROCESSING With its nutritional value confirmed, and its possibilities recognised, soya flour found its way into smallgoods as a binder, emulsifier and protein extender. It is used in the baking industry to increase protein content of baked goods, breads in particular, and included in batters for coating foods such as fish in food processing industries.

VARIETIES
There is a non-fat soya flour containing higher levels of protein, carbohydrates and minerals than the full fat variety.

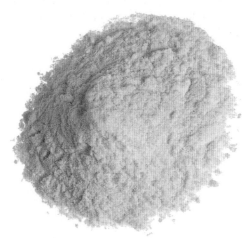

Sponge Flour

also called Cake flour, High-ratio cake flour

NUTRITIONAL INFORMATION No nutritional analysis available. These flours have a slightly lower protein content than domestic flour. See White Flour.

DESCRIPTION Selected flours with fine particle sizes are blended together and chlorinated to yield white, soft flour with the ability to absorb higher levels of fat, sugar and liquid than those normally used in domestic cookery.

BUYING AND STORAGE Available in bulk from flour mills and in smaller quantities in the supermarket in some states.

PREPARATION AND USE Used mainly for packet cake mixes. For domestic use, follow instructions on packet.

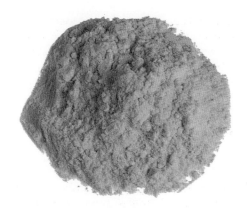

Unbleached Flour

NUTRITIONAL INFORMATION No nutritional analysis available. Unbleached flour would have a similar nutrient content to white flour.

DESCRIPTION Creamy-coloured wheat flour which has not been through the bleaching process. In Australia flour is frequently bleached by the addition of benzoyl peroxide in small amounts as permitted by Pure Food Regulations. Bleaching improves the colour and, more importantly, the baking quality of flour. During prolonged storage of flour natural bleaching or conditioning will take place.

ORIGIN AND HISTORY As for white flour.

BUYING AND STORAGE As for white flour.

PREPARATION AND USE Used for baking some yeast and quick breads.

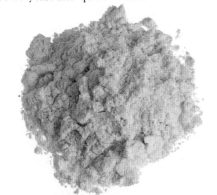

White Flour

MAJOR NUTRIENTS			PLAIN
			SERVE SIZE 40 G
Energy	590 kJ	Iron	0.5 mg
Protein	5 g	Magnesium	14.5 mg
Fat	1 g	Zinc	0.4 mg
Carbohydrate	31 g	Thiamin	0.1 mg
Dietary Fibre	1 g	Niacin Equiv.	1.5 mg
Sodium	0	Riboflavin	0
Potassium	45 mg	Cholesterol	0

NUTRITIONAL INFORMATION A good source of thiamin; moderate source of pro-

tein, niacin and iron. Also contains fibre and zinc.

Australian white flour retains 76–80% of the wheat grain (known as the extraction rate) while wholemeal flour retains 90–95% of the protein, 50% of the thiamin and niacin, 30–60% of the minerals and 30% of the dietary fibre.

Flours from the USA and the UK are milled at lower extraction rates and hence contain fewer nutrients. These flours are enriched with vitamins and minerals.

VARIETIES

Self-raising
The main difference between white plain flour and white self-raising flour is that self-raising flour contains 360 mg of sodium in the same serve size; and less potassium (40 mg).

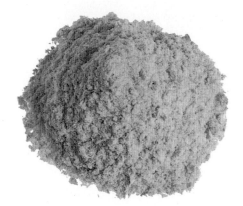

Wholemeal Flour

also called Wheatmeal flour, Wholemeal Flour, Whole wheat flour, Wheatmeal, Graham

MAJOR NUTRIENTS			PLAIN
			SERVE SIZE 40 G
Energy	530 kJ	Potassium	120 mg
Protein	5 g	Iron	1.2 mg
Fat	1 g	Magnesium	38 mg
Carbohydrate	26 g	Zinc	0.8 mg
Dietary Fibre	42 g	Thiamin	0.15 mg
Sodium	0	Niacin Equiv.	3 mg
Cholesterol	0		

NUTRITIONAL INFORMATION An excellent source of niacin; good source of fibre, thiamin, iron and magnesium; moderate source of protein and zinc.

In the process of flour milling, grinding and sieving does not destroy any of the nutrients of the wheat grain. Wholemeal flour has the same nutritional properties as the wheat grain from which it was milled.

While wholemeal flour does contain more vitamins and minerals than white flour, there is some uncertainty as to their availability in the body.

DESCRIPTION Flour milled from sound

grain which may contain 100% of the grain or may be a mixture of 90% whole grain plus 10% added wheat flour.

ORIGIN AND HISTORY Wholemeal flour was probably the first processed food used for human consumption. The ancient Romans, like the early inhabitants of Tuscany (then called Etruria), pounded the grain in a rough form of mortar and pestle. In honour of this occupation they were given the surname Piso, after pistores (grinders). The Romans invented a new goddess in honour of the development of millstones and called her Mola, the protectress of mills and millstones. The early Egyptians used grinding stones, and evidence in some of the tombs has shown that the teeth of some of the very early Egyptians were well worn, indicating that besides those from gnawing bones, there were probably plenty of chips from the stone fragments in that early flour. With the development of more sophis-ticated milling techniques, white flour became available to the rich and wholemeal products became the food of the poor — a practice that has only recently been reversed.

BUYING AND STORAGE Wholemeal flour is available in household-sized packets from all supermarkets and in larger quantities from flour mills. Buy in small quantities, store in a clean airtight container in a cool dry place and use as soon as possible, especially in hot weather.

PREPARATION AND USE Wholemeal flour is used to make bread and other yeast-raised baked products such as cakes, biscuits, pastries and pasta, and for general cooking. Wholemeal flour may be substituted wholly or partly for white flour but the texture of some products will be rather crumbly, so it may be necessary to adjust moisture and fat levels in some recipes when all wholemeal flour is used.

PROCESSING In Australia, flour is usually milled by the straight run method, which means all flours are milled for white flour and then the main components are blended back in the same proportions occurring in the natural grain. Stoneground flour, which, as the name suggests, is pulverised between two millstones, is also available and sometimes a combination of stoneground and roller-milled wholemeal flours is sold in 1 kg packets. Wholemeal flour may be finely or coarsely milled.

VARIETIES

Self-raising The major difference between wholemeal plain flour and wholemeal self-raising flour is that the self-raising flour contains 360 mg sodium in the same serve size.

PASTA AND NOODLES

PASTA

Pasta is a generic name for an international range of foods made from a basic mixture of wheat flour or semolina (preferably durum semolina) and water. Eggs may be used in place of water to give a firmer texture and a yellower colour. Wholemeal and vegetable-flavoured varieties are also available.

Historians are divided on its origin. It is a staple food in many cultures, so it is doubtful that any one person or culture 'invented' pasta. A bas-relief on an Etruscan tomb dated about 400 BC provides an early Italian connection, as it depicts equipment for pasta making. Four centuries later, pasta made an appearance in the writings of Cicero, who was known to be extremely fond of tagliatelle. Thus, although Marco Polo was supposed to have brought noodles or pasta back to Italy from Cathay, it is clear that both the Chinese and the Italians were familiar with it long before his time.

Pasta may be divided into four types: small shapes for soup, extruded long pieces for boiling and saucing, sheet pasta for baking, and shapes that can be filled with stuffing.

Fresh pasta can be bought by weight from specialty shops; it will keep refrigerated for three or four days, or may be frozen for up to one month (it becomes brittle after this). Dried pasta is sold mainly in 350 gram or 500 gram cellophane packs; it will keep indefinitely in a cool dry place. Dried 'instant' canneloni and lasagne are also available. Follow manufacturer's instructions for cooking.

General hints are to allow one litre of water for every 100 g of pasta. Bring water to a rapid boil in a large saucepan. Add salt at the user's discretion (this toughens the protein), return the water to the boil, add pasta all at once, bring water back to the boil as quickly as possible, and cook until pasta is firm to the bite — al dente. Drain thoroughly and use as required. Cooking times will vary depending on size and shape. Five hundred grams of fresh pasta serves four and the same amount of dried serves six.

Pasta made from durum semolina is considered to be superior to that made from flour. The semolina is kneaded with water or egg to form a crumbly mixture which is forced through dies to form the various shapes, cut into lengths to suit, then cooked fresh or dried. Homemade products are made the same way, or they may be rolled into a sheet by hand or by passing through the rollers of a hand-turned machine before being cut into the desired shapes.

Many different shapes are made from the traditional pasta dough. Most shapes come in a variety of sizes and many may be either ribbed or plain. When buying always check the product for shape rather than relying on the name on the packet, as there may be different regional names for the same product. Buy only the best quality pasta, 'arano dore' (durum semolina), which will hold its shape after cooking and have the very best texture.

Rigati — ribbed pastas — are better for meat saucing, while lisci — the smooth varieties — are better for cream or cheese sauces and for tossing with butter and cheese.

As well as the usual plain or wholemeal products, pastas flavoured with herbs and spinach, tomato, or other vegetable purees are popular.

Boiled pasta has a higher moisture content than bread, but 100 g of boiled pasta contain approximately the same protein, carbohydrate, dietary fibre, iron and kilojoules as 50 g of bread. Pasta, however, contains relatively less of the water-soluble thiamin, riboflavin and niacin, because of losses during boiling. One advantage which pasta has is that salt is usually not added during the manufacture, so that salt can be added at the user's discretion.

The non haem iron in pasta is not as well absorbed as the iron in flesh foods, but the absorption is improved by serving the pasta with a food containing vitamin C or with small amounts of meat.

Wholemeal pastas provide more dietary fibre and more vitamins.

Some pastas also contain vegetables and some include soya flour. This would affect the nutritional properties, according to the ingredients added.

Pasta is often thought of as 'fattening', but the sauces served with it frequently provide more kilojoules than the pasta itself. It is worthwhile to make a recipe collection of low fat sauces, based on tomatoes, tomato paste, mushrooms, and other vegetables including dried peas, beans and lentils, seafoods, lean meat, chicken, herbs, spices and wine, with only small amounts of oil. Some of the low fat or reduced fat cheeses may be added.

Pastas and noodles come in a variety of shapes and sizes, but most are made from the same basic ingredients, and have similar nutritional values. The visual interest they add to meals has an effect on nutrition, because it provides pleasure and stimulates the appetite. Watching an expert chef prepare a batch of noodles by hand in a good Chinese restaurant provides an almost magical sight which greatly enhances the excitement of the meal to come.

Noodles are made from flour which is much finer than semolina. Noodles are also produced from the flours of buckwheat, mung beans, soya beans and rice, and may contain the addition of seaweed. Eggs are also added to a number of noodles.

Despite the enormous variety of forms that pasta takes, the nutritional data remain very similar. Pasta falls into a number of categories, the nutritional details for which are given below, which avoids repetition within the individual entries.

Similarly, only the relevant headings are included in each entry, since the origin and history of most pastas is already noted in this introduction. Where the origin, buying or preparation of a pasta are of particular interest, these will be included after the description.

White Pasta

MAJOR NUTRIENTS		SERVE SIZE 80 G	
Energy	1180 kJ	Potassium	190 mg
Protein	10 g	Iron	1.5 mg
Fat	2 g	Magnesium	41.5 mg
Carbohydrate	59 g	Zinc	1.5 mg
Cholesterol	0	Thiamin	0.25 mg
Dietary Fibre	5 g	Niacin Equiv.	3 mg
Sodium	10 mg		

NUTRITIONAL INFORMATION As with all pasta, the main source of energy is from carbohydrate. An excellent source of fibre, thiamin and niacin; a good source of protein, iron and magnesium; a moderate source of zinc. The minerals in pasta (including iron) are poorly absorbed by the body.

Only the endosperm is used for making white pasta. It is therefore not inherently rich in B group vitamins unless the flour from which it is made is fortified with these vitamins. Moreover, the B vitamins are all soluble in water and heavy losses of these vitamins occur when the pasta is boiled and/or washed.

Pasta Made with Eggs

MAJOR NUTRIENTS		SERVE SIZE 80 G	
Energy	1090 kJ	Potassium	140 mg
Protein	12 g	Iron	1.5 mg
Fat	2 g	Magnesium	57.5 mg
Carbohydrate	49 g	Zinc	1.5 mg
Cholesterol	115 mg	Thiamin	0.15 mg
Dietary Fibre	3 g	Niacin Equiv.	3.5 mg
Sodium	15 mg		

NUTRITIONAL INFORMATION An excellent source of niacin; a good source of protein, fibre, thiamin, iron, and magnesium; a moderate source of zinc. Contains cholesterol.

The B vitamins are all soluble in water and heavy losses of these vitamins occur when the pasta is boiled and/or washed.

In nutrient content, pasta made with eggs is very similar to white pasta. The major difference is the cholesterol content.

Pasta with Fillings

NUTRITIONAL INFORMATION For filled pasta, such as tortellini and ravioli, there is no nutritional analysis available. The analysis would depend upon whether the pasta was white, wholemeal or made with eggs (see above), and the fillings used.

Vegetable-flavoured Pasta

There is no nutritional analysis available for vegetable-flavoured pasta. The nutrient analysis would vary depending upon the type of vegetable puree and amount of puree used.

Wholemeal Pasta

MAJOR NUTRIENTS		SERVE SIZE 80 G	
Energy	1100 kJ	Potassium	310 mg
Protein	10 g	Iron	3 mg
Fat	2 g	Magnesium	96 mg
Carbohydrate	53 g	Zinc	2.5 mg
Cholesterol	0	Thiamin	0.8 mg
Dietary Fibre	10 g	Niacin Equiv.	6.5 mg
Sodium	100 mg		

NUTRITIONAL INFORMATION Except for wholemeal spaghetti, there is no nutritional analysis for wholemeal pasta, but it is likely that other wholemeal pasta will have a similar nutrient content.

An excellent source of fibre, thiamin, niacin, zinc and magnesium; a good source of protein and iron.

The minerals in pasta (including iron) are poorly absorbed by the body, while the B vitamins are all soluble in water and heavy losses of these occur when the pasta is boiled and/or washed.

Wholemeal spaghetti has more than four times as much thiamin and twice as much niacin as white spaghetti, but the vitamins and minerals in white spaghetti may be better absorbed as wholemeal spaghetti contains more phytate (which hinders absorption) than white spaghetti.

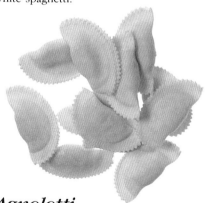

Agnolotti

DESCRIPTION Semicircular stuffed pasta resembling ravioli, but slightly larger.

ORIGIN AND HISTORY Traditionally made to use leftovers, agnolotti originated in Piedmont, where early recipes suggest they had meat or vegetable fillings. The name, originally spelt agnelotti, means 'little fat lambs'.

BUYING AND STORAGE Usually homemade. Open freeze agnolotti and then pack in a rigid container.

PREPARATION AND USE Agnolotti are usually filled with very finely chopped mixtures of vegetables and minced meat such as beef, veal or pork, brains, prosciutto or pancetta. After boiling, agnolotti are sautéed in butter and then served with cheese or a meat sauce.

PROCESSING See Ravioli.

SEE ALSO Ravioli.

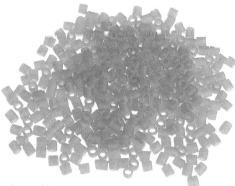

Anelini

DESCRIPTION There are at least two different pastas called anelini. Sicilian anelini are small ring shapes, served with sauces. The second variety is one of a range of pastina (generic name for tiny pasta, usually cooked in soups), and consists of very tiny rings not more than 5 mm in diameter.

PREPARATION AND USE Add to soups.

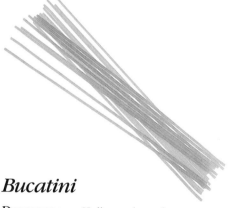

Bucatini

DESCRIPTION Hollow tubes of pasta.

ORIGIN AND HISTORY Bucatini are supposed to have originated in Sicily, where they are one of many different pastas still made in the home.

BUYING AND STORAGE Buy the dried variety in packets in the supermarket. Store in a cool dry place where it will keep indefinitely. Fresh bucatini may be bought from stores specialising in selling fresh pasta.

PREPARATION AND USE Homemade bucatini are made from pasta dough rolled into a thin rope and cut into short lengths. A knitting needle is then pushed through the centre to form a hollow tube. Boil the tubes in plenty of salted water, drain and serve with a tomato sauce flavoured with oregano. Dried bucatini are cooked whole and served with sauces or broken into 2 cm lengths and added to vegetable soups.

VARIETIES

Dried (see Spaghetti) and homemade.

SEE ALSO Spaghetti, Macaroni.

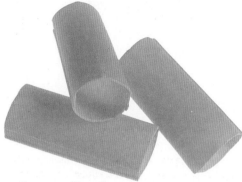

Canneloni

DESCRIPTION Large tubes, approximately 10 cm long and 2–3 cm in diameter. They may be ridged or plain.

PREPARATION AND USE Boil, then stuff with a ricotta, spinach or meat mixture; sauce with a tomato ragout and then bake.

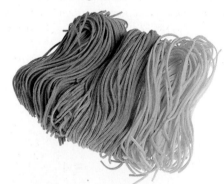

Capelli di Angelo

DESCRIPTION Long strands of dried pasta resembling capellini.

ORIGIN AND HISTORY Originally from Tuscany, capelli di angelo are very fine strands of pasta (the name means 'angel's hair'). They are coiled into nests for drying to prevent them from breaking.

PREPARATION AND USE Boil in plenty of salted water until al dente, drain well and serve with a light sauce, perhaps made from fresh ripe tomatoes, a little olive oil and basil. Add fresh butter, grated parmesan and extra basil if desired.

PROCESSING Made from pasta dough, with or without eggs. The dough is extruded, coiled into nests and allowed to dry.

SEE ALSO Capellini, Spaghetti.

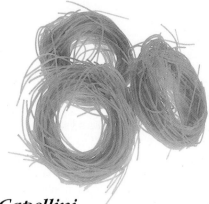

Capellini

also called **Fedelini, Vermicelli**

DESCRIPTION Thin and long, usually coiled into nests.

PREPARATION AND USE For soup. Break into short lengths.

SEE ALSO Capelli di Angelo, Spaghetti.

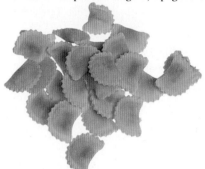

Cappelletti

DESCRIPTION Small curly rings of pasta resembling tortellini in shape.

ORIGIN AND HISTORY Cappelletti means 'little hats'.

PREPARATION AND USE Cappelletti are usually stuffed with a filling of veal, pork or ham and served with tomato sauce or soup, or tossed with butter and cheese.

SEE ALSO Tortellini.

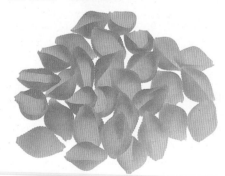

Conchigliette *(small)*, Conchiglie *(medium-sized)*, Conchiglioni *(large)*

also called **Lumache**

DESCRIPTION Shell-shaped (lumache means snails). They may be ridged or plain.

PREPARATION AND USE For conchigliette: add to soups. Conchiglie: boil, add sauce. Conchiglione: boil until al dente, stuff with savoury mixtures, bake.

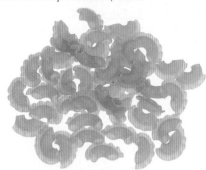

Creste di Gallo

DESCRIPTION 'Cock's Crests' are named for their resemblance to a cock's comb. About 3 cm long, they are slightly curved with a curly longer edge.

PREPARATION AND USE For soup.

Diamantini

DESCRIPTION Small diamond-shaped pasta.

PREPARATION AND USE For soup.

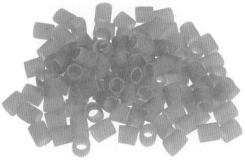

Ditalini

DESCRIPTION Short, straight hollow tubes resembling macaroni.

ORIGIN AND HISTORY Ditalini, or 'little fingers', originated in the region surrounding Genoa where they were probably preceded by broken pieces of semihollow or hollow pasta as a thickener for soups.

PREPARATION AND USE The tubes are cooked in boiling soup. Minestrone alla Genovese is one of the many types of soup that may contain ditalini.

BUYING AND STORAGE Buy in packets from supermarkets specialising in Italian foods. Stored in a cool dry place, they will keep for two to three years.

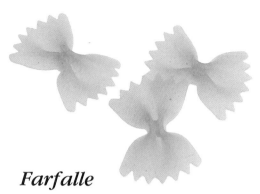

Farfalle

*also called **Butterflies, Bow ties***

DESCRIPTION Bow ties of rolled pasta dough usually 2–3 cm long.

ORIGIN AND HISTORY These thick, flat pieces of pasta were originally shaped into bow ties or butterflies by ingenious home cooks from Northern Italy.

BUYING AND STORAGE Although still made at home, farfalle are now also available from supermarkets and Italian food markets. Store in a cool, dry place.

PREPARATION AND USE Cook in plenty of boiling salted water until just tender. Drain well and serve with a meat or vegetable sauce or toss with cream and cheese. Very good for cold pasta salads.

SEE ALSO Farfallini.

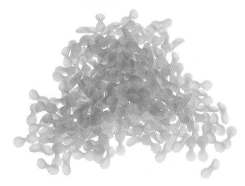

Farfallini

*also called **Farfalline, Fiocchetti***

DESCRIPTION Tiny butterfly-shaped dried pasta with serrated edges.

ORIGIN AND HISTORY From Northern Italy, these small pasta shapes were traditionally made at home. Farfallini means butterflies.

BUYING AND STORAGE Buy from supermarkets or Italian grocery stores. Store in a cool, dry place.

PREPARATION AND USE Add dry farfallini to boiling soups, where they will cook quickly to thicken the broth. Farfallini may be made at home by cutting small ovals or rectangles from thinly rolled pasta dough with a serrated cutter. The pieces should be about 1 cm wide and 1.5 cm long. Pinch the dough in the centre to form small butterflies. Dry slowly and store, or cook in soups. Fiocchetti are made in the same way, and flavoured with lemon juice.

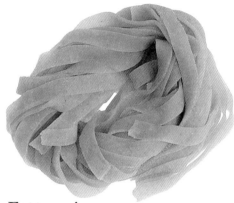

Fettuccine

*also called **Fettuccini***

DESCRIPTION Long, flat ribbons of pasta up to 1 cm wide, narrower and thicker than tagliatelle. Sometimes flavoured and coloured with tomato or spinach.

ORIGIN AND HISTORY Originating near Rome, fettuccine (a Roman name for noodles) closely resemble tagliatelle. They are made with an egg-rich pasta dough rolled into sheets and cut into strips. They are regarded as the pasta most typical of Rome. Fettuccine all' Alfredo is one of the best known dishes featuring this pasta. Alfredo, the man who made the dish famous, used a golden spoon and fork to toss each serving of fettuccine with butter, cheese, a pinch of nutmeg and a grinding of pepper before it went to the diner in his Roman restaurant.

PREPARATION AND USE Boil, use for saucing. See Tagliatelle.

SEE ALSO Linguine, Tagliatelle.

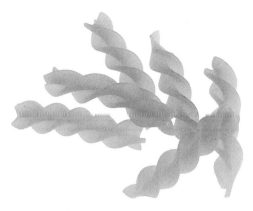

Fusilli, Fusilli Bucati

DESCRIPTION Extruded pasta which has been twisted into spirals. The name fusilli is applied to various traditional shapes. Fusilli bucati are hollow, spiral-shaped spaghetti. Fusilli means spindles.

BUYING AND STORAGE Buy in packets from supermarkets and Italian food stores. Fusilli come in various lengths depending on the brand. Store in a cool dry place.

PREPARATION AND USE Break into 3 cm lengths (see note below) and boil in plenty of salted water, then drain and serve with tomato or meat sauce. Cook broken pieces in soups. Sometimes used in place of farfalle in recipes. NOTE: This variety can be very messy to eat unless the strands are broken into shorter 3 cm lengths.

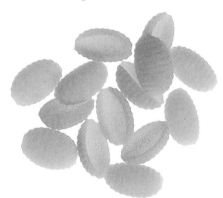

Gnocchetti Sardi

DESCRIPTION Made only in Sardinia, these small dumplings resemble conchigliette, but are much thicker.

PREPARATION AND USE They are made by thumbing small pieces of dough onto finely ridged glass. Usually boiled and sauced.

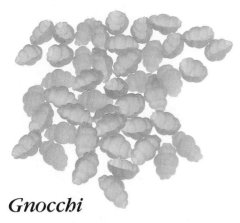

Gnocchi

DESCRIPTION Variously shaped 'dumplings' of pasta dough.

ORIGIN AND HISTORY In the days of Imperial Rome, gnocchi were made from semolina; they were fried and served with honey. Single pieces of gnocchi were called gnocco (in dialect), which means pudding-head or dullard. The early Romans also made gnocchi as one large mixture with a texture between a soufflé and a porridge which was cooked over hot water in an early form of double boiler. The early Romans also made gnocchi from semolina, milk, egg yolks and cheese.

PREPARATION AND USE Although some shell-shaped dried pastas are sold labelled as gnocchi, the more usual varieties are homemade. One way of preparing homemade Roman-style gnocchi is to make a very thick porridge from semolina and milk or water, enriched with egg yolks. The mixture, often flavoured with cheese, is then allowed to cool, flattened on a cold surface and cut into discs. These are arranged in overlapping rows in a shallow buttered dish, topped with melted butter and grated cheese, then baked in the oven until heated through. Gnocchi are usually served before a meat or poultry course and may be flavoured with tomato or mushrooms.

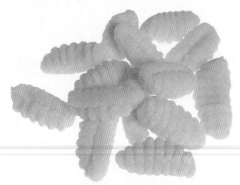

Gnocchi di Patate

DESCRIPTION Small curved shapes made from potato dough, with a rough outer side.

ORIGIN AND HISTORY Gnocchi di patate are one of the few really important uses for potatoes in Italy. Potatoes first arrived in Europe from Peru during the early part of the 16th century and by the end of that century they were grown in Italian gardens as an ornamental plant. The tuber was probably used to augment the more expensive wheat flour when it was in short supply. Flavoured gnocchi di patate are particularly popular in Tuscany, while a Genoese version is served with pesto.

PREPARATION AND USE Mashed potato, egg, salt and butter are made into a dough. The dough is formed into long rolls 2 cm in diameter, cut into 2 cm lengths and ridged by pressing the pieces with a thumb against the tines of a fork or the blunt side of a medium coarse grater. Drop a handful into plenty of boiling salted water and in a short time they will float to the top of the pan. Remove with a slotted spoon and place in a greased heated dish, add a little of the sauce to be served with them, toss well and keep hot while cooking the remaining gnocchi in two or three batches. When cooking is completed, add remaining sauce and reheat before serving. The sauce may be fresh tomato, ham and cream, or very simply fresh butter and grated cheese.

SEE ALSO Gnocchi.

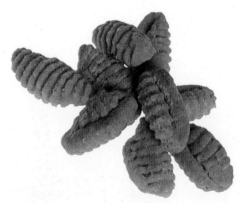

Gnocchi Verdi

DESCRIPTION Dumplings that are made with dough, spinach, cheese and sometimes eggs. May be served in a broth or dressed with cheese and butter or tomato and cream sauce. Often served before the main course. There is a version from Piedmont made with chard, spinach and gorgonzola cheese.

SEE ALSO Gnocchi.

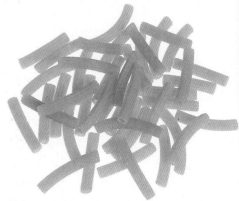

Gramigna, Gramigna Rigata

DESCRIPTION Long tubes of pasta about 1 cm in diameter. Gramigna rigata is ridged.

PREPARATION AND USE Should be boiled and sauced.

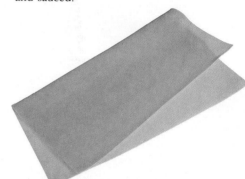

Lasagne, Lasagne Verde, Lasagnette

DESCRIPTION Sheets of pasta dough 10–12 cm wide, often with rippled or curly edges. Lasagne verde are spinach-flavoured. Lasagnette are small lasagne with a 4 cm side.

PREPARATION AND USE Boiled then layered in a shallow ovenproof dish with meat or vegetable sauce and bechamel sauce, topped with cheese and then baked. 'Instant' lasagne are made from partially precooked lasagne sheets. Lasagnette are served sauced.

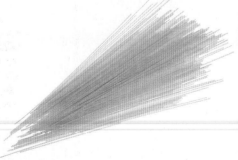

Linguine

DESCRIPTION Long thin strips of pasta dough with square-cut edges.

Origin and History Campania, where Southern Italy begins, is the home of linguine, where they have long been made in the home and by the early spaghetti factories. They are not a very common dish in Italy, but they migrated with people from the area around Naples to America, and there became more popular.

Buying and Storage Buy the dried linguine in packets from the supermarket. Store in a cool dry place.

Preparation and Use Boil in plenty of salted water until al dente. Drain and sauce as desired.

See Also Fettuccine, Tagliatelle.

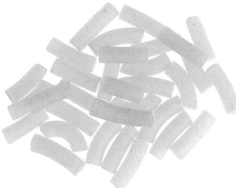

Macaroni
also called Rigatoni, Tubetti, Ziltoni

Description Thick, long hollow shapes, often broken into 3 cm lengths for baking.

Preparation and Use Boil, sauce and serve immediately or bake, depending on size.

See Also Bucatini.

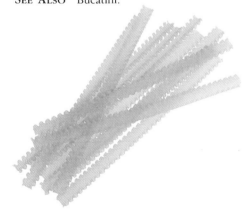

Mafalde
also called Fesonati

Description Long strips of dried pasta usually 3–5 cm wide, with curly edges, sometimes spinach-flavoured.

Origin and History Originally from the north of Italy.

Buying and Storage Buy in long packets or boxes from supermarkets or Italian food stores. Store in a cool dry place.

Preparation and Use Boil in plenty of boiling salted water, drain well and serve sauced, or layer in a casserole with meat or vegetable and cheese sauces (see Lasagne). Small broken pieces may be added to soups.

Processing Not usually made at home.

See Also Tagliatelle.

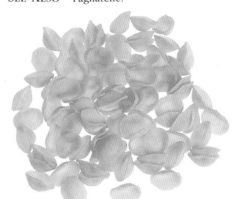

Orecchiette

Description Small shapes resembling ears (the name means 'little ears').

Origin and History This homemade pasta from Apulia (Puglia) is well suited to this highly flavoured region where chilli is popular and anchovies seem to feature in most dishes.

Buying and Storage Dried orecchiette are available from Italian food stores. They will keep almost indefinitely in a cool, dry place. The fresh homemade variety may be left to dry carefully at room temperature, then stored as above.

Preparation and Use Orecchiette are made from a mixture of durum semolina, flour and water. Made without eggs, this pasta has a chewier, firmer texture than varieties from other districts. The dough is rolled out into a 3 mm thick sheet, then cut into small 18 mm diameter discs. Each disc is shaped by placing it in the palm of one hand and rotating the thumb of the other hand in the centre of the disc until it resembles a mushroom cap 25–30 mm in diameter. Cook in plenty of boiling salted water (it will take much longer than egg pasta), then serve with a typical Apulian sauce, perhaps broccoli and anchovy.

Penne

Description Thick, hollow tubes like the stems of feathers, with ends cut at an acute angle.

Preparation and Use Served with a sauce.

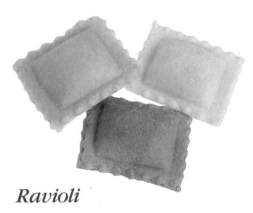

Ravioli

Description Small squares of pasta dough stuffed to resemble pillows with savoury or sweet filling, served in a sauce, usually garnished with grated parmesan cheese.

Buying and Storage Buy fresh from specialist food stores or frozen from supermarkets. Fresh ravioli will keep in the refrigerator for two or three days, but are best used as fresh as possible. Freeze for up to four months.

Preparation and Use To make ravioli 'pillows' from two sheets of pasta dough, place small mounds of filling 5 cm apart on one sheet, cover with the second and seal the pasta between the filling mounds. Cut into squares and cover with a damp cloth. Bring a large pan of water to the boil, add salt and then the ravioli, and boil rapidly until tender (approximately 8–10 minutes). Drain thoroughly and serve in a sauce — usually a light tomato sauce — or toss in butter and sprinkle with cheese.

Processing May be made at home (see above). Special pans and rolling pins for making ravioli are available at Italian equipment stores.

VARIETIES

Ravioli may be made with meat, vegetable, cheese or fish fillings, or combinations of these.

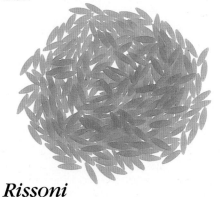

Rissoni

DESCRIPTION Small rice-sized, rice-shaped pasta.

PREPARATION AND USE For soups.

Spaghetti

DESCRIPTION Long cylindrical dried pasta of varying thicknesses and diameter, solid or hollow. The name 'spaghetti' is also used as a generic term for all long strings of extruded pasta.

ORIGIN AND HISTORY Arab invaders are thought to have introduced spaghetti to Sicily long before Marco Polo.

Pontedassio, in the province of Liguria, houses Italy's Spaghetti Museum where ancient and modern pasta machines are displayed along with documents dating back to the 13th century.

The three-pronged fork developed for spaghetti eating came into use in the late 18th century. It was a modification of the older two-pronged table fork, invented in Venice for use by rich merchants.

Many spaghetti and macaroni dishes were developed in the south of Italy, an area closely identified with tubular pasta. The modern product labelled spaghetti seems to be much thinner than earlier varieties.

BUYING AND STORAGE Buy in long packets from supermarkets. Store in a cool dry place.

PREPARATION AND USE Some traditional dishes are made with either macaroni or spaghetti depending on the district. Spaghetti (or macaroni) al sugo (with meat sauce) or al pomodoro (with tomato sauce) and the popular pommarola 'n coppa — pasta topped with a sauce of fresh tomatoes, with onions, bacon and garlic browned in olive oil — are now favourites with many pasta lovers.

VARIETIES

Hollow (in descending order of thickness): zite, mezzani, perciatelli, perciatelloni.
Solid (very fine strands): capellini, fedelini, spaghettini.

SEE ALSO Capellini, Macaroni.

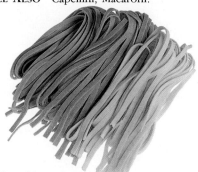

Tagliarini

DESCRIPTION Homemade fettuccine.

BUYING AND STORAGE Usually this is made when required. Store in freezer.

PREPARATION AND USE Roll the prepared pasta dough into a large thin oval by hand, or into a long sheet by machine. Roll dough up tightly and cut into thin strips with a knife. Unroll and allow to dry slightly, then cook in plenty of boiling salted water. Drain well and sauce as required.

SEE ALSO Fettuccine.

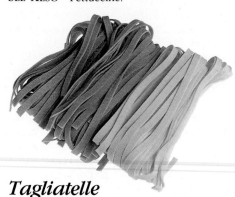

Tagliatelle

DESCRIPTION Long flat ribbon pasta. Tagliatelle may be plain, tomato or spinach flavoured.

ORIGIN AND HISTORY From the Emilia Rogno district and known as one of the best of Bolognese pastas. Tagliatelle (the name of which comes from a verb meaning to cut), according to local legend, were first presented at the home of a Bolognese nobleman by a cook who was inspired by the flaxen hair of the principal guest (uncooked tagliatelle should have the lightness suggested by fine blond hair). The guest's name was Lucrezia Borgia.

PREPARATION AND USE Prepare as for fettuccine. The term casareccia, meaning homemade, is often used for this type of pasta, which points to the ideal location for its manufacture — the family kitchen.

SEE ALSO Fettuccine, Linguine.

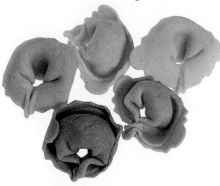

Tortellini

DESCRIPTION Small rounds of pasta dough filled with finely chopped meats (e.g. grated mortadella), parmesan and nutmeg, then sealed and shaped into rings.

PREPARATION AND USE Cook in chicken or beef broth.

SEE ALSO Cappelletti.

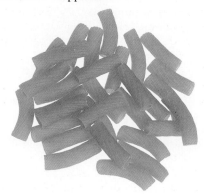

Tortiglioni

also called *Cavatappi, Elicoidali*

DESCRIPTION 3 cm lengths of twisted pasta.

PREPARATION AND USE Cooked in soups or sauces.

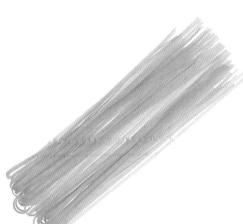

Trenette

DESCRIPTION Flat, thin, long strips of pasta.
PREPARATION AND USE Boil and sauce.
SEE ALSO Fettuccine, Linguine, Tagliatelle.

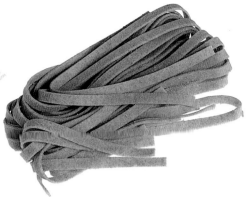

Wholemeal Pasta

*also called **Wholewheat pasta***

DESCRIPTION Pasta made with varying proportions of flour milled from the whole wheat grain and white flour.

ORIGIN AND HISTORY Wholemeal pasta is a fairly recent commercial product made popular by the worldwide interest in increasing the amount of fibre in the diet. Small quantities have always been made in the home, but recorded history does not seem to mention it.

BUYING AND STORAGE Buy in packets or boxes from supermarkets or fresh from specialist pasta shops. Wholemeal pasta is usually available as tagliatelle or fettuccine, ravioli and spaghetti, although most rolled pasta shapes can be made with wholemeal dough.

PREPARATION AND USE Combine equal quantities of plain and wholemeal wheat flours and mix to a dough with eggs and water. Knead thoroughly and allow to rest. Roll dough out to a rectangle 1.5 cm thick and use as desired (see entries for the various shapes of pasta). Cook in plenty of boiling salted water, drain, and sauce as desired.

NOODLES

Although noodle shapes do not vary as fantastically as those for pasta, the choice of these attractive foods is very wide. The background and associations of each type are discussed in the individual entries.

As for pasta, the nutritional categories for noodles are few. The tables below provide a reference when consulting the individual entries.

Noodles are generally made by mixing flour with water and common salt or alkaline salt until a homogeneous dough of crumbly consistency is produced. The mixture is formed into a sheet by passage between a pair of steel rollers. The dough structure is then developed mechanically, by passing the dough sheet between steel rollers of successively decreasing clearance. Once the dough sheet has been rolled out to the desired thickness, it is cut into noodle strands by passage between a pair of cutting rollers. Alternatively, a hand-mixed dough can be formed into a coherent mass by stamping or by compression with a bamboo pole, then reduced in thickness with a rolling pin. Finally, the dough is cut into noodle strands with a knife. Another method consists of alternately twirling and folding a length of dough by hand, until noodle strings are produced. The noodles are then either sold raw, or processed further before sale, depending on the type of noodle being produced.

The origin of Asian noodles seems to have been lost over the centuries, but it is generally recognised that the Chinese were eating noodles by the 1st century AD. During the period 960–1280AD, special shops selling noodles are said to have been familiar to the people of northern China. Noodles come in a range of sizes and shapes, from flat ribbons to thin strips — but they are always made long, as they are a sign of longevity.

Raw noodles are sold fresh, and should be kept refrigerated for a maximum of three to four days, and cooked as soon as possible.

Dried noodles are raw noodles which have been hung out to dry in the sun or in drying cabinets. They will keep indefinitely in a cool dry place.

Wet noodles are those which have been parboiled. They need to be boiled again, or fried, immediately prior to consumption.

Steamed and dried (traditional instant) noodles are steamed for 1–3 minutes, then dried, either in the sun or in special drying cabinets; they will keep indefinitely in a cool dry place.

Steamed and fried (modern instant) noodles are cut to form into a wave pattern, then assembled into oblong blocks, which pass through a steaming chamber, and then into a hot bath of oil. Excess oil is drained away after frying and the noodles are wrapped, along with a sachet of flavouring concentrate. These are generally immersed in boiling water for 2–3 minutes prior to serving. They are the most common type of noodle found in supermarkets.

Of the many different kinds of packaged noodles, some only need soaking before being added to dishes, some are cooked without soaking and some are deep-fried to provide a crisp texture. They should be cooked according to the directions (always to 'al dente' stage).

Rice Noodle, Dried

MAJOR NUTRIENTS		SERVE SIZE 80 G	
Energy	1200 kJ	Sodium	100 mg
Protein	4 g	Potassium	5 mg
Fat	0	Iron	1.2 mg
Carbohydrate	65 g	Thiamin	0.05 mg
Cholesterol	0	Niacin Equiv.	2.5 mg
Dietary Fibre	n/a		

NUTRITIONAL INFORMATION These are a good source of niacin and iron; a moderate source of protein and thiamin. Heavy losses of the water-soluble B vitamins occur when the noodles are boiled and/or washed.

Wheat Noodle, Raw

MAJOR NUTRIENTS		SERVE SIZE 80 G	
Energy	1320 kJ	Potassium	185 mg
Protein	9 g	Iron	1 mg
Fat	5 g	Magnesium	37.5 mg
Carbohydrate	60 g	Zinc	1 mg
Cholesterol	0	Thiamin	0.3 mg
Dietary Fibre	4 g	Niacin Equiv.	4 mg
Sodium	0		

NUTRITIONAL INFORMATION The nutrient analysis of plain wheat noodles is similar to that of white pasta. An excellent source of thiamin and niacin. A good source of protein, fibre and iron. A moderate source of magnesium and zinc. The minerals in wheat noodles (including iron) are poorly absorbed by the body. The B vitamins are all soluble in water and heavy losses of these vitamins occur when the noodles are boiled and/or washed.

Wheat Noodle, Steamed and Dried

MAJOR NUTRIENTS		SERVE SIZE 80 G	
Energy	1190 kJ	Cholesterol	n/a
Protein	9 g	Dietary Fibre	n/a
Fat	2 g	Sodium	n/a
Carbohydrate	60 g	Potassium	n/a

NUTRITIONAL INFORMATION This is the traditional instant noodle. There is no vitamin and mineral analysis available, but the vitamin and mineral content is likely to be similar to that of plain noodles. Heavy losses of B vitamins occur when the noodles are boiled or washed.

Wheat Noodle, Steamed and Fried

MAJOR NUTRIENTS		SERVE SIZE 80 G	
Energy	1570 kJ	Cholesterol	n/a
Protein	8 g	Dietary Fibre	n/a
Fat	17 g	Sodium	n/a
Carbohydrate	50 g	Potassium	n/a

NUTRITIONAL INFORMATION This is the modern instant noodle. A high-fat food: in these noodles, in contrast to other types of noodle and pasta, a large percentage of the kilojoules comes from fat. There is no vitamin and mineral analysis available, but the vitamin and mineral content is likely to be similar to that of plain noodles. Heavy losses of B vitamins occur when the noodles are boiled or washed.

Asian Wheat Noodle

also called **Bamee, Mee, Mein, Mie, Ramen**

DESCRIPTION Yellow (alkaline) or white (salted). Asian noodles are thick strips of dough generally cut from a rolled dough sheet made from flour, water and alkaline and/or common salt. Some have egg added for firmer texture. They come in a range of sizes and shapes from flat ribbons to thin strips, but always long as they are a sign of longevity.

ORIGIN AND HISTORY Asian noodles are a traditional food of China, Japan and Southeast Asia. Their origin seems to have been lost over the centuries but it is generally recognised that the Chinese were eating noodles by the 1st century AD. During the period 960–1280 special shops selling noodles are said to have been familiar to the people of Northern China.

BUYING AND STORAGE Asian wheat noodles may be bought raw, dried, wet, steamed and dried, or steamed and fried.

Raw noodles are sold fresh. Keep refrigerated for three to four days. Cook as soon as possible.

Dried noodles — raw noodles which have been hung out to dry in the sun or in drying cabinets — will keep indefinitely in a cool dry place.

Wet or Hokkien noodles — noodles which have been parboiled — are reboiled or fried immediately before consumption. These are the most popular type of noodle in Southeast Asia. Keep refrigerated up to two days. Cook as soon as possible.

Steamed and dried noodles (traditional instant) — noodles which have been steamed for 1–3 minutes, then dried either in the sun or in special drying cabinets — will keep indefinitely in a cool, dry place.

Steamed and fried noodles (modern instant) are noodles cut and formed into a wave pattern and then assembled into oblong blocks which pass through a steaming chamber, then into an oil frying bath. Excess oil is drained away and the noodles are wrapped along with a sachet of flavouring concentrate to be added when they have been boiled and drained. They are the most common type of noodle found in Australian supermarkets.

PREPARATION AND USE Of the many different kinds of noodles, some only need soaking before being added to dishes, some are cooked without soaking and some are deep fried to provide crisp texture. Cook according to package directions (always to al dente stage). A bowl of Chinese noodles in broth flavoured with small pieces of meat or fish and vegetables is one of the most common and popular Chinese meals.

PROCESSING Noodles are generally made by mixing flour with water and common salt or alkaline salt until a homogeneous dough of crumbly consistency is produced. The mixture is formed into a sheet by passage between a pair of steel rollers. The dough structure is then developed mechanically by passing the dough sheet between steel rollers of successively decreasing clearance. Once the dough sheet has been rolled out to the desired thickness it is cut into noodle strands by passage between a pair of cutting rollers.

Alternatively, a hand-mixed dough can be formed into a coherent mass by stamping or by compression with a bamboo pole, then reduced in thickness with a rolling pin; after this the dough is cut into noodle strands with a knife. Another method consists of alternately twirling and folding a length of dough by hand until noodle strings are produced. The noodles are then either sold raw or processed further before sale, depending on the type of noodle being produced.

VARIETIES

In addition to the different types of precooking (see under Buying and Storage), Asian noodles may be classified as somen (very fine) or udon (thick).

Somen

DESCRIPTION Fine white Japanese wheat flour noodles usually made with water, but sometimes with egg yolk. The noodle known as miswa in the Philippines is the same, as are several types now marketed in Chinese stores.

ORIGIN AND HISTORY Of Chinese origin, being akin to the earliest forms of noodle manufactured there.

BUYING AND STORAGE Sold in short sticks in small, attractively packed bundles which keep indefinitely if stored away from moisture.

PREPARATION AND USE Lightly cooked somen are eaten cold with a dipping sauce in Japan, but are also suitable for adding to soups.

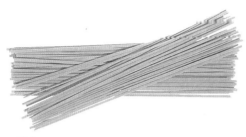

Udon

DESCRIPTION Thick wheat flour noodles very similar to the Shanghai thick noodle in appearance, although buff in colour.

ORIGIN AND HISTORY This noodle is made by a technique adopted from ancient China. It is popular in Japan as a quick snack sold at roadside food stalls where the precooked noodles are placed in bowl-shaped wire baskets which are lowered into bubbling stock, or held under a stream of boiling water until heated through, then served into a bowl with broth, slivers of meat and vegetables.

BUYING AND STORAGE Sold fresh or dried. See main entry.

PREPARATION AND USE Udon noodles are boiled in soup broth as a warming, informal snack.

SEE ALSO Egg Noodles, Shanghai Noodles, Silver Pin Noodles.

Banh Trang Rice Paper Wrapper

DESCRIPTION The Vietnamese equivalent of the spring roll wrapper: stiff, round, transparent sheets made from rice, salt and water.

ORIGIN AND HISTORY Much that is Vietnamese today originated in the Chinese cuisine, and it is probable that this did too. But it is an arguable point, as in earlier times

rice was more extensively used in Vietnam than in China.

BUYING AND STORAGE Sold in packs of 10 or so, they come in several sizes. Treated with care to prevent breaking, banh trang wrappers will last indefinitely, provided they are kept away from damp.

PREPARATION AND USE They are used as a wrapper for Vietnamese-style spring rolls, cha gio, which are eaten raw or deep fried. The wrappers must be softened before they can be used, by wiping over with a damp cloth. They can also be brushed with a thin sugar-water solution which will cause them to darken and crisp when fried. The larger, round wrappers should be cut in quarters before rolling up, using the rounded edge first and ending with the point.

PROCESSING A dough of rice flour, salt and water is thinly spread, cut into round shapes, then placed on bamboo trays to sun-dry. The trays leave their characteristic cross-hatch imprint on the wrappers.

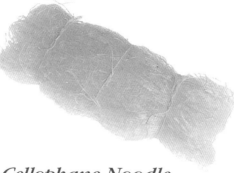

Cellophane Noodle

DESCRIPTION Shiny, thin and translucent noodles made from mung beans. When cooked in soups they develop a slippery texture and absorb the flavours of other foods.

ORIGIN AND HISTORY Traditional Asian noodles.

BUYING AND STORAGE Buy dry in 100 g packets at Asian supermarkets. They are usually tied together in bundles, then wrapped in cellophane. They will keep indefinitely in a cool dry place. Once they have been soaked they must be used as soon as possible.

PREPARATION AND USE Soak for ten minutes in hot water until soft, then drain well before frying. They may be stir fried or deep fried, forming an inexpensive extender to meat, fish or seafood dishes. They do not need prior soaking when added to soups.

VARIETIES
Bean thread, soya bean vermicelli, Japanese 'spring rain' noodle.

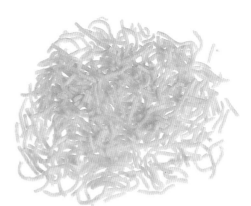

E-Fu Noodle

also called **Yi noodle**

DESCRIPTION Thin, yellow, egg and wheat flour noodles which have been dried and formed into large, tangled bundles. The noodles are prefried before drying. They have a rich flavour which makes them suitable for use in simple dishes with few additives.

ORIGIN AND HISTORY A type of noodle favoured along the southern coastal area of China, particularly the province of Fukien where they have been used for centuries. A similar type of noodle made in the Philippines is known as pancit canton.

BUYING AND STORAGE Both fried and dried e-fu noodles are sold in large bundles from the dried goods section of Asian stores. They can be kept for many months in dry conditions.

PREPARATION AND USE They require only a short cooking time and are generally used in soups and braised dishes, but are also sometimes served cold as an appetiser with a sesame-based sauce and shredded cold meat.

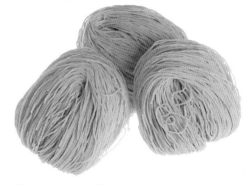

Egg Noodle

DESCRIPTION A noodle made from a dough of wheat flour and eggs. Egg noodles may vary in thickness from fine strands, to pieces as thick as a shoelace. They are a light golden colour and have a texture and taste similar to spaghetti, being made with the same ingredients. Many of the 'instant' noodles sold today are precooked and dehydrated egg noodles.

ORIGIN AND HISTORY Cantonese cooks

in the south-eastern area of China made the first known egg noodles at least four centuries ago; previously Chinese noodles were simply made from flour and water.

BUYING AND STORAGE Egg noodles are sold in several ways. Dried noodles are usually formed into small bundles, each roughly one serve, but they may also be in skeins rather like wool. Fresh noodles are piled together to be weighed out to order. Dried noodles keep indefinitely in dry conditions. Fresh noodles can be kept for about four days in the refrigerator, or several weeks in the freezer.

PREPARATION AND USE To serve noodles soft in a soup or stir-fry they should be boiled in simmering salted water until just cooked through, but still holding their shape and retaining their texture. To cook crisp, soften briefly in hot water, drain thoroughly and then fry in a very hot wok with a small amount of vegetable oil.

SEE ALSO Asian Wheat Noodles.

European Noodle

DESCRIPTION These soft, white strips or tubes of dough are usually made from wheat flour or a starch equivalent such as potatoes.

ORIGIN AND HISTORY The origin is as obscure as that of pasta, and they probably entered Europe at the same time, being a softer version than the durum semolina varieties of pasta.

BUYING AND STORAGE They can be made at home, but some varieties are available at supermarkets as packets of dried noodles.

PREPARATION AND USE This is different according to the variety, and can include a sauce or the addition of meat and vegetables.

VARIETIES

Holvshki (Czechoslovakian) Premixed with cooked, chopped cabbage; hot bacon fat is poured over.

Metelt (Hungarian) Small squares of cooked dough served with roast meat and gulyas. Fresh egg noodle ribbons are also traditionally served with gulyas.

Nouilles (French) Served in much the same way as pasta in Italy, with sauces or cheeses. Often an accompaniment to roast lamb, pork or veal. They are a particularly

important addition to the dishes of Alsace and Provence.

Nudeln (German) Tossed with butter or bacon fat, and served with a sprinkling of poppy seeds or paprika. Sometimes the noodles are stuffed with meat and served in soups.

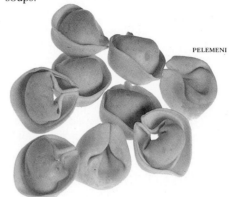

PELEMENI

Pelemeni (Russian) Stuffed dumpling noodles which are filled with beef and pork, served in soup or boiled and served with sour cream.

Pirogi (large) and Pirozkki/piroshki (small) (Polish) Yeast dough pieces stuffed with mixtures of meat, mushrooms, cabbage or fish and deep fried or baked, then served with melted butter and a tomato sauce or topped with sour cream.

Spätzle (German) Noodles made by forcing dough through a sieve into boiling soup.

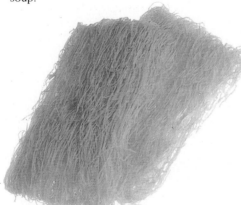

Rice Noodle, Dried

*also called **Bi-sun, Long rice, Rice stick;** numerous other regional names*

DESCRIPTION Noodles made from a pasta of ground rice and water are extruded in several forms. The flat, wide rice noodle is known as a rice ribbon, and is probably more

often sold fresh. In varying widths and thicknesses, rice ribbons are used throughout China and in Malaysia and Vietnam, most popularly in soups. They have a more distinctive flavour than cellophane noodles, and also readily absorb the flavours that accompany them.

Rice sticks also come in several sizes, are generally thinner and narrower than rice ribbons and are packaged in short flat bundles.

The finest rice noodles are known as rice vermicelli or transparent rice noodles; they resemble bundles of semitransparent whitish strands.

ORIGIN AND HISTORY Rice noodles have been known in Vietnam from its early history, with various permutations of rice noodles in soup accounting for a major part of the cuisine. Similarly the southern, rice-growing areas of China use rice for noodle making, although their rice noodles are more often sold fresh. Rice vermicelli are an integral part of the Indonesian and Malaysian curry dish known as laksa.

BUYING AND STORAGE All types of dried rice noodle can be kept indefinitely in a cool, dry store cupboard. They come in large tangled, cellophane-wrapped bundles, or neat little stacks wrapped in coloured paper.

PREPARATION AND USE Soak the noodles before use, then drain and add to the dish to continue cooking. Rice noodles should not be overcooked as they will break apart. Add to soup stock or stir-fries. Rice vermicelli can be added to curry sauces, or may be quickly deep-fried to make them expand dramatically into crisp white puffs to use as a crunchy noodle bed for stir-fried dishes, or as a garnish. They burn easily and should be cooked in small quantities for a few seconds only. They can also be soaked and fried in a double frying basket to make edible serving 'nests'.

Rice Noodle, Fresh

*also known as **Kway tiow, Sar hor fun, Bun pho***

DESCRIPTION Thick, soft, white rice

noodles that have a subtle flavour but an agreeable texture and readily absorb the flavour of accompanying seasonings and ingredients.

ORIGIN AND HISTORY First used in the southern part of Southeast Asia, in particular Canton and Vietnam, and by Chinese in the Malay Peninsula and Thailand.

BUYING AND STORAGE Fresh dough is sold in plastic packs and can be kept for about three days in the refrigerator. It can be frozen, but the texture tends to become too soft when defrosted. At home, the dough is cut crossways into ribbons of over 1 cm width.

PREPARATION AND USE Noodles should be steeped very briefly in boiling water, drained and then carefully stir-fried in oil in a wok with vegetables and meat, over intense heat. They are often served with oyster sauce. Avoid overcooking, as the noodles will break up.

PROCESSING Made by steaming a thin dough of ground rice and water over fine cloth in wide wooden tubs until firm. The sheets of dough are brushed with oil to prevent them sticking, and stacked together. Sold in rolls.

Seaweed Noodle

also called **Yang fun (Chinese)**

DESCRIPTION Thinner, more transparent and more gelatinous than cellophane noodles, these noodles are made from various types of seaweed.

ORIGIN AND HISTORY An Asian delicacy.

BUYING AND STORAGE Available in packets at Asian food stores. Sold dry. Will keep indefinitely in a cool dry place.

PREPARATION AND USE Cover with boiling water and soak for about 20 minutes. Rinse in cold water. Use to add texture to cold dishes and as an economical extender for more expensive foods.

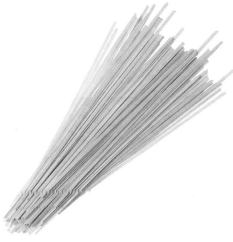

Shanghai Noodle

DESCRIPTION There are two distinct types of Shanghai noodle, the more important being the thick, spaghetti-like noodle which is usually sold only in fresh form. It is yellow in colour and heavy-textured. The other is known as thin Shanghai noodle and is a white flour and water noodle about the thickness of regular egg noodles and a creamy white in colour. It is dried.

ORIGIN AND HISTORY The cuisine of the province of Shanghai is one of strong, robust tastes in heavy, warming and nourishing foods. The large, almost chewy noodles absorb bold flavours and have been an integral part of the Shanghai diet for centuries.

BUYING AND STORAGE Fresh Shanghai noodles can be kept in the refrigerator for up to four days, or may be frozen. They are sold by weight, often premeasured into plastic bags and usually tossed with oil to prevent them drying out. Dried noodles keep indefinitely away from moisture.

PREPARATION AND USE Boil noodles in salted water until partially tender, then drain. Add sauce and braise until the noodles are tender and the sauce is absorbed.

Shirataki Noodle

DESCRIPTION Transparent noodles made from the starchy tuberous root konnyaku ('devil's tongue'). The name means 'white waterfall', which aptly describes the appearance of a forkful of the cooked noodles.

ORIGIN AND HISTORY The starchy plant called 'devil's tongue' is unique to Japan, although it resembles other starchy, fibrous roots like cassava, taro and tapioca. It is intriguing that the Japanese persist with the tedious process necessary to make this unpalatable root into edible products: the stringy konnyaku, the fine shirataki and also compressed cakes.

BUYING AND STORAGE Buy in cans from Asian food suppliers and use within two days of opening, or purchase dry. Dried filaments can be stored indefinitely in dry conditions. Fresh cakes can be kept for several days in fresh cold water.

PREPARATION AND USE Drain liquid from can and cut noodles into short lengths. Add to soups and one-pan dishes traditionally cooked at the table, e.g. sukiyaki. If dried, boil for a long time, until tender and gelatinous, and absorbing the flavours of the sauce in which cooked. Cakes should be drained and cut into strips. Simmer in well flavoured soup stocks and sauces. They are said to ease indigestion.

Silver Pin Noodle

DESCRIPTION Short, plump, silver-white, near-transparent noodles made by hand-rolling small knobs of dough made from gluten-free wheat flour.

ORIGIN AND HISTORY When the technology which allowed the gluten to be extracted from flour was achieved, it resulted in two important new food products in China. Kau fu or wheat gluten — a globular, doughy mass — became a major ingredient for vegetarians, and the refined flour which remained could be made into a crisp-tender clear dough which was used to wrap various types of steamed 'dim sum', as well as to make these particular noodles. They are named for their appearance, looking like overlarge dressmakers' pins.

BUYING AND STORAGE Usually made at home, they can occasionally be purchased from specialist Asian stores. They should be used on the day of production, and are never sold dried.

PREPARATION AND USE To use, steep briefly in boiling water, then drain. Stir-fry with shredded meats and vegetables, adding oyster or soya sauce and a thickened stock.

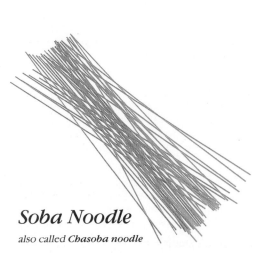

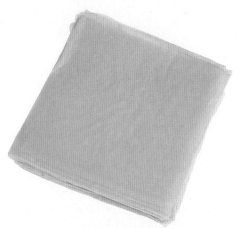

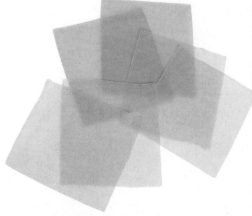

Soba Noodle

also called ***Chasoba noodle***

DESCRIPTION These are Japanese noodles, made from ground buckwheat and wheat flour. The thin beige noodles are approximately 30 cm in length. They have square edges and may be any width from 5 mm to 1.5 cm.

ORIGIN AND HISTORY Soba is rarely used elsewhere in Asia, despite its extensive use in its native land. The grain itself was brought to Japan from China, and the Chinese had in turn transported it from Tibet where it was used in making a thick, flat bread-cake.

BUYING AND STORAGE Soba noodles, both plain and green, are readily available from Japanese stores, packed, in the true Japanese tradition, in attractive paper wraps. They will keep for many months. Soba can also sometimes be bought fresh; in this case, cook as soon as possible. Freeze up to two weeks; the noodles tend to become brittle with longer freezing.

PREPARATION AND USE Cook until barely tender in boiling water, then cool under running water. Often served cold (over ice) with a soy-based dipping sauce during the hot summer months, sometimes topped with small pieces of vegetable or seafood. They can also be served as a soup–noodle snack with a dashi-flavoured soup stock.

VARIETIES
Green (green tea is added to the dough to colour it and give it a subtle, unique flavour), or pink, flavoured with beetroot.

Spring Roll Wrapper

DESCRIPTION Tough, thin, white sheets of wheat flour pastry used to encase pork or chicken and vegetables in many combinations to make rolls 1–2 cm in diameter and approximately 5–10 cm long.

ORIGIN AND HISTORY Traditional Asian food.

BUYING AND STORAGE Buy fresh from Asian food stores.

PREPARATION AND USE Dust any excess starch from the surface, then place a spoonful of filling in a strip along one end. Fold base of wrapper over filling, then fold in sides and roll up. Seal the edge with a little beaten egg white. Shallow- or deep-fry until golden.

PROCESSING Made from a wheat flour or wheat flour and tapioca batter which is poured in a thin film onto a hot-plate. When cooked it is cut to size, stacked and sold wet.

Wonton Wrapper

also called ***Egg roll wrapper, Sao mai***

DESCRIPTION Thin pieces of pliable, dry pasta dough, usually used to wrap well-flavoured savoury or sweet fillings for dumplings or snack rolls.

ORIGIN AND HISTORY A traditional food of China for thousands of years. Much appreciated by all Chinese, particularly in the northern regions.

BUYING AND STORAGE Available fresh from Asian food stores. Store in the refrigerator for three to four days. Freeze for longer storage.

Also available filled, ready for final cooking, fresh from Asian food stores or frozen from supermarkets.

PREPARATION AND USE Keep wrappers covered to prevent drying out. Fill, using meat, fish or vegetable mixtures. Boil in soup, shallow-fry, steam or braise and serve with a dipping sauce.

PROCESSING Wheat flour, eggs, water and salt are made into a dough. This is kneaded well, then rolled out into very thin sheets (1 mm thick). Cut into shapes, they are dusted with rice flour, stacked and packed, usually in airtight plastic wrap.

SALTS AND BAKING AGENTS

Most of the items in this section are used in small quantities, and few make any significant positive contribution to the nutrients in the diet. Many are important, however, because they make food more appetising and varied. A number of the foods enjoyed daily could not be produced without these ingredients.

The amount of sodium in some of the items is a definite disadvantage. In population studies, a link is shown between sodium intake and the prevalence of high blood pressure. Most of the sodium in the diet comes from salt (sodium chloride), but other sodium compounds such as sodium bicarbonate are also used in baking powder. Sodium benzoate and monosodium glutamate (MSG) are frequently used in cooking and processing.

It has been estimated that about 75% of the sodium in the Western diet comes from processed foods. Much of it comes from important staple foods such as bread, butter, margarine, cheese and breakfast cereals.

It is encouraging to see the expanding range of 'no added salt', 'salt-free', 'low salt' and 'reduced salt' products on the supermarket shelves. It is useful to remember that before a product can be classified as low salt it must contain no more than 120 mg sodium per 100 g, and buyers should read the nutrition information on the label.

Some people buy rock salt or 'natural' sea salt, or vegetable salts, in the belief that these have a health advantage: in fact they are all sodium chloride, in slightly different forms.

Thickening and gelling agents act by absorbing water and expanding. When flour, cornflour, arrowroot, rice flour or potato flour are used, it is the starch which absorbs the water. When pectin or agar agar are used, it is another complex carbohydrate, the soluble dietary fibre, which absorbs the water. In the case of jam making, the added sugar and the acid in the fruit react with the pectin to form the gel. In the case of gelatine mixtures, it is the protein which absorbs the water and expands. The gels formed from meat, chicken and fish stock are gelatine-based.

Food scientists have produced a number of efficient thickening agents which form stable sauces, gravies and other foods. These include the modified starches, in which the size of the starch molecule is larger, to increase its capacity to absorb and hold water.

Raising agents include yeast and baking powder. Yeast, under certain conditions, ferments the sugar in a mixture and produces carbon dioxide, which expands under warm conditions and leavens the dough.

Baking powder made up in the home usually consists of a mixture of sodium bicarbonate and cream of tartar (potassium bitartrate). When moistened and heated, the cream of tartar reacts with the sodium bicarbonate to release carbon dioxide. Most commercial baking powders use phosphates such as calcium salts, instead of cream of tartar. The sodium, calcium and phosphorus content of baking powders will vary according to the ingredients used in a particular brand.

In a traditional sponge made with plain flour, or a mixture of flour and/or cornflour or arrowroot, and no raising agent, the aeration depends upon incorporating the air into the mixture by whipping the egg white and sieving the flour. It is the properties of the albumin, the protein in egg white, that make this whipping possible. The added sugar stabilises the mixture.

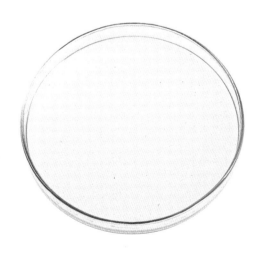

Acetic Acid

NUTRITIONAL INFORMATION Makes no significant nutritional contribution to the diet. Food Additive Code Number 260.

DESCRIPTION A colourless acidic liquid with the pungent odour of vinegar.

ORIGIN AND HISTORY Historically, this is the first acid produced deliberately and used by people. It is the substance that causes wine to go sour and is the main component of vinegar.

BUYING AND STORAGE Not readily available from food shops.

PREPARATION AND USE Used in confectionery, in the cooking of sugar and in wine or malt vinegars.

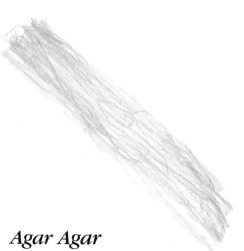

Agar Agar

also called **Bengal isinglass, Ceylon moss, Japanese moss, Kanten**

NUTRITIONAL INFORMATION Makes no significant nutritional contribution to the diet.

DESCRIPTION A flavourless gelatinous product used to set mixtures at room temperature; often described as 'vegetable gelatine'.

ORIGIN AND HISTORY Produced from red seaweeds indigenous to the seas surrounding many South-East Asian countries. History unknown.

BUYING AND STORAGE Buy from Asian food stores, as either a powder or threads. Agar agar will keep indefinitely at room temperature in an airtight container.

PREPARATION AND USE Soak the powder in hot water, stir until dissolved and use like unflavoured gelatine. The thread variety is left to swell in cold water, then dissolved in boiling liquid. It is particularly suitable for use in cooking and for setting desserts and jellies, as it is flavourless but has the ability to pick up the flavours of the dish to which it has been added. It will gel at 50°C, so dishes will stay set in very hot weather. It is favoured by the Japanese and often used to make very rigid cut shapes for garnishing platters of food. One tablespoon of powder will usually thicken 4 cups of liquid. It is useful for setting mixtures containing fresh pineapple as it cuts easily and does not crush.

Some find that agar agar gel is soothing to the stomach and bowel and aids digestion. It is much favoured by vegetarians.

PROCESSING Agar agar is made by freeze-drying certain varieties of seaweeds (in particular the 'tengusa' variety) which are found in South-East Asia.

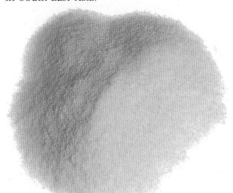

Albumen

also called Egg white mix, Pavlova mix

MAJOR NUTRIENTS		SERVE SIZE 100 G	
Energy	155 kJ	Sodium	190 mg
Protein	9 g	Potassium	150 mg
Fat	0	Phosphorus	35 mg
Carbohydrate	0	Riboflavin	0.4 mg
Dietary Fibre	0	Niacin Equiv.	1.6 mg

NUTRITIONAL INFORMATION An excellent source of riboflavin; good source of protein; moderate source of phosphorus and niacin.

An important, easily assimilated protein source which also contains 40% of daily riboflavin requirements.

DESCRIPTION White powder made from dried egg white.

ORIGIN AND HISTORY Early records show that an American patent for dehydrating eggs was granted in 1880. In the early 1900s China was a plentiful source of low cost eggs, so the Germans and Americans (along with others) developed processes to produce low cost dried egg products and set up plants in China. The exceptional quality of the pan-dried egg white that was produced was not recognised until many years later. Dried albumen was not produced in Australia until World War II, and even then a plant designed for powdering milk was used. Albumen is now produced in a very sophisticated plant, freeze-dried or frozen.

BUYING AND STORAGE Frozen albumen is available from supermarket freezer cabinets, in packs containing three 100 g sachets. Store in the freezer until required; thaw in refrigerator before use. Frozen albumen will keep for up to 1 year, but after thawing use within 24 hours.

Dried albumen is usually sold as pavlova mix in supermarkets. Store in a cool dry place.

PREPARATION AND USE The ability of egg whites to whip and incorporate air to form a stable foam is important to most cooks. Follow manufacturer's instructions for use. Use as a thickener for mousses and bavarois and in pavlovas, meringues and confectionery.

PROCESSING Egg whites are blended with vegetable gum, pasteurised and dried or frozen.

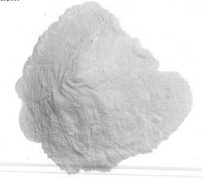

Ammonium Carbonate

also called Carbonate of ammonia

NUTRITIONAL INFORMATION No analysis available.

DESCRIPTION A white powder smelling of ammonia.

ORIGIN AND HISTORY The forerunner of ammonium carbonate was a very old form of baking powder originally called hartshorn because it was made from the ground antlers of deer; it was also an ingredient in sal volatile (smelling salts). Hartshorn has now largely been replaced by purified ammonium carbonate. Both products were very early forms of leavening common in Europe. Ammonium carbonate is still used in Europe, particularly Germany, where it is preferred because it gives a beautiful crisp texture to biscuits.

BUYING AND STORAGE Available from health food stores in small packets. Stored in a cool dry place, it will keep for years.

PREPARATION AND USE The product is used in baking, and is particularly used in Greek cooking where it gives a rich flavour to cakes. The ammonia smell and taste are strong while the cake is hot, but dissipate on cooling.

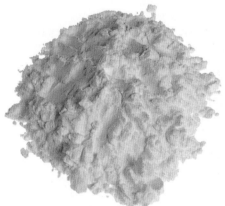

Arrowroot

also called Araruta, Bermuda arrowroot, Chok wo, Maranta starch

MAJOR NUTRIENTS		SERVE SIZE 5 G	
Energy	75 kJ	Total Sugars	0
Protein	0	Dietary Fibre	0
Fat	0	Sodium	0
Carbohydrate	5 g	Potassium	
			less than 1 mg

NUTRITIONAL INFORMATION Arrowroot is mostly composed of carbohydrates. Other nutrients are present, but in insignificant amounts.

DESCRIPTION This is a bland, slightly nut-flavoured, starchy flour which has a mealy texture when cooked. It is ground from the tuber of a plant.

ORIGIN AND HISTORY Arrowroot is made from several species of *Maranta*, but principally *M. arundinacea*, a plant from Central America and northern South America. The word arrowroot is said to be derived from the

American Indian word araruta, meaning flour-root. History books relate that it was once used to treat poisoned arrow wounds, and some types of these tubers are in fact poisonous themselves if eaten raw. Arrowroot has been cultivated in Jamaica since the 17th century, and most of the world's supply comes from the British West Indies.

BUYING AND STORAGE Readily available from supermarkets. Store airtight in a cool dry place.

PREPARATION AND USE Use to thicken sauces and glazes that require a clear glossy appearance and as an addition to wheat flour in cakes and biscuits. The thickening power of arrowroot is greater than that of maize starch or maize flour, and about equal to that of wheat flour. Use 1 teaspoon of arrowroot to thicken 1 cup of liquid. Slake the powder in a little cold liquid, then stir gradually into the boiling liquid until it reaches the desired consistency. Do not boil these sauces for too long, as arrowroot will lose its thickening power if cooked too much.

Arrowroot is also used as a digestive aid, stirred into warm milk or milk puddings.

PROCESSING Starch is extracted from washed and pulped tubers less than 1 year old. Fibres are wrung out and the liquid is sieved and allowed to settle. The sediment is rinsed with fresh water, then dried in the sun. The tubers yield about one-fifth their own weight in starch.

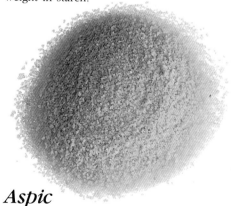

Aspic

MAJOR NUTRIENTS   BEEF STOCK, BAKED
SERVE SIZE 50 mL

Energy	50 kJ	Carbohydrate	1 g
Protein	2 g	Sodium	50 mg
Fat	0	Potassium	50 mg

NUTRITIONAL INFORMATION Makes no significant nutritional contribution to the diet.

DESCRIPTION A clear savoury jelly used to coat and decorate cold food.

ORIGIN AND HISTORY The early Greeks assembled foods in jellied moulds shaped like

bucklers or shields (aspis) and coiled snakes (asps), so the name, which originally described the whole dish, is thought to have derived from these words. It is now also used for the setting agent.

BUYING AND STORAGE Buy powdered aspic from commercial caterers and pastry-cook suppliers. Sometimes smaller packets of imported aspics are available from specialist delicatessens. In each case, follow the manufacturer's directions for use. Store in an airtight container in a cool, dry place.

PREPARATION AND USE Reduced stock should set of its own accord, provided it is made from the gelatinous joints of beef, chicken or veal.

PROCESSING Cracked animal (e.g. beef, veal) or poultry bones are simmered for hours in water or stock to extract collagen (see Gelatine). The liquid is then clarified with egg white and/or crushed egg shells, strained thoroughly, flavoured, coloured if required and used as desired. Homemade aspic may be made from gelatine dissolved in well-flavoured clear stock. The quantity of gelatine will vary depending on the end use for the aspic. Check the manufacturer's instructions before use.

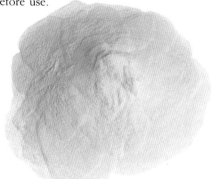

Baking Powder

MAJOR NUTRIENTS   SERVE SIZE 2 G

Energy	7 kJ	Sodium	235 mg
Protein	0	Potassium	
Fat	0		less than 5 mg
Carbohydrate		Calcium	225 mg
	less than 1 g	Phosphorus	170 mg

NUTRITIONAL INFORMATION An excellent source of calcium and phosphorus. Contains large amounts of sodium and would have to be used with discretion on a low sodium diet.

DESCRIPTION A mixture of acid and alkaline salts which, when moistened and heated, gives off carbon dioxide so that the mixture to which it has been added becomes aerated or light-textured.

ORIGIN AND HISTORY The first record of chemical leavening seems to be about 1835 when potassium bitartrate was used to make cream of tartar and then combined with bicarbonate of soda to leaven or raise cakes. Baking powder was being manufactured in Melbourne in the late 1870s. In 1938 the first patent for baking powder was taken out in England.

Modern baking powders are made from bicarbonate of soda and a mixture of food phosphates which have the ability to release carbon dioxide in two stages (double action). The first set of bubbles appears as soon as the powder is added to the batter and the second set is released later, during baking. Glucono-delta-lactone is also used as one of the acid ingredients in some baking powders. All baking powders contain a filler in the form of food starch which prevents premature release of carbon dioxide during storage.

BUYING AND STORAGE Baking powder is available in cans of varying sizes, the most common being 100 g. Stored in a cool, dry place, tightly sealed, it will keep for years.

PREPARATION AND USE Use in recipes in quantities as directed. Baking powder is usually sifted with the dry ingredients for cakes, quick breads and other baked products. The quantity varies depending on the other ingredients in the mixture. The equivalent of 1 teaspoon of baking powder may be made by combining ¼ teaspoon of bicarbonate of soda with ½ teaspoon of cream of tartar (it is not necessary to add the starch filler) and sifting this with the dry ingredients. Bake mixtures immediately, as the gas for leavening is liberated as soon as it comes in contact with liquid in the recipe.

VARIETIES

Sodium-free Baking Powder

DESCRIPTION A mixture of potassium bitartrate (cream of tartar), potassium bicarbonate, cornflour and tartaric acid. One level teaspoon weighs 2.5 g; 1½ teaspoons is equal to 1 teaspoon of ordinary baking powder.

ORIGIN AND HISTORY Developed in the mid-1980s for people requiring sodium-free diets.

BUYING AND STORAGE Available from health food stores where it is sold in 200 g sealed plastic bags. After opening, store in an airtight container in a cool, dry place.

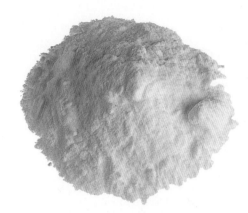

Bicarbonate of Soda

also called Baking soda, Sodium bicarbonate

MAJOR NUTRIENTS   SERVE SIZE 2 G
Sodium   300 mg

NUTRITIONAL INFORMATION This contains large amounts of sodium: would have to be used with discretion in a low sodium diet. Food Code Additive Number 500.

DESCRIPTION A fine white powder used as the alkaline component in baking powder.

ORIGIN AND HISTORY Bicarbonate of soda seems to have been used in conjunction with sour milk or buttermilk as a raising agent during the late 18th century. The first record of its being manufactured in commercial quantities seems to date back to 1835 in the USA: called saleratus, it was used in conjunction with cream of tartar as a leavening agent for cakes.

BUYING AND STORAGE Buy in small packets from supermarkets. Stored in a cool, dry place, it will keep indefinitely.

PREPARATION AND USE When used for baking it is either dissolved in the liquid in the recipe or sifted with the flour and other dry ingredients. In combination with acid ingredients such as sour milk or cream of tartar it will leaven or raise batters and doughs. In Victorian times it was mixed with water and taken as a stomach soother.

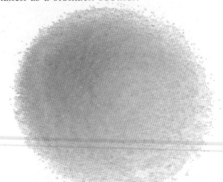

Citric Acid

NUTRITIONAL INFORMATION Makes no significant nutritional contribution to the diet. Food Code Additive Number 330.

DESCRIPTION The predominant acid in lemons, oranges and limes; also found in gooseberries, raspberries etc. and in some other plants. It is extracted from lemon or lime juice or prepared commercially by a special fermentation of glucose. It takes the form of fairly large fragile crystals and has an agreeable but acid flavour. It is highly soluble in water.

ORIGIN AND HISTORY The modern product is simply a more convenient form of concentrated lemon or lime juice, whose value has long been known in cooking.

BUYING AND STORAGE Available in some specialty health food stores. Easily kept in the dry state in an airtight container, but a solution of citric acid can be rapidly invaded by moulds.

PREPARATION AND USE Used in preserving fish, in colouring vegetables and in the manufacture of jams, pastries, lemonade, orange and lemon syrups, fruit drinks and carbonated beverages. It acts as an acidulant.

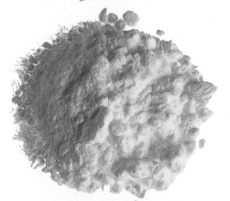

Cream of Tartar

also called Potassium acid tartrate, Potassium bitartrate

NUTRITIONAL INFORMATION Makes no significant nutritional contribution to the diet. Food Additive Code Number 334.

DESCRIPTION Purified, crystallised potassium bitartrate, used as the acid component of some fast-acting baking powder mixtures.

ORIGIN AND HISTORY Manufacture of cream of tartar dates back to 1835, when it was first used in the USA in conjunction with bicarbonate of soda as a commercial leavening agent. Potassium bitartrate present in the juice of fruits such as grapes, pineapples and mulberries was used to make cream of tartar; it was also manufactured commercially as a by-product of the wine industry.

BUYING AND STORAGE Buy in packets from supermarkets. Cream of tartar has an indefinite shelf life if kept dry.

PREPARATION AND USE Use ½ teaspoon of cream of tartar in combination with ¼ teaspoon of bicarbonate of soda to make 1 teaspoon of baking powder. Cream of tartar is often added to stabilise the foam and firm the texture of whipped egg whites.

SEE ALSO Baking Powder.

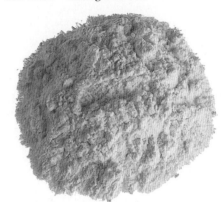

Custard Powder

MAJOR NUTRIENTS		SERVE SIZE 10 G	
Energy	150 kJ	Carbohydrate	10 g
Protein	0	Sodium	30 mg
Fat	0	Potassium	5 mg

NUTRITIONAL INFORMATION A carbohydrate-based thickening agent that can be used to eliminate the use of eggs. Contains food colourings. Food Code Additive Numbers 102, 110.

DESCRIPTION A powdered mixture of starch (wheat or corn), artificial flavouring and colouring agents.

ORIGIN AND HISTORY Custards are traditionally made with eggs, milk, sugar and a flavouring such as vanilla. The most famous custard powder, developed by Birds in the late 19th century, did not however contain eggs, despite its yellow colour. Such powders are still in use and require added milk.

BUYING AND STORAGE Store as for flour, in dry conditions.

PREPARATION AND USE Cook according to manufacturer's directions: usually the required amount of powder is mixed with a little cold milk, then stirred into the remaining sweetened hot milk, reheated to boiling and simmered for several minutes. The custard is served as a dessert sauce or used as an ingredient in desserts. Custard powder is also sometimes added to biscuit and cake mixtures.

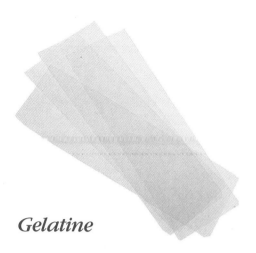

Gelatine

MAJOR NUTRIENTS

	SERVE SIZE 5 G	
Energy	70 kJ	Carbohydrate	0
Protein	4 g	Sodium	0
Fat	0		

NUTRITIONAL INFORMATION As, can be seen from the table above, gelatine contains mainly protein.

DESCRIPTION Powdered gelatine is creamy and granular in colour. Sheet gelatine is transparent with a faint crosshatched texture.

ORIGIN AND HISTORY Gelatine seems to have originated in western Europe and the UK during the time of Charles II. It was discovered that when meat cooked for soup had cooled, the cooking liquid gelled and, after clarifying, yielded a fairly clear jelly which could in turn be flavoured with herbs and wine.

The first commercial gelatine appeared in the 19th century in the UK, Europe and America. Powdered gelatine has been manufactured in Australia since 1917.

BUYING AND STORAGE Powdered gelatine is available in packets of varying sizes from supermarkets. Some packets contain a number of 10 g sachets or envelopes. Leaf or sheet gelatine is available from some specialty shops or chef's warehouses, either loose (buy the number of sheets required) or in 10 g packets, each containing 6 sheets. Gelatine will absorb moisture and odours, so it is important to place it in an airtight container for prolonged storage.

PREPARATION AND USE Gelatine is always dissolved before being added to mixtures. Follow instructions on the packet or in the recipe, or sprinkle gelatine on top of a small amount of the measured hot liquid, stir briskly until dissolved, then add to the main liquid. Each sachet is equal to 3 scant teaspoons (metric), sufficient to set 2 metric cups or 0.5 L of liquid to a medium strength jelly. Leaf gelatine sheets vary in weight but, as a general guide, 10 g will set 0.5 L of liquid.

Soak sheets in cold water for 5 minutes, squeeze out excess water and add the softened sheets to hot liquid. Gelling properties will be impaired if gelatine is boiled. Used to thicken, aerate or set mixtures.

PROCESSING Animal tissue is treated to produce pure collagen (protein) in solution, then evaporated to a highly concentrated gelatine liquor. The soft jelly formed after evaporation is further dried, then crushed, blended and screened to ensure even particle size before packaging. Sheet gelatine contains some water plus sulphur dioxide. A vegetarian alternative to gelatine, agar agar, is available from health food stores.

VARIETIES
Powdered, sheet, leaf.

SEE ALSO Agar Agar, Aspic.

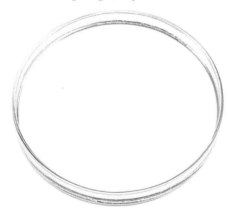

Glycerine

also called **Glycerol**

MAJOR NUTRIENTS

	SERVE SIZE 10 G	
Energy	370 kJ	Carbohydrate	0
Fat	10 g	Sodium	0
Cholesterol	0		

NUTRITIONAL INFORMATION Contains significant amounts of naturally occurring salicylates and amines. Food Additive Code Number 422.

DESCRIPTION A sweet, colourless, odourless, syrupy liquid.

ORIGIN AND HISTORY Glycerine is a by-product of soap manufacture and can be extracted from most fats. It is found in all wines and beers in varying degrees because of the fermentation of sugar by yeast.

BUYING AND STORAGE Sold as a liquid in bottles or cans in specialty food stores. Keeps indefinitely if kept tightly covered.

PREPARATION AND USE Regarded as a valuable substitute for sugar in the sweetening of diabetic food. It is used to retain moisture in some types of confectionery, and in cake icing to prevent excessive hardening.

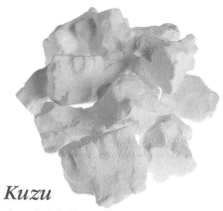

Kuzu

also called **Kudju**

MAJOR NUTRIENTS

	SERVE SIZE 2 G	
Energy	35 kJ	Total Sugars	0
Protein	0	Dietary Fibre	0
Fat	0	Sodium	0
Carbohydrate	2 g	Potassium	
			less than 1 mg

NUTRITIONAL INFORMATION Makes no significant contribution to the diet.

DESCRIPTION Powdered, lumpy, starchy material from the tuberous root of the Asian kuzu vine (very like tapioca).

ORIGIN AND HISTORY History unknown.

BUYING AND STORAGE Buy from specialist stores that stock a wide variety of Japanese food ingredients. Not readily available in Australia.

PREPARATION AND USE Grind with mortar and pestle or sift lumps. Use the resulting powder to thicken sauces, especially sweet ones. Slake the powder in water or liquid from the recipe, then add to the mixture to be thickened. Kuzu has twice the thickening power of arrowroot. For an extra-crisp crust on deep-fried food, dip the food in the powder first. Used for invalids and babies who have problems with swallowing or digesting food.

SEE ALSO Arrowroot.

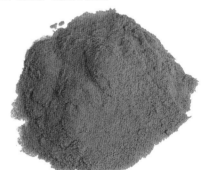

Lotus Root Starch

also called **Lotus root flour, Ou fen**

MAJOR NUTRIENTS

	SERVE SIZE 5 G	
Energy	75 kJ	Sodium	less than 5 mg
Protein	0	Potassium	
Carbohydrate	5 g		less than 5 mg

NUTRITIONAL INFORMATION A carbohydrate-based thickener.

DESCRIPTION Fine flour milled from dried lotus root.

ORIGIN AND HISTORY Unknown.

BUYING AND STORAGE Buy from Asian supermarkets in 250 g packets. Imported from China.

PREPARATION AND USE For thickening soups and sauces, mix to a smooth paste with cold liquid, then stir into simmering liquid until thickened to the required consistency. Boiling the soup or sauce after thickening will cause it to break down. When dipped in lotus root flour, deep-fried foods will have a crisp, very brown coating.

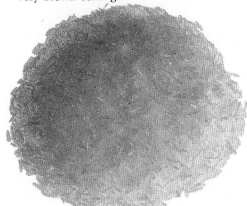

Monosodium Glutamate

also called Aji-no-moto, Ve-tsin

NUTRITIONAL INFORMATION This contains large amounts of sodium. Food Additive Code Number 621.

DESCRIPTION A natural substance found in many foods, but in greater amounts in meat, poultry, fish and vegetables. It is the sodium salt of glutamic acid, an amino acid, and is readily soluble in water.

ORIGIN AND HISTORY First discovered in the Orient, this white powder stimulates the taste buds and enhances the flavour of many foods, though it has no individual taste itself.

BUYING AND STORAGE Available in powder form in several commercial brands. Keeps indefinitely if stored in an airtight container in a cool dry place.

PREPARATION AND USE Used in small amounts in meats, soups and sauces to emphasise the natural flavour of the food.

PROCESSING Produced through fermentation processes, chiefly from molasses, though it can be made from white or maize gluten and soya protein.

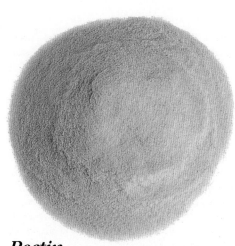

Pectin

NUTRITIONAL INFORMATION Makes no significant nutritional contribution to the diet. Food Additive Code Number 440.

DESCRIPTION A gumlike substance (acid hemicellulose) occurring as a constituent in certain fruits and vegetables in varying quantities. It causes their pulp, when boiled with sugar in the presence of sufficient acid, to set as a jelly, and is an essential ingredient in jam making. Because the pectin content varies according to the ripeness and acid content of fruit, it is often necessary to add pectin-rich fruits or a pectin extract to certain jams.

ORIGIN AND HISTORY Pectin is found in the skin and pips of citrus fruits, grapes, plums, apples and quinces, and also in split peas and lentils.

BUYING AND STORAGE Commercial pectins can be obtained in liquid or powder form. They will keep some time if stored in an airtight container.

PREPARATION AND USE If adding commercial pectin to such fruits as strawberries, cherries or rhubarb, cook the fruits until soft before adding sugar. Add 3–6 tablespoons of liquid or about 8 g of powdered pectin to each 500 g of fruit. This will bring the pectin content of the fruit up to the average level. The flavour of the jam will be lost if too much pectin is added, and its use is unnecessary when making jam from fruits which set well. The fruit in the jam will be hard if not cooked sufficiently beforehand, or if too much pectin is added in an endeavour to get a quick set.

PROCESSING An extract can be made by the long boiling of fruits such as sour apples, cranberries, gooseberries, underripe blackberries and raspberries, blackcurrants or redcurrants. Such extracts can be bottled and stored. Commercial pectin is usually prepared from apple peels and cores, or from the pips and pith of citrus fruits.

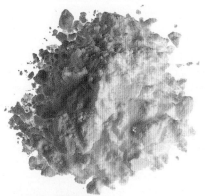

Potato Flour

also called Potato starch

MAJOR NUTRIENTS		SERVE SIZE 5 G	
Energy	75 kJ	Sodium	less than 5 mg
Protein	0	Potassium	
Carbohydrate	5 g		less than 5 mg

NUTRITIONAL INFORMATION A carbohydrate-based thickener with little protein. Useful for those who have to avoid gluten-containing flours.

DESCRIPTION A white powder prepared from potatoes.

ORIGIN AND HISTORY A product developed and principally known in Europe.

BUYING AND STORAGE Buy from supermarkets and health food stores. Stored in an airtight container, it will keep for many months.

PREPARATION AND USE Potato starch, like most root starches, has greater thickening power than cereal starches, so smaller quantities are required to thicken soups and sauces. Use also in cakes, biscuits (particularly in Jewish and European cookery) and for those on special diets.

PROCESSING Dried potatoes are ground into flour. Processing is not carried out in Australia.

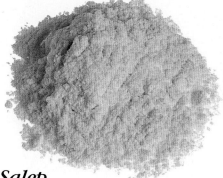

Salep

also called Salepi, Sahlab

NUTRITIONAL INFORMATION No data are available.

DESCRIPTION Salep is a light brown powder from the dried tubers of various species of orchids. It is used for its gelatinous qualities rather than its flavour and food value.

ORIGIN AND HISTORY Just when man-kind found that the tuberous roots of certain orchids could be used as a food is lost in the passage of time. Orchid species from which salep is derived are native to Europe, Asia, Asia Minor and North Africa, and it is any-body's guess who started using them. The finest salep today comes from Turkey; Greece and Macedonia produce and use it; the Persians made a jelly from it which was the probable predecessor to Turkish delight; the Syrians use it for ice cream; it is known in the Himalaya and Kashmir regions; the English and Irish used it until the 19th century.

Generally it is used to make a hot drink also called salep (or names which sound very like it in the various languages of the countries where it is known today). In Turkey and Greece, a glass of hot salep is still favoured on a cold night, sweetened with sugar and dusted with cinnamon, perhaps with a few crushed pistachios added. It was also used as a hot drink in England and Ireland before coffee became fashionable, based on water with cream, egg yolks, sugar and cinnamon added according to whim, and a dash of something alcoholic too — an early eggnog.

BUYING AND STORAGE Purchase pow-dered salep in small packages from Greek and Middle Eastern food stores and store in a sealed jar in a cool, dry place.

PREPARATION AND USE It is used in much the same way as cornflour and arrow-root, two relative newcomers which have largely replaced salep even in countries where it was traditionally used. However its gelati-nous properties are stronger and 1 teaspoon salep should replace 1 tablespoon cornflour or arrowroot when experimenting. Mix the salep to a thin paste with water or milk and stir in some of the hot liquid, then return to the pan and keep stirring until the liquid thickens and bubbles gently. For hot drinks, the consistency should be like a thin custard. Make a thicker custard for an ice cream base.

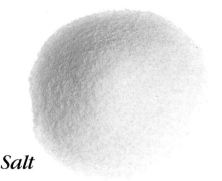

Salt

NUTRITIONAL INFORMATION See under Varieties.

DESCRIPTION Sodium chloride, a white crystalline powder with a strong salty flavour.

ORIGIN AND HISTORY Salt comes from two sources: underground seams of rock salt, which must be mined; and salt water, from the sea or from inland brine springs.

It seems that our appetite for salt grew as our ancestors settled into farming communi-ties and learned that salt preserved food as well as flavoured it, and that, in many cases, salt pickling was preferable to drying. Prehis-toric communities clearly made use of natural surface deposits or saltpans and classical writers including Pliny and Herodotus wrote about brine springs, salt lakes and salt rivers.

BUYING AND STORAGE Available in many forms (see Varieties) from general and health food stores. Being inorganic, salt will keep indefinitely and does not always require airtight storage. However, it will absorb moisture from the atmosphere and in humid climates it will soon become damp and not flow. Silica gel or a few grains of rice will help keep it dry.

PREPARATION AND USE The use of salt is universal in savoury dishes, and even in sweet baking a small pinch is often useful to bring out other flavours. It is used as an antiseptic and preservative in bacon, salt beef, herrings and kippers, and other foods which are pre-pared by curing with salt and brines. Salt has a toughening action, which is why it is used initially on pickles for a crisp texture. It is also used to draw out the bitter juices of such vegetables as zucchini and eggplants prior to cooking.

VARIETIES

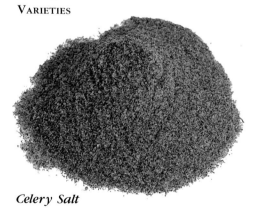

Celery Salt

MAJOR NUTRIENTS		SERVE SIZE 1 G
Energy	0 Sodium	300 mg

NUTRITIONAL INFORMATION Contains large amounts of sodium salts, so should be used with discretion in sodium-controlled diets.

DESCRIPTION A mixture of salt with ground celery seed. Celery seed is the dried fruit of *Apium graveolens* (see Celery). It is a tiny seed, brown with pale ridges. The aroma is characteristic and the flavour is warm and slightly bitter.

ORIGIN AND HISTORY Flavoured salts have always been possible to make simply by mixing ingredients. Today such products are available in supermarkets.

BUYING AND STORAGE Bottled celery salt is readily available in food stores and will keep for several months if kept tightly capped in a cool dark place.

PREPARATION AND USE Ground seed can be added to ordinary table salt and used to flavour soups, stews, savoury food and salads.

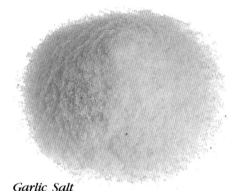

Garlic Salt

MAJOR NUTRIENTS		SERVE SIZE 1 G
Energy	0 Sodium	300 mg

NUTRITIONAL INFORMATION This con-tains large amounts of added sodium chloride, so should be used with discretion in sodium-controlled diets.

DESCRIPTION A mixture of pure garlic pow-der and free-running table salt. Starch is some-times added to prevent caking. Garlic powder is the ground powder of dehydrated garlic. It has a strong, heavy, persistent aroma and taste which gives added flavour to plain salt.

ORIGIN AND HISTORY As for celery salt.

BUYING AND STORAGE Can be purchased ready-mixed from food stores. Store in a closed container; otherwise it will become lumpy and hard.

PREPARATION AND USE To make garlic salt, rub a cut clove of garlic over coarse white table salt, or mix in the required quantity of garlic powder.

Often used in addition to or instead of plain salt in tomato juice, any meat or vegetable dish, stews, French salad dressing or salads. Garlic salt is especially handy for outdoor cookery and can be added to steaks just before cooking.

Kitchen Salt

MAJOR NUTRIENTS		SERVE SIZE 1 G
Energy	0	Sodium 355 mg

NUTRITIONAL INFORMATION Contains large amounts of sodium.

DESCRIPTION Usually a fairly coarse, free-running refined salt which may or may not have magnesium carbonate added to help it to flow freely. Also available as block salt.

ORIGIN AND HISTORY See Salt.

BUYING AND STORAGE Can be bought in coagulated bricks or blocks, generally available in health food shops. Also available in containers from food stores. Both forms must be stored in a moisture-proof atmosphere.

PREPARATION AND USE Brick or block salt must be powdered before use in cooking or as a condiment.

Kosher Salt

MAJOR NUTRIENTS		SERVE SIZE 1 G
Energy	0	Sodium 355 mg

NUTRITIONAL INFORMATION This contains similar levels of sodium to regular salt, so should still be used with discretion in sodium-controlled diets.

DESCRIPTION A highly purified, evaporated salt with a large jewellike crystal. Because the large kosher salt crystals absorb moisture very slowly, if at all, this salt is an excellent product in very humid weather.

ORIGIN AND HISTORY Kosher is a term indicating that a substance conforms to Jewish dietary laws.

BUYING AND STORAGE Sold in kosher delicatessens and food stores, this salt can be stored in a container ready for use.

PREPARATION AND USE It is perfect for salads, as greens are less apt to wilt, and for meats and fresh fruits, because they stay juicier.

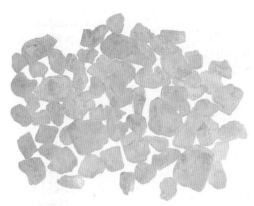

Rock Salt

MAJOR NUTRIENTS		SERVE SIZE 1 G
Energy	0	Sodium 355 mg

NUTRITIONAL INFORMATION This contains similar amounts of sodium to regular salt. If it is added to food by means of a grinder, it is easier to control the total amount added.

DESCRIPTION The common name for halite (the mineral form of sodium chloride). It is hard and crystalline and comes in large lumps. (N.B. In America the name 'rock salt' is used to describe freezing salt which is inedible.)

ORIGIN AND HISTORY A naturally occurring mineral.

BUYING AND STORAGE Not readily available.

PREPARATION AND USE Needs to be ground before use. Useful for freezing ice cream.

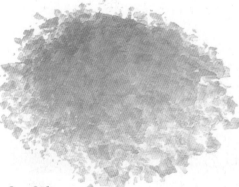

Sea Salt

MAJOR NUTRIENTS		SERVE SIZE 1 G
Energy	0	Sodium 250 mg

NUTRITIONAL INFORMATION Contains magnesium and calcium as well as sodium salts.

DESCRIPTION A mixture of salts produced by the evaporation of sea water. Also known as bay salt, sea salt takes the form of small chunks or flakes which are quite brittle.

ORIGIN AND HISTORY Salt has been extracted from the sea from time immemorial. Large saltpans are still in use in many countries, such as Thailand, where the salt is left behind as the tide recedes. In Malden, Essex, England, sea salt is still produced; it is used extensively in England.

BUYING AND STORAGE Health stores and specialty food stores stock sea salt. It should be kept free of moisture.

PREPARATION AND USE Sea salt should be crushed in a mortar or a salt mill before use in cooking or as a condiment. It has a stronger taste than refined rock salt, so less is needed.

PROCESSING The salt water must be heated by the sun, or artificially by fires, to evaporate it. The higher the temperature, the finer and whiter and less flavourful the salt. When the water barely bubbles or moves, the salt precipitates into larger, tastier crystals.

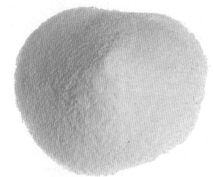

Saltpetre

*also called **Nitre**, **Potassium nitrate**, **Salitre***

NUTRITIONAL INFORMATION Makes no significant nutritional contribution to the diet, but contains potassium which, if it is used in large amounts, will make a significant contribution. Food Additive Code Number 252.

DESCRIPTION Potassium nitrate, a white crystalline salty substance that is readily soluble in hot water. Saltpetre is odourless, and has a piquant, slightly bitter taste. It is used as a meat preservative, usually with salt, and is responsible for the fine pink colour of bacons, hams, salamis, and other preserved meats and pâtés.

ORIGIN AND HISTORY Saltpetre during history has had a number of applications, including gunpowder. It is not used in the domestic kitchen.

BUYING AND STORAGE Difficult to buy, but may occasionally be bought from a fish market or a butcher. It must be kept in a cool, dry place.

PREPARATION AND USE Used in salting industries because it gives an agreeable red colour to meat, but only in small amounts because it also toughens. Preserves and colours foods such as hams, sausages and dried meats.

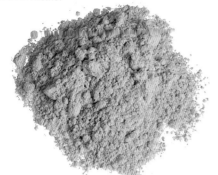

Slaked Lime

also called **Calcium hydroxide**

NUTRITIONAL INFORMATION No significant nutritional contribution to the diet. Contains significant amounts of naturally occurring monosodium glutamate, salicylates and amines. Food Additive Code Number 526.

DESCRIPTION An anticaking agent, firming agent and nutritive supplement in food such as grain products and soft candy, slaked lime is a product of limestone. When limestone, chalk or marble (calcium carbonate) is strongly heated, quicklime (calcium oxide) is formed, a caustic and potentially dangerous substance. When water is added, the quicklime gets very hot and turns into a crumbly mass of slaked lime. If quicklime is exposed to air, natural humidity will produce the same result in a few days.

ORIGIN AND HISTORY Not generally used in the domestic kitchen.

BUYING AND STORAGE Can be bought from a chemist. Keep dry.

PREPARATION AND USE Slaked lime dissolves rather sparingly to give limewater. In Belgium, Holland and Germany, dried fruit is soaked in it. To crisp watermelon rind, soak it in limewater for 3 hours before pickling.

Limewater is also the liquid in which maize is traditionally boiled to remove the horny yellow seed coat in making Mexican nixtamal, the first stage in producing masa for tortillas. Limewater softens the seed coat to the point where it can be rubbed off.

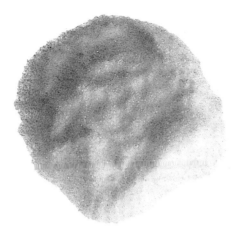

Tartaric Acid

NUTRITIONAL INFORMATION Makes no significant nutritional contribution to the diet. Food Additive Code Number 334.

DESCRIPTION An acid found in a large number of fruits and which is extracted from the lees of wine.

ORIGIN AND HISTORY Not to be confused with cream of tartar, this powder is occasionally used in the domestic kitchen.

BUYING AND STORAGE Sometimes available in specialty health food stores. It must be kept in an airtight container.

PREPARATION AND USE Used to prepare mineral drinks, syrups and effervescent powders. Also, in winemaking, added to must which lacks acidity.

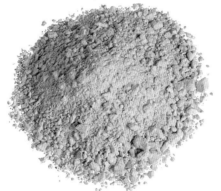

Water Chestnut Powder

also called **Water chestnut starch**

MAJOR NUTRIENTS		SERVE SIZE 5 G	
Energy	75 kJ	Sodium	less than 5 mg
Protein	0	Potassium	
Carbohydrate	5 g		less than 5 mg

NUTRITIONAL INFORMATION A gluten-free carbohydrate thickener.

DESCRIPTION A ground starchy powder with a slightly sweetish flavour.

ORIGIN AND HISTORY An Asian product.

BUYING AND STORAGE Buy from Asian

supermarkets in 250 g or 500 g packets. Stored in a cool, dry place, it will keep indefinitely.

PREPARATION AND USE Use to thicken sauces and soups — see Lotus Root Starch.

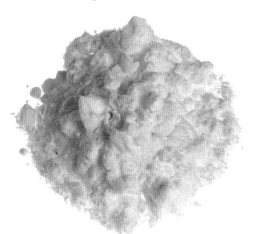

Yam Flour *Dioscorea*

also called **Yam Starch**

NUTRITIONAL INFORMATION See Yam in the chapter on Vegetables.

DESCRIPTION Fine powder ground from a starchy tuber.

ORIGIN AND HISTORY The name yam is often loosely and confusingly applied to almost any tropical crop and in America it is often used for sweet potatoes. Some species of yam are grown in Asia, particularly Vietnam, Cambodia and Laos, while others are grown in China and Africa.

BUYING AND STORAGE It is available only from Asian food suppliers. If not available substitute arrowroot or cornflour. Store in a cool dry place.

PREPARATION AND USE The tuber skin is peeled and the flesh is diced, then boiled in water until soft. After draining, the pieces are pounded in a mortar and pestle to break down some of the cellular material and starch granules, forming a stiff glutinous dough called 'fufu' in West Africa where it is eaten with stews. To make starch, the dough is dried, then powdered by pounding again.

SEE ALSO Yam in the chapter on Vegetables.

Yeast (Baker's)

MAJOR NUTRIENTS

COMPRESSED
SERVE SIZE 50 G

Energy	110 kJ	Potassium	310 mg
Protein	5 g	Phosphorus	195 mg
Fat	less than 1 g	Iron	2.5 mg
Carbohydrate		Zinc	1.5 mg
	less than 1 g	Thiamin	0.3 mg
Dietary Fibre	3 g	Riboflavin	0.8 mg
Sodium	10 mg	Niacin Equiv.	5.4 mg

NUTRITIONAL INFORMATION An excellent source of phosphorus, iron, thiamin, riboflavin, niacin and folate. Yeast has been a traditional vitamin and mineral supplement food. The balance of the nutrients above is thought to make them well absorbed by the body.

DESCRIPTION Yeast is a fungus, *Saccharomyces cerevisiae*, a microscopic single-celled organism which reproduces by a 'budding' process. It ferments sugars to produce carbon dioxide, which leavens flour mixtures.

ORIGIN AND HISTORY The use of yeast to leaven bread doughs has been known since some time during the second millennium BC, when wild yeast in the air became incorporated into the dough of an early Egyptian baker and made it rise. People then learned to save a piece of dough from one mix to the next and also to use the froth that rose to the top of the popular alcoholic beverages of the day. By the early 19th century women were preparing their own yeast. Compressed yeast was being sold in American grocery stores by the 1870s. Bottles containing homemade yeasts were part of every family kitchen. Some developed particularly pleasing flavours and were much prized.

It was not until Louis Pasteur recognised yeasts as the organisms responsible for fermentation that their action began to be understood.

BUYING AND STORAGE Buy yeast from health food stores and specialty delicatessens. Fresh or compressed yeast is usually sold in kilogram blocks to stores which, in turn, sell it in smaller quantities. Buy only good quality fresh yeast with a smooth texture, pleasant smell and cream to pale grey colour. Instant active dried yeast is sold in packets (usually 500 g vacuum packed) suitable for domestic use or in sealed containers of various sizes (sometimes combined with an improver). A combination of dried yeast plus malt flour and, sometimes, bread improver is principally available in country areas (follow manufacturer's instructions). Store yeast in the refrigerator in a sealed container. Dried yeast has a shelf life of up to 1 year. Compressed yeast must always be refrigerated in a screw-topped jar or in an airtight plastic bag; it keeps for up to 2 weeks. Compressed yeast contains 60–70% water and therefore does not freeze well under domestic conditions.

PREPARATION AND USE Mix compressed yeast with a little of the liquid from the recipe, then add with the remaining liquid to the dry ingredients. Dried yeast should be blended with a little sugar and five times its own weight of water from the recipe at 40°C. (Dried yeasts are able to tolerate higher temperatures than compressed yeast.) Let the mixture stand for 10 minutes to allow fermentation to commence. Instant active dried yeast is added directly to dry ingredients. Two metric teaspoons of dried yeast is equal to 30 g of fresh compressed yeast.

Yeast is an important leavening or raising agent for a wide range of breads, cakes and pastries.

VARIETIES

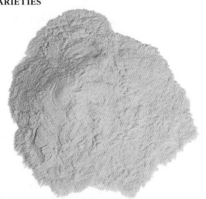

Brewer's Yeast Also a strain of *S. cerevisiae*. Beers and other alcoholic beverages have been made using yeast for thousands of years. During fermentation some yeasts rise to the top as froth and these are known as 'top yeasts' (ale process); others fall to the bottom of the vat as sediment and these are generally known as 'bottom yeasts' (lager process). Brewer's yeast has a high vitamin B content, and is therefore also used as a food supplement.

Red Yeast A variety of dried yeast used in Asia to ferment oriental vinegars. It is not readily available in Australia.

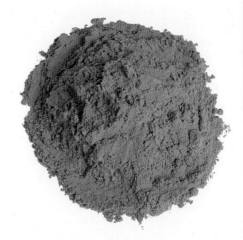

Torula Yeast *Torula utilis* or *Candida utilis* is from a large range of food yeasts used to modify other food products. It is not related to baker's yeast. Buy dry torula yeast in jars from health food stores. Usually taken as a health drink.

CAKES AND PASTRIES

Most cakes and pastries are energy-dense foods. This means that they have a high kilojoule yield per unit of weight, as illustrated by the following figures: Bread normally yields from 1000–1200 kilojoules per 100 grams; cakes, such as fruit, sponge and plain cake, yield 1250–2000; the different varieties of pastry yield 1400–2400. The shortening and the sugar in cakes and pastries are the major contribution of the extra kilojoules. When the nutrients provided by a food are compared with the energy, bread would be a more valuable source of thiamin, riboflavin and niacin, than cake or pastry. This is because most of the energy from bread comes from flour, a valuable source of these nutrients.

Cakes and pastries can also be a significant source of sodium. There may be salt (sodium chloride) in the butter or margarine, and sodium bicarbonate in the baking powder or self-raising flour. Salt is also sometimes added as an ingredient, but this can be omitted. If cakes and pastries are made in the home, salt-free butter or margarine can be used.

There has been a change in the recipes provided for cakes in cookbooks and magazines. The emphasis on dietary fibre has resulted in a greater use of wholemeal flour, and many recipes include dried fruit, fresh fruit, vegetables, nuts, sunflower seed, wheat bran, oat bran, sesame seeds and wheat germ. There are also recipes with less fat and sugar.

Pastry depends on shortening for texture so that there are limitations to the possible reductions in fat. Filo pastry, before it is layered with shortening, has a low fat content. Some people are being innovative in using a few sheets of filo as a pastry case for suitable drier fillings.

There is no reason why healthy, active people should not enjoy occasional cakes and pastries, meanwhile using the lower fat fruit loaves in preference to iced and cream-filled cakes.

Those who are overweight, or trying to reduce their blood cholesterol levels, would do well to put aside the pastries and be very selective about the cakes they eat.

CAKES

The array of cakes that can be made and bought may seem bewildering, but variety in cakes really comes chiefly from the method of mixing, rather than from the ingredients used. The types of plain cake containing principally flour, fat, eggs and sugar can be categorised broadly in the following terms — those that have the fat and sugar *creamed*, those that have the fat *rubbed in* to flour, those that have the fat *melted* before combining with other ingredients and those where eggs are *whisked* to give a light-textured result.

The creaming method is used for cakes that usually have a high proportion of fat to flour. Creaming — beating the fat until it reaches a soft, creamy consistency — makes it easier to mix in the remaining ingredients. For some creamed cakes the eggs are added whole, while for others the yolks are added first and later the beaten egg whites. The latter method incorporates more air into the mixture and produces a lighter, finer-textured cake.

Among examples of this method are what are known simply as butter cakes, even when margarine replaces the butter. These may be flavoured merely with vanilla, a fruit juice or citrus zest, or they may have melted chocolate, cocoa or coffee added. A butter cake might have a small quantity of dried fruit or even fresh fruit added as the flavouring, for example, mashed banana or crushed pineapple. Another example is what used to be called a pound cake: the name had nothing to do with the weight of the cake, but rather with the equal weight of the main ingredients — the flour, sugar, fat and eggs each weighing an imperial pound. It is from this type of mixture that lamingtons were made, though sponge cake is also frequently used.

In more economical cakes, where there is a smaller proportion of fat to the other ingredients, the fat is usually rubbed into the flour before other ingredients are added. The texture of the cake will not be as fine as in the creaming method, but though a little coarser and perhaps not so large in volume, these cakes can have a pleasant texture. Some rock cakes and light fruit cakes are made by this method.

The melted fat method is by far the quickest way to make a cake: butter is melted and added to the other ingredients and the lot folded evenly together. The fat can also be oil or margarine. With the increased popularity of carrot cake and similar cake batters with grated or mashed vegetables and fruit (zucchini, banana and pineapple), and the increasingly busy lifestyle of home-makers, this type of cake has proved most popular.

Whisked cakes are the lightest of all, and within the category there are several different methods of preparation. The first has the whole eggs beaten with sugar, sometimes over a saucepan of hot water (as for European gateau), and the mixture is then combined with flour. A variation of this method has all the ingredients beaten together with butter softened or melted in a little hot milk or water. The second method has the egg yolks alone beaten with the sugar, the whites being whipped separately and folded into the first mixture with the flour. The first method makes a softer, slightly sticky sponge while the second produces a firmer consistency, often with a more crusty top. The latter method is the more suitable for preparing a Swiss roll, in that it provides more flexibility for rolling than the all-in-together method. A third method uses only the whites of eggs, and ground nuts in place of flour.

The cakes listed in this chapter have been chosen as good representatives of the four principal types which can be made or bought today.

Entries on Biscuits and on Icings and Fillings are included to round off this chapter, which has the potential to expand into many volumes on its own.

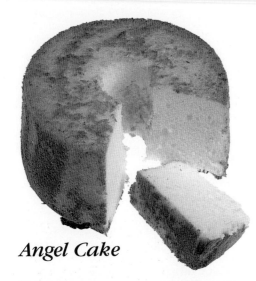

Angel Cake

MAJOR NUTRIENTS SERVE SIZE 30 G

Energy	340 kJ	Total Sugars	12 g
Protein	2 g	Dietary Fibre	0
Fat	0	Sodium	85 mg
Cholesterol	0	Potassium	25 mg
Carbohydrate	18 g		

NUTRITIONAL INFORMATION A low energy light cake which contains no cholesterol or fats.

DESCRIPTION Angel cake is a very light, airy cake which is a little dry in comparison with more commonly baked cakes. It is always cooked in a tube pan, which means it is ring shaped. It is pale in colour, having no egg yolks or fats to give it the creamy-yellow common to most plain cakes. It is a whisked cake.

ORIGIN AND HISTORY It is difficult to trace the origin of this cake, but it is fair to assume that it was probably first made in the USA, possibly in the last hundred years. Its inventor may have wanted to bake a cake that excluded egg yolks and fats of any kind, perhaps for reasons of economy or restricted diet.

BUYING AND STORAGE Because of the lack of ingredients which would normally keep a cake moist for a period, this type of cake should be covered well and preferably eaten soon after baking.

PREPARATION AND USE As well as plain flour (and almost always cream of tartar), the dry ingredients can vary with the addition of a little cornflour. These dry ingredients must be very well sifted for best results. Egg whites are whisked with caster sugar and then the dry ingredients are folded in very carefully but thoroughly and the mixture turned into an ungreased tube pan or special angel cake pan. A cake pan with a hollow centre is necessary to avoid having the outside of the cake overcooked and dried out while the centre, in a normal cake pan, would still require further baking. Baking is done in either a slow or a moderate oven and the cake

pan is inverted on a cake cooler for several hours before turning out. This is a very sweet cake, and somewhat dry. It can be served with tart fruit such as raspberries, and whipped cream.

Biscuits

DESCRIPTION Biscuits can vary from the soft, cakelike texture of bar or finger biscuits to the airy crispness of brandy snaps or anzacs, or the blow-away lightness of macaroons.

ORIGIN AND HISTORY One of the chief difficulties in trying to date the first biscuit making is the fact that for a considerable time after the making of bread was first documented, the term 'bread' covered not only bread itself but often cakes and pastry as well. It would appear from medieval writings that some of these offerings would, in our nomenclature, be rightly called 'biscuits'.

It seems that in medieval times the day's leftover pastry was handed down to the pastry cook's most junior apprentices to be used as best they could. Their creations were then hawked on the streets at the end of the day. Most cooks would probably consider that adding a few nuts and maybe some spices, then a quick roll and a biscuit cutter could do the trick very satisfactorily. Logically, in other words, one could expect that biscuits would be the likely outcome of such a situation. An ancient pagan rite associated with southern Germany has led to a now traditional biscuit called Springerle. Originally to mark the winter solstice, sacrifices of animals were made and later tokens baked from dough in animal shapes. The tradition remains but always now in the form of biscuits.

Another interesting biscuit was inspired by the bell shape of ladies' petticoats in the early 18th century. Called 'petticoat tails', it is a traditional rich Scottish shortbread.

BUYING AND STORAGE All biscuits should be kept in airtight containers away from heat and humidity.

PREPARATION AND USE The main basic methods of biscuit making are

1. Creamed fats and sugar (for melting moments)
2. The rubbing-in method (water biscuits)
3. Melting the fat with sugar and other ingredients (anzacs and brandy snaps)
4. Beating egg whites for a meringue base (macaroons).

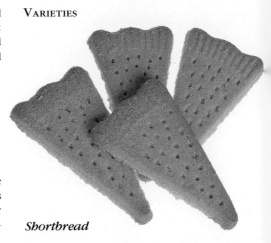

Shortbread

MAJOR NUTRIENTS SERVE SIZE 50 G

Energy	1050 kJ	Sodium	135 mg
Protein	3 g	Potassium	45 mg
Fat	13 g	Calcium	45 mg
Cholesterol	45 mg	Phosphorus	40 mg
Carbohydrate	35 g	Iron	0.7 mg
Dietary Fibre	0	Vitamin A	175 µg

NUTRITIONAL INFORMATION An excellent source of carbohydrate and vitamin A; moderate source of phosphorus, calcium and iron.

Contains large amounts of fat, cholesterol; moderate source of sodium. B vitamins are destroyed during cooking.

The high fat to flour and sugar ratio makes shortbread a particularly energy-dense biscuit for the nutrient levels present.

PREPARATION AND USE Though two different methods are used for making shortbread — the creaming technique and the rubbing-in method — it is agreed that speedy mixing with the minimum working of the ingredients results in the best shortbread. If mixed with a heavy hand the shortbread will be tough and chewy instead of short and melt-in-the-mouth as tradition demands. The traditional ingredients are butter, sugar, flour and a little rice flour or ground rice. Traditionally baked in a round pan, a pattern is usually marked on the shortbread before baking. Candied peel and halved almonds are sometimes pressed into the mixture before baking. After cooking, the colour of the shortbread should not be deeper than pale biscuit.

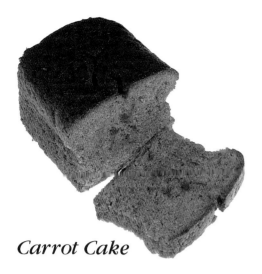

Carrot Cake

MAJOR NUTRIENTS	WITH CREAM CHEESE ICING SERVE SIZE 100 G		
Energy	1820 kJ	Potassium	120 mg
Protein	5 g	Calcium	30 mg
Fat	20 g	Phosphorus	130 mg
Cholesterol	70 mg	Iron	1 mg
Carbohydrate	60 g	Zinc	1 mg
Dietary Fibre	1 g	Vitamin A	445 µg
Sodium	290 mg	Thiamin	0.08 mg

NUTRITIONAL INFORMATION An excellent source of carbohydrate, phosphorus and vitamin A; good source of iron; moderate source of calcium, zinc and thiamin. Contains large amounts of fat, cholesterol and sodium.

Some B vitamins are destroyed during cooking.

As cake is very dense, a 100 g slice is not large. Although it contains carrots, the mixture is made with significant amounts of oil and the cream cheese icing is also energy-dense. The carrots do not make a major contribution to the nutrient profile.

DESCRIPTION This cake has a pleasantly moist, textured appearance when cut. Its comparatively healthy list of ingredients gives it a degree of substance that makes just one slice a very satisfying sweet snack. It is usually topped with a cream cheese icing. This cake is of the melted-fat variety.

ORIGIN AND HISTORY This must be classed as a comparative newcomer in the cake category, with no real history to speak of, but definitely a future.

BUYING AND STORAGE Both commercial and homemade varieties of this cake can be of very good quality. Though generally moist in texture, the cake is best eaten soon after baking.

PREPARATION AND USE Oil is used in this cake in place of traditional fats. Formerly an unusual ingredient, oil is now replacing butter and margarine in a range of cakes. All the ingredients are mixed together as the first and only step in the cake's preparation. These include eggs, sugar (often raw or brown), part wholemeal and part plain flour, walnuts or pecans, grated carrot and frequently drained crushed pineapple, sultanas or raisins and spices.

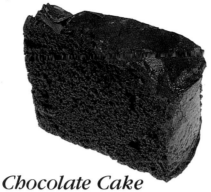

Chocolate Cake

MAJOR NUTRIENTS		WITH ICING SERVE SIZE 100 G	
Energy	1542 kJ	Potassium	155 mg
Protein	4 g	Calcium	70 mg
Fat	16 g	Phosphorus	130 mg
Cholesterol	70 mg	Iron	1 mg
Carbohydrate	56 g	Zinc	1 mg
Dietary Fibre	1 g	Vitamin A	480 µg
Sodium	235 mg		

NUTRITIONAL INFORMATION An excellent source of carbohydrate, phosphorus and vitamin A; good source of iron; moderate source of calcium and zinc.

Contains large amounts of fat and cholesterol and moderate amount of sodium. B vitamins are destroyed during cooking.

One 100 g slice is not a large slice, and often chocolate cakes are made with heavier mixtures which would have increased levels of fat, cholesterol and therefore kilojoules.

Fillings and icing will alter total energy and nutrient content. A cream or butter filling and icing can almost double energy levels. Jam or conserve fillings would be nutritionally more appropriate.

DESCRIPTION This member of the creamed family is commonly known as a plain or butter cake. It is a fairly fine-textured, moist cake and, naturally, chocolate coloured.

ORIGIN AND HISTORY For some time after its arrival in Europe chocolate was treated purely as a beverage, so it is likely that chocolate did not find its way into baking perhaps until the 18th century.

BUYING AND STORAGE Whether bought or homemade, this cake should be stored in a well-covered container in a cool, dry place. Best eaten no more than several days after baking.

PREPARATION AND USE Either chocolate or cocoa dissolved in hot water may be used to flavour the cake. First butter (or margarine) is creamed with sugar, eggs are added and then the sifted dry ingredients. Finally milk and the chocolate or cocoa mixture are stirred through. The cake is baked in a moderate oven and, when cool, may be decorated with a chocolate icing, or filled with jam and cream.

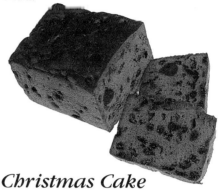

Christmas Cake

MAJOR NUTRIENTS		SERVE SIZE 40 G	
Energy	560 kJ	Dietary Fibre	1 g
Protein	1 g	Sodium	70 mg
Fat	4 g	Potassium	25 mg
Cholesterol	20 mg	Iron	0.6 mg
Carbohydrate	23 g	Vitamin A	50 µg
Total Sugars	14 g		

NUTRITIONAL INFORMATION Contains good amounts of vitamin A; moderate amount of iron.

Although it contains fruit, there is not enough to contribute significant nutrients in one slice. Although it may taste heavy, only 26% energy is from fat.

DESCRIPTION This is usually a fairly large cake, always filled with dried fruits. It may be undecorated or have a pattern of nuts pressed into the cake's surface, or be iced with a simple icing or with a more elaborate combination of marzipan and fondant. It is made by the creamed method.

ORIGIN AND HISTORY One of the early forerunners of the rich fruit cake could well have been satura, a cake prepared in Roman times, which was a mixture of barley mash, dried raisins, pine kernels and pomegranate seeds laced with condiments and honeyed wine. Another Roman cake described by the writer Apicius carried the following instructions — 'Grind pepper with garum, honey, undiluted wine, rue, pine nuts, mix boiled spelt and crushed walnuts with these ingredients and add toasted hazelnuts' — not exactly a close relation to today's rich fruit cake but certainly reflecting the future mix of ingredients.

By the 14th century German bakers were taking advantage of the increasing trade in spices to enhance their wares. The availability of ginger, cinnamon, nutmeg, almonds, rose water, citron and orange in conjunction with their own local honey, resulted in the invention of a new exciting Kuchen (cake). This popularity was such that two centuries later a Christmas market specialising in its sale was established and still exists today.

BUYING AND STORAGE Bought Christmas cakes should be stored in accordance with their use-by date. Homemade Christmas cakes should be stored in a well-covered container in a cool, dry place. Under these conditions a cake should keep for several months. Leave at least several weeks before cutting, if at all possible. The life of the cake will be extended if alcohol is used to soak the fruit prior to mixing and/or sprinkled over the cake just after cooking. This inhibits the growth of mould which might otherwise occur, particularly in humid conditions. Cakes so treated have been known to keep in good condition for a number of years.

PREPARATION AND USE For best results soak the dried fruits in rum or brandy for some hours before mixing the cake ingredients. Butter and sugar are creamed very well before adding eggs, dry ingredients and fruit along with the soaking alcohol. The cake is baked in a well-lined cake pan in a slow oven for several hours. Extra alcohol may be poured over the cake after it comes out from the oven. The cake should then be well wrapped, first in a tea towel and then in several layers of newspaper. When cool, remove the wrappings and store in a plastic bag in a well-sealed cake tin.

Icings and Fillings

DESCRIPTION These substances, usually containing sugar, fats or both, are spread over or between layers, to moisten and sweeten a cake or biscuit.

ORIGIN AND HISTORY Icings and fillings have been in vogue since baking began, the first sweetener being honey.

BUYING AND STORAGE They are usually made at home, though prepared products such as soft icing are available.

PREPARATION AND USE The preparation varies depending on the richness and consistency required. Most icings are put on a cake or biscuit shortly before consumption, and lose their appeal if left to dry out.

VARIETIES

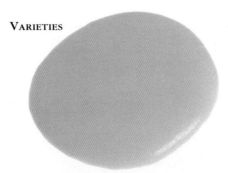

Butter Filling Containing sugar syrup and egg yolks, beaten with butter and flavoured with essences or alcohol.

MAJOR NUTRIENTS		SERVE SIZE 10 G	
Energy	460 kJ	Total Sugars	10 g
Protein	0	Dietary Fibre	0
Fat	8 g	Sodium	90 mg
Cholesterol	23 mg	Potassium	
Carbohydrate	10 g		less than 5 mg
		Vitamin A	75 µg

NUTRITIONAL INFORMATION A high energy filling. Good source of vitamin A. Contains significant amounts of cholesterol and large amounts of fat.

Cholesterol level may be reduced by the use of vegetable margarine as a fat source. Sodium level may be reduced by the use of unsalted fat.

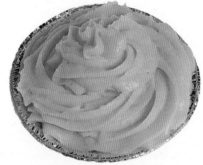

Crème Pâtissière A stiffly whipped egg white is folded through a rich egg custard and the mixture cooked gently and flavoured with vanilla essence. This is used as a filling for flans and small pastry items, sometimes in conjunction with other ingredients such as fruits.

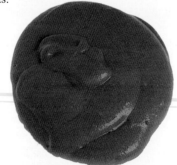

Dark Chocolate Icing Containing melted chocolate, butter, vanilla essence and icing sugar.

MAJOR NUTRIENTS		SERVE SIZE 40 G	
Energy	620 kJ	Dietary Fibre	
Protein	1 g		less than 1 g
Fat	9 g	Sodium	75 mg
Cholesterol	20 mg	Potassium	44 mg
Carbohydrate	18 g	Phosphorus	50 mg
Total Sugars	9 g	Vitamin A	75 µg

NUTRITIONAL INFORMATION A good source of vitamin A; moderate source of phosphorus. Contains large amounts of fat.

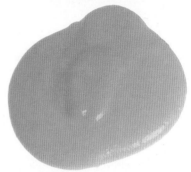

Frosting Containing water, sugar, egg whites and cream of tartar.

MAJOR NUTRIENTS		SERVE SIZE 10 G	
Energy	130 kJ	Total Sugars	40 g
Protein	less than 1 g	Dietary Fibre	0
Fat	0	Sodium	70 mg
Cholesterol	0	Potassium	10 mg
Carbohydrate	40 g		

NUTRITIONAL INFORMATION This is a non-fat icing.

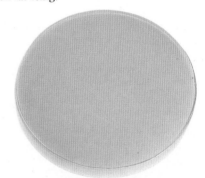

Glacé Icing Two teaspoons of soft butter are added to a cup of icing sugar mixture, flavoured with vanilla essence and blended with 1 tablespoon of boiling water. The icing is beaten well and spread immediately over a cake.

SEE ALSO Fondant in the chapter on Confectionery.

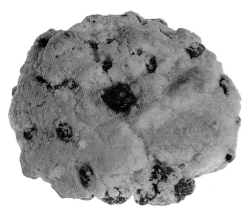

Rock Cake

MAJOR NUTRIENTS   SERVE SIZE 100 G

Energy	1658 kJ	Sodium	480 mg
Protein	4 g	Potassium	210 mg
Fat	16 g	Calcium	140 mg
Cholesterol	70 mg	Phosphorus	150 mg
Carbohydrate	60 g	Iron	1 mg
Dietary Fibre	1 g	Vitamin A	180 μg

NUTRITIONAL INFORMATION An excellent source of carbohydrate, phosphorus, calcium and vitamin A; good source of iron.

Contains large amounts of fat, cholesterol and sodium.

A dense type of product, so a normal cake may be larger than this 100 g serve. Although it contains some dried fruit, this does not make a significant contribution to the nutrient profile.

DESCRIPTION These individual cakes, rather rough or rocklike in appearance, have a 'short' or firm texture, because they are made by the rubbed-in method. They almost invariably contain dried fruits and sometimes chopped nuts.

ORIGIN AND HISTORY Cakes of a similar appearance have no doubt been made over the past few centuries, particularly before the advent of cake pans and when cake mixtures had to be cooked directly on top of a stove or inside an oven not regulated, as modern ones are, with thermostatic controls. Certainly there are early records of fruits and spices being included in cake mixtures before refined flour became available. These conditions could well have resulted in something similar to rock cakes.

BUYING AND STORAGE The same cool, dry storage conditions apply to rock cakes as do to cakes of any description.

PREPARATION AND USE The rubbed-in method requires chilled butter or margarine to be chopped into small pieces and rubbed into flour with the fingertips until the mixture somewhat resembles breadcrumbs. Sugar and dried fruit are added and lastly an egg and milk stirred through. Mounds of the mixture are baked on an oven tray in a moderately hot oven. Spices, grated lemon rind, and fresh or crystallised mixed peel may be added.

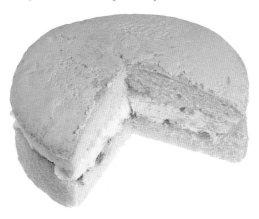

Sponge

MAJOR NUTRIENTS   SERVE SIZE 30 G

Energy	380 kJ	Dietary Fibre	
Protein	3 g		less than 1 g
Fat	2 g	Sodium	25 mg
Cholesterol	80 g	Potassium	35 mg
Carbohydrate	16 g	Phosphorus	50 mg
Total Sugars	9 g		

NUTRITIONAL INFORMATION A moderate source of phosphorus. Contains large amounts of cholesterol.

Relatively low energy cake — little fat content. Fat content comes from egg yolk which is also the source of the significant level of cholesterol. If a low fat topping is used this makes a very good choice of cake for a fat-controlled diet.

DESCRIPTION A cake produced by the whisked method, which is distinguished by its fluffy lightness of texture.

ORIGIN AND HISTORY In the mid-17th century a cookbook was published in France which is now thought to be among the most rare and valuable in the world. It was written by François Pierre de la Varenne. His culinary contribution to the world was principally in the simplification of food preparation — a turning away from the rich and often complicated recipes of the time. In addition to simplifying sauces and treating vegetables as a food in their own right, he included in his book a number of delicately spiced batters of egg and sugar, in fact the types of sponge from which sweet cakes later developed. How close they were to today's sponge cakes is not absolutely clear, but it is certain that he was a trailblazer extraordinaire in the realm of baking.

BUYING AND STORAGE Bought or homemade sponges are best eaten within a day or two of making. However, keeping qualities vary according to the ingredients used and the method of preparation. Butter or margarine in the mixture will produce a richer cake which will not dry out as quickly as a mixture lacking fat.

PREPARATION AND USE Eggs are separated, the whites beaten until fairly stiff, then sugar added gradually and beaten until the mixture is thick. The yolks are stirred through, then flour is folded in lightly. Butter or margarine, melted in hot water, is quickly and lightly stirred through. The mixture is divided between two sandwich tins and baked in a moderate oven. When cool, the cakes are sandwiched with jam, jam and cream, or a mixture of fruit such as sliced strawberries and cream, and often the top is dusted with icing sugar.

PASTRIES

Pastry has been known as a food since the days of antiquity. For example, as early as the 12th century BC, the Egyptian upper classes had no fewer than 40 different types of bread and pastry from which to choose, though the quality would not necessarily have compared favourably with the pastries we have today. Though we have no record of the actual recipes, we do know that some were made with honey, some with milk and others with eggs. Five or six centuries later the Greeks were baking pastry from flour, honey and sesame seeds. Similar recipes are recorded in medieval transcriptions of the oldest surviving cookbook, which contains the recipes of Apicius, a Roman gourmet of the 1st century AD. In the middle of the 16th century we see the famous philosopher Nostradamus in a different light — that of the cookbook writer. He tells us, among other things, how to go about 'making pear preserves, Spanish nougat and marzipan tart'. This era seemed to mark a high period, culinarily speaking, but apparently it was not to last, as in the first decade of the 17th century there were to be found recipes for 'bacon pasties and herb pasties in which ground almonds, bacon, stewed leeks and egg yolks are mixed with sugar and an excessive quantity of cinnamon', reflecting the worst excesses of medieval cooking. Fortunately by the middle of the century the situation was improved markedly with the advent of two cookbooks by François Pierre de la Varenne. These listed all the basic pastry recipes — shortcrust, puff, choux made with oil, and raised pie pastry.

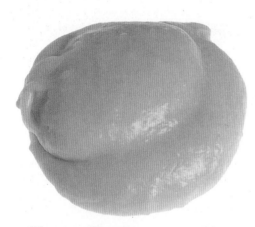

Choux Pastry

MAJOR NUTRIENTS   SERVE SIZE 30 G

Energy	440 kJ	Dietary Fibre	0
Protein	3 g	Sodium	130 mg
Fat	7 g	Potassium	40 mg
Cholesterol	35 mg	Phosphorus	130 mg
Carbohydrate	10 g	Vitamin A	70 µg

NUTRITIONAL INFORMATION An excellent source of carbohydrate and phosphorus; moderate source of vitamin A.

Contains large amounts of fat, cholesterol and a moderate amount of sodium. B vitamins are destroyed during cooking.

Contains lower fat levels than other forms of pastry, so if substituted in a recipe would reduce total energy of finished product.

DESCRIPTION Of all pastry this is probably the most unusual in terms of its preparation. It is in fact cooked twice — once in the combination of the ingredients and again to dry out the pastry ready for filling or assembling.

Probably the most recognisable forms of cooked choux pastry are cream puffs and chocolate eclairs.

ORIGIN AND HISTORY We know that choux pastry was being made at least by the middle of the 17th century as recipes for this and many other still popular pastries were collected at the time in a cookbook entitled *Le Pâtissier François*, written by François Pierre de la Varenne. It is noted that this choux pastry was made with oil.

BUYING AND STORAGE Cooked choux pastry will keep well for several days if kept in an airtight container, providing any uncooked dough is scraped out of the pastry shell before storing.

PREPARATION AND USE Butter and water are brought to the boil and flour is added away from the heat. The batter is beaten until it is smooth and leaves the sides of the saucepan. It is then allowed to cool. Eggs are whisked and added, a little at a time, to the batter. When finished, the paste should be smooth and shiny. Unlike other pastries, this one cannot be rolled but must be spooned or piped onto a baking tray. For tiny puffs, make the balls of pastry walnut size. They are cooked in a hot oven for 15–20 minutes. To help the balls to dry out, it is a good idea to pierce each with a fork shortly before they are fully cooked to release the build-up of steam inside them. When cooled, the balls may be filled with pastry cream or sweetened whipped cream.

VARIETIES

Cream puff, chocolate eclair, croquembouche (a pyramid of balls of choux pastry held together with toffee), profiteroles (balls topped with chocolate, coffee or caramel sauce and filled with cream).

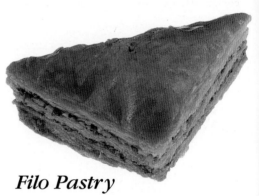

Filo Pastry

*also called **Phyllo pastry, Yufka***

MAJOR NUTRIENTS   SERVE SIZE 50 G

Energy	730 kJ	Dietary Fibre	2 g
Protein	6 g	Sodium	500 mg
Fat	1 g	Potassium	85 mg
Cholesterol	0	Phosphorus	70 mg
Carbohydrate	35 g	Iron	0.7 mg
Total Sugars		Thiamin	0.10 mg
less than 1 g			

NUTRITIONAL INFORMATION A good source of phosphorus, iron and thiamin. High sodium content.

A very low fat pastry. If added fats are limited in the cooking process, this is a nutritionally excellent pastry to use, but many traditional foods containing filo pastry are prepared with the addition of more fat than would be found in a puff pastry.

DESCRIPTION A tissue-thin, pliable pastry, made with high-gluten white flour, a little oil, salt to improve shelf life, and water.

ORIGIN AND HISTORY As filo's popularity began when Greek migrants introduced it into their adopted countries, it is regarded as a Greek pastry. Its popular name is from the Greek and means leaf. It is also widely used in Turkey, Lebanon and Syria. Filo was always made by hand, a process requiring great skill; special machinery is now used by large manufacturers.

BUYING AND STORAGE Filo can be purchased chilled or frozen from supermarkets and delicatessens. Chilled filo keeps for many months in the refrigerator, providing it is well sealed to prevent it drying out. Frozen filo should be held in the freezer until required for use; any left over should be stored in the refrigerator and used within 1 month.

PREPARATION AND USE Thaw unopened, frozen filo at room temperature for 2–3 hours; bring chilled filo to room temperature for 1–2 hours. Open pack and open filo sheets out in a stack onto a dry cloth. Cover with a thick sheet of plastic, or a dry cloth topped with a lightly moistened one, to prevent pastry drying out. Do not put a moist cloth in direct contact with the pastry or the sheets will stick together.

Use melted unsalted butter, clarified butter, ghee or good quality margarine for brushing sheets; olive or maize oil can be used for savoury dishes. For fat-controlled cooking, use only a small amount of chosen fat or oil.

Use for pastry appetisers and pies, for wrapping savoury and sweet foods, and for traditional Greek and Middle Eastern pastries. Prepared foods may be brushed with fat, frozen, then packed, sealed and returned to freezer for later use.

Flaky Pastry

MAJOR NUTRIENTS		UNCOOKED, COMMERCIAL SERVE SIZE 50 G	
Energy	1120 kJ	Total Sugars	
Protein	3 g		less than 1 g
Fat	20 g	Dietary Fibre	1 g
Cholesterol	15 mg	Sodium	230 mg
Carbohydrate	23 g	Potassium	45 mg

NUTRITIONAL INFORMATION Contains a large amount of fat and a moderate amount of sodium.

Although a good source of complex carbohydrate, over 65% of total energy comes from fats.

If egg used to glaze pastry, cholesterol and fat levels will increase.

DESCRIPTION This is a simplified puff pastry, using a combination of puff and shortcrust, most recipes using all butter, but some a mixture of butter and lard.

ORIGIN AND HISTORY The origin of flaky pastry is tied in with the origin of puff pastry. No doubt someone along the way — perhaps a busy cook, pressed for time — cut short a step here and there and found that the result, though not perfect, was good enough.

BUYING AND STORAGE Good quality

flaky pastry is available at the supermarket these days. Treat it as you would the homemade variety. It may be stored for short periods in the refrigerator, but for more than several days, store in the freezer. If the package has been opened, cover well before storing.

PREPARATION AND USE Butter is softened slightly until workable and divided into four equal portions. One portion is rubbed into flour and water is added to make the first dough. After 30 minutes' rest, it is rolled into a rectangle, dotted with a second portion of butter and folded in three, enclosing the butter pieces. The butter must be soft but cool. If too firm it would tear the pastry, too soft and it will melt as you roll the dough and escape out the sides of the pastry. Rolling, buttering and folding is repeated twice more until all the butter has been incorporated in the pastry. A rest in the refrigerator is necessary between foldings. Though it will not rise as well as true puff pastry, this version is suitable for pies, flans, fruit turnovers and vanilla slices.

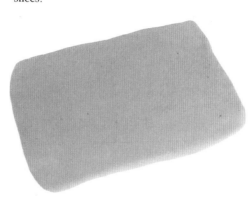

Hot Water Pastry

MAJOR NUTRIENTS		SERVE SIZE 50 G	
Energy	895 kJ	Total Sugars	0
Protein	4 g	Dietary Fibre	1 g
Fat	10 g	Sodium less than 10 mg	
Cholesterol	80 mg	Potassium	50 mg
Carbohydrate	27 g		

NUTRITIONAL INFORMATION Contains large amounts of fat.

High fat crust. Low in sodium if no salt is added in the preparation.

DESCRIPTION Hot water pastry is used mainly for meat and game pies and is unusual in that boiling water is poured onto flour and the dough used while still warm.

ORIGIN AND HISTORY Used in the elaborate pie dishes popular in the Middle Ages, hot water pastry has a long history.

BUYING AND STORAGE Hot water pastry

is made at home, and eaten soon after cooking.

PREPARATION AND USE An egg yolk is added to sifted plain flour and salt. Lard and water are heated until the lard melts. When the mixture comes to the boil it is poured into the flour. It is very important that the water should be boiling, otherwise it will be difficult to mould the pastry and it may crack during cooking. The pastry is mixed with a wooden spoon until all streaks of egg yolk have disappeared and the dough is smooth. The pastry should then be covered and allowed to rest in a warm place for 30 minutes.

The best-known use for this type of pastry is in the English Melton Mowbray pie.

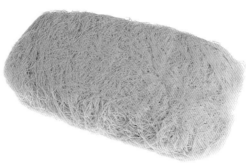

Kataifi Pastry

also called **Kadaif, Konafa**

MAJOR NUTRIENTS		SERVE SIZE 128 G	
Energy	1600 kJ	Cholesterol	9 mg
Protein	6 g	Sodium	120 mg
Fat	12 g	Iron	2.4 mg
Carbohydrate	62 g	Magnesium	27 mg

NUTRITIONAL INFORMATION An excellent source of iron; good source of protein and magnesium; moderate source of fat.

Moderate sodium content. A concentrated source of energy.

DESCRIPTION Strands of dough which resemble very fine, soft vermicelli. Kataifi is made with a batter prepared from very low-gluten (sponge) flour, oil, salt and water, mixed to a cream consistency. The batter is poured through a perforated container onto a revolving heated copper plate where the strands dry slightly, then scooped up, cooled and packed.

ORIGIN AND HISTORY With kataifi mentioned in *The Thousand and One Nights* by its Arabic name, konafa, it can be assumed that this unusual pastry has been made in the Middle East for a few hundred years at least. Its origins could be Persian or Arabic, even Greek, for all three cultures had exchanges in one form or another from ancient times.

BUYING AND STORAGE Purchase from Greek and Middle Eastern food shops; some supermarkets and delicatessens also stock it. It is packed in plastic bags, boxed by some manufacturers. Store in the refrigerator, well sealed, and use within 3 months.

PREPARATION AND USE Leave in packaging and bring to room temperature for 1–2 hours. Squeeze and knead kataifi in its unopened bag until strands loosen, then turn into a bowl and use as directed in recipes.

Besides being used for traditional Greek and Middle Eastern pastries, kataifi can be moulded into nest shapes in suitable containers, dabbed with butter and baked until crisp; use for sweet or savoury fillings and garnishes (small nests). When using kataifi, keep two facts in mind: uncooked kataifi dissolves in liquid; and it does not absorb fat, so use as little as you need to do the job.

Puff Pastry

MAJOR NUTRIENTS		SERVE SIZE 50 G	
Energy	1120 kJ	Total Sugars	
Protein	3 g		less than 1 g
Fat	20 g	Dietary Fibre	1 g
Cholesterol	15 mg	Sodium	230 mg
Carbohydrate	23 g	Potassium	45 mg

NUTRITIONAL INFORMATION Contains significant amounts of sodium and large amounts of fat.

Although a good source of complex carbohydrate, over 65% of total energy comes from fats.

If egg is used to glaze pastry, cholesterol and fat levels will increase.

DESCRIPTION Puff is considered to be the finest of all pastries, blending flour, fat (usually butter) and water in a special folding and rolling technique to give a light, airy, layered texture.

ORIGIN AND HISTORY In the nineteenth century historians believed that Claude Lorraine, the 17th century landscape painter, was the inventor of puff pastry. However it is recorded that the Bishop of Amiens had mentioned it as early as 1311.

BUYING AND STORAGE Since not many cooks these days are prepared to give the time to making their own puff pastry, it is fortunate that it is available commercially. For short periods it may be stored in the refrigerator, but if storing for more than several days, it is wiser to freeze the pastry. If partly used, cover well before storing in freezer or refrigerator.

PREPARATION AND USE The dough for puff pastry is made with flour and water with fat added in a whole block (French method) or in small pieces (English method). The dough is folded over the fat, rolled, rested and then the same procedure repeated 6 times. It is then cut to the desired shape and baked in a hot oven until crisp and golden. The interleaving of fat with pastry causes quite spectacular rising, resulting in a wonderfully crisp and light texture. The pastry has many uses — in pies, flans, tortes, cakes and millefeuille (a thousand leaves).

VARIETIES

Rough Puff Pastry

NUTRITIONAL INFORMATION The same as for puff pastry.

DESCRIPTION This variation of puff pastry is the simplest of the short cuts. It will rise, though not as well as puff or flaky pastry.

ORIGIN AND HISTORY The origin of this pastry is the same as that of puff pastry. The variation is no doubt the invention of an enterprising cook who could see that this less refined method of distributing butter through a dough would give rising of sorts, though not as successfully as with puff or flaky pastry.

BUYING AND STORAGE Refrigerate if storing for only a couple of days, otherwise store in the freezer.

PREPARATION AND USE For this really simple variation of puff pastry the proportion of butter to flour is flexible. You may use from half, up to the same, weight of butter to flour. The butter is cut roughly into the flour with two knives until the mixture resembles large crumbs. Cold water is added to make a dough which is then rolled and turned a number of times to enclose the butter as far as possible in the dough. For best results the dough should be rested in the refrigerator between rollings. Use in the same way as flaky pastry.

Shortcrust Pastry

MAJOR NUTRIENTS		COMMERCIAL SERVE SIZE 50 G	
Energy	1270 kJ	Dietary Fibre	1 g
Protein	3 g	Sodium	320 mg
Fat	20 g	Potassium	50 mg
Cholesterol	17 mg	Phosphorus	40 mg
Carbohydrate	27 g	Iron	0.7 mg
Total Sugars		Vitamin A	185 µg
	less than 1 g		

NUTRITIONAL INFORMATION Excellent source of vitamin A and good source of iron. Contains significant amounts of sodium and large amounts of fat.

Lower fat and therefore energy level than puff and flaky pastry.

DESCRIPTION Shortcrust is one of the most popular and easiest to prepare of all the pastries. It has a firm but pleasantly short texture and, though mostly used for tarts and pies, it is sometimes used as the base for cakes or slices.

ORIGIN AND HISTORY There is evidence that pastry was made in Egypt in the time of the pharaohs and in ancient Greece and Rome. Gradually, over the centuries, techniques were refined until pastry recipes similar to those known today appeared in the cookbook Le Pâtissier François, produced by François Pierre de la Varenne in the mid-17th century. Apparently the book was inspired by an Italian publication produced in Venice almost a century earlier. It also mentions a typical tart, filled with pastry cream, flavoured with cinnamon and rose-flower water, Corinth raisins, pine nuts and candied lemon zest. These ingredients reflected the influence of Islamic cuisine.

BUYING AND STORAGE Like several other popular pastries, shortcrust can be conveniently bought from the supermarket, frozen and ready rolled. It may be kept in the refrigerator for several days, but for longer periods it needs freezing.

PREPARATION AND USE Shortcrust is made from flour, butter or margarine, water and a pinch of salt, usually with half the weight of butter to flour. The butter is rubbed into the flour with the fingertips to keep the mixture as cool as possible. Add only enough water, gradually, to have the dough hold together. The coolness of the ingredients and the speed with which the pastry is prepared are important to the success of the finished pastry. The butter should be chilled and chopped into fairly small pieces prior to rubbing in and the water kept icy cold. Overworking the fat and flour, excessively humid weather or clammy hands can cause the pastry to become oily and hard when cooked. These problems could be overcome with the use of a food processor or perhaps using a pastry blender or two knives to cut in the fat instead of using the fingers. The two knives technique will not blend the fat as evenly with the flour as the other methods. Larger pieces of fat remaining through the mixture will produce a flakier pastry. The dough should be chilled for about 15 minutes before using to allow the gluten to relax and make the pastry easier to roll. Cover during the holding period with plastic wrap, aluminium foil or greaseproof paper. Use for pies, flans, biscuits or as a base for some cakes and slices.

VARIETIES

Rich Shortcrust

DESCRIPTION Rich shortcrust pastry, as the name implies, is similar to ordinary shortcrust pastry, but enriched with eggs (and sugar if a sweet pastry is required).

ORIGIN AND HISTORY The origin of this particular pastry is of course linked with that of plain shortcrust. The addition of eggs and sugar to enrich the original pastry could well have come some 50–60 years after the publishing of La Varenne's book *Le Pâtissier François*. At this time there was a great increase in the quantity of sweet flavourings used in all baking and a much greater emphasis on refining techniques.

BUYING AND STORAGE The pastry should be kept chilled and well wrapped to avoid drying out of the surface which makes rolling the pastry very difficult.

PREPARATION AND USE The method of preparation is similar to that of plain shortcrust, but the sugar (if a sweet shortcrust is required) is usually added with the flour and the egg combined with a little chilled water to be worked into the flour mixture.

The pastry is used for sweet or savoury pies or flans. The sweet variety is also used in slices or as a base for certain cakes.

Savoury Shortcrust
With added cheese or herbs.

Sweet Shortcrust
With added sugar.

MAJOR NUTRIENTS		SERVE SIZE 50 G	
Energy	1150 kJ	Total Sugars	3 g
Protein	3 g	Dietary Fibre	1 g
Fat	20 g	Sodium	230 mg
Cholesterol	15 mg	Potassium	45 mg
Carbohydrate	25 g		

NUTRITIONAL INFORMATION Contains large amounts of fat.

Although a good source of complex carbohydrate, over 65% of total energy comes from fats.

If egg or butter is used to glaze pastry, cholesterol and fat levels will increase.

Wholemeal Pastry
Made with all or some wholemeal flour. It makes a good pizza base.

MAJOR NUTRIENTS		SERVE SIZE 50 G	
Energy	1120 kJ	Dietary Fibre	3 g
Protein	3 g	Sodium	230 mg
Fat	20 g	Potassium	90 mg
Cholesterol	15 mg	Phosphorus	40 mg
Carbohydrate	23 g	Iron	0.8 mg
Total Sugars		Thiamin	0.1 mg
	less than 1 g	Niacin Equiv.	1.2 mg

NUTRITIONAL INFORMATION Contains large amounts of fat. Good source of iron. Moderate source of phosphorus, thiamin and niacin.

Increased levels of dietary fibre, phosphorus, iron, thiamin and niacin compared to plain flour pastry. Although a good source of complex carbohydrate, over 65% of total energy comes from fats.

If egg or butter is used to glaze pastry, cholesterol and fat levels will increase.

Strudel Pastry

MAJOR NUTRIENTS		SERVE SIZE 50 G	
Energy	1120 kJ	Total Sugars	
Protein	3 g		less than 1 g
Fat	20 g	Dietary Fibre	1 g
Cholesterol	15 mg	Sodium	230 mg
Carbohydrate	23 g	Potassium	45 mg

NUTRITIONAL INFORMATION Contains significant amounts of sodium and large amounts of fat.

Although a good source of complex carbohydrate, over 65% of total energy comes from fats.

If egg or butter is used to glaze pastry, cholesterol and fat levels will increase.

DESCRIPTION Unlike most pastries, this is a flexible dough with ingredients slightly warmed during its preparation rather than chilled. It is finally stretched until it is almost transparent and is used to enclose fillings.

ORIGIN AND HISTORY Since strudel pastry needs high quality white flour for any degree of success it is unlikely that this delicious confection was developed more than several hundred years ago.

PREPARATION AND USE A soft dough is prepared with an egg, melted butter and water mixed together and stirred into flour. When the dough forms a cohesive mass it is turned onto a floured surface and kneaded until it is no longer sticky. The dough is finally rolled and stretched on a large floured cloth and kept moist during the stretching by brushing with a little melted butter. When it has been rolled and stretched until almost transparent, it is then used to enclose the chosen filling. Apple is no doubt the most popular filling but another favourite is a filling of cream cheese served with a hot cherry sauce.

Suet Crust Pastry

MAJOR NUTRIENTS		SERVE SIZE 50 G	
Energy	895 kJ	Total Sugars	0
Protein	4 g	Dietary Fibre	1 g
Fat	10 g	Sodium less than 10 mg	
Carbohydrate	27 g	Potassium	50 mg

NUTRITIONAL INFORMATION Contains large amounts of fat and cholesterol.

High fat crust. Low in sodium if no salt is added in the preparation.

DESCRIPTION The appearance of this pastry is different from most other types. The uncooked mixture is similar to a light scone dough. It is most commonly used to line a pudding basin for a steak and kidney pudding.

ORIGIN AND HISTORY In Roman times the word bread was used to cover what today we call cakes, pastry and biscuits. We learn that suet bread was part of the Roman diet and since it is known that the breads were mainly eaten as an accompaniment to meat or dunked in wine or goat's milk, suet 'bread' may have been just one step away from the simple steak and kidney pudding that we know.

Centuries ago, pies and tarts were among the pastries in the French pastry cook's repertoire as they could be baked on the hearth without an oven. The pastry was made with fine wheat flour, probably with lard and water, and usually contained a savoury filling, fruit fillings being unknown at that time.

PREPARATION AND USE Self-raising flour and salt are sifted together; suet is added and mixed in well. The light but dry dough is mixed with water, turned onto a floured board and kneaded well.

DESSERTS AND PUDDINGS

Perhaps the first authenticated existence of cooked desserts was revealed when an Egyptian tomb, dated at early in the third millennium BC, was excavated. Among the items found were cakes, stewed figs and uncooked berries. The Egyptian tradition of leaving, among other items of value, sufficient food to keep the tomb's occupant going until the other world was reached, provided a valuable, tangible record of life in those distant centuries.

Ancient Greece and Rome saw the development of greater refinements in the area of desserts. We discover in the writings of Apicius what could well be the first recipe for a sweet omelette: a mixture of eggs, milk and oil, cooked in an oiled pan, turned out and served moistened with honey and sprinkled with pepper.

A considerable time jump in our search for desserts brings us to an early 16th century banquet in Rome for a member of the Medici family. Included among the hors d'oeuvres were cakes made of pine nuts and marzipan, sweet cup custards and figs. A variety of preserves and candied fruits were among the desserts.

Yet another Roman banquet, this time for King Charles VI, had as part of its third course 'jelly' and what is thought, on translation, to be bread and jam. However since the other items were all savoury, the jelly may not have been the traditional set piece that we all know so well, but something more like an aspic. The banquet's third course is more easily recognised as dessert, with pear pastries, almonds and sugared tarts.

What becomes clear after research is the fact that during the 15th and 16th centuries Italy stood out among the countries of Europe for its increased refinements in many aspects of food service. It can also be credited, during this period, with the invention of pastry and sweetmeats.

A publication on good manners during the 17th century carries the rather quaint recommendation that 'One should not carry away in one's handkerchief or one's muff sweets that are served as dessert.' At 17th century dinner parties doggy bags were obviously not quite the thing.

Most people enjoy something sweet at the end of the main meal of the day, and most national cuisines have their typical desserts and puddings.

The dessert may be a simple fruit dessert or milk pudding, or a hearty steamed fruit pudding, or treacle tart and custard. The energy (kilojoule) and nutritional value will vary according to the ingredients.

In a well planned meal, the dessert provides a balance with the other course or courses. It can offer a contrast in flavour, colour and texture. Nutritionally, the dessert can also provide a balance, making a significant contribution to the value of the meal.

There are fashions in desserts, as there are in other foods. Some of the old family favourites such as bread and butter custard, and fruit crumble, have almost disappeared from home menus, but are now being revived in many up-market restaurants, and are taking on a new image.

The search for quickly prepared home meals has helped boost the popularity of ice cream and other frozen ice desserts, as well as canned fruit and some of the more exotic fresh fruits. Yoghurt is another popular dessert.

Food laws stipulate a percentage of milk fat in ice cream, usually 10%, but there are lower fat milk ice confections on the market that taste very similar to ice cream. Some of these have as little as 1–2 grams of fat per serving. Combined with fruit, these provide a popular low fat dessert which also makes a worthwhile contribution to nutrition.

To enjoy desserts and puddings, it is best to give priority to those based on fruit, milk and yoghurt, including the low fat varieties; starchy foods such as rice and semolina; or crumble toppings made from rolled oats or wholemeal breadcrumbs or flour, with moderate numbers of eggs and small amounts of sugar or fat. The high sugar, high fat desserts are for more occasional use, such as a weekend treat or a special celebration.

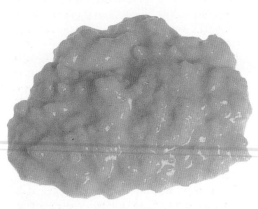

Cereal Dessert

MAJOR NUTRIENTS		RICE PUDDING SERVE SIZE 100 G
Energy	390 kJ	Dietary Fibre	0
Protein	3 g	Sodium	50 mg
Fat	3 g	Potassium	140 mg
Cholesterol	10 mg	Calcium	90 mg
Carbohydrate	15 g	Phosphorus	80 mg
Total Sugars	11 g	Riboflavin	0.1 mg

NUTRITIONAL INFORMATION An excellent source of calcium; good source of phosphorus; moderate source of riboflavin. High carbohydrate type of dessert, which contains significant levels of the major nutrients found in milk, so a useful way to include extra calcium and riboflavin in the diet. Dried fruit can be added which will alter the total carbohydrate level, but would not contribute significant nutrients in the quantities consumed.

DESCRIPTION Cereals featuring in desserts include rice, sago, tapioca, semolina and oats. Rice offers a very wide range of recipes for desserts, from the simplest creamy rice pudding to the quite exotic. Nutritious, creamy desserts may be prepared from any of the cereals. Two of the better known desserts once popular but now rarely included in family fare are lemon sago and tapioca cream. However, rice desserts, probably due to the ongoing promotion of their product by rice growers, continue to win friends in combination with fresh, canned and dried fruits, candied citrus peels, nuts and praline. Two dessert recipes showing the versatility of rice are the simple creamy rice pudding and the somewhat extravagant and delicious Rice Imperial.

ORIGIN AND HISTORY Though it is no doubt likely that rice was being combined with milk or other liquids to provide foods of substance for centuries, there are few available recipes for rice puddings before the Middle Ages. However a rice pudding was part of a 16th century menu prepared for Pope Pius V. The third of the four courses included 'Turkish-style rice with milk, sprinkled with sugar and cinnamon' — a dish that could well be closely related to our rice pudding.

BUYING AND STORAGE Ideally buy rice or other cereal as required. If you have an oversupply and there is danger of insect infestation, store in the freezer if space permits. If kept in the pantry, store in the unopened package or in a jar with a well-sealed lid.

PREPARATION AND USE For a simple rice pudding, rice is cooked in milk flavoured with vanilla essence in a double saucepan until soft and creamy — about 2 hours — stirring from time to time. Sweeten to taste and if desired, when cool, fold in whipped cream. Delicious if served with fresh or frozen raspberries or strawberries.

To make *Rice Imperial*, use about ⅔ cup of raw rice to 3–3½ cups of milk and when almost cold, stir through about 3 tablespoons of chopped glacé fruit which have been soaked for some hours in kirsch. Add ¾ cup of rich egg (stirred) custard and finally, just before serving, fold in a cup of whipped cream.

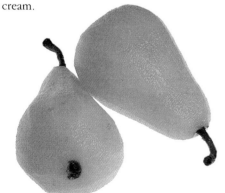

Fruit Dessert, Cooked

DESCRIPTION Desserts such as poached fruit, fruit compotes, flambéed fruit, caramel bananas and apple snow, are all comparatively simple to prepare and generally present fruits in a form where their flavours are preserved in close to 'fresh fruit' condition.

ORIGIN AND HISTORY Stewed fruit certainly has a long history. Stewed figs were discovered with the excavation of an Egyptian tomb dating from the third millennium BC. The fruit, along with other items of value, were traditionally placed in the tombs of the rich and famous of ancient Egypt to bring them comfort on their journey to the next world. We tend to treat stewed fruit with a little less reverence these days although this simple dessert never seems to go out of fashion. With very little added effort these simple dishes can be transformed into a dessert fit for a king.

PREPARATION AND USE *Poached fruit and fruit for compotes* are simmered gently in either a sugar and water or sugar, water and wine syrup, sometimes flavoured with spices or the zest of citrus fruit. They are generally served chilled.

Flambéed fruit are first simmered and then sprinkled with sugar before adding warmed brandy which is then ignited with a burning taper. The fruits and syrup must be hot but not boiling to achieve success.

Fruit soufflés may be prepared in several different ways. One of the simplest is to puree the fruit (or use fruit juices), separate eggs and cook the yolks over simmering water with sugar until slightly thickened, add softened gelatine and when cool add pureed fruit or fruit juice to the mixture. Egg whites are whipped and combined with whipped cream and finally combined with the fruit mixture. All are folded together very gently and chilled before serving.

Caramel bananas are peeled, sliced lengthways and fried gently in butter until lightly browned but not too soft. Transfer to serving dish and add brown sugar, brandy or dry sherry and sufficient butter to the pan to make a smooth syrup — simmer, stirring constantly for a minute or two. Pour syrup over bananas and serve hot with pouring cream or ice cream.

Apple snow is made by simmering sliced apples with sugar, lemon zest and very little water. The apples are then blended or pushed through a sieve and when chilled, combined with stiffly beaten egg white. If the apples are cooked by microwave there is no need to add any cooking water. This will allow the addition of a little lemon juice in place of the lemon zest, if preferred. Chopped candied peel may be stirred through the apple, if desired.

Fruit Dessert, Uncooked

MAJOR NUTRIENTS

		FRUIT SALAD, CANNED SERVE SIZE 100 G	
Energy	405 kJ	Dietary Fibre	1 g
Protein	less than 1 g	Sodium	less than 5 mg
Fat	0	Potassium	120 mg
Carbohydrate	25 g	Vitamin C	3 mg
Total Sugars	25 g		

NUTRITIONAL INFORMATION A good source of vitamin C. The canning process retains the majority of nutrient present in the fresh fruit, so fruit salad is a rich carbohydrate with significant vitamin C.

DESCRIPTION Fruit salads, fruit coulis, toffee-glazed fruits, chocolate-coated bananas — all involve uncooked fruits.

ORIGIN AND HISTORY Uncooked fruits have featured in the very earliest documented menus. Toffee glazing would probably have begun some time in the 19th century or even earlier, when experiments in confectionery were a popular culinary art in Europe.

PREPARATION AND USE *Fruit salads* are among the simplest but most popular of all fruit desserts. A combination of almost any fruits makes a successful fruit salad but care should be taken to ensure that each fruit can be recognised easily. A salad that is made up of pieces of fruit so small that they cannot be identified is boring and quite unappetising. Its main attraction should be the definite splashes of colour of whole strawberries, slices of kiwi fruit and banana, small wedges of red-skinned apple and so on. The addition of tiny mint sprigs or a scattering of pretty blue borage flowers (edible, if you feel adventurous) will add interest. Do not overchill fruits in a salad — this tends to blunt their full flavour.

Fruit coulis is pureed fruit, usually served as a sauce for other fruits or sometimes with savoury foods. It may be thinned with a little fruit juice if desired. A berry fruit coulis may need to be sweetened a little before serving. Mango coulis needs no sweetening and has a particular affinity with cold chicken in much the same way as pureed apple has for long been a successful companion for pork when served hot or cold.

Toffee-glazed fruits are a spectacular finale to serve with coffee after a meal. Strawberries are particularly successful in this role. The berries are washed and dried but not hulled — leave a little of the stalk as a handle. They should not be left to stand for long after glazing or the fruit's juices will begin to soften the crisp toffee coating. A sugar syrup is boiled until a pale gold colour and the fruits are dipped in the toffee and placed on a tray greased with butter for easy removal when set. Setting takes only a very few minutes. Cherries and seedless grapes (all with their own 'handles') are also successful as glazed fruit.

Chocolate-coated bananas are usually quite a hit with children. Chocolate is melted very carefully over hot but not boiling water, preferably using the special easy-melt chocolate. The bananas, cut in half lengthways, rest on a wire cake cooler and after being coated with chocolate may have a sprinkling of chopped nuts to add to their desirability. They are ready to eat when the chocolate sets.

VARIETIES
Those above are used as examples: the possibilities are endless.

Fruit Pudding

DESCRIPTION This category covers a wide variety of puddings, diverse in both appearance and method of preparation: crumble-topped fruit puddings, fruit puddings topped with dumplings or pastry pinwheels, fruit cobblers, baked fruit roly-polies, upside-down fruit puddings. All provide methods of extending and/or enhancing the fruits involved.

BUYING AND STORAGE There are many frozen varieties of fruit pudding available.

ORIGIN AND HISTORY During the 16th century at least two books containing recipes for making 'fruit preserves' appeared in France. In one, the noted prophet Nostradamus explains 'the manner and fashion of making preserves of several sorts, in honey as well as in sugar and cooked wine' and also 'preserving whole little limes and oranges, quinces in quarters with sugar, making cotignac [a fruit paste]' and 'a way of making jelly of guignes [a variety of cherry] that is very delicate but expensive and for

noblemen'. It is obvious that we have broadened the use of fruit in desserts considerably in the last few hundred years, but the simple recipes of past centuries are in no way dated or considered out of fashion.

PREPARATION AND USE *Crumble-topped puddings* are amongst the simplest to prepare. Stewed fruits are topped with a mixture of flour, rolled oats or a combination of the two into which butter or margarine is rubbed with or without the addition of sugar and spices. The dish is then baked until the fruits are cooked and the topping lightly browned and crisp. A similar type of pudding has a cooked fruit base with a topping of either *dumplings* made with a scone-type mixture or *pinwheels* made by rolling a scone or pastry dough thinly and spreading with mixed fruits and spices or jam. The mixture is rolled, Swiss-roll fashion, and cut into pinwheels which are placed on top of the fruit. Both dumplings and pinwheels should be used over fairly juicy fruits; the dumplings, particularly, cook best when in a very moist environment.

Fruit cobblers are prepared with a cooked fruit base, once again with a good proportion of juice, covered with a rich, thinly rolled scone dough, and baked in a hot oven.

Baked fruit roly-polies are made with a pastry base rolled thinly and covered with thinly sliced fruit or fruit conserve. This is rolled up, Swiss-roll fashion, and placed in a casserole; a sugar, water and butter syrup is poured over and the roll baked until cooked and well glazed.

Upside-down puddings are made with a cake topping poured over a mixture of melted brown sugar and butter into which fruits (usually in a set pattern) are pressed. After cooking, the pudding is turned out and served upside-down.

VARIETIES
The types of fruit puddings are endless: one variety is given below as an example.

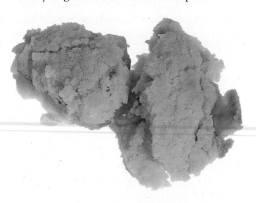

Apple and Rhubarb Crumble

MAJOR NUTRIENTS		SERVE SIZE 120 G	
Energy	1050 kJ	Sodium	85 mg
Protein	2 g	Potassium	120 mg
Fat	8 g	Phosphorus	40 mg
Cholesterol	6 mg	Vitamin A	100 µg
Carbohydrate	44 g	Thiamin	0.05 mg
Total Sugars	27 g	Niacin Equiv.	1 mg
Dietary Fibre	3 g	Vitamin C	7 mg

NUTRITIONAL INFORMATION An excellent source of vitamins A and C; moderate source of phosphorus, niacin and thiamin. High carbohydrate dessert, with less than 30% of energy coming from fat sources. If served with large amounts of cream or ice cream, energy value will increase dramatically.

DESCRIPTION Apple and rhubarb crumble is a baked fruit dessert of sliced apple and rhubarb with a crisp topping.

ORIGIN AND HISTORY Could it be that cooks of more ancient times first considered making what we now call a 'fruit crumble' for the very same reason that many present-day cooks choose this method rather than a fruit pie? The attraction for today's cook is no doubt twofold — we use a much lower proportion of pastry with a crumble, thus adding fewer kilojoules to the family meal, and, perhaps an even more attractive inducement, it is so much easier and quicker to prepare. It is doubtful that kilojoules played any part in the decision of past generations, but there could have been an economic consideration instead — the fruits were often home-grown, but the pastry ingredients were purchased.

BUYING AND STORAGE This dessert is intended to be made at home and eaten immediately.

PREPARATION AND USE The apples are peeled, cored and sliced along with the rhubarb. Sugar is added with or without a preferred spice (ground ginger is particularly compatible with these two fruits). The topping is made by rubbing butter or margarine into either flour or a mixture of flour and rolled oats and adding sugar and more spice if desired. The fruit may be partly cooked before adding the topping, or fruit and topping cooked at the same time. A fairly high heat is required to crisp the topping. Should the fruits be very juicy, it may be better to thicken the mixture with a little flour sprinkled on the fruits prior to cooking, or, if the topping is to be added after the fruit is cooked, the juices may be thickened with a little blended cornflour before adding the topping. This will help prevent the topping from sinking into the juices and losing some of its crispness. The dessert may be served hot or cold with custard, cream or ice cream.

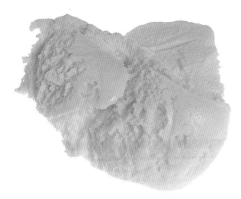

Ice Cream and Sorbet

MAJOR NUTRIENTS		ICE CREAM, VANILLA SERVE SIZE 50 G	
Energy	420 kJ	Sodium	40 mg
Protein	2 g	Potassium	90 mg
Fat	6 g	Calcium	70 mg
Cholesterol	20 mg	Phosphorus	50 mg
Carbohydrate	11 g	Vitamin A	65 µg
Total Sugars	10 g	Riboflavin	0.1 mg
Dietary Fibre	0		

NUTRITIONAL INFORMATION A good source of phosphorus and calcium; moderate source of vitamin A and riboflavin. Although 50% of energy comes from fat sources ice cream is a useful source of calcium in the diet as the calcium is well absorbed from this source. New super premium ice creams are much higher in fats than regular ice cream and so should be eaten in moderation. Ice confections, although their fat is non butter fat, tend to have almost the same level of fat as regular ice creams and contain similar nutrient levels.

DESCRIPTION Ice cream and water ice are frozen desserts, some made with cream as a base (ice cream), some with water or fruit juice (sorbet, sherbet). Many, but not all, of both the cream and water-based ices have whipped egg whites among their ingredients.

ORIGIN AND HISTORY Ices or sorbets as we know them today almost certainly first saw the light of day in China some 3000 years ago. There exist recipes from early India (date of development unknown) and from ancient Persia for iced sherbets made from mixed fruit juices. The people of ancient Turkey were known to have found sherbet a popular refreshment also. Towards the end of the 17th century there was a great movement towards increased consumption of ices and sherbets. This no doubt led to recipe variations which ultimately added cream to the confection. The question is, who put the cream into ice cream? Various authorities credit different sources — one source insists ice cream was born in 16th century Tuscany, others say Spain or Sicily. One seemingly indisputable fact appears to be that Catherine de Medici

was responsible for introducing the confection to France on her arrival from Italy to marry France's Henry II. Catherine had brought her own Florentine cooks with her and they prepared a different flavoured ice cream for each day of her wedding festivities. An interesting story about that strange ice cream dessert called baked Alaska brings us closer to home. A brilliant American-born scientist, Benjamin Thompson, later knighted by King George III and ultimately to become Count Rumford, claimed that baked Alaska was an inadvertent invention of his own, resulting from his experiments in 1804 into the resistance of stiffly beaten egg whites to the induction of heat.

BUYING AND STORAGE It is now possible to buy an incredible range of iced desserts. Premium quality supermarket ice creams may well be persuading the former home ice cream makers to put away their favourite recipes; however it is still cheaper to prepare your own. Always store ice cream in an efficient freezer, preferably with a door that is separate from the main door of the refrigerator. Without an efficient freezer it is not possible to achieve the smooth, velvety texture of a good ice cream or the fine, quick-frozen crystals of a good water ice.

PREPARATION AND USE Ice creams may be made from a number of basic recipes. Some have a custard-type base, others have as their chief ingredient cream or evaporated milk, some rely on beaten egg whites to help achieve the texture they are looking for. You may also use a commercial ice cream churn, hand- or electrically operated.

VARIETIES
These are too numerous to mention and depend of course on the flavour used. Two examples are given.

Coffee Ice Cream
This is a delicious but simple ice cream. Powdered instant coffee is added to egg whites which are beaten with sugar until thick and foamy. The mixture is combined with whipped, sweetened cream and turned into a cake pan or ice cream container to set. There is no second beating. For variety, toasted slivered almonds may be folded through just before freezing, or try folding through roughly chopped pecan or walnut praline. For a more economical ice cream, try one with a full-cream powdered or evaporated milk base. Chocolate, caramel, pureed fruit or fruit juices are some of the popular flavouring ingredients to choose from.

Lemon Water Ice (Sorbet)

MAJOR NUTRIENTS		SERVE SIZE 50 G	
Energy	260 kJ	Dietary Fibre	0
Protein	less than 1 g	Sodium	10 mg
Fat	0	Potassium	12 mg
Carbohydrate	7 g	Vitamin C	4 µg
Total Sugars	7 g		

NUTRITIONAL INFORMATION If made with half a lemon, it is a high vitamin C containing dessert, which is relatively low in energy and contains no fat.

DESCRIPTION A syrup is prepared with sugar and water, lemon juice and sometimes gelatine is added, with grated lemon zest for added flavour. When cool, strain and pour into ice cream trays to set. Stir from time to time for even freezing. When it is still a little mushy, remove from freezer and beat lightly for just a few seconds. Have ready a beaten egg white sweetened with sugar, and fold through the lemon mixture quickly but evenly. Return to freezer and freeze until firm.

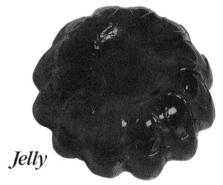

Jelly

MAJOR NUTRIENTS		SERVE SIZE 50 G	
Energy	130 kJ	Dietary Fibre	0
Protein	less than 1 g	Sodium	less than 5 mg
Fat	0	Potassium	
Total Sugars	7 g		less than 5 mg

NUTRITIONAL INFORMATION A low energy, easy to prepare dessert. If made with low energy sweeteners, will contain less than 5 kilojoules per serve.

DESCRIPTION Jellies are transparent or semi-transparent, softly solidified desserts coloured either artificially or by the particular ingredients used (usually fruit juices).

ORIGIN AND HISTORY During the Middle Ages and indeed almost up to the 16th century the wealthy frequently dined, particularly when entertaining, in a manner we would call, at the very least, excessive. There were many courses and many dishes in each course but it is interesting to note that on these occasions every course would include a 'sotelte' (subtlety), which was a jelly or pastry.

In 1555 in Lyon, France, a rather remarkable cookbook became available, written by the celebrated prophet, Nostradamus, containing some gems of useful information, one of those being 'a way of making a jelly of guignes (cherries) that is very delicate but expensive and for noblemen'! Just 100 years later, in what purported to be a contemporary exposé of the royal kitchens of the House of Stuart in England, one is asked to believe that royalty was fed, among other things, no doubt, 'Banbury tarts, quaking pudding and gooseberry fool'.

The 18th century saw the development of menus on a grand scale. Even folk a little down the social scale such as the urban upper middle class entertained in some style. An English parson records that for a formal dinner he served, in addition to a lengthy list of fishes, chicken, mutton, pigeon, veal and sweetbreads — 'apricot tart and in the middle a pyramid of syllabubs and jellies.'

A famous jelly brand name of more recent times is indisputably Australian. In 1927, a Mr Appleroth was out road-testing his new car when a rather unusual sound overhead caused him to stop, get out of his car and look skywards. The uncommon sight of an aeroplane flying overhead on that day was inspirational — Mr Appleroth immediately turned to family members and said — 'That's what I'll call my new company — *Aeroplane,* above all!'

BUYING AND STORAGE Most jellies are commercially packaged and require only the addition of boiling water. Though they have a long shelf life, watch use-by date. After preparation they should be refrigerated except under very cold conditions.

PREPARATION AND USE If you plan to make your own jellies from scratch, do not expect to achieve the same clarity and jewellike colours as a commercially packaged jelly. If you do not mind a cloudy jelly it is simply a matter of combining strained fruit juice, sugar and water with soaked gelatine and heating until the sugar and gelatine are dissolved. The mixture is then chilled until set.

A shortcut towards clarity involves an additional step. After heating until the sugar and gelatine are dissolved, the lightly beaten white of an egg, together with the crushed, washed shell, is added and the mixture allowed to come to the boil. The pan is removed from the heat for a minute or two and then allowed to come to the boil twice more. Some of the solids in the liquid adhere to the egg white and shell and when these are skimmed from the liquid, the result is a clearer jelly.

For a really clear, sparkling colour, the same technique is used but the jelly is poured several times through a special cloth jelly bag. Fruits may be set in or stirred through jellies before setting, but avoid fresh pineapple and kiwi fruit which will not allow jellies to set. With all fruit, pat dry before adding to jelly for best results.

VARIETIES
There are many, including jelly whip, one of the simplest ways of making a delicious light dessert. To prepare it, you will need to have chilled in advance 1½ cups of cream or evaporated milk. Make up a commercial jelly with half the recommended water (usually 1 cup) and chill until the jelly is wobbly but not quite set. Whip the cream or evaporated milk until thick, then beat in the not-quite-set jelly. Chill until quite set.

Milk Pudding

MAJOR NUTRIENTS

		CUSTARD, NO EGGS SERVE SIZE 50 ML	
Energy	250 kJ	Sodium	35 mg
Protein	3 g	Potassium	85 mg
Fat	3 g	Calcium	70 mg
Cholesterol	8 mg	Phosphorus	55 mg
Carbohydrate	8 g	Vitamin A	20 µg
Total Sugars	5 g	Riboflavin	0.1 mg
Dietary Fibre	0	Niacin Equiv.	1.2 mg

NUTRITIONAL INFORMATION A moderate source of calcium, phosphorus, vitamin A, riboflavin and niacin. Useful product to increase daily food intake. Can be made with reduced fat milk or skim milk to reduce total fat and cholesterol levels.

DESCRIPTION Milk puddings are set during cooking by the action of eggs or by adding junket (rennet) tablets. Various ingredients and flavourings are added to give a wide range of results in these desserts.

ORIGIN AND HISTORY Though some may bear little resemblance to today's recipes, it is clear that puddings made with milk have played a part in the human diet for many centuries. We read that in the early Middle Ages a wealthy Indian might have as his final course a drink made by boiling milk to reduce it somewhat and then adding sugar and honey and colouring with saffron. In Europe during the Middle Ages a commonly prepared item was a milky jelly called 'frumenty', made by soaking husked wheat in hot water. This was sometimes eaten with milk and honey, providing a nourishing item in a diet which one

is forced to admit was otherwise rather uninspiring.

As the centuries passed, milk became an important ingredient in much more refined desserts. By the mid-17th century the value of the formerly humble egg had been acknowledged. It can be assumed that recipes combining these two basic ingredients brought about the development of many of the desserts we still prepare today.

PREPARATION AND USE All milk puddings must be cooked with care to avoid spoiling their delicate texture. Those using eggs to set them are particularly sensitive to overheating. The flavour, consistency and smoothness of a custard depends on the egg yolk. If overheated, the coagulated egg albumen hardens and the mixture separates or curdles. Junket, using rennet as the setting agent, will separate if the milk is not at the correct blood heat when it is poured on the dissolved junket tablet.

A basic *baked custard* is a simple mixture of eggs, milk, sugar and usually a flavouring essence such as vanilla. Like all baked custards it is cooked in a dish which sits in another dish containing water (a water bath) to better regulate the gentle heat required to set a custard successfully.

As its name suggests, *bread and butter custard* has small pieces of buttered bread floating on top of a prepared custard, buttered side up. Sultanas are sometimes added to the basic custard mixture. The custard is placed in a water bath and is cooked when set and the bread lightly browned and hopefully a little crisp around the edges of the dish. A little butter dabbed around the edge of the dish before cooking will sometimes encourage the crisping of the outside pieces of bread.

Crème brûlée is a very rich custard indeed. Made with cream instead of milk and with 4 egg yolks to little more than 2 cups of cream, it is cooked in a double saucepan and not allowed to reach boiling point at any stage. It is strained into a fireproof dish and allowed to stand for some hours. The cream is then dusted with a thin layer of caster sugar which is allowed to caramelise slightly under a heated griller. When cool it is usually served with cooked fruit as it is rather rich to eat on its own.

VARIETIES
Apart from the desserts mentioned above, and the countless variations available worldwide, the following are given as examples.

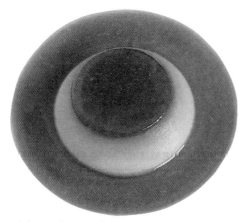

Crème Caramel

MAJOR NUTRIENTS SERVE SIZE 75 G

Energy	420 kJ	Potassium	110 mg
Protein	4 g	Calcium	70 mg
Fat	4 g	Phosphorus	90 mg
Cholesterol	95 mg	Iron	0.5 mg
Carbohydrate	13 g	Niacin Equiv.	1 mg
Total Sugars	13 g	Vitamin A	45 μg
Dietary Fibre	0	Riboflavin	0.15 mg
Sodium	56 mg		

NUTRITIONAL INFORMATION An excellent source of phosphorus; moderate source of protein, calcium, iron, vitamin A, niacin and riboflavin. Contains large amounts of cholesterol from eggs and whole milk. If made from whole milk and eggs, fats contribute about 35% of total energy. With controlled portion size this type of dessert is often lower in total energy than other common specialty products. If cream is added to milk, fat levels will increase. Can be made with fat-reduced milks if sugar levels are maintained.

DESCRIPTION This is a rich custard which, when cooked and chilled, is turned out into a serving dish to reveal a caramel syrup surrounding the custard.

ORIGIN AND HISTORY The Roman writer Apicius gave a recipe for tripartina (so called because it consisted of three ingredients) made with milk, honey and eggs, to be cooked over a slow fire until thickened. This obviously describes what we would call a custard and is probably one of the earliest of such recipes available. The fact that it is recommended that the finished dish should be peppered before serving does strike a strange note with us but does not alter the fact that it is still a custard.

Crème caramel, with its delicate but delicious flavour, was probably invented some time later, possibly during the early 19th century when sugar, and the confectionery that could be prepared with it, was all the rage. Caramelised sugar would no doubt have been recognised as an ideal flavouring for various desserts and particularly those made with milk.

BUYING AND STORAGE A type of commercial caramel custard is sometimes available but though a good product, it is vastly more satisfying to make your own. Always store custards in the refrigerator. However, they tend to lose their initial fine texture on standing, so are best eaten the day they are made.

PREPARATION AND USE The caramel base for the custard is prepared by melting caster sugar until it begins to change colour. It is then stirred until a good even brown. Taking care to protect the hands (the dish will be very hot indeed), pour the caramel into a heated soufflé dish or cake pan. Quickly turn the dish about to coat the bottom and sides evenly with the caramel. A rich egg custard is made and poured into the prepared dish. Stand the dish in a water bath, cover loosely with a piece of baking paper and bake in a moderately slow to moderate oven until set. Refrigerate for several hours or overnight before turning out. Serve alone or with a little pouring cream.

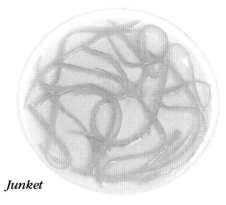

Junket

MAJOR NUTRIENTS SERVE SIZE 100 G

Energy	380 kJ	Potassium	150 mg
Protein	3 g	Calcium	120 mg
Fat	4 g	Phosphorus	95 mg
Cholesterol	14 mg	Vitamin A	35 μg
Carbohydrate	10 g	Riboflavin	0.2 mg
Total Sugars	5 g	Niacin Equiv.	1.1 mg
Dietary Fibre	0	Vitamin C	1.5 mg
Sodium	50 mg		

NUTRITIONAL INFORMATION An excellent source of phosphorus and calcium. Good source of riboflavin and moderate source of niacin, vitamins A and C. Easily digested dessert, which contains all the nutrients of the milk used. Energy level and cholesterol content can be reduced by using lower fat milk. Additional flavours such as cocoa powder will slightly alter the total energy value.

DESCRIPTION Junket is made by setting milk to a very soft consistency with rennet in the form of junket tablets.

ORIGIN AND HISTORY Rennet is made from the lining of the stomach of unweaned calves, and since it is known that in prehistoric times milk was sometimes carried by itinerants and shepherds in dried pouches made of such things, it is entirely possible that the first junket was made inadvertently.

BUYING AND STORAGE It is unlikely that junket has ever been marketed in any form other than its chief ingredient, rennet or junket tablets. Once prepared, junket should ideally be kept at room temperature, though a hot climate requires that it be eaten shortly after its preparation. Refrigeration tends to toughen the curds in junket and allow it to disintegrate to some extent.

PREPARATION AND USE The best possible advice on the first step towards the perfect junket comes from Constance Spry and Rosemary Hume in *The Constance Spry Cookbook*: 'Ideally the milk should be warm from the cow.' We may rarely get this great opportunity but should it present itself we have the perfect blood-heat temperature at which to begin. A junket tablet is quickly crushed with a little cold water in the bowl in which the junket will be served, and the milk, at blood heat and lightly sweetened, is poured immediately onto the dissolved tablet. A quick stir, then the dish is left undisturbed in a reasonably warm place to set — not with applied heat, but away from cold draughts.

Traditionally junket was never flavoured, but most cooks now add a little vanilla and a sprinkling of grated nutmeg. Some old recipes suggest adding a dash of brandy. Others suggest pouring over the junket a little thick cream once the junket is set. These last two suggestions begin to remove this simple dessert from its sometime category of invalid food.

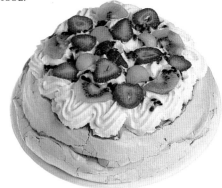

Pavlova and Meringue

MAJOR NUTRIENTS MERINGUE
SERVE SIZE 30 G

Energy	110 kJ	Total Sugars	27 g
Protein	less than 1 g	Sodium	10 mg
Fat	0	Potassium	10 mg
Carbohydrate	27 g		

NUTRITIONAL INFORMATION Contains no fat and no cholesterol. The main energy contribution comes from cream or ice cream fillings, which are added on to the base analysed above.

If filled with mainly fruit mixes and moderate amounts of ice cream, it makes an interesting, low fat dessert.

DESCRIPTION Pavlovas and meringues are light, airy desserts made by cooking combined egg whites and sugar and are usually served with either fruits, sweet sauces or flavoured cream. Floating Island calls for the uncooked meringue to be poached, rather than baked.

ORIGIN AND HISTORY Perhaps the greatest ever devotee of the sweets course would be Queen Elizabeth I of England. It has been written that she was a sweet-tooth extraordinaire and always carried candies with her in the folds of her gown. It seems that she doted on meringues, which became known as 'kisses' because she kissed the 'faire cloth' of the table that held them.

There are two theories concerning the inventor of the Pavlova. By far the most popular is that Herbert Sachse, a former shearers' cook but then chef at the now demolished Hotel Esplanade in Perth, was requested to prepare something very special for an elegant afternoon tea. The year was 1935, and with memories of the visit of the famous ballerina Pavlova to Perth in 1929, he decided to prepare something worthy of the lady's name. He experimented for a month and the now famous Pavlova dessert was the result. The second theory is that Pavlova was the invention of a New Zealand chef.

BUYING AND STORAGE Both pavlovas and meringues may be bought, though the homemade variety is almost invariably superior. Whether bought or homemade these rather delicate items can be kept, well covered in a dry atmosphere, for a few days.

PREPARATION AND USE There are two schools of thought about the best method of preparing meringues. Some recipes suggest beating egg whites until stiff but not dry, adding first a little sugar and beating well until the sugar dissolves, then adding the remaining sugar and beating until it also dissolves completely. Other recipes toss all ingredients into the bowl and beat until the mixture is thick and satiny. Cream of tartar or a little salt is sometimes added to help strengthen the egg whites. Most methods of cooking suggest a moderate oven to commence, with reduced heat for the bulk of the cooking time. Others recommend a very slow oven for the entire

cooking time. Meringues may be lightly coloured if desired and flavoured with vanilla, almond or other essences. When joined together with whipped cream they are known as kisses. The surface of cooked meringues should be crisp and not sticky.

Pavlova recipes are many and varied. The main ingredients of a traditional pavlova are always egg whites and sugar and usually one or more of the following — cream of tartar, cornflour, vinegar and lemon juice. By contrast, the all-in-together pavlova has the added ingredient of boiling water. The cornflour is added to prevent the mixture from running and to produce the typical crisp crust with the pleasantly soft, marshmallowy centre. Vinegar and lemon juice also help to produce the marshmallow centre of the pavlova.

Pavlova is usually topped with a quantity of whipped cream and fresh or canned fruit. Fruits that have a pleasant tartness such as berries and passionfruit are a perfect foil for the sweetness of pavlova.

VARIETIES
Among the many possibilities is Floating Island, a delicately flavoured dessert, part of which is a simple meringue mixture of egg whites and sugar, with the sugar gradually beaten into the well whipped egg whites. The meringue is poached in milk which has been flavoured with vanilla and sweetened with sugar. A rich stirred custard is prepared in advance and cooled. The 'islands' of poached meringue are floated on the custard. The dish is chilled, then sprinkled with toasted slivered or flaked almonds before serving.

Pie and Tart

DESCRIPTION A dessert pie is a dish or plate of fruit enclosed in, or simply covered by pastry and baked in an oven. In place of a pastry lid, a pie may be covered by a crumble-type topping or meringue. Baklava, while not exactly a pie, has certain similarities which qualify it for inclusion here. Made from layers of filo pastry, this Middle Eastern delicacy is usually cut in diamond shapes. Strudel is a Bavarian dessert now popular the world over. Few people these days make their own strudel pastry, using commercial filo pastry instead. Like a Swiss roll, the pastry is rolled up to enclose the filling. The tart is a layer of pastry covered by fruit or other filling and left uncovered.

ORIGIN AND HISTORY An interesting fact

to be learned from the Roman era is that pastry, or rather the pie, tended to serve a dual purpose. Since most Romans ate with their fingers, sauces could be a problem. A good practical example of using pastry like a spoon is included in writings of the time describing a tart served 'with a mixture of some wonderful Spanish wine and hot honey.' A guest took a 'fat helping of the tart and scooped up the honey generously.'

Medieval pies were equally interesting. We read of a herring pie — a stew composed of pickled fish, raisins, currants, dates and cinnamon placed in a 'coffin', that is, a pastry blanket, and baked. Another, served in the court of Charles VI of France, consisted of three partridges, six quails, a dozen skylarks, thrushes and diced bacon mixed with 'verjus' — a kind of vinegar made of green grapes or apples.

We read of pies served at banquets, which, when the crust was removed, revealed live birds, which — happily — flew out and about the banquet table much to the delight of the guests. Even more bizarre was the pie served at a 15th century 'pheasant feast' which contained twenty-eight live persons playing different instruments!

As the centuries passed, with greater refinements in not only the flour, but also the recipes and the ovens in which the pies were cooked, it was the Italians who were credited with turning pastry making into a fine art, but the English who were acknowledged as Europe's finest pie makers. During the Elizabethan era pies as we know them would not have rated a mention. Pies for an Elizabethan banquet were masterpieces of architectural beauty — sometimes 'whole castles of pastry'.

BUYING AND STORAGE Pies and tarts can be bought frozen, or ready made and hot. Check the use-by date.

PREPARATION AND USE For a *two-crust pie* a little more than half the pastry is usually used as the base, the filling is added and the remaining pastry becomes the top, covering the filling. Baking is usually in a hot oven.

For a *single crust pie* the filling is placed in the pie plate and covered by a single sheet of pastry.

A *crumble-topped pie* has a base of pastry but in place of a pastry top it has a covering of either a mixture of a fat rubbed into flour with added sugar and spices, or, in place of the flour, a cereal — either raw (rolled oats) or cooked (corn flakes, rice bubbles, biscuit crumbs) — or possibly coconut combined with an egg and sugar.

A tart is made with pastry, sometimes previously baked, then topped by fruit.

VARIETIES

The varieties of dessert pies and tarts are too numerous to mention. They include cheesecake, flan, baklava and strudel — every country having its range of delicacies. The example below is just one of many.

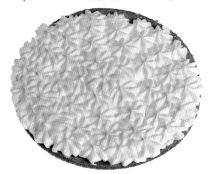

Lemon Meringue Pie

MAJOR NUTRIENTS		COMMERCIAL, PACKET SERVE SIZE 75 G	
Energy	1020 kJ	Dietary Fibre	
Protein	3 g		less than 1 g
Fat	11 g	Sodium	150 mg
Cholesterol	70 mg	Potassium	60 mg
Carbohydrate	34 g	Phosphorus	65 mg
Total Sugars	18 g	Vitamin E	0.5 mg
		Vitamin D	0.5 μg

NUTRITIONAL INFORMATION A moderate source of vitamins E and D; high in fat and cholesterol. Contains a range of important nutrients, but fat contributes 40% of energy and so this is a dessert to use after a lighter main course. May contain food colouring, usually 102 and 110, and permitted emulsifiers and thickeners.

DESCRIPTION This is a pie with a pastry base and a cooked filling covered with a meringue topping.

ORIGIN AND HISTORY The method for preparing this kind of pie is as old as that of making pastry. For these pies the pastry is often baked first, the filling being cooked separately and then poured into the pie shell.

BUYING AND STORAGE Mixtures for desserts such as this are sold in packets, and they are also available frozen. When a pastry shell is baked without a filling it is best baked 'blind'. The pastry is pressed into the pie plate, covered with a sheet of crumpled greaseproof or baking paper and weighted with dried beans or rice. After baking in a hot oven the pastry is cooled and the filling added. Sugar and cornflour are blended with water (sometimes milk) and lemon juice and cooked until thickened. After removal from the heat, egg yolks and lemon rind (and in some cases a little butter) are stirred through, giving a little extra beating to melt the butter, if added. Cool the filling a little before pouring into the cooked pie shell. The egg whites are beaten with sugar to form the meringue which is spread evenly over, completely covering the filling. The meringue should touch the pastry crust all round, or else the meringue may shrink.

The pie is then baked in a moderate oven for 10–15 minutes until set and lightly browned.

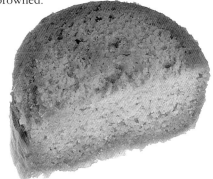

Self-saucing Pudding

MAJOR NUTRIENTS		SERVE SIZE 75 G	
Energy	780 kJ	Sodium	325 mg
Protein	5 g	Potassium	65 mg
Fat	5 g	Phosphorus	150 mg
Cholesterol	85 mg	Iron	0.5 mg
Carbohydrate	32 g	Vitamin A	75 μg
Total Sugars	16 g	Thiamin	0.05 mg
Dietary Fibre		Niacin Equiv.	1.1 mg
	less than 1 g		

NUTRITIONAL INFORMATION An excellent source of phosphorus; good source of vitamin A; moderate source of protein, iron, thiamin and niacin. Popular family dessert which is not excessive in kilojoules or fat content. Other flavours will have similar nutrient content, except chocolate will be slightly higher in fats and iron.

DESCRIPTION Self-saucing puddings consist of a cake topping with sauce beneath.

ORIGIN AND HISTORY The strange method of preparing this type of pudding leads one to speculate on how it came about that a quantity of liquid should be added at the last minute to what must surely have looked already like a finished mixture. Could it be that the forgetful cook incorrectly added a second quantity of liquid with the result that it settled out as a sauce, sinking to the bottom of the pudding?

BUYING AND STORAGE Packaged self-saucing puddings are available in supermarkets. Store in a cool, dry place and check use-by date. Homemade puddings are best eaten the day they are cooked and while still warm.

PREPARATION AND USE A simple cake mixture is prepared and turned into an ovenproof dish. The desired flavouring is sprinkled over the top of the cake mixture and then hot water, fruit juice or tea is poured over, depending on the flavouring used. When cooked, the dessert has a moist cake topping with sauce beneath.

For *chocolate sauce pudding* a mixture of brown sugar and cocoa is sprinkled over the pudding mixture, followed by hot water. Brown sugar and hot coffee produce the *coffee sauce pudding*. For a fruit variation, either chopped prunes or dates are included in the actual cake mixture and to provide the sauce, brown sugar is sprinkled over the cake and strong, hot tea poured over.

VARIETIES

Chocolate; coffee; fruit; packaged varieties.

Soufflé and Mousse

NUTRITIONAL INFORMATION The nutritional value of a soufflé depends upon the number of eggs used. If a mousse is cream-based, it will be very high in energy, fat and cholesterol. Mousses can be almost entirely fruit-based, and produced with a lower kilojoule level.

DESCRIPTION Soufflé and mousse are light-textured desserts which owe their considerable volume to eggs. They may be served hot straight from the oven or chilled, depending on the preparation method. Their chief flavouring ingredient may be fruit, fruit juice, a puree of nuts, chocolate, coffee, one of a variety of essences, a liqueur or spirits.

ORIGIN AND HISTORY A foretaste of the simple fruit mousse of today is reflected in a recipe from a publication of 1658 by the physician to England's king, Charles I. The recipe, apple cream, uses sweetened spiced apples cooked in rose wine, pureed and set with gelatine. When they begin to set, whipped cream is folded through and the dessert chilled until firm.

Baked soufflés similar to those of today were apparently being served late in the 18th century in one of the most prestigious of Paris restaurants, La Grande Taverne de Londres. In earlier centuries soufflé making was difficult until Count Rumford, an American-born scientist, greatly acclaimed in Europe for his innovative approach to all things culinary, finally developed an oven which, with the use of flues, dampers and other attachments (soon to be part of all household ranges), solved the problem of uneven heat. After that the soufflé could be baked with much improved chances of success.

BUYING AND STORAGE These desserts are made at home and usually served at once.

PREPARATION AND USE Though the fine line between the mousse and the soufflé has become rather blurred, if one were to describe the traditional difference it would be that a mousse would have a smoother, more creamy texture than a soufflé. This is the result of the combination of egg yolks with proportionately more whipped cream and frequently less egg white — sometimes, none at all. Soufflés are frequently baked and served hot; a mousse recipe, though it may have some of the ingredients cooked briefly (eggs or fruit), is not usually baked. Either may be served in one or several individual dishes, often with a 'collar' which helps the soufflé to rise evenly during cooking and the uncooked mousse mixture to be poured above the rim of the dish; the collar is removed once the gelatine mixture is set.

VARIETIES

Apricot Soufflé This soufflé, made by a much simpler method, uses only the whites of eggs and results in a rather more delicate mixture which will not stand after preparation and must be eaten as soon as it comes from the oven.

Dried apricots are soaked until plump in hot water, then pureed. A light meringue is made with egg whites and sugar, the apricots are stirred through and the mixture turned into a greased soufflé dish and cooked in a moderate oven. Serve immediately.

Chocolate Soufflé The method of preparation for this baked soufflé involves stirring flour into melted butter in a double saucepan. Milk is added and heated until thickened. Grated chocolate and sugar is stirred through and the mixture allowed to cool a little. Beaten egg yolks are added, followed by separately beaten egg whites. The mixture is poured gently into a greased dish with a collar and the soufflé is baked in a moderate oven.

Note: This soufflé may be prepared ahead of time and refrigerated, uncovered, or frozen, covered with foil or plastic wrap. The refrigerated soufflé will need about 15 minutes extra cooking time and if frozen, about 20 minutes longer.

Lemon Mousse (or Soufflé) This is an unbaked mixture, though egg yolks are cooked briefly on the range top over a gentle heat with sugar, lemon juice and rind until thickened. Dissolved gelatine is added, followed by lightly whipped cream and lastly, whipped egg whites. The mixture is poured into the usual collared dish and allowed to set. When the collar is removed, this type of mousse is often decorated on top with cream and may have chopped nuts pressed into the sides above the edge of the dish.

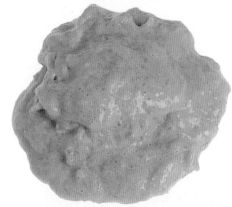

Mango Mousse The simplest form of this dessert requires none of the ingredients to be cooked. Only the gelatine is heated to dissolve it before it is combined with mango pulp. Fruit juice may be added — orange, or a mixture of orange and lemon are the most popular. As the mixture thickens, sweetened whipped egg white and cream are stirred through. Chill to set.

Steamed or Boiled Pudding

DESCRIPTION Steamed puddings are traditionally cooked in covered basins in a water bath. Their appearance and colour will depend on the ingredients used, varying from rich fruit puddings (Christmas or plum pudding) to light steamed puddings (ginger pudding).

ORIGIN AND HISTORY All steamed puddings would appear to be distant relatives of the original plum (or Christmas) pudding. The ingredients of the latter were no doubt beyond the purse of most and the result seems to have been the gradual shedding of the more expensive items until it has become little more than a cake or sponge mixture imaginatively flavoured with ingredients within the reach of all.

BUYING AND STORAGE Good quality canned fruit puddings are available in supermarkets. Store in cool, dry conditions and check the use-by date. Light steamed puddings are best eaten the day they are cooked. To store, cover well and refrigerate.

PREPARATION AND USE These puddings usually have the basic ingredients of plain or self-raising flour, a fat (butter, margarine, oil or, more rarely, suet), sugar, eggs (though not always), dried or fresh fruit and sometimes grated carrot or apple. Spices may be added, or a variety of flavouring ingredients such as vanilla or other flavouring essences, coffee, cocoa, fruit juices or syrups. The fats may be rubbed into dry ingredients or creamed with sugar. For steamed puddings the final mixture is usually turned into a well-covered pudding basin. Small moulds for individual serves may also be used. The pudding basin is placed in a very large saucepan or boiler with a quantity of water and steamed.

When a Christmas pudding is cooked in a cloth instead of a basin, it is boiled directly in water. The same method is used for what is now probably a rarely cooked family dessert — jam roly-poly. A pastry roll, filled with jam, is wrapped in a cloth and boiled. If made now, it is usually baked in the oven with a sugar syrup, jam or fruit sauce poured over during cooking to give a pleasantly crisp crust.

VARIETIES

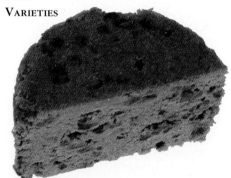

Christmas Pudding

MAJOR NUTRIENTS			**SERVE SIZE 50 G**
Energy	700 kJ	Sodium	85 mg
Protein	2 g	Potassium	220 mg
Fat	6 g	Iron	0.8 mg
Cholesterol	30 mg	Niacin Equiv.	1 mg
Carbohydrate	29 g	Vitamin A	65 µg
Total Sugars	23 g	Vitamin E	0.5 mg
Dietary Fibre	2 g		

NUTRITIONAL INFORMATION A good source of iron; moderate source of niacin, vitamins A and E. Rich traditional pudding but, although filled with dried fruit, this does not contribute significant vitamins and minerals in the quantity of pudding consumed.

DESCRIPTION A Christmas pudding, also called plum pudding, is traditionally dark in colour and rich with dried fruits. Its appearance and texture will depend on the particular ingredients added. The same mixture may be cooked in small, individual pudding moulds.

ORIGIN AND HISTORY The original Christmas pudding started life in the Middle Ages as a type of porridge, served as a first course with meats. Gradually its consistency became thicker until it finally moved to the dessert end of the meal, minus meat but retaining the suet which traditionalists still use instead of the now more popular butter. The first published recipe for plum pudding that we would recognise appeared in 1675. It is interesting to note that the Puritans outlawed the pudding as being 'sinfully rich'. No mention of the addition of silver coins is found in the 17th century version of the recipe.

BUYING AND STORAGE Canned Christmas puddings may be bought and should be stored in a cool, dry place. Remember to check the use-by date. Homemade Christmas puddings should keep for some time after cooking, particularly if some spirit (rum, brandy) has been added. However the pudding should be kept in a cool, airy place. Those cooked in a pudding cloth should be hung suspended in mid-air.

PREPARATION AND USE For best results soak dried fruits in rum or brandy for some hours or overnight. If grated suet is used, it is added to the flour with the spices, sugar (brown or white) and prepared fruit, along with the spirits in which they were soaked. The eggs should be well beaten before adding to the mixture, and the breadcrumbs (if used) and nuts stirred through. Some recipes include grated carrot or apple. If using the creaming method with butter or margarine in place of suet, this should be the first operation; eggs are then beaten in one at a time, followed by flour and spices, breadcrumbs and nuts and finally the soaked fruit with the spirits. If using breadcrumbs, the mixture should be allowed to stand for at least half an hour. Use a pudding basin lowered into boiling water in a very large saucepan. Cover and boil gently for the length of time given in the recipe. To reheat for serving, the pudding should be lowered into boiling water, covered and boiled for an hour. Serve with brandy or hard sauce, rich egg custard or cream.

Ginger Pudding

MAJOR NUTRIENTS		SERVE SIZE 75 G	
Energy	1080 kJ	Sodium	230 mg
Protein	4 g	Potassium	65 mg
Fat	12 g	Calcium	160 mg
Cholesterol	80 mg	Phosphorus	140 mg
Carbohydrate	34 g	Iron	1 mg
Total Sugars	17 g	Vitamin A	120 µg
Dietary Fibre	0	Niacin Equiv.	1 mg

NUTRITIONAL INFORMATION An excellent source of calcium and phosphorus and vitamin A; moderate source of protein and niacin. Contains large amounts of fat and cholesterol. A high carbohydrate dessert, with fat levels contributing over 40% of energy.

DESCRIPTION This is a light pudding. Steaming rather than baking gives this style of pudding a pleasantly spongy texture.

ORIGIN AND HISTORY This type of steamed pudding probably evolved as a scaled-down version of the traditional Christmas pudding.

BUYING AND STORAGE Leftovers tend to dry out quickly. If possible reheat very briefly by microwave for best results. Otherwise serve heated with a little custard or fruit sauce.

PREPARATION AND USE This type of pudding is prepared by creaming the fat and sugar, adding one or two well-beaten eggs, flavourings or spices, and folding in flour and liquid alternately before turning into a greased mould, covering with several layers of greased paper or foil and steaming. The powdered ginger used to flavour this pudding could be replaced by finely chopped glacé or crystallised ginger. Serve hot with custard or cream.

MILK PRODUCTS

All mammals produce milk in one form or another. Those utilised worldwide by man are very diverse, and include milk from cows, sheep, goats, horses, reindeer, yaks, water buffalos and camels.

It is impossible to identify when the use of animals' milk as a food source commenced, but it is reasonable to assume it coincided with the domestication of animals, around a million years ago. Milk is a complex mixture of fats, proteins, sugar and various other elements. Variations in the milk content of animals relate to the needs of their offspring. When buying milk, check the use-by date and the condition of the packaging. Milk purchased in bottles and plastic containers should not be left exposed to light even in cold conditions, as light and oxygen can act to the detriment of the product. Generally it is best to purchase milk daily and to store it away from strong-smelling foods, with the container properly closed.

Serve or use straight from the refrigerator, without allowing the milk to stand in warmth, or bright light.

Milk is an excellent source of readily absorbed calcium and phosphorus. Milk, cheese and yoghurt provide up to 75% of the calcium in Western diets. Two to 3 glasses of milk are recommended daily, particularly for growing children, and for pregnant and lactating women. The calcium–phosphorus balance in milk is ideal for building strong bones and teeth. In addition, milk is a good source of high quality protein, vitamins A and B (especially riboflavin) and moderate amounts of magnesium, zinc and sodium.

Whole milk is high in saturated fat and contains moderate amounts of cholesterol. For control of blood cholesterol, milks with reduced fat are recommended. Processing such as pasteurising, homogenising, sterilising (as in long life milk), drying or evaporating, has little effect on nutritional value. Pasteurising, a short heat treatment to kill harmful bacteria, is necessary for all milks. Pasteurised milk is produced by heating milk to 72°C for 15 seconds and then rapidly cooling to 4°C. The pathogenic (disease-carrying) organisms are destroyed and the milk will keep for about 1 week in the refrigerator. Ultra heat treated (UHT) products are heated to 142°C for 2 seconds. This destroys more micro-organisms than pasteurisation. UHT products, unopened, have a shelf life of several months without refrigeration. Once opened they should be refrigerated and treated in the same way as the pasteurised products.

Some people suffer an intolerance to lactose and while avoiding milk they may tolerate fermented milk products such as cheese, yoghurt and buttermilk.

It is a widely held belief that milk produces mucus; it is thus avoided by many people who suffer from congestion in the nose and bronchial tubes. But research has not detected any association between milk and mucus production. Milk drinks are considered to be sleep-promoting, and research has indicated that there are substances in milk and other foods which influence sleep.

One point which needs to be emphasised is that it is extremely difficult to reach the recommended dietary intake of calcium without including milk, cheese and/or yoghurt in the diet. The dairy industry has responded to the need for lower fat levels, and a range of foods which have less fat is available, with nutritional information provided. There is no reason to avoid dairy products in order to reduce fat intake, as these foods are the major source of calcium and riboflavin in the diet.

This chapter includes milk products other than butter and cheese. A separate chapter is devoted to cheese, and butter is included with the fats and oils.

Aerosol Cream

also called Pressure pack cream

MAJOR NUTRIENTS — SERVE SIZE 40 G

Energy	380 kJ	Cholesterol	30 mg
Protein	1 g	Sodium	20 mg
Fat	9 g	Vitamin A	75 µg
Carbohydrate	1 g		

NUTRITIONAL INFORMATION For nutritional information see Cream.

DESCRIPTION Reduced (25% butterfat) cream, sterilised and packed under pressure. The air pressure within the can creates the soft 'whipped' appearance of the cream.

ORIGIN AND HISTORY The idea came directly from the USA to New Zealand, in the early 1960s, and then to Europe. It has remained popular because of its convenience. However, it has never been marketed strongly in Australia, and nowadays aerosol cream is imported from New Zealand.

BUYING AND STORAGE Make sure the can is sealed and undamaged. Check the use-by date, and store in the refrigerator, as for regular cream.

PREPARATION AND USE Aerosol creams are generally used for decoration purposes and are an ideal convenience cream for quick and easy aerated cream patterns as required.

Refrigerate until required and use well chilled. Always shake the can well before use.

Buttermilk

MAJOR NUTRIENTS — SERVE SIZE 250 ML

Energy	400 kJ	Potassium	390 mg
Protein	9 g	Calcium	295 mg
Fat	2 g	Phosphorus	220 mg
Carbohydrate	11 g	Magnesium	35 mg
Cholesterol	n/a	Thiamin	0.1 mg
Sodium	210 mg	Riboflavin	0.4 mg

NUTRITIONAL INFORMATION Similar in nutritional value to skim milk except the fat content may be slightly higher, varying from 0.2% to 0.8%. In processing, the protein in buttermilk is partially digested, so buttermilk is preferred by some people with digestive problems. For nutritional information see Skim Milk.

DESCRIPTION A cultured milk product made from pasteurised skim milk. Low fat. Mildly acidic with a creamy taste and thick consistency.

ORIGIN AND HISTORY Buttermilk must have been discovered long ago during the churning of naturally soured cream to make butter. It was the liquid that remained once the butter was formed — hence its name. These days, because commercial butter is made from sweet cream (i.e. fresh cream as it comes off the separator), buttermilk is made by adding special cultures to skim milk; hence it is usually sold as 'cultured buttermilk'.

BUYING AND STORAGE It is sold in cartons. Always check the use-by date of the carton and ensure it is correctly sealed. Buttermilk will last unopened in the refrigerator for approximately 15 days. Once opened it should be used within a week or so. Buttermilk should have a refreshing acidic taste. It must be kept sealed to avoid tainting by other stronger foods.

Do not shake the carton and do not freeze, since the curd will be broken and its texture altered.

PREPARATION AND USE Keep refrigerated until needed. Use for blending low kilojoule milkshakes containing fresh fruits in season, or use in soups. Blend with fruit juices. Especially good with orange, strawberry, lemon and pineapple. It may be used as a milk substitute in baking of, e.g., breads or cakes.

Canned Reduced Cream

NUTRITIONAL INFORMATION This cream has a reduced fat content of 25%.

DESCRIPTION Canned reduced cream is a long life product which is canned and sterilised. The temperature used during sterilisation acts to thicken the cream by coagulating some of the protein.

ORIGIN AND HISTORY Before World War II, cream was sterilised in glass bottles and had 45% fat content. In 1951, a new canned cream was introduced with a minimum of 23% fat, which tasted less 'oily'. Canned reduced cream is one of Nestlé's oldest products on the market and is now the only long life reduced cream sold in Australia.

BUYING AND STORAGE Look for cans that are clean and properly cared for (e.g. undented), on supermarket shelves. As it is a long life product, it may be stored in the pantry or cupboard for many months without refrigeration until opened. Once opened, however, store as for fresh cream and keep it in the refrigerator. Use within a few days.

PREPARATION AND USE Canned reduced cream is a handy convenience dairy product to keep in the pantry. Chill before opening and serving.

Despite its unique thick consistency, this product will not whip easily. It can be used in hot dishes, where the usual rules for cooking with cream will apply. Use also as a reduced fat topping for desserts, on fruit salads, or with savoury dishes such as pasta.

Clotted Cream

also called Devonshire cream, Scalded cream

NUTRITIONAL INFORMATION See Cream.

DESCRIPTION A thick mass of cream with a rich nutty taste. It is cream (generally 48% fat) which has been heated to just below boiling point, then cooled.

ORIGIN AND HISTORY The famous cream associated with the ever-popular Devonshire tea is clotted cream which, needless to say, originated in Devon. The old way of making clotted cream was a slow, gentle warming of cream in earthenware bowls which were cooled on stone floors; hence a term often used in reference to clotted cream — stone-cold. In Australia, clotted cream is called scalded cream, and was initially manufactured by Jindivick, in Victoria.

BUYING AND STORAGE Today, clotted cream is no longer manufactured by Jindivick, but it may be available through specialty farmhouse outlets. Buy fresh as required. Clotted cream will last a little longer than pure or regular cream (approximately 12 days). Refrigerate and store well sealed, to prevent tainting by strong-smelling foods in the refrigerator. Look for thick cream which shows no signs of dry aging. It should have a characteristic nutty or scalded taste. It will store for several weeks unopened, and 2 weeks opened. It will not separate during storage.

PREPARATION AND USE Serve from the refrigerator. Use with fresh scones and jam, cakes and pies.

Condensed Milk

MAJOR NUTRIENTS		WHOLE SWEETENED SERVE SIZE 20 G	
Energy	270 kJ	Cholesterol	5 mg
Protein	2 g	Sodium	25 mg
Fat	2 g	Calcium	56 mg
Carbohydrate	11 g	Phosphorus	45 mg

NUTRITIONAL INFORMATION Condensed milks are not suitable substitutes for milk because of the high sugar content and because they provide only a moderate amount of calcium and phosphorus. Whole condensed milk is a moderate source of fat, while skimmed condensed milk contains negligible fat. They are a convenient food for bushwalking, as the high sugar content delays spoilage.

DESCRIPTION Condensed milk is slightly more concentrated than evaporated milk, with the addition of approximately 40% sugar.

ORIGIN AND HISTORY There are two types of condensed milk — sweetened and unsweetened, the latter commonly being called evaporated milk (see separate entry). Condensed milk was developed in the latter part of the 19th century, to provide a milk which required no refrigeration and had an extended life. Today, condensed milk is still popular as a cooking ingredient and milk alternative.

BUYING AND STORAGE Cans should be examined for damage or distortion to ensure that no contamination has occurred. Because of the natural preservative effect of sugar, this product can be stored indefinitely and once opened can be stored unrefrigerated, although reasonable care should be taken to ensure there is no contamination. It is also available in a tube.

PREPARATION AND USE Condensed milk can be reconstituted to approximate milk, using a ratio of 2 parts water to 1 part milk. Milk made in this way will be sweet owing to the added sugars. It is ideal to use in desserts, ice cream, cheesecakes, mayonnaise and some sauces (sweet and sour) because of the sweetness. It also caramelises with ease if simmered for 3–4 hours, for use in recipes requiring a caramel base.

VARIETIES
Condensed skim milk, condensed whole milk.

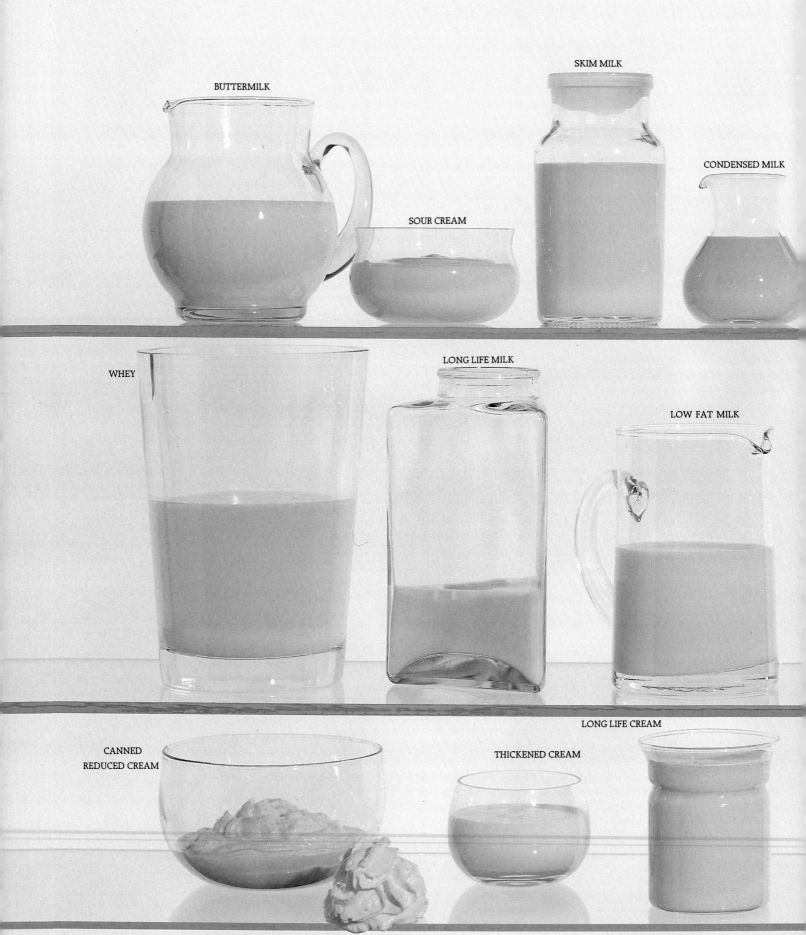

BUTTERMILK

SKIM MILK

CONDENSED MILK

SOUR CREAM

WHEY

LONG LIFE MILK

LOW FAT MILK

LONG LIFE CREAM

CANNED
REDUCED CREAM

THICKENED CREAM

AEROSOL CREAM

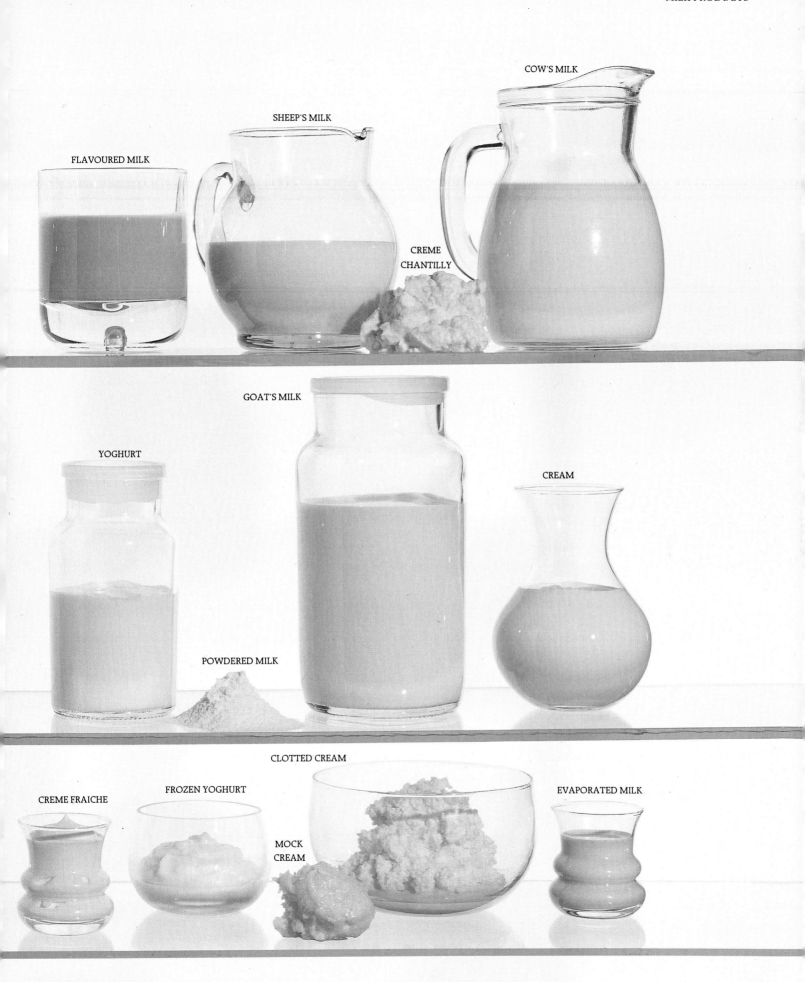

FLAVOURED MILK

SHEEP'S MILK

COW'S MILK

CREME
CHANTILLY

GOAT'S MILK

YOGHURT

CREAM

POWDERED MILK

CLOTTED CREAM

CREME FRAICHE

FROZEN YOGHURT

EVAPORATED MILK

MOCK
CREAM

Cow's Milk

Major Nutrients

Serve Size 250 mL

Energy	680 kJ	Phosphorus	235 mg
Protein	8 g	Zinc	0.7 mg
Fat	10 g	Magnesium	30 mg
Carbohydrate	12 g	Thiamin	0.1 mg
Cholesterol	35 mg	Riboflavin	0.5 mg
Sodium	125 mg	Vitamin B6	0.1 mg
Calcium	300 mg	Vitamin A	75 µg

NUTRITIONAL INFORMATION See the introduction to this chapter.

DESCRIPTION Cow's milk basically consists of water, lactose (milk sugar), proteins, fat, vitamins and minerals. It will have varying butterfat levels according to the breed of cow:

Holstein 3.4–3.7%

Jersey 4.8–5.0%

Guernsey 4.5–5.0%

Shorthorn 3.6–3.8%

Ayrshire 3.8–3.9%

ORIGIN AND HISTORY The cows used for milk production today were developed from breeds which originated in Europe. Settlers introduced them worldwide, and crossbreeding was established to suit environmental requirements. In Australia, the first dairy cattle were brought out by the First Fleet, though only five months after arriving they were lost in the bush. During the early 1800s, cows were regularly imported from Britain to Australia, with the first dairy being established by John Harris, in 1803, in Ultimo, Sydney, NSW. This became the site of one of Australia's largest dairy companies — Dairy Farmers' Co-op.

BUYING AND STORAGE Check the use-by date and the condition of the packaging. Milk purchased in bottles and plastic containers should not be left exposed to light. Store away from strong-smelling foods, with top closed. Stored at 4.5°C, milk will keep for 10 days; at 10°C, it will only last 2½ days.

PREPARATION AND USE Serve or use straight from the refrigerator, without allowing to stand in warmth. Use in drinks, soups, sauces and desserts. Cow's milk is widely used to produce numerous varieties of cheese, butter, and yoghurt.

Cream

Major Nutrients

Devonshire; Clotted or Scalded; Double or Rich Serve Size 40 mL

Energy	740 kJ	Cholesterol	56 mg
Protein	1 g	Sodium	10 mg
Fat	19 g	Vitamin A	170 µg
Carbohydrate	1 g		

NUTRITIONAL INFORMATION This small serve size (2 tablespoons) contains more energy and twice as much fat as 250 mL of whole milk. It also contains half as much cholesterol again as a glass of milk.

Major Nutrients

Light Serve Size 40 mL

Energy	300 kJ	Cholesterol	20 mg
Protein	1 g	Sodium	15 mg
Fat	7 g	Vitamin A	65 µg
Carbohydrate	1 g		

NUTRITIONAL INFORMATION The fat and cholesterol of light cream are less than half those of full cream — but compared with other foods it is still high in these nutrients.

DESCRIPTION Cream is the fat globules which separate from milk. It has, in Australia, a minimum fat content of 35%. Varieties vary in fat content as listed below.

ORIGIN AND HISTORY Since cream naturally separates, and then floats on the balance of the milk, it can be assumed that it was well known to ancient man. As well as its gastronomic use, it has also been used extensively for facials and various pharmaceutical applications.

Cream is naturally a worldwide dairy food and is used to produce not only butter, but also many varieties of cheese. Its popularity in the 1970s and 1980s may have declined with the search for healthy substitutes, such as yoghurt, but its special nature and characteristics ensure its continuing prominence on the market.

BUYING AND STORAGE Check the use-by date and examine the container for any damage. Cream is best consumed as fresh as possible, but it will keep for up to 10 days from date of purchase. It should always be kept refrigerated. Store away from strong-smelling foods and in the coolest part of the refrigerator.

PREPARATION AND USE Keep refrigerated until used. For whipping, cream should be well chilled. It is well suited for inclusion in numerous recipes, particularly noodle dishes and desserts, and is extremely versatile in the kitchen. Use in soups, pour over desserts, use in instant sauces, add to coffee. If cooking with cream, remember to add last, and do not boil.

VARIETIES

Rich cream	48% minimum fat
Pure cream	35% minimum fat
Reduced cream	25% minimum fat
Light cream	18% minimum fat
Extra light cream	12% minimum fat

SEE ALSO Aerosol Cream, Canned Reduced Cream, Clotted Cream, Long Life Cream, Thickened Cream, Whipping Cream.

Crème Chantilly

NUTRITIONAL INFORMATION Crème Chantilly is made from cream, sugar and vanilla, and the nutrients will vary according to the proportions of cream and sugar used.

DESCRIPTION Crème Chantilly is sweetened whipped cream with vanilla added.

ORIGIN AND HISTORY Chantilly takes its name from a French town near Paris, famous for its chateau and its horses. It is likely that crème Chantilly originated here, since the town is also well known for its pastries filled with sweetened whipped cream.

The word 'Chantilly' in culinary contexts indicates that whipped cream is present in a mixture.

BUYING AND STORAGE Crème Chantilly is not generally available on a commercial basis in Australia (although there are similar artificial creams). Crème Chantilly has a shelf life of 7 days once prepared.

PREPARATION AND USE Should be used straight from the refrigerator. Use with desserts, in pastries and eclairs, or as a topping.

Crème Fraîche

NUTRITIONAL INFORMATION This product is high in fat.

DESCRIPTION Crème fraîche in French means simply fresh cream, but in cookery the term has come to mean a mix of sour cream with fresh cream. Alternatively, pure cream can be mixed with buttermilk. It has a 48% fat content and is very rich.

ORIGIN AND HISTORY Crème fraîche originated in France, and has long been produced in Europe. It has become more popular in recent years in Australia and is now produced by several manufacturers.

It is easily made in the home by blending 2 parts pure cream and 1 part sour cream. Leave covered at room temperature for 5–6 hours, then cover and chill in refrigerator. It will store well for up to 10 days.

BUYING AND STORAGE Crème fraîche is available in cartons. Check the use-by date, and examine the container for any damage. Store as for regular cream or sour cream.

PREPARATION AND USE Crème fraîche does not curdle in cooking, and therefore is ideal for sauces that need reducing, and in savoury dishes such as pasta. It is an excellent substitute for yoghurt. Its richness makes it an interesting topping for desserts, fresh fruits and pies.

Evaporated Milk

MAJOR NUTRIENTS

WHOLE
SERVE SIZE 100 mL

Energy	660 kJ	Phosphorus	250 mg
Protein	9 g	Magnesium	28 mg
Fat	9 g	Zinc	1.1 mg
Carbohydrate	11 g	Thiamin	0.05 mg
Cholesterol	35 mg	Riboflavin	0.5 mg
Sodium	180 mg	Vitamin A	90 μg
Calcium	280 mg		

NUTRITIONAL INFORMATION Evaporated milk is simply milk condensed to about 40% of its original volume by evaporation, carried out at a low temperature to avoid damage to the protein, fat and sugar structures and to retain the vitamin make-up. Skimmed evaporated milk is also available, containing negligible fat.

DESCRIPTION A thick, white liquid, homogenised, canned, sterilised and sealed.

ORIGIN AND HISTORY Until the mid-19th century, milk for travellers at sea came from live animals carried on the voyage. The migration patterns and the increase in child passengers encouraged the development of evaporated milk, which has remained largely unchanged except for the introduction of the sweetened variety, listed under Condensed Milk.

BUYING AND STORAGE When purchased, the can should be checked for the use-by date and for any distortions or dents which may indicate poor handling. Canned evaporated milk will keep indefinitely, unopened. Once opened, it should be refrigerated and used fairly quickly. It is advisable to empty the contents into a sealable container to prevent flavour transfer.

PREPARATION AND USE Evaporated milk can be reconstituted by adding 3 parts water to 2 parts evaporated milk. There are slight, although noticeable, differences in colour and taste, and a loss of those vitamins sensitive to heat such as vitamin C and thiamin, but in most practical applications evaporated milk can be used in place of full cream milk. It can be used undiluted to enrich coffee and tea, as a topping, or to bind and moisten minced meat dishes. It is ideal in dips.

Flavoured Milk

MAJOR NUTRIENTS

SERVE SIZE 250 mL

Energy	970 kJ	Cholesterol	25 mg
Protein	10 g	Sodium	45 mg
Fat	4–9 g	Calcium	280 mg
Carbohydrate	27 g	Phosphorus	225 mg

NUTRITIONAL INFORMATION Although no vitamin data are available, will contain similar levels of vitamins and minerals to milk. Milk drinks are made from full cream or reduced fat milks. While they have similar nutritional value to milk they contain sugar and are higher in kilojoules. For nutritional information see the introduction to this chapter.

DESCRIPTION Regular or modified milk with the addition of flavouring substances and modifying agents, with or without sugar and allowable colouring agents.

ORIGIN AND HISTORY People have been flavouring milk for centuries, but commercial flavoured milk, as we know it, was first brought onto the market in half pint bottles in the late 1920s and early 1930s in the USA. The idea spread to Europe through the US Armed Forces during the war years, and was circulated around Europe during the late 1940s. There were numerous flavours in those days owing to the ease of bottling. In Australia, Queensland was the first state to produce flavoured milks, during the late 1960s. They were aimed originally at the teenage market and gained immediate popularity. They are now popular with all age groups, including children. Australia has had greater demand and higher sales than the USA or Europe. The most common flavours produced in Australia are generally chocolate, strawberry and coffee with occasionally new flavours such as caramel (introduced in 1988). There is also a range of long life flavoured milks available — a relatively recent addition to the market in Australia — as well as a range of low or reduced fat flavoured milks.

Interestingly, in Queensland it is the reduced fat varieties which are more popular, owing to the hot climate, whereas in NSW the regular fat flavoured milks are preferred.

BUYING AND STORAGE Look for cartons or bottles which are well sealed and check the use-by date (if applicable). Check there is no leakage and refrigerate as soon as possible after purchase. Store as for regular white milk, in the coolest part of the refrigerator at 4.5°C for best results.

PREPARATION AND USE Serve straight from the fridge, well chilled for the best results, or make into a milkshake by adding ice cream.

Frozen Yoghurt

NUTRITIONAL INFORMATION This yoghurt has 80% less fat than ice cream.

DESCRIPTION The soft serve variety, more common than hard frozen, is similar in texture to soft serve ice cream. It has a delicate creamy taste, with a tang, rather than the sweeter flavour of ice cream. Available as natural yoghurt or with fruit purees.

ORIGIN AND HISTORY Soft serve frozen yoghurt is believed to have been the brainchild of the USA, developed in 1972. It was originally called Frogurt and was introduced during the 'back to nature' craze, which peaked in the 1970s, as the result of requests from a health food shop for a healthy fresh product which would appeal to its young health-orientated customers. Soft serve frozen yoghurt really took off in the United Kingdom and the United States during 1976–1978. In 1977, tentative arrangements were made to market Frogurt in France, Germany and Scandinavia, while another soft serve frozen yoghurt, called Yogsof, appeared on the British market, and a French product called Yogglace claimed to be the best seller in Europe.

Although the soft serve type has had greater success worldwide, it was actually the hard frozen type which appeared first. Sold on a stick, it was first launched onto the market in Australia in 1968, by Oak Hunter Valley Co-op.

The soft serve style took over, and by 1977, eight or so other manufacturers had launched their products. However, the popularity of frozen yoghurt was not sufficient to support all brands, with a gradual decrease in sales. Today, frozen yoghurt has become established as a competitor to ice cream in its own right.

BUYING AND STORAGE The hard frozen style of frozen yoghurt is no longer on the market. Soft serve yoghurt is available in 100 g and 750 g cartons. Frozen yoghurt should be stored in the freezer until required, and should be treated in the same manner as ice cream.

PREPARATION AND USE Frozen yoghurt should be eaten straight from the freezer. However, if it thaws, the nutritional value will not be altered. It can be used in much the same way as ice cream, in milkshakes, with desserts, etc.

VARIETIES
Hard frozen, soft serve.

SEE ALSO Yoghurt.

Goat's Milk

MAJOR NUTRIENTS		SERVE SIZE 250 mL	
Energy	740 kJ	Potassium	450 mg
Protein	8 g	Phosphorus	275 mg
Fat	12 g	Magnesium	50 mg
Carbohydrate	11 g	Zinc	0.7 mg
Cholesterol	28 mg	Thiamin	0.1 mg
Sodium	100 mg	Riboflavin	0.35 mg
Calcium	325 mg	Vitamin A	100 μg

NUTRITIONAL INFORMATION The nutrients are similar to those of cow's milk except that cow's milk contains some folate. Because of the lack of folate, goat's milk is not recommended for infant feeding.

DESCRIPTION Goat's milk is whiter and sweeter than cow's milk. When goat's milk is used to produce cheese, the curd is soft and may need time to settle. The final cheese will be white.

ORIGIN AND HISTORY Goats have an ability to live in inhospitable areas, grazing on arid pastures, and still yield high quality milk. The Saanen breed gives the highest milk yield.

BUYING AND STORAGE In some areas goat's milk may be harder to find than cow's milk owing to the lower production level, and is sold in health food shops, rather than super-markets. It is available in cartons, and also as a powder. Storage as for cow's milk.

PREPARATION AND USE Keep refrigerated until required. Goat's milk may be used as a beverage, particularly for those who find cow's milk hard to digest. It is also used for making yoghurt and cheese.

Long Life Cream

*also called **UHT (ultra high temperature) cream***

NUTRITIONAL INFORMATION See comments on Cream.

DESCRIPTION Cream which has been heated to approximately 135°C for a very short period of time (2–3 seconds) with special care paid to sterile handling. It is packed in cartons lined with aluminium or polythene to exclude all oxygen and light.

ORIGIN AND HISTORY UHT cream was developed in the early 1960s, in the USA, then Europe. The UHT process was designed to reduce heating and therefore lessen the 'cooked' taste familiar in sterilised products. UHT milk was produced in Tasmania in the early 1960s, and by 1965 had begun to be manufactured in Queensland and then the other Australian states.

UHT cream was produced shortly after the UHT milk. It was initially used in industrial areas because of its long life, well before it was used as a commercial cream.

BUYING AND STORAGE Look for UHT cream on supermarket shelves rather than in refrigerated cabinets, since it does not require refrigeration until opened. It will store well for up to 5 months but, once opened, must be treated like fresh cream: refrigerate and use within a day or so.

PREPARATION AND USE Ideal where refrigeration is not available. Use straight from the paper carton but, if the cream is to be whipped, ensure that it is well chilled first, otherwise it is more difficult to whip. UHT cream may be used wherever regular cream is used.

Long Life Milk

*also called **UHT milk***

NUTRITIONAL INFORMATION Major nutrients similar to the original milk (full cream or skim). For nutritional information see the introduction to this chapter.

DESCRIPTION Regular milk, either full cream, low fat or flavoured, which has been subjected to the UHT (ultra high temperature) process, i.e. 135°C heat for 2–3 seconds. Packed in specially lined paper cartons to exclude oxygen and light.

ORIGIN AND HISTORY See Long Life Cream.

BUYING AND STORAGE Long life milks are generally found on supermarket shelves rather than in the refrigerated cabinets with other dairy foods. Buy as required and store in the pantry. Unopened they will last for up to 5 months. Once opened, treat as for regular milk and refrigerate.

PREPARATION AND USE Use as required, either straight from the pantry or else chilled. Ideal for isolated areas where food supplies are hard to reach daily. Because of sterile packaging, long life milk is ideal for infant feeding, where cow's milk is required.

SEE ALSO Cow's Milk.

Low Fat Milk

MAJOR NUTRIENTS		REDUCED FAT MODIFIED SERVE SIZE 250 mL	
Energy	580 kJ	Calcium	337 mg
Protein	10 g	Phosphorus	240 mg
Fat	5 g	Magnesium	32 mg
Carbohydrate	14 g	Thiamin	0.1 mg
Cholesterol	20 mg	Riboflavin	0.5 mg
Sodium	150 mg	Vitamin A	40 μg
Potassium	450 mg		

NUTRITIONAL INFORMATION Similar in nutritional value to milk, but processing has halved the fat and cholesterol content. This provides a flavoursome drink with moderate fat and a high calcium content. Low fat milks are not recommended for feeding of infants or toddlers. See also the introduction to this chapter.

MAJOR NUTRIENTS		LOW FAT MODIFIED SERVE SIZE 250 mL	
Energy	490 kJ	Sodium	170 mg
Protein	12 g	Potassium	500 mg
Fat	0	Calcium	408 mg
Carbohydrate	17 g	Phosphorus	315 mg
Cholesterol	0		

NUTRITIONAL INFORMATION Although no vitamin data are available, will contain other vitamins and minerals similar to skim milk. Suitable for use in low fat and cholesterol-lowering diets. It is recommended for females at high risk of developing osteoporosis. See also Skim Milk.

DESCRIPTION Regular milk with the fat taken away (in the case of Shape) or reduced (in Lite White) and with higher added solids and an increased calcium content.

ORIGIN AND HISTORY These are milks of the late 20th century, especially formulated to meet the needs of consumers who are concerned about living healthy lifestyles, reducing their cholesterol, and increasing their calcium intake, to aid in preventing osteoporosis.

There is no doubt that there is a consumer demand for fat-reduced and calcium-increased milks worldwide. Low fat milks originated in the USA, and Europe and Australia began production shortly afterwards, in the early 1950s. Popularity has remained high.

BUYING AND STORAGE Look for well-sealed cartons and check the use-by date. Refrigerate as soon as possible after purchase, in the coolest part of the fridge. Purchase daily as required and store as for regular milk.

PREPARATION AND USE Serve well chilled as a drink, or use as a substitute for regular milk when cooking. Low fat milks are ideal for thirst-quenching summer milkshakes and may be used with breakfast cereals or wherever a low fat alternative to regular milk is required. Serve straight from the refrigerator and do not allow to stand for any length of time in heat or direct light.

VARIETIES
Low fat modified milk, reduced fat modified milk.

Mock Cream

MAJOR NUTRIENTS			SERVE SIZE 40 MG
Energy	170 kJ	Carbohydrate	4 g
Protein	1 g	Cholesterol	0
Fat	3 g	Sodium	15 mg

NUTRITIONAL INFORMATION Mock cream is high in saturated fat and sugar and has little nutritional value.

DESCRIPTION Mock cream is artificial cream made by replacing dairy fats with other fats such as vegetable fats. Skim milk powder is also used in production.

Mock cream is better known in its homemade version. It is made easily by beating butter and icing sugar together, with the optional addition of an egg white, or a drop of milk. The egg white makes the mock cream more fluffy and raises the protein content.

ORIGIN AND HISTORY This product became established in Europe in the 1940s. It is doubtful that it is available in Australia on a commercial basis for retail sale, but it is often used with cakes in retail outlets.

Mock cream was originally made with butter, beaten in a bowl with ordinary sugar until light and creamy. It was then held under cold running water and 'washed' through several times.

BUYING AND STORAGE Make up batches of mock cream, fresh daily or as required. Mock cream can be frozen for up to 2 months, or kept in the refrigerator for 4–5 days. If made with added egg white, it will last 2–3 days.

PREPARATION AND USE Prepare as described above. Use chilled, before it sets.

Powdered Milk

MAJOR NUTRIENTS			WHOLE
			SERVE SIZE 30 G
Energy	620 kJ	Phosphorus	220 mg
Protein	8 g	Zinc	0.9 mg
Fat	8 g	Magnesium	25 mg
Carbohydrate	12 g	Thiamin	0.1 mg
Cholesterol	0.35 mg	Riboflavin	0.35 mg
Sodium	130 mg	Vitamin A	95 µg
Calcium	306 mg		

NUTRITIONAL INFORMATION When reconstituted with water, has similar nutritional value to whole milk. 30 g of dried whole milk powder reconstitutes to 250 mL of milk. Lecithin is added to 'instant' milk powders to allow easy reconstitution. For nutritional information see the introduction to this chapter.

MAJOR NUTRIENTS			SKIM
			SERVE SIZE 22 G
Energy	330 kJ	Calcium	262 mg
Protein	8 g	Phosphorus	210 mg
Fat	0	Zinc	0.9 mg
Carbohydrate	12 g	Magnesium	25 mg
Cholesterol	5 mg	Thiamin	0.1 mg
Sodium	120 mg	Riboflavin	0.35 mg

NUTRITIONAL INFORMATION When reconstituted with water, has similar content to skim milk. 22 g of dried skim milk powder reconstitutes to 250 mL of milk. For nutritional information see Skim Milk.

DESCRIPTION Concentrated milk solids produced by eliminating almost all moisture from the original milk, resulting in increased life of the product. The resultant product may be modified for particular uses, e.g. infant formulas, or instant powders designed for ease of reconstitution.

ORIGIN AND HISTORY Powdered milks originated as a means to overcome supply problems associated with a short life product such as regular milk.

The 'drying' process was a natural extension of the condensing process. The original process involved spraying the milk onto steam-heated rollers, with the powder being scraped off and collected. This process, although still used in limited applications, was unable to avoid damage to the delicate protein structure and flavour balances. This led to the development of such processes as spray and freeze drying.

BUYING AND STORAGE Milk produced under these conditions, if packed in sealed cans, keeps for more than 12 months. Once opened it should be resealed carefully and stored in a cool, dry area. Powders purchased in packet form should, on opening, be placed in an airtight container to avoid spoilage. When purchasing, the use-by date should be noted and the containers checked to ensure there is no visible damage and that they are correctly sealed. Selection should be based on your requirements, keeping in mind such factors as fat, protein and calcium levels.

PREPARATION AND USE Details of preparation vary and are given on the packaging. Use in baking, sauces, soups, drinks, custards, meat loaves, various toppings, ice creams and desserts. They are an ideal binding agent and lend themselves to numerous cooking applications.

VARIETIES
Full cream powdered milk, full cream instant powdered milk, skim milk powder, instant skim milk powder.

Rennet

MAJOR NUTRIENTS			SERVE SIZE 10 G
Energy	50 kJ	Cholesterol	n/a
Protein	0	Sodium	2230 mg
Fat	0	Calcium	350 mg
Carbohydrate	2 g		

NUTRITIONAL INFORMATION Rennet contains a large amount of sodium and is an excellent source of calcium. However, as it is normally used in small amounts, it has little nutritional significance. 'Vegetarian' cheese can be made from milk coagulated with rennet not obtained from animals.

DESCRIPTION Rennet is the name given to the agent used to bring about coagulation of milk, resulting in a solid curd mass.

ORIGIN AND HISTORY Originally rennet was extracted from the abomasum (4th stomach) of a young ruminant, giving a mix of the enzymes rennin and pepsin. The use of vegetable rennet was first recorded in the 3rd century AD by a writer advocating the use of extracts from the teasel flower or fig. Nowadays extensive use is made of microbial rennet owing to the lack of high quality animal rennet and the increased quality control exercised over the production process.

PREPARATION AND USE Rennet's main use is to coagulate milk, although it does also bring about a breakdown of milk proteins, which is an essential component of the ripening process in cheese making.

VARIETIES
Animal, microbial, vegetable.

Sheep's Milk

NUTRITIONAL INFORMATION Sheep's milk has twice the fat content of cow's milk and is therefore frequently used in cheese making.

DESCRIPTION Sheep's milk is richer than cow's milk and is whiter in colour and sweeter in taste.

ORIGIN AND HISTORY Sheep have been milked for thousands of years in the Mediterranean countries, Africa and the Middle East. Sheep and goats were the first milk-producing animals to be domesticated, long before cows, and a solid milk industry was established in ancient times in Greece, France, Spain, Czechoslovakia and Italy. Dairy breeds of ewes vary according to country and are too numerous to list; for instance, one particular Spanish breed is called Manchega and its milk is used to make the famous Spanish cheese of the same name.

In more recent years, countries which have never been traditional sheep's milk producers are entering the industry. These include the USA, Canada, New Zealand and latterly Australia.

In Australia the first sheep dairies began in the mid-1960s in Victoria; however, they ceased, owing to the high labour costs of producing traditional cheeses. During the 1970s, research programmes operated on a stop–go basis depending on funding. In 1986 the NSW Department of Agriculture built a sheep research dairy in the Riverina district of NSW. A small dairy was also built to milk 200 ewes and thus began the development of a cheese factory at Leeton and an alternative industry for the Murrumbidgee Irrigation Area of NSW.

BUYING AND STORAGE Sheep's milk is generally used to make milk products such as cheese, smaller amounts of yoghurt and on occasions butter, rather than as a commercial beverage.

The same storage principles apply as for cow's milk.

PREPARATION AND USE Sheep's milk is most commonly used to make different varieties of cheese according to country of production, e.g. Spanish manchega; French roquefort; Greek fetta; Italian pecorino. It is also on occasion used to produce butter, but the end product is much more oily than that made from cow's milk. A small amount of ewe's milk is used for yoghurt production.

Skim Milk

MAJOR NUTRIENTS		SERVE SIZE 250 ML	
Energy	360 kJ	Calcium	325 mg
Protein	9 g	Phosphorus	250 mg
Fat	0	Magnesium	30 mg
Carbohydrate	12 g	Zinc	1 mg
Cholesterol	0	Thiamin	0.1 mg
Sodium	130 mg	Riboflavin	0.5 mg

NUTRITIONAL INFORMATION An excellent source of high quality protein, calcium and phosphorus; good source of vitamin B, especially riboflavin; contains moderate amounts of magnesium, zinc and sodium. As fat, cholesterol and vitamin A are removed during processing, skim milk is highly suitable for cholesterol-lowering diets.

Skim milk, particularly in the concentrated powder form, is the ideal supplement when high protein is required in the diet. It contains high levels of all essential amino acids and is the best and cheapest amino acid supplement for building body tissues.

DESCRIPTION Milk with a butterfat content below 0.15%. It is produced by removing the cream from the whole milk.

ORIGIN AND HISTORY Skim milk takes its name from the old process of allowing the milk to stand until the cream rises to the surface and can be skimmed off. This process is now replaced by mechanical separation.

Skim milk originated from the need to obtain the cream component of milk to make butter and cheese. In affluent areas, skim milk was used as animal feed, but it has no doubt always been a drink for the less wealthy populace. In modern times, particularly the 1980s in Australia, skim milk has become an important dietary drink for those concerned about healthy lifestyle.

BUYING AND STORAGE Buy fresh daily and check the use-by date. Refrigerate as soon as possible after purchase, and store at 4°C for up to 10 days, unopened.

PREPARATION AND USE Serve chilled as a low fat drink. Do not allow to stand before use. Use in hot and cold drinks, and generally where regular milk is used, for a reduction in overall fat intake in the diet.

SEE ALSO Low Fat Milk.

Sour Cream

NUTRITIONAL INFORMATION Major nutrients are the same as for the cream from which it is made. This is normally light cream (18% fat). See Cream.

DESCRIPTION Thicker than pure or sweet cream, sour cream is cream to which a special culture has been added, to give it a slightly sour taste.

ORIGIN AND HISTORY In the days before pasteurisation, cream was often left to sour naturally in farmhouse kitchens. Today, pasteurisation kills all the naturally occurring bacteria, and therefore a special culture has to be added to produce sour cream.

It is believed that commercial sour cream as we know it today was first developed in Denmark and Holland, during the early 1950s. In Australia, sour cream was first produced in Victoria during the late 1950s and from there other states took up production. Today it is widely available in Australia. UHT sour cream was produced in the early 1960s, but was not successful.

BUYING AND STORAGE Sour cream will remain at its peak for up to 15 days. Check the use-by date and ensure the container is undamaged with a well-sealed lid. Refrigerate as soon as possible after purchase and store away from strong-smelling foods in the fridge.

PREPARATION AND USE Use it straight from the fridge. If adding sour cream to soups or other hot recipes, add at the end of the cooking time and gently reheat without boiling.

Ideal for soups, savoury sauces, dips and jacket potatoes as well as with desserts.

Sour cream can be used to make a good substitute for mayonnaise, with less fat.

VARIETIES

Sour light cream (18% butterfat).

Thickened Cream

also called **Cream mixture**

MAJOR NUTRIENTS		SERVE SIZE 40 ML	
Energy	550 kJ	Cholesterol	40 mg
Protein	1 g	Sodium	15 mg
Fat	14 g	Vitamin A	120 µg
Carbohydrate	1 g		

NUTRITIONAL INFORMATION All creams are high in saturated fat and have a moderate to large amount of cholesterol. Apart from being an excellent source of vitamin A, they have little nutritional value and are high in kilojoules. Cream should be used sparingly, particularly by people wanting to control blood cholesterol levels.

DESCRIPTION This is a 35% fat cream, to which 1% of a thickening agent (e.g. gelatin, rennin, alginate) is added. It has a smooth, thick, pouring texture, suitable for whipping.

ORIGIN AND HISTORY It is believed that thickened cream is a product of modern times, based on the popularity of the Devonshire clotted creams. It has gained in popularity thanks to its ability to be whipped into a larger volume and to maintain its volume for use. In Australia, it was first produced in the early 1900s, and numerous brands are now on the market.

BUYING AND STORAGE Check the use-by date and the container for any damage. Thickened cream is best used fresh; however, it will keep for 10 days in the refrigerator. Store in the coolest part of the fridge away from strong-smelling foods.

PREPARATION AND USE Best used straight from the refrigerator. It will whip up more easily than other creams, with a reduced chance of curdling or separation.

Use whipped for cakes, pavlovas and other dessert toppings.

SEE ALSO Cream, Clotted Cream, Whipping Cream.

Whey

MAJOR NUTRIENTS		SERVE SIZE 250 ML	
Energy	270 kJ	Calcium	125 mg
Protein	2 g	Phosphorus	130 mg
Fat	1 g	Magnesium	25 mg
Carbohydrate	12 g	Thiamin	0.05 mg
Cholesterol	n/a	Riboflavin	0.35 mg
Sodium	n/a		

NUTRITIONAL INFORMATION Whey is a low fat milk drink. It contains only a third of the calcium and protein of skim milk. The high lactose (milk sugar) makes whey a flavoursome energy drink, providing calcium and phosphorus, moderate amounts of high quality protein and a good source of vitamin B, especially riboflavin. 20 g of whey powder reconstitutes to 250 mL liquid whey.

DESCRIPTION Whey is the liquid part of the milk drained off the curd during cheese making. A valuable by-product, whey contains one-fifth of the milk proteins.

ORIGIN AND HISTORY Whey has been an integral part of cheese making since time began. Varieties of cheese differ according to the amount of whey drained off, the manner of manipulating the curd and the ripening process. It is believed to have been a common occurrence for the whey to have been drained off and discarded or given to the animals; however in the days during the first discovery of cheese by the wandering nomad tribes there is little doubt that the whey was found to be an acceptable drink and the curds were pleasant to eat. The first cheeses to be produced from whey were most likely from goat's milk whey (see gjetöst cheese), sheep's and cow's milk. Whey became popular for producing ricotta cheese, but more recently milk is added.

BUYING AND STORAGE Whey is not commonly sold on a commercial basis.

PREPARATION AND USE It is used primarily to produce cheese (ricotta, gjetöst). Some whey-based drinks have also been developed.

Whipping Cream

NUTRITIONAL INFORMATION See Cream.

DESCRIPTION 'Whipping Cream' as a term means cream which when beaten long enough will form peaks which retain their shape. Used on a label, the phrase may describe creams of differing fat content. In the state of Queensland, Australia, Whipping Cream consists of the rich cream (48% fat content) which is known in other places as Thickened Cream. In Western Australia, on the other hand, the Whipping Cream sold corresponds to pure cream (35% fat content). In the United Kingdom, the two creams with high fat content are known as Double and Single Cream.

ORIGIN AND HISTORY Use of the term in labelling originated in Europe, where it described a product halfway between single and double cream. It has been extremely popular in Europe for decades and is gradually gaining popularity in Australia.

BUYING AND STORAGE Examine the container for dents or damage and check the use-by date. Whipping cream can be stored for 10 days in the refrigerator, but is best used fresh. Store away from strong-smelling foods.

PREPARATION AND USE Use straight from the refrigerator, and, once whipped, keep chilled.

Use to decorate cakes, pies and desserts. Also use as a topping or in hot drinks.

Yoghurt

also called **Dahi, Mast, Mazum, Yogurt**

MAJOR NUTRIENTS		PLAIN (NATURAL) SERVE SIZE 200 G	
Energy	650 kJ	Calcium	330 mg
Protein	9 g	Phosphorus	280 mg
Fat	8 g	Magnesium	30 mg
Carbohydrate	12 g	Zinc	1.2 mg
Cholesterol	30 mg	Thiamin	0.1 mg
Sodium	140 mg	Riboflavin	0.5 mg
Potassium	440 mg	Vitamin A	72 µg

NUTRITIONAL INFORMATION Nutritionally, yoghurt is similar to milk, being an excellent source of calcium and phosphorus, and a good source of high quality protein and vitamin B, especially riboflavin. Depending on the ingredients used to make the yoghurt it may be high in saturated fat and contain moderate amounts of cholesterol. Low fat yoghurts are recommended for controlling blood cholesterol. Flavoured yoghurt, including frozen yoghurt, is high in sugar, containing varied amounts of added sugar (7–15%). Sugar increases the kilojoules with no other nutritional benefits.

Yoghurt, particularly the acidophilus variety, is widely acclaimed as a health food. It contains small amounts of healthy bacteria such as *Lactobacillus acidophilus* which are normally present in the intestines. These may be destroyed by infections or by drugs such as penicillin. Eating yoghurt may assist in restoring any imbalance of the healthy organisms in the gut. During processing the fat and protein in the yoghurt are partially digested, and lactose is broken down into lactic acid, so yoghurt may be easier to digest than milk in certain disorders and gastric infections.

Fermenting of milk to make yoghurt provides a safe drink, particularly in hot climates where milk is not pasteurised or refrigerated. Harmful bacteria are destroyed during fermentation. This accounts for past generations of people eating yoghurt being healthier and living longer than people drinking unpasteurised milk.

Low fat yoghurt is similar to plain yoghurt except for negligible fat, cholesterol and vitamin A and lower kilojoule content (about two-thirds).

Flavoured and fruited yoghurt has a similar nutritional value to plain yoghurt but contains a large amount of sugar and is higher in kilojoules (almost twice the amount).

DESCRIPTION Yoghurt is a creamy product made by warming milk of various fat levels and introducing a special culture of bacteria. Milk sugars are broken down, releasing lactic acid which acts to coagulate the milk into the familiar curd consistency. Plain or natural yoghurt has a fresh tangy taste, while the fruited varieties are sweeter.

ORIGIN AND HISTORY Before the days of refrigeration, it was discovered that the goodness of milk could be preserved by fermenting it into yoghurt. It originated in the Balkans and was introduced into Europe during the 18th century from the region around Turkistan. Yoghurt is the anglicised Turkish word for fermented milk. It was credited with a range of medicinal and remedial properties, some of which have re-emerged and been debated more recently, e.g. the *Lactobacillus acidophilus* debate. (It is believed that this is the only bacterial culture which will survive the passage through the digestive system to the lower gut and thus re-establish the vital flora which is essential to the absorption phase of the digestive process. It is therefore claimed to be particularly valuable following any surgical procedure which requires evacuation of the bowel and lower intestine.)

In Europe, yoghurt is made in the home as well as for commercial sale, but in Australia commercial manufacture is the norm. Yoghurt in Australia has only been enjoyed since the late 1930s; however, its popularity is increasing, recently by 10–20% each year.

BUYING AND STORAGE Check the use-by date, and ensure the container is undamaged and the seal intact. If the product has been stored incorrectly, the seal cover may bulge, indicating problems. Yoghurt should be stored in the refrigerator and, once opened, should be resealed with its own lid if available or plastic cling wrap. It has a shelf life of around 7–10 days.

PREPARATION AND USE Keep refrigerated until required. No preparation is necessary before use, except draining off any excess whey. Use on its own for a snack, dessert or lunch with fresh fruits in season. Use in sauces and toppings as a low kilojoule alternative to cream. Stir through mashed potatoes in place of butter or milk.

VARIETIES
Natural, flavoured or fruit, low fat or skim milk.

SEE ALSO Frozen Yoghurt.

CHEESES

The first type of cheese produced would undoubtedly have been a sour milk cheese, forerunner to today's group of fresh, unripened cheeses such as cottage and cream cheese.

It was a very short time after the discovery of sour milk cheese that the wandering nomads discovered better keeping qualities for cheese by removing the moisture, pressing the curd, salting it and drying it in the sun — thus beginning the production of firm hard cheeses. This method of making firm cheese is said to still exist in Arabia and is called kishk.

At this point in history individual recipes were adopted, produced and handed down through families. Several countries needed cheeses with good keeping qualities to travel without their quality being impaired. One such cheese which travelled worldwide, due to the Dutch merchant ships dominating the Mediterranean, was edam. Another was cheddar. The cheddaring technique developed in the 19th century led to a widespread reform of cheese making. It involves cutting, stacking, turning and folding the curd, releasing as much moisture as possible, then milling, stirring, salting and pressing it into a mould.

Cheeses are of five main types. The first, curd cheese, coagulates because of acids in the milk from which it is made. Cream-based cheeses are coagulated by acids or by rennet. The soft cheeses are made from milk which is coagulated by rennet. The fourth kind of cheese is semihard. This may be pressed lightly but unscalded, like caerphilly, or all mould ripened, like stilton, and possibly both pressed and scalded. Hard cheese, such as cheddar, is both pressed and scalded.

Hard cheeses are generally varieties that have been pressed, cooked and have a moisture level lower than 40%. They have the lowest moisture level of the cheese groups and vary from hard to very hard cheese. In some countries the term hard is a classification which indicates a group of cheese ranging from cheshire and cheddar to romano and parmesan. All have good keeping qualities due to low moisture levels. The Italian term for hard cheese is grana. Under the classification charts one country may classify cheddar as firm, whilst another calls it hard.

A number of terms used in this chapter require explanation. A natural cheese is one which is allowed to ripen and mature to its peak, without any further manufacturing or heat treatment.

Processed cheese is made by stopping the ripening action at a given point by heat treatment. As a result, the cheese remains constant and uniform in taste and texture throughout its entire life.

Unripened cheeses are the freshest of varieties, which have no ripening, maturing or cooking processes involved. They are generally very moist and have the shortest life.

Ripened cheeses are those which over time reach their own unique texture and taste (typical to that variety), through complex chemical and physical changes.

Surface ripened, surface mould ripened, surface smear ripened and washed rind cheeses are ripened by the action of special bacteria, moulds or yeasts applied to the surface of the cheese.

Internal mould ripened cheese is ripened internally by the introduction to the cheese milk of special *Penicillium glaucum* or *Penicillium roqueforti* spores, used in the production of blue vein cheeses.

A cheese can also be surface *and* internal mould ripened, by a combination of internal 'blue vein' spores and surface moulds.

Soft ripened cheese is either made with a soft creamy centre to begin with, or develops as such, through surface ripening.

Double cream cheese is cheese produced with a fat content of approximately 60% (this may vary by country). Triple cream cheese is produced with a fat content of approximately 74% (this may vary by country).

Pasta filata is a group of cheeses whose curd is manipulated by kneading and stretching under hot water or whey.

Brined cheeses, such as fetta, are ripened and dipped into a salt and water solution.

There is a range of smoked cheeses, most of them produced in Germany and Austria. Commonly sausage-shaped, and orange-brown in colour with a shiny rind, they have a smooth texture and smoky flavour and are often processed. However, some varieties such as smoked provolone (affumicato provolone) are natural cheeses, smoked. The smoked flavour is induced by either genuine smoking or the addition of a smoked essence.

When there is heat treatment involved during the cheese-making process (other than pasteurisation), cheeses can be classified as uncooked or raw (i.e. temperature does not exceed 40°C); scalded (temperature does not exceed 48°C) or cooked (temperature exceeds 48°C). The amount of whey varies according to these temperatures and the length of heating.

There can be a wide range of fat content between manufacturers for any variety of cheese. When a legal minimum fat content is required for Australian cheese, this is noted under the food entry. Labelling for fat content is confusing, as cheese originating in Europe states the fat content as percentage of dry matter and the figures appear very high. Percentage of fat on other labels represents percentage for the whole cheese. English varieties of cheese such as cheddar are usually higher in fat than continental varieties. New Zealand cheddars will frequently have higher fat than English and Australian varieties. Sapsago, a hard cheese made from a mixture of skim milk and buttermilk, may have fat content as low as 5%. Production of low fat cheeses is a continuing industry.

Cheese traditionally contains a variety of ingredients not stated on the label: e.g. salt, colours and bleaching agents. Salt content can vary from 1–5%. The highest amount of salt is found in blue cheeses, very hard cheeses (e.g. parmesan) and brined cheeses such as fetta. Swiss-style cheese tends to be low in salt. Smoked and processed cheeses and cheese spread are similar to hard cheeses in nutritional value. Smoking is used to impart a savoury flavour and aid preservation.

Because hard cheeses have minimal lactose (milk sugar) and low moisture they remain fresh for extended periods. This makes cheese an ideal concentrated protein food for trekking etc. When eaten at the end of a meal it assists in the prevention of dental caries because of its alkaline content. Cheeses, especially matured and blue varieties, contain tyramine which may precipitate a migraine in susceptible people.

Despite a wide variety of flavours and textures, the nutritional value of hard cheeses is very similar. They provide an excellent source of calcium and phosphorus, a moderate source of protein and vitamin A. They are high in saturated fat with moderate amounts of cholesterol. Nutritionally 30 g of hard cheese is similar to 250 mL of milk except that a large amount of salt (sodium) is added and vitamin B is removed during the process of making hard cheese. The high saturated fat and sodium require cheese to be restricted for people wanting to control hypertension and blood cholesterol levels.

The very hard cheeses such as parmesan, romano and sbrinz have a very low moisture content when compared to softer varieties of cheese such as brie and camembert. The harder cheeses will therefore contain more protein, fat and minerals but usually they are eaten in small portions — 5–10 g.

Cheeses made from goat's milk and buffalo's milk will always be white as they contain no carotene unless they are artificially coloured. Cheeses made from these milks will have a distinctive flavour due to different types of fatty acids in the milk. Like cow's milk, the fat is saturated fat and the only relevant nutritional factor is the amount of fat in the cheese.

Some cheeses have reduced fat or sodium content, for people concerned about the possible adverse effects of saturated fat on blood cholesterol levels and high sodium influencing blood pressure control. Australian jack cheese is made with no added salt (sodium), and nimbin has approximately half the sodium content of other hard cheeses. Salt-free cheese will not keep fresh over an extended period.

Cheeses with reduced fat or ones made partially from skim milk frequently remain high fat products: e.g. reduced fat cheddar can contain a maximum of 27% fat. This is less than normal cheddar, with a minimum fat of 31%, but is high compared to many continental cheeses.

For manufacture of filled cheeses, milk fat has been replaced with polyunsaturated oils (soya bean oil and sunflower oil). These oils contain essential fatty acids which have a slight lowering effect on blood cholesterol. Filled cheeses are high in fat and need to be eaten in moderation.

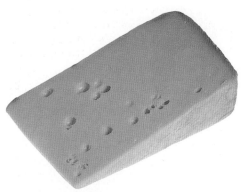

Appenzeller

also called Appenzell

NUTRITIONAL INFORMATION Minimum fat is 25%.

DESCRIPTION Swiss cheese similar to emmental and gruyère, but with a more fruity, spicy taste and a higher moisture content. Pale golden in colour, with a smooth brown rind, it has only a few scattered holes.

An important characteristic of this particular cheese, which is responsible for its more tangy flavour, is the tradition of washing the rind with white wine, pepper and spices.

ORIGIN AND HISTORY Appenzell takes its name from the Swiss canton or province of the same name, and has been produced for over 700 years.

BUYING AND STORAGE Look for appenzeller with a smooth dry rind, hard and brown, sometimes waxed. It is a large flat wheel or disc shape, bulging slightly at the sides. Cut surfaces of appenzeller should show an interior with well-spaced 'eyes' or holes, glistening with butterfat. The eyes should be cherry-sized and the butterfat indicates a cheese ripened to maturity.

Store refrigerated with all cut surfaces firmly wrapped in cling wrap. Correctly stored, it should last for 3 weeks in the refrigerator. Trim away any slight outside moulding that may occur and rewrap.

PREPARATION AND USE Like gruyère and emmental, appenzeller is a good fondue cheese. Well ripened appenzeller lends a fruity mature flavour to fondues.

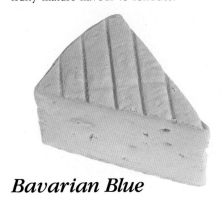

Bavarian Blue

also called Bavariablu

NUTRITIONAL INFORMATION Major nutrients similar to Danish blue.

DESCRIPTION Bavarian blue is a double cream soft blue cheese encased in a white surface rind similar to camembert. It is a surface and internal mould ripened cheese. Its flavour is aromatic and lightly piquant.

ORIGIN AND HISTORY Bavarian blue is believed to be the first of the combined blue–camembert styles developed in 1973 in Germany. Rather than being a cheese steeped in old traditions and history, it is a relatively new-age style reflecting the mix and match attitudes of the 20th century. Bavarian blue originated when the German cheese producer Bergader achieved the combination of ripening cheese with white surface flora (as for camembert) and internal blue mould (as for regular blue vein cheeses).

BUYING AND STORAGE Buy in quantities as needed. The rind of the cheese should be snowy white, sometimes with slight reddish pigmentation. It should never be dull brown or grey, nor have a darkened or slimy appearance. Stored at 4°C in the refrigerator it should last for 2–3 weeks. It must be securely wrapped around all exposed surfaces to prevent loss of moisture. Store away from the other dairy foods to avoid tainting.

Never freeze Bavarian blue. Its texture will spoil and it could cross-flavour other foods. On thawing it will quickly go bad.

PREPARATION AND USE Remove from the refrigerator 1½ hours before serving to allow the cheese to develop its true character and flavour, and use a separate knife to cut and serve it. Use for dessert cheese platters with fresh fruits, in canapés, for cheese balls or logs.

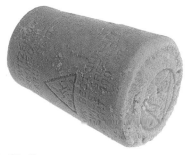

Bellelay

also called Tête de moine

DESCRIPTION This is a hard cheese, pale in colour with an aromatic spicy taste. Tête de moine means monk's head, and in many cases the cheese will be referred to thus. In Australia, it is produced by a small farmhouse cheese maker in Tasmania.

ORIGIN AND HISTORY It was originally made 800 years ago in an abbey at Bellelay.

BUYING AND STORAGE As for other hard cheeses.

PREPARATION AND USE It is traditionally 'shaved' with a sharp knife or cheese-cutter, to produce curls of fine cheese.

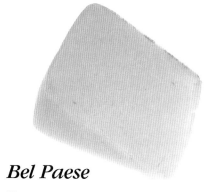

Bel Paese

NUTRITIONAL INFORMATION Despite its soft texture, this is typical of a hard cheese in its nutrient value.

DESCRIPTION A mild Italian cheese with a medium soft texture and sweetish flavour, encased in a smooth shiny golden rind.

ORIGIN AND HISTORY Bel paese, meaning beautiful country, was developed in the 1920s, styled on Saint Paulin.

The wrapper shows a famous picture of an elderly cleric and a map of Italy. A friend of the original cheese maker had written a well-known children's book, *Il bel paese* (beautiful country), which inspired the naming of the cheese.

BUYING AND STORAGE This cheese should be free of fermentation spotting, with a smooth velvety texture, mild flavour and light smell. Buy as needed and store in the refrigerator away from milk, butter and cream. It should keep for 1–2 weeks.

PREPARATION AND USE Remove from the refrigerator an hour before serving to allow it to reach room temperature. Allow a separate knife to cut and serve. Use as a table cheese on cheese boards, or in savouries, open sandwiches or cheese pastries.

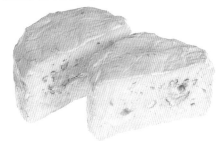

Bleu de Bresse

also called Bresse bleu

NUTRITIONAL INFORMATION Major nutrients similar to Danish blue.

DESCRIPTION A small, soft cheese with a white rind and delicate blue veining, creamy and sweet. It is an internal mould ripened cheese. Bresse bleus are styled on the Italian gorgonzola, though milder in taste.

ORIGIN AND HISTORY Regarded as one of France's best 'bleus', bleu de Bresse originated in eastern France. It comes from the rich country between Jura and Saone and is particularly soft and creamy in the spring. French blue cheeses often take the name of the district where they are produced as their varietal name. Such is the case with bleu de Bresse, created in the Bresse region near Lyon in 1950.

BUYING AND STORAGE Bleu de Bresse should be honey-coloured and creamy inside with a thin off-white rind, sometimes speckled with orange-brown pigmentation. It should show no signs of sharpness, sticky rind or pinkish colour inside. It should be rich, creamy and spreadable.

It is sold foil-wrapped and boxed. Store in the refrigerator and use within a few days as it quickly becomes overripe.

PREPARATION AND USE Remove from the refrigerator 1½ hours before serving. Keep covered and away from heat and light. Use a separate knife to cut and serve.

Bleu de Bresse is a table cheese. Use for cheese boards, dessert platters and cocktail nibbles, for stuffed fruits and with nuts. Serve with grapes and celery and assorted breads.

VARIETIES

Pipo bleu, pipo crem, pipo nain, unibresse.

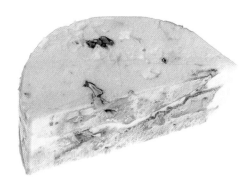

Blue Castello

NUTRITIONAL INFORMATION Major nutrients similar to Danish blue.

DESCRIPTION Blue castello is a double cream cheese with blue veins and a white moulded surface, similar to Bavarian blue. It is a surface and internal mould ripened cheese.

ORIGIN AND HISTORY This is one of Scandinavia's most popular cheeses; blue castello originated in Denmark. Believed to be the result of experimentation in the 1950s and 1960s with blue and white mould cheeses, blue castello is one of the varieties that have gained solid export markets. Similar cheeses produced elsewhere are camzola, Danish blue brie, lymeswold, brizola and Bavarian blue.

BUYING AND STORAGE Buy as needed since it has a limited life (it is considered to be at its peak around 5 weeks old). Blue castello should have a mild blue flavour, rich and creamy. It should show no signs of a grey or sticky surface, nor a darkening of the blue-veined interior. It should appear fresh without signs of dryness and should have a smooth texture.

Store refrigerated, securely wrapped in foil, for as short a time as possible.

PREPARATION AND USE Remove from the refrigerator a good hour before serving. Use as a table cheese, with fruit platters for dessert or in luncheon platters with plain crackers. Use a separate knife to cut and serve to avoid transfer of flavours to other cheeses. Most fresh fruits will go well with it.

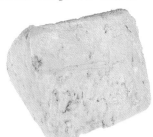

Blue Shropshire

also known as Shropshire blue

NUTRITIONAL INFORMATION This is a typical hard cheese.

DESCRIPTION A fine, smooth-textured cheese, delicate in colour with natural blue veining. Full-fat and hard-textured. An internal mould ripened cheese.

ORIGIN AND HISTORY One of Britain's newer cheese varieties, created to fill the flavour gap between blue cheshire and stilton. Blue shropshire was originally produced in Inverness by Andy Williamson, well versed in the art of stilton manufacture. It was sponsored by a London company who marketed it as 'shropshire blue'. Production ceased in spring 1980 when the Marketing Board of North Scotland closed the factory. In 1981, however, it was resurrected by another dairy and it is now once more available.

BUYING AND STORAGE Buy as required. Look for a cheese free of any grey patches, dullness or dryness. Store at low temperatures in the refrigerator with all exposed surfaces wrapped in foil. Shropshire should last 2 to 3 weeks. Change the wrapping regularly to avoid tainting other foods in the refrigerator. Keep away from butter, milk and cream. Smaller wedges have a maximum life of 6 weeks, while whole cheeses last 8 weeks providing storage temperature is 2°C.

PREPARATION AND USE Remove the cheese from the refrigerator 1½ hours before serving, to allow its true character and taste to develop. Always use a separate knife to cut and serve. Use on a cheeseboard or as a table cheese. It melts well under the griller, and crumbles well. It makes a good filling for jacket potatoes, or an addition to green salads.

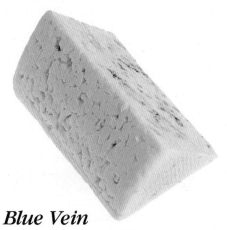

Blue Vein

also called Blue cheese, Bleu

NUTRITIONAL INFORMATION Nutritionally, Danish blue is typical of most blue vein cheeses. See the entry for that cheese.

DESCRIPTION Blue vein cheeses are generally rich and piquant in flavour, with varying textures, colours and rinds, depending on the variety and brand. The network of veining

may be blue or green. They are internal mould ripened cheeses.

ORIGIN AND HISTORY The term 'blue vein' originated in the USA (alternative terms are blue cheese or, in French, bleu). Generally all blue vein cheeses are based on one of the three great blues (roquefort, gorgonzola and stilton). Produced worldwide, roquefort is the oldest, followed by gorgonzola and stilton. Experiments to produce blue vein cheese in the USA came to fruition in 1918; meanwhile over in Denmark developments were underway to produce a roquefort-style cheese. In Australia blue vein manufacture on a commercial scale commenced well into the 20th century. Maczola was an early blue vein cheese produced on the north coast of NSW, taking its name from that of the Macleay River combined with 'gorgonzola'; however, production ceased in the 1950s. Today there are three blue vein varieties produced in Australia, each quite different.

BUYING AND STORAGE Buy as required. The veining should be even and clear of any dullness or grey appearance. There should be no trace of pink mould, nor any stickiness. Store in the refrigerator well wrapped to avoid tainting of other foods and keep at a low temperature — around 4°C. It should last for 2–3 weeks (depending on the size).

PREPARATION AND USE Remove the cheese from the refrigerator an hour ahead of the serving time, keeping it covered and away from heat to allow it to gradually reach room temperature and develop its true character. Strong, pungent cheeses will dissipate their flavour slightly as the balance of the cheese's character returns. Use a separate knife to cut and serve blue vein cheeses, to ensure the flavour is not transferred. Blue vein is ideal to use crumbled in salad dressings, or creamed with a little extra cream to make cheese cocktail balls; it is also served in the classical manner on a cheese board with raspberries, blueberries or other fresh fruits, dried or fresh figs, muscatels etc. Blue vein is also a versatile cheese in cooking.

VARIETIES

Bavarian blue, blue castello, bleu de Bresse, blue cheshire, blue shropshire, blue wensleydale, Danish blue, fourme d'Ambert, gorgonzola, mycella, roquefort, stilton: see separate entries. (Australian brands — Unity Blue, Gippsland Blue, Milawa Blue.)

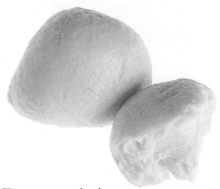

Bocconcini

NUTRITIONAL INFORMATION Major nutrients similar to mozzarella.

DESCRIPTION Young fresh mozzarella cheeses similar in size to small tomatoes, small and white in colour; soft, moist and fresh, mildly sweet in flavour. A pasta filata (stretched curd) cheese.

ORIGIN AND HISTORY Originating in Italy, mozzarella is more commonly eaten whilst fresh and moist, and the small mozzarellas take the name of bocconcini. As a fresh unripened cheese which only takes 24 hours to make, bocconcini are sold and stored in bags containing the natural whey, to keep them moist. In overseas countries where the Italian mozzarella has become established, it is best known for its use in pizzas. It was originally made in southern Italy from buffalo's milk, however most cheese manufactured on a large scale is now made using cow's milk. In some instances bocconcini also refers to a recipe in which the cheese is sliced finely, then sprinkled with olive oil and freshly cracked black pepper.

BUYING AND STORAGE Buy as required. Stored in the refrigerator at 4°C they should last up to 3 weeks, ripening during that time to become firmer and drier like the large pizza mozzarellas.

Bocconcini should be white in colour, moist and tender with a mild fresh taste. They should show no sign of yellowing.

PREPARATION AND USE Serve from the refrigerator whilst cool and moist. Slice bocconcini into thin slices and sprinkle with freshly ground black pepper and pure olive oil. Use in salads, e.g. with tomatoes and shredded lettuce.

SEE ALSO Mozzarella.

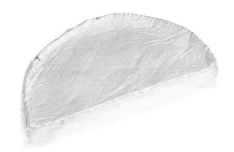

Brie

MAJOR NUTRIENTS			SERVE SIZE 20 G
Energy	280 kJ	Sodium	120 mg
Protein	4 g	Calcium	102 mg
Fat	6 g	Phosphorus	60 mg
Carbohydrate	0	Vitamin A	75 µg
Cholesterol	19 mg	Thiamin	5 mg

NUTRITIONAL INFORMATION Minimum fat 16%. Despite its soft texture, the nutritional value of brie is typical of the hard cheeses.

DESCRIPTION A soft creamy cheese encased in a velvety white surface rind. Creaminess and depth of flavour will vary between countries. Brie is traditionally made in the shape of a large flat disc. It is a surface mould ripened soft cheese.

ORIGIN AND HISTORY First mentioned in the Court of Champagne Records around 1217, brie was possibly the first of the famous French cheeses. Known as the 'Jewel of the Ile de France', brie achieved worldwide fame overnight during the Vienna Congress of 1814 and 1815, when Talleyrand proclaimed a competition to find the best cheese-producing country attending the congress. Brie de Meaux was proclaimed to be the best of the 60 cheeses involved and was crowned 'Roi de Fromages' (King of Cheeses). Originally a farmhouse cheese taking its name from the province of Brie, brie cheese in France also carries the name of the district of production on the label (e.g. brie de Meaux). Brie produced outside France may use the name provided the country of origin is indicated.

BUYING AND STORAGE Brie should not appear misshapen nor excessively dried and grey at the edges. Some coloration across the surface rind is common. Young, milder bries will have a snowy white surface. Look for a cut cheese which has a creamy honeylike centre bulging from the rind. Avoid cheese which has dark patches, dry shrunken appearance or an excessively ammoniated smell. Its taste should be rich and fruity. Store wrapped in its original wrapper if possible, or in foil or plastic cling wrap. Do not store other heavier foods on top of the cheese. Small wedges of brie will not store successfully for long: they are best used within a day or so.

PREPARATION AND USE Remove from the refrigerator 2 hours before serving unless the brie is fully ripened, then allow 1 hour to reach room temperature. Keep the cheese covered loosely until serving. Young brie may need to be left at room temperature through the preceding night to soften.

Use on cheese boards. Serve at the end of meals. Use in brie tortes for desserts. Best served with fresh berry fruits in season, walnuts and fruit breads, nuts, grapes and avocado.

Use overripe brie for deep frying.

PROCESSING Brie may be tinned and heat-treated to extend its life. The resultant product is uniform in flavour and texture and does not require refrigeration until opened.

VARIETIES

Double cream, triple cream, brie de Meaux, brie de Coulommiers, brie de Melun; brie flavoured with pepper, herbs, mushrooms.

SEE ALSO Coulommiers.

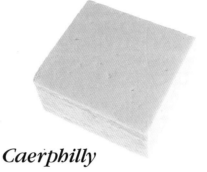

Caerphilly

NUTRITIONAL INFORMATION Major nutrients similar to cheddar.

DESCRIPTION A semisoft fresh cheese in block form. White with a crumbly porous texture and a light, mildly sour taste similar to buttermilk.

ORIGIN AND HISTORY Originating in Wales, caerphilly takes its name from the Welsh village where it was first produced near Cardiff. During the 1800s it was the mainstay of Welsh farmers, with almost every farmhouse along the 11 km stretch north of Cardiff following the tradition of twice daily (morning and evening) making caerphilly. As demand increased production began in England in Somerset. Generations of miners in Wales found that caerphilly's saltiness (due to brining) helped against the loss of body moisture down in the mines and that it also remained deliciously fresh and moist to eat underground.

Caerphilly is a fresh cheese ready to eat after 10 days, and cannot be kept for long periods of time. As a result it lapsed in production during the war years and until 1954.

Today, caerphilly enjoys popularity amongst a new generation of cheese eaters, both in England and overseas countries.

BUYING AND STORAGE Buy as required and use within a week or so. It has 10–30 days' life from manufacture. Choose fresh-looking cheese without dryness (a sign of age). It should be white with a fairly open porous texture, and should slice easily. The flavour should be mildly lactic with a slight tartness. Store well wrapped away from strong-smelling foods in the refrigerator.

PREPARATION AND USE Remove from the fridge an hour before serving. The cheese should be kept covered during that time to keep the moisture in. As caerphilly can flake or crumble, use a hot sharp knife to cut cleanly and quickly for cheese board displays. Serve with celery, capsicums, tomatoes, crusty fresh bread or salted crackers. An ideal lunch cheese. Use in fondue for a tasty touch without over-richness.

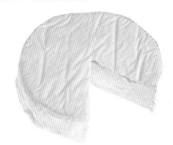

Camembert

MAJOR NUTRIENTS			SERVE SIZE 20 G
Energy	220 kJ	Sodium	130 mg
Protein	4 g	Calcium	95 mg
Fat	5 g	Phosphorus	60 mg
Carbohydrate	0	Vitamin A	60 µg
Cholesterol	19 mg	Thiamin	5.5 mg

NUTRITIONAL INFORMATION Minimum fat 16%. Despite its greater moisture content, the balance of nutrients is similar to that of a hard cheese.

DESCRIPTION A small surface mould ripened soft cheese with a white downy surface (some red speckling on occasions); soft and creamy in consistency to the point of flowing when fully ripe. Camemberts will vary according to the country of origin and varying milk fat levels.

ORIGIN AND HISTORY Believed to date back to 1791, camembert is named for the village of Camembert in the department of the Orne. Tradition credits Marie Harel as the creator of camembert and a statue was erected in her memory at Vimoutiers; however, the style of cheese was already known and described in the 17th century. It is most likely, in fact, that the cheese was well known and liked by William the Conqueror, under the name of 'Angelot' cheese. Angelot is now the local name for pont l'évêque.

Marie Harel can, nevertheless, be recorded as the inventor of a 'modern' camembert, since she was the first one to establish a regular and controlled mould flora. Factory production is enormous today, not only in France, but in countries all over the world, including more recently Australia and New Zealand. (There is a small camembert on the Australian market called a Little Bertie.)

A real camembert should not be confused with its tinned counterpart (processed for export).

BUYING AND STORAGE   Choose camembert according to your taste: young cheese has a mild taste and some firmness of body; fully ripened cheese has a stronger, fruitier flavour with creamy, almost flowing, consistency. There should be no excessive hardening, no grey or dark patches, nor too much reddish pigmentation.

Correctly stored in the refrigerator covered in its original wrapper it should last 3 weeks approximately, but it will continue to ripen and lose moisture. Best eaten within a few days to a week.

PREPARATION AND USE Remove from the fridge 2 hours before serving to allow the full character of the cheese to develop. Use a separate knife to cut and serve. Underripe cheese may be left at room temperature away from light and heat for 24 hours to ripen and soften. Camembert is primarily a table cheese. Use as a dessert cheese, in savoury appetisers and dips, for tortes, or deep fried. Also good in jaffles.

PROCESSING Camembert is often tinned and heat-treated to extend its life span. It is uniform in texture and taste and will keep unrefrigerated until opened.

VARIETIES
These include Geramont and pepper camembert.

Normandy has two other famous cheeses: while neither is strictly a variety of camembert, they are dealt with below because of their common region of origin, and because both are, like camembert, soft cheeses.

Livarot Livarot is not for the faint-hearted, since its aroma is powerful; however, the springy soft golden body of the cheese is quite mild in taste, once the brownish rind is cut off.

Pont L'Evêque Originally called angelot, until in the 17th century it was renamed pont l'évêque. It is generally made in small flat square shapes, with a golden brown rind. It has a tangy pronounced flavour.

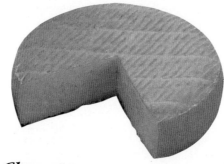

Chaumes

NUTRITIONAL INFORMATION No detailed data available.

DESCRIPTION Chaumes is a washed rind cheese with a shiny golden rind. It has a soft texture and a strong aroma similar to munster.

ORIGIN AND HISTORY It is one of a range of soft cheeses with washed rinds, exported from France under a variety of labels. Apart from chaumes, there are vacheral, Saint Albray and vieux pané.

BUYING AND STORAGE Buy chaumes that is soft, but not 'runny'. Keep away from delicate foods, and cling wrap the cut surfaces. It is best eaten soon after purchase.

PREPARATION AND USE A good contrast if served on a platter with milder cheeses.

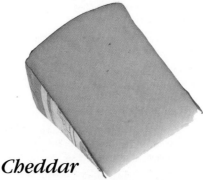

Cheddar

also called Tasty cheese, Matured cheese

MAJOR NUTRIENTS		SERVE SIZE 20 G	
Energy	340 kJ	Calcium	160 mg
Protein	5 g	Phosphorus	105 mg
Fat	7 g	Zinc	0.8 mg
Carbohydrate	0	Vitamin A	70 µg
Cholesterol	20 mg	Thiamin	4 mg
Sodium	20 mg		

NUTRITIONAL INFORMATION   Minimum fat 30%. A typical hard cheese.

DESCRIPTION A hard cheese varying in age and taste from mild to mature to vintage. Its colour will vary from the palest yellow to a

deeper hue according to its place of production, specific recipe and ripening. Flavour can be mild and mellow, rich and nutty, or strong and clean. A hard scalded curd cheese.

ORIGIN AND HISTORY Believed to be the biggest and best cheese in England during the first Queen Elizabeth's reign, cheddar originated in Somerset and was named after the village of the same name. It is most likely that the original cheddars were produced from ewe's milk, but production from cow's milk was certainly established by Tudor times. Those subjects of old English folksongs, the dairymaid and the milkmaid, were the 'stars' of cheese production in the good old 'hit or miss' days, and the old saying 'The bigger the dairymaid, the better the cheddar' refers to the ability of the dairymaid to press the whey out of curds using her full weight.

As production on farms in the Cheddar district increased in the 17th century, neighbouring districts began pooling their milk and cooperative dairy production began; healthy cheddar trade developed across England and abroad. Towards the latter half of the 19th century Joseph Harding began teaching the cheddaring process and factory skills were well on the way to replacing much of the farmhouse production. Cheddar is now the most widely copied cheese variety, produced in factories right around the world.

Today in Australia, cheddars are regaining the interest of consumers, but their availability is now limited. It is to be wondered whether the wheel will turn the full cycle. Robertson is a cheddar named after its home town in NSW, Australia.

BUYING AND STORAGE Choose a cheddar which is free of dryness and cracks on the outer surface and has a clean appearance. Prepacked cheeses should show no trace of air traps (e.g. blown up packs).

Stored in the refrigerator wrapped across all exposed surfaces with cling wrap, cheddar should keep well for several weeks. Change the wrapping regularly and trim any traces of mould which appear on the surface.

PREPARATION AND USE Remove from the refrigerator a good hour before serving and allow it to come to room temperature. For cooking, grate, dice or slice from the cold block straight from the fridge. Use a hot knife for easy cutting. Use cheddar cheese for sandwiches, snacks or savouries, toasted, or on cheese boards. Use also in cooking.

PROCESSING Cheddar is often processed to extend its life and for convenience. It is then uniform in texture and taste.

SEE ALSO Processed Cheese.

Cheedam

NUTRITIONAL INFORMATION A typical hard cheese. Minimum fat 23%.

DESCRIPTION Pale yellow in colour, cheedam, a firm cheese, is a cross between edam and cheddar. Mild in flavour, with a clean taste, slightly creamy.

ORIGIN AND HISTORY Originating in Australia, cheedam is in fact one of the very few Australian cheeses developed especially for that country. Although Australia produces over 40 varieties of cheese, most of them take their origin from other countries. Cheedam, however, was developed by the CSIRO's Dairy Research Division for production in Victoria and Tasmania. The purpose of the development was to produce a cheese similar to Dutch edam but without the costly equipment and labour-intensive process of manufacture that edam requires. Because the process of manufacture was best suited to those factories producing cheddar, the resulting variety was a cheddar-type cheese with edam characteristics. In 1983–84, 798 tonnes were produced.

BUYING AND STORAGE Cheedam has good keeping qualities, like cheddar and edam. Purchase in quantities as required and keep the cheese well wrapped at all times to prevent loss of moisture. Look for cheese which is a clean firm block without any signs of dryness or sweating.

PREPARATION AND USE Remove the cheese from the refrigerator an hour before serving unless it is to be used in recipes calling for grated or finely sliced cheese, in which case cut or grate straight from the fridge whilst still cold. Use as a snack or sandwich cheese or wherever a firm cheddar style with a mild taste is required.

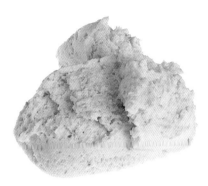

Cheese Spread

MAJOR NUTRIENTS		SERVE SIZE 20 G	
Energy	230 kJ	Sodium	235 mg
Protein	4 g	Calcium	102 mg
Fat	5 g	Phosphorus	90 mg
Carbohydrate	0	Vitamin A	40 µg
Cholesterol	15 mg	Thiamin	4 mg

NUTRITIONAL INFORMATION Despite processing, the nutrients remain those of hard cheese in general.

DESCRIPTION Soft cheese of a spreadable nature, sometimes with the addition of herbs or spices. A processed cheese.

ORIGIN AND HISTORY Cheese spreads are generally made to create a delicious new cheese from an already established variety. Commercial spreads are often seen as a subprocess to the production of processed cheese, which is believed to have originated from the habit of using fondue leftovers. Cheese spreads are processed by modifying the fat and protein components and increasing the moisture content, then applying varying heat treatments. They generally utilise a variety of cheeses mixed together to produce a smooth-textured spread.

BUYING AND STORAGE Buy in quantity or as required and store in the refrigerator once opened unless directed otherwise on the pack or jar. Check the use-by date.

Look for correctly sealed packs. Unopened, cheese spreads should have a long shelf life.

PREPARATION AND USE Use in cooking, for spreads (mix with extra herbs if you wish) or for dips; or make instant sauces by heating in the microwave.

Homemade spreads can be made by mixing the cheese with spices or herbs in a food processor until smooth (this takes 3–5 minutes); then place in a covered container and refrigerate until ready to use. Varieties of cheese suitable for using in spreads are cheshire, leyden, blue leicester, emmental, gruyère, sharp cheddar.

VARIETIES
Adler brand spreads with herbs or chives, mushrooms, salami. Gruenland spreads with garlic, herbs, black pepper. Bayernland spreads with rum, mushroom.

SEE ALSO Processed Cheese.

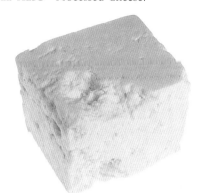

Cheshire

NUTRITIONAL INFORMATION Major nutrients similar to cheddar. Minimum fat 27%.

DESCRIPTION Light, crumbly and loose-textured cheese, white or red in colour, with a lightly salty tang. A semihard scalded curd cheese.

ORIGIN AND HISTORY Cheshire originated in England, taking its name from the county of Cheshire. The oldest named cheese in Britain, it was often called 'chester' by the French after the capital where the cheeses for export were sold. Produced in three types — red, white and blue — it is said to be held in high esteem by Union Jack patriots.

Red and white cheshire are very similar. Red cheshire was originally coloured with carrot juice, but these days annatto (a natural vegetable dye) is used.

Mentioned in the 'Domesday Book' as an already established cheese, cheshire is believed to have been the cheese enjoyed by the 20th Legion Roman soldiers garrisoned in Chester.

BUYING AND STORAGE White and red cheshire will turn bitter and rank if too old. Look for cheese which displays a clean appearance free of dry edges or discoloration.

Buy as required and store in the refrigerator, wrapped in cling wrap. Change the wrapping often to avoid build-up of stale butterfat. Cheshire should keep for about 2 weeks, depending on the size of the piece of cheese.

PREPARATION AND USE Remove from the refrigerator 1 hour before serving to allow the taste and texture of the cheese to develop. Use as a table cheese, for cheese boards, ploughman's lunch, Welsh rarebit. Cheshire melts well and can be used in cooking. Use a hot, dry knife for cutting, as the cheese tends to crumble.

Varieties

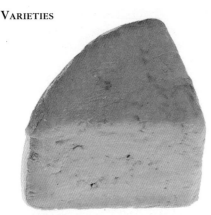

Blue Cheshire

Nutritional Information Major nutrients similar to other hard cheeses.

Description A 'technicolour' cheese with green veins scattered across a golden mass. Soft and buttery taste with a delectable bite. An internal mould ripened cheese.

Origin and History Once the rarest of blue cheeses and at first an accident of nature, blue cheshire originated in England. Openings left in white cheshire cheeses after draining the whey were ripe for mould development, resulting in the odd cheese spontaneously turning blue. To start with much of the blue cheese was thrown away, a little was kept to treat sores and infected wounds in the primitive days of medicine, and the remainder was sold off cheaply to the cheese markets.

These cheeses were originally called 'Green Fade' and remained a rare prize until 1968. As factory production commenced with the purpose of actively inducing the blue veins in cheshire cheese, one of Britain's rarest blues became its newest commercial cheese: blue cheshire.

Buying and Storage Buy as needed. Blue cheshire should have a rind free of grey patches, dryness or a clammy appearance. Look for a golden orange colour with a mass of greenish-blue veins. The veining should be well distributed and even in colour. The cheese should have a crumbly texture with a rich, creamy, fragrant bite.

Stored in the refrigerator well wrapped in foil it should keep for 2 weeks. Keep it away from milk, butter, cream or other delicate foods to avoid tainting.

Preparation and Use Remove the cheese from the refrigerator a good hour prior to serving to allow its taste and texture to develop. Use a separate knife to cut and serve to avoid flavour transfer. Blue cheshire is best served as a table cheese rather than used in cooking; however, it can be used in recipes calling for a crumbly rich fragrant blue. For cheese boards, serve with black grapes, dried fruits and whole nuts.

Red Cheshire This has the same characteristics as white cheshire, except for its colour.

Chester Chester is the French version of England's cheshire cheese; it is orange in colour. It was first produced shortly after World War II, taking its name from Cheshire's capital city.

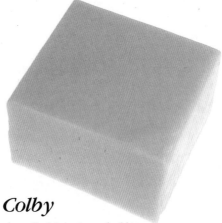

Colby

*also called **American cheddar***

Major Nutrients		Serve Size 20 g	
Energy	330 kJ	Sodium	120 mg
Protein	5 g	Calcium	130 mg
Fat	7 g	Phosphorus	100 mg
Carbohydrate	0	Vitamin A	70 µg
Cholesterol	20 mg	Thiamin	5 mg

Nutritional Information Minimum fat 30%. A typical hard cheese.

Description Similar to cheddar but softer in texture with more moisture and a sweeter, creamier, nuttier taste. A washed curd cheese.

Origin and History An American cheese, colby originated in Wisconsin, in 1882. It takes its name from the township of Colby. (American cheddars take on the name of the town where they are produced.) A large percentage of America's cheese production is cheddar — the cheese industry in America began in 1851 with the first cheddar factory being established in New York state. The majority of American cheese today is produced in Wisconsin.

Colby is a very popular American cheese which is now also produced in Australia, New Zealand, Canada and Denmark. New Zealand colby is exported to Australia and the USA. Colby matures much more rapidly than cheddar and is easier to manufacture, making it a popular variety with cheese makers. In some cases, it is sold as mild cheddar.

Buying and Storage Buy as required. Colby will not store as well as cheddar because it is higher in moisture and lower in salt. It is often available prepacked from the dairy case of supermarkets. Look for packs which are well sealed without any air traps, moulding or bulging of the package.

Once cut, store rewrapped securely in plastic wrap in the refrigerator. It should keep for 2–3 weeks.

Preparation and Use Remove from the refrigerator an hour before serving. Keep the cheese covered and away from direct heat or sunlight and allow it to reach room temperature. (Grate whilst the cheese is cold for easier grating.) Colby has a mild flavour ideal for children, and is suitable for salads, snacks, sandwiches or cheese platters. Serve with apples, pears or other fresh fruit.

Colby is also a good melting cheese.

Varieties Brand names include New Zealand colby, Devondale colby, Draft colby, United Dairies colby.

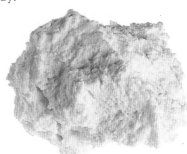

Cottage Cheese

*also called **Curd cheese, Dutch cheese, Farm cheese, Popcorn cheese, Pot cheese, Quark, Schmierkäse***

Major Nutrients		Creamed Serve Size 20 g	
Energy	100 kJ	Cholesterol	5 mg
Protein	3 g	Sodium	40 mg
Fat	1 g	Thiamin	5 mg
Carbohydrate	0		

		Baker's, continental-style, quark Serve Size 20 g	
Energy	70 kJ	Cholesterol	2 mg
Protein	3 g	Sodium	90 mg
Fat	1 g	Thiamin	8 mg
Carbohydrate	0		

Nutritional Information The high moisture content of cottage cheese results in low levels of kilojoules and of all nutrients. Cottage cheese is sometimes eaten in large quantities (100 g) and, while it may then provide a good source of protein, it is low in calcium and phosphorus and therefore not suitable as a milk substitute. In general cottage cheeses contain moderate amounts of fat and sodium. The fat content of creamed cottage cheese and other curd-style cheeses can vary from 4–10%. Baker's or continental-style cheese varies in fat content from negligible to 12%. Quark is similar to baker's cheese and usually has cream blended to make it 10% fat. Because of the saturated fat in cottage cheeses, the brands containing high fat should be used with caution. However, these cheeses do provide a low fat alternative to cream cheeses. Salt-free varieties are available.

DESCRIPTION Fresh, white, unripened curd cheese, resembling a mass of curd particles.

ORIGIN AND HISTORY Cottage cheese originated in Central Europe. It was the first crude cheese, discovered quite by accident. Legend has it that a nomadic herdsman travelling through the desert stopped to drink milk from his pouch and found a lumpy solid mass in a watery liquid. Unwittingly he had created the right conditions to produce cheese — his pouch, made from the stomach of a young animal, still contained the digestive enzyme rennin, which acted on the milk (warmed by the sun and shaken by the ride through the desert) to produce crude 'cheese'.

Many countries worldwide produce their own cottage cheese varieties. They are fresh cheeses which do not travel well. The commercial term 'cottage cheese' originated in the USA, where large quantities are produced. It takes its name from the practice of producing it in local cottages.

BUYING AND STORAGE After buying, refrigerate as quickly as possible. Cottage cheeses are delicate, high moisture cheeses with a short life. For peak quality use within 4 days. When buying tubs or packs, look for correctly sealed lids and check the use-by date. Cottage cheeses should be white, clear of any yellowing, and moist. The size of the curd particles varies according to type.

PREPARATION AND USE Cottage cheeses are best served straight from the fridge. They are the one group of cheeses that may be served cool rather than at room temperature.

VARIETIES

Continental-style has a finer, pastelike appearance; fat composition varies from non-fat to full cream. Farm-style is a small-grained creamed cottage cheese. Granular or American-style is skim milk cottage cheese dressed with a light cream dressing; sometimes sold with gherkin, pineapple or other flavours. Quark and baker's cheese are varieties of skim milk unsalted cottage cheese.

Liptauer is a fresh cheese often homemade from quark with paprika, butter and chopped onions mixed into it to form a spread. It was originally purely the name for the basic pot cheese produced in Hungary from ewe's milk,

but in many other countries, liptauer refers to the spread. Other types of seasonings or spices may be added.

Paneer is a soft, Indian cottage cheese with a texture like beancurd and a subtle curd-cheese flavour.

Anari is the cottage cheese of Cyprus. It is a whey cheese made like ricotta, with a slightly sweetish flavour and a fine, moist texture.

SEE ALSO Mizithra.

Cotto

MAJOR NUTRIENTS		SERVE SIZE 20 G	
Energy	180 kJ	Sodium	150 mg
Protein	5 g	Calcium	190 mg
Fat	2 g	Zinc	0.5 mg
Carbohydrate	0	Thiamin	6 mg
Cholesterol	10 mg		

NUTRITIONAL INFORMATION A dietary modified cheese with reduced fat and salt content.

DESCRIPTION A skim milk cheese, creamy white in colour and wheel-shaped. Cotto has a fresh, delicate, bland taste with a firm block texture, fairly soft but sliceable. It is available plain, smoked or with chives.

ORIGIN AND HISTORY Cotto was developed in Australia by United Dairies in NSW in response to consumer demand for a block cheese suitable for specific dietary needs. It was originally endorsed by the National Heart Foundation as one of a number of foods recommended for cholesterol-lowering diets. It has a low fat and salt content and remains the only block cheese produced from skim milk in Australia. There are, however, a number of other cheeses produced with reduced fat and salt levels.

BUYING AND STORAGE Buy in small or large quantities. Look for cheese free of dry edges or discoloration, and mould-free. Store wrapped in cling wrap in the refrigerator and use within a week or so for best quality. The reduction in fat and salt means that cotto will not store as long as cheddar.

PREPARATION AND USE Remove from the

refrigerator an hour before serving and use a knife to cut into thin slices. Cotto melts well. Use in sauces, melted over vegetables, in rice or salads, cubed, or added into recipes that call for a cheddar-style cheese, to reduce the overall fat content of the dish.

SEE ALSO Dietary Modified Cheese.

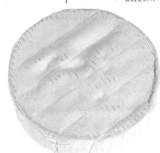

Coulommiers

also called **Brie de Coulommiers, Petit brie**

NUTRITIONAL INFORMATION Major nutrients similar to brie.

DESCRIPTION A small brie 300–500 g in size. A surface mould ripened cheese, coulommiers is popular eaten fresh and unripened (i.e. at the first sign of the white surface flora). At this stage it is delicate and mild in flavour. Left to ripen, it resembles a camembert in flavour.

ORIGIN AND HISTORY Originating in the Ile de France, coulommiers is generally larger than camembert and smaller than brie. It takes its name from the town where it was first produced; however, it is now made elsewhere.

BUYING AND STORAGE Look for white-surfaced cheese without any grey or dark patches, nor signs of ageing and drying, and check the use-by date. Coulommiers will keep in the refrigerator, depending on its degree of ripeness when purchased, but it is best eaten as soon as possible. If storing in the fridge, ensure that there are no heavy weights on top of the cheese. Store in the original wrapper if possible; otherwise wrap in foil.

PREPARATION AND USE Remove from the refrigerator an hour and a half before serving. Loosen the wrapping but do not uncover. Allow the cheese to reach room temperature. Serve on cheese platters as a whole cheese garnished with fresh berry fruits or whole nuts, fruit breads, avocado and melon slices. Always allow a separate knife to cut and serve to avoid flavour and texture transfer. Use in recipes requiring whole small bries for brie tortes, or cut into wedges and deep-fry.

VARIETIES

Chaource A small soft ripened cheese with

a downy white surface mould rind. Chaource, like coulommiers, is between a camembert and a brie in size. It takes its name from the market town in Champagne. It is rich and creamy in taste and texture, becoming saltier as it matures, with a pronounced mushroom aroma developing.

SEE ALSO Brie.

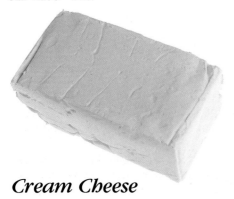

Cream Cheese

MAJOR NUTRIENTS			SERVE SIZE 20 G
Energy	360 kJ	Cholesterol	20 mg
Protein	1 g	Sodium	60 mg
Fat	10 g	Vitamin A	85 µg
Carbohydrate	0	Thiamin	5 mg

NUTRITIONAL INFORMATION Cream cheese is high in saturated fat and has a moderate amount of cholesterol. While a good source of vitamin A, it has little nutritional value and is high in kilojoules with at least 33% fat. Continental-style cottage cheese and ricotta may be substituted in recipes for cream cheese to reduce the fat. Neufchâtel contains at least 20% fat but less than 33% and also provides a reduced fat substitute for other cream cheeses. Because of the high level of saturated fat, cream cheese should be used sparingly.

DESCRIPTION Cream cheese is, as its name suggests, a fresh unripened curd cheese produced from cream. (In some cases it may be a mixture of cream with milk — e.g. neufchâtel.) Varieties differ around the world, ranging from the original fresh unripened mass of smooth cream (e.g. mascarpone), so thick it can be cut, to a firmer-bodied smooth cream cheese with a longer shelf life (e.g. philadelphia).

ORIGIN AND HISTORY Cream cheese is one of the oldest of cheeses, produced throughout Europe and England. The exact origin is uncertain. It is these fresh unripened cheeses that are most likely to have been enjoyed as a staple part of the diet back in the Dark Ages, because they were simple and quick to make. However, the best and richest of milks were required, rendering them a cheese for the lords of society in England, rather than for the peasant.

There are several recipes for producing cream cheese. The curd may be uncooked or cooked. The uncooked method is simply to add a special starter to cream, then allow it to stand for several hours until a solid curd forms. This is then placed in a cheesecloth and hung for several more hours, until all the whey is drained off.

France, Italy and England (to name just three countries) all have their own special fresh cream cheeses, but it was America that revolutionised cream cheese production in the 1880s with the introduction of the 'hot-pack' method (i.e. packaging the hot curd). This doubled the maximum life of the cheese to 60 days.

BUYING AND STORAGE Buy short-life fresh cream cheese as needed daily and store in the coolest part of the refrigerator away from strong-smelling foods. Cream cheese with a longer life (e.g. philadelphia) may be purchased in advance in larger quantities. Check the use-by date of individual brands. Cream cheese may also be purchased in bulk or packaged in tubs, cylindrical sausage shapes or foil packs. Look for cheese which has a fresh, moist, unblemished appearance without signs of dryness, dullness of colour or yellowing. It should have a rich creamy smooth texture and light acidic flavour.

PREPARATION AND USE Keep refrigerated until needed. Cream cheese may be served chilled as a dessert cheese with fresh fruits in season or used as a base for savoury appetisers or dips. Use for cheesecakes, in cheese rolls, logs or balls and for crepe fillings.

PROCESSING Cream cheese is sometimes used to make fruit cheese logs; usually it is neufchâtel which is used.

VARIETIES
Caboc, mascarpone, neufchâtel, philadelphia: see separate entries. Also petit suisse and its close relative, gervais.

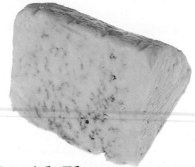

Danish Blue

also called Danablu

MAJOR NUTRIENTS			SERVE SIZE 20 G
Energy	320 kJ	Sodium	155 mg
Protein	4 g	Calcium	110 mg
Fat	7 g	Phosphorus	60 mg
Carbohydrate	0	Vitamin A	60 µg
Cholesterol	20 mg	Thiamin	9 mg

NUTRITIONAL INFORMATION Minimum fat 27%. A typical hard cheese.

DESCRIPTION Pale straw to white in colour with even blue-green veining. Strong and fairly tangy in flavour. Sliceable consistency. An internal mould ripened cheese.

Danablu is soft-textured with a buttery consistency, easy to spread and slice, with a pronounced savoury flavour and stronger than mycella, or 'Danish gorgonzola'. The other Danish blue vein cheese produced more recently is blue castello.

ORIGIN AND HISTORY Originated in Denmark in the early 1900s. It was styled on roquefort, but it is produced from cow's milk rather than ewe's milk. It was invented by Marius Boel, who introduced a bread mould culture into high fat cheese made from homogenised milk. The name danablu is a blend of two words meaning 'Denmark' and 'blue'.

BUYING AND STORAGE Look for milk-white cheese with an even distribution of blue veins. Avoid any greyness of colour, dullness or dry appearance. Store well wrapped in foil in the refrigerator away from delicate foods which could be tainted by its strong aroma. Correctly stored, it should last for 2–3 weeks. Check the use-by date and be aware that the smaller the piece of cheese, the shorter the amount of time it may be stored without excessive drying and moulding.

PREPARATION AND USE Remove from the refrigerator 1½ hours before serving to allow the cheese to develop its true character and taste. Loosen its wrapping during this time and keep away from direct sun and heat. Serve with a separate knife. If cutting slices of cheese, use a hot, dry knife for clean cutting without sticking. Use as a table cheese after dessert. It may also be used in salad dressings, and as a filling mixed with cream cheese for open sandwiches and cocktail savouries.

SEE ALSO Blue Castello, Mycella.

Dietary Modified Cheeses

NUTRITIONAL INFORMATION See under Varieties.

DESCRIPTION Dietary modified cheeses are cheeses that have been developed and produced with an altered fat and/or salt content. The various varieties may have either reduced or low amounts of fat or salt, or altered structure resulting in an overall low cholesterol product (e.g. lo-chol).

ORIGIN AND HISTORY A product of the modern day, dietary modified cheeses evolved as a result of increasing interest in the state of overall diet, particularly in relation to cholesterol. As consumers' knowledge and awareness of nutritionally balanced diets increased, significant technological investment was made to develop cheeses with an acceptable taste but reduced or altered fat and salt levels.

Countries such as France and Italy appear not to have set a trend in these varieties, with any serious cheese lover discounting them as unreal 'cheeses', whereas in Australia a market exists for low cholesterol products as well as for cheddar styles with reduced levels of fat and salt.

BUYING AND STORAGE In many cases these cheeses are available from health food shops, as well as supermarkets and delicatessens, depending on the variety and brand.

The skim milk cheeses (such as cotto) and low cholesterol cheeses (such as lo-chol) have an almost white colour. The reduced fat and salt cheddars, on the other hand, are in appearance the same as regular cheddar with its varying degrees of yellow. Their appearance should be fresh and clean without any trace of moulding, excess moisture or dryness. Cheddars with reduced fat and salt content last on average 6–8 weeks less than regular cheddars. Best purchased fresh, as required, and used within 2–3 weeks.

PREPARATION AND USE Use in recipes as a substitute for cheddar or other firm cheese to reduce the overall fat and/or salt content. Cheese varieties melt more easily with a better result if they are higher in fat content. However, the dietary modified cheeses will melt quite well, varying according to brand. Their flavour will be unassuming and mild, able to blend well with appropriate herbs and spices. As with regular cheese, remove from the refrigerator an hour before serving. Use for sandwiches, snacks and salads and in cooking.

VARIETIES
Apart from the varieties listed below, a reduced fat and salt cheddar is also available. Cotto, a skim milk cheese, has its own entry elsewhere.

Lo-Chol

MAJOR NUTRIENTS		SERVE SIZE 20 G	
Energy	330 kJ	Carbohydrate	0
Protein	5 g	Cholesterol	0
Fat	6 g	Sodium	150 mg

NUTRITIONAL INFORMATION No data available on vitamin and mineral content.

DESCRIPTION A reduced cholesterol cheese. Lite-chol is the name of a new Australian variety of Lo-chol.

Nimbin

MAJOR NUTRIENTS		SERVE SIZE 20 G	
Energy	320 kJ	Cholesterol	n/a
Protein	5 g	Sodium	72 mg
Fat	6 g	Calcium	160 mg
Carbohydrate	0	Thiamin	8 mg

NUTRITIONAL INFORMATION Apart from the lower salt content, this is a typical hard cheese.

DESCRIPTION An Australian brand of low salt cheese.

Reduced Fat Cheddar

MAJOR NUTRIENTS		SERVE SIZE 20 G	
Energy	280 kJ	Cholesterol	15 mg
Protein	5 g	Sodium	140 mg
Fat	5 g	Thiamin	8 mg
Carbohydrate	0		

NUTRITIONAL INFORMATION Contains less fat than regular cheddar.

Saint Otho One of Switzerland's best low fat cheeses (around 4% fat). It is firm-textured, pale ivory with an orange rind, and has small holes dotted throughout the body of the cheese. It has a mild flavour and is used for snacks or sandwiches.

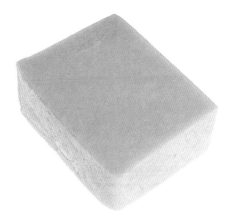

Double Gloucester

NUTRITIONAL INFORMATION Major nutrients similar to cheddar.

DESCRIPTION A hard block cheese, bright orange in colour with a smooth satiny texture and full flavour. A hard uncooked curd cow's milk cheese.

ORIGIN AND HISTORY An ancient English cheese steeped in festive spring traditions adapted from the 8th century May Day custom of rolling the cheese down the slopes of the Cotswolds. A 1911 tale describes gloucester cheeses decked with spring flowers heralding the start of spring with a grand parade into a church at Randwick. Afterwards the flowers were removed and the magnificent wheel-shaped and tough-crusted cheeses were rolled around the churchyard three times, then dressed again with flowers and taken into the village to be cut and distributed to the parishioners for eating.

Up to 1945 there were two varieties of gloucester: single and double. Double gloucester remains in production, but the single variety now lies dormant. The bright orange colour characteristic of double gloucester was originally due to the addition of carrot juice, but now the natural vegetable dye annatto is used.

BUYING AND STORAGE Double gloucester should be bright orange in colour with a satiny smooth texture. Avoid cheese which appears sweaty or cracked. Prepacked cheeses should show no signs of air bubbles or blown packaging. Double gloucester has excellent keeping qualities. Store in the refrigerator, making sure all the exposed surfaces are wrapped in cling wrap. Leave the rind uncovered, as this will allow it to breathe. Should any traces of mould appear, trim the cheese and rewrap. Its flavour should be full and savoury, without bitterness. Correctly stored, it should keep for several weeks.

PREPARATION AND USE Remove from the refrigerator 1 hour before serving. Keep the cheese wrapped or place under a cheese dome with a sugar cube to prop up the cover (this will absorb moisture given off). Double gloucester has a full, mellow flavour. It is good for slicing for sandwiches, on toast, over steaks or with apple pie. Also serve with pickles or fresh apples and pears.

VARIETIES
Cotswold is double gloucester cheese which has been flavoured with chives and onions.

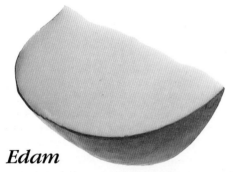

Edam

also called Tête de mort, Tête de maure, Manbollen, Katzenkopf, Moor's head

MAJOR NUTRIENTS   SERVE SIZE 20 G

Energy	300 kJ	Calcium	165 mg
Protein	5 g	Phosphorus	105 mg
Fat	5 g	Zinc	0.8 mg
Carbohydrate	0	Vitamin A	5 µg
Cholesterol	15 mg	Thiamin	2 mg
Sodium	195 mg		

NUTRITIONAL INFORMATION Minimum fat 21%. A typical hard cheese.

DESCRIPTION A round cannonball-shaped cheese coated in red wax, with a firm texture and mild buttery taste. An uncooked semifirm cheese.

ORIGIN AND HISTORY Edam is one of Holland's most famous cheeses, dating back to the Middle Ages. It originated in northern Holland and takes its name from the town of Edam. Unique worldwide as the only cheese to be completely round like a cannonball, edam was one of the early cheeses carried in the hulls of the ships when the Dutch became the dominant freight carriers in the Mediterranean in the late 1300s. Thanks to its shape and wax coating, it transported easily without damage and had good keeping qualities. As a result the bright red balls of edam are well known worldwide. In Holland itself, however, edam is often unwaxed or coated in yellow wax: the red-waxed edams are all exported. Legend has it that the cannonball shape evolved to enable the edam balls to be rolled from the warehouses to the wharves nearby and then down into the hulls of the freight ships.

Edam is widely copied. Some varieties are spiced with cumin.

BUYING AND STORAGE Look for well-shaped cheeses free of any cracks or splits on the red or yellow wax coating. Edam may have a few tiny holes in its body, but generally should have a smooth texture, sliceable and pliant. Edam has exceptional keeping qualities. Wrap all exposed surfaces of the cheese with cling wrap, leaving the waxed rind uncovered.

PREPARATION AND USE Remove the cheese from the refrigerator an hour before serving to allow it to reach room temperature and develop its smooth texture and mellow flavour. Keep the cheese covered during this time to prevent drying out. Use as a breakfast or lunch cheese, or where a mild delicate flavour is required. Edam is a good all-round cheese suitable for slicing, dicing or grating. Use in sandwiches, for snacks, and on cheese boards with apples and pears. It has poorer melting qualities than cheddar owing to its lower fat content.

PROCESSING Edam can sometimes be bought as prepacked slices.

VARIETIES
Edam may be classifed by size as baby edam (880–1100 g), commissie (3–4.5 kg), middlebare (5–6.5 kg).

Molbo is a round cheese produced in Denmark resembling Dutch edam with its red rind and yellow body. Molbo has a mild taste and is believed to be a reasonably good copy of edam.

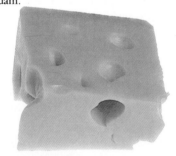

Emmental

also called Emmentaler

NUTRITIONAL INFORMATION Minimum fat 25%. Major nutrients typical of hard cheese.

DESCRIPTION A firm yellow cooked curd cheese with round 'eyes'. It has a sweet-dry flavour with a nutty aftertaste and a hazelnut aroma.

ORIGIN AND HISTORY One of Switzerland's most famous cheeses, emmental originated in the canton of Bern. It takes its name from the Emme Valley (emmental meaning 'Valley of the Emme'). A true Alpine cheese, it was originally made by the alpine herdsmen (Sennen) in their mountain huts which they used as dairies. They not only tended the cattle, milked them and made cheese, but also carried their cheeses on donkeys to the markets in the valleys to sell to the public.

These first emmentals were quite small. It was not until the 16th century that the Sennen learned how to make larger cheeses that could store longer. Swiss cheese production increased rapidly during the first half of the 17th century and eventually small cheese dairies were established in the valleys to cope with the extra demand in the 18th century. As little distinction could be made between the cheese made up in the alpine huts and that produced in the valleys, more dairies started production until eventually almost every village had its own.

BUYING AND STORAGE Look for emmental with a smooth dry rind, hard and golden yellow, sometimes waxed. It is a large flat wheel or disc shape, bulging slightly at the sides. Cut surfaces of emmental should show an interior with large well-spaced 'eyes' or holes, glistening with butterfat. The eyes should be cherry-sized and the butterfat indicates a cheese ripened to maturity.

Store refrigerated with all cut surfaces firmly wrapped in cling wrap. Correctly stored, it should last for 3 weeks in the refrigerator. Trim away any slight outside moulding that may occur and rewrap.

PREPARATION AND USE For table use, sandwiches and cheese platters, ensure the cheese has been removed one hour before serving to allow it to reach room temperature and develop its true characteristics of flavour and texture. Use also in cooking. Emmental tends to draw threads when melted, so blend it with gruyère for traditional fondues. Good in cheese or savoury pastries and rice dishes. Serve cubed in salads, or grated over chicken, vegetables, veal or egg dishes.

PROCESSING Emmental is often processed and used as a base for flavoured processed cheeses.

VARIETIES

Herrgärdsöst Produced in Sweden, herrgärdsöst is styled on emmental, but has a milder character. There is a full fat version available in Sweden called hergard elite. Another popular breakfast version is called drabart; it is foil-ripened and mild in taste.

Herrgärdsöst enjoys the same storage principles and uses as emmental.

Montasio Produced in Italy, montasio is similar in texture and taste to emmental until it ages and hardens, when it becomes more like asiago and is used for grating.

Saint Claire Australia's own version of emmental. Saint Claire, produced in traditional large wheels and coated in thin wax, is rich yellow in colour. It has a distinct nutty flavour. It has many large eyes and is an ideal melting cheese. As it ages, it gains in flavour.

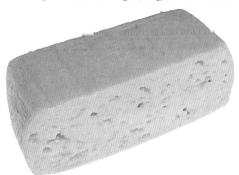

Esrom

NUTRITIONAL INFORMATION No detailed data available. Being a full cream cheese, it would have a high fat content.

DESCRIPTION A full cream oblong cheese with a firm texture and spicy flavour. Golden yellow in colour with small holes, it has a washed rind. A semihard uncooked curd cheese.

ORIGIN AND HISTORY Esrom takes its name and origin from the monastery town of Esrom in Denmark. It was originally copied from the recipe for port salut and was made by monks at Esrom. It later died out and was for a time forgotten until the Danish Dairy Research Institute rediscovered it and production commenced. This new cheese is believed to be richer and creamier than the original. It was renamed Esrom when Danish authorities decided to take a step towards establishing a Danish range of cheeses. Esrom is now well entrenched as a cheese in its own right.

BUYING AND STORAGE Esrom should have a smooth thin rind with a supple sliceable body dotted with small holes. It should not show any signs of dryness, nor darkening. It should have a distinctive aroma. Buy as required and store wrapped in foil in the refrigerator at a maximum temperature of 6°C for 2–4 weeks.

PREPARATION AND USE Remove from the refrigerator an hour before serving and keep covered until served. Serve as a snack cheese or for open sandwiches and hors d'oeuvres. Esrom slices well. Generally used as a table cheese rather than in cooking.

VARIETIES
Esrom may sometimes be spiced with onions, herbs, garlic or pepper.

Biarom Semisoft Bavarian cheese which may be spiced with caraway, peppercorns, paprika or onion. It is commonly foil-wrapped, and is styled on esrom. Biarom is sometimes called port salut.

SEE ALSO Port Salut.

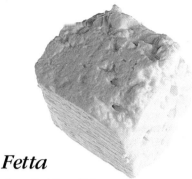

Fetta

*also called **Feta, Telemes***

MAJOR NUTRIENTS		SERVE SIZE 20 G	
Energy	200 kJ	Sodium	220 mg
Protein	5 g	Calcium	70 mg
Fat	3 g	Phosphorus	80 mg
Carbohydrate	0	Thiamin	3 mg
Cholesterol	12 mg		

NUTRITIONAL INFORMATION Minimum fat 19%. Despite the higher moisture content, the nutrients are similar to those of hard cheese.

DESCRIPTION Fetta is white in colour. It is an uncooked soft cheese 'pickled' by maturation in brine, giving it a characteristic salty taste.

ORIGIN AND HISTORY The ancient ancestor of modern fetta was undoubtedly a cheese made in Greece. The subject of Greek myths, it appears in several tales including Homer's account of the hero Odysseus, who enters the cave of the cyclops to find row upon row of white cheeses and casks overflowing with whey.

Made by shepherds in the mountains near Athens, fetta was traditionally made from ewe's milk and sometimes from goat's milk too. Fetta has been produced in the Balkans for centuries and is made worldwide in countries such as Australia, America and Denmark. These countries generally use cow's milk to produce their fetta. Bulgaria also produces fetta, using ewe's milk.

Fetta takes its name from the word *fetes* meaning large blocks or slices: the curd is cut into such blocks before being ripened and stored in brine.

BUYING AND STORAGE Fetta is sold either in bulk from delicatessens, or in large tins, buckets or prepacks. Choose clear, moist-looking cheese, white in colour, in block form. Young fetta will be softer with

occasional holes. It will store very well, particularly if purchased in large quantity buckets or tins (2.5–3 kg), since it may then be kept in the brine solution. Prepacks are best bought as required and used quickly to avoid drying out. Store in the refrigerator, preferably in some of the cheese's own brine solution. Sealed cans have a life span of about 4 months.

PREPARATION AND USE Remove the amount of cheese blocks required from the tin or bucket (if purchased in large quantity), carefully resealing the lid. Drain the cheese blocks to avoid brine leaking over the plate, by lifting them out of the tin, bucket or prepack and placing onto a clean cloth. Use diced or crumbled in salads, for stuffing mixes, spinach pies, mixed with other cheeses for cooking. Fetta may be used as a table cheese but is most frequently used in cooking.

VARIETIES
Bulgarian, German and Australian Attiki brand fetta are creamy and slightly salty with sweet overtones. Italian, Greek and Danish fetta are coarser and saltier. American fetta has a sharp and pronounced taste.

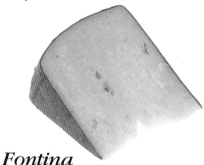

Fontina

*also called **Fontal***

NUTRITIONAL INFORMATION With major nutrients similar to gouda, this is a typical hard cheese.

DESCRIPTION A semihard flat round cheese with a dark golden brown brushed rind. It has an ivory interior with a smooth texture and a few tiny holes. Faintly nutty, sweet and buttery in flavour with a smooth creamy texture. A scalded curd semihard cheese.

ORIGIN AND HISTORY Many connoisseurs place fontina amongst the six great cheeses of the world. Known as the 'delicious gift of Piedmont', and cited as one of Italy's best cheeses in a dairy encyclopaedia in 1477, it was served to the dukes of Savoy. Fontina Val d'Aosta was originally made in the Valley of Aosta in the province of Piedmont; dating back to the 13th century, it was made from ewe's milk. Modern-day fontina, however, has become an important source of income for cattle owners in the area, with village factories and larger concerns producing the cheese from cow's milk.

Fontina takes its name from Mount Fontin and the name is restricted by Italian law to cheese produced in the Aosta Valley. Because of this, almost identical cheeses made in other parts of northern Italy are called fontal.

It is a widely copied variety of cheese produced in other countries under different names or variations of the name. Danish fontina has a sourer taste, whilst the Swedish variety has a fuller flavour. French fontal is softer and sweeter with buttery overtones. In the USA and Australia a variety called fontinella is produced. All of these types are generally softer in texture than fontina.

BUYING AND STORAGE Italian fontina has a brown rind whilst the French, Danish and Swedish copies all have red waxed rinds. Avoid cheese with a sandy texture, a swollen appearance and an exaggerated hole formation. The cheese should have a delicate, slightly fruity flavour with very little aroma. It should be supple and smooth, showing tiny holes, with a thin, almost smooth rind. Store in the refrigerator covered in cling wrap and change the wrapping regularly. It should last 1 or 2 weeks.

PREPARATION AND USE Fontina is the basis of the Italian dish called fonduta in which butter, milk, melted cheese and beaten egg yolks are mixed together and topped with thin slivers of white truffles, then served over polenta.

SEE ALSO Pastorello.

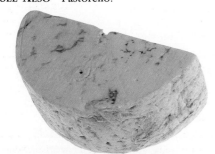

Fourme d'Ambert

also called Fourme de Montbrison, Fourme de Pierre-sur-Haute

NUTRITIONAL INFORMATION This is a typical hard cheese.

DESCRIPTION A cow's milk soft cheese, shaped into tall cylinders. It has a dark grey dry rind, dotted with bright red and light yellow pigments, and a pale yellow interior scattered with blue veins. An internal mould ripened cheese, it has a crumbly texture and

a strong, salty taste.

ORIGIN AND HISTORY One of the French 'bleus', originating in Auvergne, central France. It is a cheese of high repute in France and is ripened in the very damp atmosphere of cellars for up to 5 months. The best seasons for production are summer and autumn. It is often known as, or referred to as, fourme de Pierre-sur-Haute. 'Fourme' is a genetic term for a group of cheeses (mostly produced in Auvergne). Fourme d'Ambert is styled on the French roquefort but produced from cow's milk. It differs from imitations made elsewhere in France in that the salt is mixed into the curd rather than rubbed into the surface.

BUYING AND STORAGE Choose cheese which has a clean homogeneous surface free of cracks or stickiness. Fourme d'Ambert has a pronounced bitterness, but it should not be excessively bitter, nor have a grainy texture. Store wrapped in foil or cling wrap in the refrigerator and keep away from milk, butter and cream. It should keep for 1–2 weeks, but is best purchased as required.

PREPARATION AND USE Best served at the end of meals. Allow an hour at room temperature with the cheese covered over for its character to develop. Use a separate knife to cut and serve. Slice with a hot, dry knife for a clean, easy cut. Serve with celery and grapes. It will blend well in flavour with rich cream cheeses such as mascarpone, thanks to its strong flavour. Use in cocktail nibbles, cheese balls, and with dried fruit and whole nuts.

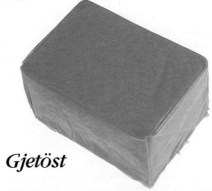

Gjetöst

MAJOR NUTRIENTS		SERVE SIZE 20 G	
Energy	390 kJ	Sodium	120 mg
Protein	2 g	Calcium	80 mg
Fat	6 g	Phosphorus	90 mg
Carbohydrate	8 g	Riboflavin	0.2 mg
Cholesterol	20 mg	Thiamin	4 mg

NUTRITIONAL INFORMATION Gjetöst and mysöst are whey cheeses which contain the carbohydrate lactose (milk sugar) and whey proteins. They are excellent sources of calcium and phosphorus. Gjetöst is a good source of riboflavin and is high in saturated

fat. These cheeses traditionally have iron added in their manufacture. They provide an excellent energy source as well as some high quality protein. Combined with crispbreads they provide Scandinavians with a healthy convenience food highly suited to their cold climate. These cheeses need to be kept well chilled for freshness.

DESCRIPTION A golden brown to orange, firm, small oblong block cheese with a sweet caramelised taste. A whey cheese.

ORIGIN AND HISTORY Originally a cheese of expediency, gjetöst is one of Scandinavia's oldest cheeses, originating in Norway. Because cow's milk was used to produce butter in Norway, the whey cheeses (such as gjetöst) were made from the whey of goat's milk. (Whey is liquid drained off the curd during cheese making.)

Originally it was made by poor farmers who boiled the whey into a brown paste, which was then used as a spread for bread. Eventually cream or milk from either cow's or goat's milk, or a combination, was added, resulting in gjetöst cheese. It is now prepared from a mixture of 10% goat's milk and 90% cow's milk. Ekte gjetöst is made totally from the whey of goat's milk and has a darker colour and richer taste. Kvit gjetöst is a blend of 95% goat's and 5% cow's milk. It is white and firm-textured and has a mild goat cheese taste (earthy).

Gjetöst is not widely copied by other countries — America is believed to be the only other country producing its own gjetöst whereas other whey cheeses such as ricotta are widely produced.

BUYING AND STORAGE Gjetöst is most often referred to by the brand name Ski Queen. It should be a small brick-shaped cheese, dark orange in colour, with a smooth, almost glossy surface. When tasted it should resemble peanut butter in texture and have a sweet caramel taste. Store wrapped in cling wrap or foil in the refrigerator. Buy in quantities as required rather than storing for any long period of time.

PREPARATION AND USE Remove from the refrigerator and serve in wafer-thin slices on crispbread or crackers topped with jam or marmalade. Gjetöst is an acquired taste owing to its fudgelike caramel sweetness. It is a staple part of the Norwegian diet, very popular for breakfast with strong black coffee.

VARIETIES
Ekte gjetöst, kvit gjetöst (see Origin and History). The most common brand is Ski Queen.

SEE ALSO Mysöst.

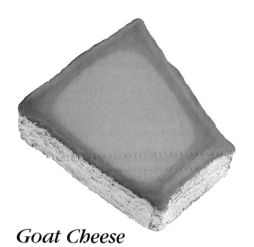

Goat Cheese

*also called **Chevres, Zieger***

NUTRITIONAL INFORMATION Major nutrients similar to equivalent types of cow's milk cheese.

DESCRIPTION Any type of cheese made using goat's milk rather than cow's milk.

ORIGIN AND HISTORY Goat cheese, renowned for its musky full taste, is well established in France and Italy, and also widespread in India, Africa, Turkey and Iran. A somewhat new industry is evolving in Australia. It is likely that in the pre-Viking era, many countries relied on goat's milk, rather than cow's milk, for cheese making.

In early Roman times it was goats, along with ewes, that were the most domesticated of animals, providing a diet of milk and cheese made by curdling their milk with the latex of the fig tree. One of the most famous early cheeses in the 1200s was marzoline, produced in Tuscany from goat's and cow's milk together.

BUYING AND STORAGE The single common feature to look for is the colour of the cheese (beneath the coating if there is one): it should be chalk-white without any appearance of dryness around the edges. Avoid cheese with a smell of ammonia. Buy as required, since refrigeration tends to dry these delicate, moist cheeses. Store no longer than 2 weeks. The rind or skin may vary from bluish-grey (ash-coated) to off-white.

PREPARATION AND USE Remove from the refrigerator and sprinkle young chevres with thyme and olive oil for serving. Once prepared, however, do not refrigerate again as the oil dressing will discolour and harden the cheese — it must be used immediately. Young cheeses are milder; serve an older chevre if a pronounced earthy taste is required. Serve as a table cheese with dates.

VARIETIES
There are 400 or so varieties of goat's milk cheese, too numerous to list. They are produced from either pure goat's milk or a combination of goat's and cow's milk. Most are soft varieties, either with a bloomy rind or surface-smeared, and the shape and size vary — cones, pyramids, balls, small round discs. Some are covered in ash.

Brand names include: Baron, Chabichou, Valencay, Sainte Maure, Bucheron, Dougon White Pyramid.

Saint Marcellin is a soft French cheese originally made from goat's milk, but now mostly made from either a mix of cow's milk and goat's or entirely cow's milk. It has a moist soft texture, with a piquant taste. It may be mixed with herbs and olive oil, and sold in jars. It is then called 'Le Pitchou'.

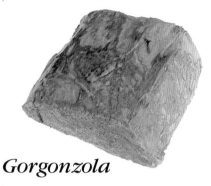

Gorgonzola

NUTRITIONAL INFORMATION Despite its texture, the major nutrients of gorgonzola are those of a hard cheese.

DESCRIPTION A soft, moist cheese, creamy in colour with blue-green veining. Has a rich, mellow flavour and creamy texture. An internal mould ripened cheese.

ORIGIN AND HISTORY Originating in Italy, gorgonzola is called after the village of the same name in Milan. Produced as far back as the 9th century, it was originally called stracchino gorgonzola. *Stracco* means tired, referring to the tiring journey of the dairymen of Lombardy moving their cows to summer pastures. Gorgonzola was the place they broke their journey for a rest and to milk the cows — hence the milk used to make gorgonzola cheese was 'tired' milk.

Gorgonzola is one of the three great blue cheeses copied worldwide. In Italy it is matured in caves. It is creamier than stilton or roquefort (the other two great blues).

BUYING AND STORAGE Buy as required. Try to avoid storing for any length of time, as the potent aroma of gorgonzola may taint other foods in the refrigerator. If it must be stored, wrap the cheese securely and keep away from lighter, more delicate foods. It should keep for about 2 weeks, depending on the size of the cheese.

Gorgonzola should have an almost smooth reddish-grey rind with a white interior. Avoid cheese which has hardened and sharpened in flavour, or which has very few veins. It should be tender and soft in texture, almost to the point of running. Aged cheese has a heavy moulding and is strong, dry and crumbly.

PREPARATION AND USE Remove from the refrigerator 1½ hours before serving, loosen wrapping and allow the cheese to reach room temperature. Use a separate knife to cut and serve.

Serve with fresh peaches or pears. Layer with mascarpone, or basil. Stuff pears, figs, dates, nuts, dried apricots, grapes.

Crumble aged cheese into salads. Melt over steaks, jacket potatoes. Gorgonzola may also be used in cooking. It is creamier and less salty than the other blues.

VARIETIES
Dolcelatte is the brand name of a factory-made gorgonzola. Pannarone (gorgonzola bianca) is a white gorgonzola. This variety is highly salted, without mould except on the crust (and this is washed off before marketing). It acquires a piquant, slightly bitter taste.

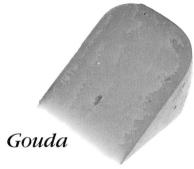

Gouda

MAJOR NUTRIENTS		SERVE SIZE 20 G	
Energy	320 kJ	Calcium	160 mg
Protein	5 g	Phosphorus	115 mg
Fat	6 g	Vitamin A	65 µg
Carbohydrate	0	Thiamin	4 mg
Cholesterol	20 g	Zinc	8 mg
Sodium	130 mg		

NUTRITIONAL INFORMATION Minimum fat 26%. A typical hard cheese.

DESCRIPTION A firm, sliceable cheese with a buttery taste which deepens as the cheese matures. It is produced in wheels with a yellow waxed rind. Creamier than edam. A semihard uncooked curd cheese.

ORIGIN AND HISTORY One of the oldest Dutch cheeses (and from all accounts the principal variety), gouda originated in the heart of Holland, near Rotterdam. Legend claims that the first cheese was produced in the village of Stolwijk and in fact the stamp of Stolwijk still guarantees a really tasty gouda cheese. The name comes from the town of Gouda, which has always been famous for excellent cheese and milk as well as for freight and trade. Gouda cheeses were compared to the English derby cheeses back in the 13th century. At that time six-monthly cheese markets were held for merchants from Scotland and England to buy and sell cheese.

Traditionally, gouda was always made on farms by the womenfolk. It is the cheese responsible for the rustic country dish called kaasdoop in which gouda is melted and cooked with milk and eaten similarly to Swiss fondue with the exception that brown bread is used rather than crusty white, or potatoes.

Leyden is a close relative and there are many matured cheeses, such as mona lisa, made in the gouda style.

BUYING AND STORAGE The red or yellow waxed rind should be free of splits or cracks. The interior should be cream to pale yellow in colour, firm and smooth with a few tiny holes, irregular in size. Gouda has good keeping qualities, so large quantities may be purchased and stored in the refrigerator. Ensure all cut surfaces are securely wrapped in plastic film. Aged gouda will have a dryness under the rind and its colour should be a darker yellow. Correctly stored, gouda will keep for several weeks.

PREPARATION AND USE Remove the cheese from the refrigerator an hour before serving. Use a hot knife to cut. It is a good slicing cheese and is essentially used as a table cheese in sandwiches and open sandwiches, on cheese boards and with crusty bread and quince jelly. It is also versatile in the kitchen and may be used for melting over vegetables, veal, chicken etc.

VARIETIES

Sveciaöst Sveciaöst is the Swedish version of gouda. When aged for 12 months, it has a full flavour, whereas young cheeses are mild. Occasionally they may have the addition of cumin or caraway. There are several family types of sveciaöst, all based on gouda, but with varying fat levels, some aged and some young, some spiced, others plain.

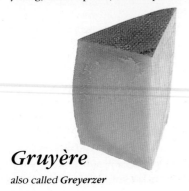

Gruyère

also called Greyerzer

NUTRITIONAL INFORMATION Gruyère is a typical hard cheese. Minimum fat 27%.

DESCRIPTION A hard amber yellow cheese with only a few holes or eyes the size of peas, enclosed in wrinkled brownish rind. A relative of emmental, it has more moisture with a stronger fruity flavour and is much smaller in size. A cooked curd hard cheese.

ORIGIN AND HISTORY Gruyère originated in the canton of Fribourg, Switzerland, where the black and white Swiss cattle are found. The first court of Gruyère is said to have levied taxes payable in cheeses of the region back in 1115. Years later in the 1600s, the cheese was found in Italy and Lyon.

The origins of gruyère stretch across the French–Swiss border. Both France and Switzerland were granted the right to use the name 'gruyère' by the Sesa Convention. In France, it was born out of the need for a cheese with long keeping qualities. The Swiss gruyère is sweeter than the French one. Cheese called gruyère is also produced in other countries, including Australia.

BUYING AND STORAGE The rind of gruyère should be dark gold to brown, hard with some degree of dryness under the rind. The interior should be pale amber, scattered with tiny holes ranging from pea to cherry size. The rind should be intact without any signs of splitting. It should taste nutlike, fruity and flavoursome without excessive sharpness; it is sometimes salty. Gruyère has an assertive aroma: store in the refrigerator with all cut surfaces wrapped in cling wrap and keep away from milk, butter and cream. It should keep for several weeks; during this time it may become stronger and lose some of its moisture.

PREPARATION AND USE Gruyère is a good after-dinner cheese: serve with dates, dried fruits and whole nuts. Use also in traditional fondue, mixed with emmental. Gruyère has a richer flavour and more moisture than emmental. It is an excellent melting cheese which draws hardly any threads. Use in salads, classical sauces and a variety of hot dishes, as well as open sandwiches and savouries.

PROCESSING Gruyère may also be processed to create a variety called grappe, which is processed gruyère covered in grape seeds. Or it can be processed with either kirsch or cherry extract blended into it: this variety is called gourmandise or fromage fondu.

VARIETIES

Gruyère de comte is French gruyère; it is sometimes called comte. Gruyère is also made in the Beaufort region of the Savoie Moun-

tains and is called gruyère de Beaufort. Comte bears a stronger resemblance to the Swiss original than does Beaufort. It has a delicate nutty aromatic taste and has a scattering of small holes.

Vacherin fribourgeois is produced in Switzerland. The name refers to the herdsmen of Fribourg, who first made the cheese. It is a Swiss cheese without holes, although it does have small cracks. It has a creamier, more pronounced taste than gruyère, smooth in texture. It is believed to have developed from gruyère and is a specialty of the region of Fribourg in Switzerland. It is not commonly seen outside the country. It makes a stronger fondue than the other Swiss cheeses.

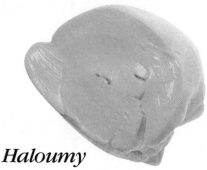

Haloumy

also called Halloumi

MAJOR NUTRIENTS		SERVE SIZE 30 G	
Energy	200 kJ	Calcium	180 mg
Protein	5 g	Phosphorus	130 mg
Fat	3 g	Vitamin A	60 µg
Carbohydrate	0	Thiamin	4 mg
Cholesterol	10 mg	Zinc	0.8 mg
Sodium	600 mg		

NUTRITIONAL INFORMATION An excellent source of calcium; good source of protein, vitamin A and phosphorus; high source of fat, predominantly saturated. Contains a high sodium content and moderate cholesterol.

DESCRIPTION A sheep's milk cheese, firmish and string-like in texture, creamy white in colour, and a little like fetta cheese in flavour. It is a cooked cheese, with the drained, gently compacted curd being cut in portions and boiled in its own whey until it floats. These pieces of curd are removed, sprinkled with dried mint flakes or black cumin seeds and salt, then folded in three to hold in the flavouring. It is normally matured in a brine pickle for at least 6 weeks, but can be eaten freshly made.

ORIGIN AND HISTORY Haloumy is a specialty of Cyprus, Lebanon and Syria, dating back some 2000 years, and used throughout the Middle East. It began as a cheese made in the home, and is still frequently homemade; cow's milk may also be used. The Cypriot version uses mint as the flavouring; the Lebanese and Syrian versions use black cumin seeds.

BUYING AND STORAGE Available in blocks of 200 g from Middle Eastern, Greek and Cypriot food stores, where it is likely to be taken from a bucket of brine. However, vacuum packing has made haloumy easier to purchase and store, and some supermarkets, delicatessens and specialty cheese shops now also stock the cheese. Store bulk haloumy in brine in a cool, dark place for a few weeks, or in plastic wrap in the refrigerator for 1–2 weeks. Vacuum-packed haloumy can be stored in the refrigerator for some months until it is opened, after which it should be used within a week or so. Haloumy is one cheese which freezes well without loss of flavour or texture.

PREPARATION AND USE Wipe dry and slice thickly across the narrow end where the folds are visible. It is an excellent cheese for grilling on a heated, lightly oiled griddle; serve the grilled cheese with barbecued lamb or pork, smoked pork in particular. It can also be coated with flour and shallow-fried in hot olive oil until browned, with a squeeze of lemon added. Fried cheese is taken to the table in its pan, and portions are taken up with pieces of bread (it comes away in strings).

Use also as it is with bread or crackers, or dice and add to green salads. Serve haloumy with Greek wines such as retsina, with fruity red wines, or with ouzo (aniseed liqueur).

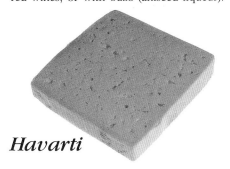

Havarti

MAJOR NUTRIENTS			SERVE SIZE 20 G
Energy	330 kJ	Sodium	160 mg
Protein	4 g	Calcium	100 mg
Fat	7 g	Phosphorus	80 mg
Carbohydrate	0	Vitamin A	60 µg
Cholesterol	25 mg	Thiamin	8 mg

NUTRITIONAL INFORMATION Minimum fat 22%. A typical hard cheese.

DESCRIPTION Havarti has a supple body, holes, and a fairly mild taste. Havarti made in Australia may be plain, or spiced with caraway or pepper, like buetten, produced in Victoria.

ORIGIN AND HISTORY Havarti is styled on tilsit, from East Prussia. It was developed by Hanne Nielsen, an important cheese pion-

eer, who discovered tilsit whilst producing gouda in East Prussia. On returning to her homeland, Denmark, she called the cheese 'havarti' after her farm. It is one of Denmark's most famous cheeses, exported worldwide.

BUYING AND STORAGE The body of havarti should have a smooth homogeneous appearance with a few tiny holes and a thin smeared rind of a darker hue than the body of the cheese. It should have a clean look, free of stickiness or slime. The flavour should be fruity, acquiring sharpness as the cheese ages. A few cracks in the cheese are acceptable and common. Store in the refrigerator, well wrapped in foil or plastic wrap, away from other dairy foods. It should keep for up to two weeks.

PREPARATION AND USE Use as a table cheese in cheese platters, open sandwiches, snacks. Mild havarti is good with fresh fruits and salad vegetables. Mature havarti goes with pickled fish and rye breads; it melts well and is useful in sauces and pasta.

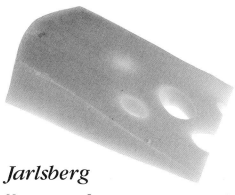

Jarlsberg

NUTRITIONAL INFORMATION Major nutrients typical of hard cheese.

DESCRIPTION A rich yellow cheese with large eyes encased in a deeper yellow waxed rind. Similar to emmental but with a more buttery delicate taste, somewhere between gouda and emmental. A scalded curd hard cheese.

ORIGIN AND HISTORY Jarlsberg originated in the area of Norway where the Vikings first settled, on the west bank of Oslo Fjord; its exact date of origin is uncertain. At one time the cheese virtually went out of existence until Norwegian experiments gradually recreated the original product, and in 1959, jarlsberg as we know it today was born. Jarlsberg bears a close resemblance to emmental, which is produced in different countries worldwide, but Norwegians are adamant that it is a variety in its own right.

BUYING AND STORAGE Select a cheese which has a surface rind completely intact and free of cracks, splits or lifting. The interior of

the cheese should be smooth and light golden with well spaced eyes or holes, glistening with butterfat. Watch out for excessive dryness, small clusters of tiny holes and splits.

Store with only the exposed surfaces covered with cling wrap; this allows the rind to breathe, protecting the cheese inside at the same time. Jarlsberg has good keeping qualities and should last for several weeks.

PREPARATION AND USE Remove from the refrigerator 1 hour before serving; keep covered to avoid drying, and away from direct sunlight or heat. Use a cheese plane for serving, so that thin slices may be cut or curled for decoration. Use in sandwiches, cheese boards, fondues, breads, croissants with ham, fruit salads, green salads, sauces, or macaroni bake; melt over hamburgers.

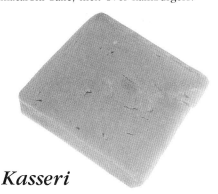

Kasseri

NUTRITIONAL INFORMATION No detailed data available.

DESCRIPTION A hard, pressed uncooked curd cheese made from goat's or sheep's milk. Creamy white in colour and firm in texture, with only a few small holes, it has the tangy flavour one associates with sheep's or goat's milk cheeses.

ORIGIN AND HISTORY Kasseri originates from Greece, where similar cheeses have been made from classical times. The ancient Greeks were true diplomats in that, when accreditation for a gastronomical discovery was deemed necessary, a deity received the honours. In the matter of cheese, Aristaeus, a son of Apollo and Cyrene, was the acknowledged creator.

BUYING AND STORAGE Kasseri is made in large wheels about 9 kg in weight. Purchase cut in wedges from Greek food stores, some delicatessens and specialty cheese shops. Wrap in plastic film and store in the refrigerator for 3–4 weeks, changing the wrap every 2 days. If the cheese shows signs of mould, cut it off and wrap in fresh plastic.

PREPARATION AND USE Besides being a good table cheese, kasseri may be grated for serving with pasta; it also melts nicely and can be cut in small dice for topping special lamb and macaroni dishes cooked in the oven — add towards end of cooking. Flour-coat fairly thick slices of the cheese and shallow-fry in hot olive oil, adding a squeeze of lemon juice; serve straight from the pan, using bread to scoop up the cheese.

Use also for cheese boards with fresh fruit or crisp vegetables. Serve with dry white wine or beer, depending on how the cheese is prepared.

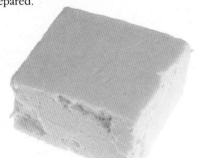

Lancashire

NUTRITIONAL INFORMATION Lancashire is a typical hard cheese.

DESCRIPTION Lancashire is a firm cheese, white in colour, loose-textured with a buttery taste and a mild flavour which sharpens with age. An uncooked curd hard cheese.

ORIGIN AND HISTORY Lancashire originated in England and takes its name from the county of the same name. Originally it was grouped with cheshire cheese; it is mentioned as such in the 'Domesday Book'. By the 18th century it was most certainly identified in its own right. Until recently it was often called 'Leigh toaster' by many people in the cheese producing area, after the village of Leigh and in reference to its excellent toasting qualities. It was traditionally produced on farms; the first dairy to produce lancashire was in the village of Chipping in 1913, and others followed.

True lancashire cannot be successfully copied in factory production, resulting over the years in most of the cheese sold commercially being nothing like the original farm-produced cheese. The factory varieties were thus called 'new lancashire' during the 1970s; in 1980 the word 'new' was dropped and replaced with 'single-acid'. They are a drier, longer-lasting cheese than the original soft loose-textured variety. The traditional lancashire cheese can, however, still be found in England, but is unlikely to be seen outside that country.

BUYING AND STORAGE Care should be taken to select a cheese showing the distinct curd texture and consistency, described

above. Excessively dry or moist cheeses should be avoided and there should be no trace of mould contamination. In colour it should range between white and ivory. Wrap securely in cling wrap and store in the refrigerator. It should keep for approximately 10 days or longer, depending on the care taken.

PREPARATION AND USE Use as a table cheese for cheese boards, or for lunch platters with cold meats and salad vegetables, pickles and fresh breads. Remove the cheese from the refrigerator an hour before serving and allow it to reach room temperature. Keep the cheese covered during this time to stop it from drying out. Lancashire gently heated develops a delicate custardlike consistency and at 3 months of age will spread like softened butter. Use as an accompaniment to biscuits and toast (Welsh rarebit), or sprinkle into soups, sauces etc.

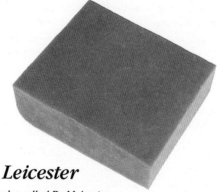

Leicester

also called **Red leicester**

NUTRITIONAL INFORMATION Leicester is a typical hard cheese.

DESCRIPTION A hard red-russet cheese with a grainy yet moist texture. It has a mellow mild taste with an open buttery texture. An uncooked curd hard cheese.

ORIGIN AND HISTORY Originating from the green heartland of England in Leicestershire, surrounding the village of Melton Mowbray, leicester cheese owes much of its origin to both cheddar and cheshire. However, regional influences are evident when the cheese is compared to the double gloucester which it resembles. Its red colour, coming originally from carrot juice, is now achieved by the addition of annatto. The first factory was established in 1875, with farmhouse production going into a decline.

Up to World War II a blue leicester was produced which rivalled stilton; subsequently, however, rationalisation of the industry led to its demise.

BUYING AND STORAGE Look for a good red·colour without any trace of dryness,

cracks or splits in the rind or body of the cheese.

As it matures, leicester reduces its moisture levels and develops a full nutty flavour. The age of leicester cheeses varies between 3 and 9 months. The crust is edible and can be assisted in the hardening process by leaving the cheese unwrapped in a dry atmosphere.

Store in the refrigerator with all cut surfaces wrapped in cling wrap. Should any moulding occur, trim away and rewrap. It should keep for several weeks.

PREPARATION AND USE Remove from the refrigerator 1 hour before serving and allow the cheese to come to room temperature. Serve as a table cheese with fresh salad vegetables or fruits. Leicester melts well and may be used for cooking. Use in sandwiches, savouries, or where the red colour will enhance recipes requiring cheese. Use a hot knife for clean and easy cutting without crumbling.

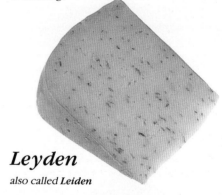

Leyden

also called **Leiden**

NUTRITIONAL INFORMATION Leyden is a typical hard cheese.

DESCRIPTION A hard, close-textured cheese with whole cloves, cumin or anise (or a combination) added. It has a distinctive taste and aroma, salty and spicy, more acidic than gouda.

ORIGIN AND HISTORY Originating in Holland, leyden is one of the lesser-known Dutch cheeses. It originally arose as a farmhouse cheese made from skim milk and buttermilk. Cumin seed was kneaded into the curd by the farmer, who would tread the curd with his feet (which had been cleaned beforehand in whey). This gave a very special character to the cheese; needless to say, however, the practice of treading the curd is now considered unhygienic and has ceased. Modern manufacture still requires an intensive working of the curd with the spices added in layers. The red rind of leyden is stamped with the symbol of two crossed keys, signifying the coat of arms of the City of Leyden.

BUYING AND STORAGE Leyden should

have an intact surface rind without any trace of cracks or splits. The spices should be evenly spread and the cheese should not appear moist nor discoloured. Buy as required and store in the refrigerator with all exposed surfaces securely covered with cling wrap. It has fairly good keeping qualities and will keep refrigerated for several weeks. Any trace of surface mould should be trimmed away and the cheese should be rewrapped.

PREPARATION AND USE Remove from the refrigerator an hour before serving and allow the cheese to regain its full character. Keep it covered and away from direct heat. Serve with a cheese slicer or plane to cut thin slivers. Leyden is a table cheese, but it may also be used in cooking to give the desired herb flavour to a range of dishes. Use in sandwiches, salads, jaffles.

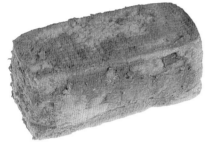

Limburger

also called Limbourg

NUTRITIONAL INFORMATION No detailed data available. Fat content is variable.

DESCRIPTION A rectangular or cube-shaped cheese with a thin, smooth reddish-brown washed rind. Inside it is yellow in colour, smooth with small irregular holes. It has a strong, distinctive, rank aroma and a pungent taste. A soft uncooked curd cheese. Consistency varies with the fat content.

ORIGIN AND HISTORY Often mistakenly thought to be of German origin, limburger in fact originated in Belgium during the Middle Ages. One of the world's great 'smellies', it takes its name from the province of Limburg where it was first produced by monks. Adopted by the Allgauer cheese makers in the 1800s, it is now one of Germany's major cheese varieties. Modern limburger is more solid than the original, with differences of manufacture being adopted as cheese technology has advanced (e.g. dry salting by hand replaced with brine baths).

BUYING AND STORAGE Best purchased in small quantities for immediate use, as the strong aroma from limburger will permeate other foods in the refrigerator unless it is well sealed and stored in a separate compartment.

The cheese should appear close-textured with a shiny red-brown rind. Do not be misled by the unpleasant smell into thinking the cheese is past its prime.

PREPARATION AND USE Limburger is a table cheese, rather than one used in cooking. Serve at room temperature, allowing an hour between refrigeration and serving. A certain amount of the cheese's strong smell will dissipate, restoring a balance to the cheese's character. Serve with dark breads and vegetables such as radish and shallots.

VARIETIES

Backsteiner Backsteiner is one of a number of variations of limburger. Most of the limburger cheese exported worldwide comes from Austria, Switzerland and Germany, rather than its native place of production.

Hervé Hervé was originally made by monks at Liège and there are several varieties made, including a low fat type, and others which have chives, parsley or thyme. Remoudou is one of the most popular hervé cheeses. It is velvety, supple in texture, golden in colour with a reddish-brown rind.

Romadur A mild version of limburger, produced in Bavaria, Austria and Czechoslovakia. It is oblong in shape with a washed rind surface, ripened with a smooth texture. As with many washed rind or surface ripened cheeses its flavour is strong and fruity. Romadur aged past its prime becomes either dry and hard, or runny and sticky.

Weisslacker Bierkäse This is a variety of limburger, excellent with beer, as indicated in its name bierkäse (beer cheese). A small cheese with a white waxy skin, it is firm-textured, with a piquant taste reminiscent of bacon.

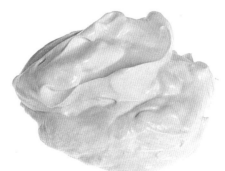

Mascarpone

NUTRITIONAL INFORMATION This cheese is high in saturated fat and has a moderate amount of cholesterol. While a good source of

vitamin A, it is of little nutritional value.

DESCRIPTION A fresh, unripened smooth triple cream cheese resembling thick clotted cream. It has a rich sweet taste, slightly acidic.

ORIGIN AND HISTORY This lush cream cheese, sometimes so similar to cream that it hardly seems to merit the name of cheese, originated in Lodi, 20 km from Milan, Italy, more than two centuries ago. The name derives from *mascherpa*, meaning 'creamy product'. It is made (in the winter and autumn months) from cream and sometimes lemon juice. In Italy it is sold in muslin bags with sweetened fruits to complement it. It may also be seen aged, when it becomes firm and a deeper butter colour; the aged mascarpone may be grated.

The Trieste area of Italy is responsible for the practice of mixing mascarpone with gorgonzola, anchovies, mustard, caraway and leeks, resulting in a cheese similar to the Hungarian lipto.

BUYING AND STORAGE Refrigerate at 4°C for no longer than 5 days. Mascarpone looks like a mass of thick clotted cream and is available either loose or in tubs. It should look moist and creamy without yellowing or dryness. Best purchased fresh daily.

PREPARATION AND USE Use in appetisers, cheesecakes, desserts; layer with blue cheese (e.g. gorgonzola), mustard and anchovies. It is usually served with fruit and sugar and liqueurs (e.g. Strega) for dessert. Most definitely a dessert cheese.

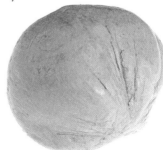

Mizithra

NUTRITIONAL INFORMATION Major nutrients similar to cottage cheese. Only a small amount of salt is used to make mizithra.

DESCRIPTION A fresh, unripened cottage cheese made with whole cow's milk. It is a sweet-tasting cheese, without the tang one associates with cottage cheese. It is slightly off-white in colour with a fairly smooth, creamy texture.

ORIGIN AND HISTORY A Greek cottage cheese made from classical times in the home with goat's or sheep's milk. In the earliest days of making this cheese, the coagulant was the latex of the fig plant. Whole milk, heated to lukewarm, was stirred gently with a freshly broken, sappy twig from a fig tree until curds began to form. These were drained in special moulds, lightly weighted, then turned out. Any cheese not used within a day or two was salted, drained further, then dried and used as a table or grating cheese.

Today mizithra is mostly made with cow's milk and rennet is used as the coagulant, although fig latex is still widely used. While it is still made in the home, it is also manufactured.

BUYING AND STORAGE Purchase from Greek food stores and delicatessens stocking Greek foods'. Dried mizithra is also available from these outlets. Store fresh mizithra in a covered dish in the refrigerator and use within 3 days. Wrap dried mizithra in plastic film and store in the refrigerator.

PREPARATION AND USE Fresh mizithra is excellent spread on fresh bread. Serve also with fresh fruit — figs and grapes are particularly good with it. Use in any recipe which calls for cottage cheese. Dried mizithra is excellent for pasta dishes.

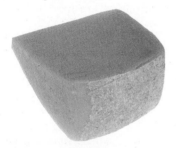

Monterey Jack

also called Jack, Monterey

MAJOR NUTRIENTS			SERVE SIZE 20 G
Energy	320 kJ	Cholesterol	n/a
Protein	5 g	Sodium	0
Fat	6 g	Calcium	160 mg
Carbohydrate	20 mg	Thiamin	4 mg

NUTRITIONAL INFORMATION Minimum fat 28%.

DESCRIPTION A creamy white, firm, supple-textured cheese, similar to colby but softer and with more holes. A scalded and semihard cheese.

ORIGIN AND HISTORY Originating in California, monterey originally evolved from an old monastery recipe and was exclusively made by Spanish padres in the 18th century — they called it queso del pais. Monterey jack is named after David Jacks who in fact shipped a new cheese evolved from the old Monterey with his name on it (Jacks) and that of the port of shipping (Monterey). Hence the

two names became entwined although the cheeses were quite different. It is often termed 'Californian Jack'.

BUYING AND STORAGE Monterey Jack is made in a wheel or loaf shape and should be creamy white in colour, either rindless or with a natural fine rind. It is mild, bland and buttery. Wrap securely in cling wrap and store in the refrigerator; it should keep for 2–3 weeks. When purchasing, look for cheese which shows no signs of dryness or yellowing.

PREPARATION AND USE High moisture jack (see Varieties) is ideal in or on top of baked dishes; it has a pliant consistency. Used as a table cheese, high moisture Jack is good for snacks or sandwiches. Remove from the refrigerator an hour before serving to allow it to reach room temperature. The aged version is a little like cheddar with a richer, saltier taste. Grate straight from the refrigerator while still cold.

VARIETIES

High moisture Jack (also called Teleme jack or cream jack), Sonoma jack (often flavoured with herbs, spices, garlic, pepper), dry jack (a hard grating cheese made from skim milk).

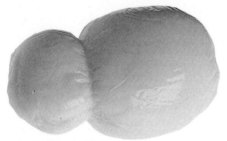

Mozzarella

also called Pizza cheese

MAJOR NUTRIENTS			SERVE SIZE 20 G
Energy	270 kJ	Calcium	165 mg
Protein	5 g	Phosphorus	100 mg
Fat	5 g	Vitamin A	50 µg
Carbohydrate	0	Thiamin	4 mg
Cholesterol	15 mg	Zinc	0.8 mg
Sodium	75 mg		

NUTRITIONAL INFORMATION Minimum fat 20%. Nutrients typical of hard cheeses.

DESCRIPTION A smooth white cheese produced in a variety of shapes including round, oval, pear-shaped and block. It has a mild flavour, vaguely sweet and milky. A pasta filata (stretched curd) cheese.

ORIGIN AND HISTORY It is to be wondered which came first, the pizza or the cheese. Mozzarella, famous for its use in the ubiquitous pizza, originated in Italy. It was first produced from water buffalo's milk and then later from a mix of buffalo's milk with

cow's milk. The herds of water buffalo came from India during the 7th century, but today their numbers are small in southern Italy, hence much of the cheese is produced from cow's milk.

It is traditionally mozzarella whose whey (drained off during manufacture) is used to make ricotta. Mozzarella is quick to produce and as a fresh cheese is generally made for local consumption, with each country making its own. In Australia, for instance, several different cheese companies manufacture mozzarella around the country.

BUYING AND STORAGE Always look for mozzarella which has a fresh clean white appearance without any signs of dryness. It should be shiny smooth, creamy white in colour. There should be no holes and the texture should be giving and elastic. Store in the coolest part of the refrigerator, wrapped in plastic wrap to prevent loss of moisture. It should last for approximately 1–2 weeks, but is best bought as required.

PREPARATION AND USE Remove from the fridge and slice, grate or dice according to the requirement. Mozzarella is primarily used in cooking, and is suitable for a variety of dishes, particularly Italian cuisine: veal, pizzas, melted over steaks, with chicken. Fresh, tender, moist mozzarella (such as bocconcini), however, is a table cheese to be finely sliced and served with fresh tomatoes and basil, sprinkled with black pepper and olive oil.

VARIETIES

Bocconcini, manteca, mozzarella affumicata, scamorze.

Treccia is an Italian cheese similar to mozzarella, except in shape — it is shaped in a plait. Its characteristics and flavour are basically the same as for mozzarella. It is mild in flavour and forms long threads when used in cooking. Ideal for pizza.

SEE ALSO Bocconcini.

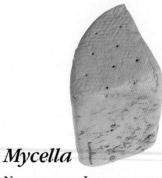

Mycella

NUTRITIONAL INFORMATION This is a typical hard cheese.

DESCRIPTION A cow's milk blue cheese with a pale yellow interior scattered with greenish-blue veins, in a deep round shape. An internal mould ripened cheese.

ORIGIN AND HISTORY Mycella originated in Denmark. It was known as, and called, Danish gorgonzola until 1951 when the Sesa Convention established a restriction on the use of certain names of the varieties, gorgonzola being one. As a result the name mycella (taken from the type of mould used to produce the cheese — *Mycelium*) was born. It was during the 1800s that Denmark along with other European countries began producing foreign cheeses for its own domestic market. Most of the Danish varieties eventually took on their own district names (e.g. Danish emmental became samsoe) and were recognised at the Sesa Convention.

Mycella, styled on the Italian gorgonzola with the same creamy colour, is considered by Scandinavians to be a good substitute for stilton.

BUYING AND STORAGE Buy as required and use within a short time to avoid cross-flavouring and tainting of other foods in the refrigerator. Look for cheese which shows no signs of greying or dullness of colour, nor excessive pungency. Wrap securely in foil and refrigerate to store. Keep it away from other dairy foods such as milk and cream. Correctly stored it should last 1–2 weeks, but small pieces will dry more quickly than larger blocks.

PREPARATION AND USE Remove from the refrigerator 1½ hours prior to serving, loosen the foil and allow the cheese to reach room temperature and develop its true taste and texture. Use as a table cheese on cheese boards at the end of meals. Supply a separate knife to cut and serve. Use in cocktail cheese balls mixed with cream cheese and rolled in crushed nuts. Serve with grapes, whole nuts, figs, dates, rye breads, damper.

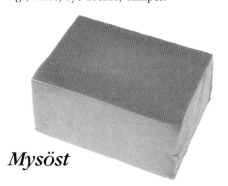

Mysöst

MAJOR NUTRIENTS   SERVE SIZE 20 G

Energy	210 kJ	Sodium	n/a
Protein	1 g	Calcium	212 mg
Fat	0	Phosphorus	90 mg
Carbohydrate	10 g	Thiamin	3 µg
Cholesterol	n/a		

NUTRITIONAL INFORMATION A whey cheese containing the carbohydrate lactose, and whey proteins. It is an excellent source of calcium and phosphorus and is high in saturated fat. Iron is traditionally added in the manufacture.

DESCRIPTION A light brown to orange firm block cheese with a sweet caramelised taste, made from goat's or cow's whey and sometimes containing cloves, cumin, cinnamon and brown sugar. There are a number of styles.

ORIGIN AND HISTORY Mysöst originated in Norway. One of the most popular cheeses in its own homeland, it was originally a cheese of expediency. It is believed to have been the cheese that the Vikings carried with them for energy and endurance. A high energy cheese, mysöst is considered to be an essential beginning for a busy day. It takes its name from the words Myse (whey) and Öst (cheese).

Like so many ancient cheeses, mysöst was formerly made on mountain farms and originally from goat's milk since cow's milk lacked butterfat in its whey, having been used to produce butter. When mysöst is made from the whey of goat's milk it is called gjetöst (Gjei being the Norwegian word for goat). All of the mysöst varieties have the same general characteristics — brown colour, caramelised sweet taste and a firm texture.

BUYING AND STORAGE Mysöst varieties should appear brown-orange in colour with a smooth and firm texture. It should not appear dry. Buy as required and use within a short time.

PREPARATION AND USE Mysöst cheeses are noted for their use in the famous open sandwiches and are ideal for use in sauces. They are often combined with a selection of meat, salad or fish for the arm's length sandwich called 'landgang' in Norway.

Remove from the refrigerator and cut into thin slices with a sharp hot knife or a cheese plane.

VARIETIES
Mysöst made with goat's milk is called gjetöst — see separate entry.

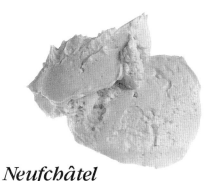

Neufchâtel

*also called **Low fat cream cheese***

MAJOR NUTRIENTS   SERVE SIZE 20 G

Energy	220 kJ	Cholesterol	18 mg
Protein	2 g	Sodium	60 mg
Fat	5 g	Vitamin A	40 µg
Carbohydrate	1 g	Thiamin	5 mg

NUTRITIONAL INFORMATION See Cream Cheese. Cream cheese generally has 33% fat; neufchâtel is lower at 25%.

DESCRIPTION A fresh unripened cream cheese shaped in cylinders, rectangles, small discs or heart shapes. Fresh neufchâtel has a soft creamy texture and light, refreshing taste. In France it is often eaten surface-ripened, whereas in America and Australia it is eaten fresh.

Neufchâtel may be made from either skim milk or whole milk or a mix of cream and milk. Similar varieties are petit suisse and petit carre.

ORIGIN AND HISTORY Neufchâtel comes from the area of Paris that sports some of the finest dairy country, called Pays de Bray. English merchants first purchased this famous cheese as long ago as the 15th century and took it home for the Christmas market. It is believed that this is one cheese that has changed very little over the centuries.

BUYING AND STORAGE Best purchased fresh for use as required. Look for cheese which has a clear, fresh, moist appearance without yellowing, dryness or coarseness. Neufchâtel resembles a soft cream mass and should have a light, refreshing tang. Some varieties have fruits added. Store like cream cheese, well wrapped to avoid loss of moisture and away from strong-smelling foods in the refrigerator. Correctly stored, it should keep for up to 10 days; however, check the use-by date, as brands may vary.

PREPARATION AND USE Essentially a dessert cheese. Keep refrigerated until required. Use as a base for cheesecakes, mousses, icings, cake toppings. Use also with fresh fruits in season. Cheese logs or cocktail nibbles can be made with it.

VARIETIES
Plain, chocolate and strawberry; neufchâtel with fruits (fruit logs).

Boursin

NUTRITIONAL INFORMATION Major nutrients similar to cream cheese.

DESCRIPTION A fresh unripened triple cream cheese produced in the shape of low cylinders of about 100 g. Snowy white in colour with a light, mild, fresh taste and creamy, buttery texture. It is often flavoured with herbs, garlic or pepper.

ORIGIN AND HISTORY A relative youngster amongst the numerous cheese varieties for which France is renowned worldwide, boursin is a form of neufchâtel which comes from the area surrounding Paris. Many of the cheese varieties here are not known outside their place of origin. Boursin, however, is widely exported to other areas and enjoys fame as a refreshing cream cheese likely to set the pace for fresh cream cheese production in other countries. It is believed to be as popular in France as yoghurt and is often eaten in a similar fashion as a snack. One local French cheese maker in Australia released a boursin-style cheese onto the Australian market several years ago, but it is not now available.

BUYING AND STORAGE Buy in small quantities as required. Boursin is sold in small cylindrical shapes wrapped in foil. It is a high fat cheese and should have a rich creamy flavour and soft texture. Avoid cheese which has any signs of dryness or is a dull colour. It should be smooth, white and rindless.

Store in the cool part of the refrigerator, well wrapped in foil, and use within a few days.

PREPARATION AND USE Remove from the refrigerator just before serving. Use a separate knife to serve. Boursin is a fresh, rich cream cheese best served as a table cheese rather than used in cooking. Use as a filling for cold cocktail nibbles.

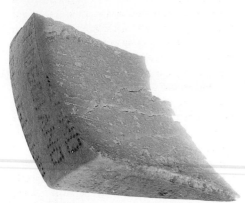

Parmesan

also called **Mantua, Grana, Parmigiano, Parmigiano reggiano, Romano**

MAJOR NUTRIENTS		SERVE SIZE 20 G	
Energy	340 kJ	Calcium	220 mg
Protein	7 g	Phosphorus	155 mg
Fat	6 g	Zinc	1 mg
Carbohydrate	0	Vitamin A	80 µg
Cholesterol	18 mg	Thiamin	3 mg
Sodium	150 mg		

NUTRITIONAL INFORMATION Minimum fat 22%. A typical hard cheese.

DESCRIPTION A hard granular cheese with a grainy texture. Its colour is straw-yellow and its flavour is distinctive and sharply piquant yet fruity. Most commonly known as the world's most popular grating cheese, it is a hard cooked curd cheese of the type known as grana.

ORIGIN AND HISTORY Parmesan takes its name from Parma in northern Italy, where it originated as long ago as AD 1200. It is one of the few cheese varieties whose ancient formula has remained the same since its characteristics were first described. It has for centuries been the pride of Italy and can only carry the stamp 'parmigiano reggiano' if it comes from particular areas of northern Italy.

Parmesan cheese can attribute its fame to its rich flavour and ability to be used in cooking (without forming strings as some cheeses do). Because of these qualities it was in ready demand for export by the monks of Chiaravalle. In 1666, during the Great Fire of London, legend has it that an enormous pit was built especially to conceal and protect a store of this great Italian cheese from the intense heat of the fire.

The name 'parmesan' was passed as a generic term by the Italian Government as a result of rivalry between Italian towns producing parmesan.

BUYING AND STORAGE Italian parmigiano reggiano is aged for 2–3 years and takes the form of large deep wheels with the name stamped on the rind. Look for a cheese which is hard and granular in texture, pale straw-yellow in colour, with a full fruity to sharp taste and crumbly texture. It should melt in the mouth and not be overly sharp nor rancid. There should be no evidence of large cracks or splits internally. Parmesans will store exceptionally well at low temperatures for long periods of time, almost indefinitely, thanks to their low moisture content and hard texture.

PREPARATION AND USE Parmesan may be enjoyed as a table cheese, particularly when young. It is primarily a hard grating cheese. Use in cooking with pasta or rice, and in minestrone, pies, sauces and antipasto dishes. Serve the younger table cheese with apples, figs, peaches or grapes. Serve in small squares

as an accompaniment to cocktails.

PROCESSING Some varieties are grated and prepackaged.

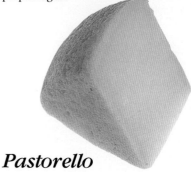

Pastorello

NUTRITIONAL INFORMATION A typical hard cheese.

DESCRIPTION A large, flat, round wheel-shaped cheese with a natural pale yellow-brown rind. It has a smooth firm texture with a mild buttery taste. A soft cheese.

ORIGIN AND HISTORY Pastorello originated in New South Wales, Australia. Styled after the Italian fontina but quite different owing to certain differences in manufacture, pastorello is one of the few Australian varieties to have its own name and is protected by its registered trade name. Developments of pastorello began in the 1960s when the United Dairies group of companies launched into cheese production, under the careful guidance of Dr Lostia. Pastorello was perfected after his return to Italy in the 1970s. The cheese is allowed to develop its own natural rind which protects it during maturing. It takes 6 weeks to ripen, at which time the rind is washed and the cheese is packed. It may be matured for 6 months, but is generally aged for 6–8 weeks.

BUYING AND STORAGE Pastorello should have an ivory to pale yellow body with a creamy smooth texture. It should not have any surface or interior cracks. It has a mild, slightly nutty taste, buttery and smooth. Store with the cut surfaces wrapped securely in cling wrap and refrigerate. It has good keeping qualities and will last for several weeks. Should slight surface moulding develop, this may be trimmed away and the cheese rewrapped.

PREPARATION AND USE Pastorello must be allowed to reach room temperature before serving, to allow its creamy smoothness to develop, so remove it from the refrigerator an hour before serving. Use as a table cheese, on cheese boards and with luncheon platters of cold meats and fruits. Suitable as a mild cheese for children. Use in salads and sandwiches, or use in cooking, melted over

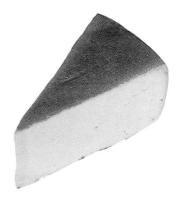

chicken, veal or vegetables. An excellent fondue base and a good melting cheese.

SEE ALSO   Fontina.

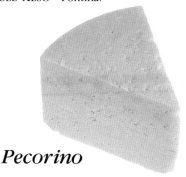

Pecorino

MAJOR NUTRIENTS		SERVE SIZE 20 G	
Energy	300 kJ	Sodium	185 mg
Protein	6 g	Calcium	162 mg
Fat	5 g	Phosphorus	110 mg
Carbohydrate	0	Vitamin A	65 µg
Cholesterol	15 mg	Zinc	0.7 mg

NUTRITIONAL INFORMATION   Minimum fat 25%. A typical hard cheese.

DESCRIPTION   The name pecorino is generic for cooked curd hard cheeses produced from sheep's milk. They are similar in type and texture to parmesan. Pecorino is the hard grating cheese of southern Italy (parmesan comes from the north). Pecorino pepato has peppercorns added to the curd. Pecorino fresco is a young fresh pecorino, whilst romano is an aged hard pecorino. Pecorino romano and pepato are close cousins of parmesan.

ORIGIN AND HISTORY   An ancient cheese, the true shepherd's cheese, pecorino originated in southern Italy as long ago as the 1st century AD. Pecorino remained a shepherd's cheese right up until the last century when small dairies took over, which in turn led to larger, more progressive factories being built.

As demand for pecorino grew, much of the milk from the Sardinian sheep was used in its production, thus threatening extinction for fiore sardo (the shepherd's cheese). However, it did survive.

Pecorino romano is the oldest and most often the best of the range. Pecorino follows closely on the heels of parmesan as the two important Italian cheese exports to the USA.

Pecorino cheeses in Australia were made solely from cow's milk until the development of the sheep's milk industry during the latter half of the 1980s.

BUYING AND STORAGE   Pecorino romano should be sharp and hard and without an excessive grainy texture. It should not be bitter. It may be fairly brittle and when it is grated it can be mistaken for parmesan. Like parmesan, it will last almost indefinitely, correctly stored under refrigeration. Keep away from delicate foods in the refrigerator as it may have a strong permeating aroma.

PREPARATION AND USE   Young pecorinos are good as table cheeses, whilst the hard stronger cheeses are suitable for grating and for use in cookery. Young pepato and romano may be served as full flavoured cheese board cheeses.

VARIETIES

Pecorino fresco, pecorino pepato, pecorino romano, pecorino sardo (also called fiore sardo and made from ewe's milk).

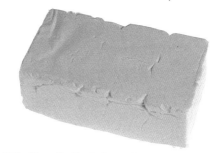

Philadelphia Cream Cheese

NUTRITIONAL INFORMATION   Major nutrients similar to cream cheese.

ORIGIN AND HISTORY   Originating in South Edmeston, philadelphia cream cheese was developed by a New York dairyman who named it after Philadelphia in the late 1800s. It became the largest-selling packaged cheese. It was popular in stores and homes because of its ease of handling (thanks to its silver foil wrapping) and its ability to store well.

BUYING AND STORAGE   Philadephia is packaged in silver foil and boxed; the soft variety is packaged in tubs. Check the use-by date and buy in quantities as required. The cheese should be creamy white in colour, smooth and homogeneous without any yellowing or dryness around the edges. Store wrapped in its own foil wrapper in the refrigerator. It should keep for up to 2 months.

PREPARATION AND USE   Soft philadelphia spreads easily from the refrigerator. Remove block philadelphia from the fridge 15 minutes or more before use to allow it to soften for easier blending. Use in cheesecakes, cheese logs, stuffed vegetables, dips, pâtés, quiches, omelette fillings. If using in cubes, cut or slice whilst cold from the fridge.

VARIETIES

Soft philadelphia with fruits.

SEE ALSO   Cream Cheese.

Port Salut

also called Abbaye, Entrammes, Port du Salut

NUTRITIONAL INFORMATION   Major nutrients similar to gouda. A typical hard cheese.

DESCRIPTION   A deep orange, washed rind cheese with a golden interior, smooth with a few tiny holes. Its taste is savoury and smooth. A surface smear ripened cheese.

ORIGIN AND HISTORY   Port salut originated in France, where it was first produced by Trappist monks who had returned to Brittany after their years of exile following the French Revolution. Port salut means 'port of salvation', which was the name given to the abbey in Brittany by the monks.

It was introduced to Paris in 1870 and instantly became a success. From that point on, it was widely copied. Monks producing the cheese called it entrammes. Because they could not keep pace with demand, they sold the brand name of Saint Paulin to a commercial dairy after World War II. Port salut and Saint Paulin are similar and in fact are difficult to tell apart when factory-made. Many countries copy port salut. Denmark eventually renamed their copy esrom; it now stands on its own as a variety. Port salut tends to vary in taste, texture and maturity according to the location where it is made.

BUYING AND STORAGE   Port salut should have a supple, tender texture and a smooth, thin reddish-orange skin. It should cut easily without any clamminess and should taste velvety smooth and mild (depending on the maturity) with a light lactic fermentation aroma.

Buy in small quantities as required and wrap in cling wrap. Keep in the refrigerator and change the wrapping regularly. Port salut should keep for 1–2 weeks, depending on the size.

PREPARATION AND USE   Remove from the refrigerator an hour before serving to allow it to reach room temperature. Use as a table cheese, on cheese boards, and in cheese pastries, sandwiches and savouries. The rind may be eaten or not as desired. Use a hot knife to cut.

SEE ALSO   Esrom, Saint Paulin.

Processed Cheese

MAJOR NUTRIENTS		SERVE SIZE 20 G	
Energy	260 kJ	Sodium	270 mg
Protein	4 g	Calcium	120 mg
Fat	5 g	Phosphorus	55 mg
Carbohydrate	0	Vitamin A	50 µg
Cholesterol	17 mg	Zinc	0.7 mg

NUTRITIONAL INFORMATION Despite processing, the nutrient values remain similar to those of hard cheese.

DESCRIPTION One or more types of cheese, grated, heated to pasteurisation level and mixed with emulsifiers into a homogeneous mass. The flavour and texture are uniform and unchanging during the life of the cheese. Heat treatment ensures long life and easy storage.

ORIGIN AND HISTORY The method of processing cheese by heat treatment was developed in the 1890s by cheese makers in southern Germany and Switzerland. The first processed cheese was cheese in cans (heated and preserved in the can). Preserving of camemberts started in 1914, using canning and heat treating. In Australia, potted cheese evolved in the early 1900s. In the pre-war years, West German, Swiss and Australian cheese makers were well on the way to developing processed cheese. The largest commercial venture was established by Kraft Foods.

BUYING AND STORAGE Because of their long life and uniform character, processed cheeses will store well and may be purchased in advance and stored until needed. Once opened, they must be treated like natural cheeses and kept in the refrigerator. Check the use-by date on the package and wrap in plastic film once opened to prevent mould development and dehydration.

PREPARATION AND USE There are many different varieties of processed cheeses. They are all ideal snack makers, convenient and easy to store. Use prepacked cheese slices for toasted jaffles and hamburgers, melted over veal, chicken or steak, or on top of shepherd's pie. Grate the block processed cheddar for use in sauces, hamburger mixes, pizza snacks, pasties and pastries. Tinned camemberts may be deep-fried either whole or in cocktail wedges. Processed cheeses with the addition of nuts (walnuts or pecans), chives or herbs, smoked etc., generally are cut off large blocks and need to be put into refrigeration. Remove them an hour before serving, as for natural cheese. These may be served as table cheeses with dried fruits and nuts, celery and shallots.

VARIETIES
Cheese slices, processed logs (Cradle Valley brand), canned camemberts, cheese spreads, Kaese canned bries, Kraft cheddar (brand).

SEE ALSO Cheese Spread.

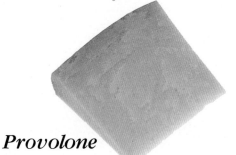

Provolone

MAJOR NUTRIENTS		SERVE SIZE 20 G	
Energy	300 kJ	Sodium	200 mg
Protein	5 g	Calcium	150 mg
Fat	6 g	Phosphorus	110 mg
Carbohydrate	0	Zinc	0.8 mg
Cholesterol	20 mg	Vitamin A	35 µg

NUTRITIONAL INFORMATION Minimum fat 25%.

DESCRIPTION Golden yellow in colour with a smooth shiny skin, sometimes waxed. Young provolones are tender and mild. As they age they become sharper in taste. Quite often they are lightly smoked. A pasta filata (stretched curd) cheese.

ORIGIN AND HISTORY A common sight to herald the start of the Christmas season in Italy is row upon row of provolones hanging outside the delicatessen stores.

Originating in Campania, southern Italy, provolone belongs to the spun curd cheeses well known in ancient Roman times. Provolone, meaning 'large oval', took its name from a local round cheese which was called provva. As production spread up to northern Italy and into Latin America and the USA, provolone started to take on all kinds of shapes: melons, sausages, pears and cones. Cheeses are commonly tied so that they can be hung and are often lightly smoked.

Provolone was originally produced from the milk of water buffaloes, and its two close relations provolo and provahira are still produced from buffalo's milk in Italy. Up to 9 months of age they are used as a table cheese, while the aged, stronger cheeses are more commonly used for grating. Provolone is similar to caciocavallo and mozzarella.

BUYING AND STORAGE Provolone has a smooth, homogeneous, close, dryish texture with a full flavour. It is a firm slicing cheese and should show no signs of moulding. It will store reasonably securely for 2 weeks. It should have a golden glossy rind. Wrap in cling wrap and store in the refrigerator.

PREPARATION AND USE Use provolone in fondues or to make savoury fillings to season chicken. Grate into sauces, over steak and over schnitzels (grate whilst still cold from the refrigerator). For melting, slice thinly with a hot knife. Use smoked provolone as a table cheese on cheese boards, served with fruit.

VARIETIES
Provolone affumicato is smoked. Provolone dolce is mild, while provolone piccante is piquant.

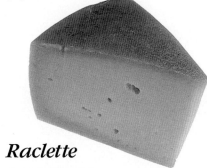

Raclette

also called **Groviera**

MAJOR NUTRIENTS		SERVE SIZE 20 G	
Energy	310 kJ	Sodium	175 mg
Protein	5 g	Calcium	110 mg
Fat	6 g	Phosphorus	90 mg
Carbohydrate	0	Vitamin A	70 µg
Cholesterol	19 mg		

NUTRITIONAL INFORMATION This is a typical hard cheese.

DESCRIPTION A firm wheel-shaped or square cheese with a light reddish-brown rind. It has a full, fragrant, creamy taste, excellent for melting, particularly as it ages. It is a scalded curd semihard cheese with eyes.

ORIGIN AND HISTORY Mountain cheeses such as gomser and bagnes, known collectively as raclette cheese, originated in Valais, Switzerland. Raclette takes its name from the word *racler*, meaning to scrape, referring to the age-old tradition among mountain farmers of melting large hunks of cheese over an open fire and scraping the bubbling cheese onto a plate with white onions, sour gherkins and new potatoes. This dish is called raclette and is as popular on one side of the Swiss mountains as fondue is on the other; bubbling raclette is a common sight in Swiss cafes.

Raclette was introduced to Minnesota University before World War II by Swiss balloonist Jean Picard. It is also produced in other countries outside Switzerland.

BUYING AND STORAGE Raclette should have a light brown rind and a pale amber interior dotted with tiny holes. It should have a mild fruity flavour, not too dominating, but distinctive. It should not be chewy in texture, and there should be no evidence of cracks or splits in the cheese. Store well wrapped to avoid tainting of other light dairy products.

PREPARATION AND USE Use in the traditional raclette dish or in sauces or soup toppings. It can also be used as a table cheese. It melts well without too much drawing of threads. For table use or the cheese board, remove from the refrigerator an hour before serving. Do not cook on a high heat. It should keep for several weeks.

VARIETIES
Anivier, bagnes, conches, gomser, orsières, Swissfield (brand).

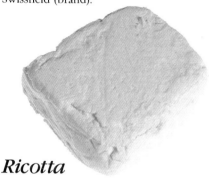

Ricotta

MAJOR NUTRIENTS		SERVE SIZE 20 G	
Energy	105 kJ	Cholesterol	0
Protein	2 g	Sodium	35 mg
Fat	2 g	Thiamin	6 mg
Carbohydrate	0		

NUTRITIONAL INFORMATION The high moisture content of ricotta results in low levels of kilojoules and all nutrients. It mainly provides moderate amounts of protein and fat. The fat content of ricotta varies in accordance with the amount of skimmed or whole milk added to the whey during manufacture. The fat content can be as low as 1% or as high as 20%. The lactose (milk sugar) imparts a sweet flavour and sodium content is very low. It makes an ideal substitute for cream cheese in desserts when a lower fat content is desired.

DESCRIPTION Ricotta is a high moisture, fresh, delicate cheese made from the whey of the milk, sometimes enriched with extra milk or cream. It has a mild sweetish flavour, a moist texture and a snowy white colour.

ORIGIN AND HISTORY Originally a product of expediency forced by poverty, ricotta originated in Italy. It was traditionally made

from cow's milk whey which was drained off during the manufacture of mozzarella. The coagulated curd is skimmed off the surface and placed into perforated baskets for draining.

In Italy today ricotta is prepared from the whey of either sheep's milk (ricotta pecora) or cow's milk (ricotta vaccina) and is named after the region of production, e.g. ricotta siciliano, ricotta romana, etc. There are three types: unsalted unripened (called tipo dolce); salted, dried and firm (called tipo molitemo) and matured in long containers (called tipo forte).

Ricotta is believed to be the cheese referred to in Calo's *De Agricultura*, where he lists a recipe for a cake called *libum* enjoyed by the Romans. Libum would have been a cheesecake baked on leaves in an earthenware dish. It is still popular in cheesecakes.

Fresh unripened ricotta cannot be exported owing to its delicate nature and short life; however, many countries now produce their own ricotta. Its popularity in Australia has become stronger in line with the trend towards healthy eating and reducing overall fat in the diet. In Germany there is a similar product called Ziger.

BUYING AND STORAGE Outside Italy, ricotta is most commonly sold fresh in bulk with the basket weave pattern clearly seen on the curdy mass of cheese, or packed in parchment packs or tubs. Ricotta is a fresh short-life cheese and should be purchased daily as required. Avoid cheese which shows signs of dryness or discoloration. It should be snowy white and moist, with a fresh appearance. Keep it in the cool of the refrigerator and use within a day or so.

PREPARATION AND USE Serve straight from the fridge as a dessert cheese with fresh fruits, or use as a base for cheesecakes, stuffings and fillings, and in baking. Mix with gorgonzola for a savoury spread. Use in pancakes or canneloni. Drain off any excess whey.

VARIETIES
Ricotta pecora, ricotta vaccina.

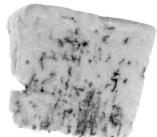

Roquefort

NUTRITIONAL INFORMATION This is a typical hard cheese.

DESCRIPTION A rich creamy-textured cheese produced from ewe's milk. It is creamy white in colour with greenish-blue veins and a thin orange-yellow skin. An internal mould ripened ewe's milk cheese.

ORIGIN AND HISTORY Roquefort takes its name from the village of Roquefort-sur-Soulzon in southern France, where it originated quite by accident. Legend tells the story of a herdsman leaving some fresh curd cheese with a loaf of bread in the local caves only to find on his return that the cheese had turned mouldy. Instead of discarding it he tasted it and found it so good that local farmers began to mature their cheeses in the same way. Roquefort is totally protected against any other country's imitating it and calling the cheese roquefort or even roquefort-style — thanks to its unique manner of being ripened in the limestone caves of the region. It has, however, enjoyed a long export history from the 18th century when it was first sent across the Alps. It was a popular cheese with the Romans, well known to Emperor Charlemagne and praised by Casanova.

The best production season is February through to July; however, roquefort is produced all year round now. The cheeses may be made as far away as Sardinia, but they must always go into the limestone caves near Roquefort to be ripened.

BUYING AND STORAGE Roquefort should be smooth and firm with a distinctive bouquet and the pronounced flavour unique to sheep's milk. The rind should be unblemished and the veining inside should be uniform throughout. The inside should not be too white with sparse veins. There should be no grey patches, nor excessive sharpness. Buy as required and refrigerate carefully wrapped in foil. Store away from milk, butter and cream. Use within 2 weeks.

PREPARATION AND USE Remove from the refrigerator an hour before serving to allow the taste, texture and aroma to develop. Keep the cheese covered during this time. Serve on a cheese board with fresh figs, grapes and nuts, or use in canapés, in salad dressings, on open sandwiches, to stuff grapes or dried apricots, or to make cheese cocktail balls or logs.

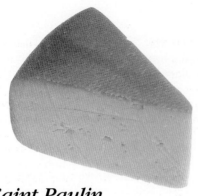

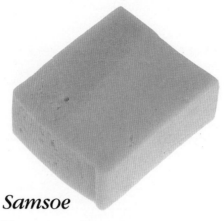

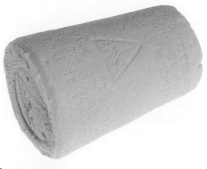

Saint Paulin

NUTRITIONAL INFORMATION Despite its softness, this is typical of hard cheese in its nutrient value.

DESCRIPTION Saint Paulin has a semisoft creamy texture with a taste ranging from mild and buttery to full, tangy and rich. It is made in the shape of small wheels and has a thin reddish-orange washed rind.

ORIGIN AND HISTORY Saint Paulin originated in France. It is the descendant of port salut and is in fact the generic name for cheeses styled on that cheese but produced in factories outside the protected area. The monks of Entrammes responsible for port salut were unable to keep up with demand, so they sold the name of Saint Paulin to a commercial dairy soon after World War II and as a result the Saint Paulin varieties are now more commonly produced and are known worldwide. The most common variety is bonbel. The Norwegian variety is called ridder.

Port salut and Saint Paulin are difficult to tell apart when produced in factories, although Saint Paulin is generally a little milder.

BUYING AND STORAGE Saint Paulin should have a smooth reddish-orange rind, free of fermentation spotting, with a smooth velvety texture, mild flavour and light smell. Buy as needed and store in the refrigerator away from milk, butter and cream. It should keep for 1–2 weeks.

PREPARATION AND USE Remove from the refrigerator an hour before serving to allow it to reach room temperature. Allow a separate knife to cut and serve. The outside rind may or may not be eaten, depending on individual tastes. Use as a table cheese on cheese boards, or in savouries, open sandwiches or cheese pastries.

SEE ALSO Port Salut.

Samsoe

NUTRITIONAL INFORMATION A typical hard cheese.

DESCRIPTION A mild, supple cheese with a pale colour.

ORIGIN AND HISTORY Samsoe was originally thought of as a Danish emmental, until it developed its own character and reduced size, and Denmark took steps to rename several foreign-inspired varieties.

BUYING AND STORAGE Look for samsoe with a smooth dry rind, hard and golden yellow, sometimes waxed. It is a large flat wheel or disc shape, bulging slightly at the sides. Cut surfaces should show an interior with large well-spaced 'eyes' or holes, glistening with butterfat. The eyes should be cherry-sized and the butterfat indicates a cheese ripened to maturity.

Store in refrigerator with all cut surfaces firmly wrapped in cling wrap. Correctly stored, it should last for 3 weeks in the refrigerator. Trim away any slight outside moulding that may occur and rewrap.

PREPARATION AND USE For table use, sandwiches and cheese platters, ensure the cheese has been removed one hour before serving to allow it to reach room temperature and develop its true characteristics of flavour and texture. Use also in cooking. Samsoe tends to draw threads when melted, so blend it with gruyère for traditional fondues. It is good in cheese or savoury pastries and rice dishes.

VARIETIES

These take their names from the place of production: cheeses produced in Fyn, Thy and Mols are named fynbo, tybo and molbo.

Danbo also belongs to the samsoe family: it is a mild, supple cheese with small, regular holes, and is occasionally spiced with caraway.

Svenbo is another Danish cheese, resembling fynbo. It is a firm cheese, with a characteristic nutlike, slightly sweet flavour. Svenbo is a yellow-white firm cheese with large round holes. It is produced with or without a rind of yellow paraffin wax.

Sapsago

*also called **Glamer schabzieger, Hobelkäse***

MAJOR NUTRIENTS		SERVE SIZE 20 G	
Energy	300 kJ	Sodium	155 mg
Protein	5 g	Calcium	130 mg
Fat	7 g	Vitamin A	65 µg
Carbohydrate	0	Thiamin	6 mg
Cholesterol	20 mg		

NUTRITIONAL INFORMATION A typical hard cheese.

DESCRIPTION A hard grana cheese, cone-shaped, with a greenish interior and strong pungent taste and smell. It has no rind and has a dry, hard texture.

ORIGIN AND HISTORY Sapsago originated in Switzerland and has been made for over a thousand years in the canton of Glarus. It is believed to have been one of the cheeses produced by monks and used not only as food in the monasteries but also as a medicinal treatment for stomach problems. Produced from skimmed milk, it has a unique pungent herbal flavour. Its green colour is due to the dried clover which is added to the curd along with other herbs.

After the cheese has ripened for 2 weeks it is finely ground and mixed with the herbs, then pressed into the cone shapes for sale or drying. If it is dried, it is eventually rubbed to a powder and used for sprinkling into salads or soups. The dried variety was given the title of 'poor folks cheese' because (with its strong taste) so little was needed to flavour bread.

BUYING AND STORAGE As it is one of the hard cheeses, sapsago will keep almost indefinitely in a cool, dry place. Refrigerate but wrap well to avoid tainting other foods. Keep it away from milk, cream and butter. Look for cheese which has a grainy, hard texture. It should be cone-shaped with a greenish interior and a strong, pungent smell and taste.

PREPARATION AND USE Use as a grating cheese. Use in salads or as a condiment to replace grated parmesan over pasta. Use a solid, sharp, hot knife for easier cutting, or break the cheese to grate it.

VARIETIES

Younger softer cheeses are called spalen.

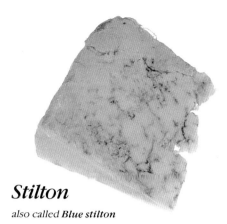

Stilton

also called **Blue stilton**

MAJOR NUTRIENTS SERVE SIZE 20 G

Energy	320 kJ	Sodium	155 mg
Protein	5 g	Calcium	72 mg
Fat	7 g	Phosphorus	60 mg
Carbohydrate	0	Vitamin A	80 µg
Cholesterol	25 mg	Thiamin	9 mg

NUTRITIONAL INFORMATION Nutritional value similar to that of other hard cheeses.

DESCRIPTION A creamy white to amber cheese with a marbling of blue veins and a crinkly outer crust. Deep cylindrical shape, on occasion precut. Ripe stilton should be reminiscent of pears in its aroma.

ORIGIN AND HISTORY Wymondham, south of Melton Mowbray, England, is the place of origin of one of the world's three great 'blues' — stilton. Stilton is named after the village of the same name in Little Huntingdonshire where the first great pile of cheeses was sold outside the Bell Inn. Stilton was a staging post for coachloads of visitors eager to partake of this wonder among cheeses. As a result its fame soon spread far and wide. Stilton is the only English cheese with a trade copyright and is not widely copied. An Australian cheese maker by the name of Saxelby did, however, produce a cheese of the stilton style in the 19th century.

BUYING AND STORAGE Buy as required. Look for even veining across the cut surface of the cheese, creamy white texture and a firm dry coat or rind. The rind may be deep gold and rough-textured, or smoother and thinner with a paler colour.

Store refrigerated with the cut surfaces securely covered with cling wrap, leaving the rind free to breathe; it should last 2–3 weeks. Whole cheese carefully handled will last 6–8 weeks.

PREPARATION AND USE Remove from the refrigerator 2 hours or more before serving; loosen wrappings but keep covered. Essentially a table cheese for use at the end of meals or for lunch, for snacks, or with cocktails. Stilton is not as salty as roquefort nor as creamy as gorgonzola. It has a rich piquant taste with cheddar characteristics. Always use a separate knife to cut and serve.

VARIETIES

White stilton, which is marketed young before blue veining has developed, does not have the same rough stilton coat and is white in colour.

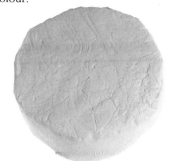

Stracchino

NUTRITIONAL INFORMATION Despite its softness, this is typical of a hard cheese in its nutrient value.

DESCRIPTION This is a rindless soft white cheese with a melt-in-the-mouth texture and a tangy flavour.

ORIGIN AND HISTORY Originating in Lombardy, Italy, stracchino takes its name from the Italian word 'stracca', meaning tired. There is a range of stracchino cheeses, which are quick to ripen (or 'tire'), delicate and soft. Crescenza is the creamiest of all.

Other varieties of cheese like stracchino are robiola and taleggio. Descending from robiola are a range of soft Italian cheeses called italico. These may or may not have a surface flora and the best-known variety is bel paese. Stracchino is also produced in Australia.

BUYING AND STORAGE As a fresh, moist cheese, it is best purchased fresh and used within a few days.

PREPARATION AND USE A fresh, white cheese that is a good accompaniment to fruit.

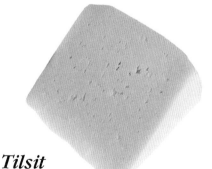

Tilsit

also called **Tilsiter**

MAJOR NUTRIENTS SERVE SIZE 20 G

Energy	300 kJ	Sodium	180 mg
Protein	5 g	Calcium	140 mg
Fat	6 g	Phosphorus	105 mg
Carbohydrate	0	Vitamin A	70 µg
Cholesterol	28 mg	Thiamin	4 mg

NUTRITIONAL INFORMATION Minimum fat 22%. A typical hard cheese.

DESCRIPTION A firm, smooth cheese, pale yellow with a washed rind that is yellow-orange in colour. Mild to medium-sharp piquancy with a prominent aroma. Its flavour is somewhere between mild limburger and port salut. A washed rind surface-smeared cheese.

ORIGIN AND HISTORY Tilsit originated in East Prussia (Sovetsk, now in the USSR) and takes its name from the city of Tilsit. It is believed that Dutch cheese maker Hanne Neilsen, studying cheese making abroad, accidentally created the tilsit variety while producing a batch of gouda in East Prussia. The cellar where the cheeses were stored was too damp and they turned soft and sharp and cracked. Thus was a brand new variety of cheese born. Hanne Neilsen later on returned to her own country and reproduced the recipe for tilsit, calling it havarti, which explains the link between those two cheeses, and their similarities.

Tilsit is now copied worldwide and the modern variety is no doubt much milder. The recipe has travelled to Australia and America and as far north as Norway. In central Europe it is made under the name of ragnit. Australia produces havarti and tilsit.

BUYING AND STORAGE The body of tilsit should have a smooth homogeneous appearance with a few tiny holes and a thin smeared rind of a darker hue than the body of the cheese. It should have a clean look, free of stickiness or slime. The flavour should be fruity, acquiring sharpness as the cheese ages. A few cracks in the cheese are acceptable and common. Store in the refrigerator well wrapped in foil or plastic wrap, away from other dairy foods. It should keep for up to two weeks.

PREPARATION AND USE Use as a table cheese in cheese platters, open sandwiches, snacks. Mild tilsit is good with fresh fruits and salad vegetables. Mature tilsit goes with pickled fish and rye breads; it melts well and is useful in sauces and pasta.

VARIETIES

Ansgar, made in West Germany, is a milder variety. There is also a skim milk variety and one containing caraway seeds.

Royalp is a Swiss cheese similar to tilsit in its method of manufacture. Wheel-shaped and firm-textured with a reddish-brown rind, it has a mild buttery taste, lightly aromatic and not as strong as tilsit.

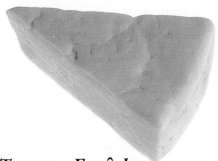

Tomme Fraîche

NUTRITIONAL INFORMATION Despite its greater moisture content, this is typical of a hard cheese in nutrient value.

DESCRIPTION Partially cured cantalets. A soft fresh partially ripened cheese.

ORIGIN AND HISTORY Tomme fraîche originated in France, and is a partially cured small French cheddar (cantalet). Cantal is the name of the French cheddar, cantalets being small cheddars.

Few, if any, tomme cheeses are likely to be seen outside France; however, they may be copied and produced in overseas countries for local consumption. Tomme fraîche is a relatively new variety to be produced in Australia. It tends to be something like a cross between unripened brie and cheddar. It is soft and creamy with a refreshing tang.

BUYING AND STORAGE Buy in small quantities as required, fresh daily. If stored these cheeses will lose their moisture and dry out. Cover in cling wrap and store in the refrigerator away from pungent or strong-smelling cheeses. Use within a week.

PREPARATION AND USE Remove from the refrigerator an hour before serving, keeping the cheese covered but loosening the wrapping. Serve as a table cheese between main course and dessert to freshen the taste buds. Serve with fresh fruits such as melon, avocado, kiwi fruit, pawpaw, fresh figs.

VARIETIES
Tomme d'aligot.

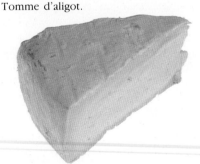

Triple Cream Cheese

NUTRITIONAL INFORMATION This is high in saturated fat and contains a moderate amount of cholesterol. While being a good source of vitamin A, it has little nutritional value.

DESCRIPTION Triple cream cheeses are rich and creamy, usually made in the shape of cylinders, wheels, discs and oblongs. They have the appearance of brie and sometimes have a sourish tang and a lightly piquant taste. Usually creamy-white in colour. These are the creamiest of cheeses and highest in fat (75%). They are soft ripened cheeses.

ORIGIN AND HISTORY Double creams originated in Normandy at the end of the 19th century. Types include caprice des dieux. Triple creams originated in France as the next logical step after double creams. Italy has a fresh unripened triple cream called mascarpone (70% fat). Many countries worldwide are now starting to produce triple creams, Australia included with Jindivick Supreme and Timboon Triple Cream.

BUYING AND STORAGE Buy fresh as required and use within a day or so. Keep refrigerated, wrapped in foil to keep the light out, as well as air. Foil allows the soft ripened cheese to breathe better. Look for cheese without dry or hard edges and with an evenly strong aroma. It should look like cream — buttery yellow, rich and shiny.

PREPARATION AND USE Remove from the refrigerator 2 hours before serving. Use a separate knife to cut and serve. Use on cheese boards after dinner in place of dessert with berry fruits in season — blueberries, strawberries, raspberries, figs and pecan nuts. Walnut and fruit breads blend well with these cheeses. Too exotic to be used for cooking, although brie tortes could utilise one of these if need be.

VARIETIES
Saint André; Jindivick Supreme, Timboon Triple Cream (Australian brand names). French brand names include Brillat-Savarin and Suprême.

SEE ALSO Mascarpone.

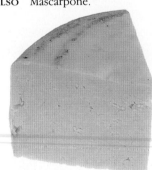

Wensleydale

NUTRITIONAL INFORMATION This is a typical hard cheese.

DESCRIPTION White: A quick-ripening, mild, crumbly, lightly salted cheese. It is white and firm but flaky, with a lingering honey taste.

Blue: Blue wensleydale is rich and full flavoured, creamy and tangy — a rival to stilton. Takes 6 months to mature.

ORIGIN AND HISTORY The cheese renowned for its excellent partnership with apple pie is wensleydale. It originated in Yorkshire, England, and most likely gave rise to the popular saying 'Apple pie without cheese is like a kiss without a squeeze'. Of ancient lineage, it is believed to have been made by Cistercian monks from an old Norman recipe. It could as a result claim ancestry to the French bleu de Bresse; it was originally, however, a closer relative to roquefort, being made from ewe's milk.

During the 16th century the monasteries were dissolved and the monks taught their skills to the wives of local farmers. Around this time wensleydale changed from ewe's milk to cow's milk cheese.

White and blue wensleydale are produced, but the white cheese is now more common than the blue. It is sold young with a flavour similar to caerphilly. Plentiful before World War II, blue wensleydale became a casualty of wartime rationing; cheese makers had to put the younger white cheeses onto the market, leaving none to produce the blue variety from. As a result blue wensleydale is still less common than the white variety.

BUYING AND STORAGE White wensleydale is younger than the blue and should be lightly sour, reminiscent of buttermilk in flavour and similar to caerphilly. Blue wensleydale should be fairly mild with a soft texture and creamy flavour. The white cheese should have a flaky texture and both cheeses should be free of dryness or yellowing. Sourness or yellowness indicates an overaged cheese. Buy as required and store for as short a time as possible at 4–7°C.

PREPARATION AND USE Wensleydale is famous for its partnership with apple pie: it blends well with apple thanks to its honeylike aftertaste. Serve at room temperature, allowing up to an hour for the character of the cheese to develop before serving. Essentially an after-dinner cheese, wensleydale blends well with fruits, with ham and with wheatmeal biscuits.

VARIETIES
Blue, white.

PULSES

Pulses or legumes are the edible seeds of plants from the Leguminosae family; these terms are usually used in association with dried peas, beans and lentils. Fresh, canned or frozen green peas, French beans and broad beans belong to the same family, but their nutritional value is different, because their water content is high and because the nutrient levels in the immature plants, when eaten fresh, are different.

The pulses grow in many soils and many climates, and feature in many traditional cuisines, including those of the Mediterranean, the Middle East, Egypt, China, Africa, Mexico, and Central and South America.

A good example of the versatility of pulses is provided by the 16 species of wild soya beans, growing in places as varied as cold mountains and deserts. The products derived from soya beans are equally varied.

Pulses are rich in protein, containing between 20–25% when dried and raw, and 6–8% after cooking. They are rich in complex carbohydrate (starch and dietary fibre), containing about 50% in the dried form and 20% after cooking. With the exception of soya beans, pulses contain very little fat. They are a valuable source of thiamin and niacin equivalents and of the minerals iron, calcium, phosphorus, zinc and magnesium. In diets which do not include animal products, such as meat and dairy foods, pulses play a very important role as a source of energy, protein, vitamins and minerals.

The iron, zinc and calcium are not as well absorbed as the iron and zinc from meat, or the calcium from dairy products, but the absorption of iron is improved by including a source of vitamin C in the meal. Like other plant foods, pulses contain no cholesterol.

The protein is rich in the essential amino acid — lysine — which is deficient in cereals; the combination of cereals and legumes results in a food with a protein quality similar to meat. Examples of such combinations are: baked beans on toast; curried lentils and rice; rice and beans; tortillas and beans; pea soup and bread.

The dietary fibre contained in pulses is rich in the soluble fibres, which help to control the level of cholesterol in the blood.

The starches in pulses are slowly digested and absorbed and they give rise to a slow, steady release of glucose into the blood. This is helpful in controlling blood sugar levels in people with diabetes.

Soya beans have been important in Oriental diets for centuries. The fat has been a valuable source of energy, and adds polyunsaturated fatty acids to diets which otherwise tend to be deficient in both energy and fat. The beans have been processed to make bean curd (tofu), noodles, oil and the fermented products, tempeh, miso and soya sauce, all of which add flavour and piquancy to other foods. Many of the pulses have been used to produce flours, pastes and fermented products.

Some pulses contain anti-nutritional enzymes which need to be denatured during the cooking process. This can be accomplished during cooking by holding the pulses at 100°C (212°F) for at least 15 minutes. If using a slow cooking appliance, or cooking the pulses slowly in the oven, boil the soaked pulses on the stove for 15 minutes before including them in the dish being prepared. Individual entries identify those pulses which require this process.

When such pulses are germinated for sprouts, the enzymes are denatured naturally, and they are also destroyed when pulses are canned.

To cook pulses, first pick them over, removing any small stones and damaged seeds. Cover with cold water, stir well, then discard any that float. While lentils and split peas do not require soaking, other pulses do. There are two methods for soaking, and individual entries indicate which can be used. Pulses which have been soaked for a number of hours take less time to cook than if quick-soaked.
Slow-soak method   Place in a bowl and add at least 3 cups of cold water to each cup of the particular pulse. Soak in a cool place for several hours. If pulses are soaked in a warm place, they will ferment, causing digestive problems later, even if water is changed. In warm weather, place the soaking pulses in the refrigerator and leave for desired length of time; in fact they can be held in this way for 2–3 days.
Quick-soak method   Place the washed pulses in a large saucepan, add cold water as above and bring to the boil. Boil for 2 minutes, remove from heat and cover pan. Leave for 1–2 hours until plump.
General notes on cooking   Do not add bicarbonate of soda to hasten cooking, as this can destroy B-group vitamins. Adding salt or acidic ingredients such as tomatoes, wine, vinegar etc. can slow down cooking; add acidic ingredients halfway through cooking, and salt towards end of cooking. Individual entries detail actual cooking methods and times.

An excellent range of canned pulses is available, including 'no added salt' varieties. These foods are ready for use in salads, soups and entrées and they are excellent as meat extenders when added to stews and casseroles, meat loaves and meat balls.

Many people suffer from flatulence and wind when they eat legumes. This is in part explained by the presence of two carbohydrates — raffinose, consisting of 3 sugar molecules, and stachyose consisting of 4 sugar molecules. These carbohydrates are not broken down in the upper digestive tract, but by the action of bacteria in the large bowel. This gives rise to the production of gases. Soaking of the beans and long cooking after discarding the water, will reduce the levels of raffinose and stachyose.

Pulses are highly nutritious foods, and are particularly important in the diets of vegetarians. They are a useful alternative to meat, and their low fat content is a bonus in a healthy diet.

In general, they contain lower levels of protein, vitamins and minerals than animal products, but they are excellent foods in a mixed diet and for many people they provide the best available supplement to the staple cereals.

Note that, unless otherwise stated, the major nutrients given in the individual entries are those of the raw forms of these pulses.

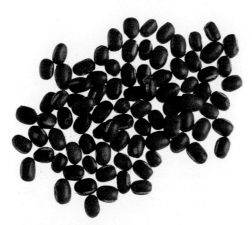

Adzuki Bean *Phaseolus angularis*

also called **Aduki bean, Azuki bean, Hong dow, Tientsin red bean**

MAJOR NUTRIENTS		SERVE SIZE 50 G	
Energy	650 kJ	Potassium	335 mg
Protein	12 g	Magnesium	39 mg
Fat	1 g	Iron	4 mg
Carbohydrate	27 g	Zinc	2 mg
Cholesterol	0	Thiamin	0.25 mg
Dietary Fibre	6 g	Riboflavin	0.1 mg
Sodium	20 mg	Niacin Equiv.	3 mg

NUTRITIONAL INFORMATION An excellent source of iron, thiamin and niacin; good source of magnesium, zinc and potassium; moderate source of riboflavin and folate. Also contain copper.

An excellent source of protein, these beans make a valuable contribution to nutrient intake in a vegetarian regime. They are a good source of the essential amino acid lysine.

The bean is low in fat and cholesterol free, while providing good quality vegetable protein and dietary fibre.

DESCRIPTION The tiny reddish-brown bean, almost oblong in shape, when cooked is unusually sweet for a bean.

ORIGIN AND HISTORY Grown on a bushy annual, native to China, the adzuki bean is now extensively cultivated in Japan. Since the Han dynasty in China (206BC–AD220) the red bean has meant good luck, and so is always included in any festive meal. Japanese continued this tradition using the red bean in the form of an, a smooth or crunchy red bean paste, sarashi-an, a flour made from ground red bean, and whole cooked beans. Dried beans are put out to ward off evil spirits at Chinese New Year.

The red bean is served with rice, used for a sweet porridge, jelly and confectionery, ground into a flour for pastry, and made into a sweet bean paste for filling steamed buns (ma yung bao — China).

BUYING AND STORAGE Purchase from Asian or natural food stores. The bean should be smooth and shiny, with little evidence of damage. Store in a sealed container in a cool, dry place and use within a year.

PREPARATION AND USE Prepare as for all pulses and slow-soak for 2–3 hours only. Change water, bring to the boil and boil for 15 minutes, then simmer, covered, for 45 minutes to 1 hour until tender. Adzukis can also be pressure-cooked for 15 minutes.

Adzuki beans have become popular outside Japan and China as a sprouting bean; the sprouts are available at greengrocers and natural food stores, and are often included in salad sprout mixes.

The beans may be served on their own, added to soups and stews where the sweetish flavour would complement other ingredients, or in salads. Use the sprouts raw, or lightly cooked in stir-fried dishes.

In Japan, the whole boiled beans are served over ice with fruit or ice cream as a dessert; the puree is made into a dessert, or ice cream, and is used as a sweet filling for cakes. In China the beans are boiled with sugar and water and served hot or cold as a sweet soup, and the sweetened puree is used as a filling for sweet buns and pastries. They can also be cooked and seasoned to serve as a savoury side dish in the same way as lentils are used.

PROCESSING Sweetened red bean paste — azuki (Japan), hong dow (China) — is available in cans. Adzuki flour is also available.

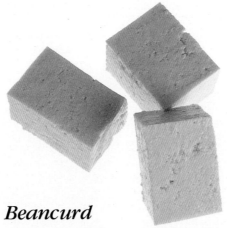

Beancurd

Also called **Tahu, Tofu**

MAJOR NUTRIENTS		SERVE SIZE 100 G	
Energy	290 kJ	Potassium	120 mg
Protein	7 g	Dietary Fibre	0
Fat	4 g	Calcium	500 mg
Carbohydrate	1 g	Phosphorus	120 mg
Cholesterol	0	Iron	2.4 mg
Sodium	5 mg	Zinc	0.7 mg

NUTRITIONAL INFORMATION Excellent source of magnesium, calcium, phosphorus and iron; good source of protein; moderate source of thiamin, folate and potassium; no fibre Compared to other legumes, tofu is relatively high in (mainly polyunsaturated) fat, and contains more calcium and iron.

DESCRIPTION A white, firm custardlike preparation made from soya beans. It has a bland flavour and little aroma. Tofu, the Japanese name, has replaced 'beancurd' to a large extent in Western nomenclature.

ORIGIN AND HISTORY Believed to date back to the Han Dynasty, 206BC to AD220, it was, and is still, one of the most important by-products of the soya bean because of its high nutritional value.

To make the beancurd, soya beans are soaked in water until they soften — about 4 to 6 hours. After draining, sufficient fresh water is added to enable beans to be ground to a puree. More water is added according to the amount of beans used, and the puree is strained to yield a soya bean 'milk' which is boiled and a coagulant added, setting the liquid into a junketlike mass. The curds are strained through cheesecloth and pressed to form cakes of fresh beancurd. Further processing, fermentation and drying produces other beancurd products for a variety of cooking uses.

BUYING AND STORAGE Traditional fresh beancurd or tofu is available at Asian and natural food stores, cut into squares and packed in water. Such beancurd is stored in the refrigerator and will keep for 3–4 days, with water changed each day.

PREPARATION AND USE Depending on cooking use, beancurd is cut in small cubes, shredded, stuffed, even pureed — according to traditional uses or vegetarian recipes. Since it is bland, a variety of flavourings, seasonings and additional ingredients can be added to produce nutritious meals.

Use for stir-fry dishes with vegetables and flavourings as a meat substitute or extender, for omelettes, add to soups, puree for a vegetable or salad dressing, shred or cube and add to salads.

PROCESSING A variety of beancurd products is available at Asian food stores, such as yellow or red beancurd and dried beancurd in sheets, sticks or twists. With the discovery of beancurd by those following natural food or vegetarian diets, many beancurd and tofu products are available, such as silken tofu, tofu ice cream, dry tofu mix and tofu cheese.

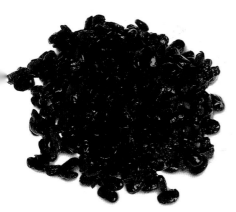

Black Bean, salted *Glycine max; G. soja*

also called Dow see

NUTRITIONAL INFORMATION No specific analysis is available for black bean, but nutrient levels should be similar to those of soya bean, except for an increased sodium content due to salting.

DESCRIPTION The black soya bean is fermented and salted, and available dried (in packs) or moist (in cans or jars). The dried bean is actually fairly moist and is small and wrinkled. The bean from jar or can is plump and shiny. When used sparingly, it imparts a deliciously savoury flavour and aroma to foods.

ORIGIN AND HISTORY Nearly 2500 years ago Chinese discovered that the beans of a native plant, the soya bean, were edible and highly nutritious, and the seeds could be dried and fermented with salt to make a versatile appetite-stimulating seasoning. Texts and drawings retrieved from ancient tombs depict the beans as an important seasoning food, and actual beans, still in a recognisable state of preservation, have been uncovered. In most rural households, particularly in southern China, a crock of homemade salt-fermented soya beans had pride of place in the kitchen as main seasoning. Strangely, Szechuan cuisine, which specialises in robust seasonings, omits the black bean from its fiery seasoning pastes and sauce.

BUYING AND STORAGE After dry-packed beans have been opened, reseal and store in the refrigerator; they keep indefinitely. Transfer canned beans to a jar after opening and float a little peanut oil on top to prevent drying; do likewise for jar-packed beans — store in the refrigerator for up to 6 months.

PREPARATION AND USE Soak the dry-packed beans in warm water for 10 minutes, then rinse well. Other salted beans need only be rinsed in cold water. Mash well with a fork

before using. About 1–2 tablespoons of black beans is sufficient for an average dish.

Use in combination with other flavouring ingredients for stir-fried meat and seafood dishes, and for steamed fish.

PROCESSING Black bean and hot black bean (or chilli bean) sauce combine salted black beans with other flavourings, with ground, hot chillies added for the hot variety. The salted beans are also a component in some Westernised Chinese-style sauces.

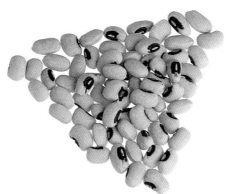

Black-eyed Bean *Vigna sinensis; V. catjan*

also called Black-eyed Pea, Cowpea, Catjang

MAJOR NUTRIENTS		SERVE SIZE 75 G	
Energy	1080 kJ	Calcium	36 g
Protein	17 g	Phosphorus	320 mg
Fat	1 g	Magnesium	170 mg
Carbohydrate	46 g	Iron	4.5 mg
Cholesterol	0	Thiamin	0.75 mg
Sodium	5 mg	Riboflavin	0.15 mg
Potassium	770 mg	Niacin Equiv.	1.5 mg
Dietary Fibre	9 g		

NUTRITIONAL INFORMATION The black-eyed bean has all the virtues of pulses: low fat, no cholesterol, high protein and the presence of fibre.

DESCRIPTION Small, cream, kidney-shaped beans with a distinctive black or yellow 'eye', depending on the variety. They have a pleasant, slightly sweet flavour when cooked.

While 'cowpea' is an alternative name for black-eyed bean, there is another cowpea available (*Vigna unguiculata*); it is principally used as a cover or summer forage crop, but the seeds are used for sprouting and included in mixed salad sprouts. The cowpea is very tiny, tan in colour with a small white 'eye'.

ORIGIN AND HISTORY Native to tropical Africa and Asia, the black-eyed bean has been used as a food since ancient times, featuring in Central African, Greek, Middle Eastern, and Indian cooking. Black-eyed beans feature in the 'soul food' cooking of the deep south of the USA, and in Jamaica, travelling to the new world via the slave trade.

BUYING AND STORAGE Size depends on region in which beans were grown, and is not an indication of quality. The beans appear very slightly wrinkled and dull, with a clear 'eye'. Store in a sealed container in a cool, dry place, and use within 6 months.

PREPARATION AND USE Prepare in the usual way and slow-soak for 2–3 hours, or quick-soak as detailed in the introduction. Change water, bring to the boil, then simmer, covered, for 1 hour until tender. Can also be pressure-cooked for 10 minutes.

Use for bean soups and stews and in bean salads. Raw beans, slow-soaked for 8 hours, can be ground in a food processor with fresh ginger, chilli, garlic, onion and seasoning, and deep-fried in hot oil for the bean fritters of Central Africa (akara) and Jamaica (akkra). Do not attempt to make such fritters with cooked beans.

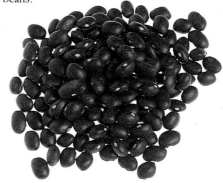

Black Kidney Bean *Phaseolus vulgaris*

also known as Turtle bean

NUTRITIONAL INFORMATION No specific analysis is available, but nutrient levels would be similar to those of red kidney beans. A good source of vegetable protein, and exceptionally rich in dietary fibre. The bean needs to be boiled for at least 10 minutes to remove anti-nutritional factors, which slightly reduces the amount of vitamin B.

DESCRIPTION Shiny black kidney-shaped dried bean, with a pleasant flavour and smooth texture when cooked.

ORIGIN AND HISTORY Native to the Americas, they were first cultivated in Mexico, and have long been a staple food item, particularly in Mexico, Central America, Brazil, and the Caribbean. Size varies according to region where grown.

BUYING AND STORAGE Beans should be shiny and smooth. They are difficult to find outside Latin America, the Caribbean, and the USA (popular in the southern states and California), but are often included in pulse mixes sold in natural food stores. Store in a sealed container in a cool, dry place, and use within a year.

PREPARATION AND USE Slow-soak for 8–10 hours, or quick-soak as detailed in the introduction. Change water, bring to the boil and boil for 15 minutes, then simmer, covered, for 2–3 hours until tender. Can be pressure-cooked in 15–20 minutes.

Use in Mexican bean dishes, particularly for frijoles refritos, refried beans. Use also in chilli con carne, and for bean soups, stews and salads.

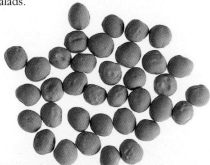

Blue Pea *Pisum sativum*

*also called **Whole dried pea***

MAJOR NUTRIENTS

		COOKED SERVE SIZE 200 G	
Energy	880 kJ	Calcium	50 mg
Protein	14 g	Phosphorus	220 mg
Fat	1 g	Magnesium	60 mg
Carbohydrate	38 g	Iron	3 mg
Cholesterol	0	Zinc	2 mg
Sodium	5 mg	Thiamin	0.2 mg
Potassium	540 mg	Riboflavin	0.15 mg
Dietary Fibre	10 g	Niacin Equiv.	2 mg

NUTRITIONAL INFORMATION The blue pea provides good quality vegetable protein, dietary fibre, and B group vitamins. As the blue pea is low in fat and cholesterol-free, it helps to provide a balance when eaten in the traditional form with meat pies.

DESCRIPTION Whole dried peas with a bluish tinge and slightly wrinkled skins, blue peas are the dried seeds of the matured common garden pea, not to be confused with the freeze-dried, quick-cooking peas packaged in small quantities. While the blue pea has a definite pea flavour, it tends to cook to a mush.

ORIGIN AND HISTORY Dating back to prehistoric times, the pea most probably originated in middle Asia; seeds found in the 'Spirit Caves' near the Burmese border of Thailand have been carbon-dated to 9750 BC. Finds in the Near East are thought to date from some 2000 years later. Archaeological finds have placed them at Stone Age sites in Hungary and Switzerland, at France and northern Greece Bronze Age sites, and the Iron Age site at Glastonbury, England.

BUYING AND STORAGE Look for even colour; skins should be only slightly wrinkled. Store in a sealed container in a cool, dry place, and use within a year.

PREPARATION AND USE See Pulses for preparation and slow-soak for at least 8 hours. Change water and bring to the boil. Cover and simmer gently for 1 hour until tender, adding a little sugar, and salt and mint if desired, towards end of cooking.

Blue peas often cook to a mush, and are known as mushy peas in England; a favourite use is to serve these with fish and chips, or pour them over hot meat pies. Because of this quality, the blue pea can be used in soups. If the variety purchased retains its shape after cooking, serve tossed with a knob of butter as a fresh pea substitute.

PROCESSING Roasted, spiced blue peas are available at Indian food stores and are excellent as a snack food.

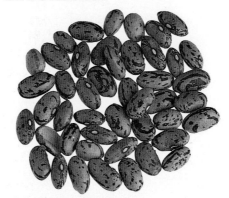

Borlotti Bean *Phaseolus vulgaris*

*also called **Roman bean, Romano bean, Cranberry bean, Saluggia bean***

NUTRITIONAL INFORMATION Nutritionally, the borlotti bean is similar to the brown bean. Like all pulses this bean is a good source of protein, fibre and B group vitamins. Small amounts of the latter are lost in cooking.

DESCRIPTION The borlotti bean is varied in colouring from beige, attractively speckled with burgundy-coloured markings, to a pale brown with similar markings, to an even deeper background colour with the markings almost covering the bean. The latter is often labelled as the cranberry bean. The saluggia bean is regarded as a different bean, but its difference is only in size — it is smaller. All have the same smooth texture and hamlike flavour when cooked.

ORIGIN AND HISTORY Native to tropical America and introduced to Europe via the Spaniards. In 1528, some beans were sent to Pope Clement VII, who passed them on to

Canon Pietro Valeriano in Florence. He planted them, liked his first crop, and passed them around. Whether the first beans introduced into Italy were the borlotti or the cannellini of today is not known, but from the time of their introduction, the Tuscans were tagged mangiafagioli (bean eaters). Because they are so favoured in Italy, borlottis are widely regarded as Italian; the immature beans are a popular Italian vegetable in their season.

BUYING AND STORAGE Look for smooth beans; slightly wrinkled skins indicate staleness, and such beans require longer cooking. Store in a sealed container in a cool, dry place, and use within a year.

PREPARATION AND USE See Pulses for preparation and slow-soak for 8–10 hours or quick-soak. Change water, bring to the boil and boil for 15 minutes, then simmer, covered, for 1–1½ hours until tender. Borlottis can be pressure-cooked in 15 minutes.

Use for bean soups, stews and casseroles, or for salads. Very good mixed with tuna, raw onion rings, parsley, olive oil and vinegar for a cold salad.

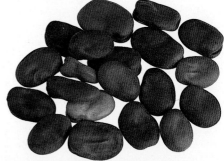

Broad Bean (dried) *Vicia faba*

*also called **Fava bean, Windsor bean***

MAJOR NUTRIENTS

		SERVE SIZE 75 G	
Energy	1030 kJ	Calcium	76 mg
Protein	19 g	Iron	3.2 mg
Fat	1 g	Thiamin	0.35 mg
Carbohydrate	43 g	Riboflavin	0.15 mg
Cholesterol	0	Niacin Equiv.	2 mg
Sodium	5 mg		

NUTRITIONAL INFORMATION The broad bean provides an excellent source of vegetable protein, a variety of minerals, B group vitamins and good dietary fibre. No specific amounts are available for the fibre, zinc or phosphorus present in the beans. Small amounts of vitamin B are lost in cooking. Eating broad beans causes favism in susceptible people of Middle Eastern origin. Favism is a disease which leads to weakness, pallor and fatigue due to a type of anaemia.

DESCRIPTION A large, flat bean, roughly oval in shape, it can be green, beige or brown in colour. When cooked, texture is smooth and creamy, flavour is strong, but the skin is quite tough. Flavour improves if the bean is skinned before cooking.

ORIGIN AND HISTORY Native to the Mediterranean, the broad bean is one of the most ancient old world cultivated food plants. Bronze Age and Iron Age relics of the British Isles, Europe and the Mediterranean region indicate their use as a food from those times. Early Greeks and Romans used the bean for balloting — the white bean signifying agreement, the 'black' bean, opposition.

BUYING AND STORAGE Green and beige-coloured beans signify a new season's crop, however a purchase of broad beans may contain a variety of hues. Skins should be relatively smooth. Store in a sealed container in a cool, dry place and use within a year.

PREPARATION AND USE Prepare as usual and slow-soak for 12 hours. Change water, bring to the boil and boil for 15 minutes, then simmer, covered, for 2–2½ hours until tender. Can be pressure-cooked for 25 minutes.

In Italian, Greek and Middle Eastern cooking, the broad bean is soaked for 48 hours with frequent changes of water, and the creamy centres popped out of the skins. This bean is used for soups, purees, or ground (uncooked) with other ingredients for the bean patties tameya (Egypt) and falafel (Lebanon). Do not make patties with cooked beans or they will disintegrate during frying.

Toss whole boiled broad beans with parsley sauce and serve with ham, or use in soups, stews and salads.

PROCESSING Skinned broad beans may be found in Greek and Middle Eastern food stores. They are preferred for many traditional recipes as they require less preparation and take less time to cook.

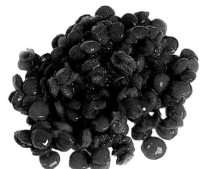

Brown Bean *Phaseolus vulgaris*

also called Dutch brown bean, African brown bean

MAJOR NUTRIENTS		SERVE SIZE 75 G	
Energy	1060 kJ	Calcium	101 mg
Protein	17 g	Phosphorus	315 mg
Fat	1 g	Magnesium	125 mg
Carbohydrate	46 g	Iron	5.9 mg
Cholesterol	0	Thiamin	0.4 mg
Sodium	5 mg	Riboflavin	0.15 mg
Potassium	780 mg	Niacin Equiv.	1.5 mg
Dietary Fibre	8 g		

NUTRITIONAL INFORMATION The brown bean provides an excellent source of vegetable protein, a variety of minerals, and B group vitamins, plus good dietary fibre. While zinc is present in the beans, specific levels are not available. Small amounts of vitamin B are lost in cooking. The bean must be boiled for at least 10 minutes to remove anti-nutritional factors.

DESCRIPTION A rich brown version of the haricot bean, kidney-shaped and a little larger than the haricot, but still a small bean.

ORIGIN AND HISTORY Originated in the Americas. Because the brown bean is particularly favoured in the Netherlands, it may have reached Holland via the Dutch in South Africa, as the bean is also used in Africa.

BUYING AND STORAGE Look for the smooth-skinned, shiny bean of medium size, as it is more likely to be the right bean. There is a tendency to package many beans without adequate identification, and purchase from a food store specialising in Dutch foods is recommended. Store in a sealed container in a cool, dry place, and use within 6 months.

PREPARATION AND USE Prepare as usual and slow-soak for 6–8 hours or quick-soak. Change water, bring to the boil and boil for 15 minutes, then simmer, covered, for 1½–2½ hours. Can be pressure-cooked for 15–20 minutes.

Follow the Dutch lead and use for bean pots, or simply boil, drain, and toss with diced and fried smoked speck, fried onions and the rendered speck fat. Dill-pickled cucumbers are a traditional accompaniment. Use also in bean soups, stews and salads.

PROCESSING Canned Dutch brown beans are available at food stores stocking Dutch foods.

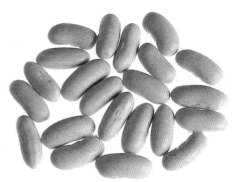

Cannellini Bean *Phaseolus vulgaris*

also called Great Northern bean

MAJOR NUTRIENTS		COOKED SERVE SIZE 200 G	
Energy	990 kJ	Dietary Fibre	3 g
Protein	16 g	Calcium	100 mg
Fat	1 g	Phosphorus	270 mg
Carbohydrate	42 g	Iron	5.5 mg
Cholesterol	0	Thiamin	0.3 mg
Sodium	5 mg	Riboflavin	0.15 mg
Potassium	830 mg	Niacin Equiv.	1.5 mg

NUTRITIONAL INFORMATION This bean contains good quality protein, fibre, B group vitamins and a range of minerals including zinc, though no analysis for zinc is available. Must be boiled for at least 10 minutes to remove anti-nutritional factors.

DESCRIPTION A white bean, kidney-shaped and larger than the haricot bean, mild-flavoured and fluffy in texture when cooked. A true cannellini bean is somewhat angular at each end, while the Great Northern is rounded, but the latter, being grown in greater quantities, is often sold as cannellini.

ORIGIN AND HISTORY Native to tropical America, the cannellini bean was first cultivated by the Incas. Cannellini is the most popular white bean in Italy, while the Great Northern has become an important bean crop in North America for canning and export. (See Borlotti Bean for additional historical information.)

BUYING AND STORAGE Look for the smooth-skinned bean with a slightly off-white colour. There is little difference between cannellini and Great Northern as far as flavour is concerned. Store in a sealed container in a cool, dry place, and use within a year.

PREPARATION AND USE Prepare as usual and slow or quick-soak. Change water, bring to the boil and boil for 15 minutes, then simmer, covered, for 1–1½ hours until tender. Cannellinis can be pressure-cooked for 15 minutes.

Use for soups, stews, casseroles, bean pots such as the French cassoulet, and salads.

PROCESSING Available canned on their own or in bean mixes.

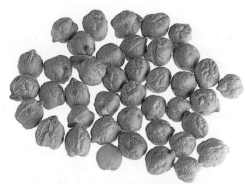

Chickpea   *Cicer arietinum*

also called Garbanzo bean, Bengal gram, Desi chickpea, Kaala chana, Kabli chana

MAJOR NUTRIENTS		SERVE SIZE 75 G	
Energy	1010 kJ	Calcium	110 mg
Protein	15 g	Phosphorus	225 mg
Fat	5 g	Magnesium	120 mg
Carbohydrate	38 g	Iron	4.8 mg
Cholesterol	0	Zinc	1.8 mg
Sodium	30 mg	Thiamin	0.35 mg
Potassium	600 mg	Riboflavin	0.1 mg
Dietary Fibre	11 g	Niacin Equiv.	1 mg

NUTRITIONAL INFORMATION The chickpea provides good quality vegetable protein, B group vitamins, and many minerals, including copper. An excellent source of dietary fibre unless skinned, and, unlike most pulses, it contains a small but significant amount of oil. Small amounts of vitamin B are lost in cooking.

DESCRIPTION A beige-coloured pea, round and rough-textured, with a pointed 'beak' at one end. Nutty in flavour with a mealy texture when cooked. Bengal gram (desi chickpea or kaala chana) is much smaller and medium to dark brown in colour.

ORIGIN AND HISTORY The seed of a plant native to west Asia, chickpea is used extensively in the Middle East and in Spain and France. In northern Africa it is crushed to a meal and used in making a dip called hommos. The chickpea has grown in India throughout its history. These little golden pellets are revered as an important protein vegetable, being used as grain and to make a heavy flour, besan. The dry roasted chickpea, flavoured with salt, spices and chilli is perhaps one of the most popular snack foods in India. The chickpea is rarely used in other parts of Asia.

Introduced to the New World by the Spaniards.

BUYING AND STORAGE Look for even colour and smooth skins. Kaala chana is not very uniform in colour, with a 'withered' appearance. Store in a sealed container in a cool, dry place, and use within a year.

PREPARATION AND USE Prepare as usual and slow-soak for 12 hours or quick-soak.

Drain, add fresh water and boil gently for 1–1½ hours until tender. May be pressure-cooked for 15 minutes, but it is advisable to boil the peas uncovered for 15 minutes, skim well to remove froth and add a tablespoon of oil before bringing to pressure.

To remove skins from the chickpeas (required in some recipes), slow-soak and rub beans in a cloth, floating off the skins.

Use for purees (Middle Eastern hommos), Indian dals, soups, stews, casseroles and salads. Also ground, after slow-soaking, to make Middle Eastern bean patties, falafel; if cooked chickpeas are used, they disintegrate when fried.

In India the chickpea is cooked with chilli and tart spices to serve as a spicy side dish to serve with curries, or to stuff into fried bread called puris. The cracked grain is cooked into a kind of meal used as a filling for savoury-fried snacks.

PROCESSING Besan, a flour of ground chickpeas with a distinctive nutty flavour, is used in Indian and Pakistani cooking. Roasted chickpeas, a snack food, are available salted, unsalted or spiced.

SEE ALSO Besan.

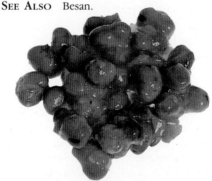

Ful Medami   *Vicia faba* var. *minor*

also called Egyptian Brown bean, Ful, Fava, Tick bean

NUTRITIONAL INFORMATION This bean provides an excellent source of vegetable protein, a variety of minerals, B group vitamins and good dietary fibre. No specific amounts are available for the fibre, zinc or phosphorus present in the bean.

DESCRIPTION A variety of broad bean, smaller and more rounded than its more commonly known relative. Colour ranges from beige to brown. Finer-skinned and with a more refined flavour than the broad bean, its texture is smooth and creamy when cooked. Commonly known by its Arabic name, ful medami, from the Egyptian specialty of that name. Ful is often transliterated as fool and foul.

ORIGIN AND HISTORY Native to the Mediterranean, the bean probably dates back to pre-Pharoah times. It is a staple food in Egypt, with its preparation of such importance that a special metal cooking vessel, the idra, was developed. This vessel has a bulbous body with a narrow neck to conserve moisture during cooking.

BUYING AND STORAGE Look for the smooth-skinned bean. Store in a sealed container in a cool, dry place, and use within a year.

PREPARATION AND USE Prepare as usual and slow-soak for 12 hours or quick-soak. Change water and bring to the boil. Simmer, covered tightly, for 3–3½ hours. The long, slow cooking develops the flavour and its colour changes to a purplish-brown. The bean can be pressure-cooked in 25–30 minutes.

Use for purees, soups, casseroles and salads. For ful medamis, mash the cooked beans with cooking liquid, serve in deep plates with olive oil and lemon juice. Excellent for ground bean patties, falafel or tameya — slow-soak for 12–24 hours, but do not remove skins, and do not cook beforehand or the patties will disintegrate when fried.

PROCESSING The dried beans are ground for a packaged dry falafel mix, available from Middle Eastern and natural food stores.

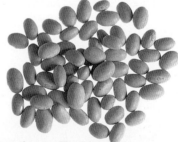

Haricot Bean   *Phaseolus vulgaris*

also called Navy bean, Pea bean, Soisson

MAJOR NUTRIENTS		COOKED SERVE SIZE 200 G	
Energy	790 kJ	Calcium	130 mg
Protein	13 g	Phosphorus	240 mg
Fat	1 g	Magnesium	90 mg
Carbohydrate	33 g	Iron	5 mg
Cholesterol	0	Zinc	2 mg
Sodium	0	Thiamin	0.25 mg
Potassium	640 mg	Niacin Equiv.	1 mg
Dietary Fibre	15 g		

NUTRITIONAL INFORMATION This bean is an excellent source of vegetable protein and dietary fibre while being low fat and cholesterol-free. A serve of haricot or baked beans will provide half the recommended daily fibre intake. Baked beans with toast are an excellent fast food for any meal.

DESCRIPTION A small white bean, oval in shape. Some varieties are almost round like a pea. Soissons are named for the town where the haricot was first grown in France, and are particularly large. All haricots have a smooth texture with a rather bland flavour when cooked. As they absorb other flavours well, haricots are the most widely used beans for canned baked beans.

ORIGIN AND HISTORY Native to Central and South America and first cultivated by the Aztecs, the French word haricot is derived from the Aztec, ayacotl. The haricots found their way into the cooking pots of the early North American settlers. The New England specialty of Boston baked beans popularised dried beans on the Western table; canned baked beans owe their beginnings to this humble bean pot. The dried haricots were essential supplies for the USA navy, giving yet another name to this bean.

BUYING AND STORAGE Choose the smooth-skinned bean with a creamy-white colour. Wrinkled and dark cream beans indicate old stock. Store in a sealed container in a cool, dry place and use within a year.

PREPARATION AND USE Prepare as usual and cold-soak for 2–3 hours, or quick-soak and leave 1 hour until plump. Change water, bring to the boil and boil for 15 minutes, then simmer, covered, for 1–1½ hours until tender. Can be pressure-cooked for 15 minutes.

Use for the traditional Boston baked beans, for cassoulet, and in soups, stews, casseroles and salads.

PROCESSING Canned baked beans, available with a variety of flavours added to the basic tomato sauce.

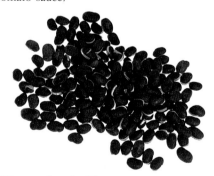

Hyacinth Bean *Dolichos lablab*

also called Lablab, Lubia, Bonavist, Val

MAJOR NUTRIENTS SERVE SIZE 75 G

Energy	1070 kJ	Calcium	66 mg
Protein	15 g	Iron	2.6 mg
Fat	1 g	Thiamin	0.45 mg
Carbohydrate	46 g	Riboflavin	0.15 mg
Cholesterol	0	Niacin Equiv.	1.5 mg
Sodium	25 mg		

NUTRITIONAL INFORMATION This bean contains good-quality vegetable protein, dietary fibre and B group vitamins. As well as iron this bean provides fibre, phosphorus and zinc although specific amounts are not available. The hyacinth bean must be boiled for at least 10 minutes to remove anti-nutritional factors. Boiling also slightly reduces vitamin B content.

DESCRIPTION A brown or black bean with a distinctive white line running along one side. The bean contains a poisonous glucoside, but cooking destroys this. The skins are fairly thick even when cooked, but not inedible. They have a mealy texture and bland flavour.

ORIGIN AND HISTORY Native to India, but used today mainly by the inhabitants and expatriates of the Indian state of Gujarat. Also used in Egypt and the Sudan as they grow well in arid tropical regions.

BUYING AND STORAGE The hyacinth bean is difficult to obtain but is available from some Indian food stores under the name of val. While Indians prefer the light brown beans, the black beans are also acceptable. Store in a sealed container in a cool, dry place.

PREPARATION AND USE Prepare as usual and slow-soak for 24 hours. If desired, the skins may be removed by rubbing the soaked beans in a cloth, then floating them off. Check beans after soaking; some hyacinth beans are from sources where growing conditions affect quality, and a few of the beans refuse to take up water, remaining small and hard. These should be picked out and discarded.

Add fresh water and bring to the boil. Boil for 15 minutes, cover and simmer for 30–45 minutes until tender.

Use the skinned beans for dal, soups or purees, the whole beans for spicy stews with tomato added. Meat may also be added.

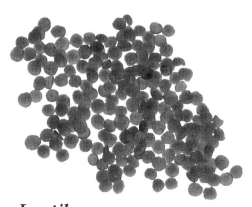

Lentil *Lens esculenta*

also called Continental lentil, Red lentil, Masoor dal

MAJOR NUTRIENTS COOKED
SERVE SIZE 200 G

Energy	840 kJ	Dietary Fibre	9 g
Protein	15 g	Calcium	40 g
Fat	1 g	Phosphorus	150 mg
Carbohydrate	34 g	Magnesium	50 mg
Cholesterol	0	Iron	4.8 mg
Sodium	30 mg	Zinc	2 mg
Potassium	420 mg	Thiamin	0.2 mg

NUTRITIONAL INFORMATION The lentil is an excellent source of vegetable protein, fibre, and the B vitamins — thiamin, niacin and vitamin B6; good source of potassium, magnesium and zinc. Brown lentils are a good extender for mince dishes, providing extra protein, while being low in fat and cholesterol-free.

DESCRIPTION The lentil varies in colour from green to brown; it is often referred to as the continental lentil and is rather bland in flavour. The orange-coloured lentil is tiny and already skinned and split when purchased; more commonly known as the red lentil, it has a subtle spicy flavour.

ORIGIN AND HISTORY Used from prehistoric times, the lentil probably originated in southwest Europe and temperate Asia. Archaeological discoveries date its use by humans as far back as 6750 BC at Qalat Jarmo (Iraq). A Hindu proverb says 'Rice is good, but lentils are my life'. The red lentil is the oldest known variety of these beans. Chinese archaeologists uncovered containers of red lentils from Han tombs. Although it is not included in the list of 'five important ancient grains', from accompanying drawings and its presence in the tomb, it is evident that the red lentil was in use in China as a food well over 2000 years ago. Ancient Egyptians used red lentils and they have also been discovered in Bronze Age lake settlements in Switzerland, indicating their presence and use were widespread.

BUYING AND STORAGE The continental lentil should be smooth-skinned. Store in a sealed container in a cool, dry place.

PREPARATION AND USE Pick over lentils and remove small stones. Rinse in a sieve to remove grit. They do not require soaking, but continental lentils can be soaked in cold water for 1–2 hours if desired.

Place lentils in a pan with at least 3 times their volume of water and bring to the boil. Skim off surface froth, partly cover and simmer gently for 30 minutes (red lentils) or 1–1½ hours (continental lentils). To prevent lentils sticking to base of pan, do not stir during cooking.

Use for soups, purees and casseroles; use red lentils for Indian dal. The continental lentil can be used in salads and is also suitable for sprouting. Either type may be used for vegetarian loaves and crumb-coated patties.

PROCESSING Lentil flour is available for vegetarian and Indian cooking.

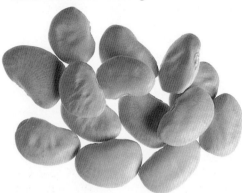

Lima Bean *Phaseolus lunatus*

also called *Butter bean, Calico bean, Sieva bean, Madagascar bean*

MAJOR NUTRIENTS
COOKED
SERVE SIZE 190 G

Energy	770 kJ	Dietary Fibre	9.5 g
Protein	13 g	Phosphorus	165 mg
Fat	1 g	Magnesium	65 mg
Carbohydrate	32 g	Iron	3.2 mg
Cholesterol	0	Zinc	1.9 mg
Sodium	30 mg	Thiamin	0.25 mg
Potassium	760 mg	Niacin Equiv.	1.5 µg

NUTRITIONAL INFORMATION This bean contains good vegetable protein, excellent fibre, a variety of minerals, and B group vitamins. The lima bean must be boiled for at least 10 minutes to remove anti-nutritional factors. The exceptionally high fibre results in flatulence in susceptible people.

DESCRIPTION The flat, kidney-shaped bean can be white or green, large or small. It has a floury texture and a pleasant, slightly sweet flavour when cooked. The large white lima is more frequently called butter bean, calico bean, or Madagascar bean after the country which produces a particularly large variety. The small green lima is also used fresh.

ORIGIN AND HISTORY Native to central South America, the bean was named for Lima, capital of Peru, where it was first cultivated. Its use in the North American succotash, a dish attributed to the Algonquin Indians of present-day Canada, indicates the bean had travelled far long before European settlement of North America.

BUYING AND STORAGE Choose the smooth-skinned bean with a dull sheen. Store in a sealed container in a cool, dry place and use within a year.

PREPARATION AND USE Prepare as usual and cold-soak for 4–6 hours, or quick-soak

and leave 1–2 hours until plump. Change water, bring to the boil and boil for 15 minutes, then simmer, covered, for 1–1½ hours until tender. Can be pressure-cooked for 15 minutes. Boil the fresh lima bean in lightly salted water for 15 minutes.

Use for soups, stews, casseroles and salads. Green limas, both fresh and dried, may be tossed with butter and served as a vegetable accompaniment, particularly for roast lamb. A good substitute for the flageolet bean, which is difficult to obtain.

PROCESSING The small green lima bean is available frozen and canned; butter beans are canned on their own; green limas are included in canned bean mixes.

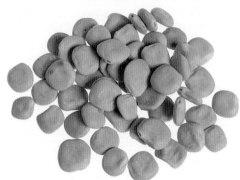

Lupin *Lupinus luteus*

NUTRITIONAL INFORMATION No reliable analysis is available.

DESCRIPTION A squarish flat white seed which can be large or small, depending on variety. Because of the high alkaloid content, this seed needs special preparation to make it edible.

ORIGIN AND HISTORY Certain lupins have been used as a food in the Mediterranean region from 2000 BC. Once New World beans became established in the region, lupins remained in Italian and Middle Eastern kitchens purely as a snack food. They are called lupini in Italian, troumis in Arabic.

BUYING AND STORAGE The smaller lupins are considered sweeter than the larger variety, and both are available from Italian, Greek and Middle Eastern food stores. Store in a sealed container in a cool, dry place.

PREPARATION AND USE Lupins must be soaked to rid them of the bitter alkaloids, with the larger lupins (favoured by Italians) requiring a more prolonged treatment than the small.

Soak any lupin in plenty of cold water in a cool place for 12 hours. Change water, bring to the boil and simmer, covered, for 2 hours or until the point of a knife penetrates easily. Drain, add cold water and leave until cool.

Drain, place in a bowl and add 3 cups water and 1 tablespoon salt for each cup of dried lupins.

For large lupins, leave in a cool place and change salted water twice each day for 6–7 days until lupins taste sweet without a trace of bitterness. Put into fresh salted water and store in a sealed jar in the refrigerator. Small lupins do not require the brine to be changed. Drain to serve as a snack; serve plain or with a squeeze of lemon juice. Skins may be eaten or discarded.

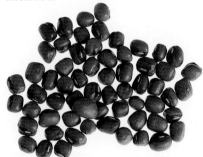

Mung Bean *Phaseolus aureus*

also called *Green gram, Golden gram, Moong dal*

MAJOR NUTRIENTS
COOKED
SERVE SIZE 200 G

Energy	990 kJ	Calcium	120 mg
Protein	22 g	Phosphorus	360 mg
Fat	1 g	Magnesium	170 mg
Carbohydrate	36 g	Iron	8.1 mg
Cholesterol	0	Thiamin	0.45 mg
Sodium	30 mg	Riboflavin	0.2 mg
Potassium	850 mg	Niacin Equiv.	9 mg
Dietary Fibre	20 g		

NUTRITIONAL INFORMATION The mung bean contains good quality vegetable protein and fibre, and is an excellent source of magnesium, iron, folate, niacin and thiamin. In Asian countries the mung bean is used as a beri beri preventative, especially during pregnancy.

DESCRIPTION Tiny moss green beans, used whole or skinned and split. Split mung beans are creamy in colour. Flavour is mild when cooked. Mung beans are most widely used for sprouting.

ORIGIN AND HISTORY Native to tropical Asia and one of the most widely cultivated pulses in India and China, used from ancient times. In India, the skinned split mung is known as moong dal. In China, the whole mung bean is sprouted, and when skinned, is ground into a powder and used in the making of sweets and cellophane noodles (full see).

BUYING AND STORAGE Look for smooth, shiny beans. Store whole or split beans in a sealed container in a cool, dry place and use within a year.

PREPARATION AND USE Prepare as usual, washing well as the mung bean does not require soaking. Pick over moong dal well to remove any small stones, and rinse in a sieve to remove grit. Add water and bring to the boil. Boil for 15 minutes, reduce heat, cover and simmer for 30–45 minutes, adding salt towards end of cooking.

Use in soups, stews and salads, and for a side dish in Indian cuisine, called dal like the lentil itself. Sprouts can be used raw or lightly cooked in stir-fried dishes.

VARIETY

Mouth/Mowth Dal

NUTRITIONAL INFORMATION Like all pulses the red mung bean is high in vegetable protein, making it a valuable addition to the diet of vegetarian Indians.

DESCRIPTION A red mung bean.

ORIGIN AND HISTORY Although, like its green cousin, it grows throughout India, the red mung is most popular in the Indian states of Rajasthan and Gujarat.

BUYING AND STORAGE Usually available only from specialist Asian stores, in dried form and sold by kg. The red mung bean should be rinsed thoroughly and can be cooked whole, or sprouted in damp, warm conditions.

PREPARATION AND USE Used in Indian cooking as a dal and sprouted to cook as a vegetable.

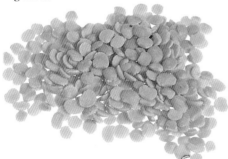

Pigeon Pea *Cajanus cajan*

also called **Gunga pea, Congo pea, Red gram dal, Toor dal**

MAJOR NUTRIENTS			SERVE SIZE 75 G
Energy	960 kJ	Calcium	80 mg
Protein	15 g	Phosphorus	235 mg
Fat	1 g	Magnesium	90 mg
Carbohydrate	40 g	Iron	6 mg
Cholesterol	0	Thiamin	0.2 mg
Sodium	20 mg	Niacin Equiv.	5.5 mg
Potassium	825 mg	Folate	75 µg
Dietary Fibre	11 g		

NUTRITIONAL INFORMATION This pea contains vegetable protein, excellent dietary fibre, B group vitamins, and minerals including zinc, though no specific level is available for zinc. Cooking will slightly reduce the vitamin B content.

DESCRIPTION The pigeon pea is a pea-shaped pulse, beige in colour with tan to brown speckles or blotches. It has a smooth texture and slightly sweet flavour when cooked.

ORIGIN AND HISTORY Native to tropical Africa, the pigeon pea has been grown in the Nile Valley and other parts of Africa since ancient times. Skinned and split, as in the picture on the left, it is also important in India where it is known as toor dal. As this pulse is also popular in the West Indies, where it is known as gunga pea, it undoubtedly travelled there via the slave trade.

BUYING AND STORAGE Select smooth-skinned pigeon peas to ensure they are of the new season's crop. Store in a sealed container in a cool, dry place for 6–8 months. Toor dal (red gram dal) is stored in the same way, but should be used within 2 months.

PREPARATION AND USE Prepare as usual and slow or quick-soak. Change water, bring to the boil, then simmer for 30 minutes to 1 hour. Can be pressure-cooked in 10–15 minutes. Red gram dal should be picked over thoroughly to remove any small stones, then rinsed in a sieve to remove grit. Place in a pan with water and bring to the boil, then simmer, covered, for 30–45 minutes until soft.

Use pigeon peas in soups, stews, casseroles and salads. They are used in Indian cooking to make a spicy side dish with a tart flavour introduced from tamarind, lemon juice or green mango. Split chickpeas or yellow split peas can be substituted.

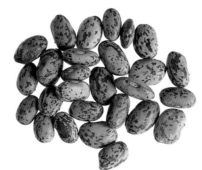

Pinto Bean *Phaseolus vulgaris*

MAJOR NUTRIENTS			SERVE SIZE 75 G
Energy	1100 kJ	Dietary Fibre	12 g
Protein	17 g	Calcium	101 mg
Fat	1 g	Phosphorus	340 mg
Carbohydrate	49 g	Iron	4.8 mg
Cholesterol	0	Thiamin	0.65 mg
Sodium	20 mg	Riboflavin	0.15 mg
Potassium	735 mg	Niacin Equiv.	1.5 mg

NUTRITIONAL INFORMATION Like all pulses the pinto bean is rich in vegetable protein, fibre, and B group vitamins. Zinc is present in these beans though no specific amount is available. Boiling will slightly reduce the vitamin B content. Borlotti can be substituted for the pinto bean.

DESCRIPTION A plump, kidney-shaped bean, beige in colour and speckled with brown. It cooks to a pleasant salmon pink colour with an appetisingly savoury flavour and smooth texture.

ORIGIN AND HISTORY Native to the Americas and first cultivated by the Aztecs. It is one of the most widely used beans in Mexico, particularly for frijoles refritos, refried beans, and through the Mexican use of the beans, the pinto became particularly popular in the southern states of the USA. Cowboys call them 'Mexican strawberries'.

BUYING AND STORAGE The bean should be smooth skinned with a dull sheen. Store in a sealed container in a cool, dry place, and use within a year.

PREPARATION AND USE Prepare as usual and slow or quick-soak. Change water, bring to the boil and boil for 15 minutes, then simmer for 1½–2 hours until tender.

Use for soups, stews, casseroles, refried beans, salads and Mexican and American chilli-spiced bean dishes. Meats such as beef and pork combine well with the pinto bean.

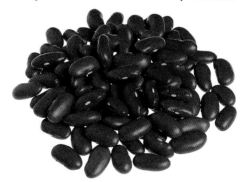

Red Kidney Bean *Phaseolus vulgaris*

also called **Raajma**

MAJOR NUTRIENTS			SERVE SIZE 75 G
Energy	870 kJ	Calcium	105 mg
Protein	17 g	Phosphorus	310 mg
Fat	1 g	Magnesium	135 mg
Carbohydrate	34 g	Iron	5 mg
Cholesterol	0	Zinc	2.1 mg
Sodium	40 mg	Thiamin	0.41 mg
Potassium	870 mg	Riboflavin	0.15 mg
Dietary Fibre	19 g	Niacin Equiv.	1.5 mg

NUTRITIONAL INFORMATION The red kidney bean is a good source of vegetable protein, and exceptionally rich in dietary fibre.

Excellent source of potassium, magnesium, iron, thiamin, niacin and folate; moderate source of calcium, zinc and riboflavin; contains copper. The bean must be boiled for at least 10 minutes to remove anti-nutritional factors. The exceptionally high fibre results in flatulence in susceptible people. Cooking slightly reduces the vitamin B content.

DESCRIPTION The kidney-shaped bean can be either elongated or plump in shape, and range in colour from dusky pink (sometimes called the pink bean) to a deep red. It is floury in texture and has a pleasantly sweet flavour when cooked.

ORIGIN AND HISTORY Native to the Americas and cultivated by the Aztecs. It is one of the most used beans in Mexico, and became popular in the Western kitchen through the North American chilli con carne, a dish with Spanish, Mexican and American-Indian origins.

BUYING AND STORAGE Look for shiny, smooth-skinned beans. Size and depth of colour varies according to where the beans were grown. Store in a sealed container in a cool, dry place, and use within a year.

PREPARATION AND USE See Pulses for preparation, and slow or quick-soak. Change water, bring to the boil and boil for 15 minutes, then simmer, covered, for 1–1½ hours until tender.

Use for soups, stews, casseroles, purees such as refried beans, and for salads.

The red kidney bean is popular, although not extensively used, in Indian cooking, but is favoured in the states of Punjab and Rajasthan, where it is made into a thick curry with tomatoes.

PROCESSING Canned red kidney beans are widely available, either packed on their own, or in canned bean mixes.

Soya Bean Glycine max; G. soja

also called *Soy bean*

MAJOR NUTRIENTS

			COOKED SERVE SIZE 200 G
Energy	1090 kJ	Calcium	145 mg
Protein	22 g	Phosphorus	360 mg
Fat	11 g	Iron	5.5 mg
Carbohydrate	18 g	Zinc	2 mg
Cholesterol	0	Thiamin	0.4 mg
Sodium	5 mg	Riboflavin	0.2 mg
Potassium	1080 mg	Niacin Equiv.	11 mg
Dietary Fibre	9 g		

NUTRITIONAL INFORMATION The soya bean provides the best quality protein of all pulses. While containing some starch it also has a high amount of fat in the form of poly-unsaturated oil. It also provides dietary fibre, some B group vitamins, and a range of minerals. The bean requires soaking and boiling for at least 10 minutes to remove anti-nutritional factors.

Soya drinks, soya 'cheese' and tofu have major nutrients similar to soya beans, except that because of the method of processing, tofu is an excellent source of calcium. This is important in Asian-style eating as there are few other good calcium sources in the normal Asian diet.

Lecithin extracted from the soya bean is used commercially because it promotes smooth blending in food products. It is also sold as granules, but has no special health benefit.

DESCRIPTION The small, oval soya bean is about the size of the common pea, with the most common variety creamy-yellow in colour, but it can also be red or black. The bean takes a long while to cook, and has a floury texture and bland flavour.

ORIGIN AND HISTORY The bean originated in temperate and tropical Africa and Asia.

One of the 'five ancient grains' of China, the soya bean was known to have been grown for food in China over 2000 years ago. When the famed Han tombs, which dated from between 175 and 145 BC, were opened in 1972 it was discovered that the contents were in an excellent state of preservation. Among the remains unearthed were 48 bamboo cases and 51 pottery vessels each containing items of food, spices, fruits, seeds, meats, and vegetables. There was a quantity of soya beans. They were destined to become one of the most important food crops in the world, for their high vegetable protein content makes them the choice candidate as a substitute for meat protein.

Introduced into Japan via Korea before 200 BC, into Europe in the 17th century, and the USA in 1804. The soya bean is of great importance in Asian diets because of its by-products more than the bean itself. Because of these by-products, modern by-products, and the nutritional value of the beans, soyas are the most commercially exploited beans today.

BUYING AND STORAGE Choose smooth-skinned beans and store in a sealed container in a cool, dry place.

PREPARATION AND USE Prepare as usual and slow-soak for 8 hours or longer so that cooking time may be shortened. Change water, bring to the boil and boil for 15 minutes, then simmer, covered, for 3–4 hours until tender. Can be pressure-cooked in 30–35 minutes.

Use in soups, stews, casseroles and salads. Soya bean sprouts should always be lightly cooked in stir-fry dishes or blanched before using in salads.

Usually cooked whole, in Japan and Korea black soya beans are boiled and served with a dressing usually containing sesame oil or sesame seeds. Natto is made by fermenting and mashing cooked soya beans, and is used in Japan as a salad dressing. Chinese cook, sweeten and mash black soya beans to make a filling for sweet buns and pastries.

VARIETIES

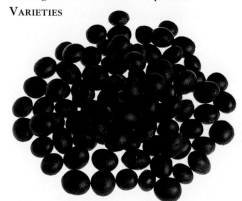

Black Soya Bean

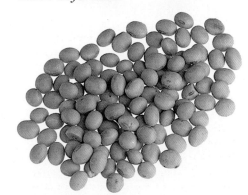

Yellow Soya Bean

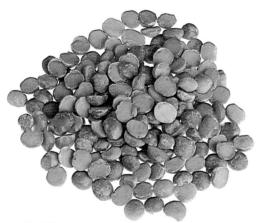

Split Pea *Pisum sativum*

also called Matar dal, Harhardal

MAJOR NUTRIENTS

COOKED
SERVE SIZE 200 G

Energy	1010 kJ	Phosphorus	240 mg
Protein	17 g	Magnesium	60 mg
Fat	1 g	Iron	3.5 mg
Carbohydrate	44 g	Zinc	2.5 mg
Cholesterol	0	Vitamin C	94 mg
Sodium	30 mg	Thiamin	0.2 mg
Potassium	540 mg	Niacin Equiv.	2 mg
Dietary Fibre	10 g		

NUTRITIONAL INFORMATION The split pea contains good quality vegetable protein, excellent fibre, vitamin C and iron, some B group vitamins, and minerals, including copper.

DESCRIPTION The split pea is prepared from the field pea, a variety of the common garden pea. It can be yellow or green, with husks removed.

ORIGIN AND HISTORY Most probably originated in middle Asia, and certainly used since prehistoric times. Peas found in the 'Spirit Caves', near the Burmese border of Thailand, have been carbon-dated to 9750 BC. Finds in the Near East are thought to date from some 2000 years later. Archaeological finds have placed them at Stone Age sites in Hungary and Switzerland, at France and northern Greece Bronze Age sites, and the Iron Age site at Glastonbury, England.

BUYING AND STORAGE Look for split peas with a strong colour, whether green or yellow, which denotes better quality. Store in a sealed container in a cool, dry place, and use within a year.

PREPARATION AND USE Pick over peas to remove tiny stones. Wash well, drain and place in a heavy pan with at least 3 times by volume of water. Bring to the boil, skimming off grey froth. Partly cover and simmer gently for 45–60 minutes until very soft. To prevent peas sticking to base of pan, do not stir during cooking. Add salt at end of cooking. Can be pressure-cooked in 15 minutes, with a little oil added after skimming.

Use for pea soups with ham or bacon bones added if desired, and for pease pudding served with boiled salt pork. Purees can have a little butter stirred in to serve as an accompaniment, or use as a basis for crumbed vegetable patties. Use yellow split peas for Indian dal.

PROCESSING Canned pea soup is an easy way of including this nutritious pulse in the diet.

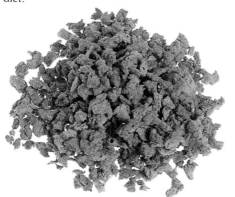

Textured Vegetable Protein

also called TVP

MAJOR NUTRIENTS

SERVE SIZE 100 G

Energy	1300 kJ	Phosphorus	730 mg
Protein	49 g	Calcium	560 mg
Fat	2 g	Magnesium	250 mg
Cholesterol	0	Iron	10 mg
Carbohydrate	19 g	Zinc	30 mg
Dietary Fibre	7 g	Thiamin	5.2 mg
Sodium	170 mg	Riboflavin	0.8 mg
Potassium	190 mg	Niacin Equiv.	9.7 mg

NUTRITIONAL INFORMATION Excellent source of protein, potassium, calcium, iron, zinc, thiamin, riboflavin and niacin. Contains large amounts of sodium. This bland product, which is low in fat and high in essential vitamins and minerals, has large amounts of added sodium to improve texture and taste.

DESCRIPTION Brown, rough granules produced from soya beans as a meat substitute for cooking uses. The brown TVP and a bleached version are used in food manufacturing industries as protein extenders.

ORIGIN AND HISTORY The Archer Daniels Midland Co. of Illinois, USA, was the pioneer in the extraction of soya flour from soya beans in 1930. By the late 1960s, circumstances caused the company to look at the further possibilities of soya flour; meat prices were rising and diet-related health problems were receiving wide publicity, with meat bearing the brunt of the criticism. The company's food technologists discovered the means to process the flour further to produce a meat substitute minus cholesterol and saturated fat, and in 1970, Textured Vegetable Protein was patented by the company.

Soya flour is mixed with water and extruded through a high-pressure chamber in a similar manner to pasta making. It is then cooked in ovens and milled to coarse granules. More recent technology allows simultaneous extrusion and cooking. TVP is brown when dried, further processing gives a 'roast' flavour, and it is marketed for consumer use or in food manufacturing. A bleached TVP is used in the manufacture of poultry products.

BUYING AND STORAGE TVP is available in packages at supermarkets and natural food stores. Store at room temperature in a sealed container.

PREPARATION AND USE Easy-to-follow directions are on the packs, and all that is required for making hamburgers and patties is the addition of water and flavouring ingredients of your own choice. It can also be used in casseroles, for savoury pie and crepe fillings, vegetable loaves, stews and pasta sauces.

SEE ALSO Soya Bean, Soya Flour.

SEEDS AND NUTS

Seeds are contained in the fruits of plants, and when the fleshy part of the fruit has fallen away or been consumed, allow the plant to reproduce.

Nuts are dry, hard-shelled fruits with a single seed. Some popular nuts are cashews, almonds, pistachios, coconuts, pecans, walnuts, Brazil nuts and hazelnuts. Pine nuts are not so widely used, but feature in Middle Eastern and some Mediterranean dishes.

Peanuts are actually legumes, but they are usually considered along with the nuts, which they resemble in physical characteristics and nutritional value.

Other seeds commonly eaten as foods are sunflower seeds, pumpkin seeds, sesame seeds, caraway seeds and poppy seeds. Some are used in bakery to flavour breads, biscuits and cakes. Sunflower seeds and pumpkin seeds are used as ingredients in foods such as muesli and are eaten alone as snacks.

Seeds and nuts have a similar nutrition profile: they are rich in fat (40–60%) and dietary fibre (5–15%), with moderate amounts of protein (2–25%), and small amounts of starch (up to 10%). Chestnuts are an exception, containing about 30% starch and only 3% fat.

The fats in seeds and nuts are predominantly monounsaturated and polyunsaturated. The exceptions are those in coconut and palm nut, which are predominantly saturated. Being plant foods, seeds and nuts contain no cholesterol.

They contain significant amounts of minerals, including calcium, phosphorus, iron, zinc and magnesium. The calcium, iron and zinc are not as well absorbed as they are from dairy products and meat.

Most seeds and nuts contain significant amounts of vitamins, thiamin, riboflavin, niacin, folate and vitamin E.

These foods have been gathered since the times of the hunter-gatherers. They feature in many traditional cuisines, and have been used as ingredients in savoury dishes and desserts.

Some flours, pastes and butters are made from nuts and seeds, which also provide important raw materials for vegetable oil, the residue after the extraction of oil being used as animal fodder.

Nuts and seeds contain very little natural sodium, and they have a high content of potassium. This ratio of sodium to potassium is recommended in a diet for the control of blood pressure. Unfortunately, most nuts are salted before they are used as snack foods and the ratio of sodium to potassium is altered. It is easy to overconsume these foods, and in so doing to take in a lot of salt and fat.

Used in moderate amounts, in unsalted forms, these are nutritionally valuable foods.

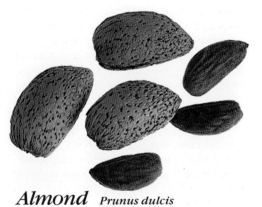

Almond *Prunus dulcis*

MAJOR NUTRIENTS   SERVE SIZE 30 G

Energy	700 kJ	Calcium	75 mg
Protein	5 g	Phosphorus	130 mg
Fat	16 g	Magnesium	80 mg
Carbohydrate	1 g	Iron	1.3 mg
Cholesterol	0	Zinc	1 mg
Sodium	5 mg	Thiamin	0.05 mg
Dietary Fibre	4.5 g	Riboflavin	0.3 mg

NUTRITIONAL INFORMATION   Almonds are high in oil, the oil being 87% unsaturated, mainly monounsaturated. They are an excellent source of dietary fibre, vitamin E, and several minerals. Vitamin E acts as a natural antioxidant which helps protect the nuts from rancidity. Roasting the nuts destroys most of the thiamin.

DESCRIPTION   The almond is a flat nut with pointed ends and a smooth texture. Creamy white, it is covered with a brown skin and is encased in a flat, pitted, light brown shell.

ORIGIN AND HISTORY   The almond has been cultivated around the Mediterranean since ancient times. The exact origin is obscure but it is mentioned often in the Bible, being common in biblical lands. In the 17th chapter of the book of Numbers, the Rod of Aaron is placed in the Tabernacle by Moses and brings forth flowers and ripe almonds, signifying God's special commission to the house of Levi.

Some botanists believe that the almond cultivated today is the ancient natural hybrid of three species of wild almonds found in the arid mountains of central Asia: one, a small tree in Russian Turkestan; another, a shrubby tree in Armenia; and the third, a shrub in central Asia. It is still found wild in Algeria, in countries at the eastern end of the Mediterranean and near the Black Sea.

Cultivated almonds are the kernels of the fruit of the almond tree. Half the world's supply is cultivated in California, the rest is produced in Spain, Italy, Portugal, Morocco, Iran and (a small quantity) in Australia.

BUYING AND STORAGE   Almonds are available all year round though the crop peaks in summer and autumn.

Buy nuts in the shell for maximum flavour and for longer storage. Store in an airtight container in the refrigerator or in a cool place.

Shelled and blanched almonds should be free from damage or weevil moths. Blanched almonds, whether whole, sliced, flaked, slivered, chopped or ground, are best purchased in airtight clear packaging so that the oil content is retained. Shelled nuts should be stored in their sealed package or in a glass jar in the refrigerator so that the oil content will not turn rancid.

Almond paste should be evenly caramel coloured with a firm texture, and hygenically packed in airtight clear packaging. Store in the refrigerator.

PREPARATION AND USE Blanch almonds to remove the skin. The simplest method is to place almonds in a bowl, cover with boiling water and stand for 3 minutes. Pour the hot water off and cover with cold water then, by pressing the nuts one at a time, between the thumb and forefinger, the skin will slip off. Dry on a clean tea towel before use.

Almonds may be used whole, chopped, slivered or ground, in cakes, biscuits, pastries, praline, confectionery and ice cream. Use whole or slivered in savoury or fruit salads, in casseroles, savoury stuffings, savoury rice, pasta dishes or nut cutlets. Use flaked almonds for cakes, biscuits, pastries and decoration. Use ground almonds for marzipan, almond paste or for thickening soup or fish and chicken casseroles.

PROCESSING Whole almonds are processed into halved, flaked, slivered, ground, roasted and salted forms. They are used in snack foods, marzipan, almond paste and confectionery, as well as for almond oil, liqueur and essence.

VARIETIES

While there are several botanical varieties of almond, the varieties which concern the consumer are: almonds in the shell; natural shelled almonds, in their skin; whole blanched almonds, with skin removed; sliced (flaked) natural almonds; sliced (flaked) blanched almonds; blanched, slivered almonds; blanched, chopped almonds; blanched, ground almonds; almond paste, a commercial mixture of ground almonds, sugar and egg used in confectionery and baking, and for the first layer of icing on a fruit cake, underneath the royal or fondant icing.

SEE ALSO Bitter Almond.

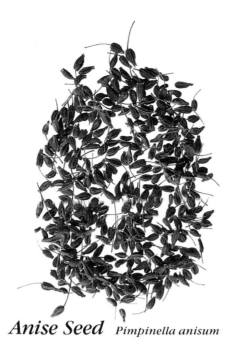

Anise Seed *Pimpinella anisum*

MAJOR NUTRIENTS		SERVE SIZE 2 G	
Energy	29 kJ	Cholesterol	0
Protein	0	Sodium	0
Fat	0	Iron	0.7 mg
Carbohydrate	1 g		

NUTRITIONAL INFORMATION Because these seeds are eaten in small amounts they provide few nutrients other than a moderate amount of iron.

DESCRIPTION Anise seeds come from anise, a plant similar to parsley but twice as tall, with serrated leaves and clusters of flat white flowers. The brown seeds are small, aromatic and oval with an aniseed flavour. They appear after flowering is completed. Anise grows in sunny, sheltered places in well-drained, light soil.

ORIGIN AND HISTORY Anise is native to the Middle East. It was known thousands of years ago and was cultivated by the ancient Greeks and Romans, the latter using the seeds in spiced cakes served at the end of a meal to aid digestion. Anise seeds are mentioned in the Bible and became known in Europe during the Middle Ages for their digestive properties.

BUYING AND STORAGE Buy anise seeds from a reputable spice shop or health food shop, or buy recognised brands in clear, sealed containers from the supermarket.

Store in airtight glass jars in a dry area away from direct sunlight. Check on freshness after one year.

PREPARATION AND USE To collect seeds from the plant, cut the flower heads off when the seeds have turned brown, place flowers in a single layer in a shallow cardboard box and dry in the sun. Shake the dry flowers to obtain the seeds, then sieve the seeds before storage.

Use anise seeds to flavour biscuits, cakes and bread. Use as an alternative to caraway seeds to flavour cabbage dishes and root vegetables such as carrots, turnips and swedes.

The fresh leaves of the plant can be added to salads.

PROCESSING Anise seeds are used primarily in the preparation of anisette liqueur. They are also used to flavour cough medicines and lozenges for the relief of bronchial irritation. Aniseed flavoured sweets are popular. The seeds used to brew herbal tea are an antidote for indigestion.

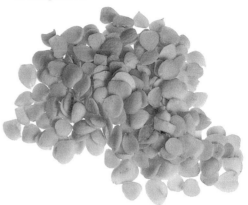

Bitter Almond *Prunus armeniaca*

NUTRITIONAL INFORMATION No reliable analysis is available, but probably similar to almond.

DESCRIPTION Cream-coloured, brown skinned seeds resembling sweet almonds, but smaller and somewhat flat. They have a distinctive medicinal aroma and bitter flavour.

ORIGIN AND HISTORY The sweet almond, imported from Turkestan, was being cultivated in China in the late T'ang Dynasty (AD 619–907), but it never had the appeal of the strongly flavoured local bitter almond, which was in fact the kernel of the native apricot. This same apricot was taken to Europe and its fruit is now enjoyed all over the world. It is used in Chinese medicines for respiratory dysfunctions. The bitter almond kernel is toxic in its raw state and must be carefully handled prior to eating or cooking. It should be boiled briefly, then parched in a warm oven for at least 20 minutes.

BUYING AND STORAGE Sold in small packs, or loose by weight, in Chinese stores and herbalists. They will keep indefinitely in a covered jar in dry conditions.

PREPARATION AND USE Used primarily in Chinese desserts, the most popular being the wobbly almond jelly which is also known as almond beancurd. Ground and boiled with water or milk it makes a delicious hot sweet soup.

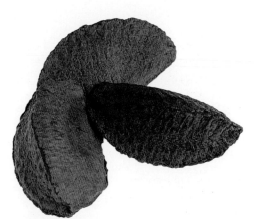

Brazil Nut *Bertholettia*

MAJOR NUTRIENTS SERVE SIZE 30 G

Energy	760 kJ	Calcium	55 mg
Protein	4 g	Phosphorus	175 mg
Fat	18 g	Magnesium	125 mg
Carbohydrate	1 g	Iron	0.5 mg
Cholesterol	0	Zinc	1 mg
Sodium	0	Thiamin	0.3 mg
Dietary Fibre	2.5 mg		

NUTRITIONAL INFORMATION Brazil nuts have a high oil content which is 70% unsaturated, consisting of similar amounts of polyunsaturated and monounsaturated oils.

DESCRIPTION Brazil nuts are long, three-sided creamy-coloured nuts with a dark brown skin, enclosed in a three-sided, tough, dull brown-grey shell.

ORIGIN AND HISTORY Brazil nuts are native to the tropical region of South America and surprisingly they are not cultivated yet. All the world's supplies are still gathered from wild trees, the majority of which grow in wet, waterfront locations along the river Amazon from the Atlantic coast to the mountains of Peru, a distance of 3000 km. The nuts develop in 2 concentric rings around a central core, inside a large, round, tough, brown, heavy pod 10 cm in diameter, which has a 1.2 cm lining of hard fibres. The pods grow in groups of 3 or 4, on enormous trees which often grow to 30 m tall. The pods fall down like cannon balls when the nuts are ripe. The momentum of their fall is so great that they are often embedded in the ground and can kill or badly injure the Indian labourers who gather them. The Brazil nut pods are broken open with an axe and the nuts are gathered into baskets, then loaded onto the Indian canoes for transportation to the jungle traders. The local monkeys also love the nuts.

BUYING AND STORAGE Available in autumn and winter. Buy in the shell and store in a cool place or in a container in the refrigerator. If buying shelled Brazil nuts make sure they are not dry or rancid.

PREPARATION AND USE Shell nuts and serve fresh with dessert fruits or cheese. Use whole in festive fruit cakes. Blanch and chop for use in cakes, biscuits, nut cutlets, stuffing and salads. Use ground nuts in pastry, cakes, petit fours and confectionery.

PROCESSING Brazil nut oil is used in salad dressing.

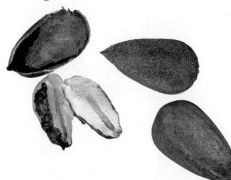

Bunya Bunya Pine Nut
Araucaria bidwillii

MAJOR NUTRIENTS SERVE SIZE 50 G

Energy	350 kJ	Dietary Fibre	5 g
Protein	15 g	Sodium	5 mg
Fat	1 g	Iron	2.5 mg
Carbohydrate	35 g		

NUTRITIONAL INFORMATION The bunya bunya pine nut is low in fat and has less energy than most nuts. Its main contribution is as a source of complex carbohydrate (starch). In composition and usage it is more similar to potatoes than to nuts.

DESCRIPTION The nuts from the female pine cone can be up to 2.5 cm long and 2 cm wide and are encased in a thin but woody shell.

ORIGIN AND HISTORY The Bunya bunya pines are endemic to Australia but prior to 1788 trees were restricted to the area around Brisbane and Rockhampton. The nuts were an important food for Aborigines in these areas as ceremonial and feasting food.

BUYING AND STORAGE Choose nuts with unsplit shells. Store in an open weave bag in a refrigerator.

PREPARATION AND USE Shelled nuts can be eaten raw or cooked by boiling. Unshelled nuts can be boiled or roasted and while the nuts are still hot the shell can be removed using a sharp knife. The shell will harden on cooling. Boiling for at least 30 minutes is the method of choice and is easier to control. Boiled and shelled nuts can be fried in butter and flavoured with either pepper or sugar or added to stews and soups. Minced nuts can be added to quiches, damper, scones, pancakes, cakes and biscuits.

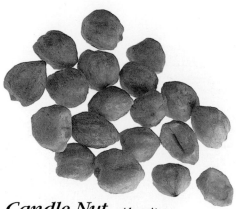

Candle Nut *Aleurites moluccana*

*also called **Kemiri (Indonesia), Buah keras (Malaysia)***

MAJOR NUTRIENTS SERVE SIZE 30 G

Energy	790 kJ	Cholesterol	0
Protein	6 g	Sodium	0
Fat	19 g	Iron	0.6 mg
Carbohydrate	2 g		

NUTRITIONAL INFORMATION These nuts are a concentrated energy source because of their high fat content.

Limit the amount of these nuts, and always roast, as raw ones have been known to cause sickness.

DESCRIPTION The candle nut is a round, laterally flattened, mottled grey to black nut, 5 cm in diameter, with a thin, papery husk containing one or two rough-coated inner seeds or nuts.

ORIGIN AND HISTORY The candle nut comes from the candleberry tree native to Indonesia and Malaysia. It grows also in the Philippines and Sri Lanka and throughout the South Pacific. The name derives from the early use of the nuts in Indonesia for burning as an illuminant. The nuts were ground to a paste with copra (coconut fibre) and used to make candles. Traditionally the Javanese have roasted the nuts for eating.

BUYING AND STORAGE Candle nuts are gathered by hand. Readily available from Asian food stores, they can be kept for several months.

Store in a cool, dry place.

PREPARATION AND USE Candle nuts are roasted when only half ripe to extract their oil for lighting purposes. Fully ripe candle nuts are roasted before extracting their oil for cooking. Ripe candle nuts are roasted then pounded to a meal and mixed with salt, chillies and shrimp paste to make a relish or they are mixed with green vegetables and boiled rice. They can be added to spicy condiment mixtures and served with curries.

PROCESSING Crudely processed to produce oil for lighting and cooking.

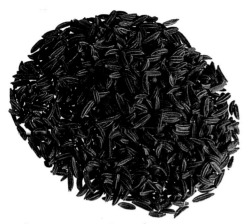

Caraway Seed *Carum carvi*

MAJOR NUTRIENTS		SERVE SIZE 2 G	
Energy	30 kJ	Carbohydrate	1 g
Protein	0	Cholesterol	0
Fat	0	Sodium	0

NUTRITIONAL INFORMATION Caraway seeds have no nutritional value because they are eaten in small amounts. However, they improve palatability and aid salivary flow, thus assisting in the digestion of food.

DESCRIPTION The caraway seed is a tiny, aromatic, crescent-shaped, brown-black seed with a strong, aromatic flavour. Caraway seeds come from the caraway plant, which grows to 60 cm tall, with feathery green leaves and pink-tinged white flowers. Caraway grows in sunny sheltered places in well-drained, loamy soil.

ORIGIN AND HISTORY Caraway is native to Europe, particularly around the Mediterranean and in North Africa. The Romans, ancient Greeks and Egyptians used it for its healing properties and it was also used in love potions to prevent the loved one from straying. It was once widely used in England, served with baked apples, to prevent flatulence.

BUYING AND STORAGE Buy caraway seeds from a reputable spice shop or health food shop or buy a recognised brand in a clear, sealed container from the supermarket.

Store in an airtight glass jar in a dry area away from direct sunlight. Check freshness after one year.

PREPARATION AND USE Allow the caraway blooms to fade and the petals to fall, so that the seeds can form. Harvest the heads of seeds when they turn brown, then sieve them to remove any chaff before storage.

Use caraway seeds in traditional English seed cakes, Hungarian goulash, with boiled onions and root vegetables.

The fresh leaves may be added to a green salad or cooked with spinach. The roots may be cooked and eaten as a vegetable.

PROCESSING Caraway is used to make kümmel liqueur, kümmel being the German word for caraway. Ground caraway seeds and the oil extracted from them are both used in medicines to aid digestion, prevent flatulence and reduce body fluids. Caraway seed is also added to cheese in Europe.

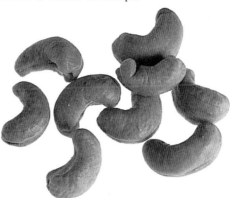

Cashew Nut *Anacardium occidentale*

*also called **Gajus (Malaysia), Monkey nut***

MAJOR NUTRIENTS		SERVE SIZE 30 G	
Energy	700 kJ	Sodium	0
Protein	5 g	Magnesium	80 mg
Fat	14 g	Iron	1 mg
Carbohydrate	8 g	Thiamin	0.1 mg
Cholesterol	0		

NUTRITIONAL INFORMATION Cashews are high in oil which is 74% unsaturated, mainly monounsaturated. They have good quality vegetable protein and some minerals including zinc, though no specific figures are available for zinc.

DESCRIPTION Cashews are cream-coloured, kidney-shaped nuts, approximately 1 cm long, in kidney-shaped shells.

ORIGIN AND HISTORY Originating in the West Indies and native to the north of Brazil, Portuguese explorers took the cashew to India and Malaya, as well as Mozambique in Africa where it is now cultivated and is an important commercial industry. The hard-shelled nut develops inside the cashew apple, a fleshy receptacle 10 cm long and 5 cm wide, on a tall tree. When mature, the apple turns bright red or yellow and the nut protrudes from the end. The tree is a member of the poison ivy family and precautions must be taken when extracting the nuts from the shells. The shell contains an oil which irritates the skin, so the nuts are heated to render the oil less caustic. The smoke or steam produced may also irritate the skin and eyes and precautions should be taken. When heated, the nuts are harmless and may be extracted safely from their shells.

BUYING AND STORAGE Available all year round. Always buy shelled cashew nuts, preferably those which are sold in airtight packaging.

Once the seal of the package is broken, store in a glass jar in the refrigerator to keep oil content fresh.

PREPARATION AND USE Use whole for snacks; chop and add to salads, nut cutlets or stuffings.

PROCESSING May be roasted, or roasted and salted for use as a party snack food.

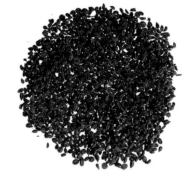

Celery Seed *Apium graveolens*

NUTRITIONAL INFORMATION In the quantities in which they are used, celery seeds are not nutritionally significant.

DESCRIPTION Celery seeds are the dried fruits of the celery vegetable. They are small and brown with a strong flavour.

ORIGIN AND HISTORY Today's cultivated celery originated from a pot herb known as smallage or wild celery. Around 2200 BC the Egyptians gathered wild celery from large areas of protected marshland. It is thought that the Italians and French were the first to cultivate it, and Americans in the state of Utah developed the thicker, juicy, stringless celery stalks of today.

BUYING AND STORAGE Buy recognised brands of celery seeds in clear, sealed containers from the supermarket.

Store in airtight glass jars in a dry area away from direct sunlight. Check on freshness after one year.

PREPARATION AND USE Allow the celery plant to seed, then gather the seed tops and dry in a single layer in cardboard boxes in the sun. Sieve seeds away from husks before storage.

Use celery seeds to flavour soups, casseroles, sauces, tomato juice, seafood sauce and dips. Add to pickled cucumbers and pickled onions, sprinkle on homemade bread, add to fish and vegetable dishes.

Celery seeds are useful for the relief of rheumatism.

PROCESSING Commercial celery salt is a popular flavouring in dehydrated soups, sauces, pasta and rice dishes.

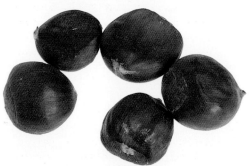

Chestnut *Castanea mollissima*

MAJOR NUTRIENTS		SERVE SIZE 100 G	
Energy	720 kJ	Dietary Fibre	7 g
Protein	2 g	Calcium	46 mg
Fat	3 g	Phosphorus	75 mg
Carbohydrate	37 g	Magnesium	35 mg
Cholesterol	0	Iron	0.9 mg
Sodium	0	Thiamin	0.2 mg
Potassium	500 mg	Riboflavin	0.2 mg

NUTRITIONAL INFORMATION Chestnuts are a starchy nut with little oil content. They contain excellent dietary fibre, several minerals and B group vitamins.

DESCRIPTION Chestnuts are large, round, grey-white fleshy nuts, pointed at the top, with a thin brown skin inside a smooth, glossy brown, soft shell.

ORIGIN AND HISTORY Chestnuts are thought to have originated in southern Europe and in Persia. They are mentioned in Virgil's writings, and it is said that the children of Persian nobility were fattened on chestnuts. The chestnut tree, similar in size to an apple tree, is now cultivated in Georgia, USA, in Victoria, Australia, and also in France, Italy, Spain, China and Malaysia.

BUYING AND STORAGE Available during autumn and winter. Buy chestnuts in the shell. Choose nuts that are heavy for their size with undamaged shells.

Store in a cool place for up to a week or in a container in the refrigerator for longer storage.

PREPARATION AND USE The skins may be removed by boiling, baking or roasting over red-hot coals. Boil gently in a pan of water for 20 minutes, drain and remove shells. Alternatively, slit shell at point of chestnut, then bake in a hot oven at 220°C for 10 minutes, cool and remove shell. To roast, slit points of chestnuts then place over red-hot coals until shells split open and nuts are golden brown.

Use in soups, savoury soufflés, and in turkey stuffing. Sauté with vegetables, chop and use in nut cutlets, or puree and use in desserts or ice cream. Grind to a flour and use in bread and porridgelike puddings.

PROCESSING May be canned whole or as a puree, glacéed, preserved in brandy, or processed as crème de marron puree. Chestnuts are also made into flour, which is starchy, with a low fat content.

VARIETIES
There are many varieties, the best-known being Chinese, American, Spanish, Japanese and Chinquapins.

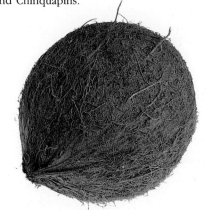

Coconut *Cocos nucifera*

MAJOR NUTRIENTS		COCONUT MEAT SERVE SIZE 15 G	
Energy	220 kJ	Cholesterol	0
Protein	0	Sodium	0
Fat	5 g	Dietary Fibre	2 g
Carbohydrate	1 g		

NUTRITIONAL INFORMATION There are no significant nutrients in a small piece. When eaten in large amounts as in the Pacific Islanders' diet, it is a moderate source of iron. Coconut is high in fat which is 87% saturated.

Because of the high cellulose fibre it is a good dental cleanser.

Desiccated coconut is a more concentrated source of the above nutrients.

Coconut cream is a rich energy food, with high levels of saturated fat.

Coconut milk (or coconut water) is an excellent source of vitamin C (2 g per 100 ml) and contains natural sugars. Because the liquid is sterile, it is safe to drink in the tropics. It can be used as a substitute for fruit juice in infant feeding.

DESCRIPTION The coconut is the fruit of a palm tree which has an edible kernel and therefore qualifies as a nut. It has a large, thick green pod, enclosing a brown fibrous husk around a brown shell, which contains a layer of soft white flesh and clear milk in the centre.

ORIGIN AND HISTORY Native to Malaysia, the Philippines and Brazil, the coconut is the most important nut in the world commercially. It is valued for its flesh and milk; the shell is used as charcoal; the fibrous husk is used to make rope, cloth and brushes; the trunk is used as building material; and the leaves are used for thatched roofs.

BUYING AND STORAGE Available all year round. Buy coconut as fresh as possible with soft flesh when buying at the source of production, otherwise choose coconuts which are heavy for their size.

Store fresh coconut in the refrigerator.

PREPARATION AND USE Insert a metal skewer into juice 'holes' and hit gently with a hammer making two holes, then pour coconut milk out. Crack shell open, then scoop or scrape out white flesh.

Use coconut milk in drinks, curries, marinades and Malaysian dishes. Use soft coconut flesh in desserts or add to fruit salad or ice cream. Serve hard coconut flesh on the shell as a snack or scrape off, grate or chop finely and use in ice cream, curries, Malaysian dishes.

PROCESSING Coconut flesh may be shredded or desiccated, used in commercial ice cream, confectionery, biscuits and cakes. Coconut juice/milk may be canned, frozen or processed as coconut cream or paste.

VARIETIES
There are several varieties, usually classified according to the country of origin.

Macapuno

DESCRIPTION A mutant form of coconut which does not become firm and white when ripe, but fills with a greyish, gelatinous substance.

ORIGIN AND HISTORY Much prized in the Philippines as a dessert ingredient. It is also known there as 'sports coconut', perhaps owing to the fact that being solid, unlike a normal coconut, it can be used for play without fear of splitting.

BUYING AND STORAGE Sliced fresh is

available in bottles, packed in sweetened water. It has a slightly fermented taste, similar to that of the liquid inside a fresh ripe coconut.

PREPARATION AND USE Eaten straight from shell or bottle.

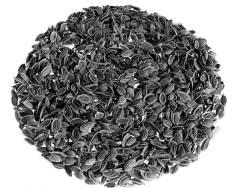

Dill Seed *Anethum graveolens*

MAJOR NUTRIENTS			SERVE SIZE 2 G
Energy	30 kJ	Carbohydrate	1 g
Protein	0	Cholesterol	0
Fat	0	Sodium	0

NUTRITIONAL INFORMATION The seeds have little nutritional value because they are eaten in small amounts.

These pungent seeds produce a medicinal oil used in Asian medicine for its calmative effect. Dill water is used in Western medicine as an anti-colic agent for infants.

DESCRIPTION The khaki-coloured dill seeds are flat, oval and aromatic. The dill plant is grown for its fernlike, green-blue foliage used as a herb as well as for its seeds. The seeds follow the yellow flower heads which spread out like an umbrella.

ORIGIN AND HISTORY Dill originated in the Mediterranean countries of Europe then spread north to the colder parts of Europe as a wayside weed. Today it grows all over the world and still grows wild near waterways in suitable ground soil. Dill seeds became known as 'meetin'' seeds in America where they were given to children to eat during long Sunday sermons! The Norse people gave dill water to babies to calm them when suffering from flatulence.

BUYING AND STORAGE Buy dill seeds from reputable spice shops or health food shops or buy recognised brands in clear, sealed containers from the supermarket.

Store in airtight glass jars in a dry area away from direct sunlight. Check for freshness after one year.

PREPARATION AND USE To collect dill seeds from the plant, cut the flower heads after the petals have dropped and lay them in a box. Dry in direct sunlight, then shake out the seeds and sieve them to remove the husks.

Store seeds in an airtight glass jar.

Use dill seeds in dill pickled cucumbers to aid digestion. Add to gas-forming vegetables such as cabbage, Brussels sprouts and pulse legumes to aid digestion and prevent flatulence. Sprinkle on homemade bread and bread rolls, add to fish, potato, veal, pork and vegetable dishes. The fresh leaves are used as a herb with fish, cream cheese, lamb, veal and chicken, and in potato salad.

PROCESSING Dill seeds are added to commercial dill pickled cucumbers, pickles, chutneys, canned sauerkraut, bread and pastries. Oil of dill is processed and sold by pharmacists for digestive problems.

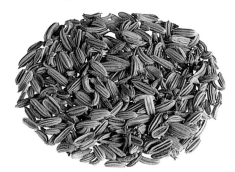

Fennel Seed *Foeniculum vulgare dulce*

MAJOR NUTRIENTS			SERVE SIZE 2 G
Energy	30 kJ	Cholesterol	0
Protein	0	Sodium	0
Fat	0	Iron	0.4 mg
Carbohydrate	1 g		

NUTRITIONAL INFORMATION Apart from a small amount of iron, these seeds provide few nutrients.

Fennel seeds are used in Asian medicine to prevent flatulence.

DESCRIPTION Fennel seeds are aromatic, oval and brownish-black, similar to but fatter than dill seeds, with a slight aniseed flavour.

ORIGIN AND HISTORY Fennel seeds come from the fennel plant which is native to the Mediterranean region. The two best known varieties are the perennial fennel which grows wild along country hedgerows and the annual Florence fennel which has a crisp, bulbous, edible stem which looks like a squat head of celery. The seeds form when the flower has dropped its petals.

The Romans introduced fennel to the rest of Europe. It is mentioned in Anglo-Saxon herbal documents and was said to guard against unseen evil. Chaucer and Shakespeare referred to it and Longfellow implied that fennel could restore lost vision. It was also an old-fashioned treatment for losing weight, perhaps because the seeds are now known to help digest starchy food.

BUYING AND STORAGE Buy from a reputable spice shop or health food shop or buy a recognised brand from a supermarket.

Store in clear, airtight glass jars in a dry place out of direct sunlight. Check on freshness after one year.

PREPARATION AND USE Cut the flower heads off the fennel plant once the petals have dropped, and dry in shallow cardboard boxes in direct sunlight. Sieve before storing.

Use fennel seeds as for dill and caraway seeds or add to cabbage dishes, Brussel sprouts, cauliflower and onion to prevent flatulence. Add to curries, fish, rabbit, pork, liver and kidney dishes. Sprinkle on homemade bread and rolls, add to cheese dips.

The fresh fennel leaves may be added to fish dishes, pasta, rice, potatoes, salad dressings and soups.

PROCESSING Fennel seeds are added to commercial curry powder and pastes, and to pickles. Fennel seed oil is used in liqueurs, cordials, soap and perfume.

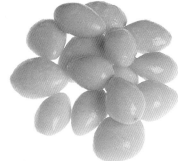

Ginkgo Nut *Ginkgo biloba*
also called **Maidenhair tree**

MAJOR NUTRIENTS			SERVE SIZE 15 G
Energy	120 kJ	Cholesterol	0
Protein	1 g	Sodium	0
Fat	0	Vitamin C	4 mg
Carbohydrate	6 g		

NUTRITIONAL INFORMATION Ginkgo nuts are an excellent source of vitamin C and when eaten in large amounts they provide several minerals.

Roasting will destroy the vitamin C.

DESCRIPTION When ripe and fresh, ginkgo nuts are covered by a pulpy yellow substance which must be removed as it rots quickly after harvesting. Beneath is a smooth, very hard, cream-coloured ovoid shell. This contains a kernel which has a brown skin. Raw ginkgo nuts are a creamy white colour but turn green when cooked.

ORIGIN AND HISTORY The ginkgo is a prehistoric tree which survives as a wild tree only in China. There is a petrified forest of ginkgo trees on the bank of the Columbia River in Washington state which shows they were growing there 15,000,000 years ago, before the formation of the Rocky Mountains.

The fruit resembles a tiny plum but has a foul smell. The Chinese wait for the smelly hull to fall off, then paint the nuts and use them in festoon decorations and finally crack them open and eat the kernel.

BUYING AND STORAGE The Chinese gather the nuts by hand and store them in a cool, dry place. They are sold in the shell by weight and also canned in water.

PREPARATION AND USE In Japan and Korea, gingko nuts are threaded onto skewers and grilled, and used in various dishes and soups, as a vegetable and a garnish. Popular in Chinese vegetarian dishes.

PROCESSING Not processed commercially.

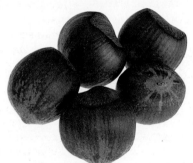

Hazelnut Corylus avellana

also called Cob nut, Filbert

MAJOR NUTRIENTS   SERVE SIZE 30 G

Energy	470 kJ	Sodium	0
Protein	2 g	Dietary Fibre	2 g
Fat	11 g	Phosphorus	70 mg
Carbohydrate	2 g	Thiamin	0.01 mg
Cholesterol	0		

NUTRITIONAL INFORMATION The high oil in these nuts is 87% unsaturated, mainly monounsaturated, and they are an excellent source of vitamin E.

Vitamin E is a natural antioxidant and helps protect the nuts from rancidity.

DESCRIPTION Small, light brown, round nuts with a point at the top, hazelnuts have a thin brown skin, inside a smooth, hard shell with a rough round area at the base.

ORIGIN AND HISTORY Native to both North America and Europe, it is called hazelnut in Europe and filbert in the USA. Hazel comes from the Anglo-Saxon haesel meaning a hood or bonnet. Some say filbert comes from Saint Philibert, whose feast falls on 22 August, corresponding to the ripening of the earliest nuts in the northern hemisphere. Grown commercially in Oregon and Washington states, around the Black Sea and the Mediterranean, the hazelnut grows on a shrub which forms thickets in cool, deciduous woodlands.

BUYING AND STORAGE Available all year round although the season peaks in the autumn. Preferably select nuts which are a good size with an undamaged shell.

Store both unshelled and shelled nuts in a glass jar in the refrigerator.

PREPARATION AND USE Remove nuts from shell with a nutcracker. Use hazelnuts whole or chopped for snacks, in cakes, biscuits and stuffings, or grind in a blender or food processor and use in petit fours, pastry, confectionery, ice cream and desserts.

PROCESSING Used in commercially baked products and ice cream.

VARIETIES
There are a total of 15 species in the world.

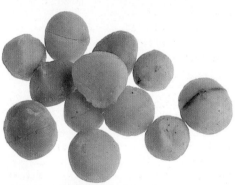

Macadamia Nut
Macadamia integrifolia, M. tetraphylla

also called Queensland nut

MAJOR NUTRIENTS   SERVE SIZE 30 G

Energy	750 kJ	Sodium	0
Protein	2 g	Dietary Fibre	7 g
Fat	19 g	Phosphorus	100 mg
Carbohydrate	2 g	Iron	1 mg
Cholesterol	0		

NUTRITIONAL INFORMATION Macadamias are high in oil, the oil being 78% unsaturated, mainly monounsaturated. They are also an excellent fibre source.

DESCRIPTION The macadamia is a light brown, smooth, spherical nut, 2–3 cm in diameter, with a very hard, smooth, brown shell, covered with either a smooth or a slightly rough brown husk.

ORIGIN AND HISTORY The macadamia nut is native to the coastal rainforest and scrubland of Queensland in northeast Australia. It was an important food for the Aborigines of the region, and white settlers were quick to adopt the nut also. In 1888 macadamia trees were planted in Hawaii, where, thanks to hybridisation and careful cloning, the nuts became a valuable commercial crop, sold under the name 'Hawaiian nut'. The macadamia is now enjoying commercial cultivation in Australia, the only native Australian food to do so.

It is also now cultivated in South Africa, Zimbabwe, Malawi, parts of South and Central America and California.

BUYING AND STORAGE The nuts fall off the tree when ripe. After collection they are husked, then air-dried to reduce their moisture content to a low level and prevent them from going mouldy and rancid. Once treated thus, the nuts will store well in their shell for 12 months.

When buying shelled nuts, select nuts in an airtight package. Once opened, store in the refrigerator.

PREPARATION AND USE A special type of macadamia nutcracker or a hammer is essential for opening the nuts in their shell. Serve nuts whole for a snack or use to decorate cakes. Chop nuts and use in desserts, or with savoury pasta, rice or rissoles. Grind nuts finely and use in confectionery or add to ice cream.

PROCESSING Macadamia nuts are roasted and salted for snack foods and coated with chocolate for commercial confectionery. They are also processed into macadamia nut butter.

VARIETIES
Only two of the five Australian species have become important commercial food producers. Five other species are found in New Caledonia, Sulawesi and Madagascar. Another large type grows in Australia but these nuts contain cyanide. They are eaten by Aborigines only after special treatment to remove the poison.

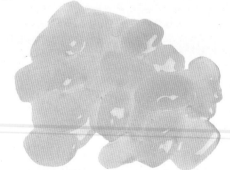

Palm Nut Borrassus flabellifer

also called Siwalan

NUTRITIONAL INFORMATION No reliable data are available. The fat is predominantly saturated.

DESCRIPTION From the hard, shiny layered-husked nut of the palmyra palm comes a sweetish transparent sap with a gelatinous texture.

ORIGIN AND HISTORY The palmyra palm, which has been used since prehistory, provides one other valuable ingredient, palm sugar.

BUYING AND STORAGE Both canned and bottled palm nuts are available. They will keep for many months unopened. Once opened they can be kept in the refrigerator for several days.

PREPARATION AND USE They are used in Indonesian cooking in soups and desserts.

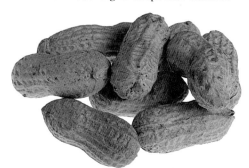

Peanut *Arachis hypogaea*

also called Goober, Groundnut, Monkey nut

MAJOR NUTRIENTS		SERVE SIZE 30 G	
Energy	710 kJ	Dietary Fibre	2.5 g
Protein	7 g	Phosphorus	110 mg
Fat	15 g	Magnesium	55 mg
Carbohydrate	3 g	Thiamin	0.25 mg
Cholesterol	0	Niacin Equiv.	5 mg
Sodium	0		

NUTRITIONAL INFORMATION Peanuts are high in oil, the oil being 76% unsaturated, mainly monounsaturated. Peanuts, being a legume, are an excellent source of protein.

Whole nuts are not recommended for children under 3 years because of the possibility of inhalation of the nuts. Aflatoxin can be generated on mouldy nuts, especially peanuts, so careful storage is essential as aflatoxin is toxic and in some cases carcinogenic.

DESCRIPTION The peanut is not a true nut. It is the seed of a leguminous plant with a straw-coloured soft pod, about 5 cm long and as thick as a pencil. Each pod contains 2 to 4 cream-coloured kernels or seeds covered with a reddish-brown skin. The nuts grow on long tendrils below ground, hence the alternative name of groundnut.

ORIGIN AND HISTORY The peanut is native to Brazil. They have been found in South American tombs dating back to 950 BC. It is now grown throughout the tropics with the largest population in India and China. It was introduced from the New World into West Africa where it soon adapted well and has displaced the native 'ground peas' of the same family. Nigeria is the largest exporter of peanuts today and they are also important to the economy of Senegal and Gambia. They are also grown in the USA and in Queensland, Australia.

BUYING AND STORAGE Available all year round. Buy peanuts in their shells if required to store for a long time. Otherwise buy shelled raw peanuts, roasted or salted, in airtight packages.

Store peanuts in an airtight container in a cool place or in the refrigerator. Peanuts may be frozen for long storage periods.

PREPARATION AND USE Remove the skin by pressing the peanut between forefinger and thumb. Blanch nuts if skin is difficult to remove.

Roast or fry, sprinkle with a little salt and serve as a snack. Chop nuts and add to salads, meat, poultry and fish dishes, rice and pasta, biscuits, cakes and ice cream. Grind nuts and use in a satay sauce.

PROCESSING The most popular processed peanut product is peanut butter, which is made by removing the skin and germ and grinding the roasted nuts. Oil is extracted from peanuts and sold as peanut oil for cooking and salad dressing, and is also used for packing canned sardines and in manufacturing some varieties of margarine. The residue left after oil extraction is used to make oilcakes for animal fodder.

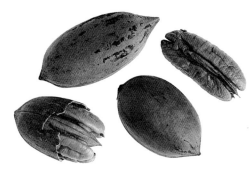

Pecan Nut *Carya illinoinensis*

also called Mississippi nut

MAJOR NUTRIENTS		SERVE SIZE 30 G	
Energy	870 kJ	Sodium	0
Protein	3 g	Phosphorus	100 mg
Fat	22 g	Iron	1 mg
Carbohydrate	4 g	Thiamin	0.2 mg
Cholesterol	0		

NUTRITIONAL INFORMATION Pecans are high in oil, the oil being 85% unsaturated, mainly monounsaturated. Unlike most nuts they are low in fibre.

Because they are a concentrated energy source and low in fibre they are the one natural food used by American astronauts in space.

DESCRIPTION The pecan is a 3–4 cm long elliptical nut with a thin, brown shell, sometimes with black stripes, covered by a husk. The kernel is ridged lengthways and resembles a 'stretched', smooth walnut in appearance. The nut is the fruit of a spreading tree which can grow up to 30 m tall, but is pruned to a more practical height for harvesting when cultivated.

ORIGIN AND HISTORY The pecan is the most important native nut tree of North America. It was discovered by Europeans in 1541 growing abundantly on high ground west of the Mississippi swamps in what is now Arkansas. The oldest pecan variety, Centennial, was originated by a slave gardener, Antoine, on a plantation in Louisiana. The famous pecan praline appeared in Louisiana in 1762. Thomas Jefferson planted pecans at Monticello and sent nuts from his trees to George Washington who planted them at Mount Vernon in 1786, where they may still be seen as the oldest trees there. The most important pecan-producing states today form a belt from Georgia in the east to Texas and Oklahoma in the west. A pecan breeding station is maintained by the United States Department of Agriculture in Texas. On the large orchards, operations are entirely mechanised with gigantic tree shakers, nut sweepers and vacuums used for harvesting. Pecan cultivation was introduced into New South Wales, Australia, about 10 years ago with great success.

BUYING AND STORAGE Available all year round although harvested in autumn. Buy pecans in the shell if required to store for a long time, otherwise select shelled nuts in clear airtight packaging free from damage.

Store nuts in a clear airtight container in the refrigerator.

PREPARATION AND USE Use whole, chopped or ground. Whole nuts may be used in pecan pies, biscuits, fruit cakes and nutbreads. Chopped pecans may be used in cakes, biscuits and confectionery and served with ice cream. Ground nuts may be added to pastry, ice cream and used in confectionery.

PROCESSING Pecans are used in commercial pies and confectionery. The shells are used for paving paths and driveways, garden mulch and chicken litter and are ground for use as soft abrasives in soap and metal cleaners.

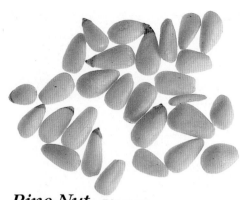

Pine Nut *Pinaceae*

also called Pinon nut, Pignolia

Major Nutrients
		Serve Size 30 g	
Energy	800 kJ	Dietary Fibre	3 g
Protein	5 g	Phosphorus	155 mg
Fat	18 g	Iron	1.5 mg
Carbohydrate	5 g	Thiamin	0.2 mg
Cholesterol	0	Niacin Equiv.	3 mg
Sodium	0		

Nutritional Information An excellent source of thiamin and phosphorus; good source of protein and iron; moderate source of niacin. The high oil in pine nuts is 81% unsaturated, containing similar amounts of monounsaturated and polyunsaturated oils. They also contain good quality protein.

These nuts are prone to rancidity and sometimes require roasting to remove a turpentine flavour.

Description The pine nut is a small, cream-coloured, soft kernel, 1–2 cm (about ½ in.) long. It is in fact a seed which is shed from the woody scales of a mature pine cone when it opens out.

Origin and History Pinea is Latin for pine nut. Pine nut shells have been found in Pompeii and in the remains of Roman camps in England. Pine nuts are referred to in the Bible in the book of the prophet Hosea. All these references refer to the Stone or Parasol pine which has been planted for centuries along the Mediterranean from the Lebanon to the east of Spain.

The Digger pine was named after the Indians who ate it in California, where it grows along the trail of the Camino Real.

Pine nuts from the Mexican nut pine have been an important staple in the diet of Mexican Indian tribes for hundreds of years. The Navajos make the nuts into a flour for cakes and pound them into a paste to be used like butter.

It has proved very difficult to establish a pine nut industry for the trees grow slowly and do not crop heavily until they are 75 years old. Spain, Italy and Greece are the main exporters of pine nuts.

Buying and Storage Usually available all year round. Select fresh, undamaged nuts with a fresh odour.

Store in a clear, airtight container in the refrigerator. Pine nuts may also be frozen for longer storage.

Preparation and Use Pine nuts may be roasted, dry fried or grilled until golden, or left plain for a more delicate flavour.

Add pine nuts to stuffings, pasta sauce, lamb, game, salads, savoury vegetable dishes, cakes, biscuits and fruit salad.

Processing May be processed into flour and used in confectionery. Oil from the broken kernels is used in soap and the cones are used for fuel.

Varieties

There are 80 different pines in the world, most of them growing in the cool latitudes of the northern hemisphere. Some of those known for their pine nuts include the Mexican nut pine, Lorean nut pine, Digger pine, stone or parasol pine, Chilgoza pine, white pine, longleaf pine, scrub pine and lodgepole pine.

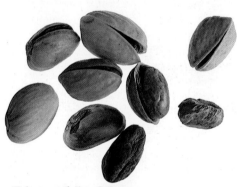

Pistachio Nut *Pistacia vera*

Major Nutrients
		Serve Size 30 g	
Energy	790 kJ	Sodium	0
Protein	6 g	Calcium	40 mg
Fat	16 g	Iron	4 mg
Carbohydrate	5 g	Thiamin	0.2 mg
Cholesterol	0		

Nutritional Information Pistachios are high in oil, the oil being 80% unsaturated, mainly monounsaturated. They are also an excellent source of iron.

Description The pistachio nut is a small, green kernel, covered with a thin, yellow-red skin, encased in a smooth, cream-coloured, brittle shell which separates from the kernel.

Origin and History The pistachio nut is the fruit of a deciduous tree originating in Asia Minor where it formed forests at high altitudes in Syria, Palestine and Persia. The nuts had great trade value to the nomadic tribes of those forests. The pistachio nut is now cultivated extensively in India where it is hawked in the streets, and also in the Far East, north Africa, Europe, Mexico, southern USA and California.

Buying and Storage Available all year round. The pistachio nut is sold either in its shell, or shelled and blanched. Select fresh undamaged nuts with a good fresh colour. Select shelled nuts in airtight packages.

Store in a clear, airtight container in the refrigerator.

Preparation and Use Remove the shell by crushing in the fingers, then remove skin by blanching. To preserve green colour, blanch by covering with water. Bring to the boil, then strain and cover immediately with more cold water. Remove the skins and dry slowly.

Serve salted pistachios for a snack, use plain pistachios in pâtés and terrines, add to game, use in desserts, confectionery, for decorating cakes, pastries and cold soufflés, and add to ice cream.

Processing Used in commercial ice cream and pâtisserie.

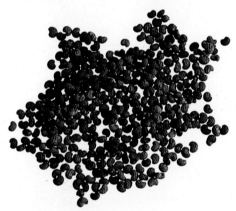

Poppy Seed *Papaver rhoeas*

Major Nutrients
		Serve Size 3 g	
Energy	70 kJ	Cholesterol	0
Protein	1 g	Sodium	0
Fat	1 g	Calcium	43 mg
Carbohydrate	1 g		

Nutritional Information As poppy seeds are eaten in small amounts they provide few nutrients other than a moderate amount of calcium.

In China, poppy seeds are used in the treatment of nausea and vomiting.

Description Poppy seeds are tiny, round and slate-blue to black with a strong nutty flavour.

Origin and History The poppy seed is produced by an annual poppy flower. It is native to Asia but was carried by travellers to Europe centuries ago, where it now grows profusely, both wild and in many gardens.

The poppy plant is a source of opium from the unripe heads, but the poppy seed is free of narcotic ingredients.

BUYING AND STORAGE Buy poppy seeds from a reputable spice shop or health food shop or buy recognised brands from the supermarket. Store in an airtight glass jar in a dry area away from direct sunlight. Check for freshness after one year.

PREPARATION AND USE Hang bunches of poppies upside down to dry, then shake the seeds from the poppies. Dry in sunlight and sieve before storing.

Use poppy seeds in traditional Jewish poppy seed cakes, sprinkle on homemade bread rolls, add to potato salad and pasta dishes. Also use in pastries and curries.

PROCESSING Used in commercial poppy seed cake, on cracker biscuits and bakers bread. Poppy seed is also crushed to produce oil.

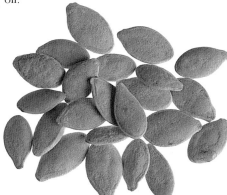

Pumpkin Seed Curcurbita

also called **Pepita**

MAJOR NUTRIENTS		SERVE SIZE 15 G	
Energy	350 kJ	Sodium	0
Protein	4 g	Phosphorus	170 mg
Fat	7 g	Iron	1.5 mg
Carbohydrate	2 g	Vitamin C	10.5 mg
Cholesterol	0		

NUTRITIONAL INFORMATION These seeds are a good source of iron, zinc, and vitamin C. Specific figures for zinc are not available.

DESCRIPTION Pumpkin seeds are dull green, flat, oval-shaped kernels enclosed in creamy white shells.

ORIGIN AND HISTORY The seed is found inside a ripe, mature pumpkin. The pumpkin is native to South America and has spread to North America, Australia and parts of Asia. Although introduced to Europe, it has not flourished there owing to climatic differences.

The pumpkin seed is a popular healthy snack food in South America and is gaining popularity in Australia.

BUYING AND STORAGE Buy pumpkin seeds from health food stores.

Store in a clear glass, airtight jar in the refrigerator to retain freshness for up to 6 months.

PREPARATION AND USE Gather pumpkin seeds from the pumpkin and dry in direct sunlight or in a microwave oven. Store as directed above. Roast in oil if liked before serving.

Use as a snack food, in salads, in vegetarian dishes, sprinkled in soups and casseroles. Add to fruit and nut cakes, tea bread, biscuits and slices.

PROCESSING Used in commercial health bars and salted as a snack food.

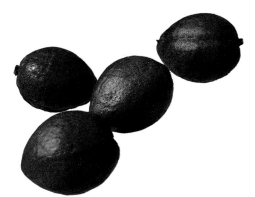

Red Bopple Nut Hicksbeachia *pinnatifolia*

MAJOR NUTRIENTS		SERVE SIZE 50 G	
Energy	640 kJ	Dietary Fibre	3 g
Protein	4 g	Sodium	10 g
Fat	3 g	Calcium	260 mg
Carbohydrate	29 g	Iron	2.5 mg
Cholesterol	0		

NUTRITIONAL INFORMATION This nut is particularly low in fat and energy compared to other nuts. It could make a useful contribution to calcium intakes; good source of potassium and other trace metals.

DESCRIPTION The red bopple nut is about the size of a hazelnut surrounded by a woody husk 0.5–1 cm in thickness and with a bright red outer skin.

ORIGIN AND HISTORY A relative of the macadamia nut, it was an important food for Aborigines of the east coast rainforests. The species has recently been under scrutiny as a possible crop.

BUYING AND STORAGE The nuts are fully ripe when the outer skin changes from orange to bright red. They will keep for several weeks at room temperature but slowly dry out. Shelled nuts must be refrigerated or frozen.

PREPARATION AND USE Depending upon the age of the fruit the edible nut (kernel) can be removed with a sharp knife or a nutcracker. The nuts can then be eaten raw or roasted. The low fat content makes this a slimmer's nut.

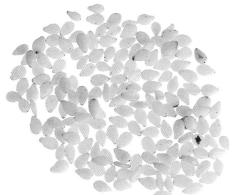

Sesame Seed Sesamum indicum

also called **Benne, Gingelli**

MAJOR NUTRIENTS		SERVE SIZE 15 G	
Energy	370 kJ	Cholesterol	0
Protein	3 g	Sodium	0
Fat	8 g	Phosphorus	90 mg
Carbohydrate	3 g		

NUTRITIONAL INFORMATION Sesame seeds contain a large amount of oil. The oil is 86% unsaturated, containing 44% monounsaturated and 42% polyunsaturated oils.

Sesame seeds are normally hulled. If they are not hulled they contain calcium; this calcium is not as well absorbed by the body as the calcium from milk. They also contain vitamin E, magnesium, phosphate and zinc, though specific figures for these are not available.

DESCRIPTION Sesame seeds are the very small, flat, cream-coloured seeds of the sesame herb, a plant which grows 1 m high, with white flowers that are followed by pods which dramatically pop open when touched, scattering the seeds. The seeds have a nutty aroma which is accentuated when they are baked or roasted.

ORIGIN AND HISTORY Sesame is one of the oldest and most nourishing herbs known. It is native to Indonesia where it has been cultivated for over 4000 years. Most countries of the Old World have grown it for its seed. Records of sesame production in the Tigris and Euphrates Valleys date back to 1600 BC. African slaves took sesame seeds with them to America. It has been associated with fables such as Ali Baba, Sanskrit literature, Egyptian records and Hebrew writings. Marco Polo wrote that the sesame oil he sampled travelling through Persia was the best flavoured oil he had tasted on all his travels and Cleopatra is thought to have used it as a skin oil.

BUYING AND STORAGE Buy sesame seed from a reputable spice shop or health food shop, or buy recognised brands from a supermarket. Store in glass, airtight jars in a dry area out of direct sunlight. Check on freshness after one year.

PREPARATION AND USE Toast sesame seeds by gently frying in a dry pan. Add to salads, vegetable dishes, casseroles, meat loaves, cottage cheese loaves, quiches and stuffings. Use raw sesame seeds mixed with breadcrumbs to coat fish or veal or savoury rissoles, in savoury biscuits, sprinkled on scones, loaves and bread rolls. Add to any food that will brown while baking. A paste can be made from the seeds as a substitute for butter.

PROCESSING Sesame seeds are used to manufacture tahini, a sesame seed paste which is used as a spread or in Middle East dishes such as hommos and halvah. Ground seeds are sold as sesame meal in health food shops for vegetarian recipes. They are used in manufactured health bars, biscuits and yeast products, and are pressed to make sesame seed oil, an important source of polyunsaturated fats, which is used in Oriental recipes and salad dressings.

VARIETIES
Black or brown sesame (*sesame orientale*).

SEE ALSO Sesame Oil, Tahini.

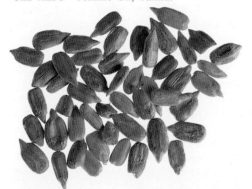

Sunflower Seed *Helianthus annuus*

MAJOR NUTRIENTS		SERVE SIZE 15 G	
Energy	350 kJ	Sodium	0
Protein	4 g	Phosphorus	125 mg
Fat	7 g	Iron	1 mg
Carbohydrate	3 g	Vitamin C	7.5 mg
Cholesterol	0		

NUTRITIONAL INFORMATION These seeds are a good source of iron, zinc, and vitamin C.

Specific figures for zinc are not available.

DESCRIPTION Sunflower seeds are small, flat, oval-shaped, beige-coloured kernels covered with a fawn and black striped shell.

ORIGIN AND HISTORY Sunflower seeds come from the sunflower, a tall plant which produces a large single yellow flower head with a large seed-bearing centre. They are native to Central America and Peru, where the Indians cultivated them. They are now grown extensively in Russia as well as in the USA, Europe, Africa and Australia.

BUYING AND STORAGE Buy from a reputable health food shop. Care should be taken to ensure that there is no insect infestation. Store in a glass, airtight jar in the refrigerator for up to 6 months.

PREPARATION AND USE Muslin bags slipped over the flowers prevent seed loss. The bag also catches ripe seeds as they fall. Once the flower heads have shrivelled and dried, the seeds can be threshed and stored in an airtight container. Use raw, roasted or boiled, or grind to a powder. Use raw in savoury vegetarian dishes such as soups, stir-fries, rice and pasta. Roasted sunflower seeds can be added to green, savoury or fruit salads, sprinkled over dressed vegetables or served as a snack. Boiled sunflower seeds can be used in baked products such as cakes, biscuits and puddings.

PROCESSING Sunflower seeds are crushed to produce sunflower oil used for salads, cooking and for the manufacture of polyunsaturated margarine. The substance left after crushing the seeds is called sunflower meal; it is sold in health food stores.

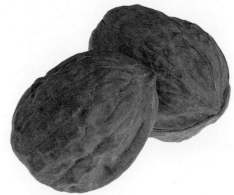

Walnut *Juglans*

MAJOR NUTRIENTS		SERVE SIZE 30 G	
Energy	650 kJ	Phosphorus	155 mg
Protein	3 g	Magnesium	40 mg
Fat	15 g	Iron	0.5 mg
Carbohydrate	2 g	Zinc	1 mg
Cholesterol	0	Thiamin	0.1 mg
Sodium	0		

NUTRITIONAL INFORMATION Walnuts are high in oil, being especially rich in linoleic acid, an essential polyunsaturated fatty acid.

Because of their large amount of polyunsaturated oil they are prone to rancidity.

DESCRIPTION The walnut is the fruit of the walnut tree. The nut has a smooth, outer green husk, covering a creamy-brown round shell, shaped in two hemispheres which encase the two lobes of the ridged, 'butterfly'-shaped, light brown kernel.

ORIGIN AND HISTORY The walnut is related to the hickory and the pecan. There are 15 different kinds of walnut, scattered from the Mediterranean to eastern China and from North America to the Andes in South America. They vary from the white butternut to the yellow-brown Persian walnut and the dark brown or black walnut, but the yellow-brown one is the most popular. The walnuts from Persia were introduced into Italy before Christianity. A huskless variety grows in China. In France, the Titmouse variety has a shell so thin that a bird can break the shell and eat the nut. Now grown commercially in California, and also in Australia.

BUYING AND STORAGE Buy walnuts in the shell, preferably, as they are fresher. Store in a cool place or in the refrigerator for up to 6 months. When buying shelled nuts, choose airtight packages or cans and store after opening in an airtight glass jar in the refrigerator.

PREPARATION AND USE Remove shells from walnuts with a nutcracker or a clean hammer. They may be eaten from the hand or walnut halves may be added to salads, fruit desserts and fruit cakes. Chopped nuts can be used also in biscuits, stuffings and salads. Ground walnuts can be added to pastry and biscuits, fruit tarts and confectionery.

PROCESSING Walnuts are crushed to extract walnut oil which is prized for salad dressings as well as cooking. Walnut kernels are canned.

FATS AND OILS

Fats and oils are extracted from a variety of different plants and animal products.

Generally the solid fats are extracted from animals, for example: lard (from pigs), tallow or suet (from cattle and sheep), butter (from cow's milk) and dripping (from roast meat). The oils are generally extracted from seeds and nuts.

They may be further modified by processing. This is well illustrated by the manufacture of margarine, which can be produced from a variety of oils and fats which are quite different in their physical, chemical and flavour characteristics.

The products included in this chapter are those most easily obtainable. As oil production continues, those such as cottonseed oil and rice bran oil may become more widely used.

The oils and fats provide more kilojoules per unit of weight than any other food. An extra teaspoon of butter or margarine on bread or on vegetables, or extra oil in a mayonnaise or vinaigrette, may boost the kilojoules more than a little extra bread, vegetable or salad in a diet. It is very easy to overconsume these high fat foods, and become overweight in the process.

Oils are 100% fat, while butter, dairy blend and margarine are 80% or more fat.

The demand for less fat in the diet has led to the production of spreads which contain less fat than butter or margarines. These have been available in Europe and the U.S.A. for many years but they became available only recently in the Pacific region.

Legislation provides for products with 30–50% fat, and it is certain that other products with even less fat will become available. It is important to read the food label to check on the amount and variety of fat in the products purchased.

Most fats consist of triglycerides, which are combinations of glycerol and three fatty acids. The saturated, monounsaturated and polyunsaturated fatty acids, and their different functions, are discussed in the Introduction to this book.

Fats and oils are made up of a mixture of fats containing varying amounts of saturated, monounsaturated and polyunsaturated fatty acids, and foods are usually classified according to the fatty acids which predominate. The individual entries below give details of the predominant fatty acids for each oil or fat.

The animal fats are predominantly saturated, and most of the vegetable oils available are predominantly polyunsaturated or monounsaturated. It is important to note that coconut oil and palm oil, two vegetable oils widely used by food manufacturers, are predominantly saturated.

The heating of polyunsaturated fats can cause structural changes, but in normal domestic use the changes in colour and odour of the oil results in the oil being discarded before significant changes occur. If food is fried, it is better to use shallow rather than deep frying, and not to re-use the oil or fat.

The vegetable oils are free of cholesterol while the animal fats contain significant levels of cholesterol.

Vegetable oils contain only negligible amounts of sodium, but butter, margarine, dairy spreads and reduced-fat spreads usually have salt (sodium chloride) added in processing. A range of reduced-salt products is available and the label will provide details of the sodium content of the product.

The oils and fats contain the fat soluble vitamins A, D and E. Butter contains varying amounts of vitamin A, depending on the carotene in the animals' feed, and varying but small amounts of vitamin D. In Australia, table margarine, dairy blend and reduced fat spreads must contain not less than 850 micrograms of vitamin A, and 5.5 micrograms of vitamin D per 100 grams. Cooking margarines may have added vitamin A and D, but this is not required by law. The consumption of butter has been falling steadily over decades, and the consumption of table margarine has increased, although together these foods have seen a fall in consumption.

The amount of vegetable oils and fats used by the food industry has increased, and in spite of the drop in butter and margarine consumption and the drop in the consumption of meat, the fat intake of consumers remains steady. More fat consumed is now coming from the fats and oils in processed foods such as potato crisps and other snack food, biscuits, pastries, cakes, fried foods and takeaways.

Increased affluence usually results in an increase in fat consumption, and a high fat intake has been associated with an increase in prevalence of nutrition-related conditions and disease such as obesity, high blood cholesterol levels, heart disease, high blood pressure and stroke, non-insulin-dependent diabetes and certain types of cancer.

There is a wide acceptance of the need to reduce the fat intake in Western diets. In order to do this, it is important to control the use of fats and oils in the home, but it is just as important to use fewer foods to which the manufacturers have added fats and oils.

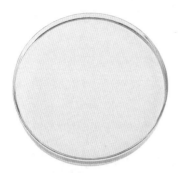

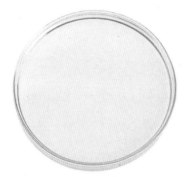

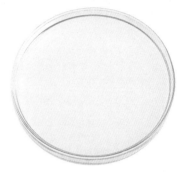

Almond Oil

MAJOR NUTRIENTS · SERVE SIZE 18 G

Energy	660 kJ	Cholesterol	0
Protein	0	Dietary Fibre	0
Fat	18 g	Sodium	0
Carbohydrate	0		

NUTRITIONAL INFORMATION The fat in almond oil is predominantly mono-unsaturated. It is an excellent source of vitamin E.

DESCRIPTION The oil extracted from the dried kernels of the almond tree, *Prunus amygdalus*.

ORIGIN AND HISTORY As an edible oil, almond oil is not currently of commercial significance, since the almond is an expensive raw material and therefore infrequently used to produce oil. It is more frequently used externally, as a gentle moisturiser, which the ancient Egyptians valued highly as a treatment for the prevention of wrinkles.

BUYING AND STORAGE Available from some specialty food outlets. It should be bland in flavour and colourless, free from rancidity and other undesirable flavours.

Store in a sealed container at room temperature and out of direct light. The oil may be refrigerated after opening.

PREPARATION AND USE Use as a salad oil or for general cooking and baking.

PROCESSING The oil is extracted from the dried kernels by cold pressing, or heat pressing/solvent extraction plus refining for edible use.

Apricot Kernel Oil

MAJOR NUTRIENTS · SERVE SIZE 18 G

Energy	660 kJ	Cholesterol	0
Protein	0	Dietary Fibre	0
Fat	18 g	Sodium	0
Carbohydrate	0		

NUTRITIONAL INFORMATION Apricot kernel oil is predominantly made up of mono-unsaturated fats. It is an excellent source of vitamin E.

DESCRIPTION The oil extracted from the dried kernels of the apricot tree, *Prunus armeniaca*.

ORIGIN AND HISTORY This oil is very similar in characteristics and composition to almond oil. Apricot kernel oil is produced as a by-product of the fruit juice industry in some countries, and is not currently of commercial significance.

BUYING AND STORAGE Available from some specialty food outlets. It should be bland in flavour and colourless, free from rancidity and other undesirable flavours.

Store in a sealed container at room temperature and out of direct light. The oil may be refrigerated after opening.

PREPARATION AND USE Use as salad oil or for general cooking and baking.

PROCESSING The oil is extracted from the dried kernels by cold pressing, or heat pressing/solvent extraction plus refining for edible use.

Avocado Oil

MAJOR NUTRIENTS · SERVE SIZE 18 G

Energy	660 kJ	Cholesterol	0
Protein	0	Dietary Fibre	0
Fat	18 g	Sodium	0
Carbohydrate	0		

NUTRITIONAL INFORMATION The fat in avocado oil is predominantly mono-unsaturated. It is an excellent source of vitamin E.

DESCRIPTION The oil extracted from the fruit of the avocado pear, *Persea americana, Persea gratissima*.

ORIGIN AND HISTORY The avocado is a native of Central America and the West Indies. It was introduced into Australia late in the 19th century. The fruit is not currently an important commercial source of oil, although it contains 15–30% oil, which has been utilised mainly in the cosmetic industry as a skin-care agent, many finding it useful for the relief of sunburn. The refined oil has only recently been introduced to the world food market.

BUYING AND STORAGE The crude oil is available from normal health product outlets. It has a green colour, similar to that of olive or grapeseed oil and a slight, unpleasant flavour and odour. The product is marketed as a skin-care product. The refined oil may be obtained from some specialty food outlets. It is generally a pale straw colour and should be free from rancidity or other undesirable flavours.

The crude oil is very sensitive to oxidation when exposed to light. Store the refined or crude oils in a sealed container, at room temperature and out of direct light. Some of the natural components may solidify on storage, particularly at lower temperatures.

PREPARATION AND USE The crude oil is used as a skin-care agent. The refined oil currently has limited commercial applications in the food industry.

PROCESSING The oil is extracted from the

pulped fruit by mechanical means or with solvent. It may then be refined. It may also be 'winterised' to remove higher melting components.

Butter

MAJOR NUTRIENTS		SERVE SIZE 19 G	
Energy	580 kJ	Cholesterol	45 mg
Protein	0	Dietary Fibre	0
Fat	16 g	Sodium	160 mg
Carbohydrate	0	Vitamin A	190 µg

NUTRITIONAL INFORMATION Butter must not contain less than 80% milk fat by law. As butter is an animal fat, the fat is predominantly saturated, and contains a large amount of cholesterol. It is an excellent source of vitamin A and contains a moderate amount of sodium. Use a thin scrape on bread/toast as part of a low-fat diet. A low salt or unsalted variety is preferable.

DESCRIPTION A mixture of milk fat (derived from cow's milk) and water, prepared by churning cream. May contain added salt.

ORIGIN AND HISTORY Butter is thought to have been developed in the cooler lands, where milk carried by travellers did not curdle because it was accidentally churned in the container during transport. Butterfat is one of a relatively small number of fats and oils that are prized for their individual flavour and used with little or no purification.

Butter flavour may vary from country to country, depending on local custom. In Europe, butters containing little or no salt and prepared from cultured (soured) cream, are popular. Australian butters generally contain higher levels of salt (1% or 2%) and are prepared from fresh cream. Most countries specify a legal minimum butterfat content of 80% and maximum water content of 16%.

There has been a trend away from butter towards the use of vegetable fats (particularly polyunsaturated fats) due to its high cholesterol and saturates content.

BUYING AND STORAGE Check use-by date on the packaging. Australian butters generally have a use-by date of 6 months from the time of production. Butter should be free of rancidity, with a characteristic, pleasant flavour and aroma. Store at or below 5°C (refrigerator temperature) for improved keepability. Butter can also be frozen. Store in protective wrapping or sealed container to avoid absorbing food odours.

PREPARATION AND USE Generally used as a spread (for example, on bread), for general cooking, baking, shallow frying, and so on.

Remove from the refrigerator 15–30 minutes before use or warm slightly in a dish by standing in warm water to improve spreadability. Butter may also be softened by placing in the microwave on High for approximately 20 seconds.

PROCESSING The cream is separated from cow's milk and whipped (churned) until most of the water has separated from it. The remaining semi solid is butter, which is salted to taste and chilled.

For commercial butters in Australia, the cream must be pasteurised. Unpasteurised cream is used to prepare 'farm butter'.

VARIETIES

Compound butter

MAJOR NUTRIENTS No specific nutritional analysis is available.

NUTRITIONAL INFORMATION Fruit butters are prepared from butter, eggs, sugar, water and flavouring from the fruit named. They may contain other additives, for example colouring.

DESCRIPTION A combination of the ingredient of choice creamed with butter: savoury butters such as mustard, curry, nuts, garlic, capers, herbs, cheese, anchovy; and sweet butters such as honey, golden syrup, cinnamon, fruit, brown sugar.

ORIGIN AND HISTORY Compound butters were developed to use as a spread (for example, for bread, sandwiches, canapés) or to add flavour to cooked food such as steaks or fish.

The sweet butters provide a tasty topping for waffles, pancakes, crumpets and muffins.

BUYING AND STORAGE Some prepared compound butters can be purchased from the supermarket cold cabinets (for example, garlic butter).

Store in a sealed container or protective wrapping at or below 5°C (refrigerator temperature).

PREPARATION AND USE For savoury butters, use either salted or unsalted butter and add salt to taste. Prepare the ingredient of choice, for example finely chopped herbs, grated cheese. Cream butter with added ingredient (a rough guide is 125 g butter to 2 tablespoons of fresh herb, cheese, mustard). Form into a roll, cover in plastic wrap and refrigerate. Cut into serving slices when firm.

For sweet butters, cream unsalted butter and beat in the ingredient of choice, a little at a time. Add ingredient to taste. Melt over hot waffles, pancakes, etc.

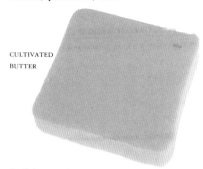
CULTIVATED BUTTER

Cultivated or ripened butter Produced to give a rich flavour.

Farm butter A richly flavoured product.

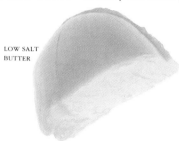
LOW SALT BUTTER

Low salt butter Useful for those conscious of sodium in their diet and for the baking of sweet cakes and desserts.

MAJOR NUTRIENTS		SERVE SIZE 19 G	
Energy	580 kJ	Cholesterol	45 mg
Protein	0	Dietary Fibre	0
Fat	16 g	Sodium	75 mg
Carbohydrate	0	Vitamin A	190 µg

NUTRITIONAL INFORMATION Using a low salt butter can significantly reduce the sodium in the diet.

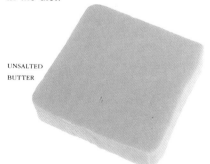
UNSALTED BUTTER

Unsalted butter Has the same uses as low salt butter.

NUTRITIONAL INFORMATION The nutrient value of unsalted butter is identical to that of low salt butter, except that there is no sodium content.

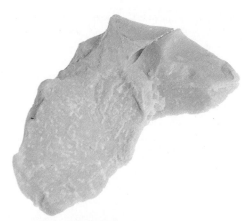

Cocoa Butter

also called Cacao butter, Theobroma oil

NUTRITIONAL INFORMATION No details are available on the nutritional value of this product, but it is a saturated fat.

DESCRIPTION The fat obtained from the kernel of the cocoa bean (from the tropical plant *Theobroma cacao*).

ORIGIN AND HISTORY Cocoa butter belongs to the family of fats referred to as vegetable butters. It is hard and non-greasy at ordinary temperatures, with a melting point about 10°C below body temperature. Its melting properties, and its characteristic flavour make it very suitable as a coating fat for confections (it is ordinarily blended with chocolate). Africa is the major source of cocoa.

BUYING AND STORAGE Not available to the consumer as a pure, edible fat but is present in many prepared foods.

PREPARATION AND USE Cocoa butter is used chiefly in the manufacture of chocolate confections, in coatings for chocolates and candies and in cosmetics. It is used to some extent as a component in suntan preparations.

PROCESSING The butter is obtained primarily by the pressing of kernels of cleaned, roasted, beans. No refining is necessary unless to reclaim poorer quality fat from damaged beans.

SEE ALSO Cocoa.

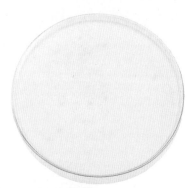

Coconut Oil

also called Copha

MAJOR NUTRIENTS		SERVE SIZE 17 G	
Energy	630 kJ	Cholesterol	0
Protein	0	Dietary Fibre	0
Fat	17 g	Sodium	0
Carbohydrate	0		

NUTRITIONAL INFORMATION The fat in copha is predominantly saturated. As coconut oil is from a plant, it is cholesterol free. Coconut oil (like palm oil) is one of the few plant oils that is not unsaturated. This is why it is solid/semisolid at room temperature, rather than liquid as are the other plant oils. Coconut oil is used extensively in the food industry — often in vegetable fat based foods, for example, confectionery, margarine, cooking oils.

DESCRIPTION The oil derived from copra (dried coconut meat), from the coconut palm, *Cocos nucifera*.

ORIGIN AND HISTORY The coconut palm is of unknown origin but is thought to have spread across Polynesia from the Indian Ocean and today is found in the coastal belts of all tropical countries. Local inhabitants use the oil for cooking, lighting and as a hair dressing oil. Together with the oil palm, the coconut palm is the most important oil-bearing tree in terms of world trade. Copra contains typically 63–70% oil, which is a white solid at temperatures below 20°C.

BUYING AND STORAGE Pure coconut fat can be purchased from the refrigerated cabinets in Australian supermarkets. It should be a clean, white solid, free of rancidity (indicated by a 'soapy' flavour). Store at or below 5°C (refrigerator), or freeze.

PREPARATION AND USE Coconut fat is used in the manufacture of margarine, cooking oils and fats, ice cream, confectionery (for example, chocolate), imitation dairy products. It is also used in soap manufacture and the cosmetics industry.

PROCESSING The coconut is harvested, split and sun-dried. The oil is then extracted by crushing the dried coconut meat. It is refined and may be hydrogenated before inclusion in edible products.

SEE ALSO Coconut.

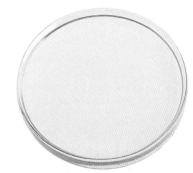

Corn Oil

also called Maize oil

MAJOR NUTRIENTS		SERVE SIZE 18 G	
Energy	660 kJ	Cholesterol	0
Protein	0	Dietary Fibre	0
Fat	18 g	Sodium	0
Carbohydrate	0		

NUTRITIONAL INFORMATION The fat in corn oil is predominantly polyunsaturated. It is an excellent source of vitamin E.

Use a small amount of this oil in preference to a saturated fat.

DESCRIPTION The oil obtained from the kernel of corn, *Zea mays*. It is predominantly polyunsaturated.

ORIGIN AND HISTORY Corn oil is a by-product of the milling of corn. Corn is one of the principal crops of the USA, which is responsible for about 70% of the world's consumption of corn oil. It is used in the same manner as other polyunsaturated oils such as sunflower. The corn germ contains up to 50% oil. The crude oil has a dark reddish-amber colour.

BUYING AND STORAGE The refined oil is generally a darker yellow colour than most vegetable oils. It possesses a characteristic corn flavour but should be free from rancidity or other undesirable flavours.

Store in a sealed container, at room temperature and away from direct light. Some solids (wax) may appear on storage, particularly at lower temperatures.

PREPARATION AND USE The pure oil is used chiefly as a salad or cooking oil. Major industrial edible uses are in margarine, cooking oil and salad oils/dressings.

PROCESSING The oil is obtained by milling of the corn, followed by pressing or solvent extraction. It is then refined to improve flavour and keepability. Corn oil contains appreciable levels of natural waxes and needs to be 'winterised' before it can perform as a salad oil. The oil may also be hydrogenated for inclusion in some margarines.

SEE ALSO Maize.

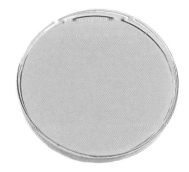

Cottonseed Oil

MAJOR NUTRIENTS		SERVE SIZE 18 G	
Energy	660 kJ	Cholesterol	0
Protein	0	Dietary Fibre	0
Fat	18 g	Sodium	0
Carbohydrate	0	Vitamin E	7 mg

NUTRITIONAL INFORMATION The fat in cottonseed oil is predominantly polyunsaturated. It is an excellent source of vitamin E.

Use a small amount of this oil in preference to a saturated fat.

DESCRIPTION The oil derived from the seeds of various species of the cotton plant, chiefly *Gossypium hirsutum* and *Gossypium barbadense*.

ORIGIN AND HISTORY The cotton plant has been cultivated for thousands of years, primarily to produce cotton fibre. Cottonseed is essentially a by-product. Serious commercial uses were only found for cottonseed late in the 19th century and by the late 1960s it was the second largest producer of vegetable seed oil. The crude oil has a strong, characteristic flavour and odour and a dark, reddish-brown colour. It is not suitable for edible use unless refined. The seeds contain 18–28% oil.

BUYING AND STORAGE Cottonseed is not generally sold as a pure oil in Australia as it forms solids at ambient temperature and will gel at refrigerator temperatures. The refined oil is a pale yellow to amber colour; odourless and bland tasting. It should be free of rancidity or other undesirable flavours. Store in a sealed container, at room temperature and away from direct light.

PREPARATION AND USE Major uses in the food oil industry are in the manufacture of margarine, cooking fats and oils.

PROCESSING Some of the oil can be extracted by mechanical pressing, but solvent extraction methods are generally used. The crude oil is refined and may be hydrogenated before use in margarine or shortenings. It is not ideal as a salad oil due to its relatively high content of higher melting solids. If intended for this purpose it needs careful winterising.

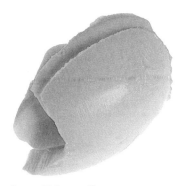

Dairy Blend

MAJOR NUTRIENTS No detailed nutritional analysis is available.

NUTRITIONAL INFORMATION Dairy Blend is a blend of milkfat (not >67%) and vegetable oil (not >20%) and water. As for butter and margarine, it must legally contain 80% fat (maximum) and 16% water (maximum). It also contains vitamins A and D added to the same levels as for margarine, plus added salt. Also available as low salt (65 mg sodium/19 g serve).

Dairy Blend was developed to have the flavour of butter and the spreadability of margarine. Use a thin scrape on bread/toast as part of a low fat diet. A low salt variety is preferable.

DESCRIPTION A table spread formed by blending butter with edible vegetable oil.

ORIGIN AND HISTORY Dairy or butter blends are of recent origin. A portion of the butter fat is replaced with liquid edible vegetable oil. This results in a product with the flavour of butter but the spreadability of margarine at lower temperatures. It is also lower in saturates and cholesterol than standard butter. The amount of vegetable oil legally permitted may vary from country to country. In Australia, vegetable oil must be 15% (minimum) and 25% (maximum) of the total fat in the product. Dairy blends may also contain added antioxidant, milk solids, colouring substances and certain other legally permitted additives.

BUYING AND STORAGE Check the Use-By date to ensure freshness. Product should be free from rancidity and other undesirable flavours. Dairy blends are available containing 2% salt or 1% salt ('low salt').

Store at or below 5°C. Can also be frozen.

PREPARATION AND USE Use as for butter or margarine.

PROCESSING The oil may be added to the milk or cream before churning, or to the butter during its working stage. The blend is mixed thoroughly and chilled.

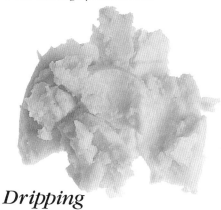

Dripping

also called *Edible tallow*

MAJOR NUTRIENTS		SERVE SIZE 17 G	
Energy	630 kJ	Cholesterol	25 mg
Protein	0	Dietary Fibre	0
Fat	17 g	Sodium	0
Carbohydrate	0		

NUTRITIONAL INFORMATION As dripping is an animal fat, it contains predominantly saturated fats. It also contains a small amount of cholesterol. Use this fat sparingly, if at all. Use a small amount of unsaturated fat in cooking in preference.

DESCRIPTION Fat derived from the meat, muscles and bones of animals belonging to the ox family (for example, beef) and/or sheep.

ORIGIN AND HISTORY People have used fat from land animals in the preparation and cooking of foods since their early hunting days. Towards the end of the 19th century, the soft (oleo) fraction of edible tallow was used in the production of the first margarines. During the mid-20th century, improved technology allowed an increasing use of edible tallow in the manufacture of shortenings. In Australia today, it is still used in the manufacture of shortenings, cooking margarines and baking products, but it is rarely used in table margarines.

BUYING AND STORAGE Can be purchased packaged from the butcher or from the cold-cabinet section of supermarkets. Dripping should be a clean, light colour, free from rancid odour and flavour.

Store in its protective wrapping or in a dry, sealed container, at or below room temperature. Store away from direct light.

PREPARATION AND USE Strain the fat from roasted meat or melt pieces of trimmed fat over gentle heat and strain to remove skin and membrane.

Use as a shortening in the preparation of dough, pastries, and so on, for frying and basting foods.

If using for frying, strain thoroughly after each use and discard immediately when rancidity or other undesirable flavours develop. Care should be taken not to heat the fat above its 'smoke point' when frying.

PROCESSING As for lard. It may also be refined and hydrogenated for incorporation in commercial edible products.

VARIETIES
Beef, Mutton.

Flavoured Oils

also called **Gourmet oils, Specialty oils**

MAJOR NUTRIENTS No specific nutritional analysis available.

NUTRITIONAL INFORMATION Nutritional value depends on the oil used in preparation — refer under specific oil type.

DESCRIPTION Oil with added herb, spice or condiment.

ORIGIN AND HISTORY Flavoured oils were developed to impart a chosen aroma and flavour to the prepared or cooked food. Any edible liquid oil can be used in their preparation. Olive oil is generally preferred and grapeseed oil is also frequently used. A large selection of herbs, spices, condiments may be added to the oil.

BUYING AND STORAGE Flavoured oils are available from some specialty or gourmet food outlets. Check the Use-By date on the packaging. The flavoured oils generally have a 6 month shelf life. They will vary in colour depending on the oil and additive, but should be free of rancidity or unpleasant off-flavours.

PREPARATION AND USE Select oil of choice. Prepare the additive as required. Add to the oil to taste (an approximate guide is 2 tablespoons of additive per 500 ml oil). Seal and store out of direct light. Allow at least 2 weeks for the flavour to develop.

Use in salad dressings, shallow frying or as desired.

PROCESSING Some additives may require processing before adding to the oil (for example, peel garlic cloves, wash fresh chillies).

VARIETIES

Bayleaf oil

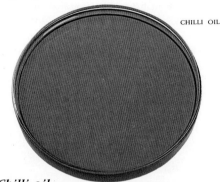

CHILLI OIL

Chilli oil

DESCRIPTION A bright red oil with an intensely hot flavour, made by steeping dried chillies in vegetable oil. It is also called lat yu.

ORIGIN AND HISTORY Chillies are an important ingredient in the cuisine of the Szechuan and Hunan provinces of China. The late Chairman Mao was known to only really enjoy those meals on which the cook lavished chilli. Cantonese have a more cautious approach to strong flavours, and so devised this sharply flavoured oil which could be used with discretion.

BUYING AND STORAGE It can be bought from Chinese food stores in small bottles with a shaker top, and should be refrigerated to retain the intense flavour.

PREPARATION AND USE Chilli oil is used as a flavour highlight, never as a cooking oil. Sprinkle over a dish as a condiment, or add to the wok when cooking stir-fries. It can be made at home by heating 1 cup of vegetable or peanut oil until very hot, without beginning to smoke. Remove from heat and stir in about 4 tablespoons of broken, dried small red Thai chillies or 2½–4 tablespoons (depending on the required strength) of hot chilli flakes. Leave to cool, stirring occasionally, then strain through a cloth and transfer to a shaker bottle. Use in the same way as Tabasco sauce, to add a dash of chilli to a dish during cooking or at the table.

PROCESSING Commercially prepared chilli oil is made by a similar process as above, the oil is filtered after steeping the chillies and occasionally a little extra red food colouring is introduced.

Garlic oil

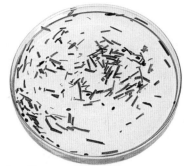

Herb oil

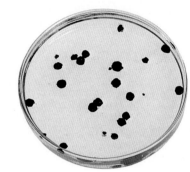

Pepper oil

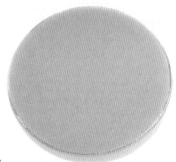

Ghee

also called **Ghi**

MAJOR NUTRIENTS		SERVE SIZE 19 g	
Energy	700 kJ	Carbohydrate	0
Protein	0	Vitamin A	75 µg
Fat	19 g	other nutritional	
Cholesterol	12 mg	analyses unavailable	
Dietary fibre	0		

NUTRITIONAL INFORMATION Ghee is an animal fat and so is predominantly a saturated fat. It is a good source of vitamin A, but is high in cholesterol.

DESCRIPTION Clarified butter, clean butter fat with the milk solids and salt removed.

ORIGIN AND HISTORY Ghee was the preferred cooking medium of the Aryan nomads, who introduced it to India about 1750 BC. It had assumed particular importance in Indian society by about 500 BC because of the sacred status of the cow, and became a part of many Indian caste and religious rituals. Panch gavya, the eating of five products of the cow (dung, urine, milk, curds and ghee) was a common form of expiation for a crime against the caste.

Hindus travelling away from home are absolved of the problems of eating food not prepared in the right caste conditions (pakki food), if the food is cooked in ghee. In 1917, high-caste Brahman Indians in Calcutta demanded a mass ritual purification ceremony on the banks of the Hooghly River when they learned that ghee used for religious offerings and cooking had been adulterated.

Ghee can be heated to greater temperatures than fresh butter without burning or spitting and is therefore used for frying. It imparts particularly good colour and flavour to the cooked food. It is used extensively in Indian and other Asian cooking where it is also produced from the milk of the water buffalo.

BUYING AND STORAGE Can be purchased from most supermarkets in tubs, cartons or tins. Should be free from rancidity and other undesirable flavours. Store in a sealed container at room temperature. It can be kept unrefrigerated for several weeks in cooler climates, and will keep for many months, refrigerated.

PREPARATION AND USE Heat the butter gently until a foam appears at the top. Cook a further few seconds, then remove from the heat and leave for a few minutes. A milky residue will sink to the bottom. The clear yellow liquid above it is the clarified butter. Pour clarified butter into a container.

In Indian cooking, it is used for the preliminary frying of ingredients for a curry. Ghee, being purer than butter, will stand higher temperatures, making it excellent — although expensive — for deep and shallow frying, particularly of breads and dessert ingredients. It gives a rich, buttery flavour to foods and so is used extensively in Indian sweet-making.

SEE ALSO Butter.

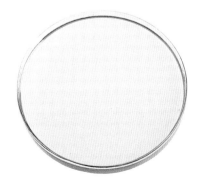

Grapeseed Oil

MAJOR NUTRIENTS		SERVE SIZE 18 G	
Energy	660 kJ	Cholesterol	0
Protein	0	Dietary Fibre	0
Fat	18 g	Sodium	0
Carbohydrate	0		

NUTRITIONAL INFORMATION The fat in grapeseed oil is predominantly polyunsaturated. It is an excellent source of vitamin E. Use a small amount of this oil in preference to a saturated fat.

DESCRIPTION The oil derived from the seeds of the grape, *Vitis vinifera*, *Vitis labrusca*.

ORIGIN AND HISTORY The production of oil from grapes was ongoing in 1560 and several factories were operating in Italy in 1790. The oil was used in paints and varnishes and as an edible cooking oil. Oil production died out towards the end of the 19th century when lower priced oils came into use but was resumed before and during World War I. The oil is produced from waste raisin seeds and as a by-product of the wine industry, the seeds containing from 6–20% oil. It is produced on a commercial scale in France and Italy.

BUYING AND STORAGE The refined oil is a pale yellow-green colour with a slightly fruity flavour. The crude oil is darker in colour with a stronger flavour. The oil should be free of rancidity and other undesirable flavours.

Store in a sealed container, at room temperature and away from direct light. Natural waxes may precipitate out on storage, particularly at lower temperatures.

PREPARATION AND USE The refined oil is used primarily as a cooking and salad oil. In its crude state it is used as an ingredient in dressings. It has a high linoleic acid content (comparable to safflower oil) and is frequently marketed as a health product.

PROCESSING The grapeseeds are recovered from pomace or wine press residues by several processes involving washing, threshing and sieving. The seeds are dried, cooked, milled and flaked before pressing or solvent extraction of the oil. The oil is generally then refined. It may also be winterised to remove waxy materials.

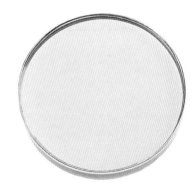

Hazelnut Oil

*also called **Filbert oil***

MAJOR NUTRIENTS		SERVE SIZE 18 G	
Energy	660 kJ	Cholesterol	0
Protein	0	Dietary Fibre	0
Fat	18 g	Sodium	0
Carbohydrate	0		

NUTRITIONAL INFORMATION The fat in hazelnut oil is predominantly mono-unsaturated. It is an excellent source of vitamin E. Hazelnut oil is one of the oils that is richest in vitamin E.

DESCRIPTION The oil extracted from the kernel of the hazelnut, *Corylus avellana*.

ORIGIN AND HISTORY The hazelnut is one of the oldest forms of cultivated plant in Europe. Currently most of the world's crop comes from Turkey, Italy, and Spain. The hazelnut, like the walnut and macadamia, is a rich source of oil, the kernel containing 50–60%. The oil is not of major commercial importance in the food industry due to the high cost of the hazelnut but is popular as a 'gourmet-style' oil.

BUYING AND STORAGE The oil can be purchased from specialty food outlets. It is generally prepared from roasted nuts and thus has a distinctive odour and flavour and a dark brown colour. The oil should be free from rancidity and other undesirable flavours.

Store in a sealed container, at room temperature, away from direct light.

PREPARATION AND USE The oil is generally used in salad dressings and as a flavoursome cooking oil.

PROCESSING For use as a flavoursome cooking oil, the oil is generally recovered by milling and pressing of the hazelnuts. The nuts may be roasted before milling; this enhances the flavour of the oil and results in a darker colour.

The oil may be solvent extracted and refined if desired.

SEE ALSO Hazelnut.

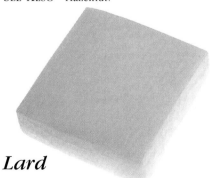

Lard

MAJOR NUTRIENTS		SERVE SIZE 17 G	
Energy	630 kJ	Cholesterol	25 mg
Protein	0	Dietary Fibre	0
Fat	17 g	Sodium	0
Carbohydrate	0		

NUTRITIONAL INFORMATION Lard is predominantly a mixture of monounsaturated and saturated fat — contains a small amount of cholesterol. Use lard sparingly if at all. A small amount of an unsaturated fat in cooking is preferable.

DESCRIPTION The clean, white fat rendered from the meat of pigs.

ORIGIN AND HISTORY The separation of lard from pork and its use in preparation and cooking of foods has been known to humans since their early hunting days. High 'shortening value' is a natural property of lard. For this reason and because of its ready availability, lard was the primary shortening agent used during the first half of the 20th century in the USA. The use of lard has decreased as the modern trend is towards vegetable fat products.

BUYING AND STORAGE Can be purchased fresh from the butcher or packaged from the supermarket cold-cabinet section. It should be free of rancidity.

Store in its protective wrapping or a sealed container, out of direct light at or below normal room temperature.

PREPARATION AND USE Trim fat from pork and melt over a gentle heat. Strain the heated liquid carefully into a container.

Use as a shortening in the preparation of doughs, pastries and so on, or as a frying and roasting medium. The fat should be strained carefully after each frying use and discarded immediately rancidity or undesirable flavours develop. Care should be taken not to heat the fat above its 'smoke-point' when frying.

PROCESSING Fats, including lard, are prepared on a large scale by a variety of processes called rendering. The fatty tissues are heated, steam sometimes being injected during the heating to aid the processing. Generally, the lower the temperature used during rendering, the higher quality fat that results.

Lard may be refined and hydrogenated for incorporation in commercial shortening or cooking fats.

SEE ALSO Pork.

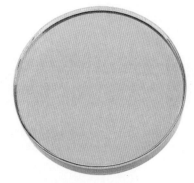

Macadamia Oil

NUTRITIONAL INFORMATION No detailed data are available. The fat content is predominantly unsaturated.

DESCRIPTION The oil extracted from the kernel of the macadamia tree, *Macadamia ternifolia.*

ORIGIN AND HISTORY The macadamia tree is a native of the subtropical rainforest of Eastern Australia. It was discovered in the mid-19th century and named after Dr John Macadam MD. The oil is unique among vegetable seed oils in that it contains a major portion of the monounsaturated fatty acid palmitoleic acid (containing 16 carbons with 1 double bond), rather than the more common oleic acid. It is not currently of commercial significance in the edible oils industry, partly owing to the high cost of the raw material.

BUYING AND STORAGE Available from some specialty food outlets. The oil is a pale yellow colour and should be free from rancidity and other undesirable flavours.

Store in a sealed container at room temperature and away from direct light. Some solids may settle out on storage, particularly at lower temperatures, due to the presence of certain naturally occurring substances.

PREPARATION AND USE Use as a salad oil and for general cooking and baking.

PROCESSING The oil may be extracted from the nut using cold pressing or heat pressing/solvent extraction methods. It may be refined for edible use.

SEE ALSO Macadamia Nut.

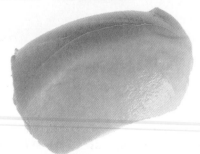

Margarine

NUTRITIONAL INFORMATION The nutrient

contents of the various margarines are discussed below.

DESCRIPTION A mixture (emulsion) of oil/fat (minimum 80%) and water (maximum 16%). Margarine may contain added antioxidant, colour, salt, emulsifiers, milk and flavours.

ORIGIN AND HISTORY Invented by the French chemist Hippolyte Mège-Mourie in 1869, margarine was developed to meet butter shortages in France and to provide a table spread with satisfactory keepability for the armed forces.

It was originally produced using the soft fraction (oleo oil) from beef fat and was in block or stick form.

Today table margarines are generally formulated using vegetable oils/fats as the major fat component and are designed to be soft and spreadable from the fridge.

BUYING AND STORAGE Look for the use-by date on the packaging to ensure product freshness. Australian margarines generally have a shelf life of 6 months, which is the time that the manufacturer expects the product, if stored correctly, to maintain good flavour and texture.

Store at or below 5°C (refrigerator temperature). Margarine can also be frozen.

Store in its sealed container or protective wrapping to avoid absorbing food odours.

PREPARATION AND USE Is commonly used as a spread (on bread) and for general cooking purposes (baking, shallow frying).

PROCESSING The processed oil is mixed with the water and other ingredients, chilled and beaten in a process similar to ice cream manufacture. The extent of chilling and beating helps determine the product texture.

VARIETIES

Cooking Margarine

MAJOR NUTRIENTS		SERVE SIZE 19 G	
Energy	550 kJ	Cholesterol	20 mg
Protein	0	Dietary Fibre	0
Fat	15 g	Sodium	220 mg
Carbohydrate	0	Vitamin A	160 μg

NUTRITIONAL INFORMATION Cooking margarines contain slightly more monounsaturated than saturated fats, plus a moderate amount of cholesterol and sodium. An excellent source of vitamins A and E, and a good source of vitamin D. The vitamins A and D are added to a minimum level by law. Use cooking margarine sparingly — a small amount of unsaturated fat is preferable.

Polyunsaturated Table Margarine

MAJOR NUTRIENTS			SERVE SIZE 19 G
Energy	580 kJ	Cholesterol	0
Protein	0	Dietary Fibre	0
Fat	15 g	Sodium	140 mg
Carbohydrate	0	Vitamin A	160 µg

NUTRITIONAL INFORMATION By law, the fats in this type of margarine must be predominantly polyunsaturated. The cholesterol content must be less than a minimum level (5 mg/100 g). It is an excellent source of vitamins A and E, and a good source of vitamin D. It contains a moderate amount of sodium.

The production of margarine from vegetable oils involves the process of hydrogenation, which hardens the oil into a spread. During this process, some polyunsaturated fats can be converted into 'trans' fatty acids, which may be potentially harmful. While the nutritional implications are not fully resolved, levels of trans fatty acids in Australian margarines are declining and may be reducing any possible health hazard.

A minimum level of vitamins A and D is added to margarine by law. Often it contains more than this minimum level (check container label). The added vitamin E is an antioxidant.

Use a thin scrape of margarine on bread/toast as part of a low-fat diet. A low salt or salt-free variety is preferable. Also available milk-free.

Polyunsaturated Table Margarine, Low Salt and Salt-free

MAJOR NUTRIENTS			SERVE SIZE 19 G
Energy	580 kJ	Dietary Fibre	0
Protein	0	Sodium low salt	75 mg
Fat	15 g	salt-free	0
Carbohydrate	0	Vitamin A	160 µg
Cholesterol	0		

NUTRITIONAL INFORMATION By law, the fats in this type of margarine must be predominantly polyunsaturated. The ratio of polyunsaturated to saturated fat must be a minimum of 2:1. The cholesterol content must be less than a minimum level (5 mg/100 g). It is an excellent source of vitamins A and E, and a good source of vitamin D. The sodium content is not significant.

Using a low salt or salt-free margarine can significantly reduce the sodium in the diet.

Also available milk-free.

Table Margarine

MAJOR NUTRIENTS			SERVE SIZE 19 G
Energy	570 kJ	Cholesterol	5 mg
Protein	0	Dietary Fibre	0
Fat	15 g	Sodium	180 mg
Carbohydrate	0	Vitamin A	160 µg

NUTRITIONAL INFORMATION Margarines contain not less than 80% fat by law. Table margarines are predominantly a mixture of monounsaturated and saturated fats. They contain a moderate amount of sodium. They are an excellent source of vitamins A and E, and a good source of vitamin D. The cholesterol content is not significant.

Vitamins A and D must be added to table margarine by law. Often they contain more than this specified level (check container label). Vitamin E acts as an antioxidant. Use a thin spread on toast/bread as part of a low fat diet. A low salt variety is preferable.

Table Low Salt Margarine

MAJOR NUTRIENTS			SERVE SIZE 19 G
Energy	570 kJ	Cholesterol	5 mg
Protein	0	Dietary Fibre	0
Fat	15 g	Sodium	75 mg
Carbohydrate	0	Vitamin A	160 µg

NUTRITIONAL INFORMATION As for table margarine. Use a thin spread on toast/bread as part of a low fat diet. Using a low salt margarine can significantly reduce the sodium in the diet.

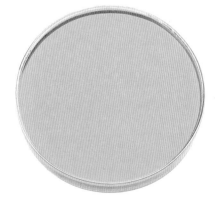

Mustard Oil

also called **Mustard seed oil**

NUTRITIONAL INFORMATION No detailed data are available. The fat content is predominantly unsaturated.

DESCRIPTION The oil extracted from the seeds of the mustard plant, including *Brassica alba* and *Brassica nigra*.

ORIGIN AND HISTORY Mustard seed oil is a close relative of conventional rapeseed oil and similarly possesses a high level (up to 50%) of erucic acid. Oils containing high levels of this fatty acid are not legally permitted for edible purposes by the authorities in many Western countries, including Australia. It is, however, still used for edible purposes in some of the Asian countries. The seeds contain approximately 25–40% oil.

BUYING AND STORAGE The oil is not legally permitted as an edible product in Australia. It varies in colour from yellow to light brown.

PROCESSING The oil may be pressed or solvent-extracted. It may also be refined.

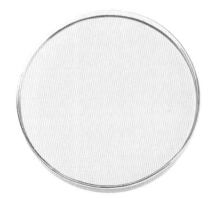

Olive Oil

MAJOR NUTRIENTS			SERVE SIZE 18 G
Energy	660 kJ	Cholesterol	0
Protein	0	Dietary Fibre	0
Fat	18 g	Sodium	0
Carbohydrate	0		

NUTRITIONAL INFORMATION Olive oil is predominantly a monounsaturated fat. It is an excellent source of vitamin E.

The observation that coronary heart disease rates are low in the Mediterranean region, where large quantities of olive oil are consumed, has led to an interest in the role of monounsaturated fats in heart disease. Further research on this topic continues.

DESCRIPTION The oil pressed from the pulp of the fruit of the olive tree, *Olea europa*.

ORIGIN AND HISTORY Cultivation of the olive appears to have originated about 6 000 years ago in the eastern Mediterranean region although it grew wild before that time. Olive oil was a major export product of Greece as far back as 3 000 BC. The olive was developed by the Syrians and Palestinians into a compact, oil-rich variety which is now grown along the entire shores of the Mediterranean and wherever a Mediterranean-type climate prevails. The largest producers of olive oil today are Spain and Italy. Unlike most other vegetable oils, good virgin grades of olive oil are consumed as a food without refining or other processing.

BUYING AND STORAGE The oil has a characteristic pleasant, fruity odour and flavour. Its colour may vary from yellow to green, depending on the region in which the olive is grown and from pale to dark, depending on the type of oil. Virgin oil has a stronger flavour and colour than refined or pure oil. Flavour and colour of the pure oils vary, depending on the relative amounts of virgin and refined oils blended together.

Olive oil is more stable to oxidation than most liquid oils owing to its low content of polyunsaturates. Store in a sealed container at room temperature, out of direct light.

PREPARATION AND USE The virgin and pure oils are used chiefly as salad and cooking oils. Residue oil, if refined, may be included in edible products such as blended vegetable oils, but legally may not be sold as 'olive' oil. The inedible residue (also known as sulphur oil or olive kernel oil) is widely used in soapmaking.

PROCESSING Olive oil is physically pressed from the fruit, the pressing occurring in 2 stages. The first pressing yields the highest grade oil. Each successive pressing yields oil of lower grade, which must generally be refined to improve the flavour and keepability.

VARIETIES

Extra virgin olive oil/Virgin olive oil The highest quality oil, obtained from the fruit using physical means only.

Olive pomace oil/Olive residue oil Obtained by solvent extraction of the olive residue remaining after mechanical expression of the virgin oil. It is made edible by refining.

Pure olive oil/Olive oil A blend of virgin and refined oils.

Refined olive oil Obtained by refining virgin olive oil.

(Olive kernel oil is obtained by solvent extraction of the soil from the seed, and is not permitted for edible use.)

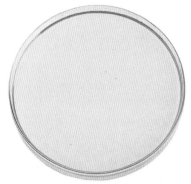

Peanut Oil

also called Arachis nut oil, Earthnut oil, Groundnut oil, Monkey nut oil

MAJOR NUTRIENTS			SERVE SIZE 18 G
Energy	660 kJ	Cholesterol	0
Protein	0	Dietary Fibre	0
Fat	18 g	Sodium	0
Carbohydrate	0		

NUTRITIONAL INFORMATION Peanut oil is predominantly a monounsaturated fat. It is an excellent source of vitamin E.

DESCRIPTION The oil obtained from the kernels of the groundnut, the plant *Arachis hypogaea*.

ORIGIN AND HISTORY The peanut or groundnut is a native of South America, where its oil has been used in cooking for thousands of years.

Today peanuts are cultivated throughout most tropical and sub-tropical areas of the world, the biggest producers being India, China, Nigeria, USA, Senegal, and Mali. Peanut oil is the most important by-product of peanut cultivation, in fact, in many countries it is the essential reason for growing the crop. A typical peanut contains 45–55% oil.

BUYING AND STORAGE The refined oil is a pale yellow to amber colour with a slight, characteristic nutty odour and flavour. The oil should be free of rancidity and other undesirable flavours.

Store in a sealed container, at room temperature and away from direct light. The oil will cloud or gel if refrigerated.

PREPARATION AND USE It is popular as a cooking oil or in salad dressings owing to its characteristic flavour. Main edible industrial uses include the preparation of margarines, shortenings, mayonnaise, cooking oils and salad dressings.

PROCESSING The oil is extracted from the chopped, blanched nuts by mechanical pressing or solvent extraction. It is then refined before incorporation in edible products. Peanuts may also be roasted prior to oil extraction. There is a substantial market for the cold-pressed oil in many European, Asian, and South American countries.

SEE ALSO Peanut, Peanut Butter.

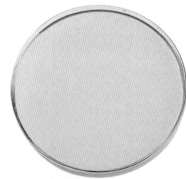

Pecan Oil

also called Pecan kernel oil

MAJOR NUTRIENTS			SERVE SIZE 18 G
Energy	660 kJ	Cholesterol	0
Protein	0	Dietary Fibre	0
Fat	18 g	Sodium	0
Carbohydrate	0		

NUTRITIONAL INFORMATION The fat in pecan oil is predominantly monounsaturated. It is a moderate source of vitamin E. Use a small amount of this oil in preference to a saturated fat.

DESCRIPTION The oil extracted from the kernel of the pecan, *Carya pecan* or *Carya illinoensis*.

ORIGIN AND HISTORY The pecan tree belongs to the same family as the walnut and hickory nut, and is indigenous to the southern states of North America. The dried kernel contains 60–70% oil which is very similar to that of the almond and apricot kernels. The edible oil is not currently of commercial importance.

BUYING AND STORAGE Available from some specialty food outlets. The oil should be free from rancidity and other undesirable flavours.

Store in a sealed container at room temperature and away from direct light. May be refrigerated after opening.

PREPARATION AND USE Use as a salad oil and for general cooking and baking.

PROCESSING The oil may be extracted from the kernels by cold-pressing or heat-pressing/ solvent extraction. It may also be refined for edible use. The pecan kernels may be roasted prior to oil extraction, resulting in a darker oil colour and enhanced flavour.

SEE ALSO Pecan Nut.

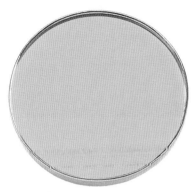

Pumpkin Seed Oil

NUTRITIONAL INFORMATION No detailed data are available. The oil is predominantly unsaturated.

DESCRIPTION The oil extracted from the seeds of the pumpkin, *Cucurbita pepo*.

ORIGIN AND HISTORY Pumpkin seeds are commonly dried, roasted and eaten as snack foods but may also be used as a source of edible oil. The seeds contain 30–40% oil, which is not currently of commercial significance but is produced on a smaller scale in a few countries, including Yugoslavia.

BUYING AND STORAGE Available from some food stores. The oil may vary in colour from pale yellow to dark brown and in flavour from bland to aromatic, depending on the processing methods used. It should be free from rancidity and other undesirable flavours.

Store in a sealed container, at room temperature and away from direct light.

PREPARATION AND USE Use for general cooking and baking.

PROCESSING The oil may be extracted by cold-pressing or heat-pressing/solvent extraction methods. It may be refined for edible use. The pumpkin seeds may be roasted before oil extraction, resulting in a dark colour and enhanced aroma and flavour.

SEE ALSO Pumpkin Seed.

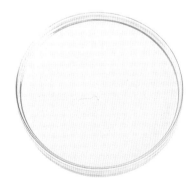

Rapeseed Oil

also called Canbra oil, Canola oil, Colza oil, Rape oil

MAJOR NUTRIENTS		SERVE SIZE 18 G	
Energy	660 kJ	Cholesterol	0
Protein	0	Dietary Fibre	0
Fat	18 g	Sodium	0
Carbohydrate	0		

NUTRITIONAL INFORMATION The fat in rapeseed oil is predominantly mono-unsaturated. It is an excellent source of vitamin E.

DESCRIPTION The oil extracted from the seeds of the rape plant, *Brassica campestris* or *Brassica napus*.

ORIGIN AND HISTORY The rape plant belongs to the 'crucifer' or 'cabbage' family. Rapeseed world production is high and the oil has been used in the past as a salad oil and for illumination. Conventional rapeseed oil, unlike other edible vegetable oils, contains a high proportion of erucic acid (considered undesirable in the human diet) and has been banned by several countries for human consumption. In the latter part of this century, varieties of rapeseed oil with little or no erucic acid have therefore been developed. These oils are also referred to as canola oil.

BUYING AND STORAGE Often sold as a constituent of blended vegetable oils and vegetable margarines.

The refined oil is a pale yellow colour, bland and odourless.

PREPARATION AND USE Major industrial culinary uses include the manufacture of cooking and salad oils, mayonnaise, salad dressings and table margarines.

PROCESSING The oil is extracted from the seed by pressing and/or solvent extraction. It is then refined before inclusion in edible products. The oil may also be hydrogenated.

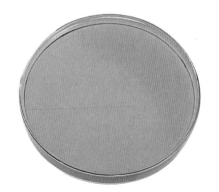

Rice Bran Oil

MAJOR NUTRIENTS		SERVE SIZE 18 G	
Energy	660 kJ	Cholesterol	0
Protein	0	Dietary Fibre	0
Fat	18 g	Sodium	0
Carbohydrate	0	Vitamin E	7 mg

NUTRITIONAL INFORMATION Rice bran oil is a mixture of both polyunsaturated and monounsaturated fats. It is an excellent source of vitamin E.

DESCRIPTION The oil extracted from the bran of the rice grain, *Oryza sativa*.

ORIGIN AND HISTORY Rice bran is about 6% by weight (on a dry basis) of rough rice and contains 15–20% oil. It is a potentially important source of oil, as rice is the world's most important crop.

The oil is produced in Japan; some has also been produced in the USA.

The oil has excellent stability towards oxidation due to the presence of several natural antioxidants, but due to a high enzyme activity, crude oil deteriorates rapidly on storage.

BUYING AND STORAGE The refined oil should be free from rancidity and other undesirable flavours.

Store in a sealed container, at room temperature.

PREPARATION AND USE Rice bran oil is very similar in physical characteristics to cottonseed and groundnut oils. The composition of rice bran oil makes it suitable for use, when refined, as a salad and cooking oil and for the manufacture of hydrogenated products, such as a cocoa butter substitute.

PROCESSING The oil is solvent-extracted promptly from the isolated rice bran and then refined to improve the colour and flavour. The product may also be 'winterised', as it contains high levels of natural waxes which solidify on storage.

SEE ALSO Rice.

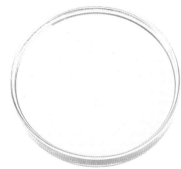

Safflower Oil

MAJOR NUTRIENTS		SERVE SIZE 18 G	
Energy	660 kJ	Cholesterol	0
Protein	0	Dietary Fibre	0
Fat	18 g	Sodium	0
Carbohydrate	0		

NUTRITIONAL INFORMATION The fat in safflower oil is predominantly polyunsaturated. It is an excellent source of vitamin E. Safflower oil is the richest oilseed source of polyunsaturated fat. Use a small amount of this oil in preference to a saturated fat.

DESCRIPTION The oil extracted from the seed of the safflower plant, *Carthamus tinctorius*.

ORIGIN AND HISTORY The safflower plant belongs to the thistle family. Safflower oil has been known since ancient times but has only gained commercial importance during the last 20 to 30 years. It has the highest linoleic acid content of any commercially produced oil and is today an important oil in the production of high polyunsaturated margarines and oils. Some of the major oil producers are India, Mexico, the USA, Spain, Portugal, and Australia.

BUYING AND STORAGE The refined oil is a very pale yellow colour, with a bland taste. The oil should be free from rancidity and other undesirable flavours.

Store in a sealed container, at room temperature and away from direct light. Some solids may appear in the oil if stored at cooler temperatures.

PREPARATION AND USE The oil is used predominantly as a salad or cooking oil.

Major edible industrial uses are in margarine (specifically 'health' brands with high polyunsaturates content) and the preparation of salad and cooking oils.

PROCESSING The oil is extracted from the seed by pressing or solvent extraction. The crude oil is not highly stable and is therefore further processed (refined) soon after extraction. Oil destined for use as a bottled oil is usually winterised to remove components that may solidify on storage.

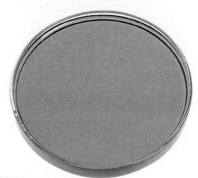

Sesame Oil

MAJOR NUTRIENTS   SERVE SIZE 18 G

Energy	660 kJ	Cholesterol	0
Protein	0	Dietary Fibre	0
Fat	18 g	Sodium	0
Carbohydrate	0		

NUTRITIONAL INFORMATION The fat in sesame oil is predominantly a mixture of polyunsaturated and monounsaturated fats. It is only a moderate source of vitamin E.

As for all oils, fat provides all the energy in sesame oil. It is one of the poorest sources of vitamin E of all the oils. Use a small amount of this oil in preference to a saturated fat.

DESCRIPTION The oil from the seed of the sesame plant, *Sesamum indicum*.

ORIGIN AND HISTORY Sesame is an ancient crop, believed to be the first annual oilseed cultivated. Domestication of the crop first occurred in ancient Persia. From there it was introduced to the Middle East, India, and finally Asia. It has been grown extensively in China and India for many centuries.

The crude oil is of a high quality, and is more stable than oils of equivalent unsaturation, due to the presence of natural antioxidants. The seed contains typically 45–55% oil.

BUYING AND STORAGE The crude oil has a distinctive flavour and an amber colour. The refined oil is a pale yellow colour, with a slight characteristic flavour. Oil should be free of rancidity and other undesirable flavours.

Store in a sealed container, at room temperature and out of direct light.

PREPARATION AND USE Sesame oil is used for much the same purposes as olive oil: for cooking, frying, salads.

In Western society, small amounts are also used in margarine, prepared salad dressings and cooking oils.

PROCESSING The oil is extracted from the seed mainly by pressing methods. It is prized for its individual flavour and may be used as a salad or cooking oil without refining. The seeds may be roasted before extracting, enhancing the flavour and giving a darker colour.

The oil is refined and hydrogenated before use in margarine and shortenings.

Shortening

MAJOR NUTRIENTS   SERVE SIZE 17 G

Energy	630 kJ	Dietary Fibre	0
Protein	0	Other nutrients depend	
Fat	17 g	on the type of fat	
Carbohydrate	0	present (see Lard)	

NUTRITIONAL INFORMATION General cooking fats are predominantly a mixture of saturated and monounsaturated fats, and contain a moderate amount of cholesterol. Pure vegetable fats contain no cholesterol. If animal fat is used, then cholesterol will be present.

DESCRIPTION Includes a wide range of cooking products made from animal and/or vegetable fats.

ORIGIN AND HISTORY The word 'shortening' was first used to describe the fat — mainly lard — used to tenderise baked foods by preventing the protein and carbohydrate components from becoming a hard, continuous mass during cooking. Today the term includes a much wider range of products and in the USA can include emulsions of water in oil (margarine-type). These products contain higher melting fats and salt levels than retail margarine and are therefore more temperature stable. In Australia, shortenings are 100% fat. Vegetable shortenings have gained popularity in the last few decades.

BUYING AND STORAGE The majority of shortenings are produced for the baking and catering industry and are not available to the average consumer. Some shortenings (lard) are available from the supermarket.

These should be stored in a sealed container or protective wrapping, out of direct light, at or below room temperature.

PREPARATION AND USE Can be used for deep frying (100% fat shortening) and in the preparation of doughs, pastries, bread, cakes, icings, and so on. Shortenings are generally used to tenderise (shorten) but also may provide exterior gloss, moisture resistance and lubrication in baked goods. Specific shortenings are also used as creaming fats (in preparation of imitation creams).

PROCESSING The 100% fat shortenings are chilled and beaten, as for margarines. The extent of chilling and beating, together with the type of fat, determines the texture of the shortening.

VARIETIES

Animal shortenings   Using animal fat.

Blended shortenings   Using both animal and vegetable fats.

Vegetable shortenings   Using vegetable oils.

SEE ALSO Butter, Dripping, Lard, Margarine, Vegetable Oil, Blended.

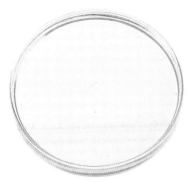

Soya Bean Oil

also called **Manchurian bean oil, Soya bean oil, Soybean oil**

MAJOR NUTRIENTS		SERVE SIZE 18 G	
Energy	660 kJ	Cholesterol	0
Protein	0	Dietary Fibre	0
Fat	18 g	Sodium	0
Carbohydrate	0		

NUTRITIONAL INFORMATION The fat in soya bean oil is predominantly polyunsaturated. It is an excellent source of vitamin E.

DESCRIPTION The oil obtained from the seeds of the soya bean plant, *Glycine max* or *G. soja.*

ORIGIN AND HISTORY The soya bean originated in Eastern Asia and has been grown by the Chinese for thousands of years, providing a versatile source of food such as soya milk, bean curd, soya cheese, sprouts, flour and oil for cooking. Today it is also the major commercial source of lecithin. Some consider that the oil, when incorporated in the diet, helps lower blood cholesterol levels. Demand for edible soya bean oil increased rapidly this century, with the introduction of the margarine, and then the fast food industries. The USA is the world's largest producer of soya beans and soya bean oil.

The soya bean contains 18–20% oil, which is a light amber colour and has a characteristic bean taste in the crude state.

BUYING AND STORAGE The refined oil is a pale yellow with a bland taste. It should be free of rancidity and other undesirable flavours.

Store in a sealed container, at room temperature and out of direct light.

PREPARATION AND USE The liquid oil is used in the home as a cooking or salad oil. Major edible commercial uses are in the preparation of margarine, shortening, cooking fats, and salad oils.

PROCESSING The oil is obtained from the soya bean by pressing or solvent extraction. It is then refined before incorporation in edible products. The oil contains significant levels of linolenic acid. It is therefore often partially hydrogenated to remove some of this fatty acid and improve the oil's flavour stability.

SEE ALSO Soya Bean.

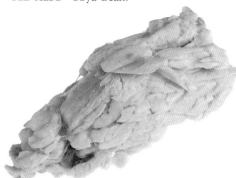

Suet

MAJOR NUTRIENTS		SERVE SIZE 17 G	
Energy	610 kJ	Cholesterol	10 mg
Protein	0	Dietary Fibre	0
Fat	17 g	Sodium	0
Carbohydrate	0		

NUTRITIONAL INFORMATION As suet is derived from animal fat, it is predominantly a saturated fat. The cholesterol content is not significant. Use suet sparingly, if at all. Cooking with a small amount of an unsaturated fat is preferable.

DESCRIPTION The hard, white fat that surrounds the kidney in beef and mutton.

ORIGIN AND HISTORY The use of animal fats in food preparation was discovered during humans' early hunting days and became important as far back as around 4 000 BC when sheep were first domesticated.

Beef suet is a harder, cleaner fat than normal dripping and can be heated up to 180°C without burning. It is also odourless and has become important in the preparation of suet pastry which is usually boiled or steamed to make a soft crust for puddings or dumplings.

BUYING AND STORAGE Can be purchased fresh from the butcher. It should be a clean, white colour, free from rancidity. Prepared mixtures of shredded suet and flour are also available from the supermarket.

Store in its packaging or a closed container, away from direct light.

PREPARATION AND USE Trim the fat from fresh kidneys and remove any skin. Grate the fat or chop it finely with a little flour to prevent sticking.

Use in the preparation of suet pastry/ pudding.

The fat can also be melted down (rendered) over gentle heat, strained and used for frying.

Remove any impurities by straining after each frying use and discard immediately rancidity or other undesirable flavours develop.

Care should be taken not to heat the fat above its 'smoke-point' when frying.

VARIETIES
Beef suet, mutton suet.

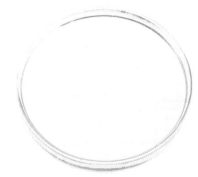

Sunflower Oil

MAJOR NUTRIENTS		SERVE SIZE 18 G	
Energy	660 kJ	Cholesterol	0
Protein	0	Dietary Fibre	0
Fat	18 g	Sodium	0
Carbohydrate	0		

NUTRITIONAL INFORMATION The fat in sunflower oil is predominantly polyunsaturated.

Sunflower oil is one of the richest oilseed sources of vitamin E. Use a small amount of this oil in preference to a saturated fat.

DESCRIPTION The oil derived from the seed of the sunflower plant, *Helianthus annuus.*

ORIGIN AND HISTORY The wild sunflower is believed to have originated in southern USA and Mexico, where it was found growing as a weed. The Spaniards took the wildflower to Spain in the 16th century, from where it spread throughout Europe.

Its cultivation as an oilseed crop began in Russia and some eastern European countries in the 19th century. Today the major sunflower seed producing countries are the USSR, USA, and Argentina. The seed contains from 20–30% oil.

BUYING AND STORAGE The crude oil is a light amber colour, with distinctive odour and flavour. The refined oil is a pale yellow colour, with a bland flavour. Oil should be free from rancidity and other undesirable flavours.

Store in a sealed container at room temperature and out of direct light. Sunflower can contain significant levels of waxes, which may settle out on storage, particularly at lower temperatures.

PREPARATION AND USE Sunflower oil is used almost exclusively for edible purposes such as cooking or as a salad oil, in margarine and shortenings. It has a very high level of polyunsaturates, which makes it particularly suitable for manufacture of polyunsaturated margarines.

PROCESSING The oil may be cold-pressed from the seed but in major commercial production is generally heat-pressed or solvent-extracted and then refined. It may also be hydrogenated for inclusion in some margarines and shortenings. If sold as a salad oil, it is usually winterised to prevent the oil clouding on storage.

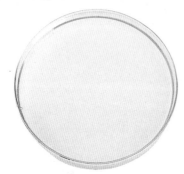

Vanaspati

*also called **Vegetable ghee***

NUTRITIONAL INFORMATION No detailed data are available on vanaspati.

DESCRIPTION A 100% vegetable fat product, designed to reproduce the coarsely crystalline, plastic texture and cooking properties of ghee.

ORIGIN AND HISTORY Ghee is an important, all-purpose cooking fat in the warmer climates, where it has much better keeping qualities than butter. Vanaspati, a hydrogenated vegetable shortening, has been developed to imitate the cooking properties of ghee. It is largely saturated, but has the advantage of containing much less cholesterol than ghee. Raw materials (oil-bearing plants) are also generally more available than the ghee raw material (milk) in the tropics. It is used where religion forbids the consumption of various animal products.

India and Pakistan are the major producers and consumers of vanaspati. Palm oil is one of the major oils used in vanaspati production.

BUYING AND STORAGE Storage conditions as for ghee.

PREPARATION AND USE Used as an all-purpose cooking medium (as for ghee). Filter/strain carefully after use as a deep-frying oil. Discard immediately if rancidity or other undesirable flavours develop.

PROCESSING The vegetable oils are refined, hydrogenated (fully or partially) and blended to obtain the desired texture, melting point and consistency. The blended oil may be mechanically processed (chilled and beaten) to obtain the desired texture.

SEE ALSO Ghee.

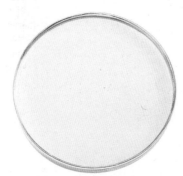

Vegetable Oil, Blended

MAJOR NUTRIENTS		SERVE SIZE 18 G	
Energy	670 kJ	Cholesterol	0
Protein	0	Dietary Fibre	0
Fat	18 g	Sodium	0
Carbohydrate	0		

NUTRITIONAL INFORMATION These oils are predominantly a mixture of polyunsaturated and monounsaturated fats. The price and availability of oils determines which oils are used in the blend.

Use a small amount of this oil in preference to a saturated fat.

The polyunsaturated type of this oil has the same nutrients as above, but the fats contained are predominantly unsaturated.

DESCRIPTION The oil extracted from the seeds or fruits of plant life. The oils vary significantly in physical and chemical properties and may be used for a variety of food and/or industrial purposes. May also be classified as 'saturated', 'monounsaturated' or 'polyunsaturated'.

ORIGIN AND HISTORY Oils and fats are essential constituents of all forms of plant life. Only about 100 varieties of plants have oil-bearing seeds with sufficient oil content to warrant commercial interest and about 22 of these are developed on a large scale. Some plants are cultivated for their oil alone, such as the flax (linseed oil) and castor (castor oil) plants. Many are a source of oil and other edible products (e.g. soya bean, coconut, peanut) and some are derived as a by-product of another major industry (e.g. cottonseed oil, corn oil, grapeseed oil).

Oil has been in demand for thousands of years for food, lighting, medicine and per-

fumed unguents. Today it is used extensively in the food industry and various non-food industries including the manufacture of cosmetics, paints, varnishes, inks, soaps and resins.

Vegetable oils have become increasingly popular in the food industry and are now frequently used in place of animal fats for health reasons. Vegetable oils contain very low levels of cholesterol in comparison to animal fats and usually contain significantly fewer saturated fatty acids (the exceptions are cocoa butter, coconut, palm and palm kernel oil). Most vegetable oils contain significant levels of natural antioxidants called tocopherols.

BUYING AND STORAGE Liquid vegetable oils can be purchased pure or as blend of various liquid oils. When purchasing check the use-by date to ensure freshness. They generally have a use-by date of 12 months from the time of packaging and may contain certain, legally permitted, added antioxidants to improve keepability.

The oils will vary in colour and flavour depending on their vegetable source and on the type and amount of processing given them. Some fats and oils are prized for their individual flavour components and are used with little or no purification (such as olive, sesame, poppy seed oils). Most commercially prepared oils are however processed to a bland flavour and pale colour. The oils, when purchased, should be free of rancidity and other undesirable flavours.

Most oils are sensitive to heat and light. They undergo a deterioration process called oxidation on storage and should therefore be stored in a clean, sealed container, at (or below if possible) room temperature and away from direct light. Salad oils may be stored in the refrigerator but other cooking oils will solidify/gel at lower temperatures.

PREPARATION AND USE The liquid oils are used in the home for general cooking purposes and as salad oils. If using for deep frying, the oil should be carefully strained after each use and discarded immediately unpleasant flavours develop.

Vegetable fats and oils are used in the food industry to manufacture margarine, cooking fats and oils, salad dressings, mayonnaise, shortenings, ice creams, confectionery, imitation cream/dairy products.

PROCESSING Oils may be cold-pressed, heat-pressed or solvent-extracted from their fruit or seed. Most commercially important oils are heat-treated and solvent-extracted to increase yields and are then refined to remove excessive colour and flavour before incorporation into food products. Some oils may also be hydrogenated to either improve their keepability or to make them more solid for incorporation into margarines, shortenings, etc.

Oils used as salad oils are normally winterised to prevent solids forming on storage.

SEE ALSO The various fruit, nut, seed and vegetable oils under their separate listings.

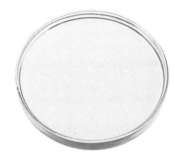

Walnut Oil

MAJOR NUTRIENTS   SERVE SIZE 18 G

Energy	660 kJ	Cholesterol	0
Protein	0	Dietary Fibre	0
Fat	18 g	Sodium	0
Carbohydrate	0		

NUTRITIONAL INFORMATION The fat in walnut oil is predominantly polyunsaturated. It is a moderate source of vitamin E.

Use a small amount of this oil in preference to a saturated fat.

DESCRIPTION The oil is extracted from the kernel of the walnut, *Juglans regia* or *Juglans nigra*.

ORIGIN AND HISTORY Oil was extracted from the walnut (as well as the olive and opium poppy) in ancient Greece. The walnut kernel contains 60–70% oil, which is recovered from walnut processing as a by-product. The crude oil is particularly popular in Europe as a cooking oil, owing to its characteristic flavour and aroma. It is not presently of commercial importance, as walnuts are expensive.

BUYING AND STORAGE The oil can be purchased from various specialty shops. The crude oil has a strong, characteristic flavour and odour and is a dark brown colour. The oil should be free from rancidity and other undesirable flavours.

Store in a sealed container at room temperature and away from direct light. Solids may settle out at lower temperatures due to the natural, high-melting components present.

PREPARATION AND USE Walnut oil is used chiefly as a cooking oil or in salad dressings.

PROCESSING For use as a flavoursome cooking oil, the oil is generally recovered by milling and pressing of the walnuts. The nuts may be roasted prior to milling; this enhances the flavour of the oil and results in a darker colour.

The oil may also be solvent-extracted and refined if desired.

VARIETIES
Black walnut oil, English walnut oil, Persian walnut oil.

SEE ALSO Walnut.

HERBS AND SPICES

Each traditional food culture includes a group of herbs and spices. Although they are used in small quantities, they bring a great deal to the various dishes. They contribute to the aroma, flavour and colour of food and they often transform bland and dull food into a delicious and interesting dish.

Many local herbs were used by Europeans in medieval times. These included basil, bay, chives, dill, fennel, juniper berries, marjoram, mint, parsley, rosemary, sage, thyme and winter and summer savory.

These foods were used to mask the foul-smelling meats and other foods which people were forced to eat during the winter months when fresh food was not available: the only way to preserve food at that time was by heavy salting or drying in the home and this did little for the flavour.

Even more highly prized in Europe than the local herbs and spices were the more aromatic Eastern spices — which did a much better job of covering the flavour of spoiled food — cardamom, cinnamon, cloves, coriander, ginger, mace, nutmeg, turmeric and especially pepper.

Spices were amongst the many foods brought back to Europe from the East by Marco Polo. The search for spices was one of the main reasons for some of the great early sea voyages, including those of Columbus and Vasco da Gama. Herbs and spices were also valued for their medicinal properties and some were used in perfumes. Poems and songs extolled their virtues.

In spite of this romantic background, these foods are of little direct nutritional value. Their value lies in the pleasure they have contributed to eating. They stimulate the jaded appetite and in this way make a valuable contribution to nutrition.

Health is more than physical health: it also means mental and social well-being, which includes the enjoyment of food.

Today, international cuisine often borrows from various traditional food cultures and creates a pleasant blend of herbs and spices. For example, there is a noticeable Asian influence in many of the popular foods in restaurants and hotels today; the use of herbs and spices is important in these dishes.

Reducing the use of heavily salted foods and avoiding the addition of salt in cooking and at the table is made easier by using herbs and spices as well as lemon juice and lime juice.

The growing range of herbs and spices on the supermarket shelves and in the fruit and vegetable market indicates that many people are using these ingredients more extensively in the foods they prepare at home.

The range of herbs and spices available today is too large to be contained in one chapter of this book. The best known varieties are discussed here, with emphasis on the culinary herbs and spices. Many plants which are cooked as vegetables or used as herbal teas can also flavour food; these include chamomile, comfrey, dandelion, rose, sweet geranium, hibiscus, marigold and nasturtium. Many mixtures of spices and herbs also exist in the cuisines of the world: quatre epices, fines herbes and bouquet garni from France; curry powders and panch phora from India; shichimi from Japan; Chinese oriental and five spice powders; baharat and za'tar from the Middle East. Many of the individual ingredients of these mixtures are examined in this chapter.

Herbs are best purchased either whole or 'rubbed', which means the leaves have been broken up when removed from the stem. The process of drying a herb, either naturally by air, artificially in an oven, or by the technologically advanced freeze-drying method, removes most of the moisture to prevent bacteria and mould proliferating.

The dried herb is a shrivelled version of the fresh, its moisture reduced and yet still retaining flavour in the cells of the dried leaves. Grinding breaks these cells, releasing a pungent aroma which rapidly dissipates, however, leaving an all but tasteless powder. For this reason, avoid buying powdered herbs.

Spices, however, are usually ground in order to make them more convenient to use in cooking. They are much higher in volatile oils and therefore do not lose their flavour and aroma as rapidly as herbs.

Packaged herbs and spices will store best if packed in airtight, screw-top glass jars and stored in a cool, dark place.

Most herbs from the garden can be air-dried. Pick the herbs in the morning, after the dew has dried and before the sun has been on the leaves for too long. Large leaves should be separated from the stalk, small leaves can be left on and rubbed off after drying.

Spread the clean, dry leaves or leaf-bearing stalks in a single layer on a piece of gauze, in a dark, well-aired place. Depending upon prevailing weather conditions, the leaves should be crisp and dry within about one week. Avoid drying herbs in damp or humid weather. Alternatively the herbs can be tied up in bunches and hung in a dark, well-aired place to dry. This method is recommended for large, thick leaves such as bay leaves.

Herbs grown at home or purchased from the fruit and vegetable shop can be successfully dried in a microwave oven. Spread the clean, dry leaves in a single layer on three folds of paper towel in the microwave oven and set to cook for two minutes on High. Then feel the leaves and remove the ones that are crisp. Repeat the procedure with the remaining leaves, this time turning them over and checking them for crispness every 30 seconds. Continue to remove the crisp leaves until the remainder covers about 4 sq cm of paper towel. Discard these or allow to air-dry.

Whichever method you have used, always store the herbs in airtight, screw-top glass jars and check for crispness and aroma at least once a month. Discard if there is any sign of mould, as this indicates the leaves were not dry enough when stored, or moisture has got into them after drying.

According to their composition, some herbs and spices can be described as 'good' sources of calcium, iron, vitamin B and carotene; and chillies and parsley, for instance, are 'excellent' sources of vitamin C. Most dishes, however, contain no more than one gram of any herb or spice per serving. These ingredients are also often used in a dried form and stored for long periods. Under these conditions there is a heavy destruction of vitamins.

The actual quantity of herbs and spices used in the diet is thus insignificant compared with that of other foods: while most meals would contain only tiny amounts of herbs and spices, they could contain hundreds of grams of meat, vegetables, fruit and so on. The exceptions are recipes requiring handfuls of fresh herbs such as parsley or basil — for example, pesto sauce, which has its own entry in the chapter on Sauces, Mustards and Pastes.

It was considered unnecessary, therefore, to list the composition of every herb and spice throughout the chapter. Nutritional information is not supplied individually, but analyses are included below — with exact figures given, since the quantities are so small — of sample herbs and spices. In each case, the quantity given represents a teaspoonful of the substance. It will be noted that spices are higher in kilojoules, fat and carbohydrate than herbs, but the quantities are of course so small that this difference is of no significance in the diet.

Crumbled Bay Leaf

MAJOR NUTRIENTS

Energy	8.0 kJ	Carbohydrate	0.45 g
Protein	0.05 g	Cholesterol	0
Fat	0.05 g	Sodium	Trace

Dried Parsley

MAJOR NUTRIENTS

Energy	3 kJ	Carbohydrate	0.15 g
Protein	0.07 g	Cholesterol	0
Fat	0.01 g	Sodium	1 mg

Ground Nutmeg

MAJOR NUTRIENTS

Energy	48 kJ	Carbohydrate	1 g
Protein	0.13 g	Cholesterol	0
Fat	0.80 g	Sodium	Trace

Fresh Chopped Chives

MAJOR NUTRIENTS

Energy	1 kJ	Carbohydrate	0.04 g
Protein	0.03 g	Cholesterol	0
Fat	0.01 g	Sodium	0

Coriander Seed

MAJOR NUTRIENTS

Energy	22 kJ	Carbohydrate	0.99 g
Protein	0.22 g	Cholesterol	0
Fat	0.32 g	Sodium	1 mg

Ground Paprika

MAJOR NUTRIENTS

Energy	2.5 kJ	Carbohydrate	1.17 g
Protein	0.31 g	Cholesterol	0
Fat	0.27 g	Sodium	1 mg

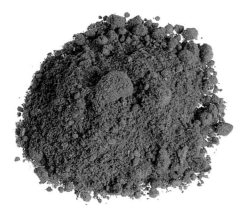

Aamchur   *Mangifera indica*

also called **Amchoor**

DESCRIPTION   An Indian seasoning powder, greenish-grey, made from finely-ground, dried, unripe mango. It has a tart, lemony taste.

ORIGIN AND HISTORY   Originally adapted in India to add a tart flavour. In the north, it may have come into use as an alternative to sumach, an ancient acidulating ingredient from China which became commonly used in the Arab world. Mangoes grow abundantly in India, and the southern Indian Tamils found the sharp flavour of unripe mango accentuated their spicy vegetarian dishes which are mostly based on bland-tasting, dried pulses and starchy vegetables.

BUYING AND STORAGE   Aamchur powder is sold commercially but it quickly loses its fresh flavour after opening, so should be kept tightly capped in a cool, dry place. Buy only in small quantities.

PREPARATION AND USE   It is used in India in some meat cooking as an acidulant and tenderiser and in southern Indian vegetarian dishes, particularly when cooking chickpeas. In the far north and Kashmir, aamchur is included in a spicy condiment mix used to dress salads and grilled meats. Sliced aamchur is also used in marinades, and the powder is added to various dishes such as samosas (fried pastries) and cooked vegetables.

2–3 tablespoons of lemon juice may be substituted for 1 teaspoon of aamchur.

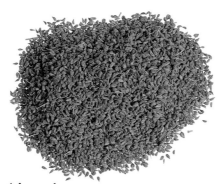

Ajwain   *Carum ajowan*

also called **Ajowan, Bishop's weed, Carom**

DESCRIPTION   Small, tear-shaped, ochre-coloured seeds from a shrub of the same family as cumin and parsley. It resembles lovage. It has a slightly harsh, strong flavour, rather like thyme.

ORIGIN AND HISTORY   Believed to be a native of India as it has been known to grow there from early times. Ajwain, or carom as it is also known, is rarely used in other cuisines. Indians are particularly fond of its distinctive flavour and a popular use, apart from flavouring curries and chutneys, is to include it in the dough used to make the crisp bread, pappadum. Medicinally, it is used in India in an infusion as a digestive, and a cure for stomach ailments.

BUYING AND STORAGE   Sold at specialist Indian food shops. In a spice jar the seeds will keep for many months. To identify them, as they rather resemble celery seeds, look for a clear ochre to light-brown colour and distinct yellow-ochre lines. When crushed with the fingers they should release a strong, fresh thymelike aroma. Do not purchase in powder form.

PREPARATION AND USE   Crush lightly to increase flavour. Use sparingly in curries, pickles and chutneys. They may be sprinkled over breads or grills. Ajwain seeds are infused to make an antibacterial drink.

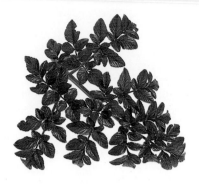

Alexanders *Smyrnium olusatrum*

also called Black lovage, Black pot-herb, Horse parsley

DESCRIPTION This sturdy herb grows 50–150 cm high, with roundish, dark-green, shiny leaves growing in groups of three. The stalks are thick and furrowed. Yellowish-green flowers bloom in summer and are followed by small black seeds.

ORIGIN AND HISTORY Native to the Mediterranean region, this herb was well known to the Greeks and Romans. It was described as a culinary herb by Pliny, Dioscorides, Columella and Galen. Its common name probably evolved when it was used by Alexander the Great. Although popular through the Middle Ages, it became unfashionable in the 18th century.

BUYING AND STORAGE Not available commercially; alexanders is best used fresh.

PREPARATION AND USE Young leaves and stems can be finely chopped and added to salads, soups and stews, while the celery-flavoured large stems can be cooked as a vegetable, served with butter or white sauce. The flower buds make an unusual salad when gently steamed for five minutes, cooled and served with an oil and vinegar dressing.

PROCESSING Young leaves can be dried in the same way as parsley and stored in an airtight container.

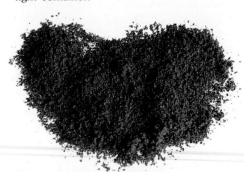

Allspice *Pimento dioica*

also called Bay rum berry, Jamaica pepper, Pimento

DESCRIPTION Allspice is the dried, unripe fruit of an evergreen tree about 10 m high, native to Jamaica. The fruit is 4–6 mm in diameter and is harvested three to four months after flowering when fully developed but still green.

ORIGIN AND HISTORY The first records occur in the journal of Christopher Columbus, and in those of early Spanish settlers to Jamaica, who exported allspice to Europe and England. Aztecs used it to flavour their national drink, chocolada. Allspice tastes like cinnamon, cloves and nutmeg, although it is not a combination.

BUYING AND STORAGE When buying ground allspice, look for a dark to medium-brown powder, packaged in an airtight container. When buying whole berries, choose smaller, rough-surfaced berries rather than plump round ones. Always store in airtight containers away from direct light.

PREPARATION AND USE Whole allspice berries are used as an ingredient of pickling spice, and in chicken or veal casseroles. Ground allspice is used in many spice blends and as a flavouring for cakes, desserts and vegetables.

PROCESSING Unripe berries are usually piled in bags or heaps for up to five days for fermentation. During this time they lose weight, and this treatment accelerates browning and drying. They are then sun-dried.

VARIETIES

Bay rum tree *(Pimento racemosa).*

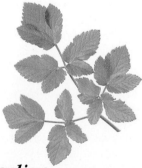

Angelica *Angelica archangelica, Archangelica officinalis*

DESCRIPTION A tall, stately herb, growing 1.5–2.5 m high, with indented, large leaves on strong, hollow stems. Umbels of tiny greenish-white flowers appear every second spring. Angelica has a delicately sweet aroma in the stems, leaves and flowers.

ORIGIN AND HISTORY Angelica is native to Lapland, Iceland and Russia and was used throughout Europe in both pagan and Christian festivals. The name comes from a legend: an angel appeared to a monk in a dream and revealed to him that angelica would cure the plague. It is an ingredient in beverages such as vermouth and chartreuse, originally prepared by monks as medicines.

BUYING AND STORAGE Most commonly available as candied or crystallised stalks. Fresh leaves can be refrigerated in water and used within three to four days.

PREPARATION AND USE The crystallised stems are used for cakes, desserts and cassata ice cream. Fresh stems can be stewed with acid fruits and added to jams and jellies. Raw stalks are delicious with cream cheese, and the young leaves in salads. Fresh roots can be cooked and eaten as a vegetable. Adds a delicate flavour to fruit punch.

PROCESSING To candy stems, cut into lengths and pour over them a boiling solution of 600 mL water and 125 g salt. Cover. Leave for 24 hours. Drain and peel. Make a syrup of 750 g sugar and 750 mL water, boil 10 minutes, add angelica for 20 minutes. Drain for four days. Boil again for 20 minutes in same syrup. Cool in syrup, drain three to four days. Strew well with sugar and store in an airtight container.

VARIETIES

A. pachycarpa.

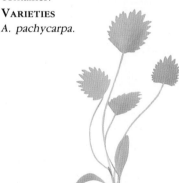

Anise *Pimpinella anisum*

also called Aniseed

DESCRIPTION Anise is a sun-loving annual plant, about 50 cm tall, with feathery, serrated leaves and delicate umbels of creamy-white flowers. The seeds are light brown, oval, and have a strong liquorice taste.

ORIGIN AND HISTORY Anise was mentioned in the Bible, and used in Roman times to flavour cakes served at the end of a rich meal to assist digestion. It is still used frequently in Europe, particularly in Germany and Austria, to flavour cakes and soups. Traditionally, anise has been used in the treatment of stubborn coughs. It is native to the Middle East and has been grown there for thousands of years. Main suppliers to the world are still India, Spain, North Africa and Italy.

BUYING AND STORAGE As anise seeds

can lose their pungency, buy in small quantities and keep in airtight glass jars away from direct sunlight.

PREPARATION AND USE Anise is famous for its use in drinks such as pernod, anisette and ouzo, and for the universally loved aniseed sweets. It can be used as a seed topping for crusty bread or added to vegetables, e g steamed carrots tossed in honey and aniseeds just before serving.

PROCESSING The seeds are threshed and dried in either outdoor trays or ovens, and turn greyish-brown. They are also distilled to yield a fragrant volatile oil for medicinal and commercial products.

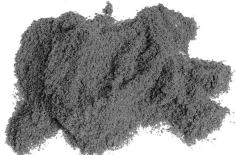

Annatto Bixa orellana

also called **Achiote, Achuete, Biji, Latkhan, Roucou, Urucu**

DESCRIPTION Annatto comes from a 10 m tall tree with heart-shaped leaves and prickly fruit pods containing slightly peppery, deep red, triangular seeds.

ORIGIN AND HISTORY Native to tropical America and the East and West Indies, annatto was brought to the Philippines by 17th century Spanish colonists. It is now widely cultivated in Asia and Africa, where it is used as an orange-red dye for food and fabric. As a spice it is known in a number of tropical countries. In the Yucatan, for instance, it is used in various pastes such as recado colorado and adobo.

BUYING AND STORAGE Annatto seeds are only generally available in specialty shops, in particular those stocking Asian or West Indian foods. The hard seeds store easily and retain their flavour and colouring attributes for two to three years when stored in airtight containers.

PREPARATION AND USE The slightly peppery taste goes well with fish, rice and vegetables. Annatto is used in the Philippines in pipian, a traditional meal of chicken and pork cubes in a spicy sauce. It is used in Jamaica in a sauce for salt cod and ackee. The characteristic colour and spicy flavour in many Mexican foods comes from annatto seeds, and

in the West it is used as a colouring agent for smoked fish and the red rinds of cheeses.

In Asian cooking annatto is used to give roast and preserved meats a characteristic colour, thought, particularly by the Chinese, to be lucky. It features on roast pork and such exotica as boiled pigs' snouts, ears and tails.

PROCESSING The recent trend for food manufacturers to use natural colourings instead of artificial colours has rekindled interest in spices such as annatto. The artificial yellow colour tartrazine (102), which causes allergic reactions in certain people, has been replaced by some manufacturers with annatto extracts (160b).

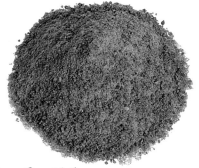

Asafoetida Ferula asafoetida

also called **Asefetida, Devil's dung, Ferule perisque, Giant fennel, Heeng, Hing, Ling, Perunkaya, Sheingho, Stinking gum, Teufelsdreck**

DESCRIPTION An edible Indian seasoning powder, obtained from the milky resin in the stems and roots of two varieties of giant fennels (similar to well-known garden fennel but not related). These tall, evil-smelling perennials have thick roots, stout, branched stems with long leaves and greenish-yellow flowers. The unpleasant smell does not transfer to food.

ORIGIN AND HISTORY Native to central and western Asia, asafoetida was known in ancient times as 'food of the gods'. The Romans used it for its medicinal purpose as an anti-flatulent, for which it is still used today. In the second century AD, it was used as a drug, and a tax was levied on it in Alexandria. Arab physicians of the Middle Ages called it hiltit. It was brought to India from the north and west and was used in many vegetarian dishes.

BUYING AND STORAGE This pungent resinous gum is sold in solid, waxlike pieces or in powder form. Store in an airtight container in a cool, dry cupboard and it will retain its aroma for many months.

PREPARATION AND USE Lump asafoetida can be moistened and attached to the inside of

the saucepan lid to release flavour during cooking. It can also be added in minute amounts directly to a braised or curried dish. It complements fish, and brings out the flavour in stews, gravies or sauces. In Iran and Afghanistan the leaves and stems are used as a vegetable. It features rarely in French cuisine and is used in Indian sauces, pickles and Worcestershire sauce.

PROCESSING The plant is cut close to the roots and the milky, white gum extracted, poured onto trays and dried in the sun. It turns a reddish-brown with a crystalline appearance. It is then broken into small pellets or ground to a powder. The dreadful fetid smell disappears on cooking.

VARIETIES
F. narthex.

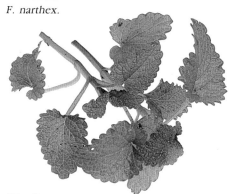

Balm Melissa officinalis

also called **Common balm, Lemon balm**

DESCRIPTION Balm is a delicately lemon-scented perennial with soft, wrinkled foliage. Although related to mint, it has a small root system and grows in a compact, leafy clump 30–80 cm tall. Taller flower stalks in summer bear clusters of tiny white blooms.

ORIGIN AND HISTORY Native to southern Europe, it later spread to England, North America and Asia. The Latin name *Melissa* means bee, which reflects the early association of bees with balm. Bee hives have been rubbed with balm for centuries to prevent bees from swarming. Paracelsus called balm 'the elixir of life', and John Evelyn, the noted English herbalist, said, 'Balm is sovereign for the brain, strengthening the memory and powerfully chasing away the melancholy.' 'Balm' is an abbreviation of 'balsam', because of its sweet aroma.

BUYING AND STORAGE Balm is best used fresh, as its aroma and food value can deteriorate after drying. It should have firm stems and leaves. Leaves can be stored in water in the refrigerator and used within two to three days.

PREPARATION AND USE The fresh balm

leaves can be used in fruit drinks, fruit salad and milk puddings. In hot weather, a balm leaf can be added to a pot of tea for extra refreshment. Mix chopped balm with yoghurt for a curry accompaniment or salad dressing. It is an ingredient of the liqueurs bénédictine and chartreuse.

PROCESSING Cut stalks and hang in bunches, or lay on wire racks in an airy, shady place. When leaves are crisp-dry, strip from stalks and store in airtight containers.

VARIETIES
Variegated balm (*M. officinalis variegata*).

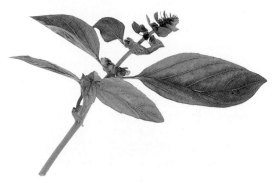

Basil *Ocimum basilicum*

also called **Sweet basil**

DESCRIPTION Sweet basil is an annual bush growing to 75 cm with curved, plump-looking, veined leaves and a sweet, pungent flavour. Bush basil is small, approximately 30 cm high, of compact shape with small, pointed leaves. Both varieties are excellent for culinary use and have small, white-lipped flowers in autumn.

ORIGIN AND HISTORY The plant's name is derived from 'basilikon phyton', Greek for 'kingly herb'. In India, tulsi (*O. sanctum*) was cherished as a sacred herb. Also known in ancient Egypt, Greece and Rome, it was introduced to Europe in the 16th century, and cultivated by monks and farmers as a popular addition to food.

BUYING AND STORAGE Commercially dried basil is generally sweet basil. Buy in an airtight glass jar, preferably pieces of leaf rather than powdered, for best flavour. When buying fresh basil, store in water in the refrigerator and drain well before use. Use within two to three days.

PREPARATION AND USE Whole leaves can be used as garnish for pasta dishes, tomato soup or sorbet. Use chopped with tomato, tomato juice, zucchini, squash or spinach, in salads, herb vinegar or herb butter.

PROCESSING Basil should be harvested in early autumn, before flowering and before it

starts to die off. (In tropical climates it grows all year and easily self-sows.) Cut branches for drying, strip off leaves and dry on wire mesh or paper in an airy, shady place. If the leaves go black while microwave drying, they will not dry properly. To dry as quickly as possible, cover a single layer of leaves with microwave paper, using weights on the corners to keep it close to leaves. Microwave on High for two to three minutes. When crisp-dry, store in airtight container. Fresh leaves can be chopped and frozen in blocks of cooking oil.

VARIETIES
Oriental basil: includes purple, hairy and Thai basil — all species of *Ocimum*, like sweet basil. Basil is an important ingredient in the cuisines of Thailand, Laos and Vietnam.

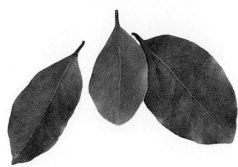

Bay Leaf *Laurus nobilis*

DESCRIPTION The bay is a dense, evergreen tree growing to 15 m. It is very slow-growing and is popular as a decorative potted tree. Leaves are strong and dark green, with glossy top sides, usually 4–8 cm long. The tree has insignificant creamy-yellow flowers in spring and summer.

ORIGIN AND HISTORY The Latin name of the bay tree comes from laurus meaning laurel, and nobilis meaning famous. Laurel wreaths of bay leaves were used to crown heroes and statesmen. The tree is native to Mediterranean countries and for centuries was used as a strewing herb for its fresh aroma and antiseptic qualities. In 1629 the herbalist John Parkinson wrote that Augustus Caesar wore a garland of bryony and bays to protect himself from lightning. He also believed that bay could be used 'to procure warmth, comfort and strength to the limmes of men and women by bathings and anoyntings out and by drinks inwards'.

BUYING AND STORAGE Bay leaves can be picked straight from the tree and used fresh. If buying dried leaves, look for good colour and unbroken leaves, and store in an airtight container away from direct light. Fresh sprays of leaves can be dried by hanging upside-down in a dark, airy place until crisp. Bay

leaves dry successfully in a microwave, by placing the dry leaves on paper towel and cooking on High for approximately ten minutes, until crisp.

PREPARATION AND USE The bay leaf is an important part of a bouquet garni, and one or two leaves flavour stocks, casseroles, soups and marinades. The leaf is usually removed before serving. They are also used in pot pourri, milk puddings, pot roasts, corned beef and pickled pork.

PROCESSING Bay leaves are still harvested by hand and air-dried as they have been for centuries. Most commercially produced dried bay leaves come from Turkey.

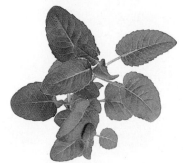

Bergamot *Monarda didyma*

also called **Bee balm, Red bergamot**

DESCRIPTION Bergamot is a perennial plant growing to 1.2 m. The oval 8–15 cm leaves are attached in pairs to a square stem. Showy tubular red flowers bloom in late summer, 4–5 cm long and full of nectar. It has a matted, spreading root system. The flowers and leaves have an orange perfume, which is why this plant is named after the bergamot orange.

ORIGIN AND HISTORY Bergamot is native to North America, and was named after 16th century botanist Nicholas Monardes. The leaves were used extensively by Oswego Indians and became familiar to American settlers, who used them as a substitute for Indian tea after the Boston Tea Party of 1773. Its subtle flavour is commonly associated with Earl Grey tea. Oil of bergamot is distilled not from this herb, but from the bergamot orange.

BUYING AND STORAGE Bergamot is most likely to be found in dried form as a herbal tea. Store in an airtight container. If fresh leaves or flowers are available, store in water for use the same day, or chop and freeze in water iceblocks.

PREPARATION AND USE Leaves can be used as a savoury herb in meatloaf, vegetarian dishes, pork and veal. Add to sweet dishes such as fruit salad and ices in the same way as mint. Flowers can be gently shredded and tossed over a green salad.

PROCESSING Harvest foliage and flowers in late summer when plant is in full bloom, and quickly air-dry on a wire rack or in a net-sling in a warm, shady place, or microwave. Store in an airtight container as soon as crisp-dry.

VARIETIES
Oswego tea, White bergamot (*M. citriodora*), Wild or Purple bergamot (*M. fistulosa*).

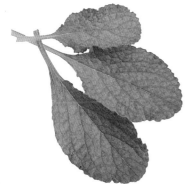

Borage *Borago officinalis*

DESCRIPTION This annual herb grows to 90 cm, with thick, soft stems and large, rough leaves, both covered in fine, bristly hairs. Star-shaped, vivid-blue drooping flowers cluster on soft racemes. The blooms are full of nectar and attractive to bees.

ORIGIN AND HISTORY Originally from Aleppo in the Middle East, borage has adapted easily to wherever it was introduced. Most historical references to borage mention its ability to make people merry, possibly because of its own merits, or because it was widely used as an addition to alcoholic drinks!

BUYING AND STORAGE Borage is not usually found in the marketplace. However, if you do find leaves available, purchase only the very young and tender leaves, otherwise the hairs will be prickly and unpleasant to eat. Store as for fresh vegetables and use within one to two days.

PREPARATION AND USE Borage flowers can be crystallised, or dipped in egg white then caster sugar for use as a garnish for fruit salads and desserts. Add the finely shredded, cucumber-flavoured young leaves to salads, soups and herb sandwiches, or dip whole leaves into light batter and fry.

PROCESSING Flowers can be preserved by crystallising or by freezing in iceblocks (three or four per cube) for adding to drinks. Leaves can be air-dried in the shade or dried in a microwave in a single layer. Cook on High for one minute at a time until leaves are crisp-dry. Store in an airtight container.

VARIETIES
White-flowering borage.

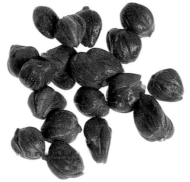

Capers *Capparis spinosa*

DESCRIPTION The caper bush is a prickly, sprawling plant 1 m high with tough, roundish, dark leaves. Pretty pink or white single flowers with long, whiskery stamens bloom and die in 24 hours. The edible capers are the unopened flower buds. Their strong, aromatic flavour is due to the capric acid, which is enhanced by pickling.

ORIGIN AND HISTORY Capers are native to the barren, dry areas of the Mediterranean, and were mentioned in the writings of Dioscorides, the Greek physician. The flower buds, pickled in wine vinegar, have been used as a condiment for centuries.

BUYING AND STORAGE Capers are always sold as a processed condiment in pickling liquid. Once opened, they should be kept refrigerated and not allowed to dry out.

PREPARATION AND USE The popular uses include addition to sauces and vinaigrettes, soft cheeses, in salads, with cooked vegetables, chicken, fish and lamb. Pickled green nasturtium seeds can be used as a substitute for capers.

PROCESSING The caper flower opens with the rising sun, therefore the buds must be harvested between daybreak and sunrise. They are wilted in the air for one day, then pickled in strong, salted, white vinegar, which allows the capric acid to develop.

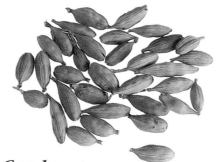

Cardamom *Elettaria cardamomum*

also called **Cardamom pods, Cardamom seeds**

DESCRIPTION A perennial plant with branched, subterranean rhizomes from which arise several erect, leafy shoots. There is a stout horizontal rhizome with numerous fibrous roots in the surface layer. Leafy shoots, 2–5 m tall, are borne in thick clumps. The leaves are long and narrow, dark green, smooth on top and paler beneath. The flowering stems spread horizontally near the ground and bear small, loose, elongated flower clusters on stalks. The fruits (cardamom pods) are thin-skinned oval capsules, beige to yellow in colour and about 1 cm long, containing 15 to 20 dark-brown, angled seeds, with a pungent, spicy, sweet flavour and an aroma like eucalyptus.

ORIGIN AND HISTORY Cardamom occurs wild in the evergreen monsoon forests of the Western Ghats in southern India and Sri Lanka. It was not cultivated until 1800. Cardamom was an article of Greek trade during the 4th century BC, and by the 1st century AD, Rome was importing substantial quantities of cardamom from India. It is mentioned by Dioscorides in his *Materia Medica* as a popular flavouring and digestive spice.

BUYING AND STORAGE The cardamom should be bought when still in the pod. The kiln-dried, greener pods are preferred in the Middle East, but this has little bearing on flavour. Store the pods in an airtight, screw-top glass jar and only remove the seeds from the pod just before using.

PREPARATION AND USE Remove seeds from the pod and crush with a rolling pin or grind in a mortar and pestle to release flavour and aroma. Cardamom is used by the Scandinavians in Danish pastries and Indians use it to flavour coffee, curries and cakes. It adds a fresh, appealing flavour to sweet potatoes, pumpkin, squash, carrots, apple and pumpkin pies, fruit sauces, biscuits, liver pâtés, beef, lamb, pork, chicken and veal dishes. Cardamom is used commercially in seasonings for smallgoods and in ice cream flavourings, confectionery, baked goods, chewing gums and some alcoholic beverages.

PROCESSING Cardamom pods are picked just before they are ripe as fully ripe pods tend to split on drying and do not give such a good colour. Freshly picked green cardamoms are washed and the stalks are clipped off. They are spread on trays in a kiln or curing room, or sun-dried. White cardamom pods have been bleached with hydrogen peroxide or sulphur dioxide to create a uniform appearance.

VARIETIES
Bastard cardamom (*Amomum xanthioides*), Bengal cardamom (*A. aromaticum*), brown or large cardamom (*A. cardamomum*),

Cambodian cardamom (*A. drervanh*), green cardamom (*E. cardamomom*), greater Indian or Nepal cardamom (*A. subulatum*), Korarima cardamom (*A. kararima*), Madagascar cardamom (*A. angustifolium*), round cardamom (*A. kepulaga*) winged Java cardamom (*A. maximum*).

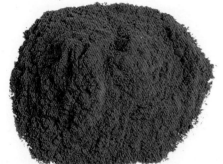

Cassia *Cinnamomum cassia*

also called **Bastard cinnamon, Cassia bark**

DESCRIPTION Not to be confused with flowering cassia, which is a legume, cassia is one of over 250 varieties of camphor laurels, fragrant evergreen trees with flame-coloured spring growth. The bark separates easily from the trunk, and is regarded as a substitute for cinnamon. Dried, unripe fruits also taste of cinnamon.

ORIGIN AND HISTORY The earliest record of cassia (kwei) was in Chinese literature of the 4th century BC, when it was regarded as the Tree of Life. Also mentioned in the Bible, it was a valuable commodity sold to the Greeks and Romans by Arab traders. The dried cassia buds were used in the Middle Ages in the preparation of a spiced wine called hippocras. Modern uses include pot pourri, confectionery and food manufacture.

BUYING AND STORAGE Whole cassia quills (curls of dried bark) should be 20–40 cm long, varying from light to dark reddish-brown with patches of grey depending on the country of origin. Freshness is indicated by a pungent, non-musty aroma. Ground cassia should be purchased in an airtight container and kept away from direct light.

PREPARATION AND USE As for cinnamon. Quills go in stews, curries, vegetables, fruit salads and percolated coffee. Ground cassia is added to cakes, pastries, chocolate, fruit coulis, and sweet snacks. Commercially, the powder, oil and oleoresin from cassia are used in manufacture of perfumes, confectionery, beverages, chewing gum, cakes, smallgoods and pharmaceuticals. It is widely used in the Middle East and Greece as a less expensive cinnamon substitute, and because the bark is firmer, it is preferred for use in dishes as it does not break up.

VARIETIES
Black cinnamon, China cassia (*C. aromaticum*), India cassia (*C. tamala*), Indonesia cassia (*C. sintok*), Java or Batavia cassia, also cassia vera or Padang cinnamon.

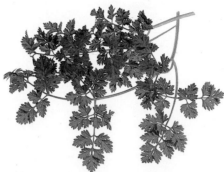

Chervil *Anthriscus cerefolium*

DESCRIPTION This small (30 cm) biennial herb has vivid green, soft ferny leaves, similar in structure to parsley leaves. They taste mildly of aniseed and pepper. White flowers in umbrella-shaped clusters bloom in summer. Chervil is sometimes referred to as 'gourmet's parsley'.

ORIGIN AND HISTORY Native to eastern Europe. In the first century AD, Pliny wrote of chervil as a seasoning and a cure for hiccoughs, also as a food used by the Syrians. It is thought to hasten the healing of bruises when used as a poultice. It was introduced to France and England by the Romans, and to Brazil in 1647 by the Spanish. It is a popular culinary herb in France, where it is an important ingredient in fines herbes.

BUYING AND STORAGE Dried chervil is hard to find commercially so it is best to use fresh. Store fresh sprays of leaves immersed in water in the refrigerator and use within five days.

PREPARATION AND USE Chervil is combined in equal proportion with chives, tarragon and parsley for fines herbes. Add chervil only for last five to ten minutes of cooking to preserve its delicate flavour. Use in scrambled eggs, omelettes, mashed potatoes, salads, sandwiches, and with poultry and fish. Add chopped leaves to soups and mornays, or use a whole spray of leaves as a garnish.

PROCESSING Chervil can be air-dried away from direct light on a wire rack or paper, or microwaved. When crisp-dry, store in an airtight container away from direct light.

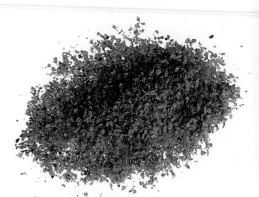

Chilli Pepper *Capsicum annuum, C. frutescens*

also called **Cayenne, Red pepper, Chilitepines, Ginnie pepper**

DESCRIPTION Chilli or cayenne pepper is one of many capsicum varieties. It is a perennial shrub growing to 2 m. The drooping pods, varying in length from a few millimetres up to 15 cm, are conical and grow on smooth, erect stems with oblong leaves. The most pungent varieties are smaller, and are generally referred to as chillies. They are dark to bright red with numerous yellow seeds. The aroma is sweet, warm and peppery at first, becoming acrid and irritating if inhaled for too long. The flavour is intensely pungent, biting hot, and can leave a lingering burning sensation deep in the throat. It is thought to be a very strong gastric stimulant.

ORIGIN AND HISTORY All species of capsicum are of American origin, and were unknown in Europe before 1494, when Chanca, Christopher Columbus's physician, described them. By 1650, they were widely cultivated as a condiment throughout Europe, Africa and Asia. There are now many hybrids and considerable variation exists in growth habit, size, colour, shape, flavour and pungency.

BUYING AND STORAGE Whole peppers can be bought fresh. As a general rule, the smaller the fruit, the hotter and more pungent the flavour. Dried chillies are sold whole or ground. Cayenne pepper is generally a blend of various grades of *C. frutescens*, mixed to achieve a uniform, desired colour and flavour. Chilli powder is traditionally a blend of several varieties of capsicums and other herbs and spices, one of the better-known styles being Mexican chilli powder. Keep in airtight containers in a cool, dark place.

PREPARATION AND USE Care should be taken when handling fresh chilli peppers, as they can cause burning irritation to the skin and eyes. Wash hands thoroughly immediately after preparation. Chilli and cayenne pepper are used in Mexican, Italian, Indian and oriental dishes to add a pungent taste, as in chilli con carne, Szechuan dishes, Thai soups and chilli prawns. Chilli adds heat to curry powder and is an excellent condiment for those who like their food hot and spicy.

PROCESSING Chilli peppers must be thoroughly dried if they are to be stored, as they are prone to mould. When the peppers are ground, the colour varies depending upon the quantity of yellow seeds within the pod.

VARIETIES

Bird pepper *(C. annuum minimum), C. chinense, C. pendulum, C. pubescens,* Tabasco pepper or Bird's eye chilli *(C. frutescens).*

Ancho Pepper A large, brown, heart-shaped chilli that is wrinkled and deep reddish-brown. This is probably the chilli most commonly used in Mexico. The flavour ranges from mild to piquant. Available only in specialist greengrocers, the chilli will dry out with age and should be used soon after purchase. Lightly toasted and torn into small pieces, the ancho pepper is used as table sauce, or relish, though it is more often ground to make the base of a cooked sauce.

Mulato Pepper A large, relatively pungent chilli, popular in Latin America. It is brownish black when dried with a wrinkled, rather tough skin. The flavour is slightly sweet. Possibly only available if home-grown as there is little demand for many of the chilli varieties. Keeps for a short time in the refrigerator. Prepare as fresh chilli. Adds a hot flavour to stews and soups.

Pasilla Pepper (*Chili negro*) A thin, 17 cm long brownish-black chilli, wrinkled in appearance. It is not too hot and has a very piquant and rich-tasting flavour. Not readily available and may have to be home-grown. Keeps as fresh chilli. Ground dry for table sauce or toasted and cooked as a sauce to eat with seafood.

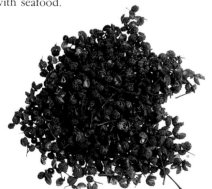

Chinese pepper Xanthoxylum piperitum

also called Fagara, Sansho, Szechuan pepper

DESCRIPTION Small red-brown, aromatic seeds resembling pale black peppercorns. They have a peppery-lemony flavour and none of the heat associated with black pepper.

ORIGIN AND HISTORY The deciduous, prickly ash tree, known also as the Japanese sansho or Chinese chiao, is native to China. The trees grow to 3.5 m and have thorn-bearing branches which bear small pods of yellowish-orange. The seeds are used as an aromatic spice. There are several varieties of the plant, which is of a group called fagara, given local names such as ch'in chiao and shu chiao. When black peppercorns were first introduced to China they were called hu chiao, because of their similarity to the chiao of China. However, apart from a short period in the 6th century when it replaced fagara as the main spice, black pepper was never completely accepted, white pepper being preferred and fairly widely used. During the first few centuries AD in China, fagara was taken in tea with clotted cream in the regions of Chekiang and Fukien.

BUYING AND STORAGE The pepper is sold in convenient shaker jars and will keep on a cool, dry shelf, if properly sealed, for up to a year.

PREPARATION AND USE The spice is sprinkled as a condiment or served as a dip to add an interesting flavour. When sprinkled on grilled chicken and eel dishes, it effectively masks the fatty taste.

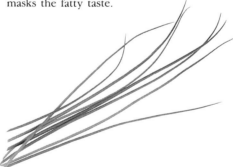

Chives Allium schoenoprasum

also called Onion chives, Rush leeks

DESCRIPTION The chive is a small relative of the onion and garlic. Onion chives resemble a clump of fine grass when young, but as they mature to a height of 30 cm, the leaves become tubular and hollow, with a distinct flavour and aroma of onion. Round pompoms of mauve flowers appear in summer. Garlic chives have flat leaves like blades of grass, and a mild garlic flavour and aroma. Clusters of small white flowers grow on tough stems unsuitable for eating.

ORIGIN AND HISTORY The Chinese are said to have used chives in about 3000 BC, and they were known in the Mediterranean lands before Christian times. Chives were listed by Emperor Charlemagne in AD 812 as one of 70 herbs in his garden. Mostly grown domestically until fairly recently, when the freeze drying method made them viable in commercial applications.

BUYING AND STORAGE Dried chives should have a bright green appearance and be stored away from light to prevent fading and loss of flavour. Fresh chives can be bought in bunches and stored immersed in water for use within four to five days, or chopped and frozen in water iceblocks for longer-term use.

PREPARATION AND USE The mild onion or garlic flavour of chives makes them a good addition to sauces, mashed potatoes, omelettes, scrambled eggs, salads, cream cheese, cottage cheese and savoury dips. Their tender texture does not take well to prolonged cooking. Chives are mixed in equal quantity with chervil, tarragon and parsley to make the fines herbes blend.

PROCESSING Fresh chives can be cut into 1 cm lengths and microwaved on a paper towel. For ½ a cup of chopped chives, microwave on High for at least five minutes, then 30 seconds at a time until dry.

VARIETIES

Garlic or Chinese chives *(A. tuberosum),* giant chive, sometimes known as bok choy.

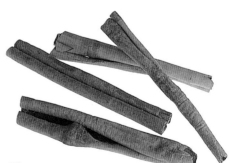

Cinnamon Cinnamomum zeylanicum

DESCRIPTION This bushy evergreen tree grows to 10 m and has thick, grey bark, strong, low-set branches, speckled greeny-orange young shoots and leathery, shiny green leaves. Cinnamon bark is the dried aromatic inner bark of the shoots. Commercially grown trees are generally 2 m tall and are bushier as a result of being cut back regularly to obtain more branches from which the bark can be cut.

ORIGIN AND HISTORY This is native to Sri Lanka, which still produces the largest quantity and best quality in the world. Cinnamon was one of the first spices to be sought after by most 15th and 16th century explorations.

BUYING AND STORAGE Whole quills of about 1 cm diameter and 10 cm length should be tightly curled, concentric layers of bark no thicker than 0.5 mm, dark reddish-brown in colour and with a mild fragrant perfume and sweet aromatic taste. The thinnest bark is the best quality. When ground, the pungency of cinnamon is greater. However, as it loses its aroma more quickly, it must then be stored in an airtight screw-top glass jar.

PREPARATION AND USE Whole quills can be used to spice coffee, mulled wine and stewed fruit. It is convenient to use as powder and gives liveliness to milk puddings, chutneys and cakes. It spices vegetables such as carrot, pumpkin and zucchini. Cinnamon is a traditional ingredient in mixed spice and curry powder.

PROCESSING The cut stems are peeled by stripping the bark and preparing quills 1 m in length from the inner bark. They are then assembled into compound quills or pipes which are rolled by hand to press the outside edges together before drying in the shade. Broken and uneven pieces are used in grinding while the best quality quills are sold whole.

SEE ALSO Cassia.

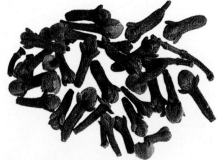

Cloves *Eugenia caryophyllata*

DESCRIPTION Whole cloves are the dried, unopened flower buds of a small, aromatic, evergreen tree reaching 12–15 m in height with dense foliage. The cloves are borne in clusters of 10 to 15 and are picked when they begin to turn red at the base. Their colour darkens after drying in the sun. Cloves have an aroma that is spicy, peppery, sweet, fruity, woody and musty, and a spicy, fruity, astringent and slightly bitter flavour with a warm, numbing effect.

ORIGIN AND HISTORY The plant is a native to the Moluccas and was introduced to China around 200 BC. Centuries before Christ,

courtiers in the presence of their emperors sucked cloves to perfume their breath. The name clove is derived from the Latin word clavus, meaning nail, which the clove resembles.

BUYING AND STORAGE Whole cloves should be uniform in size, free from stems and dark brown with a lighter top to the bud, which is intact in best quality cloves. Ground cloves lose their aroma and flavour rapidly and must be stored in airtight, screw-top glass jars.

PREPARATION AND USE Whole cloves can be used with stewed fruit, in pickles, stuck into leg ham, in percolated coffee, and are the essential component of a fruit pomander. Ground cloves used sparingly add a spicy, fresh flavour to pastries, cakes, preserves, milk puddings, various sauces and vegetable dishes.

PROCESSING Essential oil extracted from the clove buds, stems and leaves is used commercially in the manufacture of baked goods, sauces and other condiments, smallgoods, chewing gums, mouthwashes, germicides and perfumes.

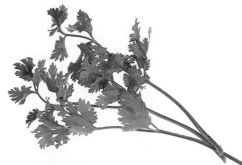

Coriander *Coriandrum sativum*

also called *Chinese parsley, Cilantro, Daun ketumber, Hara dhania, Pak chee, Yuan sai*

DESCRIPTION Coriander is an annual plant growing to 1 m, with erect stems and serrated, dark-green leaves, resembling Italian parsley. It has pink-tinged, lacy flowers and symmetrical seed clusters, from which the seeds fall when ripe. The seeds are round, bleached looking, and have an agreeable spicy flavour and fragrance when dried.

ORIGIN AND HISTORY Coriander is native to the Mediterranean region and was used in Egypt as early as 1550 BC and is referred to in the Bible and Sanskrit literature. The name coriandrum, used by Pliny, is derived from koros, meaning bug, in reference to the fetid smell of the leaves and unripe seeds. Coriander was introduced into England by the Romans and it was one of the first herbs to be grown in America by the col-

onists, having been introduced into Massachusetts before 1670.

BUYING AND STORAGE Coriander leaves are sometimes sold as Chinese parsley or cilantro, and if dried should be dark green, like parsley. The seeds can be bought whole or ground. Whole seeds store easily and retain their flavour. Ground coriander loses its aroma quickly and should be either crushed in a mortar and pestle just before using, or stored in an airtight, screw-top glass jar.

PREPARATION AND USE Leaves have a strong insectlike aroma. However, used sparingly, they add a spicy fragrance and exotic freshness to oriental food, especially Thai and Indian cuisine, where the root is also cooked. Coriander seeds are used more frequently (generally ground), to flavour fish, poultry and meat dishes. It is a useful spice in cakes, gingerbread, biscuits, pastries, bread, and sprinkled over apples, pears and peaches while baking. It is an important ingredient in curry powder and mixed spice. Chinese cooks use fresh coriander mainly as a decorative, edible garnish on seafood and other meat dishes, but also to give a unique flavour to stuffings, soups and braised dishes. It should be used with discretion. Thai cooks use the entire plant — leaves as a garnish and in salads; roots and stems in curry sauces and soups. Fresh coriander is also used in Indian cooking, giving a bright green colour and fresh taste to some curry sauces. Throughout Southeast Asia it is probably the most commonly used garnish.

PROCESSING The leaves may be picked at any time during the growing period. Spread leaf sprays on sieves in a warm, airy place, and when crisp, crumble the leaves from their stalks. They may also be microwaved. To harvest the seeds, cut off all the heads when they are about to drop, and dry in the shade on sheets of paper. Store in airtight containers.

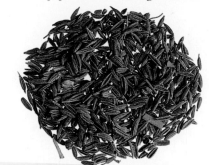

Cumin *Cuminum cyminum*

also called *Cumin seed*

DESCRIPTION A small annual plant growing to 60 cm, cumin has a slender, branched stem, the leaves divided into long narrow segments like fennel, but smaller and deep green in colour. The seed is yellowish-brown with a short stem and oblong shape, resembling caraway seed. The aroma is strong and distinctive like caraway and the taste is warm, spicy, aromatic and currylike.

ORIGIN AND HISTORY Cumin is native to the Mediterranean region. It was well known to ancient civilisations as early as 5000 BC. It was used by the Egyptians for mummifying the bodies of their kings. Among ancient Greeks, cumin was the symbol of greed and Roman misers were said to have eaten it. It is referred to in the Bible in both Old and New Testaments. In the first century, Pliny referred to cumin as the best appetiser of all the condiments. It is also said to aid digestion.

BUYING AND STORAGE Whole seeds should be clean and uniform in appearance. Ground cumin should have an oily feel and be a khaki shade. After grinding, cumin will lose its flavour very rapidly and some forms of grinding destroy much of the aroma. Store in airtight, screw-top glass jars in a cool, dark place.

PREPARATION AND USE Use whole on rye bread, in pickles, chutney, rice, cabbage and bean dishes. Ground cumin is an essential ingredient in curry powder, Mexican chilli powder and Indian vegetable dishes. Whole cumin seeds are mixed with the whole seeds of black mustard, black cumin, fenugreek and fennel to make the Indian seasoning panch phora.

PROCESSING Place seeds, gathered when the plant has finished flowering, on clean paper in a dark, warm, well-aired place. When dry (about five days) store in an airtight, screw-top glass jar. For best results, grind in a mortar and pestle just before using.

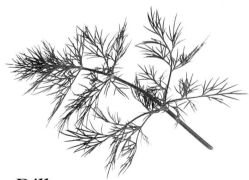

Dill *Anethum graveolens*
also called **Dill seed, Green dill**

DESCRIPTION A fragrant annual, approximately 1 m tall, it has ferny, deep-green leaves, and umbels of lacy, yellow flowers, usually from a single stalk. Similar to fennel but smaller.

ORIGIN AND HISTORY Native to Mediterranean countries and southern Russia, dill is mentioned in old Egyptian texts, Greek and Roman literature and in the Bible, also in herbals of the Middle Ages for ailments such as flatulence and colic. The name is derived from the Norse dilla meaning to lull, indicating its soothing qualities. It was considered a charm against witchcraft in the Middle Ages.

BUYING AND STORAGE Fresh dill leaves should have a good colour, although because of their softness, they will droop. Store in the refrigerator in a bowl of water or wrapped in tissue paper or foil, and use within two days. Dried seeds and green dill should be bought in airtight glass containers and stored away from direct light.

PREPARATION AND USE Fresh or dried, green dill leaves can be used to garnish soups and salads. Add to cooked seafood and to herb butter and vinegar. Dill seeds are used to make chutneys, vinegar and dill pickles (pickled cucumbers), are added to salads and soups, and can be infused to make dill water or 'gripe water' for babies.

PROCESSING Green dill can be air-dried using a net-sling or gauze to hang the leaves in a dry, airy place away from sunlight. Alternatively, spread pieces of dill (without the main stem) on paper towel and microwave on High for two minutes. Continue in shorter bursts until it is crisp. To dry seeds, allow to ripen on the plant after flowers finish, then the seeds can be shaken out onto a sheet of paper, dried and stored.

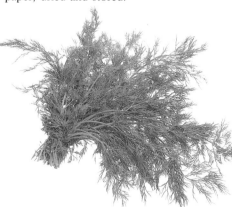

Fennel *Foeniculum vulgare*
also called **Fennel bulb, Fennel leaves, Fennel seed, Fennel stems**

DESCRIPTION Perennial sweet fennel grows tall and feathery to 1.2 m with erect stalks bearing finely divided green leaves. In early autumn it is a mass of golden flowers. The seeds are greenish-yellow-brown, up to 1 cm long, slightly oval with ridges. The flavour is like liquorice, sweet with a slightly bitter aftertaste. The lower-growing Florence fennel is similar and in more common usage.

ORIGIN AND HISTORY The fennel plant is native to southern Europe and Asia Minor. Fennel was a symbol of success in ancient Greece and was called marathon, in reference to the famous battle ground on which the Greeks gained a glorious victory over the Persians in 490 BC. It is mentioned in the early Anglo-Saxon herbals, particularly for digestive complaints.

BUYING AND STORAGE The delicacy of fennel leaves makes them unsuitable for air-drying. However, they retain their colour and flavour well with microwave drying. Fennel should be picked fresh for use the same day or chopped and frozen in water iceblocks. Fennel seeds should be pale yellow and not show signs of infestation. Ground fennel seeds will lose their flavour quickly unless stored in airtight, screw-top glass jars.

PREPARATION AND USE Florence fennel is the best variety for culinary use. The seeds go into breads and cakes, on top of rolls and fruit tarts, and in cheese mixtures and spreads. The leaves are a traditional accompaniment to fish and are used in salads, dressings and sauces. The broad white stems and bulbous base should be sliced thinly and added to green salads and can be cooked as a vegetable. Whole fennel seeds are blended with the whole seeds of black mustard, black cumin, cumin, and fenugreek to make the Indian seasoning panch phora.

PROCESSING Harvest seeds after flowering. Leaves and stems should be picked fresh. When the base of Florence fennel begins to swell, cultivate and feed the soil. Prior to harvesting the bulbous root, give the plant plenty of moisture.

VARIETIES
Bronze fennel, Florence fennel or finocchio *(F. vulgare dulce)*, sweet fennel *(F. vulgare).*

SEE ALSO Fennel in the chapter on Vegetables.

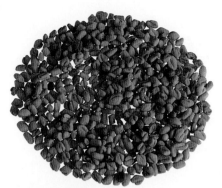

Fenugreek *Trigonella foenum-graecum*

also called **Bird's foot, Cow's horn, Goat's horn, Greek hayseed**

DESCRIPTION Fenugreek is a small, slender annual herb of the pea family, growing to about 75 cm, and similar in habit to lucerne (alfalfa). It has light-green leaves with three leaflets, yellowish-white flowers and typical legume fruits that contain the small, deeply furrowed, light-brown seeds. These seeds are the spice. Ground fenugreek has a strong maple sweetness, spicy but bitter flavour and an aroma of burnt sugar.

ORIGIN AND HISTORY Fenugreek is indigenous to western Asia and south-eastern Europe. It is one of the oldest cultivated plants, having been mentioned in medical papyri from ancient Egyptian tombs. Charlemagne encouraged its cultivation in central Europe in AD182. The Latin name Trigonella means little triangle, describing the shape of the small flowers, and *foenum-graecum* means 'Greek hay', the name given by the Romans when they brought the plant from Greece.

BUYING AND STORAGE Fenugreek seed has become readily available as it is now a popular sprouting seed. Ground fenugreek will only retain its flavour if stored in airtight, screw-top glass jars.

PREPARATION AND USE When used as sprouting seed, follow the same procedure as for alfalfa and other small seed legumes. Very few recipes call for the whole seed, therefore it is advisable to crush or powder the seeds in a mortar and pestle. It is an important ingredient in some curry blends, chutneys, stews and soups. Fenugreek adds flavour to green beans, cauliflower and salad dressing. Commercially it is used in the preparation of imitation maple syrup and rum flavours. Whole fenugreek seeds are mixed with the whole seeds of black mustard, cumin, fennel and black cumin to make the Indian seasoning panch phora.

PROCESSING Fenugreek is grown from seed, and matures three to five months later. When the seeds have matured, the entire plant is uprooted and dried, so that the seeds can be threshed, winnowed, dried once more, then stored.

VARIETIES
British species *(T. purpurascens)*.

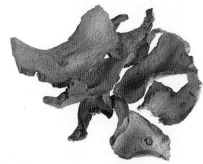

Galangal *Alpinia galanga*

also called **China root, Colic root, Galanga, Galangale, Gargaut, Greater galangal, India root, Ka, Khaa, Laos, Lengkuas**

DESCRIPTION A perennial plant with stems to 1.5 m, covered with long, narrow, bladelike leaves and orchidlike white flowers, veined with red. It has light, ochre-yellow rhizomes with firm, narrow pink sprouts and knobs. A member of the ginger family, it is commonly known as Laos or Siamese ginger as it grows profusely in Laos and Thailand, and features in their cooking. It has a peppery taste with overtones of ginger.

ORIGIN AND HISTORY Galangal is native to China and Southeast Asia. It was first recorded by a foreign traveller, Ibn Khurdadbah, in AD 869, as an article of trade from the Far East. Greater galangal was used in Europe in the Middle Ages; known as galingale, it was thought to have aphrodisiac qualities. Although the Chinese enjoyed its flavour, and included it in their medications, northern Chinese resisted accepting this 'southern Chinese' ginger for centuries.

BUYING AND STORAGE Powdered laos is readily available where Asian spices are sold. Store in an airtight jar and it will keep for many months. The fresh root can be stored for a week in the vegetable compartment of the refrigerator. Choose pale rhizomes with pink shoots or buds, firm and unwrinkled.

PREPARATION AND USE In Thailand it is added to curry pastes and, sliced, may be added to soups and stocks. A 1.5 cm piece of fresh rhizome equals 2 teaspoons of powdered laos. Young fresh ginger root can be used as a substitute but dried ginger is not of similar flavour to laos. It is popular in Indian and Eastern European cuisine and in Russia it is used commercially to flavour vinegar and the liqueur nastoika. It is used in the preparation of a tea by the Tartars, and by brewers and cordial manufacturers.

PROCESSING The branched pieces of rhizome are cut while fresh, showing a dark centre surrounded by a wider, paler layer which becomes darker on drying. The pieces must be ground finely to create a uniform powder that integrates small fibres.

VARIETIES
Lesser Galangal, a rhizome *Kaempferia pandurata* or *K. galanga*). Related to the ginger family, lesser galangal is largely unknown in the West. The tubers are brown-skinned with a pale-yellow flesh and resemble a bunch of fingers which grow downward from the main body of the rhizome. It has a milder flavour and unique taste unlike other types of ginger.

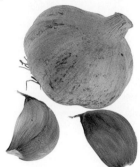

Garlic *Allium sativum*

DESCRIPTION Garlic belongs to the same family as onion and chives. Its food value lies beneath the ground in its bulb, made up of segments (called cloves) covered by a papery shell. It is a perennial with long, flattened, solid leaves 30 cm long, growing to a height of 90 cm. A flower stalk from the centre of the plant bears a mauve-white bloom.

ORIGIN AND HISTORY Garlic was probably grown in Egypt, China and India before recorded history. Several bulbs were found in the tomb of Tutankhamen, dating from *c.* 1358 BC. There is reference to garlic in the Old Testament, in Mohammedan, Roman and Greek literature and in the Talmud. Louis Pasteur reported on garlic's anti-bacterial activity in 1858, and its antiseptic qualities are renowned. Raw garlic juice was used as a field dressing during World War I. Garlic is valued in many countries as a protection against coughs and colds.

BUYING AND STORAGE Bulbs should have a plump, firm feel. Keep them away from humidity in an airy container such as a woven basket, where they will keep for several weeks. Alternatively, peel all the cloves and keep refrigerated immersed in oil in a screw-top jar. Dehydrated garlic should be a light, even colour; keep airtight.

PREPARATION AND USE Garlic is an indispensable component in many types of cooking, especially the cuisines of Mediterranean countries, Asian countries, India, Spain and Mexico. It is peeled, then chopped, minced or squeezed so that only the juice is used. Include in all types of savoury food.

PROCESSING Bulbs are ready for harvesting when the blooms and leaves wither. Dig the bulbs, shake free of dirt, and hang them by their stalks to dry and harden. Commercial garlic processing involves washing and peeling the cloves, then slicing, chopping or mincing before drying in ovens. Garlic powder attracts moisture readily, and it must be kept tightly sealed.

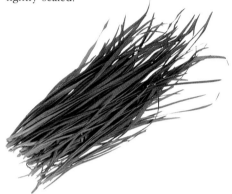

Garlic Chives *Allium tuberosum*

also called Asatuki, Chinese chives, Gow choy, Nira

DESCRIPTION A popular flavouring herb, it is grown in most parts of China, and is also cultivated in other parts of Asia. It has deepgreen, wide, flattish stems which come to a point at the top, and has the characteristic taste and smell of garlic. Variations of this include flowering chives, which have a similar appearance and slightly stronger flavour, but have rounder stems and a small bunched white flower on top. Chive shoots are of the same type again, but are grown under protection from light so that the shoots are thinner and a pale yellow-green colour.

BUYING AND STORAGE All are bought from Chinese shops in small bunches. They can be kept for several days in plastic wrapping in the vegetable compartment of the refrigerator.

PREPARATION AND USE They add a subtle flavour to soups, noodle and rice dishes and are sprinkled over other cooked dishes as a garnish and flavouring. They should never be cooked for long as they become bitter. Trim the root end to remove white root section and cut diagonally into short lengths.

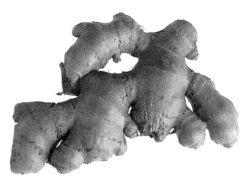

Ginger *Zingiber officinale*

DESCRIPTION Perennial, creeping plant on a thick, tuberous rhizome, producing a stem 60–120 cm high, with long, narrow lilylike leaves. It has greenish flowers marked with purple. The varieties listed have different and distinctive characteristics peculiar to the region in which they are grown.

ORIGIN AND HISTORY Ginger is native to Asia, and is now widely cultivated throughout the tropics. It was one of the first oriental spices to reach south-eastern Europe in the ancient spice trade. The Romans distributed it to all parts of their empire. Marco Polo was the first European to write of actually finding ginger in China.

BUYING AND STORAGE Whole ginger rhizomes should be clean but not peeled for storage, as removal of the skin can rupture oleoresin cells near the surface. It should be kept refrigerated wrapped in foil. Whole and preserved ginger should not be fibrous, as this indicates that it was too mature at the time of harvest. The best crystallised or preserved ginger to buy is young stem ginger. Ground ginger should be a creamy yellow, free from fibre and lumps. Minced green ginger can be bought in glass jars and should be refrigerated after opening.

PREPARATION AND USE The rhizome (or root) should be peeled and either grated or sliced thinly. Sautéed ginger, onion and garlic form the basis for most Asian dishes, including curries and stir-fries. It is also used in ginger beer, preserves and sweets. Dried ginger adds tang to biscuits, gingerbread and spice cakes, and acts as a tenderiser when applied sparingly to meat. It also contributes a freshness and distinctive heat to meat dishes.

PROCESSING The fleshy rhizome is harvested nine months after planting, then washed and sun-dried. This is known as black ginger. If the corky outer layer is scraped off before drying, it is known as white ginger. Australian-grown ginger is reputed to be the best in the world, and is grated, washed, peeled and steeped in brine for up to 12 months before being boiled in syrup, drained and packed in fresh syrup.

VARIETIES

African ginger, Australian ginger, Chinese ginger, Indian ginger (cochin), Jamaica ginger, Japanese ginger, Nigerian ginger.

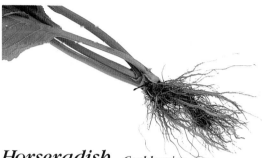

Horseradish *Cochlearia armoracia (Armoracia rusticana)*

DESCRIPTION Horseradish is a perennial member of the mustard family growing up to 1 m, with large spinachlike leaves wrinkled along the edges, and a pungent, white taproot and rhizomes. The root has a burning, sharp flavour with a biting aroma. Numerous small, white, aromatic flowers are succeeded by wrinkled seed pods.

ORIGIN AND HISTORY Native to Europe, horseradish was used in the 13th century Germany and Denmark as a medicine, condiment and leaf vegetable. It had spread to England by the 16th century, and was taken to North America by the early settlers. Bitter horseradish is eaten at the Jewish Passover, to symbolise the bitterness of their slavery to the Egyptians. Roots and pods of the horseradish tree *(Moringa oleifera)* are used in some tropical areas as an inferior substitute for the genuine horseradish.

BUYING AND STORAGE Fresh roots, if available, should be stored in a damp, dark place, or they will turn green. Dried, powdered horseradish is not as pungent as dried granules or grains, which reconstitute well in liquid, and resemble the texture of freshly grated root.

PREPARATION AND USE The fresh, raw root is grated or cut into strips to add stimulating flavour to sauces and dressings, hors d'oeuvre, seafood cocktails and mustards. Horseradish sauce is almost obligatory with traditional roast beef, corned beef, ham and tongue, and blends well with grated apples, mint and sour cream as a dressing for avocado.

PROCESSING Horseradish is ideally harvested in late autumn, as the flavour improves with cold weather. When the plant is dug, small lateral roots are cut for use, while the main taproot can be saved for replanting.

Fresh roots can be stored for some time in dry sand. Dehydrated granules of horseradish have 94% of moisture removed.

VARIETIES
Bohemian horseradish.

SEE ALSO Radish in the chapter on Vegetables.

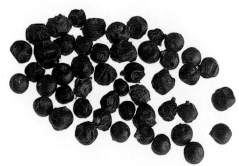

Juniper Berries *Juniperus communis*

DESCRIPTION The evergreen juniper tree is native to the northern hemisphere, and varies in size from a dense shrub to a small upright tree, 12 m tall. The aromatic berries grow to 10 mm diameter among needle-sharp, pine-scented leaves, and take two to three years to mature from green to bluish-black. While some berries are maturing, new cones are growing at the same time.

ORIGIN AND HISTORY Juniper berries were used medicinally by Greek and Arabic physicians as a diuretic. Since biblical days it has been considered a magical plant, and was popular as a strewing herb to freshen stale air. The word gin is an adaptation of jenever, Dutch for juniper, as the berries are a vital ingredient in this drink. The berries have been used as a pepper substitute.

BUYING AND STORAGE Juniper berries should only be bought in their whole state: black, shrivelled, but still plump. Be careful that there is no mould on them, as the moisture content in the dried berry is sometimes still high. Store in an airtight container in a dry place.

PREPARATION AND USE Before cooking, lightly crush the berries with a rolling pin or spoon to split the skin. Their piquant flavour is almost an essential addition to game such as duck, quail, hare, rabbit and venison, and is equally satisfactory in stuffings for chicken, goose, pork and turkey. It is a common ingredient in cabbage, sauerkraut and marinades. Herbalists advise against eating these berries when pregnant or when the kidneys are inflamed.

PROCESSING The easiest way to pick the berries from amongst the pointed leaves is to hold a dish under the ripe berries and use a skewer or chopstick to worry them loose until they fall into the dish. Spread them on paper or a wire tray to air-dry. Microwave drying is not suitable.

VARIETIES
American juniper or red cedar (*J. virginiata*), Prickly juniper or medlar tree (*Juniperus oxycedrus*).

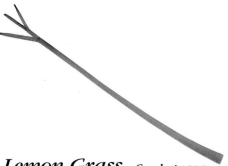

Lemon Grass *Cymbopogon citratus*

also called **Citronella, Citronelle, Heung mao tso, Serai, Sereh, Xa, Zabalin**

DESCRIPTION Lemon grass grows in a bushy clump, increasing each year. The thin blades have a rough, sticky feel and can easily make a slice in the fingers if not handled carefully. The colour at the tips can change from deep-green to yellowish or rust-red. The foliage has a delicious lemon scent. This grass has not been seen to bear flowers, and is propagated by root division.

ORIGIN AND HISTORY Known in Europe as citronelle or citronella, its other important value is as a natural insect repellant. It is a native of tropical countries and grows abundantly in Southeast Asia. Buddhist monks serve relaxing citronelle tea in their temples.

BUYING AND STORAGE Fresh lemon grass is often available at Asian specialty shops, and it can also be bought in dried form, packaged as a herbal tea. Two teaspoons of dried herb is equivalent to one stalk of fresh. Keep fresh lemon grass immersed in cold water and use within four to five days.

PREPARATION AND USE When a recipe specifies chopped, fresh lemon grass, only the bottom 6–7 cm of tender, creamy, lower stem should be used. (Remaining green blades can be steeped in boiling water to make a refreshing drink.) Lemon grass is an important ingredient in Thai cooking and, with chilli, contributes to the characteristic hot, light freshness of this cuisine. Add lemon grass to curries, steamed or baked fish, chicken, or snip a few centimetres with scissors into a pot of tea.

PROCESSING Lemon grass can be cut in autumn and either air-dried or microwaved. Although both methods are satisfactory, much of the fresh lemon appeal is lost during drying.

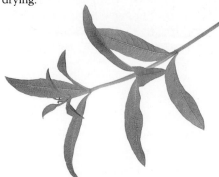

Lemon Verbena *Aloysia triphylla (Lippia citriodora)*

DESCRIPTION Having no relation to vervain (*Verbena officinalis*), lemon verbena is a small deciduous tree growing to 4 m, with strongly lemon-scented, pointed leaves. In summer, pale-mauve and white flowers mist in pyramids at the ends of leafy branches. In autumn the leaves turn yellow and fall, leaving bare branches in winter.

ORIGIN AND HISTORY Lemon verbena is a relative newcomer to our herb gardens, being virtually unknown until it was brought to England from South America in 1784. The leaves are used in Spain to make a refreshing tea thought to relieve digestive problems, and they are frequently added to pot pourri.

BUYING AND STORAGE This herb is not commercially available, and the best source of supply could be kind neighbours and friends who grow it in their gardens. Fresh branches can be kept in a vase of water.

PREPARATION AND USE Their intense lemon flavour makes the leaves a fragrant addition to baked custard and rice pudding. (Remove the leaves before serving.) Use six dried leaves or ten fresh per cup of water to make a tea. A delicious lemon tea can be made by infusing lemon grass, lemon thyme, lemon balm, and lemon verbena together.

PROCESSING Lemon verbena can be cut back hard in late summer, and the leaves stripped off before air-drying on racks or paper away from light. It also dries well when hung in bunches, but once brittle, the leaves are harder to strip from the branches. They will keep their fragrance for up to 12 months stored in a paper bag or box.

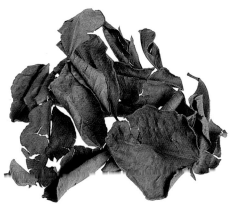

Lime Leaves *Citrus aurantiifolia*

*also called **Daun limau perut***

DESCRIPTION The lime leaves referred to have no relationship to the linden or lime tree of Europe *(Tilia europaea)* whose flowers are used as a tea. The lime is a typical evergreen citrus tree with strong, dark-green, smooth leaves and small, green, lemony fruit. The leaves are high in volatile oils, and the white blossoms are fragrant and attractive to bees.

ORIGIN AND HISTORY All citrus trees are native to Southeast Asia, and it seems likely that they were first introduced to Europe in the Middle Ages by Moorish and Turkish invaders. In northern Europe, special heated glasshouses known as 'orangeries' were built so that the citrus could withstand the colder climate. Louix XIV of France decorated his Salon des Glaces at Versailles with lemon trees in tubs of solid silver (which were melted down in the revolution).

BUYING AND STORAGE Apart from in the 'wet markets' of Asia, fresh lime leaves are not usually available for purchase, unless stocked by specialist Asian suppliers. Fresh lime leaves can be hung in bunches like bay leaves and used in varying degrees of dryness.

PREPARATION AND USE Lime leaves are best used straight from the tree for maximum freshness. They are used extensively in Asian cooking, in sambals, steamed fish, and the beef rendang (curry) of Indonesia. They add a nuance of freshness to chicken soup or fish dishes. In India, China and Southeast Asia the fruit, juice and leaves are all used in cooking.

PROCESSING Best used fresh.

VARIETIES
Mexican lime, Tahiti lime, West Indian lime (all *C. aurantiifolia*).

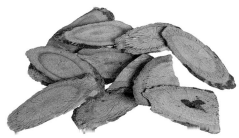

Liquorice *Glycirrhiza glabra (Liquiritia officinalis)*

*also called **Kan ts'ao***

DESCRIPTION This herbaceous perennial grows 1–1.5 m tall with a clump of straight, woody stalks. Frond-shaped leaves are set along the stems, with lilac-blue flowers growing where the leaf stalk meets the main stem. The part used is the large taproot, which can grow as long as 120 cm, with many subsidiary and transverse roots. The root is greyish-brown, with a yellow, fibrous middle, and tastes characteristically strong and sweet.

ORIGIN AND HISTORY Native to the Middle and Far East, liquorice has been known as a medicinal herb since earliest times, mainly for the relief of constipation. Its botanic name is derived from the Greek for sweet root, and the particular sweetness of this root is safe for diabetics. The Greeks and Romans drank the thirst-quenching black juice extracted from the roots. Its use as a medicine continued through the Middle Ages, and the monastery at Pontefract which first cultivated liquorice in the early 16th century later became the centre of the liquorice confectionery industry. The Chinese also valued the medicinal qualities of kan ts'ao.

BUYING AND STORAGE Available in specialty food shops as dried pieces, as black, brittle, cylindrical sticks or ground. No special storage of the dried root is required but the sticks should be kept free of moisture and the powder should be stored in an airtight container. Kan ts'ao is available in Chinese groceries or herb shops.

PREPARATION AND USE The distinctive flavour of this root is used to mask the bitter flavours of some medicines. It is an ingredient in Guinness stout, as well as chewing tobacco, snuff and confectionery. Liquorice juice is made by dissolving 30 g of liquorice stick in a glass of warm water. The roots may flavour fruit juices, syrups and dried-fruit salad.

PROCESSING Liquorice is harvested in the autumn of its third or fourth year, when the whole plant is taken up. When the roots are severed, the crowns and suckers are stored for replanting in the spring, when new roots grow. The roots are washed, trimmed and sold fresh, or dried. Processed forms include dried liquorice, extract of liquorice, block liquorice. The waste fibre after processing is used in making particle board.

VARIETIES
G. asperrima, G. echinata, G. glandulifera, G. lepidota, G. typica.

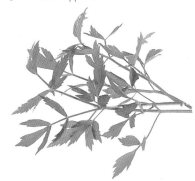

Lovage *Levisicum officinale (Ligusticum scoticum)*

*also called **Lavose, Sea parsley***

DESCRIPTION In appearance, lovage resembles angelica, although it only grows 90 cm–1.5 m tall. The straight, hollow stems bear clusters of small, sulphur-yellow flowers in summer, which are followed by seeds. The leaves have a similarity to Italian parsley, with a yeasty flavour and an overtone of celery and parsley.

ORIGIN AND HISTORY Lovage was a highly regarded herb in ancient Greece and Rome, where it was used for culinary, medicinal and cosmetic purposes. Although the rootstock is still used by herbalists because of its antiseptic qualities, the popularity of the peppery foliage has unaccountably waned.

BUYING AND STORAGE Fresh lovage can be refrigerated, immersed in water or wrapped in foil, for up to a week. It is not generally available commercially, fresh or dried.

PREPARATION AND USE Lovage leaves can be finely chopped and used in the same way as parsley. A quick sauce for fish can be made by adding 1 tablespoon of chopped lovage to 250 mL of white sauce. Lovage soup is made with chicken stock, fresh lovage, a thickening beurre manie, and milk or cream, cooked together then blended until smooth. This tasty herb can be used instead of pepper and added to most savoury foods.

PROCESSING The thick leaves of lovage are moisture rich, and are slow to dry. Cut the leaves from the stems and spread on a wire rack to dry in a dark warm place, or microwave. Store in an airtight container when quite crisp.

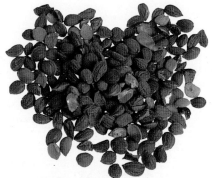

Mahlab *Prunus avium*

also called **Mahaleb, Mahlepi**

DESCRIPTION A fragrant spice from the husked kernels of a wild black cherry, with a flavour echoing the fruit. It is pale brown in colour and about the size of a peppercorn.

ORIGIN AND HISTORY The particular species of cherry from which mahlab is obtained, is native to Europe and southern Asia. The kernels were first used in the Middle East for perfumes and medicine. The major centre of production is Iran, followed by Turkey and Syria. The spice has long been used in Middle Eastern and Greek cooking to flavour sweet breads, pastries and cookies.

BUYING AND STORAGE The spice is only sold at stores stocking Middle Eastern and Greek foods. It is always sold whole, usually packed in small cellophane bags. Store in a sealed jar in a cool, dark place.

PREPARATION AND USE As only small amounts are used at a time, and the flavour is at its best when freshly ground, use a mortar and pestle to pound the seeds to a powder.

Use to flavour sweet breads, cookies, cakes and pastries. Try about ½ teaspoon in the pastry for a cherry pie, or a teaspoonful in a cherry cake to enhance the cherry flavour.

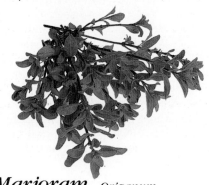

Marjoram *Origanum marjorana*

DESCRIPTION Marjoram grows as a compact bush 40–50 cm tall, with small, soft grey-green leaves. Tiny white flowers bloom in tight clusters at the tips of the stems. Both leaves and flowers have a pleasant aromatic flavour, with a gentler effect than oregano.

ORIGIN AND HISTORY In ancient Egypt, marjoram was dedicated to the sungod Osiris, and it was used in Greek and Roman temples. Marjoram was considered a symbol of happiness, and to have it growing on a grave meant eternal peace for the departed. Its tangy, fresh smell made it a popular strewing herb. It being quite similar to oregano, some producing countries sell marjoram as oregano and oregano as marjoram, depending on market demand.

BUYING AND STORAGE A fresh bunch of marjoram should be stored totally immersed in cold water for maximum freshness. Stored this way, it should be used within five to six days. The best quality dried marjoram has leaf pieces rather than powder, and should be kept in a glass screw-top jar.

PREPARATION AND USE Marjoram, along with parsley, thyme and bay leaves, makes up the classic bouquet garni, and it is also an ingredient of mixed herbs. Fresh marjoram can be sprinkled over salads, mixed into omelettes, sauces and dumplings, and added to meatloaf, fish and poultry. When using dried marjoram, use one-third the amount of fresh, to allow for the increased intensity of flavour when dried.

PROCESSING The best harvesting time is just before the flowers mature in summer. Cut long stems and hang them in bunches somewhere airy and shady until dry, then crumble the leaves into an airtight container for storage. Marjoram leaves microwave well, and can be chopped and frozen in water iceblocks.

VARIETIES Dittany of Crete *(O. dictamnus)*, knotted marjoram *(M. hortensis)*, pot marjoram *(Marjorana onites)*.

SEE ALSO Oregano.

Masala

DESCRIPTION The masalas are fine mixtures of spices found predominantly in Indian cooking.

ORIGIN AND HISTORY Masalas are traditionally part of the seasoning for a particular dish, being added in varying proportions to give an individual characteristic that meets the cook's personal preference. The best-known of masalas is garam masala, which can vary from quite hot to fragrant and slightly sweet.

BUYING AND STORAGE The spices are readily available in food shops. There is no accepted way to identify whether these are mild, fragrant or hot, therefore a certain amount of trial is needed to determine the most suitable flavour profile for individual needs. More commercial blends are mild, slightly sweet, and with a vague sharp aftertaste of pepper.

PREPARATION AND USE Use in casseroles, sprinkle over chicken, grills, shishkebabs and barbecued meats, and add to sauces, gravies and salad dressings for an exotic flavour. The aromatic character blends well with yoghurt and cucumber curry accompaniments, and ½ teaspoon added to a white sauce for cauliflower makes a delicious change.

VARIETIES

Chaat Masala A tart mixture of Indian spices, also called chat masala. The principal ingredient is dried green mango powder, aamchur, which is tart and somewhat lemony in flavour. Other ingredients are ground dried ginger and mint, with cumin, salt, chilli powder and asafoetida.

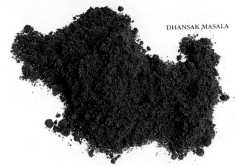

DHANSAK MASALA

Dhansak Masala A spice mixture containing toasted coriander and cumin.

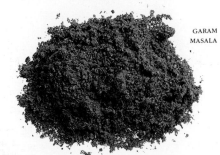

GARAM MASALA

Garam Masala An aromatic spice mixture usually brown in colour and comprising numerous spices including black peppercorns, cloves, cinnamon, cardamom, coriander, cumin and nutmeg. Some garam masala mixtures can contain over 20 different spices. Garam masala differs from commercial curry powders in the omission of the pungent, bright yellow spice turmeric. It is used in curries and on braised meats, and may also be sprinkled on cooked foods as a condiment.

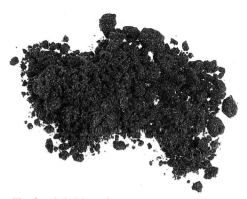

Kashmiri Masala A spice mixture used in northern India and Kashmir. It is more sweet and aromatic than garam masala, because of its high content of cardamom. Other spices include cumin, black peppercorns, stick cinnamon, mace and nutmeg.

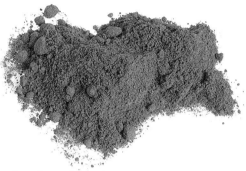

Sambar Masala A tart spice mixture comprising toasted and ground black lentils (urad dal), coriander, cumin, black peppercorns and fenugreek. A hotter variety also includes ground dried chillies, mustard seeds and curry leaves.

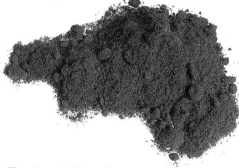

Tandoori Masala A commercial blend of spices used in Indian cooking to produce the characteristic orange-red colour and spicy flavour associated with foods cooked in the Indian tandoori oven. It comprises coriander, turmeric, mustard seeds, asafoetida, cardamom, cinnamon, ginger, salt, chilli, cloves and aamchur with a natural food colouring.

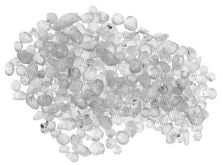

Mastic *Pistacia lentiscus*

also called **Masticha, Mistki**

DESCRIPTION Small lumps of yellow-coloured resin, faintly liquorice in flavour. Masticha, the Greek name for the resin, is also the name of a Greek liqueur.

ORIGIN AND HISTORY Mastic is derived from a small evergreen tree native to the Mediterranean region. The Greek island of Chios has been the main centre for production for hundreds of years. Small incisions are made in the bark on trunk and branches. The sap oozes out and hardens into yellow masses or drops with a spicy, bitter flavour. It is used in Greek and Middle Eastern cooking to flavour sweet yeast breads and cookies. The Greek masticha and the Turkish raki liqueurs both use mastic to flavour them, with aniseed included for raki. Both turn white when water is added. In Greece and the Balkans, the mastic is pounded and mixed with beeswax for a chewing gum. In Egyptian cooking, a small piece of mastic (mistki) is added to simmering chicken to remove unwanted flavours.

BUYING AND STORAGE Available packed in small amounts in cellophane bags, and can be purchased from Greek and Middle Eastern food shops. Put into a sealed jar and store at room temperature. Keeps indefinitely.

PREPARATION AND USE Mastic is only used in small amounts, so pound to a powder in a mortar and pestle. A quarter to ½ teaspoon is used to flavour sweet yeast breads and cookies.

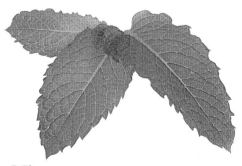

Mint *Mentha viridis, M. spicata, M. crispa*

DESCRIPTION All mints are perennial plants with a rampant creeping root system, and vary in height from the matted ground cover of pennyroyal, to 80–90 cm in most other varieties. The most commonly used is spearmint, with smooth, long pointed leaves of bright green, and a fresh 'toothpaste' flavour. Other species of spearmint have rounder, coarser leaves and may be known as common, garden or green mint. Peppermint has smaller, darker leaves and is mostly for medicinal use. All mint plants have white, mauve or purple flowers. Because mints hybridise easily with each other, there is a vast array of varieties. Like scented geraniums, sweet-scented mints can be identified by their individual aromas. The plant known as Vietnamese mint is not a *Mentha* species.

ORIGIN AND HISTORY Mint is another herb of Mediterranean origin which has been used since ancient times. Introduced to Europe and Britain by the Romans, it became popular for strewing as a room freshener and insect repellent, and had the added advantage of preventing milk from curdling.

BUYING AND STORAGE Dried mint leaf usually appears to be greenish-black. This is normal and the flavour will be good as long as it is kept in an airtight jar. Fresh mint will keep immersed in cold water for as long as a fortnight, if the water is changed every three to four days.

PREPARATION AND USE The fresh, cool flavour of mint has been adopted by toothpaste manufacturers as the epitome of cleanliness. Mint leaves are added to the famous cooling mint julep drink of southern USA, and are used to make the mint sauce and jelly accompaniments for roasted meats. A few mint leaves give freshness to herb sandwiches, salads, ice cream and cooked peas. Infused peppermint leaves make a delicious tea to drink hot or cold.

PROCESSING Mint leaves can be dried until crisp in a microwave and still retain their bright colour and fresh aroma. Although traditional air-drying is possible, microwave processing gives the best result. The dried leaves must be stored in an airtight container.

VARIETIES
Applemint (*M. rotundifolia*), eau-de-cologne or bergamot mint (*M. piperita citrata* or *M. odorata*), Japanese mint (*M. arvensis* var. *piperascens*), Mitcham peppermint (*M. piperita*), pennyroyal (*M. pulegium*), variegated applemint (*M. rotundifolia variegata* or *M. officinalis variegata*), watermint (*M. aquatica*).

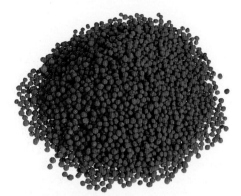

Mustard Seed *Brassica*

DESCRIPTION All varieties of mustard are annuals. Black mustard grows to a height of 2–3 m at maturity, while the white variety matures at 1 m or less. Both have bright yellow flowers, each with four petals, followed by seed pods, which, in the case of black mustard, are smooth, while white mustard seed pods are hairy. The names refer to the colours of the seeds. Brown or wild mustard seed is sometimes mixed with black. White mustard seeds are used for sprouting, often with cress.

ORIGIN AND HISTORY Mustard has been used since the earliest recorded history. It was highly regarded by Pythagoras and Hippocrates, and is referred to in the Bible as 'the greatest among herbs'. In 334 BC, Darius III of Persia sent Alexander the Great a bag of sesame seeds (symbolising the vast numbers of his army). Alexander returned a bag of mustard seeds, to imply not only the number, but the power and energy of his men. Mustard was originally included in the genus named *Sinapis* from the Greek word for mustard, but is now more commonly included in the cabbage genus, *Brassica*.

BUYING AND STORAGE Mustard seeds can be bought whole, but are usually sold as prepared mustards. The dry powder is made from a blend of black and white seeds, finely milled and sifted. Prepared wet mustard is made with finely ground seeds, vinegar and spices. The bright yellow pastes usually have turmeric mixed with the mustard. French mustards use both ground brown and black seeds and whole seeds, giving a grainy, speckled appearance. Dark seeds have a more pungent aroma and flavour.

PREPARATION AND USE Powder mustards can be mixed with varying effects: with water for a hot, sharp taste; with vinegar for a milder flavour; with wine for a spicier taste; and with beer for an extremely hot bite. Mustard is used as an accompaniment for hot or cold meats (especially corned beef), sandwiches, salad dressings, hot dogs and eggs. Young white mustard leaves can be cooked as a vegetable or added to soups. Whole seeds are an ingredient of pickling spice. Both leaves and seeds are used in oriental cooking. Black mustard seeds, combined with the whole seeds of cumin, nigella, fenugreek and fennel, make the Indian seasoning panch phora.

PROCESSING The seed pods burst on maturity, scattering the seeds. Branches should be picked when the pods are fully developed but still green, and hung in bunches to dry. When the pods are brittle, thresh out the seeds and keep in a warm, dry place until completely dry. Store in an airtight container.

VARIETIES

Black mustard *(Brassica nigra* or *B. sinapis nigra)*, brown mustard or rai *(B. juncea)*, field mustard *(B. arvensis)*, rape *(B. napa)*, white mustard *(Brassica hirta* or *B. alba* or *B. sinapis alba)*.

SEE ALSO The mustards listed in the chapter on Sauces, Mustards and Pastes.

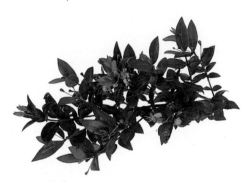

Myrtle *Myrtus communis*

DESCRIPTION The myrtle is a compact bush, growing 1–3 m high. The dark green, glossy leaves are ovate but neatly pointed, and the sweetly fragrant white flowers have long, golden stamens like exaggerated eyelashes. The flowers are followed by blue-black berries. This plant should not be confused with the crepe myrtle *(Lagerstroemia indica)*.

ORIGIN AND HISTORY Myrtle has been valued as a spice, medicine and cosmetic since before biblical times. Dried, powdered leaves made a dusting powder for babies in the Orient, and the Greeks and Romans chewed myrtle berries to fresh the breath. It has been connected in legend and tradition with love, fidelity and immortality.

BUYING AND STORAGE Myrtle is considered an attractive garden shrub, but it is not sold as a food.

PREPARATION AND USE Myrtle leaves are used in their native Mediterranean countries to flavour roasted meats and game birds. This is not done in the usual way, but by wrapping or stuffing the cooked meat with the fragrant, fresh leaves for five to ten minutes before serving. Where myrtle grows wild, branches are burnt on fires over which lamb is cooked. The dried seeds, when ground, make a peppery seasoning. A few of the gently resinous, sweet flowers can be strewn over fruit salads and desserts.

PROCESSING As the bush is perennial, the leaves may be used fresh at any time. Pick the berries when they appear and air-dry on a gauze rack or on sheets of paper in a warm, dark place. When completely dry, store in an airtight jar, and grind in a pepper grinder or mortar and pestle just before using.

Nigella *Nigella sativa*

*also called **Black cumin, Devil-in-the-bush, Fennel flower, Love-in-a-mist, Wild onion seed***

DESCRIPTION This attractive plant grows 30–50 cm high, and its dark green, feathery foliage and starburst blue flowers make it a popular cottage garden herb.

ORIGIN AND HISTORY There is no mention of nigella in ancient literature, nor in medieval English herbals. However, it is known that it was taken to America by the early settlers, who used it as a seasoning. The seeds have a peppery, almost nutmeglike flavour, and in India they are sometimes called kala jeera (black cumin). In France, nigella has been called quatre épices (four spices).

BUYING AND STORAGE Nigella seed is not commonly available, although it is sometimes sold as onion seed. The genuine onion seed has little flavour, and although the plump, tear-shaped black seeds look similar, the taste is quite different.

PREPARATION AND USE The whole dried seed is used in the spicy food of Egypt, the Middle East and India, and can be sprinkled over crusty bread or cakes. Nigella is blended with the whole seeds of black mustard, cumin, fenugreek and fennel to make the Indian seasoning panch phora (five spices). This spice tends to be overshadowed by more easily available and tastier spices.

PROCESSING Nigella flowers should be picked as they reach maturity but before they start to die. Hang heads-down in a bunch, with a tray below to catch the seeds as they dry and fall. Sieve out leaves before storing in an airtight container.

VARIETIES
White flowering ornamental variety.

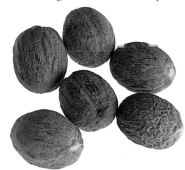

Nutmeg and Mace
Myristica fragrans (also known as
*M. officinalis, M. moschata,
M. aromatica,* and *M. amboinensis*)

DESCRIPTION Nutmeg and mace are contained in a yellow to light-brown fleshy fruit resembling a peach, that grows on a 15 m high, densely foliaged evergreen tree. Nutmeg is the inner seed removed from its hard protective shell. The reddish, lacy tissue clinging to this hard shell is known as mace. The nutmegs are greyish-brown, oval, and average 2–3 cm in diameter. The appearance is wrinkled, but it is smooth to the touch. Although it appears hard, it can be grated or sliced to reveal many brown veins containing the aromatic oil of nutmeg. Mace when dried is reddish-brown and made up of fat, shiny branched pieces with a fragrant, nutmeglike aroma and warm taste.

ORIGIN AND HISTORY The histories of nutmeg and mace are intertwined, starting in the eastern islands of the Moluccas. Neither nutmeg nor mace appear to have been known to the ancient Greek and Roman civilisations. There is a record of the spice in Constantinople about AD 540 by Detius, and it must have reached India before this time. Well-preserved anecdotes of British and Dutch colonials tell of those in power in Europe, unaware that both spices come from the same tree, requesting growers in Indonesia and Grenada to destroy the nutmeg trees and increase mace production, as mace was scarce and more lucrative than nutmeg.

BUYING AND STORAGE Whole nutmegs should be sound and unbroken with no borer holes. Ground nutmeg is unevenly coloured dark-brown, coarse, oily and highly aromatic. Mace (sometimes called blade mace), is usually bought in its ground form, which is paler than nutmeg and has a fuller, spicier aroma and

stronger flavour profile than nutmeg. Both must be stored in screw-top, airtight glass jars to retain their high oil content, which is incompatible with some modern packaging materials.

PREPARATION AND USE The volatile oil present in nutmeg and mace contains small amounts of myristicin and elemicin, which are narcotic and poisonous, therefore they must be used sparingly. Ground or freshly grated nutmeg flavours milk puddings, cakes, biscuits, soups, breads, oyster and fish dishes, pumpkin pie, cream sauces and nearly all beverages made with milk. Mace, being stronger, is used more sparingly in sauces for fish, pickles and chutneys, cheese dishes and vegetables such as spinach, carrots and potatoes. In some parts of Asia, a confection is made by crystallising the fleshy part of the fruit.

PROCESSING After harvesting the fruit, the nutmeg in its shell with the surrounding mace is separated from the flesh. Later, before sun-drying, the mace is detached from the nut and is flattened, care being taken to avoid breakage which would detract from its quality. After removal of the mace, the nutmegs are dried in their shells. When they have lost weight through drying, and begin to rattle within the shell, they are shelled to reveal the edible nutmeg.

VARIETIES
False or Bombay nutmeg *(M. malabarica),* Papua nutmeg *(M. argentea).*

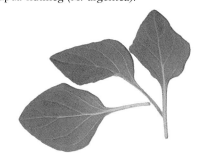

Oregano   *Origanum vulgare*

DESCRIPTION Oregano is a more robust variety of marjoram, growing to a height of 60 cm. It has an untidy, sprawling growing habit and firm, pungent leaves.

ORIGIN AND HISTORY Oregano has been popular in Greece and other Mediterranean countries since ancient times. Oregano and marjoram were both valued as medicinal herbs during the Middle Ages, and are two of the most popular culinary herbs today. Allied soldiers serving in Italy and the Mediterranean during World War II discovered the delicious flavour of oregano and made it an everyday herb in their home countries on their return.

BUYING AND STORAGE Fresh oregano should be stored immersed in cold water for maximum freshness, and used within five to six days. Dried oregano has more pungency in pieces rather than powder, and should be kept in an airtight container.

PREPARATION AND USE Oregano's lusty flavour is identified with such popular foods as pizza and pasta, and gives character to any tomato dishes. It can be added to potato, zucchini or pasta salads. The flower tops are used in the same way as the leaves.

PROCESSING Bunches hung in an airy, shady place dry well, and the leaves crumble easily off the stems once dry. Oregano can also be microwaved, which is a good way of preserving the fresh colour and flavour. The dried leaves and flowers must be stored in an airtight container.

VARIETIES

Mexican Oregano Also called Mexican marjoram.

Rigani

DESCRIPTION A popular Greek perennial herb, also called wild marjoram, which is used dried more than fresh. It is picked when the white flowers are opened as its flavour is at its best at this stage; the leaves are grey-green and more elongated than those of other oreganos. It has a pleasant though pungent aroma and flavour.

ORIGIN AND HISTORY Rigani is native to Greece, with its common and botanical names from the Greek meaning 'joy of the mountain'. It has featured in Greek remedies and cooking from ancient times. Rarely used today as a medicinal herb, in the Greek kitchen it is almost as essential as the olive oil and lemon with which it combines so well. In spring the hills and mountainsides of Greece are fragrant with its aroma, and it is gathered, tied in bunches and dried for local use and export.

BUYING AND STORAGE Can be purchased from Greek and Middle Eastern food shops in dried bunches or in small packets prepared, ready for use. If bunches are purchased, strip leaves and flower heads from stems and rub to coarse flakes by hand. Store in a sealed jar in a cool place away from direct light and use within a year.

PREPARATION AND USE If the rigani is too coarse, rub by hand to reduce the size of the flakes. Sprinkle onto roast or grilled lamb with a squeeze of lemon juice before cooking; use to flavour the marinade for souvlakia

(Greek skewered lamb); sprinkle on fish with lemon juice before grilling or baking; use in salads and sprinkle onto olives with a little olive oil and vinegar. Also try it on potatoes, sautéed or baked in olive oil with the addition of lemon juice.

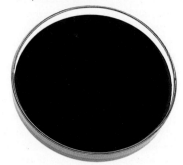

Pandan Leaf *Pandanus latifolia*

also called **Daun pandan, Rampe, Screwpine**

DESCRIPTION The screwpine tree from which pandan leaves come has stiff branches supporting themselves on stiltlike masses of aerial roots. The sharp-edged leaves are spirally arranged, and the small, decorative and fragrant white flowers are followed by large fruit heads 20 cm in diameter, looking similar to a green pineapple.

ORIGIN AND HISTORY Pandans are found in Madagascar, and throughout Southeast Asia, the Pacific Islands and tropical Australia. In older times, the tough, fibrous leaves were used for house thatching, and were woven into sails, clothing, floor mats and baskets. The evocative grass skirts worn by Pacific Island women were often made of split, bleached pandan leaves.

BUYING AND STORAGE Dried pandan leaf is sold in some shops as rampe from Sri Lanka, and as daun pandan for Malay and Indonesian dishes. Store in a cool, dark place to retain colour and flavour.

PREPARATION AND USE The flavour of pandan in Malaysia and Indonesia is as popular as vanilla is in Western countries. It is used to make the grass-green pandan cake, a favourite Asian sponge, usually topped with a green jellylike icing. Used also as a flavouring in rice and curries, strips of pandan leaves are woven into artistic baskets for serving glutinous rice or savouries. The male flower cluster of the pandan has a strong perfume that is used sparingly in Indian sweets, and is obtained as an essence or concentrate. On festive occasions, essences of rose and pandan (pictured above), are used to flavour the delicious spicy rice dish biryani.

PROCESSING The long flat leaves are either crushed or boiled to extract the flavour and colour. The leaves are air-dried and finely chopped for use in curries.

VARIETIES
Variegated screwpine *(P. veitchii)*, walking-stick palm or kewra *(P. odoratissimus)*.

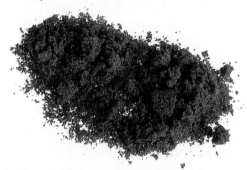

Paprika *Capsicum annuum*

DESCRIPTION Paprika is a sweet, non-pungent species of the capsicum family. It is an annual, shrubby plant with a woody stem and single white flowers. The long, tapering fruits vary in colour from a rich red to a dark reddish-brown. The powdered spice is made by drying and grinding the seeded ripe fruit with the stem removed. Hungarian paprika is bright red with a pleasant, warm, sweet taste. Spanish paprika is less red and milder in flavour, and is known to the Spanish as pimiento. The Portuguese variety is similar to Spanish.

ORIGIN AND HISTORY The origin is the same as that of chilli; however, following cultivation of *C. annuum* in Europe after 1650, the capsicums grown in different soils and climates took on modified characteristics. In Hungary the peppers that evolved, known as paprika, were much milder than their American ancestors. In Spain, they became larger in size but their pungency gradually lessened.

BUYING AND STORAGE Paprika is always purchased in its powdered form. The colour of paprika is affected by air and light, and both the colour and flavour deteriorate rapidly if stored at temperatures above 20°C. Paprika is one of the few spices best stored in the refrigerator in an airtight, screw-top glass jar.

PREPARATION AND USE Paprika is used predominantly for its colour-enhancing qualities and is suitable as a garnish on appetisers, eggs, cheese, dips, seafoods and mornays. Paprika gives Hungarian goulash its characteristic colour and flavour, and is a valuable flavouring for delicately textured foods such as crab and chicken. It may be mixed into rice dishes and shaken over split baked potatoes, hors d'oeuvre, casseroles and salads.

PROCESSING Paprika is made from the outer, fleshy portion of the fruit which is where most of the colouring matter is retained, while the inner tissues and seeds contain the pungent chemical capsaicin. Hungarian paprika is divided into five grades, from the best quality 'noble sweet', to semi-sweet 'rose' quality.

VARIETIES
Hungarian, Portuguese, Spanish.

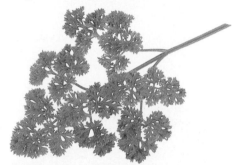

Parsley *Petroselinum crispum*

DESCRIPTION Often called curled or triple-curled parsley, this long-stemmed herb with its frills of bright green grows 25–30 cm tall. Italian parsley grows to 45 cm, and has a larger, flatter leaf structure with a mild celery flavour. Hamburg parsley's long, white taproot, like a parsnip, is sometimes cooked as a vegetable. The flowers are flattish domes of white, blooming in summer, and should be cut from this biennial herb as they appear, to prevent the plant from setting seed and dying back.

ORIGIN AND HISTORY Greek mythology says that parsley grew from the blood of Archemorous, the forerunner of death. The Greeks used it as a garlanding and funeral herb, as well as horse fodder. It was popular with the Romans, and the 9th century emperor, Charlemagne, was particularly fond of a cheese flavoured with parsley seeds. The use of Hamburg parsley root as a vegetable was fashionable in Victorian England. Parsley is known to be rich in iron and vitamins A, B and C.

BUYING AND STORAGE Fresh bunches should have firm stems and unwilted leaves for best nutrition and flavour. The leafy stems can be stored immersed in cold water for up to a week. Dried parsley should be bright green and is best kept in an airtight glass jar away from light.

PREPARATION AND USE Washed and shaken dry, fresh parsley sprigs are an ideal garnish for any savoury food. Their fresh, crisp flavour blends well with other herbs and seasonings, and parsley is one ingredient of the classic bouquet garni, for use in soups, stews and casseroles. Freshly chopped or dried parsley can be added to cooked vegetables, herb butter, salad dressing, soups and stuffings.

PROCESSING Parsley can be dried in a warm oven with the door left slightly open. It must be checked and turned regularly and taken out as soon as it is crisp, as too much heat will reduce the flavour. Parsley also microwaves well, and dries with its bright colour intact.

VARIETIES
Fern-leaved parsley *(P. crispum filicinum)*, Hamburg parsley *(P. sativum)*, Italian parsley *(P. crispum neapolitanum)*.

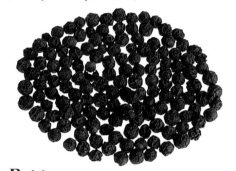

Pepper *Piper nigrum*

also called **Black, Green, Pink and White pepper**

DESCRIPTION *Piper nigrum* is a perennial vine, with dark-green shiny leaves, that grows to 10 m or more in height. Under cultivation the mature vine is trimmed to a 4 m bush. The fruit grows in long clusters of 50–60 peppercorns. The unripe fruit is green, turning greenish-yellow then red as it ripens. Black, white, green and pink peppercorns should all come from the same vine. True pepper does not come from the pepper tree *(Schinus molle)* of tropical America.

ORIGIN AND HISTORY Pepper is native to India and throughout history has been considered the most precious of spices. Peppercorns were used as currency in the Middle Ages, hence the term 'peppercorn rent', which, contrary to its modern interpretation, referred to rents paid to landlords in high priced peppercorns that were preferable to cash. Pepper was probably taken to Java between 100 BC and AD 600 by Hindu colonists. By the 17th century, it was grown commercially in the Dutch East Indies and Malaya, and by the 19th century, world production had brought the price of pepper down so that it was available to the average consumer.

BUYING AND STORAGE If whole peppercorns have stems, small stones or light (empty) berries, it is an indication that they have not been sufficiently cleaned or graded. Avoid inferior peppercorns that have evidence of mould on the surface, or have a musty smell. The true aroma is penetrating and spicy, with a hot biting and pungent taste. Green and pink peppercorns can be bought freeze-dried or in brine. Many green and pink peppercorns sold commercially come from *Schinus molle*, which is a common substitute for real pepper.

PREPARATION AND USE For best results, freshly grind this universal seasoning over food and in cooking. White pepper, which is less aromatic and has a slightly more biting heat than black, is used in foods such as white sauce where black specks of pepper would be considered undesirable.

PROCESSING Black peppercorns are the green, unripe berries harvested about nine months after flowering. They are left in heaps for a few days to ferment, then spread on mats to dry in full sunlight until they shrivel and turn dark brown to black. White pepper is produced from fully ripened, greenish-yellow berries that are soaked in water, then macerated to rub off the outer hull. They are then dried in the sun until creamy white in colour. Green peppercorns are the green unripe berries, picked and put into brine and sometimes later freeze-dried for sale. Pink peppercorns are the fully ripe peppercorns picked and preserved in brine to retain the colour.

VARIETIES
Betel pepper *(P. betle)*, Indian long pepper *(P. longum)*, Java long pepper *(P. retrofractum)*, kava *(P. methysticum)*, rough-leaved pepper *(P. amalago)*.

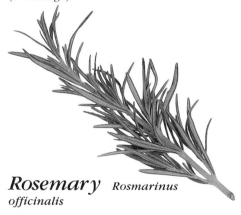

Rosemary *Rosmarinus officinalis*

DESCRIPTION This small evergreen shrub grows up to 1.5 m high, with straight upstanding branches covered in dark green, firm, narrow leaves 2–3 cm long. It has a fresh pine fragrance and tiny, two-lipped mauve-blue flowers. The prostrate variety has smaller leaves, and flowers more profusely throughout the summer.

ORIGIN AND HISTORY Literally translated, rosmarinus means 'dew of the sea', although it grows as well in dry inland areas as on the coast. Legend says that the Virgin Mary spread her cloak over a white-flowering rosemary bush while she rested. The flowers turned the blue of her cloak, and from then on the bush was called Rose of Mary. Rosemary is sometimes called the student's herb because of its stimulating head-clearing effect and was worn in head garlands by Greek scholars to improve their memories. Rosemary has been associated with remembrance and fidelity by Shakespeare and others, and is worn on Anzac Day in Australia to commemorate those who died in war.

BUYING AND STORAGE Fresh bunches of rosemary ideally have firm, flexible stems, and the leaves should not fall off easily. Store immersed in cold water and use within five to six days. The dried herb should be kept in a glass airtight container away from direct light.

PREPARATION AND USE Dried rosemary leaves are brittle and do not soften well in cooking, and it helps to break them up before adding to scones and dumplings. Fresh rosemary is traditionally added to moussaka and roast lamb. Its pungent, spicy flavour gives life to vegetables such as eggplant (aubergine), zucchini, squash and cabbage, and the chopped leaves are used in pasta sauces, pâté and terrine.

PROCESSING Rosemary branches can be hung in bunches in an airy, shady place to air-dry, after which the leaves crumble easily off the stems. Microwaving is another useful drying method. Chopped fresh rosemary can be frozen in iceblocks of water or butter.

VARIETIES
Prostrate rosemary *(R. prostratus)*.

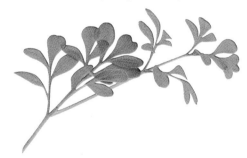

Rue *Ruta graveolens*

also called **Herb of grace**

DESCRIPTION This attractive plant grows to 1 m, and has bluish-green, lacy leaves, like a magnified maidenhair fern. The bright-yellow summer flowers have a tinge of green. It is one of the bitter herbs, although its graceful appearance belies its extraordinary bitterness.

ORIGIN AND HISTORY Native to southern Europe, rue was introduced to England by the Romans. It was used in church ceremonies, for which it earned the name herb of grace. Legend has it that a tea of rue was taken as a penance in order to achieve a state of grace.

BUYING AND STORAGE Rue is not sold commercially fresh or dried.

PREPARATION AND USE The acrid, bitter taste of rue precludes it from most cooking. However, in ancient Rome it was highly regarded as a medicinal herb, and some Italians still add a small amount of finely chopped fresh rue to salads.

PROCESSING As rue is perennial and not sought after in dried form, processing is unnecessary.

VARIETIES
Variegated rue.

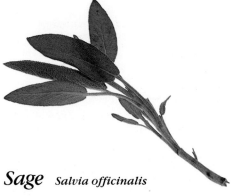

Saffron *Crocus sativus*

also called **Crocus, Karcom, Krokus**

DESCRIPTION Saffron is a dark orange-red filament which is the dried, hand-picked stigma of a mauve, autumn-flowering crocus. It is a perennial bulb with 45 cm long, grey-green, deeply ribbed leaves.

ORIGIN AND HISTORY Saffron is native to Asia Minor and the Mediterranean countries. It has been under cultivation since the 14th century in Sicily, Kashmir, China, Greece, Italy, France, Great Britain, Persia, Portugal, and Spain, which produces the finest quality. One hectare yields only 6 kg of dried saffron, and over 500 000 hand-picked stigmas are required to make up 1 kg of spice. Saffron has been prized from ancient times, when it was used medicinally, in food, in perfume and as a dye.

BUYING AND STORAGE Saffron is best purchased whole, as the powder can easily be adulterated without detection. Pliny worried in the 1st century AD that saffron was the most

frequently falsified commodity, and ever since, its very high price has led to adulteration with various cheap substitutes, from marigold petals to dyed strands of corn silk.

PREPARATION AND USE Owing to its high price and its strength as a colouring agent, saffron should be used sparingly. Crush the required number of filaments and infuse in whatever liquid is called for in the recipe. Saffron gives its character to such traditional dishes as the saffron cakes of Cornwall, the French soup bouillabaisse, and Spanish arroz con pollo (rice with chicken). It also enhances some sauces, breads, cakes, fish, chicken and Indian rice dishes.

PROCESSING Harvesting commences when the plants begin to bloom, as the flowering period may be as short as 15 days. In Spain, where the finest saffron is produced, the stigmas are 'toasted' or dried in sieves over low heat. During drying, they lose about 80% of their weight.

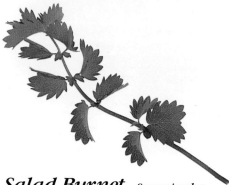

Sage *Salvia officinalis*

DESCRIPTION Sage bushes are perennial, and grow to 90 cm–1 m with square, woody stems. The long, pointed leaves have a grainy texture, and are greenish-grey with a savoury, dry aroma. In autumn, purple flowers bloom along the tips of the leafy branches.

ORIGIN AND HISTORY Originally a medicinal herb in ancient Greece and Rome, sage was believed to prolong life. It was included in Charlemagne's list of cultivated herbs in the 9th century, and became very popular with the Chinese when introduced there — they used it to help improve memory. During the 17th century, the Chinese would exchange any amount of tea for one quarter the amount of sage leaves. In recent centuries, sage has become popular as a seasoning, especially in stuffings for pork and game.

BUYING AND STORAGE Fresh sage can be kept for up to six days immersed in cold water. Dried leaves can be bought whole, 'rubbed' (crushed), or powdered, the rubbed type being the most flavoursome. Store in an airtight container.

PREPARATION AND USE Sage is a natural counterbalance for rich and fatty foods, and for this reason has become a traditional ingredient in stuffings for pork, goose and game. It is a component in mixed herbs, with marjoram and thyme. The dried herb has a strong pungency, and should be used at a rate of one-third the quantity of fresh required. A small amount can be included in herb or garlic bread, and it lends itself well to cheese and egg dishes.

PROCESSING Bunches of sage branches can be harvested at any time of year and hung to air-dry, or leaves can be stripped and spread over a mesh rack or on paper to dry in a shady place. The leaves can be microwaved. When crisp-dry, store in an airtight container.

VARIETIES
Clary sage *(S. sclarea)*, meadow sage *(S. pratensis)*, pineapple sage, red-leaved sage.

Salad Burnet *Sanguisorba minor*

also called **Garden burnet**

DESCRIPTION The perennial salad burnet has cucumber-flavoured leaves that are small, round and serrated. They are spaced about 25 mm apart in pairs of 10 or 12 on each side of a slender stem. As the stems become long and heavy, they fall outwards from the centre, giving the plant a weeping, fernlike appearance. The reddish-pink, berrylike flowers appear in summer at the top of long stalks that shoot up from the centre of the plant.

ORIGIN AND HISTORY Salad burnet is not well known today, although it was highly regarded by the ancients for its healing effects on wounds. In medieval times it was thought to ward off the plague. It is thought to have originated in the Mediterranean regions, although it grows wild throughout Europe. It was often used as a border plant in Tudor herb gardens and knot gardens.

BUYING AND STORAGE Fresh or dried salad burnet is not readily available, but it is easily grown from seed, after which leaves can be picked throughout the year.

PREPARATION AND USE Add sprays of salad burnet to a tossed green salad, or use them as a garnish for sandwiches, aspics and any dish for a buffet. Whole sprays look attractive in wine cups, punches and fruit drinks. When the small leaves are removed whole from their stem, they make an excellent filling for sandwiches, with the addition of a little cream cheese. The chopped leaves can be mixed with cream cheese or sour cream as a dip.

PROCESSING Clean, dry leaves can be air-dried on a wire rack in a shady, airy place, then stored in airtight containers. They can also be microwaved. Whole or chopped leaves can be frozen in water iceblocks.

VARIETIES
The great burnet (S. officinalis).

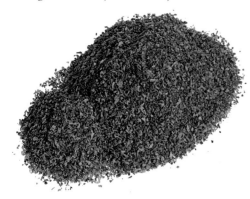

Sansho Powder

DESCRIPTION The leaves of the prickly ash (Xanthoxylum piperitum) are dried and ground in Japan to make a spice called sansho. It comes from the same tree as Chinese or Szechuan pepper, though the leaves are milder and more lemony in flavour than the berries. This is due to the citruslike aroma from the essential oils they contain.

ORIGIN AND HISTORY Japanese.

BUYING AND STORAGE Available from Japanese food shops, sansho powder should be bought in small quantities as its flavour will quickly deteriorate. Store in an airtight container in a cool, dark place.

PREPARATION AND USE As for Szechuan pepper, only a small amount of this spice should be added. It imparts a mildly hot and fragrant flavour to noodle dishes and soups.

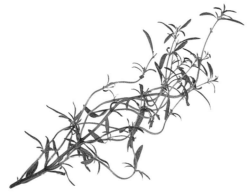

Savory   Satureia spp.

DESCRIPTION Winter savory is popular with home gardeners as it is a perennial, but the more piquant, slightly peppery flavour of summer savory is better for culinary use, especially when dried. Winter savory is a stiff, compact bush, with small, two-lipped white flowers in late summer and autumn. The glossy leaves are thin and narrow, about 12 mm long. Summer savory leaves are longer and softer, of a bronze-green, while the pale pink flowers bloom at the same time as the winter variety. Summer savory seeds prolifically and germinates easily, and has slender, erect and brittle stems.

ORIGIN AND HISTORY Savory is indigenous to the eastern Mediterranean and south-west Asia, introduced elsewhere on dry chalky soils and rocky hillsides. Once thought to be an aphrodisiac — Banckes' herbal states: 'It is forbidden to use it much in meats since it stirreth him to use lechery'. It was used in food as long as 2000 years ago, and was introduced into Europe and Britain by the Romans. The Germans have called it 'bean herb', because it complements green and dried beans so well.

BUYING AND STORAGE Savory is most often sold commercially in its dried, ground form, which is convenient as the whole leaf when dried is very hard. However, grinding herbs accelerates flavour deterioration. Always store in airtight, screw-top glass jars.

PREPARATION AND USE Both varieties of savory are used in the same way. Summer savory is an ingredient in fines herbes and the finely chopped leaves go well with all kinds of cooked beans, either with melted butter or in a creamy sauce. The nuances of summer savory enhance the flavour of poultry dishes, crumbed pork, veal and seafood, when a little powdered savory is added to the breadcrumbs. Use savory as a substitute for pepper when a milder, different flavour is desired.

PROCESSING Both savories can be air-dried in bunches with good results, having been harvested just before flowering. The crisp-dry leaves crumble easily off the stems. This herb

can also be frozen in water iceblocks or microwaved.

VARIETIES
Prostrate savory — decorative (S. repandens); summer savory — annual (S. hortensis); winter savory — perennial (S. montana).

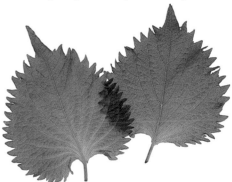

Shiso   Perilla

also called Beefsteak plant

DESCRIPTION Shiso is a leafy plant which is a member of the mint family. There are two main types, green ao-jiso, and red aka-jiso, and they have different uses in Japanese cooking.

ORIGIN AND HISTORY The plant is a native of Burma, China and the northern regions of India, particularly the Himalayan mountains, but it has been cultivated in Japan for centuries and is now rarely used in its countries of origin.

BUYING AND STORAGE Occasionally fresh shiso leaves are available in highly specialised Japanese food shops, but we are more likely to find the salted and pickled varieties.

PREPARATION AND USE The green type has a fresh, spearmint flavour and is used mainly as a garnish, either whole or chopped. It is battered and fried as a vegetable in tempura and is used in sushi. The attractive seed pod stems, when in flower, are also used by themselves as a garnish. The red leaves are of a different species, available only in midsummer in Japan, and they are used in the processing of umeboshi, the pickled sour plum so popular in Japan. They are also pickled in their own right, and are served as an accompaniment to rice. The red colour of the leaves has earned the herb the name 'beefsteak plant'.

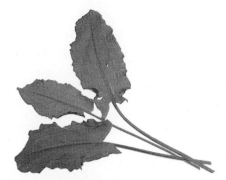

Sorrel Rumex scutatus

*also called **Dock, French sorrel, Oseille***

DESCRIPTION French sorrel is a hardy annual which grows in thick clumps similar to spinach. The broad, oval, shield-shaped leaves are about 15 cm long and 8 cm wide, with reddish stems. The small, greenish flowers appear in summer, near the top and on either side of long, scarlet-streaked stalks. Sorrel has a bitter, slightly sour taste, and the young leaves have a hint of lemon flavour.

ORIGIN AND HISTORY French sorrel is native to the south of France and central Europe, and is closely related to mountain sorrel, sheep's sorrel, English or garden sorrel and dock. The Egyptians and Romans ate sorrel to offset the richness of some foods. It is believed that French sorrel was introduced to Britain in 1596. The name is derived from the Greek word for sour.

BUYING AND STORAGE Sorrel is not readily available in fresh or dried form, but it is easy to grow from seed. Plant seeds in spring, then each autumn the plants can be increased by root division. Fresh sorrel can be stored immersed in water in the refrigerator for five to six days, or wrapped tightly in foil and frozen for four to six weeks.

PREPARATION AND USE A favourite culinary use for sorrel is to cook and eat it like spinach, with the addition of beaten eggs and butter or cream, to mellow the sharp flavour. French sorrel is popular in soup, and a white sauce with chopped sorrel added is a delicious accompaniment for poultry, fish moulds, and hot boiled potatoes. It makes an unusual filling for omelettes, and can be used in a tossed green salad. Sorrel, like spinach, should not be cooked in aluminium.

PROCESSING The fresh leaves can be gathered throughout the year in moderate climates. Dry by placing unblemished leaves flat on a wire rack in a dry, well-aired place, or microwave on paper towel in a single layer. When the leaves are crisp, store in an airtight container.

VARIETIES
Common, garden, meadow sorrel, sourgrass (*R. acetosa*).

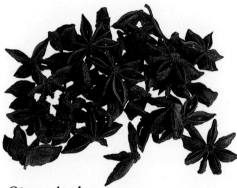

Star Anise Illicium verum

*also called **Aniseed stars, Badian, Botgok, Chinese anise, Clove flowers***

DESCRIPTION This small evergreen tree growing to 5 m with shiny aromatic leaves 7 cm long, has magnolialike greenish-yellow, unscented flowers with many petals. The fruit is star-shaped and made up of eight segments, each containing one seed which, when sundried, is woody and reddish-brown. Star anise has a pleasant, aniselike aroma and a sweet liquorice type of flavour.

ORIGIN AND HISTORY Star anise is native to the southern and south-western provinces of China and Vietnam. It is totally unrelated to anise. The star anise tree may bear fruit for 100 years or more. Traditionally the Japanese have used ground star anise bark as incense, and in Asia the seeds are chewed after meals to promote digestion and sweeten the breath. It is an essential element in the Chinese five spice blend and is used extensively throughout China. It has been adopted in most countries where the cuisine has a Chinese influence and has been in use in Europe for three centuries, via the China–Russia tea route. Star anise was known in Europe in the past as Siberian cardamom.

BUYING AND STORAGE The hard, brown, dried star-shaped fruits are generally ground for sale on the domestic market. The powder should be dark-brown and evenly coloured, with a characteristic aroma and slightly oily feel. Ground star anise should be stored in airtight glass jars to retain its quality.

PREPARATION AND USE Star anise is used in many Asian dishes. It is added whole to coffee and tea in China, and small whole pieces are used in Indian biryani rice. It complements pork and veal and can be added sparingly to stir-fried food. It is used commercially to flavour drinks and in medicine to mask bitter-tasting drugs.

PROCESSING The hard stars are broken with a hammer into small, usable pieces. The carpels which contain the seeds have a greater fullness of aroma than the seeds, and pow-

dered star anise is made by grinding the carpels and seeds together.

VARIETIES
Florida anise — ornamental (*I. floridanum*).

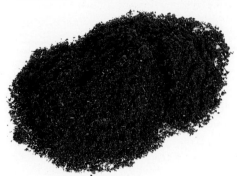

Sumach Rhus glabra

*also called **Sicilian sumac, Sumac, Sumak***

DESCRIPTION The genus *Rhus* includes some poisonous species (poison ivies and poison oaks), so care must be taken not to use the wrong one. *Rhus glabra* is a shrub 2–5 m high, with straggling branches, which grows wild throughout North America and the Middle East. It has red berries, as do all the edible varieties. It has a sour, astringent taste and is used as a substitute for lemon.

ORIGIN AND HISTORY Sumach was used by the Romans in the same way that lemons are used today, as lemons had not yet been discovered. They called it Syrian sumach. The sour seeds are used extensively in Middle Eastern cooking and in the food of the American Indians. Sumach is grown commercially in the USA and Sicily, and is used in the tanning industry. Sumach is an essential condiment for a famous Iranian dish called chelou kebab, a simple dish of lean lamb marinated in onion juice then grilled over charcoal and served with hot chelou (plain rice pilaf); an egg yolk, butter and sumach are mixed into the rice by each diner.

BUYING AND STORAGE Purchase from shops stocking Middle Eastern foods. It is available loose or packaged, and should be stored in a sealed jar in a cool place away from direct light. If you come across a sumach tree with berries, *do not* on any account pick the berries — it could well be the wrong tree as many species do have poisonous properties.

PREPARATION AND USE The berries are covered with fine hairs, which need to be filtered out through fine cloth before use. They have been used in making elderberry jam. The flavour has a rounded, fruity sourness, and the powder is used in spicy Middle Eastern dishes in the same way that tamarind is used in Indian curries. The berries of squawberry and staghorn sumach (both known as the lemonade tree) are used to make cooling summer drinks. Powdered sumach is blended with thyme and salt to make a spice called za'tar, used as a savoury sprinkle over bread.

PROCESSING The berries should be gathered with their downy covering intact, as they are not as tasty if the down has been washed off by rain. When used whole, the berries are broken, soaked in water for 15 to 20 minutes, then squeezed to extract the juice. The berries can be air-dried and then ground to make a powder.

VARIETIES
Dwarf sumach *(R. copallina)*, fragrant sumach *(R. aromatica)*, squawberry sumach *(R. trilobata)*, staghorn sumach *(R. typhina)*.

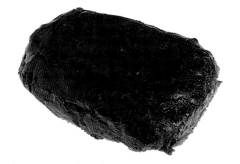

Tamarind *Tamarindus indica*

also called **Amsamgelugor, Amsam keping, Imlee, Indian date**

DESCRIPTION The tamarind is a large evergreen tree to 25 m which grows in tropical climates. The trunk is covered with shaggy, brownish-grey bark. The frondlike leaves have 20–40 small leaflets. The pale-yellow flowers have petals with red veins and grow at the ends of the branches. The fruit is a cinnamon-coloured oblong pod, 7–20 cm long, with a thin, brittle shell enclosing a soft brownish, acidulous pulp that has a bitter flavour.

ORIGIN AND HISTORY The tamarind is native to India and tropical Africa, and cultivated in the West Indies. In India it is believed that the area around a tamarind tree becomes unwholesome, and that it is unsafe to sleep under the tree owing to the acid it exhales during the night. In spite of the superstition that nothing will grow in its shade, lush gardens have been seen flourishing under tamarind trees in Bengal.

In India, probably the most refreshing drink is imli panni, or tamarind water. It is served in the Arabic countries where tamarind is known as tamr hindi (the origin of its name) and through tropical Asia it is taken medicinally to cool and cleanse the system, being particu-

larly good for the cleansing organs the liver and kidneys. Tamarind seeds rolled in sugar were the only sweet that Indonesian children knew until the Western world intervened.

BUYING AND STORAGE Tamarind is not always readily available; however, when it can be bought it is usually in the form of the whole pod, the pulp, or a ready-made tamarind paste. Some commercial preparations, called cream of tamarind, or assam powder, are made by extracting the flavour from the sticky pulp and mixing the extract with a carrier to keep it free-flowing. Store in airtight glass containers.

PREPARATION AND USE Tamarind is high in tartaric acid and it is this that gives it the sourness for which it is valued. To make tamarind water, a common curry ingredient, soak 1 tablespoon of tamarind pulp (from the pod) in ½ cup of hot water, and allow to stand for 15 minutes. Strain water into another container, squeezing the tamarind pulp as dry as possible. Discard the pulp. If a stronger sour taste is required, use more tamarind pulp when following the above procedure. The leaves are used to make a red or yellow dye, and both the leaves and flowers can be eaten in salads.

PROCESSING West Indian tamarinds are usually exported in syrup, the outer shell having been removed, and East Indian tamarinds are exported in a firm, black, shelled mass for further processing.

VARIETIES
East Indian tamarind, West Indian tamarind.

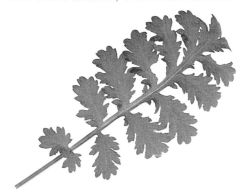

Tansy *Tanacetum vulgare*

also called **Buttons, Parsley fern**

DESCRIPTION Tansy is a spreading, perennial herb, growing to about 1 m, with a strong, creeping root system. The leaves are deeply toothed, with a bitter lemon-camphor fragrance. The late summer to autumn flowers are clustered together on one head, looking like a bunch of small yellow buttons. Tansy dies away to ground level in winter when the

roots are dormant, and sends up new growth in spring.

ORIGIN AND HISTORY Tansy is native to Europe, and over the centuries has been introduced elsewhere, especially north-east North America. It is traditionally used in tansy cakes, served at Easter as a reminder of the bitter herbs eaten at the Feast of the Passover. Tansy was a valued strewing herb in the Middle Ages, being an effective and aromatic insect repellent.

BUYING AND STORAGE Fresh or dried leaves of tansy are not readily available, however it is easily grown from seed or by root division.

PREPARATION AND USE Tansy should be used sparingly in food because of its harsh flavour. However, it is used in a modern recipe for tansy pudding, where ½ teaspoon of the chopped young leaves is an ingredient. Platters of sliced, cold meat can be garnished with decorative tansy fronds which look attractive and, when eating al fresco, serve as an effective fly repellent.

PROCESSING Tansy is best dried with the foliage still on the stalks. Hang in bunches or spread out on a drying rack in a shaded, airy place. When the leaves are crisp, strip them from the stalks and store in an airtight container. Tansy stalks begin to shrivel at the onset of winter, and should be cut back to ground level.

VARIETIES
T. crispum (larger with more finely divided leaves).

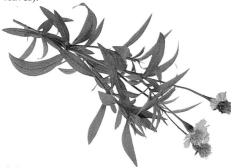

Tarragon *Artemisia dracunculus*

also called **French tarragon**

DESCRIPTION French tarragon has a low, untidy tangle of lanky stems, with straight, smooth and narrow leaves. Yellowish buds in late summer rarely come fully into bloom, making seed scarce. Russian tarragon has more robust growth, to 1.5 m tall, and a coarser, less piquant flavour. A sturdier, more compact plant is winter tarragon (pictured above), which has bright yellow flowers and a typical tarragon flavour.

ORIGIN AND HISTORY The French name estragon or 'little dragon' is thought to refer either to its coiled serpentlike root system or to its reputation for curing reptile bites. Although virtually unknown in Roman and Greek civilisations, it was mentioned in the 13th century by a botanist in Spain, and in Gerard's herbal in England in 1597. It has become a highly sought-after gourmet's herb, with its unique tart flavour and spicy aroma.

BUYING AND STORAGE Fresh French tarragon is not available in winter, although winter or Russian tarragon may be offered as an inferior alternative. Dried tarragon should have a good green colour and should be stored away from light.

PREPARATION AND USE Mixed in equal quantities with chervil, chives and parsley, it makes the classic fines herbes blend. An essential ingredient in bearnaise and tartare sauces, it can be added to chicken, turkey, game, veal, egg dishes and seafood. A fresh whole sprig can be steeped in vinegar or added to tomato juice, or chopped and added to salad dressing.

PROCESSING Cut green leaves and tender top growth once plants are well established. Remove leaves from stems and air-dry on wire racks away from sunlight, or microwave. Store in an airtight container away from direct light to preserve colour.

VARIETIES

Russian tarragon *(A. dracunculoides).*

Winter tarragon *(Tagetes minuta).*

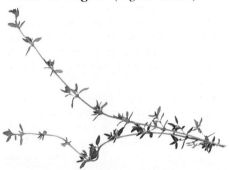

Thyme *Thymus vulgaris*

also called *Garden thyme*

DESCRIPTION The pungent, grey-leaved garden thyme grows in a compact perennial bush about 30 cm high. It has slender, densely branched stems with small, pointed leaves and white, pink or purple flowers. Lemon thyme is smaller and has slightly larger, greener leaves with a distinct lemon flavour.

ORIGIN AND HISTORY The name of this herb is derived from the Greek 'to fumigate', and it was used by the Egyptians for embalming, as well as by the Greeks as a temple incense. The Greeks considered honey from thyme blossoms a delicacy. It was introduced by the Romans into Britain and Europe, where it became popular as a seasoning and a medicine. Several modern-day cough mixtures contain oil of thyme (thymol) as it has antiseptic qualities; it is also an ingredient of the liqueur bénédictine.

BUYING AND STORAGE Fresh thyme can be stored immersed in cold water for up to a week. Because dried thyme leaves are so small, they are available as whole leaves, which are more flavoursome and attractive in food than powdered thyme.

PREPARATION AND USE Freshly picked stems can be washed and added entire to slow-cooking soups, stews and casseroles. The leaves fall off the stem as they cook, and the stem is taken out before serving. Thyme is combined with marjoram, parsley and bay leaves to make a classic bouquet garni. The flavour of thyme is a vital part of the Creole cooking of New Orleans. Its strong, sharp character goes well in moderation with stuffings, chicken, beef, herb breads, and vegetables. Lemon thyme lends a subtle lemon tang to chicken, shellfish and other seafoods, veal and potatoes.

PROCESSING Thyme dries easily when hung in bunches in a shady, airy place or spread on gauze. It also microwaves well. When crispdry, store in an airtight container away from direct light.

VARIETIES

Lemon thyme *(T. citriodorus)* and about 100 decorative varieties.

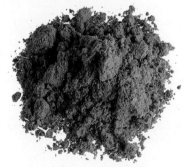

Turmeric *Curcuma domestica*

also called *Haldi, Kha min, Kunyit, Kunyit basah*

DESCRIPTION A tropical plant to 1 m high, this perennial is related to ginger. The leaves are bright green, and broad. It has pale-yellow flowers, but reproduction occurs through splitting of the rhizomes. The rhizomes have a peppery, spicy aroma and a bitter, pungent taste. When ground, turmeric is a bright yellow powder. Varieties can differ in shade.

ORIGIN AND HISTORY Turmeric is not known in a truly wild state; however, originally it came from southern Asia where it is used as a protective charm and in medicine. Marco Polo records it as occurring in China in 1280. Turmeric has now become widely distributed throughout the tropics, but its cultivation as a spice is most common in India, Southeast Asia and Indonesia.

BUYING AND STORAGE Turmeric fingers are rarely bought by domestic users, who would have difficulty in preparing them for use in cooking. Ground turmeric may be orange-yellow (Alleppey) or lemon-yellow (Madras) in colour. This does not indicate quality but the region from which it comes.

PREPARATION AND USE Turmeric is ground to a fine powder and is used mainly as a colouring. It is an essential ingredient in curry powder and is used in pickles, chutneys and mustard blends. It can be used as a substitute for saffron in rice dishes and its oleoresin is used commercially as a natural colouring.

PROCESSING Turmeric is cured by a method evolved in India, which involves boiling or steaming the fresh rhizomes in water, drying in the sun and finally peeling or polishing them for sale. There are now various methods, all with the object of killing microorganisms, preventing further growth, reducing drying time, and creating a more uniformly coloured product.

VARIETIES

Black zedoary *(C. caesia)*, bulbous central rhizomes *(C. rotunda)*, Indian arrowroot or Travencore starch *(C. angustifolia)*, temoe lawak — Indonesia *(C. xanthorrhiza)*, turmeric finger rhizomes *(C. longa)*, wild turmeric or yellow zedoary *(C. aromatica)*.

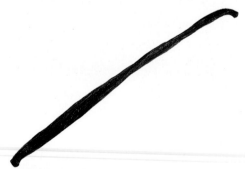

Vanilla *Vanilla planifolia*

also called *Vanilla beans, Vanilla pods*

DESCRIPTION Vanilla pods are the fruits of

the golden flowered vanilla orchid, a large, green-stemmed, climbing perennial plant with a fleshy, succulent stem, smooth, thick, oblong bright-green leaves, and numerous twining aerial roots by which it clings to trees. In its wild state, it may grow to 30 m, climbing to the tops of tall forest trees. The pods, commercially called beans, have no flavour when picked, as the flavour develops during the curing process. The beans are very dark brown and contain tiny black seeds.

ORIGIN AND HISTORY Vanilla is native to the tropical rainforests of south-eastern Mexico and Central America. When the Spanish conquistadores were in Mexico in 1520, they observed the emperor Montezuma drinking a beverage of cocoa beans, corn, vanilla pods and honey. They were so impressed that they took vanilla back to Spain and by the end of the 16th century, factories were established to manufacture chocolate with vanilla flavouring.

BUYING AND STORAGE Vanilla extract can be bought in bottles and the pods (around 10–20 cm long), bought whole, should be soft and very dark brown, almost black. A white crystalline coating on the surface is a sign of high quality as this is vanillin, the result of curing and the fragrant constituent that gives vanilla pods their flavour. Store in an airtight container.

PREPARATION AND USE Vanilla beans can be stored in a jar of sugar, permeating it with their own sweet aroma. The pod can be chopped finely or processed in a blender and used to flavour cakes, puddings, ice cream, milkshakes and many everyday sweet dishes. The whole pod can also be used to flavour custards and other liquids, taken out, dried carefully and used again up to three or four times. To flavour milk, allow one bean per 600 mL milk, bring to the boil and leave to stand for an hour.

PROCESSING Vanilla pods must be cured in order for the vanillin to be produced, which gives vanilla its flavour. Curing is performed by alternately sweating and drying the pods for up to six months until they become pliable and deep brown, with a fine white crystalline coating of vanillin.

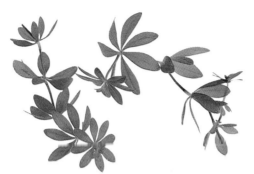

Woodruff *Asperula odorata (Galium odoratum)*

also called Sweet woodruff, Waldmeister

DESCRIPTION Woodruff, as the name suggests, is found in the woods of Europe, Asia and Africa. It is a low-growing (60–90 cm) perennial with a creeping root, delicate stems, and dark shiny leaves growing in clusters of six to eight, like spokes of a wheel. An attractive shade-loving ground cover, it has small white star-shaped flowers in spring. Its scent of new-mown hay is more prominent once the leaves are cut and dried.

ORIGIN AND HISTORY This herb is mentioned in a 13th century herbal as Wuderove — the word being derived from the French for wheel, alluding to the spoke arrangement of the leaves. Teutonic warriors believed that wearing woodruff would bring them success in battle. During the Middle Ages, garlands of woodruff were used as air fresheners, and it was used in perfumery, snuff and pot pourri. Earlier this century, it was employed in pharmacy to disguise unpleasant odours.

BUYING AND STORAGE Woodruff is not commercially available fresh or dried. If harvesting from the garden, allow to wilt for a day before using to maximise aroma and flavour.

PREPARATION AND USE Used mostly as a flavouring for drinks, woodruff is an ingredient of Maibowle, a German drink traditionally served on the 1st of May. This is made by steeping two to four wilted or dried sprigs of woodruff in a bottle of chilled white wine overnight, then combining in a punch bowl the wine, a cup of halved strawberries, and a bottle of champagne, soda water or lemonade. This herb makes a pleasant tea, and can be added to a pot of ordinary tea. Herbalists warn of undesirable side effects from overindulgence in woodruff.

PROCESSING It is necessary to dry woodruff before use to have the best aroma. Leaves and flowers should be hung in bunches or removed from the stem for air-drying or microwaving. Store in an airtight container away from light.

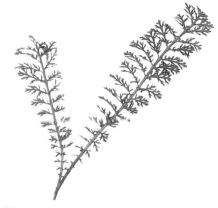

Yarrow *Achillea millefolium*

also called Bloodwort, Knight's milfoil, Military herb, Nose bleed, Old man's pepper, Sanguinary, Soldier's woundwort, Staunchweed

DESCRIPTION Yarrow is a perennial growing to 60 cm tall, with thickly matted, feathery foliage from a spreading root system. Tiny white florets mass to form flat, even flower heads on top of erect, 60 cm tall stems in summer and autumn.

ORIGIN AND HISTORY Yarrow is a wild plant of Britain and Europe. The botanical name refers to the legend that Achilles used it to staunch the blood of his soldiers' wounds. It is reputed to improve strength and stamina. Alternative names of yarrow indicate its use as first aid for wounds over the centuries. Before the use of hops, yarrow was an ingredient for brewing ale, and was used for snuff, hence the name old man's pepper.

BUYING AND STORAGE Dried yarrow is considered a medicinal herb rather than a food, and would be available through herbalists. Yarrow for eating is best picked straight from the garden and used immediately, or stored, refrigerated, immersed in water for up to four days.

PREPARATION AND USE The yarrow's pleasant, slightly bitter leaves can be steamed gently and eaten as a vegetable, made into a soup, or finely chopped and added to salads. Young leaves are more palatable than mature leaves, which have a strong, bitter flavour. It can be mixed in equal quantities with chamomile or peppermint for a refreshing tea.

PROCESSING Yarrow stems are cut and dried when in full bloom. They are air-dried then stored in an airtight container. Dried yarrow is used as a herbal remedy rather than a food, the flowers, leaves and stems all being utilised.

VARIETIES
Golden-flowering yarrow, 'Pearl' (ornamental with creamy-white blossoms).

Sugars, Syrups and Sweeteners

The Bay of Bengal is considered the most likely place of origin of sugarcane, which is a perennial grass of the genus *Saccharum*. Although sugarcane syrup was used as a sweetener in India for centuries, it did not replace honey there as the principal sweetener until the 3rd century. From India, sugarcane spread rapidly to Malaysia and Indonesia and reached Europe by about the 13th century; but it did not replace honey there until the 18th century. It was known in England in the 16th century — Shakespeare mentioned it in several of his plays — but again the transfer from honey to sugar took another two hundred years. Columbus brought sugarcane to the Caribbean during the 16th century and it was eventually cultivated there. Sugar still remained expensive for some time, however, and was certainly not a staple in the diet of the poor.

Midway through the 18th century a German chemist discovered the possibilities of using root plants such as carrots and beets to produce sugar. It was not, however, until the end of that century, with the British blockade interrupting the flow of sugarcane from the West Indies and Southeast Asia, that the theory was fully developed. The first factory to process sugar beet was established in Europe in 1801–02. When the flow of trade returned to normal, sugarcane once again became the chief source of sweetening around the world.

The basic steps through which sugarcane goes in production are shredding, rolling, heating, refining and crystallisation. Beet sugar syrup is produced by pressing beet pulp, and the raw juice is later treated. The various stages of refining these syrups produce a wide range of types of sugar.

Because the origin and history of all these sugars are mentioned above, and since buying and storage, preparation and use do not differ greatly from one product to another, the entries in this chapter contain all the relevant information under two headings, Nutritional Information and Description, alone.

The chapter includes entries for artificial sweeteners, and major fruit syrups.

The discovery of what are now known as artificial sweeteners has usually been by accident rather than design. The first of these, saccharin, was discovered by chance during laboratory experiments in 1879. The sweet properties of cyclamate were come upon in 1937, during quite unrelated scientific research.

These sweeteners have been of value in that they may replace sugar in weight-loss or diabetic diets. Medical opinion differs from country to country concerning their relative safety and benefits.

The liking for sweet foods is innate, and is usually reinforced by childhood experiences, which associate sweet foods with rewards and pleasure. In Australasia, the annual consumption has averaged between 45 and 50 kg per person throughout this century, but the pattern of sugar use has changed: in the late thirties about two-thirds of the sugar was used in the home and one-third in manufactured food. By the late seventies these figures were reversed, and two-thirds of the sugar eaten came from processed foods. This continuing trend tends to reduce consumers' awareness of the amount of sugar they are eating.

Sugar is not linked with the lifestyle diseases associated with fat, but is linked with the development of tooth decay. Sugars taken into the mouth are fermented by micro-organisms to form acids. Some of the sugars are also converted to sticky substances, which form plaques on the surfaces of the teeth. The acids accumulate around the plaques and demineralise the enamel of the teeth.

When fluoride is incorporated in the tooth enamel it is much more resistant to this acid attack. Along with improved dental care and hygiene, fluoridation of the reticulated water, introduced in the 1960s, has lowered the prevalence of dental caries in some countries.

Another disadvantage of sugar is that it is a food with a very poor nutritional balance, being a concentrated source of kilojoules, but containing no protein, dietary fibre, vitamins or minerals. When sugar is added to the diet it therefore dilutes the nutritional quality of that diet overall.

Raw sugar, brown sugar and coffee crystals contain extractives which give the foods their characteristic flavours, and traces of vitamins and minerals. The amounts of the latter are too small to give these foods any more nutritional advantage than white sugar.

Most people like sweet foods and there is no reason why small amounts of sugar should not be enjoyed. For people who need to restrict their kilojoule intake, however, either in order to lose weight or because they are inactive, sugars along with fats should be the first foods reduced in the diet.

Sugar has important properties in food apart from its sweetness. For example, it is essential in making most jams, biscuits, cakes and confectionery. The physical characteristics of sugar, and the changes which take place with heating it and mixing it with other foods, give rise to a variety of products.

The high temperature reached in some of these processes results in foods of excellent keeping quality. Low bulk artificial sweeteners cannot replace sugar in such foods.

Despite the popularity of sweeteners such as saccharin, cyclamate and aspartame, there has been no decline in the prevalence of obesity. Many people use these sweeteners, but they continue to consume energy-dense diets which are high in fat, and to consume a large amount of sugar in sweetened foods.

Sugar can be enjoyed as part of a varied diet, and those who consume high quantities should remain active to avoid becoming overweight. A sweet tooth can also be appeased by foods which have the desired sweetness, but which contain low concentrations of sugar, such as fruit.

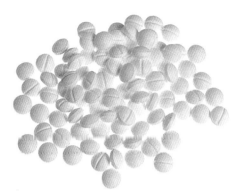

Aspartame

NUTRITIONAL INFORMATION Aspartame contains negligible energy and no carbohydrate, fat, cholesterol or sodium. It is not recommended for individuals suffering from the rare genetic disorder phenylketonuria. For other consumers, aspartame has been declared safe by the US Food and Drug Administration. Despite extensive safety tests, adverse reactions continue to be reported and these are currently being monitored.

DESCRIPTION Aspartame is a synthetic sweetener consisting of two amino acids (proteins): phenylalanine and aspartic acid. Aspartame is unstable at high temperatures and breaks down to its constituent amino acids with a subsequent loss of sweetness.

The main processing advantage of aspartame is that it does not have a bitter aftertaste.

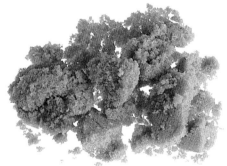

Brown Sugar

NUTRITIONAL INFORMATION Brown sugar is 95% sucrose and the remaining 5% contains glucose, fructose, a small quantity of ash, and water.

This sugar provides energy (67 kJ per teaspoon) and carbohydrate (4 g per teaspoon). Like all sugars, brown sugar does not contain fat, protein, cholesterol or sodium.

DESCRIPTION Brown sugar is a soft, moist sugar with a very fine crystal size. It has a characteristic flavour which arises from a film of molasses syrup surrounding each crystal. These properties make it especially suitable for use in baking and in fillings.

Processing does not influence the nutritional properties of brown sugar. A coarser-grained variety of the same sugar is often called 'molasses' sugar in English recipes, while a further molasses sugar is called muscovado.

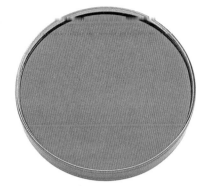

Cane Syrup

NUTRITIONAL INFORMATION Cane syrup contains energy and carbohydrate. Precise nutrient composition is unavailable; however, as cane syrup is produced in a manner similar to golden syrup and treacle, it may contain significant quantities of potassium and sodium.

DESCRIPTION Cane syrup is produced by a partial breakdown of sucrose to glucose and fructose during the refining process. A dark liquid is collected, which is then concentrated by evaporation in a vacuum pan.

Cane syrup is used as a table syrup and in puddings and sponges. Processing does not affect its nutritional properties.

Caster Sugar

NUTRITIONAL INFORMATION This has the same properties as granulated sugar.

DESCRIPTION Caster sugar is produced from special boilings of the sugar syrup which are carefully screened to the size required.

It dissolves faster than white sugar and is especially suitable for meringue, glacé fruits, cake making and puddings. Processing does not alter its nutritional properties.

Coarse, Extra Coarse Sugar

NUTRITIONAL INFORMATION Similar to granulated sugar.

DESCRIPTION These are used commercially for decoration and other special uses. The English equivalent is known as candy sugar. The United States equivalents are confectioners' AA or 'special coarse' sugar.

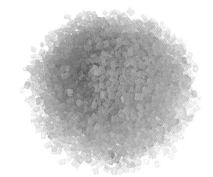

Coffee Crystals

NUTRITIONAL INFORMATION Similar to granulated sugar.

DESCRIPTION Large brown crystals with a unique flavour contributed by extractives, used for sweetening coffee. They are common to English cultures but have no equivalent in the USA.

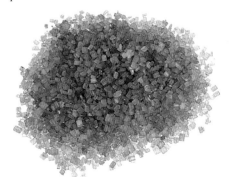

Coloured Sugar Crystals

NUTRITIONAL INFORMATION These have

the properties of granulated sugar.

DESCRIPTION Vegetable dyes are used to colour large white crystals in a variety of shades. They are used for decorative purposes on cakes, biscuits and confectionery.

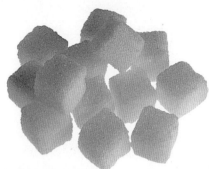

Cube Sugar

also called **Lump sugar**

NUTRITIONAL INFORMATION This has the same properties as granulated sugar.

DESCRIPTION Cube sugar is manufactured by pressing damp white sugar into moulds. The results are dried. Cube sugar is popular for beverages, enabling the exact quantity to be measured each time. Becoming more common are coloured and shaped sugars, hearts for weddings, or decoratively iced cubes. Processing does not alter their nutritional properties.

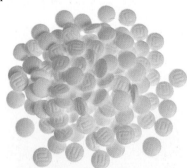

Cyclamate

NUTRITIONAL INFORMATION Cyclamate is a 'non-nutritive' sweetener. It does not contain carbohydrate, fat, protein, cholesterol or sodium. It contains an insignificant amount of energy.

DESCRIPTION Cyclamate is used in combination with saccharin to mask a bitter aftertaste when saccharin is used alone. The results of animal studies suggest that cyclamates like saccharin are cancer-causing agents of low potency when given in large amounts. As a result of these studies cyclamates have been banned in the United States. They are available, however, in Australia.

Cyclamates are stable on processing.

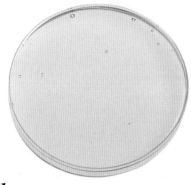

Glucose

also called **Corn syrup**

NUTRITIONAL INFORMATION Glucose contains carbohydrate and energy, 4 grams and 67 kJ per teaspoon respectively. Glucose does not offer any nutritional benefit when compared with other sugars. It is, however, less sweet than an equivalent amount of sucrose and can therefore be tolerated in larger amounts in high energy diets.

Glucose tablets or powder can be administered during diabetic hypoglycaemia. This should then be followed by portions of a complex carbohydrate such as bread or biscuits. Glucose does not contain protein, fat, cholesterol or sodium.

DESCRIPTION Glucose is a simple sugar or monosaccharide and is the main source of energy used by cells in the body. It is derived from the breakdown of glycogen, fat and protein. Very few foods contain glucose (two exceptions are honey and grapes). It can also be made from starch, for example, wheat.

The viscosity of glucose in the syrup form makes it particularly useful in the confectionery industry. Glucose is also used to flavour dairy products and beverages, particularly juices.

Liquid glucose is a heavy, colourless syrup made from a mixture of sugars and used extensively in confectionery.

Processing in these situations does not alter the nutritional properties.

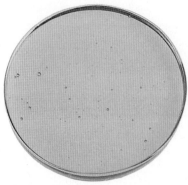

Golden Syrup

NUTRITIONAL INFORMATION Golden syrup contains energy, carbohydrate, potassium and sodium.

Per tablespoon it contains 320 kJ, 20 g of carbohydrate and 50 mg of both potassium and sodium.

Golden syrup does not contain fat or cholesterol and has only negligible amounts of protein.

DESCRIPTION Golden syrup is made from sugar syrup which has been partially broken down into glucose and fructose. It contains 27% sugar syrup (sucrose), 47% glucose and fructose, and the remaining 26% is water.

Golden syrup is widely used in baking and fillings for cakes and biscuits where it is valued for its distinctive flavour. The term 'golden syrup' features in English and English-derived recipes but not in American ones.

Processing does not alter its nutritional properties.

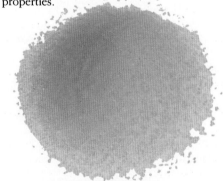

Granulated Sugar

NUTRITIONAL INFORMATION Granulated sugar is a form of sucrose which is refined from sugarcane. Sucrose provides only carbohydrate and energy; it does not contain protein, fat, cholesterol or sodium.

One teaspoon of granulated sugar contains 67 kJ, and 4 g of carbohydrate.

The safety of sugar has been extensively researched by medical scientists. The conclusion from the recent US Food and Drug Administration report on the safety of sugar is that 'sugar is safe'. Sugar should be consumed in moderation to suit energy requirements.

DESCRIPTION When we think of 'sugar' we usually think of granulated sugar, which is one type of table sugar. From the basic white granulated sugar, a wide range of sugars differing only in size are derived to suit a variety of industries. The size of the crystal is indicated by various terms such as standard, medium, medium fine, sanding fine, extra fine and 'baker's special', for example.

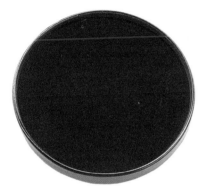

Grenadine

*also called **Dibs roman, Grenadine molasses***

MAJOR NUTRIENTS		SERVE SIZE LESS THAN 5 G	
Energy	70 kJ	Carbohydrate	2g
Protein	0	Total Sugars	2g
Fat	0	Sodium	10 mg
Cholesterol	0	Potassium	20 mg

NUTRITIONAL INFORMATION Contains significant amounts of naturally occurring salicylates, but because only a few drops are normally used in a dish, the amounts are not nutritionally significant.

DESCRIPTION A thick, dark, purple syrup made from pomegranate juice. It has a concentrated pomegranate flavour, very tart and slightly sweet.

Dibs roman (Arabic for pomegranate sugar) is the easy way to get a pomegranate flavour into traditional recipes, as any person would attest who has tried to separate the juice from the seeds. It is used to flavour the lamb filling for the Lebanese and Syrian flat pies, fatayer and sfiha. It is also used in some Middle Eastern stews where a sweet-sour flavour is called for, and is an interesting addition to marinades for lamb kebabs, a good substitute for lemon juice.

When pomegranate juice is required in a recipe and the fruit is not available, use 4 teaspoons of the syrup to 250 ml of water.

As a cordial, grenadine is very popular in Europe, where it is drunk with water or added to other drinks.

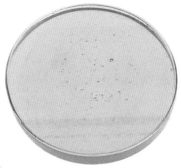

Honey

NUTRITIONAL INFORMATION The major nutrients in honey are energy and carbohydrate. Per tablespoon, honey contains 320kJ, and 20g of carbohydrate. It does not contain protein, cholesterol, sodium or fat.

Honey is often thought to be nutritionally superior to other sweeteners due to the quantities of vitamins and minerals present. However, in the context of the total diet the quantities of vitamins and minerals in honey are too small to be of any nutritional significance. The nutritional properties of honey are not changed by processing.

DESCRIPTION Honey has been a constant part of man's diet since time immemorial — first as wild honey, raided from bees' nests in the forests, then as honey produced in hives where bees were encouraged to settle. The colour varies considerably depending on the nectar foraged by the bees, and a number of processes such as creaming will determine its consistency.

Apart from its extensive use in baking, and as a spread, honey is often used to sweeten hot beverages and cereals, is used in caramelising nuts and in the confectionery industry.

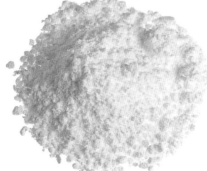

Icing Sugar

NUTRITIONAL INFORMATION This has the same properties as granulated sugar.

DESCRIPTION Icing sugar is produced by milling selected granulated cane sugar to a fine powder. Pure icing sugar has the advantage of dissolving quickly, but will turn lumpy if

stored for a long period. It is best for fine decorative work in confectionery. Icing sugar mixture has a small proportion of calcium phosphate and/or cornflour blended in to prevent caking on storage.

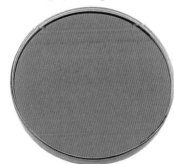

Maple Syrup

NUTRITIONAL INFORMATION No detailed data are available, but maple syrup is similar to golden syrup.

DESCRIPTION A golden sweetener made by concentrating the sap of the sugar maple tree by boiling at atmospheric pressure. It may also be concentrated at reduced pressure or by freeze-drying. The result is a sweet syrup. The characteristic flavour is derived from the volatile oil in the sap.

A product is also sold which is made by a chemical process using maple syrup, coffee flavouring extract, fenugreek extract, lovage essence and caramel.

Maple syrup is available in specialty food stores, it can be used as a syrup with ice cream, waffles, pancakes, and in confectionery.

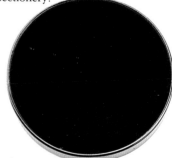

Molasses

NUTRITIONAL INFORMATION Molasses contains carbohydrate, which provides energy, but no fat, cholesterol or protein.

A precise analysis is unavailable. An approximate analysis is sucrose 34%, glucose and fructose 16%, water 21%, ash 11.3% and other sugars with gums, and traces of B vitamins, 16.3%. Ash includes calcium, magnesium, potassium, silicon, iron and phosphorus.

DESCRIPTION Molasses is the end product

of either raw sugar manufacture or refining. It is the dark, viscous liquid remaining from which no further sugar can be crystallised and economically removed by the usual methods.

Molasses is used in distilleries for the manufacture of alcohol and rum. It is generally described as inedible for human consumption and is used as a feed for farm animals, particularly cattle.

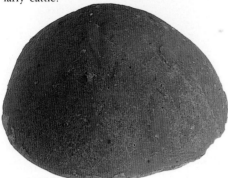

Palm Sugar

*also called **Gula jawa, Gula melacca, Jaggery***

MAJOR NUTRIENTS			SERVE SIZE 20 G
Energy	310 kJ	Dietary Fibre	N/A
Protein	Tr	Sodium	15 mg
Fat	N/A	Magnesium	23 mg
Carbohydrate	19 g	Iron	0.32 mg
Cholesterol	0		

NUTRITIONAL INFORMATION This sugar is a high carbohydrate food; it is a moderate source of magnesium and iron, and contains copper.

DESCRIPTION Jaggery is a red-brown, crumbly sugar extracted from a tree of a family of tropical and subtropical low-branched palms known as sugar or sago palms, although the dessert food, sago, is derived from the sago palm *Metroxylon sagu*, not from this particular palm. Its flavour is somewhat like treacle, for which it can be substituted in certain recipes.

The Asian palm sugar, gula jawa/java or gula melacca, is extracted from the coconut or palmyra palm, *Borassus flabellifer*.

The palms which provide sugar are native to most Southeast Asian countries, being plants which thrived in antiquity. They have never provided the sole source of sugar, as the sugarcane cultivated today grew wild throughout these regions since the earliest times. In pre-T'ang times, nearly 2000 years ago, palm sugar was used to sweeten water buffalo milk as a popular Chinese drink. The English concept of a 'hot toddy' stemmed from a milky, highly alcoholic wine made in India and Indonesia from jaggery.

Palm sugar is sold in wrapped packs compressed into block form in round, square or rectangular shapes, and also in cones or cylinders. It is also produced in coarse crystals. It will keep indefinitely in dry conditions.

Palm sugar gives a rich flavour and deep colour to sweet and savoury Indian, Malay and Indonesian dishes.

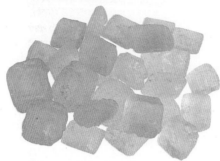

Preserving Sugar

NUTRITIONAL INFORMATION Identical to granulated sugar.

DESCRIPTION Preserving sugar is produced from special boilings, which form large crystals. This process helps to eliminate scum forming when preserves are made.

It is used for jams, sauces, chutneys, relish and other preserves. Processing does not alter its nutritional properties.

A preserving sugar known as pectin sugar is sold in England, but not in Australasia. The same result is obtained by buying the pectin and sugar separately.

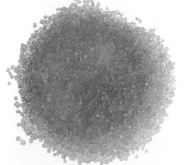

Raw Sugar

*also called **Demerara, Muscovado***

NUTRITIONAL INFORMATION Raw sugar is 98% sucrose, the remaining 2% consisting of water and ash. Ash contains calcium, magnesium, potassium and iron.

Raw sugar provides carbohydrate (5 g per teaspoon) and energy (67 kJ per teaspoon), but does not contain fat, cholesterol, protein or sodium. The ash fraction supplies quantities of minerals that are too small to be considered nutritionally significant.

Raw sugar is often thought to be nutritionally superior to other sugars: this notion is incorrect.

DESCRIPTION Raw sugar is characterised by its larger crystal size and its taste. In the home and hospitality industry, it is used primarily as a table sweetener. In the food industry, raw sugar is often used as a marketing technique, as consumers tend to consider it nutritionally superior to other sugars.

The larger crystal size makes raw sugar useful for decorative purposes, for baked goods and confectionery. Processing does not affect its nutritional properties.

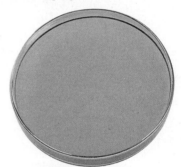

Rose Hip Syrup

MAJOR NUTRIENTS			SERVE SIZE 30 ML
Energy	297 kJ	Vitamin C	89 mg
Carbohydrate	19 g		

NUTRITIONAL INFORMATION Rose hip syrup is very rich in vitamin C. It also has a very high sugar content: 1 tablespoon provides the equivalent of almost 5 teaspoons of sugar.

DESCRIPTION Rose hips are the fruit of the rose, from which syrup is extracted. Available from supermarkets, food stores and chemists, the syrup will keep well at room temperature. It is often taken in the form of a tea when infections such as coughs and colds strike. The syrup is an excellent substitute for grenadine as a sweetening agent in cocktails and mixed drinks.

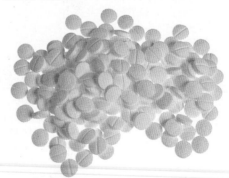

Saccharin

NUTRITIONAL INFORMATION Saccharin is a 'non-nutritive' sweetener. It does not provide carbohydrate, protein, fat, cholesterol or sodium. It provides an insignificant amount of energy.

Saccharin is intensely sweet, but suffers the drawback that approximately 30% of the population notice a bitter metallic aftertaste. To reduce this, saccharin is often used in combination with cyclamates, usually one part cyclamate to twelve parts saccharin.

Next to tobacco, saccharin may be the substance that has been most studied. The link between cancer and saccharin has been a matter of controversy among scientists. In 1985, the Council on Scientific Affairs of the American Medical Association recommended careful consideration of saccharin use by young children and pregnant women.

DESCRIPTION Saccharin is stable on processing and is incorporated into a wide range of foods. It was banned from the US market in 1969, although continuing to be available in Australia. In 1977, the US Food and Drug Administration again debated the issue, and public pressure put a moratorium on the ban. The moratorium has been renewed regularly since that time, highlighting the extraordinary consumer demand for low-kilojoule sweeteners.

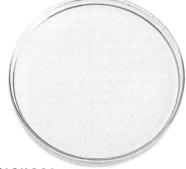

Sucrose

NUTRITIONAL INFORMATION Sucrose provides only carbohydrate energy. It does not contain protein, fat, cholesterol or sodium. One teaspoon of sucrose contains 67 kJ, and 4g of carbohydrate.

DESCRIPTION Sucrose is a disaccharide composed of two sugars, glucose and fructose. The major commercial sources of sucrose in the world are sugarcane and sugar beet. The only difference between the two is the nature of their impurities: impure cane sugar is flavoursome, while beet sugar impurities are bitter. All Australian and New Zealand sugar comes from sugarcane.

Sucrose is also found naturally in fruits and vegetables.

In acid conditions, sucrose becomes hydrolysed, forming a mixture of glucose, fructose and sucrose called 'invert sugar'. This syrup is used extensively in the food industry.

Invert sugar also occurs naturally, for instance in honey.

Sucrose enhances the palatability of a number of processed foods which contain a wide range of nutrients, for example, flavoured dairy products and juices.

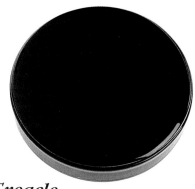

Treacle

NUTRITIONAL INFORMATION The major nutrients in treacle are carbohydrate, energy and potassium. One tablespoon of treacle contains 213 kJ, 13 g of carbohydate and 294 mg of potassium.

Treacle contains a large amount of potassium, but does not contain any fat or cholesterol, and only negligible protein and sodium. As treacle is so high in potassium, it is not recommended for individuals suffering from renal disease. For undernourished individuals, it can be added to a variety of puddings and beverages to increase energy intake.

DESCRIPTION Treacle is made from a sugar syrup and contains a mixture of sucrose (25%), glucose and fructose (50%), and water.

Treacle is produced from the liquid remaining after the refined sugar has been crystallised. It is a viscous, dark brown to black syrup. Its colour and unique flavour make it suitable for baking and for the production of confectionery, especially liquorice and toffees.

The nutritional properties of treacle do not change on processing.

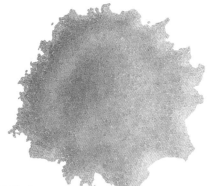

White Sugar

NUTRITIONAL INFORMATION A form of granulated sugar.

DESCRIPTION White sugar is refined to medium-sized crystals. It is used as a table sweetener and in liquid foods such as yoghurts, custards, and baked goods with sauces and syrups. Its nutritional properties are not affected by processing.

CONFECTIONERY

The world's earliest confectionery was not made, as one might expect, with sugar, but rather with honey. It is known that as early as 3000 BC a method of extracting and evaporating the juice of the sugarcane was already in use in India. The use of honey by diverse peoples around the world, however, predates the use of sugar by many centuries. Its use in the diet of so many of these early peoples is well documented, not in traditionally recorded history but rather in cave drawings, such as those by Australian Aboriginal people, illustrating the extraction of honeycomb from trees. In this respect, honey would have been considered a subsistence diet, particularly for nomadic tribes, but it is very likely that in time it would have been mixed with seeds or nuts to form into an early version of the modern 'health bars'.

Thousands of years later, but before confectionery was known throughout Europe, the Egyptians, Arabs and Chinese were preparing 'sweetmeats' made from honey and fruit juices. Egyptian records dating from around 2000 BC show the making of confectionery, but it was not until after the Crusades, which lasted from the early 12th to 14th century AD, that sugar in any quantity became available in Europe. Even then, it was largely used by apothecaries and not by the general population.

Around this period it was believed that confectionery had some medicinal value. As an example, marshmallows, originally made with an extract of the roots of the marshmallow plant, were actually sold by apothecaries as a remedy for chest ailments.

In the late 15th century, sugar refining was perfected in Italy, and for some time Italian chefs were the grand masters in Europe for the making of confectionery. Following the lead of the Italian masters of the art and despite the high cost of sugar, the art spread through Europe, and many extravagant examples began appearing on the tables of royalty and of those who could afford the services of the confectionery craftsmen.

No doubt the most famous of these was a Frenchman, Antonin Carême, chef and cookery writer extraordinaire of the early 19th century, who rose from the most modest of circumstances to be wooed by kings and statesmen for his services. His set pieces in confectionery, and particularly with pulled and spun sugar, were truly monumental, reflecting his belief that confectionery was in fact associated with architecture. He was a skilled writer and illustrator, leaving for posterity meticulously written and beautifully illustrated books on the subject. His depth of feeling is well illustrated by a sentence he wrote which was quoted by Anatole France, French novelist and critic: 'The fine arts are five in number, to wit: painting, sculpture, poetry, music, architecture — whose main branch is confectionery.'

Confectionery is an energy-dense food, 100 grams providing between 1300 and 2200 kilojoules. The kilojoules come mainly from sugars, but chocolates, toffees and caramels also contain significant amounts of fat.

Plain chocolate contains about 30% fat, carob bars contain about 25%, the fat being predominantly saturated.

Most confectionery items contain between 60 and 75% sugar. Hard, clear lollies such as boiled lollies are more than 90% sugar.

In general, confectionery does not supply protein, minerals or vitamins in the amounts which would provide a balance with the kilojoules. Milk chocolate, however, is a significant source of protein, calcium and riboflavin, and chocolate, carob, liquorice and the bars with seeds, fruit and nuts provide worthwhile amounts of iron.

Confectionery is associated with an increased risk of tooth decay. It is a concentrated source of sugar, and the sugar is in a sticky form which adheres to the teeth and stays in the mouth for a long time. Micro-organisms in the mouth convert some of the sugars to acid and these acids remove minerals from the teeth, increasing the risk of tooth decay.

As a group of foods, confectionery does not provide a good balance of energy and nutrients. For people who are not overweight, these foods can be eaten and enjoyed in small amounts. They should not displace foods with a good nutritional balance from the diet.

Boiled Sweets

MAJOR NUTRIENTS		SERVE SIZE 15 G	
Energy	235 kJ	Carbohydrate	15 g
Protein	less than 1 g	Total Sugars	15 g
Fat	0		

NUTRITIONAL INFORMATION Only contain sugars, so relatively lower in energy than other fat containing confections. Hard texture results in sweets having to be sucked, lasting longer and therefore providing greater satisfaction than softer items. Sweets are often brightly coloured and may contain tartrazine or azo dye colourings. This will be declared on the package.

DESCRIPTION Confections of varying degrees of firmness ranging from hard toffee to soft-textured marshmallow.

ORIGIN AND HISTORY Sugar in its most primitive form — the juice squeezed from the sugar cane — was known as early as 3000 BC in India. Sugar refineries were operating in Persia around the 7th century AD, but it was not until the 16th century that confectionery began to be made following the commercialisation of sugar refining.

BUYING AND STORAGE All confectionery, homemade or commercial, should be stored in well-sealed containers away from heat and humidity. Boiled sweets of the sticky type (toffee, lollipops and barley sugar) should be individually wrapped.

PREPARATION AND USE The base of all boiled sweets is a plain syrup of sugar and water. The different varieties achieve their individual characteristics through a number of variations in the method of preparation. The length of time the syrup is boiled, the way in which it is handled as it begins to set and the inclusion of various other ingredients all add to the variation in results. See individual entries for each variety.

VARIETIES

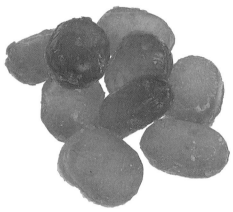

Barley Sugar

NUTRITIONAL INFORMATION See Boiled Sweets

DESCRIPTION Barley sugar, along with lollipops, is the simplest form of boiled sweet. It is usually made or bought in the form of small sweets or in strips, twisted corkscrew fashion.

ORIGIN AND HISTORY The significance of the name 'barley sugar' may be lost on many contemporary confectionery makers. Its origin is easily understood when one discovers that barley sugar was originally made from a syrup of sugar and water in which pearl barley had been cooked. Purists may still use barley water in place of plain water and probably feel the little extra preparation involved is worthwhile when taking into account the more mellow flavour and characteristic milky appearance achieved.

BUYING AND STORAGE Barley sugar should be brittle and not too sticky. If not made with barley water it should also be transparent and sparkling. Store wrapped in cellophane or plastic wrap and keep in an airtight container away from heat and humidity. If not individually wrapped, store in single layers between sheets of greaseproof or waxed paper.

PREPARATION AND USE A simple sugar and water mixture is boiled with the addition of liquid glucose, corn syrup or cream of tartar. When the sugar has dissolved, thinly pared lemon rind may be added for flavour. When the syrup has reached soft-ball stage (116°C), lemon juice is usually added. When hard-crack stage is reached (154°C), the pan should be dipped in iced water to arrest cooking. (If lemon juice is not available, a few drops of lemon essence may be added at the conclusion of cooking.) The syrup is poured slowly out onto a lightly oiled surface (preferably marble) and when slightly cooled, the edges are folded into the middle of the sheet of syrup. The two thicknesses are cut together with oiled scissors into strips and the strips held at each end and twisted into corkscrew-shaped sticks.

Bulls' Eye Bulls' eyes are a variation of pulled sugar. Two differently coloured syrups are pulled individually and then intertwined, the final result being the small hard balls of swirling red and white, responsible for the confection's name.

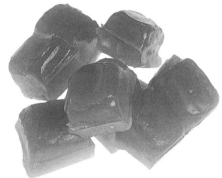

Butterscotch

MAJOR NUTRIENTS		SERVE SIZE 15 G	
Energy	400 kJ	Cholesterol	4 mg
Protein	4 g	Carbohydrate	2 g
Fat	9 g	Total Sugars	2 g

NUTRITIONAL INFORMATION The fat contained in butterscotch is a major source of kilojoules. It has a higher energy value than boiled sweets, but no significant nutrients. Generally contains caramel colour 150.

DESCRIPTION A variety of boiled sweet, not usually as clear as many of the other boiled sweets because of the addition of other ingredients which tend to cloud the toffee or syrup.

ORIGIN AND HISTORY The precise time of the first batch of butterscotch is unknown, but in all probability it would have been in the 16th or 17th century.

BUYING AND STORAGE Best individually wrapped in cellophane or plastic wrap and stored in an airtight container away from heat and humidity.

PREPARATION AND USE As the name suggests, butter is added to the basic ingredients of all boiled sweets (that is, sugar and water) and the mixture boiled to the soft-crack stage (138°C) before being poured out onto a suitable surface to cool. Butterscotch sets quite hard so must be marked into small pieces when just beginning to set and broken into pieces when quite cold.

Lollipop Lollipops are transparent flat discs of brittle toffee of varying sizes, colours and flavours with an attached stick as 'handle'. Fruit drops, a smaller variety, usually have a fruit juice included in the ingredients.

Pulled Sugar Pulled sugar, also called spun sugar, is made from a simple syrup of sugar, water and glucose syrup, corn syrup or cream of tartar. It is usually in the form of individual sweets with an attractive satiny appearance, rather like little satin pillows — the result of its somewhat unusual treatment following cooking.

This is a confection best made by the more experienced cook or, for the uninitiated, following a demonstration of sugar pulling. However, it should not be avoided as being too difficult. It can be great fun to make once confidence is boosted a little. The term 'spun sugar' usually refers to sugar which has been pulled and pulled to the stage where it resembles fine wisps of spun silk which will hold their delicate and extremely brittle shapes — but only when treated with the utmost care!

Candied Fruit

NUTRITIONAL INFORMATION The nutrients will vary according to the preparation, but all forms contain high amounts of sugar. Candying and crystallising cause an approximate sevenfold increase in the kilojoule content of the fruit being treated: for example, 100 grams of fresh apricots provide 200 kJ, whereas 100 grams of candied apricots provide 1400 kJ.

Glacé fruits have four times the kilojoule content when compared to the fresh equivalent. These three types of preserving also destroy vitamin C and, in some fruits, half the vitamin A as well.

DESCRIPTION Whole or sections of fruit are dehydrated, to an extent, of their own juices and then saturated with sugar by processing in syrup.

ORIGIN AND HISTORY Though the existence of candy in ancient Egypt is known through existing hieroglyphics, it is thought that the refinement of candying and crystallising fruits was a development of the Persians who used spices and the scents from flower petals to flavour citrus fruits in a candying process. It is interesting to note that candied fruits were part of the dessert course of a grand banquet arranged for the famous Medici family in Rome in 1513. The current vogue of the period for presenting sugared foods at several intervals during a meal of such importance is illustrated by the fact that even the hors d'oeuvre included cakes made of pine nuts and marzipan and 'sugared capons covered in fine gold'.

BUYING AND STORAGE Candied and crystallised fruit should be placed in layers between sheets of greaseproof paper in an airtight container. If kept in a dry place, the fruit should keep almost indefinitely.

PREPARATION AND USE Fruits are prepared in the usual way, cherries pitted, pineapple peeled, cored and sliced and so on. Small fruits may be crystallised whole, but should be pierced all over with a fork or fine skewer to allow the sugar to penetrate. The fruits are cooked to a certain extent to allow better absorption of the sugar syrup, and drained. Sugar is added to the reserved cooking water and some recipes advise the addition of liquid glucose at this stage. (Glucose is more readily absorbed into the fruits than sugar and this helps prevent wrinkling of the finished result.) The cooking liquid is then boiled and the resulting syrup poured over the fruit which is then left undisturbed for 24 hours. Almost every day for the next 10 days the process is repeated, with the fruit being drained and the reserved syrup strengthened by the addition of more sugar. The reason for the gradual strengthening of the syrup is that fruit subjected to the addition of a very strong syrup right at the beginning of the process would shrivel and toughen. The final drying process must also be gradual. A warm, dry place such as a sunny window would be suitable and would dry the fruit in about three days. A gas oven using just the pilot light would also be suitable and would require only four hours for the drying process. The fruits can be eaten as a confection, or used whole or chopped as an ingredient in or part of a topping for cakes, biscuits, desserts or ice cream.

VARIETIES

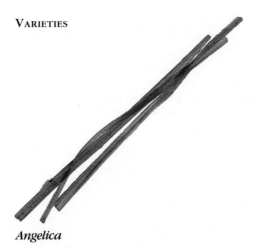

Angelica

MAJOR NUTRIENTS		CANDIED SERVE SIZE 5 G	
Energy	45 kJ	Total Sugars	3 g
Protein	0	Fibre	0
Fat	0	Sodium less than 5 mg	
Cholesterol	0	Potassium	
Carbohydrate	3 g		less than 5 mg

NUTRITIONAL INFORMATION Contains no fats so makes a lower energy decoration than cream or fat based decorations. No nutritional significance.

DESCRIPTION The angelica plant is a member of the parsley family, with sturdy stalks and very shiny, dark green leaves. When sold after processing it looks like dark green strips of what could be described as somewhat shrivelled, sugar-coated celery.

ORIGIN AND HISTORY The plant originally grew wild in the alpine regions of northern Europe. At that time it was largely valued for its medicinal properties. It is now grown primarily for its roots and stalks, the latter being used in the preparation of candied angelica and the roots in the production of liqueurs and bitters.

BUYING AND STORAGE Though the process used in preparing candied angelica reduces its moisture content considerably, look for stalks that are not too dried out in appearance. Buy only in small quantities and store in a tightly covered container just large enough to hold it.

NOTE: Angelica has become increasingly difficult to find in regular grocery outlets and so-called angelica often appears to be candied celery. Though it is in no way a suitable replacement, a jellied and candied green confection of vaguely similar appearance is sometimes available.

PREPARATION AND USE After a period of soaking in water, the stalks of the angelica plant are macerated in sugar syrup, then boiled in the syrup, drained, sprinkled with sugar and dried in a very slow oven. After processing, its colour is dark green.

Candied Peel

DESCRIPTION Candied (or crystallised) peel is made of strips of skin of citrus fruits. Put through a simple but lengthy series of processes, the peel is preserved in a semi-dried state, usually encrusted with sugar.

ORIGIN AND HISTORY The candying of fruit peel is well documented from the early 16th century. In fact during the Elizabethan era it seems few foods escaped the candying craze, with even savoury foods being 'enhanced' by the addition of sugar in some form or another. However it is likely that candying of fruits and peel was carried out by the Persians some time before its introduction to Europe.

BUYING AND STORAGE Crystallised or candied peel is available commercially but the quality is not always as good as it should be. For example, the keeping quality of well-prepared candied peel ensures it will stay in good condition for some considerable time. Peel that has been incompletely crystallised will become mouldy after a comparatively short time. Keep candied peel in an airtight container in a cool, dry place.

PREPARATION AND USE Strips of citrus fruits (oranges, lemons, grapefruit) are soaked and/or simmered in water for several hours until tender, with the cooking water changed 3 or 4 times to help remove bitterness from the peel. The peel is then added to a sugar syrup and simmered for a short time. It is then removed from the syrup and allowed to dry overnight. For the final process one of several methods may be chosen. Some recipes suggest reboiling the previous day's syrup until it reaches the hard-crack stage and dipping individual pieces of the partly prepared peel into it, then drying it out on a rack for a few minutes in a very slow oven. It may be sprinkled with sugar while it is still warm. Another method has the partly prepared peel cooked *in* the syrup the following day. When cool it is sprinkled liberally with sugar and left uncovered until completely dry before storing in a tightly closed jar.

Crystallised Fruit
Candied fruit with a sugar coating.

MAJOR NUTRIENTS — SERVE SIZE 20 G

Energy	450 kJ	Total Sugars	11 g
Protein	less than 1 g	Fibre	less than 1 g
Fat	0	Sodium	30 mg
Carbohydrate	11 g	Potassium	10 mg

NUTRITIONAL INFORMATION
All energy derived from sugar sources. No significant nutrients as fruit content is insignificant.

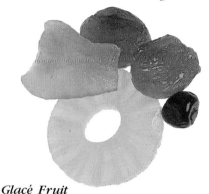

Glacé Fruit

MAJOR NUTRIENTS — SERVE SIZE 10 G

Energy	230 kJ	Total Sugars	6 g
Protein	less than 1 g	Fibre	0
Fat	0	Sodium	15 mg
Carbohydrate	6 g	Potassium	5 mg

NUTRITIONAL INFORMATION
All energy derived from sugar sources. No significant nutrients as fruit content is insignificant.

DESCRIPTION
Glacé fruit is almost the same as crystallised fruit, the only difference being that the surface of the fruit is altered slightly to give a more glazed and glossy finish.

ORIGIN AND HISTORY
The origin of glacé fruit could be said to be the same as crystallised fruit. The glazed or refined finish is unlikely to be one dating back to the 16th century (refer to crystallised fruit), however it is likely that with the advent of the great confectioners of the early 19th century this particular embellishment was added. One example is marron glacé, or glacé chestnut.

BUYING AND STORAGE
Some glacé fruits available commercially appear to have a somewhat gelatinous finish unlike the classically prepared product. However, whether bought or home-prepared, store in layers between sheets of greaseproof paper in an airtight container. If kept in a dry place, the fruit should keep almost indefinitely.

PREPARATION AND USE
The preparation for glacé fruit, short of the finished glaze, is exactly the same as for crystallised fruit. To achieve the desired glossy finish, previously prepared crystallised fruits are dipped very briefly in hot water to melt the surface and after brief draining, they are dipped in a very strong sugar syrup. The fruits are then drained and allowed to dry. The final dipping in a heavy syrup gives the fruit its traditional smooth, glossy finish.

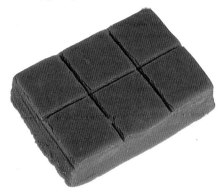

Caramel

MAJOR NUTRIENTS — SERVE SIZE 15 G

Energy	250 kJ	Total Sugars	11 g
Protein	less than 1 g	Fibre	0
Fat	2 g	Sodium	20 mg
Cholesterol	2 mg	Potassium	15 mg
Carbohydrate	11 g		

NUTRITIONAL INFORMATION
Contains fat, some of which is from milk sources, although milk content is not large enough to provide any significant nutrients. Often contains caramel colour 150.

DESCRIPTION
The addition of dairy products to the basic ingredients of a sugar syrup results in the characteristic mellow flavour and warm colour of caramel. In this it differs from many of the most common boiled sweets in that it is opaque and creamy in texture.

ORIGIN AND HISTORY
No precise time can be given for the advent of caramel on the confectionery scene but it is almost certain that the combination of ingredients that produce these delightfully mellow sweets would have been discovered by European confectioners by the 16th or certainly by the 17th century. In fact even earlier work by the confectioners of the Middle East and India could very well have resulted in the correct formula being discovered long before this time.

BUYING AND STORAGE
Caramels are best bought individually wrapped. Unwrapped, they are inclined to stick together because of their soft texture. Check that there is no sign of sugar crystals forming on the outside of the caramels and always store in a securely covered container away from light and heat.

Soft, home-made caramels are best individually wrapped and stored in the refrigerator in warm weather.

PREPARATION AND USE
Caramel recipes may call for a mixture of some of the following ingredients: white or brown sugar, golden syrup, honey, liquid glucose, butter, condensed milk, milk, cream or water. The mixture is usually boiled to the firm ball stage, however further cooking is necessary if firmer caramels are required. Regular stirring is necessary when dairy products are used in confectionery making to avoid their catching on the bottom of the container and burning. Though the creamy nature of the mixture usually ensures that unwanted crystallisation does not occur, it is wise to include what is known as an 'interfering' agent as a preventative measure. Lemon juice or cream of tartar would be effective though liquid glucose would be more reliable. When cooked the mixture should be poured into a lightly oiled container and when set, cut with a lightly oiled knife into the desired shapes.

VARIETIES
Caramel may vary in appearance and texture: a low temperature for the cooked syrup will result in soft caramel; a high temperature will give a firmer texture. Chopped dried fruits or nuts may be stirred through the mixture when cooking is completed, or chopped nuts may be pressed into the surface of the caramel immediately after the mixture has been poured out to set.

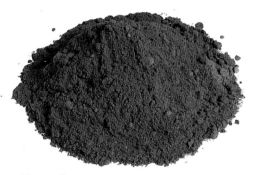

Carob *Ceratonia siliqua*
also called *St John's bread, Locust bean*

MAJOR NUTRIENTS — CAROB POWDER SERVE SIZE 4 G

Energy	50 kJ	Carbohydrate	3 g
Protein	0	Cholesterol	0
Fat	0	Sodium	0

NUTRITIONAL INFORMATION
Contains no significant vitamins or minerals. Snack foods such as carob bars usually have added fat and sugar, making them high in energy.

DESCRIPTION
While the carob is a leguminous tree, the large, long pods are used as a

food item (not the seeds, which are very hard). The pods are brown, somewhat leathery on the outside, fleshy inside. If available, they can be eaten raw and have a slightly sweet, chocolaty flavour, a quality which endears carob to those seeking a caffeine-free, low fat chocolate substitute.

ORIGIN AND HISTORY Native to the Mediterranean, the carob pod has been used as a food from biblical times. It is the 'locust' on which John the Baptist survived in his wanderings in the wilderness, hence the alternative name. In the Middle East the pods are a snack food even today, and are used for making syrup. They are ground, soaked in water and allowed to ferment for 2–3 days, and the strained liquid boiled with sugar to make the syrup called dibs.

BUYING AND STORAGE Carob powder is available at natural food stores. Store in a sealed container in a cool place and use within a year. Dibs is also available in jars from Middle Eastern food stores and will keep at room temperature.

PREPARATION AND USE Carob powder may be used in the same way as cocoa powder in cooking. Use for cakes, biscuits, desserts, confectionery and milk drinks. Plain block carob is also used as a chocolate substitute.

PROCESSING Carob is combined with lecithin, raw sugar and other ingredients to form block carob in dark, milk, nut and fruit and nut varieties, and is used in many other confections.

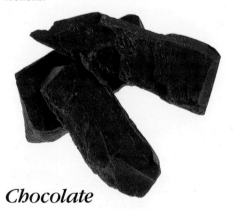

Chocolate

MAJOR NUTRIENTS

			DARK, BAR SERVE SIZE 50 G
Energy	1090 kJ	Dietary Fibre	0
Protein	2 g	Sodium	5 mg
Fat	15 g	Potassium	150 mg
Cholesterol	13 mg	Phosphorus	70 mg
Carbohydrate	32 g	Magnesium	50 mg
Total Sugars	30 g	Iron	0.9 mg

NUTRITIONAL INFORMATION An excellent source of vitamin E; good source of phosphorus, calcium, iron; moderate source of protein and magnesium. Contains large amounts of fat, providing 50% of the energy in chocolate.

DESCRIPTION Chocolate is a dark substance made from the seeds of the cacao, a tropical tree. The word comes from two Mayan words meaning warm beverage, which reminds us that even after chocolate was introduced to the New World it was used for almost 300 years only as a drink.

ORIGIN AND HISTORY The Mayan Indians of Central America and the Aztec Indians of Mexico were cultivating cacao beans when Columbus reached the Americas, but the time of their first cultivation is not known.

Chocoholics will not be surprised to learn that an aura of mystery has surrounded chocolate for centuries. Aztec legends recount the story of one of their prophets bringing the seeds of the cacao tree from paradise to plant in his garden. By eating the fruit he acquired wisdom and knowledge.

At one time the early church frowned upon chocolate because it was considered an aphrodisiac.

In the 16th century, following the conquest of Mexico by Hernando Cortès, cacao beans were introduced to Spain. By the beginning of the 17th century Italy acquired them, followed shortly thereafter by other European countries and eventually England. By the beginning of the 18th century cocoa had become a fashionable beverage in London. It took almost 300 years from the time they were introduced to Europe for cacao seeds to be transformed into the solidified form chocolate lovers know so well. Chocolate in block form was not mass-produced until the early 19th century.

BUYING AND STORAGE Chocolate is of course available in innumerable forms, and should usually be consumed as soon as possible after purchase.

PREPARATION AND USE If chocolate in its various guises survives the first sighting by the consumer, it can eventually be eaten as an accompaniment to other foods or used as a drink, sauce or filling.

VARIETIES

Chocolate Bar A filled bar is a good source of phosphorus and iron; moderate source of calcium and magnesium, and contains large amounts of fat. Higher sugar contents of fillings results in lower percentage of energy (34%) coming from fats than in whole chocolate bars. Contains caffeine, and some of the fillings may contain other food additives.

Chocolate Chips These are an excellent source of calcium, phosphorus, magnesium, iron and vitamin E; good source of niacin and protein. They contain large amounts of fat, and 63% of energy comes from fat.

Chocolate Flake A bar is an excellent source of phosphorus and vitamin E; good source of iron and calcium; moderate source of protein and magnesium. 50% of the energy in this chocolate comes from fat. Contains small amounts of caffeine.

Chocolate-coated Crunch Bar An excellent source of magnesium; good source of phosphorus and moderate source of calcium and iron. As crunch fillings contain coconut, the total fat content of a bar is over 48% of total energy. Contains lower nutrient levels than whole chocolate bars and cannot be considered a major source of these for the diet. Contains caffeine.

Cooking Chocolate This block chocolate is an excellent source of phosphorus, magnesium, iron and vitamin E; good source of niacin; moderate source of protein. Contains large amounts of fat. 63% of energy comes from fat and so it cannot be considered as a primary source of these nutrients. Contains caffeine.

Rocky Road A good source of iron and moderate source of calcium and magnesium. This is a popular light chocolate bar which contains 35% total energy from fat. Lower fat content than other chocolate bars, although still energy dense.

Sprinkles A sucrose-containing product, consumed in such small quantities that it has no nutritional significance.

Truffle This is a rich, high fat confection with 38% of energy coming from fats. Some of the more expensive varieties will be even higher in fats as centre will contain more cream. Liqueur-filled truffles will have a higher energy content due to the contribution of the alcohol.

White Chocolate An excellent source of calcium and phosphorus and moderate source of protein. Contains large amounts of fat — 50% of the energy in chocolate comes from fat — so it cannot be considered as a primary source of these nutrients. Contains very small amounts of caffeine.

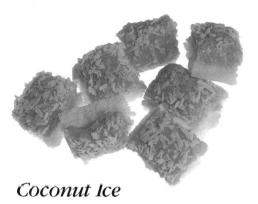

Coconut Ice

MAJOR NUTRIENTS		SERVE SIZE 20 G	
Energy	300 kJ	Dietary Fibre	
Protein	0.4 g		less than 1 g
Fat	1.5 g	Sodium	24 mg
Carbohydrate	15 g	Potassium	27 mg
Total Sugars	15 g		

NUTRITIONAL INFORMATION High sugar, non fat sweet.

DESCRIPTION Coconut ice is a firm confection of a creamy consistency with coconut as its chief ingredient. It is usually served cut into two-tone squares, half white and half pink.

ORIGIN AND HISTORY The term coconut ice appears to be confined largely to Britain and some of its former dominions (including Australia). Many countries have similar confections that are named differently. For example a similar recipe used in the USA is called coconut fudge, which is, in practical terms, a more accurate description of this type of confection. In India a confection similar to coconut ice — coconut barfi — seems to have developed as a result of the establishment of a Muslim Imperial power in India in the 16th century.

BUYING AND STORAGE Coconut ice should be stored in a covered container. If kept for more than a day or two, store in the refrigerator, particularly in warm weather.

PREPARATION AND USE A mixture of milk, sugar and either cream of tartar or liquid glucose is boiled to soft-ball stage. It is then divided into two with half the coconut and pink colouring added to one portion and the remaining coconut added to the other. One mixture is poured into a shallow cake pan and the other immediately poured on top. When cool, it is cut into squares to serve.

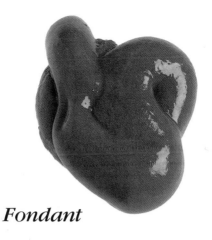

Fondant

MAJOR NUTRIENTS		SERVE SIZE 20 G	
Energy	305 kJ	Total Sugars	19 g
Protein	0	Sodium	0
Fat	0	Potassium	0
Carbohydrate	19 g		

NUTRITIONAL INFORMATION High sugar, non fat sweet.

DESCRIPTION Cooked fondant is a creamy smooth mixture which may be used as chocolate centres, moulded fruits and flowers or as an icing for cakes. Though its preparation is different from uncooked fondant, its uses are similar.

ORIGIN AND HISTORY Fondant was certainly being made early in the 19th century as history records that the celebrated French chef, Antonin Carême, used it in his splendid, architecturally-inspired confectionery masterpieces of that period. However, it is quite likely that similar mixtures had been prepared at an earlier date, possibly in Italy which is credited with being in the vanguard of confectionery making as far as Europe was concerned.

BUYING AND STORAGE Commercial fondant should be kept in an airtight container or in the package in which it was purchased. The homemade variety also needs to have all air excluded from its surface to avoid having it dry out and lose its smooth texture. When working with fondant it's wise to keep it covered with a damp cloth. Leftovers should be transferred to an airtight container.

PREPARATION AND USE The basis of cooked fondant is a sugar syrup — sugar, water and either liquid glucose or a pinch of cream of tartar. The syrup is boiled to the soft ball stage (116°C). The mixture must then stand for a few minutes until all bubbles subside. During the cooking of all sugar syrups, particularly for fondant, it is important to ensure that any crystallisation on the sides of the saucepan be removed, either by brushing down with a pastry brush dipped in cold water or by covering with a lid for a minute or two to allow the steam to do the job for you. When the bubbles have disappeared from the fondant mixture pour it out onto a damp marble slab or other cool surface and allow it to stand for 5 minutes. It should now be worked backwards and forwards with a spatula until it becomes white and opaque. Now knead until the fondant is smooth and completely free of lumps. Cover with a damp cloth if about to use, otherwise store in an airtight jar.

VARIETIES

Uncooked Fondant Egg-white, liquid glucose and flavouring (if used) are first stirred, then kneaded into pure icing sugar until a stiff paste is formed. The mixture is then kneaded on a surface dusted with icing sugar at which time colouring may be added. The fondant is ready to be used when it becomes a smooth ball without surface cracks. It may be homemade or bought.

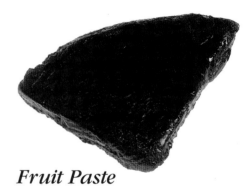

Fruit Paste

NUTRITIONAL INFORMATION The nutrient value will depend on the fruit used; the sugar content is high.

DESCRIPTION Fruit pastes are generally quite unspectacular in appearance. They are the result of boiling fruit with sugar for a considerable time. This does not, of course, always enhance the appearance of the fruit. In fact the original colour of the fruit is usually quite lost though some fruits fare better than others in this respect. However, what is lost in colour is definitely made up for in flavour. The pastes have a wonderful tangy sweetness. Pastes may also be made from dried fruits.

ORIGIN AND HISTORY By the early part of the 16th century the chefs of Italy were accepted as the innovators where confectionery was concerned. Fruit pastes were but one of their inspirations. (This is not to say that before the time of recorded history these confections were not already being made by nomadic people for whom the task of pulverising fruits and cooking them to a paste provided a more convenient form for transportation.) The trend for these pastes spread to France along with many variations of confectionery and preserves. In his book which became available in France in 1555, the famed prophet Nostradamus describes the method for making cotignac, a fruit paste.

BUYING AND STORAGE Pastes must be kept in an airtight container between layers of either waxed or special baking paper. They will keep almost indefinitely.

PREPARATION AND USE Fruit pastes are made from pureed fruits cooked with sugar until most of the moisture has been evaporated. Some fruits — quinces, pears, apples and apricots — need gentle cooking before pureeing, while soft berries such as raspberries and strawberries need only to be pushed through a sieve before they begin the lengthy cooking with sugar which ultimately turns the fruit into a firm paste on cooling. The pastes are cut into small squares or decorative shapes for serving. Fruit pastes are an ideal accompaniment for the post-meal cup of coffee or tea.

SEE ALSO Pastille.

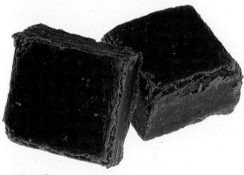

Fudge

MAJOR NUTRIENTS		SERVE SIZE 20 G PIECE	
Energy	355 kJ	Total Sugars	13 g
Protein	1 g	Dietary Fibre	0
Fat	3 g	Sodium	35 mg
Carbohydrate	13 g	Potassium	20 mg

NUTRITIONAL INFORMATION No significant nutrient contribution, from an energy dense product where over 30% of energy comes from fat. Fudges which contain nuts will have a higher percentage of energy from fats.

DESCRIPTION Fudge is similar in texture to caramel although many varieties have a more granular texture. They may differ markedly in appearance from the dark brown colour and firmer texture of a chocolate variety to the pale, creamy appearance of a softer vanilla flavoured fudge. Appearance and texture is also affected by added ingredients such as nuts and preserved fruits.

ORIGIN AND HISTORY In terms of confectionery history, fudge is probably a youngster. Its preparation seems to point to it being a distant relative of cooked fondant, which was certainly being made in France early in the 19th century. The actual birth date of fondant can't be pinpointed but it is likely that it was being made in Italy prior to its appearance in France. The variations that are represented in fudge recipes could point to the desire of early American settlers to add a variety of different ingredients to their basic fondant and caramel recipes.

BUYING AND STORAGE Unlike caramel, fudge need not necessarily be individually wrapped but should be stored in an airtight container with greaseproof or baking paper between the layers. It should keep for several weeks under normal conditions, away from heat and humidity. For best results, refrigerate in warm weather.

PREPARATION AND USE The sugar syrup for fudge is cooked to soft-ball stage. Its ingredients invariably include milk, cream or butter and often a combination of all three. Chocolate is a frequent flavouring, as are fruit juices and zest, dried and crystallised or glacé fruits and nuts. The different textures, soft or firm, are achieved by beating the mixture for different periods. For a firmer texture the mixture should be beaten just after it has reached the soft-ball stage. This results in the formation of large crystals which produce a coarse, more granular consistency and ultimately a firmer fudge on cooling. For a smoother fudge allow the mixture to cool, at which stage it begins to crystallise on its own. Beating well at this stage hastens the development of smaller, more regular crystals and the desired smooth texture.

Contrary to sugar boiling rules, occasional stirring during the cooking of the syrup is advisable as this type of mixture is likely to stick and burn if not stirred now and then. Take care not to leave fudge in the saucepan after beating as it is inclined to set at this stage. Pour immediately into a shallow pan greased lightly with oil or butter. Leave to set in a cool place, overnight if necessary and cut into squares to serve. Flavourings such as chocolate, coffee, vanilla, fruit juices and zest may be added and boiled with the syrup. Add fruit pieces and nuts after the final beating.

VARIETIES

Fudge is a comparatively soft confection which may be made with a variety of different flavourings (chocolate is a favourite) and added ingredients (such as dried or crystallised fruits or nuts).

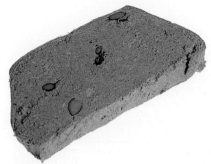

Halva

MAJOR NUTRIENTS		SERVE SIZE 25 G	
Energy	460 kJ	Sodium	20 mg
Protein	2 g	Potassium	100 mg
Fat	6 g	Phosphorus	55 mg
Cholesterol	0	Magnesium	30 mg
Carbohydrate	10 g	Iron	2 mg
Total Sugars	0	Zinc	1 mg
Dietary Fibre	1 g		

NUTRITIONAL INFORMATION An excellent source of iron, vitamin E; moderate source of phosphorus and magnesium. The fat in this product is from vegetable sources and so it contains no cholesterol. The total fat content of the product is still high, contributing 48% of total energy.

DESCRIPTION A sweetmeat or confection, light grey in colour, with a pleasant texture that is difficult to describe — light and crunchy is probably the closest. The standard halva has a pleasantly sweet sesame and vanilla flavour.

Halva, and the many variations of the word in Greek, Turkish, Arabic, Iranian and Indian languages, means sweet, and is also given to many semolina or flour-based puddings and cake-like sweets prepared in Greece, the Middle East and North Africa.

ORIGIN AND HISTORY Evidence strongly suggests that an early form of the halva confection originated in Persia around 630 AD, and its manufacture and use spread further afield through the forces of Islam. The sweetmeat is made from ground sesame seeds (tahini), sugar, glucose and an extract derived from the roots of a saponaceous tree of the eastern Mediterranean region, commonly known as halva root or wood. It is this extract which gives the halva its characteristic light, crunchy texture.

Almonds or pistachio nuts are usually added to halva, and a new flavour combination is chocolate with currants; a popular halva from Israel is chocolate-coated.

BUYING AND STORAGE Halva can be found at Greek, Middle Eastern and Jewish food stores, some delicatessens and confectionery shops. It can be purchased by weight cut from foil-wrapped blocks, in smaller foil-wrapped blocks, or in cans. Unopened cans should be stored in a cool place; once opened, remove and wrap in greaseproof paper, then wrap again with foil. For long storage (a year or more), block or canned halva should be left in the foil wrapping, wrapped again with plastic and stored in the refrigerator.

PREPARATION AND USE Most halvas crumble if not handled carefully; the exceptions are those made in Israel, as a different process is used in their manufacture. Cut in cubes or fingers and serve as a confection — excellent with after-dinner coffee. Halva is also delicious spread onto bread as a snack.

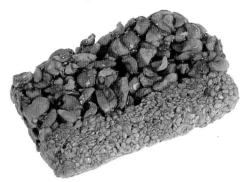

Health Bar

MAJOR NUTRIENTS			SERVE SIZE 45 G
Energy	700 kJ	Potassium	85 mg
Protein	5 g	Calcium	40 mg
Fat	12 g	Phosphorus	30 mg
Cholesterol	0	Magnesium	65 mg
Carbohydrate	11 g	Iron	1.5 mg
Total Sugars	10 g	Zinc	1 mg
Dietary Fibre	11 g	Thiamin	0.1 mg
Sodium	40 mg	Niacin	2.7 mg

NUTRITIONAL INFORMATION An excellent source of iron, magnesium, niacin; moderate source of protein, phosphorus, zinc and thiamin. Contains large amounts of fat. All nut containing bars are high in fat with over 60% of total energy coming from fats. Fruit bars may not contain fat and may contain less iron, zinc, calcium and magnesium.

DESCRIPTION Health bars are a mixture of ingredients compressed into a bar.

ORIGIN AND HISTORY The health bar is a recent invention.

BUYING AND STORAGE Whether to buy or not to buy probably hinges on whether or not one looks upon such a purchase as purely a confection or as something that can contribute to overall good nutrition.

PREPARATION AND USE Sugar and/or fat in one form or another will be present to hold the mixture together. Dried fruits, nuts, seeds, cereals and spices are among the usual ingredients.

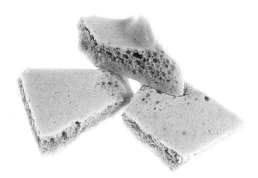

Honeycomb

MAJOR NUTRIENTS			SERVE SIZE 10 G
Energy	150 kJ	Total Sugars	4 g
Protein	0	Dietary Fibre	0
Fat	0.2 g	Sodium	20 mg
Cholesterol	0	Potassium	
Carbohydrate	4 g		less than 5 mg

NUTRITIONAL INFORMATION High sugar, non fat sweet.

DESCRIPTION Though honeycomb is basically made from a boiled sugar syrup, the addition of bicarbonate of soda turns it into a comparatively light and airy confection, with millions of tiny bubbles distributed evenly through the mixture. The result is a pleasantly crisp and crunchy texture and a colour rather like amber with a paler powdery surface.

ORIGIN AND HISTORY As with other confectionery origins, the first batch of honeycomb may well have been a case of an incorrect ingredient added at a crucial moment — say, bicarbonate of soda instead of cream of tartar. However, it appears that a similar concoction was being prepared in India several hundred years ago. 'Mysore-pak' is described as 'deliciously crisp and crumbly, honeycombed with tiny air holes'. It is interesting to note that the ingredients in the Indian recipe include roasted chickpea flour, shortening and syrup.

BUYING AND STORAGE Look for honeycomb that has been broken rather than cut. Some recipes suggest marking the mixture with a knife before the honeycomb is cold to achieve even pieces when finally broken. However this compresses the surface, making the marked edges rather chewy. Ensure that bought honeycomb is not sticky or 'sweating'. This spoils honeycomb's characteristic light and crunchy texture.

PREPARATION AND USE A sugar syrup is prepared containing water and sugar with the possible addition of glucose and a small quantity of cream of tartar. The syrup is boiled to approximately 145°C. After removal from the heat, bicarbonate of soda is added and in some recipes, butter, though the latter is the

exception, rather than the rule. When cold, the honeycomb is broken into pieces and stored in an airtight container. Glucose in the recipe will help avoid the honeycomb developing a sticky surface during storage.

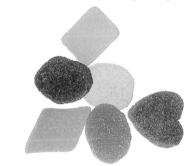

Jellied Confectionery

MAJOR NUTRIENTS		JELLY BEAN SERVE SIZE 20 G	
Energy	300 kJ	Dietary Fibre	0
Protein	0	Sodium	2 mg
Fat	0	Potassium	
Carbohydrate	19 g		less than 1 mg
Total Sugars	19 g		

NUTRITIONAL INFORMATION Contains no fat: one of the lowest energy confectionery items available.

DESCRIPTION Homemade jellies are almost always coloured and should have a reasonably firm texture. While some may be clear with an almost jewel-like sparkle, others will be clouded by the use of particular ingredients. They may be cut into any kind of decorative shape, usually squares. Sometimes they are rolled in sugar or icing sugar. Commercial jellies may be moderately soft to very hard and are generally sugar-coated.

ORIGIN AND HISTORY It is almost certain that confectionery jellies would have been made in Europe by the middle of the 16th century and possibly much earlier. In a book written by the celebrated prophet Nostradamus, reference is made to jellies made with a variety of cherry. These were possibly desserts and apparently not available to the general populace, since Nostradamus describes them as 'very delicate but expensive and for noblemen'! Though these jellies would be much softer than our jellied confectionery, it's likely that a slight miscalculation in ingredient quantities on the part of the cook could have resulted in a deliciously chewy sweet that finally became a success in its own right and the blueprint for our own jellies.

BUYING AND STORAGE Commercial jellies are less likely to be affected by light and humidity than other confectionery, but should be stored well covered as exposure to the air toughens them and may cause shrinkage. Most homemade jellies would show this effect to an even more marked degree if not kept in a sealed container.

PREPARATION AND USE Homemade jellies are one of the simplest of confections to prepare. A sugar thermometer is not required. The basic mixture is sugar, gelatine and either water or fruit juice. For jellies with a more chewy texture liquid glucose may be added. Hard jellies such as jubes and jelly beans are prepared by boiling the mixture for a longer period to make a thicker syrup. When using fruit juices, do not heat any longer than necessary to preserve the fresh fruit flavour. Fresh fruit juices give a flavour much superior to essences. For clear jellies, the juices should be passed through a fine strainer. However the juice of oranges and lemons need not necessarily be strained; the flavour will not be impaired, but the colour will be stronger and the jellies opaque. When set, the jellies are turned out and cut as desired.

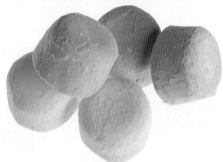

Marshmallow

MAJOR NUTRIENTS — **SERVE SIZE 10 G**

Energy	130 kJ	Dietary Fibre	0
Protein	less than 1 g	Sodium	4 mg
Fat	0	Potassium	
Carbohydrate	8 g		less than 1 mg
Total Sugars	8 g		

NUTRITIONAL INFORMATION Contains no fat and, due to whipped light nature, 10 g represents a satisfying number of sweets.

DESCRIPTION Marshmallow is a light, springy confection, cube shaped, delicately flavoured and usually dusted with icing sugar, occasionally rolled in toasted coconut.

ORIGIN AND HISTORY For a period prior to the first half of the 17th century many items of confectionery were prepared by apothecaries and considered useful on medical grounds. For example marshmallow, made at this time from an extract of the roots of the marshmallow plant, was recommended as a remedy for chest complaints. Unfortunately, modern marshmallow lovers cannot claim this

as justification for their indulgence as the marshmallow plant is no longer used and the original contention that it was beneficial to the health is highly suspect!

BUYING AND STORAGE When buying marshmallows, ensure the packs are airtight. Exposure to air results in a crustiness of the surface. Keep homemade marshmallows well dusted with icing sugar mixture to avoid having them stick together, and store in a covered container.

PREPARATION AND USE A sugar syrup, including liquid glucose, is boiled to hard-ball stage and gelatine and a flavouring agent added — traditionally rose water or orange flower water. Other less traditional essences may be added such as lemon or peppermint. The hot syrup is poured in a thin stream over whisked egg whites with beating continuing until the mixture begins to thicken but is still pourable. Turn into a shallow pan dusted with icing sugar mixture. When set, turn out onto a surface dusted with more icing sugar mixture and cut with a heavy, lightly oiled knife. Oiled scissors may be used. Icing sugar mixture gives a better coating than pure icing sugar. As an alternative the marshmallows may be rolled in toasted coconut, or after cooling, dipped in melted chocolate.

A popular American use for plain marshmallows is toasting on long forks over an open fire. The results are delicious.

VARIETIES

Chocolate dipped marshmallow; rocky road (a mixture of roughly chopped pink and white marshmallows coated in chocolate — see Chocolate).

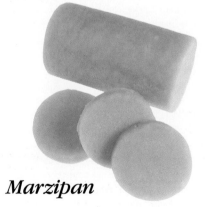

Marzipan

MAJOR NUTRIENTS — **SERVE SIZE 50 G**

Energy	930 kJ	Calcium	60 mg
Protein	4 g	Phosphorus	110 mg
Fat	12 g	Magnesium	60 mg
Cholesterol	0	Iron	1.5 mg
Carbohydrate	25 g	Zinc	0.5 mg
Total Sugars	23 g	Riboflavin	0.2 mg
Dietary Fibre	3 g	Niacin	1 mg
Sodium	6 mg	Vitamin E	4 mg
Potassium	200 mg		

NUTRITIONAL INFORMATION An excellent source of phosphorus, iron, vitamin E; good source of calcium and riboflavin; moderate source of protein. The fat in marzipan derives from the almonds. This monounsaturated fat contributes a significant 47% to the total energy.

DESCRIPTION Marzipan is a smooth but firm confectionery paste that can be moulded or cut into a variety of shapes.

ORIGIN AND HISTORY It is known that marzipan was a popular confection in Europe and India by the early 16th century; however, the recipes are known to have originated from Arabia where they could possibly have first seen the light of day several centuries earlier. According to accounts written at the time, a 16th century banquet honouring Giuliano de Medici, who had just been named a Patrician of Rome, featured a meal not only of gigantic proportions, but also exotic in the extreme. Marzipan featured in both the sweet and savoury courses, a fact not unusual at a time when sugar was presented in every possible form throughout the menus of the affluent, no doubt as a highly visible form of ancient one-upmanship. Though the marzipan undoubtedly had ground nuts as its base ingredient, it may have differed somewhat from today's variation.

BUYING AND STORAGE Marzipan should be stored between sheets of greaseproof paper in well-covered containers, preferably in a cool, dry atmosphere. If stored in the refrigerator, marzipan will keep indefinitely.

PREPARATION AND USE A sugar and water syrup is prepared to soft-ball stage. After removal from the heat, it is stirred until it becomes a little cloudy. At this stage ground almonds are stirred in with beaten egg whites. The mixture is then turned onto a surface dusted with icing sugar and when cool enough to handle, kneaded until smooth and pliable, adding a little extra icing sugar if too moist. Added flavourings and colouring may be kneaded into the mixture, some recipes suggesting this should be done while the mixture is still warm, while others suggest leaving it until cold. Marzipan may be cut or shaped as desired, but should be allowed to dry a little and firm up before serving.

VARIETIES

Uncooked Marzipan

DESCRIPTION Though often described as 'marzipan', this simple nut paste is not true marzipan but is listed here as such because it is a popular variation and one that is extremely simple to prepare. The mixture makes a relatively soft confection similar in some instances to the cooked marzipan.

ORIGIN AND HISTORY As above.

BUYING AND STORAGE Store in layers between sheets of greaseproof paper in an airtight container in a cool dry place. Unlike cooked marzipan, this variety does not have extended keeping qualities. When stored as suggested it will stay fresh for about one week. If wrapped in plastic film and refrigerated, it should keep for up to two months.

PREPARATION AND USE A mixture of ground almonds and icing sugar is formed into a paste with the addition of either egg whites, egg yolks or whole eggs. Small quantities of flavourings such as rose water or liqueurs may be kneaded into the paste before rolling, cutting or shaping. If you find the paste is too damp after the addition of any liquid flavouring, knead in a little more icing sugar. Other sugars may be used, although icing sugar gives the smoothest texture. Crystal sugar gives a grainier result while brown sugar produces a darker, stronger flavoured paste.

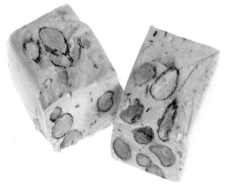

Nougat

MAJOR NUTRIENTS   SERVE SIZE 25 G

Energy	380 kJ	Dietary Fibre	0
Protein	less than 1 g	Sodium	5 mg
Fat	less than 1 g	Potassium	
Carbohydrate	24 g		less than 1 mg
Total Sugars	24 g		

NUTRITIONAL INFORMATION Mainly sugar-based confection. Some varieties contain nuts and glacé fruits. The nuts will add to the energy value per piece but there will not be enough to affect the significance of any other nutrient.

DESCRIPTION Nougat is a firm but chewy confection, opaque and of a colour which depends on the variety of ingredients which may have been added. Usually cut into small pieces in the shape of squares, diamonds or bars.

ORIGIN AND HISTORY The exact date of the first batch of nougat is uncertain but like many similar confections it was certainly eaten by the middle of the 16th century. In his cookbook which appeared in 1555 the celebrated prophet Nostradamus gives directions on how to make '. . . pignolat [pine nut nougat], sugar candy, syrups, pear preserves, Spanish nougat and marzipan tart'. Whether or not these nougat varieties had any resemblance to today's nougat recipes is unknown.

BUYING AND STORAGE Store bought or homemade nougat away from heat and humidity, preferably in an airtight container.

PREPARATION AND USE The traditional ingredients for nougat are honey, sugar, egg whites and chopped nuts. Liquid glucose or corn syrup is sometimes added. A boiled syrup is prepared and poured over beaten egg whites. Nuts and flavourings are added and the mixture is poured into a greased tin or one lined with rice paper. Some recipes call for the sugar syrup to be cooked in two stages: first to a lower temperature, at which point half is added to the beaten egg whites; the remaining half of the syrup is then heated to a higher temperature before being added to the first mixture. The honey is responsible for the characteristic mellowness of traditional nougat. Variations have additional ingredients such as cocoa or chocolate while an Italian version contains candied peel and cinnamon.

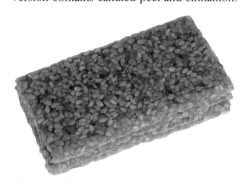

Pasteli

*also called **Sesame seed wafer, Sum-sum***

NUTRITIONAL INFORMATION Although no nutritional analysis is available, pasteli would contain a high fat and simple carbohydrate content, making it high in energy.

DESCRIPTION Crisp, toffee-coloured wafer made with sesame seeds and honey, with sugar added by some manufacturers. It is crisp and has a pleasant, nutty flavour.

ORIGIN AND HISTORY A Greek confection made from classical times. Originally it was a simple mixture of fragrant honey and roasted sesame seeds; such confections are

still made in the rural areas of Greece, with the addition of dried figs, raisins and almonds according to produce on hand. As sugar cookery techniques developed, the original simple mixture became a firm, crisp wafer.

Pasteli is not always a thin wafer; it can be slightly thicker with a topping of pistachio nuts, walnuts or almonds, increasing the flavour and appeal of the confection.

A similar confection, sum-sum, is a feature of Jewish cookery, a treat for special holidays. The mixture is formed into small squares or diamonds before it hardens.

BUYING AND STORAGE True pasteli is available at stores selling Greek foods and at natural food stores. Sum-sum can be found in stores stocking Jewish foods. Store tightly sealed in a cool place and avoid exposure to humid conditions as it will lose its crispness. Amongst the health food bars and confections developed in recent years, a softer sesame seed bar, somewhat similar to pasteli, is one of the most popular.

PREPARATION AND USE Use as a confection for the occasional snack.

SEE ALSO Sesame Seed.

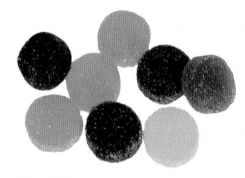

Pastille

MAJOR NUTRIENTS   SERVE SIZE 20 G

Energy	220 kJ	Total Sugars	12 g
Protein	1 g	Dietary Fibre	0
Fat	0	Sodium	15 mg
Carbohydrate	12 g	Potassium	10 mg

NUTRITIONAL INFORMATION Chewy non fat confection which would be lower in kilojoules than chewy toffee.

DESCRIPTION Pastilles are similar in appearance to fruit pastes, but usually have the addition of chopped nuts, the zest of citrus fruits and possibly spices.

ORIGIN AND HISTORY Though they may have been developed much earlier, we have an assurance that at least by the Elizabethan era, fashionable ladies of the time would not have been embarrassed to be found busy in the kitchen with a batch of pastilles.

BUYING AND STORAGE Pastilles, like fruit pastes, should be stored in an airtight container layered between sheets of waxed or special baking paper. They can keep for a considerable time if correctly stored.

PREPARATION AND USE Quinces or apples (the most commonly used fruit for pastes) are steamed in a very little water until soft. After pureeing, sugar is added to the pulp and the mixture is cooked over a low heat until very thick. A quantity of ground nuts may be added at this stage along with grated orange or lemon zest and cinnamon. The mixture is spread in a thin layer in a cake pan, chilled and cut into squares or fancy shapes, dusted with icing sugar and stored as above.

SEE ALSO Fruit Paste.

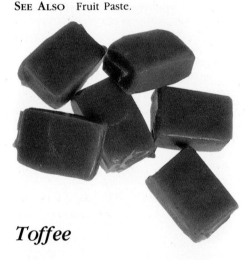

Toffee

MAJOR NUTRIENTS		SERVE SIZE 10 G	
Energy	180 kJ	Total Sugars	7 g
Protein	less than 1 g	Dietary Fibre	0
Fat	2 g	Sodium	32 mg
Cholesterol	2 mg	Potassium	21 mg
Carbohydrate	7 g		

NUTRITIONAL INFORMATION Although made with some milk, toffee is not a significant source of milk nutrients. Fat contributes 41% of total energy. If eaten in large quantities would be a significant source of energy.

DESCRIPTION A rich, sticky confection, usually a shade of brown, with a consistency varying from soft to very hard.

ORIGIN AND HISTORY There seems to be no specific time that can be pinpointed for the first toffee-making operation. It is fair to

assume that it was made by mistake and the resulting overcooked mixture of sugar and whatever was tried and not found wanting! Since that time the vogue for toffee making has become commonplace in most corners of the world. In the tropical areas where palm trees grow, the sugar ingredient for toffee would have been palm sugar.

BUYING AND STORAGE Wrap toffee pieces in cellophane or plastic wrap and store in covered containers away from heat and humidity.

PREPARATION AND USE A simple sugar using white or brown sugar is prepared with the addition of liquid glucose, corn syrup or cream of tartar and on most occasions, butter, cream or milk of one kind or another. Other ingredients such as golden syrup, lemon juice or rind, vinegar, flavouring essences and bicarbonate of soda (for honeycomb) may be used.

VARIETIES

Nut brittle; praline; toffee apple; and as an ingredient in, or adjunct to, desserts.

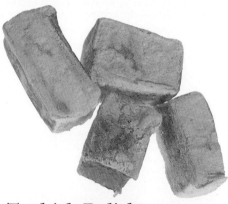

Turkish Delight

*also called **Lokum, Loukoum, Rahat lokum***

MAJOR NUTRIENTS		SERVE SIZE 20 G	
Energy	310 kJ	Dietary Fibre	0
Protein	less than 1 g	Sodium	less than 5 mg
Fat	less than 1 g	Potassium	
Carbohydrate	19 g		less than 5 mg
Total Sugars	19 g		

NUTRITIONAL INFORMATION Sucrose-containing product with no fat. Some varieties may contain nuts which will increase the energy value but not contribute significantly to other nutrients.

DESCRIPTION Cube-shaped, sugar-coated and delectable confection, pleasantly gelatinous with a melt-in-the-mouth texture. Turkish delight is made in various flavours and colours. Its Turkish name, rahat lokum, means 'giving rest to the throat' — a delightful description in itself.

ORIGIN AND HISTORY As the name implies, the sweetmeat is Turkish in origin, but the Greeks lay claim to its invention also. A Persian jellylike sweetmeat called ahbisa, from early in the second millennium AD, could well have been the predecessor to Turkish delight; it could have been made with salep or ground rice, both with gelatinous properties, and both around at the time.

However a true Turkish delight can only be made with cornflour (cornstarch) to achieve the very special texture (recipes using gelatine are poor substitutes). As cornflour would not have reached the Turkish, or the Greek, kitchen until late in the 19th century, after the refining of milled grain had been achieved, Turkish delight could have had a number of inventors, each using the new gelatinising agent to replace an earlier one.

One tradition suggests modern Turkish delight was the invention of one Hadji Bekir, whose descendants in Istanbul continued to make the confection according to a recipe whose secrecy was closely guarded.

Special equipment is required to make the confection. Cornflour, sugar and water are beaten and heated at the same time until the right consistency is reached, with glucose added during the process. Flavourings, such as vanilla, rose water, orange flower water or mint, are added with colouring, pistachios, almonds or walnuts. It is poured into oiled wooden frames, left overnight, then cut and tossed in icing sugar or coconut.

BUYING AND STORAGE Purchase from stores stocking Middle Eastern and Greek foods, from confectioners and gourmet food stores. Leave in its box or place in a sealed container. Store in a cool, dry place.

PREPARATION AND USE Needs no preparation unless humidity has caused the icing sugar coating to melt and harden; this can be scraped off and the cubes tossed in freshly sifted icing sugar. Place in little paper cases to serve with after-dinner coffee.

JAMS, SPREADS AND DIPS

Jams and conserves are cooked mixtures of fruit or fruit pieces in water and sugar. Depending on the particular fruits used and their method of cooking they may have a jellylike or syrupy consistency. Conserves differ slightly from jam in that their fruits usually remain either whole or in large pieces, while jam is usually more pulpy in texture. Jellies are the strained juices of cooked fruit, which hold their shape to some extent when spooned.

In Europe, the first references to jams and jellies occur in late medieval writings. An increase in interest in the growing of fruit trees during the 16th century was logically followed by an increase in the making of preserves of all kinds. Rose petals, orange flowers, musk, angelica and rosemary were all favoured added flavourings. It is acknowledged that the Italians were the radical innovators who led the way for the rest of Europe in the use of sugar in sweets, preserves and fruit pastes. The French also had their own outstanding innovators. Massialot, chef to a number of French noblemen and cookbook author, gives a recipe for a violet marmalade in his *Handbook of Preserves* (1692), while more than a century earlier the famous prophet Nostradamus had given a recipe for cherry jelly in his own cookbook, which also gave directions for preserving many other fruits.

The dips and spreads now available, particularly the homemade varieties, are as numerous and varied as the imagination will allow. Some which are long-established and of ethnic origin, such as taramosalata and guacamole, have become worldwide favourites, while others such as Vegemite, though loved by many, have not always translated well into the cuisines of other countries.

Although these foods are all used as spreads for bread, toast and biscuits, they are just as varied in their nutritional characteristics as they are in their ingredients and flavour. The nutrient content depends upon the ingredients used, and the changes in nutrients due to processing.

The main nutrients in the jams, conserves and jelly are sugars, with small amounts of dietary fibre. There are residual amounts of vitamins, depending on the fruits used.

The yeast extracts concentrate the vitamins found in yeast (thiamin, riboflavin, niacin and folate), and salt is also added in processing, although some manufacturers are gradually reducing salt levels.

Peanut butter is approximately 50% fat, most of which is monounsaturated. It is available in 'no added salt' varieties.

In preparing dips, it is often possible to reduce the fat levels by substituting cottage cheese, low fat ricotta cheese and low fat yoghurt for the sour cream, creamed cheese and mayonnaise when these are used as basic ingredients.

It is healthy to moderate the use of jams, dips and spreads which are high in sugar, fat and salt, and to seek out some of the low fat products.

Naturally this chapter cannot contain the great diversity that its title evokes. The entries which follow serve as a basic guide to the range of these foods.

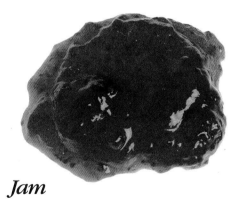

Jam

Major Nutrients		Serve Size 5 g	
Energy	60 kJ	Total Sugars	3.5 g
Protein	0	Dietary Fibre	0
Fat	0	Sodium	less than 1 mg
Carbohydrate	3.5 g		

NUTRITIONAL INFORMATION The vitamin levels vary with the fruit used and vitamin C levels are reduced in the cooking process. A moderate energy spread as it only contains carbohydrate. Both soft and stone fruit jams contribute similar nutrients.

DESCRIPTION Jam is a mixture of whole fruit or fruit pieces cooked in sugar and water.

ORIGIN AND HISTORY Possibly one of the first written references to jam came in the *Decameron*, written by Giovanni Boccaccio around 1350, in which he speaks of a group of young people who fled Florence at the time of the plague in 1348 and who ate 'sweets, preserves and jams'. There is no doubt that jams and preserves were made long before this time, but actual recipes did not begin to appear in print until some time later. In 1541 a translation of an Italian book, *The Edifice of Recipes*, introduced to France the art of making jam and preserving fruits.

BUYING AND STORAGE Store jam in a cool, dry place.

PREPARATION AND USE Jam is used as a spread, in desserts and on cakes and biscuits. To make jam, different fruits are cooked by different methods, often depending on their moisture content. While some achieve a better colour with fast cooking, others require long, slow cooking to achieve an attractive effect. There are five main methods of preparation.

1. Fruit cooked slowly in water or its own juices until tender, with sugar then added and cooked rapidly.

2. Syrup made of sugar and water or fruit juice, with fruit then added and cooked gently.

3. Sugar and fruit cooked together.

4. Prepared fruit covered with sugar overnight, then cooked gently.

5. Marmalade, using fruits with tougher skins — oranges, lemons, grapefruit — almost always has the sliced fruit soaked overnight to help release the pectin and soften the skins.

VARIETIES

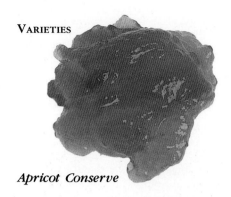

Apricot Conserve

MAJOR NUTRIENTS — SERVE SIZE 5 G

Energy	60 kJ	Total Sugars	3 g
Protein	0	Dietary Fibre	0
Fat	0	Sodium	0
Carbohydrate	3 g	Potassium	5 mg

NUTRITIONAL INFORMATION Energy almost entirely from sugars. Useful instead of added fats on breads or as dessert/cake toppings. Nutrients are the same for all types of conserve.

DESCRIPTION A jam made with fruit whole or in large pieces.

ORIGIN AND HISTORY See Jam in general.

BUYING AND STORAGE See Jam in general.

PREPARATION AND USE For this conserve an equal weight of sugar to that of fruit is required, and the fruit remains whole or in large pieces. Water and half the measured sugar are brought to the boil and cooked for a few minutes, the stoned fruit are added and the mixture cooked gently for about 20 minutes with frequent stirring. The remaining sugar is added, stirred until boiling and cooked a further 10 minutes or until a successful test for gelling has been carried out. The jam is cooled slightly then poured into heated, sterilised jars, covered and labelled.

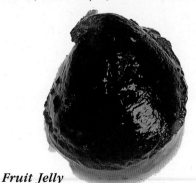

Fruit Jelly

NUTRITIONAL INFORMATION Jelly contains the same nutrients as those of jam, above.

DESCRIPTION Jellies should be clear and have good, though not necessarily deep, colour. They should hold their shape when cut and should sparkle to some degree. The best fruits for jelly-making are those rich in pectin. Fruits not so rich in pectin have lemon juice or commercial pectin added for best results.

ORIGIN AND HISTORY One of the most noteworthy jellies must surely be the one mentioned by the famous prophet Nostradamus in his book of recipes which became available in France in 1555. He explains in it 'the manner and fashion of making preserves of several sorts, in honey as well as in sugar and cooked wine.' He describes 'preserving whole little limes and oranges, quinces in quarters with sugar' and 'a way of making a jelly of guignes [a type of cherry] that is very delicate but expensive and for noblemen.' One wonders what added ingredients were used that put this obviously exotic jelly beyond the reach of all but the wealthy!

BUYING AND STORAGE Store jellies in a cool, dry place.

PREPARATION AND USE Fruit is brought slowly to the boil and simmered until soft. Using cheesecloth or a special jelly bag, the mixture is strained. The liquid must not be forced through the cloth, but allowed to drip only. Pressing on the fruit will cause the jelly to be cloudy. The resulting juice is measured and, for each cup of juice, a cup of sugar is added, the mixture heated and stirred until the sugar dissolves, then boiled briskly until a little of it gels when tested.

To test for gelling, place a teaspoonful of jelly on a cold saucer. Place in the refrigerator for a couple of minutes or until cold. Tilt the saucer — if the surface of the jam wrinkles, it is cooked; if it runs free, it requires more cooking.

Besides its use as a spread, fruit jelly is a low fat condiment useful for adding flavour to meat and poultry dishes.

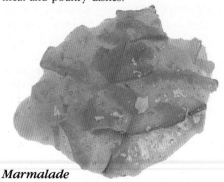

Marmalade

MAJOR NUTRIENTS — SERVE SIZE 5 G

Energy	60 kJ	Total Sugars	3 g
Protein	0	Dietary Fibre	0
Fat	0	Sodium	less than 1 mg
Carbohydrate	3 g	Potassium	2 mg

NUTRITIONAL INFORMATION A moderate energy spread, as it only contains carbohydrate. If used instead of butter or margarine on bread it can reduce total fat and energy intake.

DESCRIPTION Marmalade is similar in preparation to other jam but always uses citrus fruits — lemons, oranges, grapefruit, limes or cumquats. Sometimes a single fruit is used, sometimes two or more fruits. As most citrus skins do not break down to the same extent as other fruits used in jam making, the syrup or jellylike part of the marmalade is likely to be clearer and more sparkling than jam.

ORIGIN AND HISTORY Even though the Italians led the way in the imaginative use of sugar in the 16th century, the French also had their outstanding innovators. One, Massialot, chef to a number of French noblemen and a cookbook author, gives a recipe for a violet marmalade in his *Handbook of Preserves* (1692). Great delicacy of preparation must have been required to achieve what one imagines could have been a sparkling clear jelly with delicate violet heads suspended through it.

BUYING AND STORAGE Store marmalade in a cool, dry place.

PREPARATION AND USE According to the type of fruit used and personal taste, marmalade requires up to three times the weight of sugar to fruit. The skin is used as well as the pulp of the fruit. The pips are removed, but since they are rich in pectin (important in the gelling process of jams and marmalade) they are usually soaked in some of the measured water in advance to extract the pectin, and the water drained from the pips is used in the making of the marmalade. The whole fruit is sliced very thinly, or else the pulp is removed and chopped, and the skins finely sliced. The skins may be minced but the appearance and texture of the marmalade suffers. The prepared fruit is then covered with the measured water and allowed to stand overnight to extract the pectin. The mixture of fruit and water is then simmered until the skins are soft and the pith transparent, which could take up to an hour (the pith of lemons and some sweet oranges does not become transparent when cooked so in this case simply check for softness). The sugar is added and stirred until dissolved. Then boil rapidly until the mixture gels when tested — approximately 20 minutes. Allow to cool slightly before bottling. Once bottled, cover immediately.

Spread

NUTRITIONAL INFORMATION No average data can be obtained for spreads, since the varieties are so numerous.

DESCRIPTION Spreads have a variety of consistencies from the much loved sticky honey to smooth yeast-based spreads such as Vegemite and Marmite, and those of more body such as pastes, peanut butter, mixed nut and chocolate spreads, and pâtés.

ORIGIN AND HISTORY From the beginning of bread making, pieces of bread have undoubtedly been eaten along with some kind of fat-containing product: in most societies the palatability of bread has been considered to be improved by dipping it in oil or spreading it with a moist, fatty accompaniment. The development of the sandwich in Western society over the last two centuries has greatly increased the use of spreads, which include almost every type of food substance.

BUYING AND STORAGE Commercial products have a use-by date. Homemade items such as jam need cool storage and low humidity.

PREPARATION AND USE These will vary with the product chosen.

VARIETIES

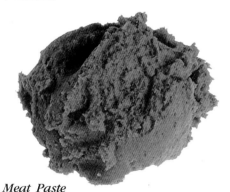

Meat Paste

MAJOR NUTRIENTS		SERVE SIZE 5 G	
Energy	40 kJ	Carbohydrate	0
Protein	less than 1 g	Sodium	35 mg
Fat	less than 1 g	Potassium	10 mg
Cholesterol	0		

NUTRITIONAL INFORMATION Low-fat, tasty spread that only contains small amounts of sodium.

DESCRIPTION Very finely minced meat and additives, which can be thinly spread.

ORIGIN AND HISTORY Potted meats have been popular for centuries (see Pâté in the chapter on Sausages and Preserved Meats).

BUYING AND STORAGE Always store in the refrigerator after opening. Will keep up to 2 weeks.

PREPARATION AND USE Mainly used on children's sandwiches, while the more sophisticated pâté is elevated to entrée status in a meal.

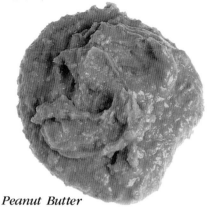

Peanut Butter

MAJOR NUTRIENTS		SERVE SIZE 10 G	
Energy	250 kJ	Dietary Fibre	
Protein	2 g		less than 1 g
Fat	5 g	Sodium	35 mg
Cholesterol	0	Potassium	70 mg
Carbohydrate	1 g	Phosphorus	35 mg
Total Sugars		Magnesium	20 mg
	less than 1 g	Niacin Equiv.	1.6 mg

NUTRITIONAL INFORMATION A good source of phosphorus, magnesium and niacin. Although this contains significant amounts of fat, which provide over 70% of energy, the fats contain no cholesterol and are high in unsaturated fatty acids. If used alone without other fat, this spread makes a suitable sandwich filling.

DESCRIPTION Roasted ground peanuts, to which some salt is added. When crushed the nuts release an oil which makes the mixture spreadable.

ORIGIN AND HISTORY A 20th century product first popularised in North America, where it is sold in a variety of textures and combinations, including peanut butter and jam.

BUYING AND STORAGE The product carries a use-by date and keeps well in the cupboard.

PREPARATION AND USE Aside from its use as a spread, it may be added to other ingredients to make homemade satay sauce.

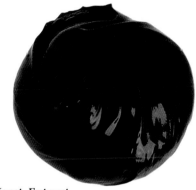

Yeast Extract

MAJOR NUTRIENTS		SERVE SIZE 2 G	
Energy	14 kJ	Potassium	50 mg
Protein	less than 1 g	Thiamin	0.5 mg
Fat	0	Riboflavin	1 mg
Carbohydrate		Niacin Equiv.	5 mg
	less than 1 g		
Sodium	65 mg		

NUTRITIONAL INFORMATION An excellent source of thiamin, riboflavin, niacin and folate.

Traditional B vitamin supplement for Australians and New Zealanders. Total sodium level has been reduced over the last few years to current levels as it is usually consumed on bread where the margarine would contain more sodium than the yeast extract.

Contains significant amounts of naturally occurring monosodium glutamate and amines.

DESCRIPTION A product made by treating yeast with acid.

ORIGIN AND HISTORY The manufacturing process was invented in Germany in the 1890s and is now used worldwide. When fresh brewer's yeast is mixed with salt it is broken down by its own enzymes. The soluble residue is evaporated under pressure to give the familiar sticky brown substance known as yeast extract.

BUYING AND STORAGE Sold commercially under proprietary names such as Marmite (UK), Vegemite (Aust.) and Savita (USA).

PREPARATION AND USE Spread yeast extracts thinly on buttered bread. They can also be used to flavour and colour casseroles and soups.

Dip

MAJOR NUTRIENTS
PACKET, SOUR CREAM BASE
SERVE SIZE 10 G

Energy	190 kJ	Total Sugars	
Protein	less than 1 g		less than 1 g
Fat	5 g	Dietary Fibre	0
Cholesterol	15 mg	Sodium	200 mg
Carbohydrate		Potassium	20 mg
	less than 1 g		

NUTRITIONAL INFORMATION If ricotta or cottage cheese is used, dip will be much lower in kilojoules and total fat level. Package dips contribute mainly sodium to the finished product. Main nutrients will depend on base mix.

DESCRIPTION A dip is any food reduced to pieces fine enough for them to be combined with a moist or oily base, so that bread, vegetables, biscuits or other food items can be used to scoop up the mixture. Dips may be of a straight liquid consistency, such as the Asian black bean sauce or soy sauce variations, or they may be soft and creamy with savoury and/or sweet ingredients added to sour cream, cottage or cream cheese, or yoghurt.

ORIGIN AND HISTORY While today we could very likely be seen dipping a cracker in a cream cheese dip, the ancient Roman would more likely be dipping a piece of coarse bread in wine or goat's milk for a quick snack.

In ancient Egypt garlic mixed with oil (the distant ancestor of mayonnaise) could well have been the favoured dip. The Romans added egg yolks to make it aioli. We perhaps consider these to be sauces, but there is no doubt that in their countries of origin they frequently served the same purpose as our modern dips.

We read that in biblical times Ruth was ordered to: 'Come thou hither and dip thy morsel [of bread] in vinegar.' We understand this was no rough vinegar, but one of a far more refined variety.

The Mayan people of Central America had been growing avocados and making guacamole centuries before the arrival of the Spanish conquistadors in the 16th century. They found a perfect partner for the delicious but mildly flavoured fruit in their own native hot red pepper.

BUYING AND STORAGE Most commercial dips have a use-by date. Particular care should be taken with products having a meat or dairy food base. Buy from reliable outlets and always store in the refrigerator.

PREPARATION AND USE Dips, like those described above, may have a wide variety of ingredients. Take care to make them of a consistency that will cling to the items being dipped. A corn chip will scoop up a relatively soft mixture but a celery stick needs a bit more body in a dip for successful eating.

VARIETIES

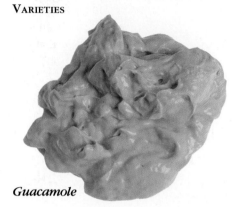

Guacamole

MAJOR NUTRIENTS
WITH CREAM AND TOMATO
SERVE SIZE 20 G

Energy	320 kJ	Dietary Fibre	
Protein	less than 1 g		less than 1 g
Fat	8 g	Sodium	5 mg
Cholesterol	10 mg	Potassium	210 mg
Carbohydrate		Iron	1 mg
	less than 1 g	Vitamin A	110 μg
Total Sugars		Niacin Equiv.	1.3 mg
	less than 1 g	Vitamin C	10 mg

NUTRITIONAL INFORMATION An excellent source of vitamins A and C; good source of iron; moderate source of niacin. High fat dip with up to 90% of energy coming from fats. Cholesterol contribution is from cream. Dip can be made with cottage or ricotta cheese which reduces the fat and energy levels and increases calcium.

DESCRIPTION A smooth, green dip whose main ingredient is pureed avocado.

ORIGIN AND HISTORY Originally seasoned by the Mayan people with their local hot red peppers, it is now usually prepared with a little finely chopped onion and tomato, and moistened with oil and lemon juice.

BUYING AND STORAGE Keep refrigerated once prepared.

PREPARATION AND USE Prepare as above. Guacamole is usually eaten with corn chips.

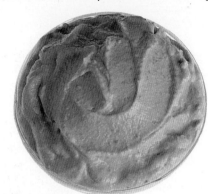

Taramosalata

MAJOR NUTRIENTS
SERVE SIZE 25 G

Energy	440 kJ	Sodium	90 mg
Protein	4 g	Potassium	45 mg
Fat	3 g	Phosphorus	70 mg
Cholesterol	50 mg	Thiamin	0.5 mg
Carbohydrate	10 g	Vitamin C	4 mg
Total Sugars	0		
Dietary Fibre			
	less than 1 g		

NUTRITIONAL INFORMATION An excellent source of thiamin; good source of phosphorus and vitamin C; moderate source of vitamin E. The cholesterol content is contributed by the roe. Fats contribute only 25% total energy, which makes this dip low in fat. Use of lemon juice provides significant vitamin C levels. If more bread is used, the energy and fat levels in the dip can be reduced.

DESCRIPTION Taramosalata is made from a base of tarama, the roe of the grey mullet, and is pink or orange in colour.

ORIGIN AND HISTORY Taramosalata is a Greek dish, used as a dip.

BUYING AND STORAGE Available ready made from delicatessens and stores selling Greek products. There are also some varieties sold in supermarkets. Store in the refrigerator.

PREPARATION AND USE The salted roe is mixed with equal amounts of stale bread which has been soaked, squeezed dry and mixed with onion, lemon juice and olive oil. Mashed potato may be used instead but the flavour is inferior. It may be served with Greek breads, crusty bread or vegetable pieces.

SEE ALSO Tarama.

SAUCES, MUSTARDS AND PASTES

Sauces have a place in a wide range of cuisines, from the simplest home cookery — when a steak is served with the juices from the pan — to the most delicate culinary engineering, inspired by the French, which goes under the name of *haute cuisine*.

A sauce may have a variety of functions. At its simplest, it serves to moisten food, as a plain butter and parsley sauce may enhance young boiled potatoes. Sauces with a bland flavour are often used as a contrast to the texture of vegetables, an example being a white sauce served over steamed fennel. When the vegetable itself is not strongly flavoured, a richer taste may be added by the sauce, an example being cheese sauce over cooked cauliflower. There are also sauces which claim almost as much attention as the foods they accompany. Often using flour and other thickeners, and with butter, wine or eggs as a base, these rich sauces should be taken into account as a food source by those who regularly use them with their meat, fish and vegetables.

The composition of dessert sauces, too, must be taken into consideration if they are to be part of a healthy diet, since they contain high quantities of sugar.

Another function of sauces is their decorative quality, which means that a well-made accompaniment to a meal may not only enhance its flavour but make it look appetising as well.

The sauces in this chapter have been chosen from amongst those most commonly found in the home and in the marketplace. It should be noted that sauces consumed in restaurants or bought from grocery shelves may have a high content of sodium. The individual entries which follow are a guide to the general content of the sauces most easily available to consumers today.

For further information about the mustards described in this chapter, the reader should refer to Mustard in the chapter on Herbs and Spices.

A number of the pastes examined in this chapter would become sauces with the addition of a little more moisture, and at the other end of the scale they may also do service as dips. Many of these are known and appreciated for their strong flavours, and even in small quantities can greatly enhance enjoyment of the foods they accompany.

SAUCES

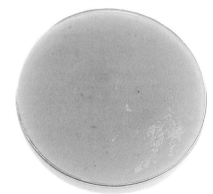

Apple Sauce

MAJOR NUTRIENTS		CANNED, SWEETENED SERVE SIZE 30 G	
Energy	122 kJ	Carbohydrate	7 g
Protein	0	Cholesterol	0
Fat	0	Sodium	0

NUTRITIONAL INFORMATION Sweetened apple sauce is mostly composed of carbohydrates. Other nutrients are present (including fibre) but not in nutritionally significant amounts.

Apple sauce, unsweetened, is about one-half the energy value of sweetened apple sauce. The ascorbic acid is easily destroyed by cooking the apples. This loss of ascorbic acid can be reduced by cooking the apples quickly in a small amount of boiling water with a tightly fitting lid.

DESCRIPTION Apple sauce is made from pureed apples, and sometimes a thickener, such as wheat or cornflour. Lemon is sometimes added if the sauce is too sweet. Butter and sugar can be other ingredients, along with nutmeg, cinnamon, ginger or mace.

ORIGIN AND HISTORY Apples have been cultivated for at least 3000 years. Twenty varieties were known and grown by the Romans. There is evidence that apples had been cultivated in Neolithic times. Apple sauce may have originated with the Romans, and is a classic English and American sauce.

BUYING AND STORAGE Preservatives are added to the commercial sauce, as well as wheat starch. After opening store in the refrigerator.

PREPARATION AND USE It is traditionally used with roast pork as a condiment. Add to the pan juices as a demiglaze or add to the gravy as flavouring. Can be used as a sauce for dessert.

SEE ALSO Apples.

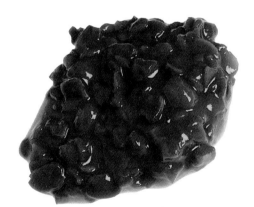

Bean Sauce

also called Yellow bean sauce

NUTRITIONAL INFORMATION No reliable data are available.

DESCRIPTION A salty Chinese seasoning sauce which comes in several varieties. It may be smooth, thick and a yellow-brown colour, or have whole yellow soya beans suspended in a very salty thin sauce, or it may be somewhat like a mixture of the two previous types.

ORIGIN AND HISTORY Salted soya beans are one of the oldest seasoning ingredients, and have been in continuous use in China for over 2000 years. Jiang (bean pickle) is frequently mentioned in ancient texts, along with shih (salted darkened soya beans), the salted and fermented black beans we know today. Jiang was the precursor of soya sauce, which is a refined and filtered version of the original salty thin bean sauce.

BUYING AND STORAGE It is sold in small cans or jars. Unopened it can be kept indefinitely. After opening, transfer unused portion to a glass jar with a non-metal top and store in the refrigerator.

PREPARATION AND USE It is added to dishes when a rich, salty flavour is required. It is rather like Japanese yellow miso, which could be used as a substitute. Used in stir-fried and braised dishes in Chinese cooking.

SEE ALSO Bean Paste; Black Bean Sauce; Soya Sauce.

Béarnaise Sauce

MAJOR NUTRIENTS		PACKET SERVE SIZE 45 G	
Energy	520 kJ	Carbohydrate	3 g
Protein	2 g	Cholesterol	33 mg
Fat	12 g	Sodium	225 mg

NUTRITIONAL INFORMATION Béarnaise sauce is high in fat and moderately high in sodium. Other nutrients are present but not in nutritionally significant amounts.

The major fatty acid present in béarnaise sauce is saturated, 64.5%. Monounsaturated fatty acids provide 30.7% and polyunsaturated provide 4.7%.

DESCRIPTION Like hollandaise and mayonnaise, béarnaise sauce is classified as an emulsion — unlike liquids held in suspension. It is flavoured with tarragon and shallots, white wine or vinegar. It contains more butter and less eggs than hollandaise sauce. The egg yolks and stock of wine and herbs are whisked together over a bain marie and the melted butter added slowly. Overheating the sauce can ruin it by coagulating the egg proteins (the vinegar or wine helps to separate them) and forming little lumps, or by the mixture separating. Packet béarnaise sauce contains vegetable starches, animal fats, dehydrated eggs and flavourings.

ORIGIN AND HISTORY As with other sauces there is some debate as to where this sauce originated, however some favour the Béarn region of France. Others disagree because Béarn is in an olive oil district and olive oil is more common in the cooking of the region than butter. Others attribute it to the chef who was in the Pavillon Henri IV at St Germain in Paris about 1835.

BUYING AND STORAGE Vacuum sealed packet béarnaise sauce can be stored in cupboard or pantry for 12–18 months. Freshly made béarnaise can be stored in the refrigerator covered for up to 3 days.

PREPARATION AND USE Used as a traditional sauce over grilled beef and over vegetables.

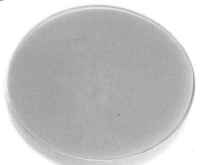

Bechamel Sauce

also called **White Sauce**

MAJOR NUTRIENTS		SERVE SIZE 45 G	
Energy	280 kJ	Sodium	185 mg
Protein	2 g	Vitamin A	45 µg
Fat	4 g	Calcium	58 mg
Carbohydrate	5 g	Phosphorus	45 mg
Cholesterol	10 mg		

NUTRITIONAL INFORMATION Bechamel sauce is high in fat and moderately high in sodium; a moderate source of vitamin A, calcium and phosphorus. Other nutrients are present but not in nutritionally significant amounts.

The fat in bechamel sauce consists of 44% saturated, 33% monounsaturated and 22% polyunsaturated fatty acids.

DESCRIPTION This is a classic French sauce made with butter and flour (white roux), mixed with milk. It is flavoured with bay leaves, thyme and nutmeg. It should be smooth, light and glossy.

ORIGIN AND HISTORY This sauce is named after Louis de Bechameil, a courtier with Louis XIV. It resulted from a revolution in sauces and cooking generally. The coarse sauces thickened with bread or ground almonds gave way to smooth, more refined sauces which enhanced and complemented the flavours of the food instead of overpowering them. Bechamel sauce with grated cheese added is called mornay sauce, after a Huguenot family. Soubise, a classic French sauce made from a puree of cooked onions mixed with a bechamel sauce, is named after a commander in the French army. Bechamel sauce is generally known in England, Australia and North America as white sauce.

BUYING AND STORAGE Can be purchased frozen or dehydrated in vacuum sealed packets. Fresh bechamel sauce should not be stored but used at once.

PREPARATION AND USE Use with fish, meats or vegetables. Mornay sauce is popular with tinned fish such as tuna. Use over pasta with cream and other flavourings such as mushrooms.

SEE ALSO Velouté.

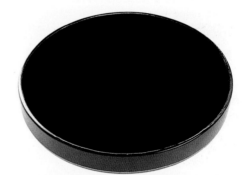

Black Bean Sauce

NUTRITIONAL INFORMATION No nutritional details are available.

DESCRIPTION Made from fermented whole and crushed soya beans. The mixture also contains water and wheat flour.

ORIGIN AND HISTORY The soya bean has been used in China for hundreds of years as a flavouring for sauces such as soya sauce and black bean sauce, and as a high protein food in its own right.

BUYING AND STORAGE Purchase from specialty stores. Keeps indefinitely.

PREPARATION AND USE Used as a flavouring in Chinese foods with meat and vegetables. Dilute with water to use as a marinade for red meats or chicken, basting the meats as they cook. A traditional Chinese dish is beef and black bean sauce.

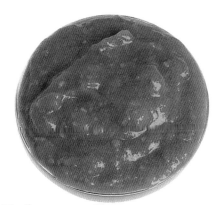

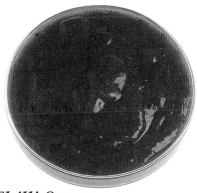

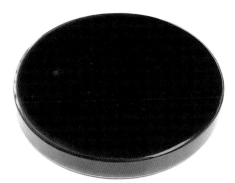

Bolognese Sauce

also called **Bolognaise**

MAJOR NUTRIENTS		SERVE SIZE 100 G	
Energy	502 kJ	Cholesterol	27 mg
Protein	8 g	Sodium	468 mg
Fat	9 g	Magnesium	22 mg
Carbohydrate	2 g	Iron	1.4 mg

NUTRITIONAL INFORMATION Bolognese sauce is a high fat food. It is high in sodium; an excellent source of iron; a moderate source of magnesium.

The fat is 33% saturated fat, 44% monounsaturated and 22% polyunsaturated. The fat content of homemade varieties can be reduced by the use of lean mince and by cooling the sauce, skimming off excess fat and reheating.

DESCRIPTION There are many versions of this sauce, but generally it consists of skinned tomatoes, mushrooms, onion, garlic, herbs, olive oil, and meats such as ham, beef or bacon. Sometimes cream is added.

ORIGIN AND HISTORY This sauce originated in the region called Emilia Romagna, in the north of Italy. Bologna is the dominant city of this region, which is very fertile, producing beef, pork, and an abundance of vegetables, hence the richness of the bolognese sauce, which often uses pork fat instead of olive oil. It is served in Bologna with tagliatelle.

BUYING AND STORAGE Can be purchased in bottles from the supermarket. Sauces manufactured, labelled bolognese and sold in bottles do not always contain meat.

Store in the refrigerator after opening, and use within 3 days, the same as for freshly made sauce. The short storage time for this sauce is because of the minced meat, which easily harbours harmful bacteria.

PREPARATION AND USE Serve with tagliatelle, spaghetti, ravioli or agnolotti. In Italy parmesan cheese which accompanies this sauce is always served in a separate bowl on the table.

Chilli Sauce

MAJOR NUTRIENTS		SERVE SIZE 20 G	
Energy	36 kJ	Carbohydrate	2 g
Protein	0.6 g	Cholesterol	0
Fat	0	Sodium	59 mg

NUTRITIONAL INFORMATION Chilli sauce is largely composed of carbohydrates. Other nutrients are present but not in nutritionally significant amounts.

Over half of the carbohydrate in chilli sauce is starch.

DESCRIPTION Chilli sauce is made from the fruits of *Capsicum frutescens* and *Capsicum annuum*. The sauce is red-orange in colour and is very hot. It contains vinegar, pepper and other ingredients as well as capsicums and chillies. Some chilli sauces have a thickener added such as wheat starch.

ORIGIN AND HISTORY Chillies originated in Central America, where this sauce is common. The Chinese make a version of chilli sauce which is served in a small dish on the table. This is usually thickened with rice starch.

BUYING AND STORAGE Purchase from specialty stores or supermarkets. Chinese versions and also versions from South-East Asia and India can be purchased from specialty stores. Chillies contain the alkaloid capsaicin which is a preservative, and the sauce keeps indefinitely.

PREPARATION AND USE The flavour of chilli sauce can be overpowered by its hotness, so use sparingly. The flavour enhances guacamole, fish dishes, and South-East Asian cookery.

Chocolate Sauce

NUTRITIONAL INFORMATION Because of the widely differing styles of manufacture, no specific analysis is available. See Chocolate in Confectionery chapter for details.

DESCRIPTION Homemade chocolate sauce is made with melted block chocolate, cream, milk and egg yolks. Bottled chocolate sauce is made with cocoa powder, chocolate flavouring, emulsifiers, sugar and water.

ORIGIN AND HISTORY Block or milk chocolate as we know it today evolved over a period of 50 years of experimentation. Conrad Van Houten invented a method of pressing the cocoa butter (the cocoa bean has more than 50% cocoa fat) out of the bean. Then Rudolph Lindt took the process further to develop block chocolate: the extracted butter was made more malleable, then cream or milk was added to some of the cocoa butter and reblended with the cocoa bean. M. Peter of Switzerland added condensed milk to some of his cocoa butter in 1875.

Chocolate sauce made with block chocolate and cream or milk was first made in the 1880s and bottled chocolate sauce was introduced in the 1900s.

BUYING AND STORAGE Commercially made chocolate sauce is stored in a cool pantry or cupboard. If the storage area is too warm, the sugar (of which there is a lot) re-crystallises. Freshly made chocolate sauce should be used immediately, however it can be re-heated to pouring consistency.

PREPARATION AND USE Commercially made chocolate sauce is usually poured over ice cream, and can be used as a flavouring for milk. Freshly made chocolate sauce is used hot or cold poured over a variety of desserts, and can be used as a filling in cakes and pastries.

SEE ALSO Chocolate, Cocoa.

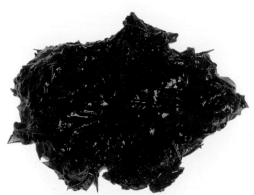

Cranberry Sauce

MAJOR NUTRIENTS		SERVE SIZE 30 G	
Energy	190 kJ	Carbohydrate	12 g
Protein	0	Cholesterol	0
Fat	0	Sodium	9 mg

NUTRITIONAL INFORMATION Cranberry sauce is mostly composed of carbohydrates. Other nutrients are present but not in nutritionally significant amounts.

DESCRIPTION Cranberries are native to North America and the Himalaya region. They are from the heath family, and are cousins to blueberries, bilberries and huckleberries. The fruits of the cranberry grow on a vine which is not a climber. They are cold tender and are grown in Massachusetts, Wisconsin and New Jersey in peat bogs where the plants are protected from the cold by being covered with water in the winter. Harvesting is by disturbing the water with something like a paddlewheel attached to a tractor. The berries float to the surface and are directed to shore by wooden booms. Cranberry sauce consists of cranberries and sugar. The sauce is made from the natural jelly because cranberries are very high in pectin. The jelly is made by cooking whole cranberries, then filtering to extract stems. High quality cranberries are added to the jelly and recooked, then it is bottled.

ORIGIN AND HISTORY Cranberries were an important food to Quinalut and Queet Indians from Oregon long before Europeans arrived. They ate them fresh and used them to make a dish called pemmican, which consisted of deer meat and berries pounded to a pulp, and shaped into cakes which were dried in the sun. Cranberries were first sent to Europe from America in 1550, but commercial production did not begin until 1811. Cranberry sauce must have been made before 1811 at home because it is a traditional accompaniment to turkey at Thanksgiving.

BUYING AND STORAGE The bottled sauce has good keeping qualities. Store in the refrigerator.

PREPARATION AND USE Used as a traditional accompaniment to turkey at Thanksgiving in America. Add some cranberry sauce to the gravy for a different flavour to enhance turkey.

SEE ALSO Cranberry.

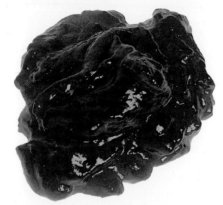

Cumberland Sauce

NUTRITIONAL INFORMATION No reliable data available.

DESCRIPTION This sauce is flavoured with port and the rind of bitter oranges, lemon and orange juice, redcurrant jelly, vinegar, cayenne pepper and mustard. Sometimes ginger is added.

ORIGIN AND HISTORY This sauce is a traditional English sauce, originating in Cumberland, England.

BUYING AND STORAGE Purchase from specialty stores and store in the refrigerator.

PREPARATION AND USE Used as a traditional accompaniment to venison.

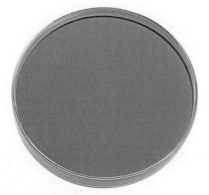

Fish Sauce

also called **Nam pla, Nuoc mam, Patis, Yu lu**

MAJOR NUTRIENTS		SERVE SIZE 15 G	
Energy	170 kJ	Carbohydrate	3 g
Protein	3 g	Cholesterol	0
Fat	2 g	Sodium	250 mg

NUTRITIONAL INFORMATION Vitamin and mineral content is negligible. A large amount of salt (sodium) is added during processing.

DESCRIPTION A thin, salty, light brown seasoning sauce with a strong fishy flavour. It is made by processing dried salted fish by fermentation, the clear liquid filtered off being the sauce. It has an unpleasant odour of putrefying seafood, which is not transmitted noticeably to a dish. It is used in many parts of South-East Asia, but in particular in Thailand and Vietnam where it is known as nam pla and nuoc mam. There are many different types and qualities of fish sauce, and variations are also made with shrimp and squid. In general, the best sauce will be clear and thin, a light ochre colour and have a clean distinct odour.

ORIGIN AND HISTORY Cooks in the ancient Thai capital recorded over 1000 years ago using a salty thin sauce made from fermented fish. Similarly in the ancient city of Angkor Wat, Cambodia, and in Laos, Vietnam and Indonesia, this is one of the most enduring of food seasonings. Also at this time, cha, an evil-smelling fish pickle, was in use in southern China, usually made with the ganoid, a fish peculiar to China and believed to have the power to transform itself into a dragon.

PREPARATION AND USE In these countries, fish sauce is indispensable in salad dressings and dips and as a condiment. It replaces the soya sauce used in China and Japan, in adding a salty, pungent flavour to many dishes.

BUYING AND STORAGE It is now readily available in Asian food stores, but can be replaced if necessary by light or tamari soya sauce, which provides the saltiness, without the characteristic fishiness.

Fish sauce can be kept in its bottle on a cool dark pantry shelf for several months. In hot climates it should be well sealed and kept in the refrigerator.

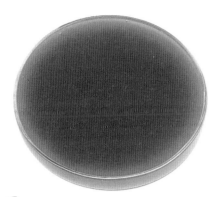

Gravy

MAJOR NUTRIENTS			PACKET SERVE SIZE 20 G
Energy	30 kJ	Carbohydrate	1 g
Protein	0.24 g	Cholesterol	1 mg
Fat	0.14 g	Sodium	110 mg

NUTRITIONAL INFORMATION Gravy, dehydrated, then reconstituted with water, is mostly composed of carbohydrates with a moderate amount of sodium.

Other nutrients are present, but not in nutritionally significant amounts. Gravy made from meat or poultry dripping, juices and flour is considerably higher in fat (saturated). This fat content can be reduced by cooling the juices and skimming excess fat from the top. Extra nutrients can be added to the gravy by using cooking water from vegetables.

Salt-reduced varieties are also available. The sodium may be reduced by as much as a half.

DESCRIPTION Meat juices from the pan, mixed with flour, are the basic ingredients of gravy. The flour is browned in the pan with some fat forming a roux, juices added and thickened with heat. It is a coarse sauce because the stock is unstrained. Other flavourings such as pepper, herbs, spices and mustard can be added to enhance the gravy. Commercial gravy powders are a combination of thickening agents, colourings and flavourings, some artificial and some natural.

ORIGIN AND HISTORY The word gravy is English, but is derived from the French word grane. It is thought that a recipe for grane was wrongly transcribed from French to English, the letter 'n' being replaced with the letter 'v'. This can be verified from identical recipes from the 14th century called grane, grave and gravy. Gravy is almost unknown in France these days but is very popular in England and many of its former colonies.

BUYING AND STORAGE Gravy mixes are purchased from supermarkets. They are packed in either boxes or tins, and should be kept airtight. They keep indefinitely if stored correctly. Freshly made gravy should be served immediately and not stored.

PREPARATION AND USE Powdered gravy mixes usually call for the addition of water, however they can be enhanced by the addition of the water left after cooking vegetables or the pan juices. Add cranberry sauce if serving with turkey. Add mustards, herbs or fruits such as apricots or peaches for a different sauce.

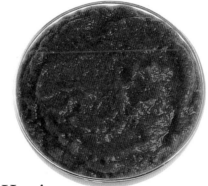

Harissa

NUTRITIONAL INFORMATION No significant nutritional contribution to the diet.

Contains significant amounts of naturally occurring salicylates.

ORIGIN AND HISTORY A fiery sauce or paste made of dried red chillies, garlic, olive oil and occasionally caraway seeds, harissa is the national spice of Tunisia and also appears in both Algerian and Libyan cuisines. In Morocco, harissa is simply red pepper, salt and oil with no caraway seeds. Sambal oelek, an Indonesian condiment, makes an excellent substitute. A similar sauce or paste, hilba, is made from fenugreek, coriander, garlic, pepper and salt, lemon juice and hot chillies.

BUYING AND STORAGE Available in small tins from Continental, Indian and Middle Eastern stores. Store for up to 2 months in the refrigerator. To prevent the sauce from drying out, cover the exposed surface with oil every time you spoon some out of the jar.

PREPARATION AND USE Mixed with lemon, cumin and fresh coriander and some of the broth left from cooking the lamb used to accompany couscous, harissa adds a touch of fire to that traditional dish. Couscous may also be served with a sauce prepared from garlic, chilli peppers and harissa and a little broth from the meat and vegetable mixture.

Thinned with lemon juice and olive oil, harissa is served as a table condiment, or as a dressing for salads.

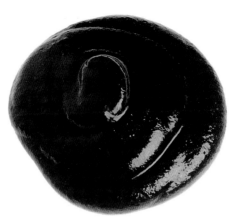

Hoisin Sauce

MAJOR NUTRIENTS			SERVE SIZE 5 G
Energy	15 kJ	Carbohydrate	
Protein	less than 1 g		less than 1 g
Fat	0	Sodium	200 mg
Cholesterol	0	Potassium	15 mg

NUTRITIONAL INFORMATION No significant nutritional contribution to the diet. Contains significant levels of sodium, naturally occurring monosodium glutamate and amines.

DESCRIPTION A thick, sweet-tasting, red-brown Chinese sauce.

ORIGIN AND HISTORY Devised by cooks in southern China to enhance the traditional banquet dish of roast suckling pig with its crisp bubbly crackling, requiring a rich, slightly sweet sauce to add a counterpoint to the sweet moist meat. Hoisin sauce combines fermented soya beans, ground to a paste, with wheat flour, salt, sugar, garlic and red rice. Red rice gives the sauce its characteristic red colour, which transfers to meat when used as a glaze when grilling.

BUYING AND STORAGE Sold in small jars and bottles, and also in cans. Unopened it can be kept indefinitely. Once opened, store in the refrigerator for up to six months.

PREPARATION AND USE Used in Chinese cooking as a dip for grilled and roasted foods. It is thinned and served as the traditional accompaniment to Peking roast duck, and used as a sweet, richly flavoured seasoning in braised dishes. It can be added to stir-fried dishes, in moderation, as its taste is slightly oversweet and cloying if used to excess. Chinese barbecue sauce can be substituted.

PROCESSING Flavour varies marginally in different brands. The basic combination of ingredients may also sometimes include chilli, star anise and Chinese peppercorns.

or fish; caper-flavoured with chicken, fish and eggs; mustard-flavoured with grilled fish or chicken. Flavoured with fresh herbs such as parsley, mint, basil or chives it complements grilled meat or chicken.

Hollandaise Sauce

MAJOR NUTRIENTS			PACKET SERVE SIZE 45 G
Energy	170 kJ	Carbohydrate	2 g
Protein	1 g	Cholesterol	9 mg
Fat	3 g	Sodium	270 mg

NUTRITIONAL INFORMATION Hollandaise sauce is high in fat and moderately high in sodium. Other nutrients are present but not in nutritionally significant amounts.

The fat in hollandaise sauce is high in saturated fatty acids, 62.9%; 32.2% mono-unsaturated; and 5% polyunsaturated fatty acids. The saturated fatty acids would mainly be contributed by butterfat.

DESCRIPTION Traditionally hollandaise sauce is made with butter, eggs, lemon juice or vinegar. It is known as an emulsion — a suspension of one liquid in another with which it would not mix normally — in this case oil in water. The egg yolks (for a serving for 4, approximately 5 egg yolks are used) are high in saturated fats, which aid in the emulsification. The vinegar helps prevent protein coagulation. It is a creamy, dense sauce.

ORIGIN AND HISTORY The gastronome Pierre François de la Varenne gives a recipe for what he called Fragrant Sauce in his book *Le Cuisinier François* published in 1651. It is very similar to a sauce developed and refined by the Huguenots when they were exiled to Holland in the 17th century.

BUYING AND STORAGE Hollandaise sauce is purchased in vacuum sealed packets. They keep indefinitely if stored in a cool dry cupboard. The ingredients vary with each manufacturer but generally the ingredients are potato starch, wheat flour or starch, lactose or milk powder, powdered eggs, lemon juice. Freshly made hollandaise contains eggs, butter and flavourings such as bay leaves and peppercorns.

PREPARATION AND USE Traditionally used as a sauce with asparagus. Lemon-flavoured hollandaise is served with chicken

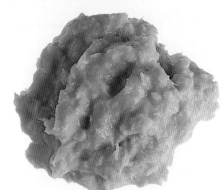

Horseradish Sauce

MAJOR NUTRIENTS			SERVE SIZE 25 G
Energy	60 kJ	Cholesterol	0
Protein	1 g	Sodium	2 g
Fat	0	Vitamin C	30 mg
Carbohydrate	3 g	Iron	0.5 mg

NUTRITIONAL INFORMATION Horseradish sauce is mostly composed of carbohydrates. It is an excellent source of vitamin C; a moderate source of iron.

DESCRIPTION Horseradish is native to southern Europe and western Asia. The outside of the taproot is grated, and the core discarded. Commercial horseradish can be a blend of horseradish root, oil, powdered milk, agar agar, vinegar, sugar and preservatives. Sulphur dioxide is used as an antioxidant.

ORIGIN AND HISTORY Horseradish is cultivated in northern Europe, North America and Australia. It is not well known around the Mediterranean, although some authorities claim it was used by the Greeks around 1000 BC. It was used in England before the Romans arrived. The Germans were known to use it and sauces containing horseradish have their origins in Germany.

BUYING AND STORAGE Processed horseradish cream and relish have lost their volatile oils which act as a preservative, therefore other preservatives must be added.

Store in cupboard or pantry and refrigerate after opening.

PREPARATION AND USE Freshly grated horseradish is exceedingly pungent. If it is cooked or heated the volatile essential oils are driven off. The pungency is reduced by adding cream, milk or lemon juice. In Scandinavian countries horseradish and cream

is popular. Recipes using horseradish usually contain vinegar or lemon juice. Eggs, white sauces and gravy are enhanced by the addition of horseradish. The relish or cream enhances fish, particularly trout and smoked fish. Use with white sauce or corned beef. Horseradish is a favourite condiment with roast beef.

SEE ALSO Horseradish (Herbs and Spices).

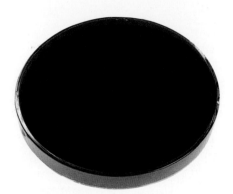

Kecap Manis

also called Bentong; Ketjap; Kecapmanis

MAJOR NUTRIENTS			SERVE SIZE LESS THAN 5 G
Energy	16 kJ	Cholesterol	0
Protein	less than 1 g	Sodium	250 mg
Fat	0	Potassium	15 mg
Carbohydrate	less than 1 g		

NUTRITIONAL INFORMATION A flavouring which contributes significant levels of sodium.

Contains significant amounts of naturally occurring monosodium glutamate and amines.

DESCRIPTION A thick, sweet type of soya sauce made in Indonesia for use as a dip, particularly with satay and grilled or roasted meats. It adds a rich flavour and sweetness to sauces, often in combination with coconut milk.

ORIGIN AND HISTORY Chinese settled in Indonesia well over a thousand years ago, bringing with them tea and many of their favourite ingredients and culinary traditions. Amongst them was soya sauce, which found limited acceptance with the Indonesians. However, they experimented with a similar process of fermentation of soya beans, and with the addition of the thick local palm sugar, produced a strong sweet sauce which they found blended with the spiciness of their cooking, and with the coconut milk which was used abundantly.

BUYING AND STORAGE Readily available in Asian food stores, it is sold in glass and plastic bottles. It can be kept indefinitely in the refrigerator or for many months in a cool cupboard.

PREPARATION AND USE In Indonesia, kecap manis is used as a table condiment and as a marinade for grilled food.

A thick soya sauce can be sweetened lightly with sugar to use as a substitute.

VARIETIES

Kecap Asin Another form of Indonesian soya sauce, this being saltier and more like Chinese dark soya sauce in taste. Used for flavouring and colouring Indonesian dishes.

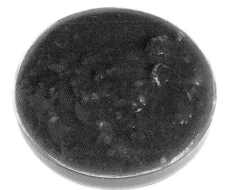

Marinara

NUTRITIONAL INFORMATION Nutrients will depend upon the ingredients used in each case.

DESCRIPTION Marinara is a mixture of seafood sometimes classed as a sauce, used with pasta. Tomatoes, basil, parsley, garlic and onions are the vegetables, the seafood traditionally being mussels, oysters, clams and fish pieces.

ORIGIN AND HISTORY Marinara sauce originated in southern Italy because of the abundant seafood along the coast, particularly oysters and mussels which are cultivated on long hemp ropes suspended from racks floating in the water.

BUYING AND STORAGE This sauce should be stored under refrigeration and used within 2 days of opening if seafood is included in the tomato base.

PREPARATION AND USE If the sauce is thick, serve with pasta. The thin sauce or soup is served with fresh crusty bread, and is usually a meal in itself.

Melba Sauce

NUTRITIONAL INFORMATION No reliable data. See Raspberry in the Fruits chapter.

DESCRIPTION Raspberries belong to the rose family, Rosaceae. Commercially made Melba sauce is made from raspberries, sugar and a thickener with a base such as currant jelly or starch. Sometimes the seeds are sieved from the sauce.

ORIGIN AND HISTORY The first documented reference to raspberries is in 1548 by Turner, the English herbalist. They are not mentioned by Greeks or Romans at all. Raspberry sauce is traditionally made from pureed raspberries with sugar added and is used in Peach Melba, where the fresh peach is poached in a vanilla syrup and served on vanilla ice cream with the raspberry sauce poured over. This combination of peach, ice cream and raspberry sauce is named after Dame Nellie Melba and was developed by the French chef Escoffier (1847–1935). Although raspberry sauce has been known for many years, the bottled raspberry sauce has been named Melba sauce by the manufacturers only relatively recently.

PREPARATION AND USE If the sauce is made from fresh berries the seeds should not be sieved with a metal strainer otherwise the acid in the fruit will react with the metal and discolour it. Use as the traditional sauce in Peach Melba, or pour over ice cream as a simple dessert. Pour over chocolate cake or chocolate ice cream, or over poached pears.

SEE ALSO Peach, Raspberry.

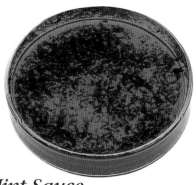

Mint Sauce

MAJOR NUTRIENTS		SERVE SIZE 30 G	
Energy	117 kJ	Carbohydrate	7 g
Protein	0	Cholesterol	0
Fat	0	Sodium	0

NUTRITIONAL INFORMATION Mint sauce is mostly composed of carbohydrate, this being in the form of sucrose. Mint jelly, which is more concentrated, is also high in carbohydrate. Other nutrients are present but not in nutritionally significant amounts.

DESCRIPTION There are several varieties of mint, spearmint being the most commonly used in mint sauce and jelly. The sauce is made from vinegar, mint and sugar, while mint jelly was originally made from a base of apple jelly with chopped mint added.

ORIGIN AND HISTORY Mint was used by the ancient Assyrians. The Greeks also used it and named a mythical character after it, Minthe. Mint sauce is of Roman origin and was introduced into England with the Roman invasion. It is used frequently by the English as an accompaniment to roast lamb.

Horsemint is a variety of mint which is common throughout the Middle East and was one of the bitter herbs with which the Paschal lamb from the Scriptures was eaten. It is commonly thought that this association with mint and lamb ultimately led to the common use of this combination.

BUYING AND STORAGE Store mint sauce in the cupboard or pantry. The vinegar preserves the mint, therefore refrigeration is not required. Mint jelly should be stored in the refrigerator after opening. Commercially made mint jelly uses sugar as a flavouring and preservative, and a starch or gelatine thickened base as the jelly.

PREPARATION AND USE To make mint jelly simply add chopped mint to apple jelly; or dissolve gelatine in hot water, add vinegar, chopped mint and sugar to taste. Mint jelly is more popular in USA and Canada than mint sauce, which is popular in England. To make a mint sauce, chop the mint leaves finely and

391

add to a mixture of vinegar and sugar. Leave for 2 hours or more before use. Mint is a traditional accompaniment to roast lamb or mutton.

SEE ALSO   Mint.

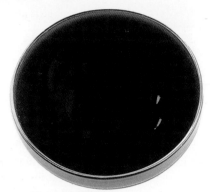

Oyster Sauce

also called Ho yo jeung

MAJOR NUTRIENTS   SERVE SIZE 25 G

Energy	85 kJ	Carbohydrate	4 g
Protein	1 g	Cholesterol	0
Fat	0	Sodium	1040 mg

NUTRITIONAL INFORMATION This sauce is composed of carbohydrate and protein and is an excellent source of vitamin B12. It is high in sodium. Other nutrients are present but not in nutritionally significant amounts. There are no data on sugar, starch, fibre and other vitamins.

DESCRIPTION A thick, dark brown Chinese sauce with a rich, meaty aroma. Processed from dried oysters, it has a slight saltiness and an intense flavour, something of a mixture of seafood and caramel.

ORIGIN AND HISTORY Oyster sauce, like its fellow Chinese flavouring soya sauce, began as a simple salty suspension of the fermented ingredient in brine. It is hardly appetising in appearance, though like all processed seafood seasonings, it has a surprising capacity for enhancing the natural flavours of food. Additions of caramel and a thickener of cornflour made a more palatable sauce from the original formula. Made in south coastal China, it quickly became a popular trade item. The pungent salty sauce brought a rare taste of the sea, plus useful minerals and iodine, to the diet of the inland Chinese.

BUYING AND STORAGE Sold in bottles and cans. Unopened it will keep indefinitely, but once opened it should be kept in the refrigerator. Transfer canned sauce to a glass jar. Avoid inexpensive brands as they invariably are of inferior quality, having a high content of food caramel colouring and often a rather metallic taste.

PREPARATION AND USE Add to braised dishes and stir fries to intensify the flavour. It is popular as a dressing on plain steamed Chinese vegetables, and will help to thicken other sauces.

PROCESSING Brine-fermented oysters are ground to a paste, thickened with cornflour and flavoured with caramel.

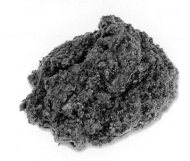

Pesto

NUTRITIONAL INFORMATION No reliable data available.

DESCRIPTION This sauce is made with fresh basil leaves, virgin olive oil, pine nuts or skinned walnuts, garlic, and parmesan or romano cheese.

ORIGIN AND HISTORY Mortar and pestle are used to crush the ingredients of pesto, from which the sauce derives its name. One of the famous sauces of the world, it originates from the region of Liguria, near Genoa in the north-west of Italy. The Genoese are proud of Genoa's history and the foods which the area produces: vegetables, basil and abundant seafoods. Genoa is a seaport and in ancient times the seamen always knew when they were nearing the city by the smell of the basil and other herbs growing on the hillsides. The Genoese traded with other countries bordering on the Mediterranean, and it is said that traders knew when the Genoese ships were arriving in port by the smell of garlic and basil on board.

BUYING AND STORAGE Pesto can be purchased in jars from specialty stores, but fresh pesto is easy to make, and tastes far better. The sauce is made by grinding in a mortar and pestle or food processor the garlic, basil, pine nuts or walnuts, and oil. The mixture can be frozen at this stage, and parmesan or romano cheese added when the required amount of basil mixture has been defrosted.

PREPARATION AND USE Serve with pasta: agnolotti, tagliatelle, spaghetti. Sometimes the sauce is a little thick, so thin with some cooking water from the pasta.

SEE ALSO   Basil, Garlic, Parmesan.

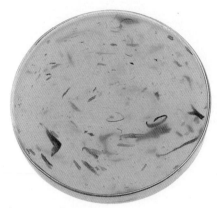

Plum Sauce

NUTRITIONAL INFORMATION No reliable analysis is available. It usually has a high sodium and sugar content.

DESCRIPTION A tart, sweet, thick, Chinese fruit sauce, with a flavour of pickled plums. In appearance it is a light red, semi-transparent, viscous sauce with suspended pieces of chopped, unpeeled plum.

ORIGIN AND HISTORY Fermented soya beans, plums and salt are the oldest form of food flavourings used in China. The ancient native plum (*Prunus mume*) is in fact what is now commonly known as the 'Japanese' apricot, used to make umeboshi, the tart Japanese pickled 'plum', which accompanies most Japanese meals. Although vinegar has been used as a seasoning in China since antiquity, it was this sour plum that gave the tartness to the original Chinese version of sweet and sour. For many centuries, salted, dried 'plums' were one of the few sweets enjoyed in China. The salt-sour taste stimulated the salivary glands and produced a sweet taste in the mouth. They are still enjoyed today.

BUYING AND STORAGE Plum sauce is sold in glass jars. It will keep indefinitely before opening, and once uncapped is best kept in the refrigerator. A piece of plastic wrap or a thin film of vegetable oil over the surface will help prevent the sauce oxidising.

PREPARATION AND USE Its most internationally known use is as a dipping sauce with Peking duck, but plum sauce can also be added sparingly to stir fries, and served as a dip with any kind of crisply fried or grilled food.

PROCESSING Plums are boiled with sugar and seasonings to a thick consistency.

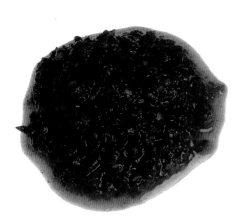

Sambal Ulek

*also called **Indonesian chilli sauce***

MAJOR NUTRIENTS		SERVE SIZE 10 G	
Energy	10 kJ	Carbohydrate	0
Protein	0	Vitamin A	100 μg
Fat	0	Vitamin C	3 mg

NUTRITIONAL INFORMATION A good source of vitamin A and a moderate source of vitamin C. No nutritional data available for minerals. Use sparingly, as it is often highly salted.

DESCRIPTION A potent, red chilli seasoning sauce used in Indonesian cooking. It combines mashed red chillies and salt in a vinegar base.

ORIGIN AND HISTORY There is dissension amongst historians as to the actual time and route by which chillies came to South-East Asia. Some hold the opinion that they came by way of Spain and Portugal, transported with those countries' navigators. Others consider that they were brought by pre-Columbians from the Americas. Whichever, it is hard not to regard the chilli as native to Indonesia, so vital is it to their cuisine. Sambal ulek is the most basic of the Indonesian 'sambals', which are the seasoning mixtures used to make Indonesian food 'pedas' (spicy hot).

BUYING AND STORAGE Sold in small glass jars, it will keep for many months in the refrigerator.

PREPARATION AND USE Used as a seasoning and as a condiment and dip for its clean, sharp chilli taste. It is often used in the rempah, the seasoning mix which forms the base of a curry sauce.

PROCESSING Ripe fresh red chillies are ground with a ulekan (stone pestle) in a mortar to a thick paste which retains some fragments of uncrushed chilli. It is salted generously and bottled.

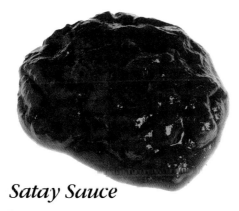

Satay Sauce

NUTRITIONAL INFORMATION No reliable data available. See Peanut.

DESCRIPTION Consists of ground roasted peanuts, soya sauce, ginger, garlic, lime or lemon juice, and spices such as coriander seed, cumin, chilli.

ORIGIN AND HISTORY The peanut was introduced into the Philippines from South America by the Spanish. It is an important source of protein and oil, therefore if it is used with vegetables (gado gado), it is almost a balanced meal nutritionally. Satay sauce is used to marinate pieces of meat such as chicken, pork or beef, which are cooked on a barbecue or under the griller on bamboo satay sticks. The remaining sauce is poured over the cooked satay. It can also be used as a dipping sauce.

BUYING AND STORAGE Can be purchased in jars, which should be refrigerated after opening. The satay should keep for at least a week because of the acid in the lemon or lime juice and the salt from the soya sauce. The meat can be marinated in the sauce for 24 hours if it is cubed (less time for mince meat).

PREPARATION AND USE This sauce can be made at home easily using peanut butter and other ingredients which are not difficult to buy. Use with beef, chicken and lamb on a skewer, or to make gado gado using fresh vegetables such as bean shoots, cabbage, onion, grated carrot etc. Rice noodles can be added for a different texture and flavour.

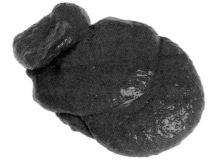

Shrimp Sauce

NUTRITIONAL INFORMATION No analysis is available. Nutritionally insignificant because it is used in small amounts, but use sparingly because of high sodium content.

DESCRIPTION A thick, creamy textured, grey-pink sauce with a strong, salty, seafood flavour.

ORIGIN AND HISTORY You always know when you are near a shrimp sauce factory, because the strong dead-fish odour is all-pervading. T'ang dynasty Chinese pharmacologists did not approve of the practice of fermenting shrimp, believing the sauce to contain a poison. This thought may have been inspired partially by the deadly smell, and partially by the danger of diseases being transferred from the faeces used to fertilise irrigation ditches in which shrimp were caught.

BUYING AND STORAGE Sold in small jars. It will keep for many months after opening, in the refrigerator. Cover the surface with a thin film of vegetable oil to prevent oxidation.

PREPARATION AND USE Particularly tasty as a flavouring for vegetables such as stir-fried spinach, and may be added sparingly to soups and braised dishes.

PROCESSING Made by salting and pulverising unpeeled baby shrimps and fermenting in large tubs.

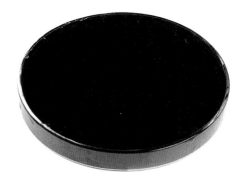

Soya Sauce

MAJOR NUTRIENTS		SOYA WHEAT SERVE SIZE 20 G	
Energy	60 kJ	Cholesterol	0
Protein	0	Sodium	1086 mg
Fat	0	Iron	0
Carbohydrate	4 g	Phosphorus	0

NUTRITIONAL INFORMATION Soya sauce is mostly composed of carbohydrate and is very high in sodium. Soya sauce made from hydrolysed vegetable protein is a good source of iron and a moderate source of phosphorus, and contains 100 kJ and more than twice the sodium of the above.

Soya sauces are close to 75% water.

There is no reliable nutritional information on the low sodium variety.

DESCRIPTION A dark, thin sauce made from

fermented soya beans. Varied processing techniques produce soya sauces with markedly different flavours. Some are thick, very dark and salty, others are light brown, thin and only mildly salty. Synthetic soya sauces are now produced using artificial soya flavour.

Japanese soya sauce goes under the name shoyu. It is generally less salty and lighter in colour and viscosity than the Chinese types. Usu-kuchi shoyu is the lightest and is amber-coloured, clean and salty tasting. Koi-kuchi shoyu is darker, has more body and is less salty. It is used in dishes where colour, rather than salty flavour, is required.

Another type of Japanese soya sauce, which is generally marketed through health food stores, is tamari. It is thick and dark with a strong flavour and is generally used as a dip or condiment. Low salt soya sauces are now available under various labels.

Chinese soya sauce also comes in light and dark types. Again the dark is thicker, more viscous and less salty, while the lighter one, which is of a mid-brown colour, is thin and salty. A well-flavoured, dark Chinese soya sauce known as mushroom soy, has excellent flavour and produces a rich brown colour.

ORIGIN AND HISTORY Soya sauce has been around almost as long as Chinese food itself. It was certainly in use in the Chou era, from the 12th century BC to 221 BC, although then it was known as shih, and was a kind of salted fermented soya bean seasoning, like a liquid bean sauce. Even then it was considered one of the necessities of life, and was well documented. In the 6th century T'ang dynasty, pickling and sauce making had been refined, and by then shih was being strained to make a sauce little changed in technique, though slightly more refined, from the one we use today. The Japanese learned soya sauce making skills from the Chinese about four centuries later, and added their own refinements, including more grain and sweeteners. Indonesians added palm sugar and thickeners to soya sauce to make their kecap manis.

BUYING AND STORAGE It is false economy to choose an inexpensive or synthetic brand of soya sauce as they are generally inferior in taste, too dark in colour and impart a metallic taste. Soya sauce is sold in bottles with a shaker top and can be kept indefinitely in dry conditions. In humid climates, store in the refrigerator.

PREPARATION AND USE Use as a marinade, as a seasoning partially replacing salt in a dish, and to add a rich flavour and colour to braised and steamed dishes. Sprinkle lightly over cooked foods for flavour enhancement, and add a dash to rice or soups.

PROCESSING Produced by a natural fermentation of roasted soya bean meal and a meal of another grain, usually wheat, with *Aspergillus* mould. After fermentation begins brine is added with a *Lactobacillus* starter and yeast. The mash is aged for up to two years, then filtered and bottled. Dark soy is tinted and flavoured with molasses.

Tabasco Sauce

DESCRIPTION A thin, red, pungent sauce made from *Capsicum annuum* and *Capsicum frutescens*, chillies from the Tabasco region in Mexico. It also contains spirit vinegar and salt. The chillies are harvested by hand, ground to a pulp and packed into oak barrels with salt. This is left to stand for four years. The seed and pulp is strained and mixed with vinegar. The resulting sauce is bottled in its distinctive bottle and sold all over the world.

ORIGIN AND HISTORY The sauce was first made by Mr Edmund McIlhenny in Louisiana, USA, in 1868. The chillies were given to him by a soldier returning from the Mexican–American campaign. It is still a family recipe.

BUYING AND STORAGE Purchase from supermarkets and delicatessens. It keeps indefinitely because of the alkaloid capsaicin which is a preservative (it also gives the peppers their fiery taste).

PREPARATION AND USE There is only one Tabasco sauce; similar concoctions are said to be inferior in taste. 1–3 drops should be used to enhance meat dishes and casseroles. Essential in Creole cuisine. Lobster and crab dishes are also enhanced with Tabasco.

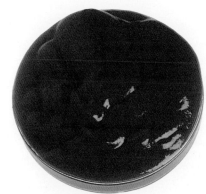

Tomato Sauce

MAJOR NUTRIENTS		COMMERCIAL AND HOME-STYLE SERVE SIZE 25 G	
Energy	105 kJ	Carbohydrate	6 g
Protein	0	Cholesterol	0
Fat	0	Sodium	280 mg

NUTRITIONAL INFORMATION Tomato sauce is largely composed of carbohydrates. The commercial variety is high in sodium. Other nutrients are present but not in nutritionally significant amounts.

The carbohydrate in commercial-style sauce is largely sugar, while there are close to equal amounts of sugar and starch in homemade sauce, which also contains much less sodium (82 mg). There is no reliable nutritional information available for low joule and low sodium sauces.

DESCRIPTION English standards for bottled tomato sauce are that the sauce should contain no less than 6% by weight of tomato solids, but a good tomato sauce should contain twice that minimum. The seeds and tomato solids are strained from that original percentage of 6%. The spices and flavourings should be only garlic, onion, cloves, pepper and paprika. Sugar is often added, 25% being the maximum. Water is added, and up to 12% vinegar. Stabilisers such as gum tragacanth or modified starch are also present.

ORIGIN AND HISTORY The bottled tomato sauce we know today is a reasonably modern condiment. The tomato was brought to Europe in 1523 from Mexico; however, the refined sauce may not have been made commercially until the 19th century because until the 1800s the tomato was considered in some countries to be poisonous.

BUYING AND STORAGE Purchase in supermarkets. The sauce will keep in a cupboard for up to 2 years, although it may discolour to a grey-brown around the top of the neck of the bottle. This is not harmful.

PREPARATION AND USE This sauce is not generally prepared at home; however, versions of it are made. The sauce is generally used as a condiment with meats such as barbecued or grilled beef. Add a tablespoon to a vinaigrette dressing for a change.

VARIETIES

Salsa di Pomodori   Tomato sauce made with peeled tomatoes, basil, onions, salt and pepper. Originating in southern Italy, it is a base sauce to which other ingredients can be added. Use on pizzas and pasta.

Velouté

NUTRITIONAL INFORMATION   No reliable nutritional information available.

DESCRIPTION   This sauce is made from the stock of unbrowned meat, vegetables and bones. The stock is reduced, then strained. It is then blended with a blond roux. (A roux is a mixture of flour and fat cooked over a low heat. A blond roux is unbrowned and is used for making white sauces. A brown roux is browned flour and fat, used for brown sauces.)

ORIGIN AND HISTORY   Sauces evolved slowly until the 1650s. They had been liable to overpower the foods with their flavourings. A sauce recipe dated 1390 uses ginger, cloves, nuts, vinegar, currants and breadcrusts. The breadcrusts were used as the thickening agent. In 1651 when Catherine de Medici married Henri II in Paris she brought with her her Venetian chefs. They used flour as a thickening agent instead of almonds and bread. The subtle flavours of the French sauces we know today had arrived.

BUYING AND STORAGE   Packet sauces are a combination of spices, herbs and thickening agents. They keep indefinitely if stored in a dry place. Frozen sauces can be kept frozen for up to one year. Freshly made white sauce should be consumed when still hot and not stored.

PREPARATION AND USE   Use white sauces over unbrowned meats such as corned beef, vegetables, fish, pasta.

White Sauce

MAJOR NUTRIENTS			SERVE SIZE 45 G
Energy	285 kJ	Cholesterol	4 g
Protein	2 g	Sodium	184 mg
Fat	5 g	Calcium	58 mg
Carbohydrate	5 g		

NUTRITIONAL INFORMATION   White sauce is largely composed of carbohydrates and fat. Savoury white sauce is moderately high in sodium and a moderate source of calcium. Other nutrients are present but not in nutritionally significant amounts. The fat is 44% saturated, 33% polyunsaturated and 22% monounsaturated.

DESCRIPTION   This is a basic sauce made in the home with butter and flour (a roux), cooked briefly over a low heat, to which heated milk is added, and finally seasonings such as salt, pepper and a little nutmeg.

ORIGIN AND HISTORY   White sauce is really a quick version of bechamel, which requires the preparation of a meat stock beforehand. Like many such sauces, it probably originated in France.

BUYING AND STORAGE   Considering its ease of preparation, white sauce is best made at home, and eaten as soon as it is ready — if left to stand the milk content will form a skin.

PREPARATION AND USE   The milk should be added carefully to the roux to avoid lumps, and the mixture simmered gently for at least ten minutes to ensure smoothness and elimination of a floury taste. Cheese and mornay sauces can be prepared from this basis. White sauce is especially popular with vegetables such as cauliflower, and is an ingredient in the preparation of such dishes as lasagne and a favourite of Australian and New Zealand children — macaroni cheese.

SEE ALSO   Bechamel Sauce.

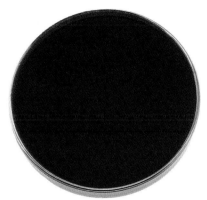

Worcestershire Sauce

MAJOR NUTRIENTS			SERVE SIZE 20 G
Energy	76 kJ	Cholesterol	0
Protein	0	Sodium	176 mg
Fat	0	Iron	0.5 mg
Carbohydrate	4 g		

NUTRITIONAL INFORMATION   Worcestershire sauce is mostly composed of carbohydrate. It is moderately high in sodium and a moderate source of iron. Other nutrients are present but not in nutritionally significant amounts.

Worcestershire sauce is 64% water, the carbohydrates being mostly sugars.

DESCRIPTION   Worcestershire sauce is a thin, black-brown sauce. The ingredients are a secret, but it is thought to contain anchovy sauce, soya sauce, molasses, chilli, ginger, shallots and garlic with over 20 tropical fruits. It is not a cooked sauce: the ingredients are marinated and blended.

ORIGIN AND HISTORY   The basis of Worcestershire sauce had its beginnings in the Roman Empire — a fish sauce, which they produced by fermenting fish liquid in wood barrels. This type of sauce is still made in South-East Asia and India in a similar way.

Worcestershire sauce was first made in Worcester, England, by accident. During Victorian times, sauces were made for individuals to personal recipes. In 1837 a retired governor, who had spent time in Bengal, India, ordered a barrel to be made up for him by one of a chain of chemists called Lea and Perrins. The sauce was not what he anticipated, and he refused to take it. The barrel was sent downstairs to storage and years later it was rediscovered. It was about to be discarded when the contents were tasted. It had matured well, so after relocating the recipe, Lea and Perrins started manufacturing. Now it is manufactured all over the world to the same recipe, and in Worcester the same Victorian machinery and vats are still used.

BUYING AND STORAGE   Purchase from

supermarkets anywhere in the world. Different makes and varieties are now available, such as relish with fruit, no anchovies etc. Keeps indefinitely.

PREPARATION AND USE Some people say there is only one Worcestershire sauce — Lea and Perrins. Other brands have a stronger molasses flavour or vinegar taste. Use on shellfish, fish, poultry and game, on grilled meats such as beef, and in stocks and soups. Mayonnaise, aspics and salad dressings all benefit from Worcestershire sauce. It is an essential ingredient in the drink Bloody Mary. Always use in moderation.

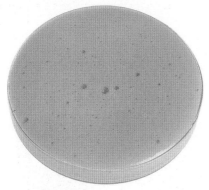

Zabaglione

*also called **Zabaione***

NUTRITIONAL INFORMATION No reliable data available.

DESCRIPTION This sauce belongs to the family of emulsified sauces, some of the others being mayonnaise and hollandaise. The ingredients are whole eggs, egg yolk, sugar and marsala. The Spanish version of this dessert sauce replaces the marsala with sherry.

ORIGIN AND HISTORY Marsala originated in Sicily, going into commercial production in 1773 under the leadership of Englishman John Woodhouse, and it is thought zabaglione originated in Sicily. The islands of Sardinia and Sicily are where distinctive Italian cuisine originated. This cuisine was imitated by the Romans BC, and exported to France when Catherine de Medici travelled to Paris to marry the future King Henri II in 1533.

BUYING AND STORAGE Zabaglione can be purchased in a jar; however, because this sauce is an unstable emulsion, thickeners and stabilisers have been added. When made fresh, it should be served immediately.

PREPARATION AND USE A very rich sauce; serve hot in a glass bowl or dish.

MUSTARDS

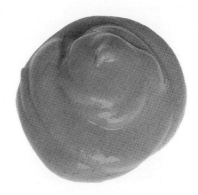

Dijon Mustard

NUTRITIONAL INFORMATION There is no reliable nutritional information available.

DESCRIPTION Dijon mustard is a pale yellow. The taste is sharp and hot, not sweet. It is made by grinding black and brown mustard seeds and using the flour from inside. White wine is used as flavouring and to aid in the preserving.

ORIGIN AND HISTORY Mustard seeds were used by the Romans, who had recipes for mustard as we know it. It is known that the city of Dijon kept the original recipe of Palladius, but it is not known when Dijon began making mustard. In the 13th century, however, Etienne Boileau, the Provost of Paris under Saint Louis, granted the vinegar makers the right to make mustards. Later, as new spices from the East were introduced to France and Europe, mustard took a temporary downward swing in popularity.

In the early 18th century Jean Naigeon, a great-grandson of one of the 23 original mustard/vinegar makers, produced a mustard containing verjuice (the unfermented juice of grapes) which caused a sensation in Paris. During 1742 a vinegar maker called Capitaine began to use white vinegar instead of red vinegar and introduced anchovies as well as capers to his mustards. In 1752 another vinegar maker called Maille introduced 24 new mustards, some of them being tarragon mustard, lemon mustard, mustard with herbs and mustard with truffles. During this time a vinegar/mustard maker called Bordin invented a mustard called 'de santé' (for the health) and 40 other mustards including mustard with champagne, with mushrooms and one with vanilla! A mustardier called Maout produced another mustard which was more pungent than the others and for more than 50

years the mustards of Maout, Bordin and Maille were placed on the table together. A mustardier called Bornibus had a factory in Paris and marketed a mustard for women, explaining that a woman's palate is more sensitive than a man's.

The best known brands of Dijon mustard are Amora, Grey-Poupon founded in 1777, and Bornibus Maille founded in 1747.

BUYING AND STORAGE Purchase from supermarkets and specialty stores. Keep airtight and discard after one year because the mustard loses its pungency.

PREPARATION AND USE Use in sauces for fish and chicken, as an accompaniment to grilled beef, and in mayonnaise and vinaigrette dressing.

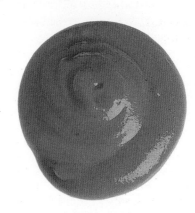

English Mustard

MAJOR NUTRIENTS		PREPARED SERVE SIZE 5 G	
Energy	30 kJ	Carbohydrate	0.28 g
Protein	0.20 g	Cholesterol	0
Fat	0.66 g	Sodium	225 mg

NUTRITIONAL INFORMATION It contains a moderate amount of sodium. Other nutrients are present but not in nutritionally significant amounts. A teaspoon (5 g) of powdered mustard contains several times the protein and fat of the above, but once again the amounts are insignificant in the diet.

MAJOR NUTRIENTS		MUSTARD POWDER SERVE SIZE 5 G	
Energy	94 kJ	Carbohydrate	1 g
Protein	2 g	Cholesterol	0
Fat	2 g	Sodium	0

NUTRITIONAL INFORMATION Mustard powder is mostly composed of fat and carbohydrates. Other nutrients are present but not in nutritionally significant amounts.

DESCRIPTION The traditional English mustard is hot and its colour is a hot yellow. Its texture is fine because the mustard seeds are ground and the husks sifted out, leaving a fine flour. It is made from black, white and brown mustard seeds.

ORIGIN AND HISTORY Mustard was introduced to England by the Romans. In medieval times it was a thick sauce, including seed husks. Tewkesbury was the centre of mustard making in England. In 1720 a woman called Mrs Clements from Lancashire found a way to separate the husk of the mustard from the centre, making a fine-textured mustard. She used to sell her mustard along the roadsides and in villages until George I discovered it and made it popular. Commercial production of mustard began in 1814, when Jeremiah Colman began marketing his powdered mustard, which is the Colman's mustard we have today. It contains wheat flour and turmeric.

BUYING AND STORAGE If the mustard is powdered, simply store in the airtight container and it will keep for up to three years. If it is prepared mustard, store for one year in cupboard or pantry.

PREPARATION AND USE England is one of the few countries where powdered mustard is sold. To prepare, just add enough water to make a paste. Leave for 10–15 minutes for the mustard to achieve its 'hotness'. The essential oils in mustard are activated by water. The enzymes produce the pungency. Add vinegar or other flavourings after this reaction has taken place; otherwise, if an acid is added to the powder, bitter oils are produced which spoil the taste.

Use with roast beef. Add some mustard to apple sauce for roast pork. Use in strong sauces to go with strong-tasting fish such as mullet or mackerel. Add to bechamel sauce for added piquancy.

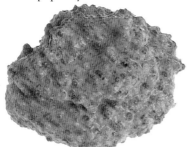

English Wholegrain Mustard

NUTRITIONAL INFORMATION There is no reliable nutritional information available.

DESCRIPTION This mustard is made from whole black and brown mustard seeds mixed with some ground mustard, white wine, allspice and black pepper.

ORIGIN AND HISTORY Wholegrain mustards were the first mustards made in England.

BUYING AND STORAGE Purchase from supermarkets and specialty stores. Keep for up to one year.

PREPARATION AND USE Use with cold meats, sausages and pork pies.

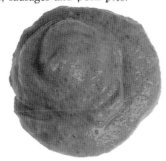

Florida Mustard

NUTRITIONAL INFORMATION No reliable nutritional information available.

DESCRIPTION A mild-tasting mustard, this is dark coloured like the Bordeaux mustard and smooth, made from seed after the husks have been removed, and mixed with wine from the Champagne region of France.

ORIGIN AND HISTORY Florida mustard comes from Champagne and was conceived by Bordin, a mustardier and vinegar maker in Paris during the 1750s who was very popular with the aristocracy of France during that time.

BUYING AND STORAGE Purchase from some supermarkets and specialty stores. Store in cool pantry or cupboard for not more than one year.

PREPARATION AND USE Use in vinaigrette dressing. Sauces are enhanced with pan juices and mustard. If used during cooking, add only at the very end, otherwise the essential oils are driven off in the heat. Use in sauces with chicken or fish, or with meats such as beef.

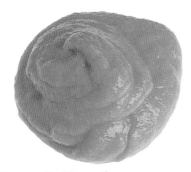

French Bordeaux Mustard

NUTRITIONAL INFORMATION There is no reliable nutritional information available.

DESCRIPTION Darker and more aromatic than the Dijon mustard because it is made from black mustard seed and husks (*Brassica nigra*), this is a sour/sweet mustard, with the addition of red wine vinegar and sugar. Tarragon is the main herb used, along with allspice.

ORIGIN AND HISTORY This mustard derives its name from the region in France where it is manufactured. Even though 80% of mustard is produced in Dijon, this is in fact the mustard known to the British as French mustard, because it is shipped from the port in Bordeaux with the wines from that region.

BUYING AND STORAGE Buy in supermarkets and specialty stores and store in cupboard for up to 12 months.

PREPARATION AND USE Use in vinaigrette dressing, with sausages or cold meats.

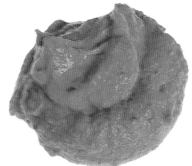

German Mustard

MAJOR NUTRIENTS		SERVE SIZE 5 G	
Energy	20 kJ	Carbohydrate	0.35 g
Protein	0.25 g	Cholesterol	0
Fat	0.28 g	Sodium	75 mg

NUTRITIONAL INFORMATION One teaspoon of German mustard contains nutrients but not in nutritionally significant amounts.

DESCRIPTION German mustard is made of a blended mustard flour and white wine vinegar. It is pungent and aromatic, not as hot as English mustard, but has an aroma like the Bordeaux. It is seasoned with herbs and spices.

ORIGIN AND HISTORY There are three areas which make mustard in Germany: Düsseldorf, Bavaria and Rhineland. Düsseldorf is the 'mustard centre' of Germany.

BUYING AND STORAGE German mustard is purchased ready made. Store in cupboard or pantry for no more than 12 months.

PREPARATION AND USE Best used in great quantities on German sausages like frankfurters; and on cold meats.

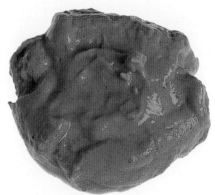

Green Peppercorn Mustard

NUTRITIONAL INFORMATION There is no reliable nutritional information available.

DESCRIPTION Green peppercorn mustard can be made with either coarse or smooth mustard as a base and crushed green peppercorns added as a flavouring.

ORIGIN AND HISTORY This mustard originated in Paris, France. It probably made its first appearance in the 18th century. It is now manufactured in Dijon, where 80% of all mustards are produced.

BUYING AND STORAGE Purchase from some supermarkets and specialty stores. The mustard will not deteriorate, because of the addition of vinegar or wine, but it will lose some of its pungency and flavour over a period of time. Use within one year.

PREPARATION AND USE Use on grilled beef or sausages as an accompaniment. To make, use green peppercorns bottled in brine. Drain thoroughly and crush. Add to the mustard. Taste and add more peppercorns if necessary after 2–3 days.

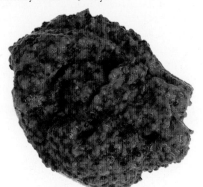

Moutarde de Meaux

NUTRITIONAL INFORMATION No reliable analysis is available.

DESCRIPTION This mustard is coarse-grained, since some of the black mustard seeds are ground and mixed with vinegar and some are left whole. It has a strong, pungent taste. Herbs and spices are added.

ORIGIN AND HISTORY The recipe for the Meaux mustard was given to the Pommeroy family of Champagne by the monks of Meaux, France, in 1790. It comes in stoneware pots, the corks sealed with sealing wax.

BUYING AND STORAGE Purchase from supermarkets and specialty stores.

PREPARATION AND USE Use on cold meats or sausages. Some suggest it is best used on humble foods such as sausages, bacon and pork pies.

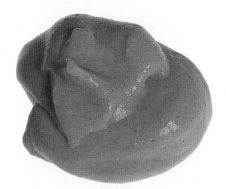

White Wine Mustard

NUTRITIONAL INFORMATION No reliable nutritional information available.

DESCRIPTION This mustard is made with white wine and black or brown mustard seeds, either hulled or whole.

ORIGIN AND HISTORY Originally mustard was made with vinegar, but about 1700 Jean Naigeon, who was a great-grandson of one of the original 23 vinegar/mustard makers of Dijon, France, added wine to his mustard. This was the turning point in the resurgence of mustards in Europe.

BUYING AND STORAGE Buy from supermarkets or specialty stores, in small quantities, and keep for no more than one year.

PREPARATION AND USE The pungency of all mustards comes from an essential oil which forms through enzyme action when ground mustard is mixed with water. Use wine mustard with grilled meats, in sauces for chicken and fish and in sauces for vegetables.

PASTES

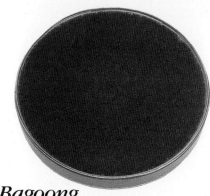

Bagoong

NUTRITIONAL INFORMATION Contains significant levels of natural monosodium glutamate and amines.

DESCRIPTION Fermented salty fish paste, usually yellowish-brown in colour.

ORIGIN AND HISTORY Bagoong is made in the Philippines from small fish or shrimps. After the heads are removed and they are cleaned, the fish or shrimps are often partially sun-dried for 3–4 days. They are then pounded to a paste. One part salt is added to three parts fish or shrimps, after which they are put in earthenware vats to ferment for 1–4 months. The paste may be further pounded and may be coloured with angkak (red colouring agent made from rice). A pickle will appear on the surface of the fermenting mass which may be removed and used as fish sauce. The solid mass left is fish paste or bagoong.

BUYING AND STORAGE The paste is sold in bottles in specialty Asian food stores and will keep for months if tightly capped and stored in a cool place.

PREPARATION AND USE Used as a condiment with rice dishes and with many other meals. Other versions are made in the Philippines, Indonesia, Malaysia, Singapore, Thailand, Burma, Laos, Vietnam, Kampuchea, Korea, Japan and China. Each area has its own type.

SEE ALSO Blachan.

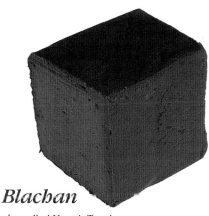

Blachan

also called Ngopi, Trasi

Major Nutrients		Serve Size 5 g	
Energy	30 kJ	Cholesterol	0
Protein	1 g	Sodium	250 mg
Fat	0	Calcium	50 mg
Carbohydrate	0		

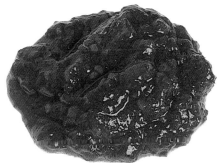

Chinese Hot Bean Paste

also called Hot bean sauce; Chilli bean paste

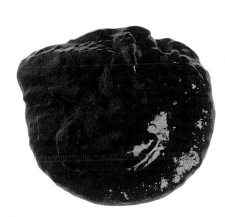

Bean Paste, Sweet

also called Chinese barbecue sauce

Nutritional Information No reliable analysis is available.

Description A thick, red-brown Chinese seasoning paste made from pureed preserved soya beans, salt, sugar and seasonings. Hoisin sauce has a very similar taste and appearance and the two can be interchanged in Chinese recipes.

Origin and History Flavourings made from fermented and salted soya beans have been made in China since antiquity. Documents from 2000 years ago describe honey and sugar as seasonings, along with soya sauce, salt and salted soya beans. The Chinese theory of yin and yang, creating balance and harmony in food — if not in life in general — meant that certain seasoning sauces need to have a sweet flavour, others tart, some salty, some hot.

Buying and Storage Sold in small bottles or cans. Unopened it will keep indefinitely; once opened transfer canned sauce to a glass container and keep refrigerated.

Preparation and Use Useful in marinades and as a seasoning in Chinese stir fries and in braised dishes. It is most commonly used as a condiment with roasted meats, particularly pork and duck.

Processing Salted, fermented soya beans are pureed and flavoured with salt, sugar and seasonings which vary with different brands but may include the Chinese spices cassia and star anise. Binders are added to make the sauce thick and smooth.

See Also Bean Sauce; Hoisin Sauce.

Nutritional Information As this paste is used as a condiment it provides few nutrients except for moderate amounts of calcium. Calcium from such sources is important in Asian-style eating when dairy foods are not available. Contains large amounts of sodium and significant amounts of naturally occurring monosodium glutamate and amines.

Description A pungent shrimp paste, blachan is a seasoning much used in Thailand and is a characteristic condiment of Burmese and Malaysian cuisines. It is made of small shrimps pounded with salt into a thick paste and then dried.

Origin and History An Asian dried prawn paste. Made of small shrimp, which are pounded with salt into a sort of thick brine, the paste is dried in the sun. It may also be made from shrimp, fresh sardines, and other small fish and chillies, which are allowed to ferment in the sun in a heap, then mashed heavily with salt. The smell has been described as 'much relished by lovers of decomposed cheese', but, nonetheless, blachan has been said to stimulate the appetite and fortify the stomach.

Buying and Storage It may be sold in bottles, jars or cans, or as flat slabs or cakes. Blachan in bottles or jars, once opened, must be stored in the refrigerator. The dried flat slabs or cakes will keep for months if tightly capped and stored in a cool, dry place.

Preparation and Use Use sparingly as it can be strong. Add to stir fries, rice, and Asian seafood dishes. ½ teaspoon of dried or 1 teaspoon liquid will usually flavour dishes to serve 4–6 people. The dried type, which must be cooked, should be minced or crumbled and roasted before adding to cooked dishes. Roll the blachan in foil before roasting (under the grill or in the oven) to prevent the smell from going through the house. It may be used in sambals to serve with rice and curries, in soups and in many Thai dishes.

Nutritional Information No nutritional details are available.

Description A pungent Chinese seasoning paste, made of fermented soya beans, salt, garlic and chilli. It may be thick and smooth and a red-brown in colour, or may be lighter coloured with some whole or broken preserved yellow soya beans in the mixture. Some are extremely hot, others of medium strength, but all have a pronounced saltiness.

Origin and History Made in the central western provinces of Szechuan and Hunan after chilli peppers had been introduced by Indian traders who had procured them through the Portuguese.

Garlic was an early introduction from the West and it grew particularly well in central China. It was used extensively in cooking, in sauces and was pickled in a sweet brine. A traveller in the Ming era describes the restaurants of Shantung serving 'a few plates of garlic and steamed bread' with wine.

Buying and Storage Sold in glass jars, which unopened will keep indefinitely. Once opened, protect the surface with a film of vegetable oil to prevent oxidation. If the jar has a metal screwtop, rinse and dry it thoroughly after use as the acids in the sauce can cause it to rust.

Preparation and Use Chilli bean or hot bean sauce gives Chinese dishes characteristic Szechuan piquancy. Use sparingly until the strength of the sauce has been established, as too much can spoil the balance of flavours.

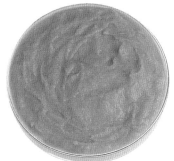

Hommos

also called Chickpea spread, Hummus

MAJOR NUTRIENTS   SERVE SIZE 30 G

Energy	230 kJ	Carbohydrate	3 g
Protein	2 g	Cholesterol	0
Fat	4 g	Sodium	200 mg

NUTRITIONAL INFORMATION Hommos is a high fat food. It is also moderately high in sodium.

DESCRIPTION Chickpeas and tahini are the main ingredients of this dish. Chickpeas are shaped like hazelnuts and are usually a light golden colour, but can be green, gold or black. They are boiled, then ground to a paste for hommos. Tahini, the ground paste of sesame seed, is then added with garlic, lemon juice and olive oil.

ORIGIN AND HISTORY Hommos is a staple food in the south-eastern and southern Mediterranean. It has been made for thousands of years in Lebanon, Syria, Cyprus, Jordan and Morocco, and chickpeas have been cultivated since 5000 BC.

BUYING AND STORAGE Can be purchased freshly made from delicatessens and specialty stores. It is easily made if the chickpeas are canned.

PREPARATION AND USE Hommos is traditionally spread onto a plate and olive oil poured onto the surface. Paprika is sprinkled on and a sprig of coriander added for decoration. It can be eaten as a 'dip' or as an accompaniment to other food, such as chicken.

SEE ALSO Tahini.

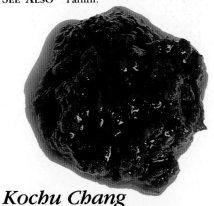

Kochu Chang

MAJOR NUTRIENTS   SERVE SIZE 5 G

Energy	16 kJ	Cholesterol	0
Protein	less than 1 g	Dietary Fibre	0
Fat	0	Sodium	250 mg
Carbohydrate	less than 1 g	Potassium	15 mg

NUTRITIONAL INFORMATION Contains large amounts of naturally occurring sodium.

Contains significant amounts of naturally occurring monosodium glutamate and amines.

ORIGIN AND HISTORY Manufactured in Korea and China, this very hot paste is made from soya beans, glutinous rice, hot peppers, soya sauce, dried beef, jujube and honey.

BUYING AND STORAGE Sometimes available in Asian food stores. Keeps indefinitely in an airtight container in the refrigerator.

PREPARATION AND USE Because of the strong flavour, use moderately in stews, soups and sauces.

PROCESSING Soya beans and red peppers are ground, then the remaining ingredients and salt brine are added. The paste is left to ferment, usually in wooden barrels, for any period from 4 months to 4 years. After the paste has matured, vinegar may be added before bottling.

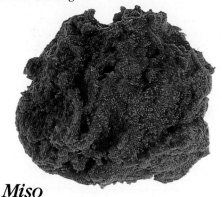

Miso

also called **Soya bean paste**

MAJOR NUTRIENTS   SERVE SIZE 17 G

Energy	120 kJ	Cholesterol	0
Protein	2 g	Sodium	500 mg
Fat	1 g	Phosphorus	50 mg
Carbohydrate	4 g		

NUTRITIONAL INFORMATION The above figures are based on one tablespoon. As a condiment soya bean paste provides mainly a large amount of sodium, some of which will be in the form of monosodium glutamate (MSG). Like all salty condiments its use should be limited.

DESCRIPTION A thick paste made in Japan from fermented and processed soya beans mixed with another grain and injected with a yeast mould. It is rich in protein and has a distinct, appealing nutty aroma and flavour. Variations in the processing method produce a number of different types of miso, which are applied to different uses, for varying effects.

Light or yellow miso is made with rice and is sweeter and a creamy yellow colour; red miso is made with barley and is very savoury; a darker miso is made with a bean known in Japan as koji and is very strong in flavour and colour.

ORIGIN AND HISTORY Miso is a derivative of the ancient Chinese bean sauce shih. Development of this salty fermented sauce took two distinct paths — into soya sauce, and into soya pastes. It is arguably one of Japan's staple foods as every Japanese is said to consume several spoonfuls each day, in one form or another. Miso has been a vital element in the Japanese diet, compensating for a low intake of animal protein. As far back as ten centuries ago there were already several kinds of miso in frequent use.

BUYING AND STORAGE It is sold in plastic packs, tubs and tubes. It should be kept in the refrigerator once opened, and will keep indefinitely if sealed and kept dry.

PREPARATION AND USE Buy miso according to use; light and sweet are good for thin soups and dressings and may be known as white shiro-miso or saikyo-miso; bright strong yellow miso is salty tasting and is used for general cooking and one-pot cooking; it is also known as shinshu-miso. Inaka-miso or sendai-miso is red in colour, good for general cooking and soups. Akadashi miso, hatcho-miso or black miso is very dark and strong. Use in strong flavoured soups.

Once miso is added to a dish, it should not be boiled, but slowly simmered or the miso will not amalgamate.

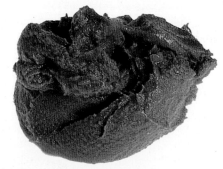

Patum Peperium

also called **Anchovy butter, Gentleman's relish**

MAJOR NUTRIENTS   SERVE SIZE 30 G

Energy	270 kJ	Cholesterol	30 mg
Protein	7 g	Sodium	1 640 mg
Fat	4 g	Calcium	50 mg
Carbohydrate	0	Phosphorus	155 mg

NUTRITIONAL INFORMATION Anchovy paste is composed of protein and fat. It is high in sodium and phosphorus and a moderate source of calcium. The data are based on the fish content only. The fatty acid composition is approximately 20% saturated, 58% mono-unsaturated and 21% polyunsaturated.

DESCRIPTION This paste is a blend of salted anchovies and butter. It is a brown colour, dense and has a strong anchovy taste. Anchovies are fished from the Mediterranean and south coasts of Spain and France and a different variety of anchovy, found off Chile, is also used.

ORIGIN AND HISTORY One of the first recipes using a similar paste was attributed to Apicius, who lived in the 1st century AD. The recipe was written in the 3rd century AD and is a sauce for shellfish: pepper, lovage, parsley, mint, bayleaf, malabuthrum (a Middle Eastern leaf), plenty of cumin, honey, vinegar and liquamen (which is a fish paste like anchovy).

BUYING AND STORAGE Patum peperium is available from specialty stores. It comes in tubes or jars and should be stored in the refrigerator after opening.

PREPARATION AND USE Patum peperium can be made at home by pounding salted anchovies which have had the salt washed off, and combining with butter. It is used as a spread and as an accompaniment to fish as well as beef and mutton. Use with pork pies.

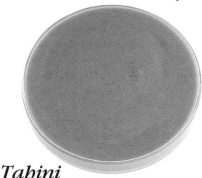

Tahini

also called Chinese sesame paste

MAJOR NUTRIENTS			SERVE SIZE 20 G
Energy	490 kJ	Sodium	15 mg
Protein	4 g	Potassium	125 mg
Fat	10 g	Calcium	280 mg
Cholesterol	0	Phosphorus	105 mg
Carbohydrate	3 g	Iron	0.9 mg
Dietary Fibre		Zinc	1 mg
	less than 1 g	Vitamin E	1 mg

NUTRITIONAL INFORMATION Excellent source of calcium and phosphorus; good source of iron and vitamin E; moderate source of zinc.

Some commercially made products may contain higher levels of fat and sodium.

Although tahini is rich in nutrients, over 70% of the total energy comes from unsaturated fats and it is a high kilojoule food.

DESCRIPTION A greyish oily paste made from toasted, ground sesame seeds. It has a nutty, slightly bitter flavour and smooth texture. Chinese sesame paste is made from sesame seeds which have been toasted to a

greater degree, changing the colour to a fawn shade, with a more defined nutty flavour.

ORIGIN AND HISTORY Sesame seeds are native to tropical Africa and Asia and have been used from ancient times. Chinese sesame paste is also used in Asian cooking. In the Middle East, tahini is used in Lebanon, Syria, Egypt, Cyprus and Turkey for sauces and dips and in cooking. Orthodox Armenians and Greeks use it during periods of fasting when foods from animal sources are not permitted.

Tahini has been popularised in the Western kitchen by those following vegetarian dishes.

BUYING AND STORAGE Purchase from stores carrying Middle Eastern, Greek and Asian foods, and from health food stores. It is usually available in tins or jars, and can be purchased in bulk. If purchased in a tin, transfer to a sterilised jar if the tin does not have a seal. Seal jars tightly after use. Store in a cool place away from direct light and use within 6 months.

PREPARATION AND USE Tahini separates on standing, and requires thorough stirring before removing the amount required. If unopened tins are stored upside down for a few days, the contents are easier to stir on opening. When making sauces and dips, water is often included in the recipe; this can cause the tahini to stiffen a great deal, but it can be 'loosened' by adding lemon juice — an ingredient usually found in most tahini recipes anyway.

Use for the popular tahini dip, in hommos (chickpea puree), mixed into cooked eggplant puree for baba ghannouj, and as a sauce for baked or grilled fish. It can be spread onto bread and used in cakes and cookies in the same way as peanut butter. In fact it is an excellent peanut butter substitute.

SEE ALSO Sesame Seed.

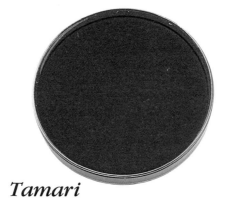

Tamari

MAJOR NUTRIENTS			SERVE SIZE 5 G
Energy	20 kJ	Carbohydrate	1 g
Protein	less than 1 g	Sodium	210 mg
Fat	0	Potassium	15 mg

NUTRITIONAL INFORMATION Contains large amounts of naturally occurring sodium so should be used with discretion in controlled sodium diets.

Contains significant amounts of naturally occurring monosodium glutamate and amines.

ORIGIN AND HISTORY Made from soya beans, it looks like a thick soya sauce. Many consider the full flavour to be superior to soya sauce. It is popular in both Japan and China. Sold in specialty Japanese and Chinese food stores, the sauce will keep indefinitely if kept tightly capped.

PREPARATION AND USE As well as using it as a flavouring, many restaurants in Japan serve it with sashimi.

PROCESSING Soya beans are soaked in water then boiled, drained and thoroughly mixed with cereal flour or meal. The mix is placed on trays and allowed to ferment for one week. Salt brine is added to form a mash which is allowed to ferment for up to one year in deep earthenware vessels. The fermented mash is filtered, pressed and filtered again.

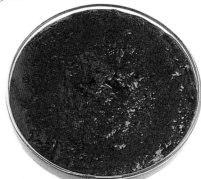

Tandoori Paste

MAJOR NUTRIENTS			SERVE SIZE 10 G
Energy	190 kJ	Potassium	190 mg
Protein	less than 1 g	Calcium	65 mg
Fat	5 g	Phosphorus	30 mg
Carbohydrate	0	Magnesium	28 mg
Sodium	50 mg	Iron	7 mg

NUTRITIONAL INFORMATION Excellent source of iron; moderate source of calcium and magnesium.

Some pastes may have added sodium chloride and so contain significant levels of sodium. Useful flavouring as generally sodium levels are relatively low. Contains significant amounts of naturally occurring salicylates.

ORIGIN AND HISTORY An Indian blend of hot and fragrant spices including turmeric, paprika, chilli powder, saffron, cardamom and garam masala. The name comes from the traditional clay oven called a tandoor in which meat and chicken are cooked.

BUYING AND STORAGE Sold by specialist food stores. Keeps indefinitely if tightly lidded and stored in the cupboard.

PREPARATION AND USE It is used to flavour chicken and beef dishes of that name.

PROCESSING Can be made by blending the spices into a paste with lemon juice and vegetable oil.

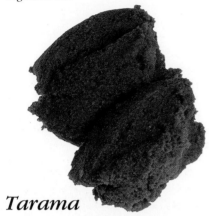

Tarama

MAJOR NUTRIENTS   SERVE SIZE 16 G

Energy	60 kJ	Carbohydrate	0
Protein	2 g	Cholesterol	112 mg
Fat	0		

NUTRITIONAL INFORMATION Contains high levels of cholesterol and sodium.

DESCRIPTION The roe of the grey mullet, found in Mediterranean waters, mixed with salt into a grainy paste. Usually a salmon pink, although some tarama is more orange in colour, depending on the source. On its own it is very salty and slightly bitter, but it is never eaten au naturel.

ORIGIN AND HISTORY Tarama is a Greek delicacy dating from ancient times, and is also popular in Turkey and Cyprus. The grey mullet are trapped in cane weirs when the female is ready to spawn. Roes that are removed intact are generally used for preparing avgotaraho (botargo), while those which are damaged have the membrane removed and salt mixed in. Excess moisture is drained off and the salty, strongly fish-flavoured grainy paste is packed in large tubs, small tins or jars. It is then stored and shipped under refrigeration.

BUYING AND STORAGE Tarama is available at Greek food stores and gourmet delicatessens. Bulk tarama is sold by weight, and this, together with tarama packed in jars, is preferable to tarama packed in tins, which tends to have a tinlike flavour. Store tarama in the refrigerator: unopened jars or tins keep for many months; bulk tarama should be used within two months.

PREPARATION AND USE Tarama is principally used for making the very popular Greek dip, taramosalata. Because of its salt content, tarama should be mixed with plenty of stale white bread (crusts removed). As a guide, use the same weight of bread as tarama. The bread is soaked in water, squeezed dry, and blended into the tarama with onion, lemon juice and olive oil. Mashed potato is sometimes used in place of the bread, but the flavour is not as good. Avgotaraho may be used instead of tarama; cut off amount required, remove skin and slice it. Soak in cold water for 15 minutes to remove some of the salt, then mix with the soaked bread and leave to stand for a while to soften. Tarama may also be mixed with mashed potatoes and other ingredients to make a type of rissole.

PROCESSING Ready-prepared taramosalata is widely available from delicatessens, packed in plastic tubs. Store in refrigerator.

SEE ALSO Botargo.

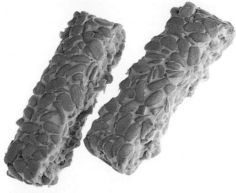

Tempeh

NUTRITIONAL INFORMATION No specific nutritional details are available.

It would make a good source of protein for vegetarian diets. This fermented food provides small amounts of vitamin B12 for the vegan diet.

DESCRIPTION A yellow-brown cake made from whole soya beans which are compressed into flat cakes and injected with a culture which causes fermentation. A soft white coating similar to that which covers a Brie or Camembert cheese forms over the cakes, holding the grains together. The taste is vegetative and slightly acrid, depending on the stage of fermentation, and the texture soft-crunchy. Nutritionally tempeh is highly beneficial as an easily assimilated, low cholesterol, vegetable protein foodstuff.

ORIGIN AND HISTORY Tempeh is thought to have been first made in Indonesia, although it is possible that the early Chinese made a similar product as a precursor to the more refined beancurd, as their fermentation techniques were highly developed.

BUYING AND STORAGE Sold packed in small flat plastic containers or bags, in the chilled food compartments of Asian and health food stores. It can be kept for several weeks in the refrigerator and freezes well.

PREPARATION AND USE Tempeh should be cut into cubes or sticks. It is usually fried to enhance the flavour before using, and readily absorbs the flavours of marinades. Tempeh requires only about 12 minutes' cooking. It is used in stir fries and may be added to curries, soups or braised dishes. Used extensively as a meat alternative in the vegetarian diet.

SEE ALSO Tofu.

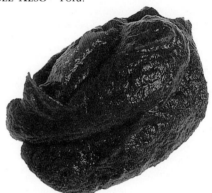

Tomato Paste

MAJOR NUTRIENTS   SERVE SIZE 100 G

Energy	290 kJ	Phosphorus	130 mg
Protein	6 g	Magnesium	66 mg
Fat	0	Iron	5 mg
Carbohydrate	10 g	Zinc	1.7 mg
Cholesterol	0	Thiamin	0.34 mg
Sodium	20 mg	Riboflavin	0.17 mg
Potassium	1 540 mg	Niacin Equiv.	4 mg
Calcium	51 mg	Vitamin C	100 mg

NUTRITIONAL INFORMATION This paste is composed of carbohydrates and protein. It is an excellent source of potassium, phosphorus, magnesium, iron, thiamin and vitamin C; a good source of zinc; a moderate source of calcium and riboflavin.

The carbohydrates in tomato paste are in the form of sugar.

DESCRIPTION A thick red paste made from tomatoes, it is a concentrated form of tomato puree. It has a strong tomato flavour and smell.

ORIGIN AND HISTORY Once tomatoes were accepted as a food in Italy, ways were soon found in which to preserve them for use through the winter months, tomato paste being one of them. Fresh, ripe tomatoes are roughly chopped and heated in a large preserving pan until soft, then rubbed through a sieve to remove seeds and skins. The juice is returned to the pan to simmer until reduced by half — tomato puree at this stage. This is spread into large dishes and left in the sun for 2–4 days to dry out. Salt is added to preserve it, and it is stored in airtight jars with a film of olive oil on top. The paste is also widely made and used in Greece, and both countries now prefer to use the fleshier plum tomatoes for its manufacture.

Through Italian and Greek influences in the kitchens of the English-speaking world, tomato paste has been adopted widely and is made by many food manufacturers. Even in countries of origin, the paste is factory-made for local use as well as export.

BUYING AND STORAGE The locally made tomato paste is available in tubes, sachets, jars and cans. Tomato paste from Italy and Greece is available from stores stocking foods from those countries, and it tends to be more concentrated. Once in use, store paste in refrigerator; if canned paste is used, transfer to a clean jar, float a little oil on top, seal and refrigerate.

PREPARATION AND USE Being a convenience food, it needs no preparation. Use a clean, dry spoon to remove amount required from jar so that jar contents do not become contaminated. If tomato puree is required, mix tomato paste with an equal amount of water.

Use in sauces, particularly for pasta, in stews and casseroles. Because of its tartness, a teaspoon of sugar added with the tomato paste improves the flavour of any dish.

SEE ALSO Tomato.

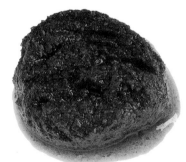

Vindaloo Paste

NUTRITIONAL INFORMATION No nutritional analysis is available.

DESCRIPTION A pungent, thick, Indian seasoning paste with a sour-hot flavour. Ingredients are ground chillies, coriander, cumin, fenugreek, mustard, fennel, cinnamon and cloves in a vinegar base.

ORIGIN AND HISTORY The fiercely hot, sour flavoured curry we know as vindaloo was created for a threefold purpose. Initially the spices and vinegar work as a preservative, useful where refrigeration is rarely available. They break down meat tissues, making tough, inexpensive cuts tender. And they make for a sensational taste combination. The genius for creation of the vindaloo can be ascribed to the south-western Indians — the rare non-vegetarians — who like their food as hot as the mouth will allow. Bold flavours demand rich, strong-flavoured meats, so most vindaloos are based on game and pork.

BUYING AND STORAGE Sold as a paste in jars by Indian or Asian food stockists. It will keep indefinitely unopened. After opening, store in the refrigerator for several months. Sometimes vindaloo spices, to which the vinegar must be added separately, are available.

PREPARATION AND USE The paste should be fried in oil before use as an instant base for vindaloo-style curries. To intensify the flavour, rub evenly over meat and allow to marinate for several hours before browning the meat in oil or ghee. Additional vinegar can be added to intensify the flavours.

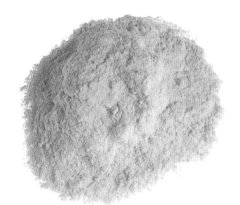

Wasabi *Wasabia japonica*

MAJOR NUTRIENTS		**SERVE SIZE 5 G**	
Energy	12 kJ	Sodium	0
Protein	less than 1 g	Potassium	25 mg
Fat	0	Vitamin C	6 mg
Carbohydrate	less than 1 g		

NUTRITIONAL INFORMATION An excellent source of vitamin C.

DESCRIPTION A hot Japanese condiment made from a locally grown root which has some resemblance to the horseradish root, but is more knobbly, with a brown skin and bright green flesh. It is sold as a pale green powder or a brighter green paste. Wasabi makes even the hottest of chilli seem mild on the tongue.

ORIGIN AND HISTORY A plant native to Japan, it is known popularly as Japanese horseradish. The Japanese name translates as 'mountain hollyhock' and the plant's natural habitat is the edge of cold mountain streams.

It does not cultivate well, but in certain parts of Japan they have been able to emulate the natural conditions favoured by the plant, for production of this invaluable ingredient.

BUYING AND STORAGE It is very occasionally sold fresh by Japanese greengrocers in Western countries. The root should be peeled and the 'eyes' scraped away before finely grating the green flesh. More commonly, wasabi is sold in paste form in a toothpastelike tube, or in powder form in small decorative cans. This should be mixed with cold water or a little sake, a few minutes before use.

PREPARATION AND USE Wasabi is a natural accompaniment to the blandness of raw fish (sashimi) and is served in a small mound at the side, to be mixed into the soya sauce dip according to personal taste. Sushi is made with a smear of wasabi paste between rice and topping.

Once opened, tubes of wasabi should be stored in the refrigerator. Keep powdered wasabi on a dry shelf and mix only the amount needed.

PICKLES AND PRESERVES

Pickling fruits and vegetables has been a method of preservation for thousands of years. Pickles, chutneys and preserves remain a popular part of the modern diet, and the range of imported foods of this kind adds considerably to the variety of condiments and accompaniments available in the diet of each country. According to official figures, pickled vegetables are more popular in the marketplace than chutneys and relishes, and amongst the latter, the vegetable-based products are purchased in greater volume than those with fruit.

When fruits or vegetables are pickled, the foodstuffs are preserved by replacing part of their normal water content by an acid. Some salt, sugar and spices may also be added.

The pickling process also produces relishes: these are sauces or mixtures which have an acid level of between 1 and 2%.

Mixed pickles are made up of a combination of chopped vegetables, pickled in vinegar. Common flavourings are mustard seeds, cider vinegar, garlic, dill and coriander. Turmeric is sometimes added for colouring.

The vegetables in pickles are firm, because they are held in brine to take out some of their liquid. When the brine is drained off, enough vinegar is poured in to cover the vegetables. Oxygen is excluded by sealing because it causes discoloration and encourages the growth of bacteria. Mixed pickles will keep for more than 12 months in a cool cupboard or pantry.

Pickles and preserves are usually used in small amounts to add flavour to the main dishes in a meal or snack. They are not an important source of nutrients, but may encourage people to eat and enjoy foods which are nutritionally important.

These foods have a high salt content, and those who are interested in eating less salt should restrict their use of pickles and preserves.

It is possible to make fresh relishes, to serve as accompaniments, from a variety of chopped fresh fruits, dried fruits and vegetables flavoured with spices, garlic, ginger and fresh herbs and mixed with a little vinegar, lemon juice or lime juice. Salt is not a necessary ingredient in such mixtures.

Included in this chapter are some items which are preserved by drying: unlike the dried fruits in the chapter on Fruits, they are not eaten alone, but serve to flavour or accompany other foods.

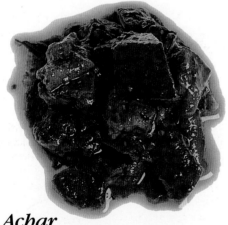

Achar

NUTRITIONAL INFORMATION No nutritional analysis is available, but the energy would be high, due to the oil content.

DESCRIPTION Indian, oil-based pickles of which the principal ingredients are limes or mangoes, pickled in mustard seed or other types of vegetable oils with spice, pepper and chilli.

ORIGIN AND HISTORY Made throughout India, most states favouring a particular style or preparation technique. The pickles of Gujerat state are fiery hot with lashings of garlic; in Maharasthra state, peanut is the base oil, giving a unique flavour; and Bengali achars

have the pungency of mustard seed oil for their distinct flavour.

BUYING AND STORAGE Commercially made pickles can be kept for many months in the refrigerator after opening, or unopened for up to 2 years in a cool, dry cupboard.

PREPARATION AND USE Serve with most Indian meals as a flavour highlight, and a digestive aid.

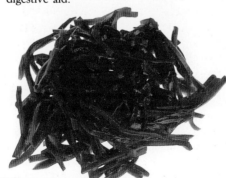

Beni Shoga

also called **Blushing ginger, Gari, Hajikami shoga, Red pickled ginger**

NUTRITIONAL INFORMATION No reliable analysis is available. Being consumed only in small amounts, it is not nutritionally significant, although those on sodium-restricted diets are warned that it is highly salted.

DESCRIPTION Rose pink to red, vinegared ginger in shreds or paper-thin shavings. The pink colour is a natural reaction of the ginger to the vinegar marinade which is applied, together with salt and sugar. Bright red colours are achieved by the addition of food dyes. Hajikami shoga are slender pink shoots of a different type of edible ginger, which are pickled.

ORIGIN AND HISTORY Ginger grows profusely in all of the Asian countries, although it is thought to be a native of tropical Asia. Its value as a medicament is legendary in every Asian culture.

Beni shoga is a Japanese vinegar-pickled ginger, referred to colloquially as gari. Hajikami shoga gives off its young shoots in spring.

BUYING AND STORAGE Beni shoga is usually sold by weight in small plastic tubs, jars or packets, in the pickling liquid. Transfer to a sealed glass jar with a non-metal lid and store in the refrigerator. It will keep indefinitely, provided the ginger is completely submerged. Hajikami shoga can be bought fresh to be pickled at home, or is sold in cans, jars and plastic tubs.

PREPARATION AND USE Ginger serves as a digestive aid, neutralises fats and enhances the flavour of bland dishes. It lends a subtle tang, and fresh taste. Beni shoga is a sushi-shop ginger. Drain and serve in small mounds as a garnish with sushi and sashimi. Use also in fillings for sushi and on toppings for rice dishes. Hajikami shoga shoots are the most popular garnish with Japanese grilled seafood.

PROCESSING Fresh young ginger roots are peeled and sprinkled with salt, then left to stand for 24 hours. They are thoroughly rinsed and marinated in a mixture of rice vinegar, water and sugar for up to 1 week, then bottled. The ginger turns pink. It is shaved into paper-thin slices along the grain, or cut into fine shreds.

There are several Chinese types of pickled ginger, which tend to be stronger in flavour than the Japanese beni shoga.

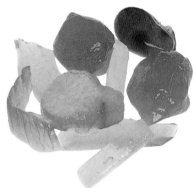

Chow Chow Pickle

also called Chinese sweet pickles

MAJOR NUTRIENTS		SERVE SIZE 20 G	
Energy	100 kJ	Cholesterol	0
Protein	0	Sodium	105 mg
Fat	0	Iron	0.5 mg
Carbohydrate	5 g		

NUTRITIONAL INFORMATION A moderate source of iron. It contains a moderate amount of sodium. No data available for other minerals and vitamins.

Use only small amounts of this food as it is highly salted.

DESCRIPTION Chinese pickled vegetables, preserved in a viscous sweet and tart syrup comprising sugar, salt and vinegar. They take on a glazed appearance and have a crunchy texture. The vegetables include carrot, celery, ginger, cucumber, melon and onion.

ORIGIN AND HISTORY This product is thought to have been created for Europeans residing in China in the last century, a kind of

bottled version of the sweet and sour sauce they favoured.

PREPARATION AND USE These pickles are a very attractive addition to stir-fried dishes, and are often combined with seafoods. Shredded chow chow pickled vegetables are added to sweet and sour sauces and occasionally scattered over steamed fish.

BUYING AND STORAGE In bottles, unopened they will keep indefinitely, and on opening can be kept in the refrigerator for many weeks.

A good substitute is ginger preserved in syrup.

PROCESSING Whole or shredded vegetables are rinsed and blanched in boiling water, then covered with a boiling mixture of vinegar, sugar and seasonings. When cool they are transferred to jars and sealed.

Chutney

also called Relish

MAJOR NUTRIENTS			FRUIT
			SERVE SIZE 25 G
Energy	185 kJ	Carbohydrate	11 g
Protein	0	Cholesterol	0
Fat	0	Sodium	39 mg
			VEGETABLE
			SERVE SIZE 25 G
Energy	89 kJ	Carbohydrate	5 g
Protein	0	Cholesterol	0
Fat	0	Sodium	35 mg

NUTRITIONAL INFORMATION Chutney and relish are mostly composed of carbohydrates, and vegetable chutney is high in sodium. The carbohydrate in chutneys is mostly sugar. Fruit chutney contains 45% sugar and relish contains 18% sugar.

DESCRIPTION Chutney is a piquant relish, consisting of spices ground to a paste, mixed with fruit, cooked or uncooked. It is preserved in an acid such as lime juice, lemon juice or vinegar, and sugar. The water level is kept to a minimum (0.5–0.8%), otherwise it would dilute the acid. Other flavourings and preservatives can be mustard, chilli and turmeric. The main preservative in Westernised chutney is vinegar.

ORIGIN AND HISTORY As chatni, it originated in India, which produces a more pungent chutney than the Westernised version.

BUYING AND STORAGE A wide range of chutneys is available, ranging from very sweet, quite liquid fruit chutneys through to the more acidic versions where the ingredients are more roughly cut, and chewy.

PREPARATION AND USE Following Indian tradition, chutney provides a piquant accompaniment to a main meal. It is also popular with meat, either in a meal or a sandwich.

VARIETIES

Too numerous to mention, although a popular variety is given below.

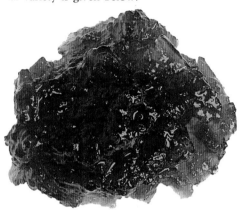

Mango Chutney

MAJOR NUTRIENTS		SERVE SIZE 25 G	
Energy	300 kJ	Carbohydrate	12 g
Protein	0	Cholesterol	0
Fat	3 g	Sodium	30 mg

NUTRITIONAL INFORMATION Other nutrients are present but not in nutritionally significant amounts.

DESCRIPTION Mango chutney is made with fresh mangoes and is flavoured with cumin, cardamom, garlic and chilli. The mango is sliced or chopped and brined. It is then mixed with preservatives such as vinegar, sugar and spices, mustard and chilli.

ORIGIN AND HISTORY Mangoes originated in India where they have been cultivated for more than 4000 years. Usually unripe mangoes are used in the Indian versions of chutney, which are not always cooked — the spices are ground to a paste and added to the chopped fruit.

BUYING AND STORAGE For the Indian version of chutney, purchase in specialty stores or Asian food stores. The Westernised versions can be purchased from supermarkets or specialty stores. Will keep in cupboard or pantry for up to 6 months after opening.

PREPARATION AND USE Use as a flavour-enhancing accompaniment to curries. Also helps tone down the fire of chillies in curry.

Use with cheeses and cold meats, with salads and with hot lamb or beef.

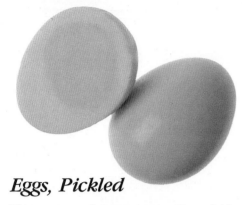

Eggs, Pickled

NUTRITIONAL INFORMATION No reliable data available.

DESCRIPTION The eggs are hard boiled and shelled, then added to a solution of white or cider vinegar. Garlic, allspice, mace and cinnamon are the main spices used as flavourings.

ORIGIN AND HISTORY The English eat them as a snack with beer. The Americans prefer the yolks to be mashed and mixed with mayonnaise and returned to the halves. They may have originated in the UK, but the Chinese also have a version of pickled egg.

BUYING AND STORAGE Store in the refrigerator for up to 6 months. If home pickled, eggs can be added at different times as long as they are constantly covered by the solution.

PREPARATION AND USE If homemade, seal the container and keep for at least 6 weeks before using. Use halved or quartered in salads, with cheese and bread, or as a snack. The Chinese use star anise as a flavouring, and turmeric gives the eggs a golden yellow colour.

SEE ALSO Eggs.

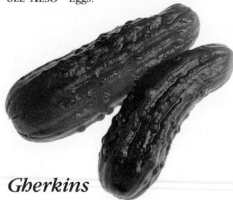

Gherkins

MAJOR NUTRIENTS		IN BRINE SERVE SIZE 25 G	
Energy	35 kJ	Carbohydrate	2 g
Protein	0	Cholesterol	0
Fat	0	Sodium	300 mg

		IN BRINE, SWEETENED SERVE SIZE 25 G	
Energy	35 kJ	Carbohydrate	2 g
Protein	0	Cholesterol	0
Fat	0	Sodium	220 mg

NUTRITIONAL INFORMATION Pickles in brine are mostly composed of carbohydrate, and are moderately high in sodium. There is no reliable nutritional information on pickles preserved in vinegar.

DESCRIPTION True gherkins come from the plant *Cucumis anguria*, a cucumber which is native to the Caribbean, although it is grown extensively in North America. The fruit is small with a firm but tender skin which is quite rough. Small varieties of other cucumbers are sometimes substituted for gherkins and are picked when still immature, before seed development. Gherkins are preserved in vinegar or brine, usually with dill flower heads and allspice as flavourings, although onions, garlic, bay leaves, cloves and tarragon are used as well. Holland is a very large producer of gherkins.

ORIGIN AND HISTORY The French call the small cucumber *cornichon*, and the Russians call it *ogurtzy*. The cucumber has been cultivated for 4000 years and was known to the Egyptians and Greeks. It arrived in France through Italy in the 9th century and it went to England in the 14th century.

BUYING AND STORAGE Purchase from most supermarkets and specialist food stores. Store in the refrigerator after opening.

PREPARATION AND USE The French serve gherkins with pâté. Sliced finely and fanned out, they make an attractive garnish for cold meats and salads.

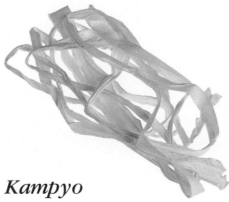

Kampyo

NUTRITIONAL INFORMATION No reliable analysis is available.

DESCRIPTION Long, thin, buff-coloured ribbons shaved from a calabash gourd and preserved by drying.

ORIGIN AND HISTORY Calabashes, or Chinese bottle gourds, have been in Asia for many centuries. The flesh is tough enough, when dried, to make into strips which can be used as edible ties for small bundles of food. Japanese traditionally like to tie food in bundles similar to the silk-wrapped bundles known as fukusa.

BUYING AND STORAGE Sold in small bundles in cellophane packs, they last indefinitely in dry conditions. To store, transfer to a covered jar.

PREPARATION AND USE Soak to soften, and rub between the fingers with salt to tenderise the fibres and increase absorbency. Rinse thoroughly, then simmer in unsalted water until softened. Once cooked, they must be handled carefully.

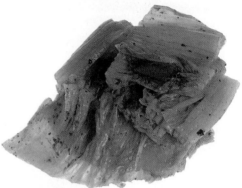

Kimchee

also called Kimchi

NUTRITIONAL INFORMATION No reliable analysis is available. It has a high sodium content as it is heavily salted. Use sparingly.

DESCRIPTION Korean pickled cabbage made with Napa/Peking cabbage pickled with salt, garlic and chilli.

ORIGIN AND HISTORY Koreans have an affinity with foods that are chilli hot, perhaps because they are a vigorous, vibrant people, perhaps as a defence against weather that can be stifling in summer and bone-chilling in winter. With few natural vegetables, they have to ensure adequate vitamins and roughage in their winter diets, so they devised this pungent, challenging pickle as a means of satisfying both taste buds and nutritional requirements. Throughout winter Korean families unearth their sealed tubs of kimchee, always ensuring there is plenty to last through the cold months.

BUYING AND STORAGE Kimchee is sold in plastic bags or tubs by weight and can be kept for many weeks, covered, in the refrigerator. Make sure it is adequately sealed, as its strong odour can taint other foods.

PREPARATION AND USE Kimchee is served with almost every Korean meal. It is particularly good with grills, and an interesting nibble to serve with drinks.

PROCESSING Chopped Chinese cabbage is salted heavily and left overnight, then kneaded to soften the vegetable fibres and impregnate with salt. Chilli and garlic are added, and the pickle is packed into large jars which are stored underground to ferment and mature. There are many versions of the basic recipe, some being quite mild, others searing hot.

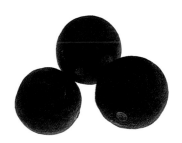

Lime, Dried *Citrus aurantifolia*

*also called **Loomi besra, Noomi, Limu omani***

NUTRITIONAL INFORMATION Nutritional data not available, but see Lime in the chapter on Fruits.

DESCRIPTION Small, round dried limes, ranging in colour from a grey-brown to almost black. They impart a pleasantly tangy flavour to foods. In the days before refrigeration, holes were punched into each end of the lime and it was added to stews and soups to remove unwanted flavours.

ORIGIN AND HISTORY This particular species of lime, *Citrus aurantifolia*, is native to the East Indies, and was introduced to the Mediterranean region by the Arabs about AD 1000. No doubt the limes were first used fresh, and it could well have been a fortunate accident that the dried lime found its way into the cooking pot.

In hot climates, limes left on the trees can eventually dehydrate to a dark, dry facsimile of the original fruit. Perhaps a curious cook wondered what they tasted like, and found the taste very pleasant indeed. Whatever the means of discovery, these limes are now left to dry on the tree. Most of such limes, used in the cooking of the Gulf States, Iraq and Iran, are grown in Iran, Iraq, and Oman and imported from Thailand. The Gulf Arabs prefer the black limes, while the Iranis and Iraqis like the lighter coloured limes.

BUYING AND STORAGE Available from Middle Eastern food stores. As humidity can affect the crispness of the fruit, store in an airtight container in a cool, dry place. They keep indefinitely.

PREPARATION AND USE Holes are punched into each end of the dried lime when adding to soups and stews in Irani and Iraqi cooking. While the original need to remove unwanted odours has ceased for the most part, the passage of the cooking liquid through the lime still imparts a pleasant, tangy flavour to the dish. In Gulf Arabic cooking, the limes are broken into pieces and added to lamb stews, chicken and fish dishes and lentil soups.

The limes also make an interesting 'spice'. Grind to a powder and sprinkle onto beef steaks or lamb chops before grilling. Add roughly crumbled lime to lamb marinades.

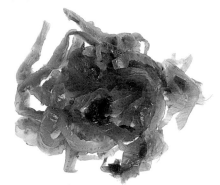

Mustard Greens, Pickled

*also called **Haam suen choy, Pickled cabbage***

NUTRITIONAL INFORMATION No reliable data are available. Contains a large amount of sodium.

DESCRIPTION A pungent, salty Chinese pickle made with the stem section and leaves of the Swaton mustard cabbage. It is packed into large pottery pots and left to mature for several months. It is crisp in texture and very salty.

ORIGIN AND HISTORY Cabbages of various kinds have provided a major source of nutrition for the people of China since early times. In the landlocked rural areas of central and northern China, where winters were harsh, pickling was the only way to ensure a supply of vegetables during the cold months.

The pungent smell of pickling cabbage was, and is still today, a familiar experience in villages all over China.

BUYING AND STORAGE In certain Asian markets, the pickle is sold by the piece from its original glazed ceramic tub, otherwise it is packed in plastic bags or tubs. It can be kept for several months, and is best refrigerated in hot and humid climates.

PREPARATION AND USE It is used in cooking to add an interesting crunchy texture and salty flavour to many types of Chinese dishes, particularly those from central and western China. It is especially good in soups. In the province of Hunan, garlic and chilli are added to salt as the pickling and flavouring agents, making the pickle very strong in flavour.

PROCESSING The fresh cabbage is trimmed and rinsed, then spread on trays and heavily salted. After several hours the vegetables are kneaded to soften fibres and allow the salt to penetrate, other seasonings are added, then the vegetable is packed into tubs, sealed and left to mature.

Olive *Olea europaea*

MAJOR NUTRIENTS			PICKLED SERVE SIZE 20 G
Energy	green	109 kJ	Carbohydrate	0
	ripe	167 kJ	Cholesterol	0
Protein		0	Sodium	490 mg
Fat	green	3 g	Dietary Fibre	0
	ripe	4 g		

NUTRITIONAL INFORMATION Energy source from fat, high in sodium. Olives are like avocados in that their energy source is from fat, not carbohydrate. This makes them quite high in kilojoules, so weight-conscious individuals should take this into consideration. The fat in fresh olives is mostly monounsaturated. It appears that monounsaturated fats may be almost as effective as polyunsaturated fats in lowering blood cholesterol levels. The fatty acid composition of olives bottled in brine is approximately 14% saturated, 73% monounsaturated and 11% polyunsaturated. Olives do not contain other useful nutrients and are high in sodium: it is recommended that people on a low salt diet should avoid consuming olives.

DESCRIPTION Oval-shaped fruit of an evergreen tree, with bitter, oily flesh clinging to the seed or stone. Green olives are picked while they are firm and almost mature; black olives when ripe, with colour ranging from mauve to dark purple. To achieve jet black olives for pickling, ripe olives are left for 24 hours before processing. Olives are treated to remove the bitterness, then pickled in brine. Green olives are also stoned and stuffed after pickling.

ORIGIN AND HISTORY With the unique

distinction of being the oldest tree in continuous cultivation in the Western World, the olive is native to the Mediterranean region. First cultivated in Asia Minor around 4000 BC and by the Minoans in Crete around 3500 BC, the fruits were first used for their oil, and archaeological finds suggest that the means of preparing olives for the table was known to the Minoans of Crete (1400 BC) and in Phoenicia (1200 BC).

Today olives are grown in many countries outside the Mediterranean region where similar climatic conditions prevail. The first olives were introduced into Australia in 1844 when a shipment of 51 plants arrived in South Australia from Marseilles, France. Australian olives received an Honourable Mention when submitted to the London Exhibition in 1851.

BUYING AND STORAGE Pickled olives are widely available packed in jars — whole green, green stuffed with pimento, almonds or anchovies, and various types of black olives. From Italian, Greek and Middle Eastern food stores, a large variety of olives is available in bulk, either pickled in brine or the 'dry' shrivelled olives — you can try before you buy. Store jar-packed olives in a cool, dark place; after opening, store in the refrigerator. Bulk olives should be transferred to a sealed jar and stored in the refrigerator.

PREPARATION AND USE Olives can be used as they are purchased. However brine-packed or shrivelled olives can be flavoured for the table. Drain off brine and replace with a mild vinegar. Add a halved garlic clove and/or sprigs of oregano or thyme, and float some olive oil on top. Seal and store in a cool place for at least a week before using.

Use any olive as a savoury nibble, in salads, as a garnish, or chopped for pizza toppings or olive bread; use whole green or black olives in vegetable, meat or chicken dishes.

PROCESSING Chopped, pimento-stuffed olives are available for use in savoury dips or pizza toppings.

VARIETIES
Botanically, these are too numerous to mention, but the three main types for purchase are listed below, in order of maturity.

Cracked Green Olives These are pickled in September in the northern hemisphere, when they have only just formed and are immature. They are always treated before use because they contain the bitter substance oleuropein. This is removed by soaking them in water which is changed every day for 2 weeks. Most of the bitterness will be washed out, but some should remain. The 'cracking'

is done by cutting them with a knife to aid in leaching out the oleuropein. They are then soaked in 10% salt brine, sometimes flavoured with fennel, bay leaves or garlic, for 2–3 months. The brine is weak enough to allow the growth of some species of bacteria which produce lactic acid — which is a preservative — and strong enough to prevent undesirable bacteria from growing — which would promote decay.

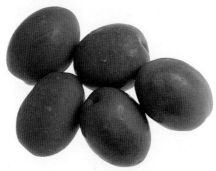

Green Olives Green olives are immature olives, picked around November in the northern hemisphere. They are more developed than the cracked green olives, therefore more oily at this stage. Since Roman times the practice has been to soak them in lye (an alkaline solution made by boiling wood ash in water) but these days a caustic soda solution is used, in which the green olives are soaked for 6 hours. The caustic solution changes the texture of the flesh. They are then soaked in frequent changes of water for 3 days (up to 15 days in Spain, which accounts for the milder flavour in Spanish olives) to remove the caustic. They then go into 10% brine, flavoured with garlic, herbs or bay leaves, and are ready to eat in a few days. The Caterian, from Italy, is green in colour when ripe, with a white flesh. The pit is oval and small.

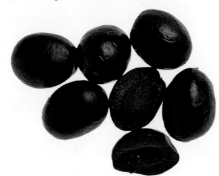

Black Olives Black olives are mature olives, prepared differently in each country, depending on whether they are for eating, for oil, or for both. There are many varieties of olives, and names vary in different regions. From Spain the Sevilla, Marelenca and Manzanete are for pickling and Manzanete also

produces a fine oil. The Manzanete is red to violet-black in colour. From Italy the Oliva di Orignola is violet-red in colour. From Greece the Kalamata, Megara and Maxcos are popular eating olives. Yugoslavia produces Obliza, which is oval, slightly curved with rough skin and is reddish-black in colour. The French produce the Liques, among many. This olive is fleshy with the pit cylindrical, curved or twisted.

In the south of France the olives are put into 10% brine solution with herbs for 9 months.

In Greece the olives are not treated in lye or caustic soda solution, so they are strong in taste. They are pickled in brine, and sometimes they are preserved in salt.

SEE ALSO Olive Oil.

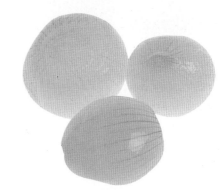

Onion, Pickled

MAJOR NUTRIENTS		SERVE SIZE 25 G	
Energy	20 kJ	Carbohydrate	1 g
Protein	0	Cholesterol	0
Fat	0	Sodium	80 mg

NUTRITIONAL INFORMATION Pickled onions are mostly composed of carbohydrate. Other nutrients are present but not in nutritionally significant amounts.

DESCRIPTION Small onions which have been soaked in brine for 24–48 hours, then preserved in malt vinegar. The vinegar is either brown or the distilled malt vinegar, which is commonly called white vinegar. The vinegar is flavoured with allspice, mustard seeds, bay leaves, peppercorns or other herbs and spices.

ORIGIN AND HISTORY Evidence that onions were pickled in ancient times has been found at Pompeii. They are very popular in England, and are sometimes eaten in pubs as an accompaniment to beer.

BUYING AND STORAGE When stored in the cupboard or pantry will keep for up to 2 years. If the pantry is cool and dark (an optimum storage area) they will keep indefinitely.

When they have been opened, store in the refrigerator, otherwise contact with oxygen encourages the growth of moulds and degrades the quality of the vinegar.

PREPARATION AND USE Preferably use small onions. Larger onions must be sliced. Store in the vinegar for 3–6 months before using. Used as an accompaniment to salads, cold meats or cheese. Small onions are used in hors d'oeuvres and are sometimes coloured artificially and called cocktail onions.

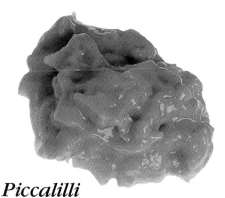

Piccalilli

also called Sweet pickle, Mustard pickle

MAJOR NUTRIENTS		PICCALILLI SERVE SIZE 25 G	
Energy	35 kJ	Carbohydrate	2 g
Protein	0	Cholesterol	0
Fat	0	Sodium	300 mg

		SWEET PICKLE SERVE SIZE 25 G	
Energy	143 kJ	Carbohydrate	9 g
Protein	0	Cholesterol	0
Fat	0	Sodium	425 mg

NUTRITIONAL INFORMATION Piccalilli and sweet pickle are mostly composed of carbohydrates. Piccalilli is moderately high in sodium and sweet pickle is high in sodium. The carbohydrate in sweet pickle is close to 37% sugar.

DESCRIPTION Piccalilli is sold and made mainly in America and England. The English version is a mixed pickle consisting of cauliflower, onions and gherkins in a thick sauce with turmeric and ground white mustard. The vegetables are brined first, then added to the thick sauce. This process is essential because the acid level in the sauce is not enough to preserve the vegetables. The vegetables are drained thoroughly of the brine, otherwise 'cracking' would occur, where the brine seeps out into the sauce. There is 4–7% sugar content in piccalilli, however there can be up to 20% sugar content when the vegetables are soaked in a sugar solution as well as the sauce. The American version is made with green tomatoes, onions, cauliflower, turmeric, sugar and cider vinegar. It has a sour/sweet taste. In both versions the vegetables should be crisp and retain their shape.

ORIGIN AND HISTORY Piccalilli originated in England when the English began returning from India and found their palates craving the stronger-tasting foods.

BUYING AND STORAGE Purchase from supermarkets or specialty stores. Will keep for up to 1 year in pantry or cupboard. Refrigerate after opening.

PREPARATION AND USE If homemade, use only good quality vegetables. In the American, use only very green tomatoes, otherwise they will lose their seeds and turn to pulp during cooking. The American version also contains a large amount of salt, which is used to draw out the liquids in the vegetables. Use with cold meats and cheeses. Americans serve piccalilli with baked beans.

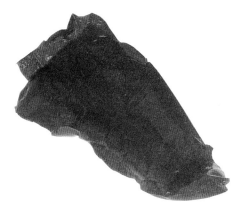

Pimento, Pickled

NUTRITIONAL INFORMATION No reliable data available.

DESCRIPTION Pimento is a long, thin capsicum, a variety of *Capsicum annuum*. The fruit is sliced and pickled in brine, then in white vinegar. The soaking in brine draws out some of the fluids in the pimento, preventing the dilution of the vinegar, which should not be less than 5% acetic acid. The different colours of pimento packed in the jar show the various stages of ripeness of the fruit: green and yellow are unripe, the red is ripe. The flavouring allspice is also known as pimento, but comes from a different family, Myrtaceae.

ORIGIN AND HISTORY The pimento was brought back from South America by Christopher Columbus in the 1600s and has been cultivated in southern Europe ever since.

BUYING AND STORAGE Store away from light and in a cool cupboard or pantry. Refrigerate after opening.

PREPARATION AND USE Use in salads or as an accompaniment to cold meats.

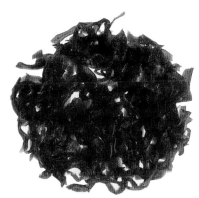

Red Pickled Cabbage

NUTRITIONAL INFORMATION No reliable data available.

DESCRIPTION Red cabbage is a purplish, round cabbage which can be shredded and soaked in brine to preserve it. It is then drained of the brine and re-pickled with a vinegar which has been spiced with flavourings such as juniper berries, pepper or caraway seeds. Sulphur dioxide helps retain the colour and the texture of the cabbage. Discolouring occurs when oxygen is present, which is mainly in the top of the jar, therefore always keep the cabbage covered with the vinegar.

ORIGIN AND HISTORY Red pickled cabbage originated in northern Europe and is popular in Holland, Germany and Denmark. In the Scandinavian countries it can contain up to 20% sucrose.

BUYING AND STORAGE Store in a dark pantry or cupboard. After opening, store in the refrigerator.

PREPARATION AND USE Do not heat the cabbage in cast iron or aluminium — it will discolour. Add chopped bacon, sliced apple and spiced vinegar. Garlic, orange juice and paprika also complement the red cabbage. Goes well with game, mutton and continental sausages.

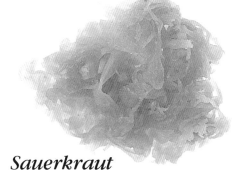

Sauerkraut

MAJOR NUTRIENTS		SERVE SIZE 100 G	
Energy	42 kJ	Sodium	355 mg
Protein	1 g	Calcium	48 mg
Fat	0	Iron	0.6 mg
Carbohydrate	2 g	Phosphorus	43 mg
Cholesterol	0	Vitamin C	20 mg

NUTRITIONAL INFORMATION The kilojoules in sauerkraut come mostly from carbohydrates. It is high in sodium but an excellent source of vitamin C. It is a moderate source of calcium, iron and phosphorus. Other nutrients are present but not in nutritionally significant amounts. Sauerkraut is close to 90% water.

DESCRIPTION Sauerkraut is fermented cabbage. The cabbage is shredded and salted with approximately 1.5% salt by weight to draw out the liquids from the cells, then soaked in a brine solution of 2.25% salt. This brine solution replaces the original liquid from the cabbage and encourages the bacterium *Leuconastoc mesenteroides* to grow, if the temperature of the solution is kept at 18–21°C. This bacterium produces lactic acid and other compounds which give sauerkraut its flavour. When the acid level reaches 1%, this bacterium declines and is replaced by *Lactobacillus pnanarum*, which increases the acid to 7% after 2–3 weeks.

ORIGIN AND HISTORY Fermented cabbage has its origins in China. The workers building the Great Wall of China relied on this food, which in those days was shredded cabbage covered by wine. There is evidence the Tartars took the idea of fermented cabbage to Europe. As the Gauls salted foods for the winter, it is possible sauerkraut originated in Europe at that time. There are recipes from the Middle Ages for sauerkraut, and it was a staple food, particularly in central and eastern Europe where it was considered a winter survival food before the potato was introduced in the 18th century. A form of sauerkraut called kimchee in Korea is a staple and is made in a few days, depending on the outside temperature, since it is buried in the ground for fermentation. It is thought that sauerkraut stimulates underactive digestion, and works well in dietary combinations with 'stodgy' foods.

BUYING AND STORAGE Canned or bottled sauerkraut is pasteurised, therefore no more fermentation occurs. After opening, store in the refrigerator.

PREPARATION AND USE If sauerkraut is too acidic it should be drained and washed under the tap until the required taste is achieved. It should be cooked in a saucepan for 25–30 minutes until almost all of the liquid has evaporated. Flavourings such as juniper berries, garlic, onion or apple can be added. Serve with fried or boiled bacon, frankfurters, or other smoked sausages, potatoes or dumplings.

SEE ALSO Kimchee, and Mustard Greens, Pickled.

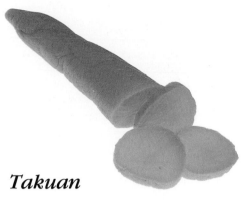

Takuan

NUTRITIONAL INFORMATION No nutritional data are available. Contains a large amount of sodium and should therefore be consumed sparingly.

DESCRIPTION Yellow Japanese radish pickle.

ORIGIN AND HISTORY A traditional Japanese pickle, it is made from the giant white radish introduced to Japan from China at least three centuries ago. Pickling is an ancient practice in Japan. Originally used as a method of preservation, it was found that the increased flavour and saltiness of pickled foods made them more suitable as side dishes. Most kinds of Japanese pickles can be made easily at home, but takuan is best store bought, as it takes several months and creates a very pervasive odour while the radishes slowly pickle in large wooden tubs filled with nuka — a mash of rice bran.

BUYING AND STORAGE Takuan is sold in jars or vacuum sealed plastic tubs, either whole, sliced or in long strips. Unopened it can be kept for many months; on opening, transfer contents to a covered jar and store on a cool shelf or in the refrigerator for many weeks.

PREPARATION AND USE It is served sliced and arranged in a small dish, often with other kinds of pickles, at the end of a Japanese meal, or to nibble with drinks. Thin strips of takuan are sometimes used in rolled sushi.

PROCESSING Unpeeled whole radishes are salted and hung to dry for several weeks, then pickled in rice bran and salt and left to mature for many weeks. They turn a bright yellow, with a crisp and chewy texture and salty flavour.

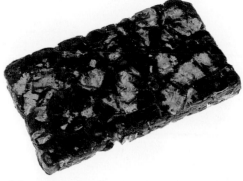

Tamarind *Tamarindus indica*

MAJOR NUTRIENTS		RAW FRUIT SERVE SIZE 100 G	
Energy	1000 kJ	Calcium	75 mg
Protein	3 g	Phosphorus	115 mg
Fat	1 g	Iron	3 mg
Carbohydrate	63 g	Thiamin	0.35 mg
Cholesterol	0	Riboflavin	0.15 mg
Dietary Fibre	5 g	Niacin Equiv.	1 mg
Sodium	50 mg	Vitamin C	2 mg
Potassium	780 mg		

NUTRITIONAL INFORMATION An excellent source of iron, thiamin and potassium; good source of phosphorus; moderate source of calcium, riboflavin, niacin and vitamin C. Usually, however, it is consumed in nutritionally insignificant quantities.

DESCRIPTION A dried pod, or a paste, made from the fruit.

ORIGIN AND HISTORY Believed to originate in East Africa, tamarind now grows wild throughout the Indian subcontinent and is cultivated in the tropics and subtropics. The word tamarind comes from the Arabic, and literally means 'date of India'. The tamarind is often spiced, and prepared into syrup and paste.

BUYING AND STORAGE Available from specialty and Middle Eastern food stores. No special storage is required. Dried pods, compressed and packaged, are available at Asian food stores.

Homemade paste will keep for up to a week in the refrigerator. Store in a glass jar.

PREPARATION AND USE Tamarind is a vital ingredient of Worcestershire sauce and its major commercial use is as a base for fruit drinks. As a juice or paste, it is used as a souring agent, particularly in curries and chutneys. Jams and jellies may often include tamarind, due to its high pectin content.

PROCESSING When a walnut-sized piece of dried tamarind is steeped in 1 cup of hot water for about 10 minutes, a dark, sour juice can be squeezed out. Alternatively, tamarind paste can be made by soaking 2–3 tablespoons of pulp in 150 ml of hot water overnight. Pass through a strainer.

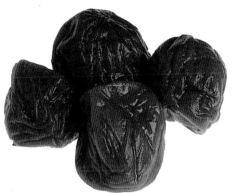

Umeboshi

also called Japanese plum pickle

NUTRITIONAL INFORMATION No reliable analysis is available. Contains a large amount of sodium, so use sparingly.

DESCRIPTION Japanese pickled 'plums', sold either in whole form or mashed. They are still unripe and yellow in colour when pickled, but the addition of red shiso leaves gives the pickle a red colour.

ORIGIN AND HISTORY The fruit used is not actually a plum but a kind of apricot (*Prunus mume*) which has grown wild in Japan and China for centuries. It is this same fruit which provided the original sour/sweet taste in Chinese sweet and sour dishes in ancient times, and in its very green stage it is used to make umeshu, the Japanese plum liqueur.

BUYING AND STORAGE Umeboshi is sold in plastic packs and small jars in varying sizes. Unopened it keeps indefinitely; once opened it is best to transfer what is not used to a glass jar with a non-metal lid. It can be kept in the refrigerator for many weeks.

PREPARATION AND USE With an interesting fruity, salt flavour it is used as an accompaniment to Japanese dinners, served by itself or with other pickles, usually at the end of the meal. Considered beneficial to the digestion, as well as an appetite stimulant.

PROCESSING Yellow ume (Japanese plums) are washed carefully and steeped in white liquor and salt for several days. Then red shiso leaves are added and the pickle put aside for one month to mature. The final stage is a series of dryings and marination of the fruit in its original liquid, now stained a bright red from the shiso leaves, to enhance the flavour of the pickle. Then comes a further one month of resting before the pickle is mature.

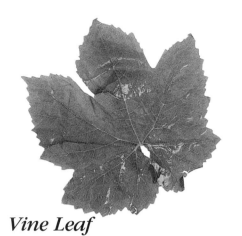

Vine Leaf

MAJOR NUTRIENTS		SERVE SIZE 10 G	
Energy	10 kJ	Sodium	220 mg
Protein	0	Calcium	40 mg
Fat	0	Vitamin C	2 mg
Carbohydrate	0	Vitamin A	38 µg
Cholesterol	0		

NUTRITIONAL INFORMATION Vine leaves are very low in energy. They are a moderate source of calcium, vitamin C and vitamin A.

DESCRIPTION Preserved leaves from the grapevine, dull green in colour, used as a wrapping for foods.

ORIGIN AND HISTORY Early Greek and Persian writings mention food wrapped in vine leaves, so the idea has been around for some two thousand years. The leaves are picked from late spring, blanched, then packed in brine for use throughout the year. Greece is the major supplier of preserved vine leaves to world markets.

Fresh vine leaves are the best to use if you have access to a grapevine not affected by sprays. Choose young, light green leaves.

BUYING AND STORAGE Preserved vine leaves are available from Greek and Middle Eastern food stores, some supermarkets and delicatessens. They are available in bulk or packed in plastic bags, jars and cans.

Canned vine leaves are disappointing, as the heat treatment required for canned products 'cooks' the vine leaves, making them difficult to work with. Vine leaves from the other sources are all easy to use. Store can- and jar-packed vine leaves at room temperature, plastic-packed or bulk purchased vine leaves in the refrigerator. They keep for many months.

PREPARATION AND USE Remove from packaging and drain well. They can simply be rinsed well in cold water. However a brief blanching is recommended to improve the flavour; blanch in small batches for 3 minutes then remove to a bowl of cold water to cool quickly. Drain well, then remove any stems with scissors. Use this same process to prepare fresh vine leaves. The leaves are placed shiny side down when wrapping food or stuffings in them.

Use with traditional savoury rice or meat and rice fillings, for wrapping fresh sardines before barbecuing them, and as a covering for oven roasted small game birds to keep them moist and complement the flavour.

SEE ALSO Canned Dolmas, in Canned and Packaged Foods.

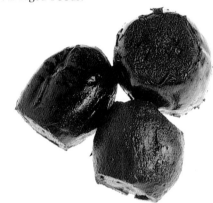

Walnuts, Pickled

NUTRITIONAL INFORMATION No reliable data available.

DESCRIPTION Immature or green walnuts are preserved in spiced vinegar. They are picked before the shell has hardened and soaked in a brine solution for 12–13 days. The walnuts are then dried and go black. They are then pickled in vinegar which has been flavoured with spices, garlic, mace or mustard.

ORIGIN AND HISTORY Pickled walnuts are in fact hardly known in Europe, where most of the walnuts are grown. Americans flavour the vinegar with sugar or honey and use cider vinegar. The result is not as strong in taste as the British mixture, which is sometimes bottled in malt vinegar.

BUYING AND STORAGE Used when they are soft, but they are best stored for 1–2 years.

PREPARATION AND USE Used as any pickle with cold meats, cheese on a platter, or as a finger food with vinegar, salt, pepper and spring onions.

EXTRACTS, ESSENCES AND COLOURINGS

Throughout history, food has been flavoured by spices, herbs and aromatic constituents of fruits and vegetables for many reasons, one of which was to disguise unpalatable flavours. Now, bakery goods, meat products, gelatine desserts, confectionery, ice creams and ices, non-alcoholic and alcoholic beverages require the addition of flavour to make them acceptable, and to satisfy continuously growing and changing demands.

Nature has provided abundant varieties of flavouring substances which can be extracted by steam distillation or solvent extraction. Others are produced by highly technical processes to duplicate aromatic substances. These can be made in unlimited quantities and are more economical to use.

Many varieties are readily available and should be stored according to directions on the container.

Flavourings can be homemade by extracting the juice from fruits and vegetables, by boiling down meats and by mixing fresh and dried herbs and spices. The base product will determine the end use.

Essences are essential flavours that are extracted by the distillation or maceration of a vegetable substance in water. There are three categories of flavouring essences:

Natural essences are made from the juices of fruits, from citrus peels, spices, beans, herbs, roots, nuts, etc.

Artificial essences such as vanillin, pineapple, rum, brandy, banana, etc. are made from various chemicals blended to give very close imitations of these flavours.

Compound essences are made by blending the concentrated juice or oil with artificial flavours.

Food essences make no significant nutritional contribution to the diet and may contain significant amounts of naturally occurring salicylates and amines.

Check whether the label states that the essence is pure or imitation. The pure is more expensive but will give much better results. Keep bottles tightly capped to prevent the flavour from evaporating and the essence should last for several months.

Essences have been used to flavour foods since early times and their use is so much part of everyday cooking it would be impossible to imagine being without them.

There are two categories of food colouring: those derived from natural sources, and those derived from chemicals found in coal tar.

The natural colours include chlorophyll, carotene, saffron, annatto (the two last are found in Herbs and Spices) and cochineal, as well as colours natural to edible fruits or vegetables such as beetroot. Another well-known colour is caramel.

The second category includes a whole range of colours which are, in general, derived from chemicals found in coal tar and are usually known as aniline colours.

Today more than 90% of all food colours used are synthetic.

Usually food colouring is purchased bottled in liquid form and should be stored, tightly sealed, in a cupboard.

Most of the commercially prepared food colourings are highly concentrated and only a small amount is needed.

Since the 1970s, when Dr Ben Feingold put forward his theories linking hyperactivity in children with the consumption of food additives, many of the foods in this section have come under fire. A great deal of research in this area has taken place, and now indicates that a very small percentage of the population has adverse reactions to certain substances which might occur naturally in foods or be added to foods. These include salicylates, benzoates, amines, monosodium glutamate, sulphur dioxide, and the azo dyes, tartrazine (yellow) and erythrosine (red). From the individual entries in this section it will be seen that many of these compounds occur in the foods listed.

Salicylates, benzoates, amines and monosodium glutamate may be added to foods, but they also occur naturally. They tend to be in higher concentrations in highly flavoured foods, including extracts and essences.

When additives are used in manufactured foods, it is mandatory for the ingredient list to identify the additive, either by the name or the approved additive number (see the table at the end of this book). These compounds have been linked with a range of conditions such as hyperactivity, migraine, asthma, urticaria (hives) and gastric disturbances.

People who suspect that they, or their children, have such a food intolerance should have a diagnosis made by a medical allergy specialist and seek dietary advice from a dietitian specialising in the area. Many people concerned about additives follow unnecessarily restrictive diets, and undermine their health in so doing; it should be emphasised that only a small percentage of the population suffers from types of food intolerance.

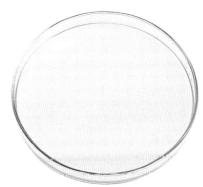

Almond Essence

NUTRITIONAL INFORMATION No significant nutritional contribution to the diet.

Contains significant amounts of naturally occurring salicylates.

DESCRIPTION A solution of oil and bitter almonds, almond essences are also made from the bitter almonds or kernels of plums, peaches, cherries and apricots. These are known as *noyaux*.

ORIGIN AND HISTORY In early medieval cooking, almond was an everyday flavouring and in Elizabethan times the fad was for 'marchpane', a combination of pounded almonds and pistachio nuts, sugar, flour and various essences including vanilla. In the Middle East, and in certain Balkan countries, many of the sweet dishes are highly flavoured with almond, as are a number of Far Eastern dishes.

BUYING AND STORAGE Available in bottles, the essence is originally colourless and will acquire a yellow colour with storage. As it will oxidise on exposure to air, keep the bottle tightly closed.

PREPARATION AND USE Usually only a small amount is required of this delicate flavouring but, if omitted for any reason, the character of the dish is changed.

It is used for flavouring puddings, cakes, sweets, ice cream, pastries and confectionery such as nougat.

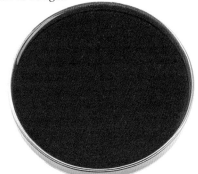

Angostura Bitters

NUTRITIONAL INFORMATION No significant nutritional contribution in the diet.

Contains significant amounts of naturally occurring salicylates.

DESCRIPTION A rum base, infused with the bitter and aromatic bark of the cusparia tree and a number of herbs and roots.

ORIGIN AND HISTORY The recipe for angostura bitters is a closely guarded secret. First made in Angostura, Venezuela, it is now made in Trinidad.

BUYING AND STORAGE Available in small distinctively labelled bottles from liquor stores, the bitters will keep indefinitely if tightly sealed.

PREPARATION AND USE Only a few drops are required when added to other beverages. It is added to gin to produce the famous Pink Gin, and is used in cocktails and mixed drinks including soft drinks. It can also be used to flavour stewed dishes, and soups and sweet dishes in the West Indies.

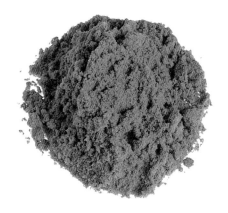

Beef Extract

MAJOR NUTRIENTS		SERVE SIZE 10 G	
Energy	70 kJ	Phosphorus	60 mg
Protein	4 g	Iron	1.5 mg
Fat	0	Thiamin	1 mg
Carbohydrate		Riboflavin	0.7 mg
	less than 1 g	Niacin Equiv.	8.4 mg
Sodium	480 mg		

NUTRITIONAL INFORMATION An excellent source of iron, niacin and folate; moderate source of protein, phosphorus and thiamin.

The iron present is in a form which means it should be well absorbed by the body. Contains significant amounts of sodium so, if used frequently, the limiting of other high sodium sources should be considered.

Contains large amounts of naturally occurring amines.

DESCRIPTION An essence made from beef, vegetables, herbs and spices.

ORIGIN AND HISTORY A traditional recipe, it was valued for its nutritive value and featured in recipes for invalid cookery.

BUYING AND STORAGE Produced commercially under several brand names, it contains yeast extract, flavour enhancers and colourings.

Available in powder and liquid form which should be kept sealed in the original container.

PREPARATION AND USE Mix 1 teaspoon in a cup of hot water for a beverage. Add to soups and stews for more concentrated flavour.

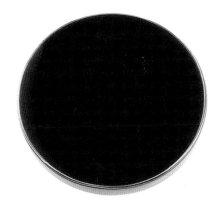

Bonox

MAJOR NUTRIENTS		SERVE SIZE 10 G	
Energy	70 kJ	Phosphorus	60 mg
Protein	4 g	Iron	1.5 mg
Fat	0	Thiamin	1 mg
Carbohydrate		Riboflavin	0.7 mg
	less than 1 g	Niacin Equiv.	8 mg
Sodium	480 mg		

NUTRITIONAL INFORMATION An excellent source of iron, niacin and folate; moderate source of protein, phosphorus and thiamin. Contains large amounts of iron.

The iron present is in a form which means it should be well absorbed by the body. Contains significant amounts of sodium so, if used frequently, the limiting of other high sodium sources should be considered.

DESCRIPTION An extract of beef and vegetables, Bonox is a thick liquid paste.

ORIGIN AND HISTORY Bonox is commercially produced.

BUYING AND STORAGE Readily available and keeps well if stored tightly capped.

PREPARATION AND USE Add 1 teaspoon to 1 cup of hot water to make a nutritious beverage. It may also be added to soups and stews.

SEE ALSO Beef Extract.

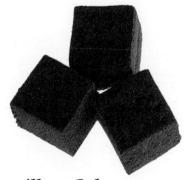

Bouillon Cube

Major Nutrients Serve Size 2 g

Energy	20 kJ	Potassium	50 mg
Protein	less than 1 g	Phosphorus	35 mg
Sodium	100 mg		

Nutritional Information A moderate source of phosphorus and folate. Adds flavour but also adds significant amounts of sodium to finished food. Contains significant amounts of naturally occurring amines.

Description Dried flavouring.

Origin and History Bouillon is one of the basic elements of French cookery.

Buying and Storage Can be bought as dried bouillon or stock cubes or as a powder in cans or jars. Keeps well in a cool dry place.

Preparation and Use Beef, veal or chicken bones are simmered with onions, carrots, celery and bouquet garni to develop a rich stock. After long, slow cooking, bouillon is strained and becomes the classic stock used in casseroles, soups and sauces.

The strained, freshly made liquid can be refrigerated for use in a few days or frozen.

Powdered bouillon and stock cubes should be dissolved in hot water before use.

See Also Consomme.

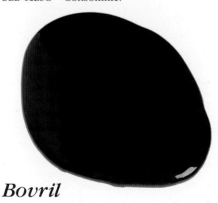

Bovril

Major Nutrients Serve Size 10 g

Energy	70 kJ	Phosphorus	60 mg
Protein	4 g	Iron	1.5 mg
Fat	0	Thiamin	1 mg
Carbohydrate		Riboflavin	0.7 mg
	less than 1 g	Niacin Equiv.	8.4 mg
Sodium	480 mg		

Nutritional Information An excellent source of iron, riboflavin and niacin. Contains large amounts of sodium. The iron, thiamin and riboflavin levels make it a very useful source of these for the diet if other sodium intakes are controlled. Contains large amounts of naturally occurring amines.

Description A commercially prepared beef essence in liquid form.

Origin and History 'Bovril' is a trade name.

Buying and Storage Readily available as a bottled essence that will keep indefinitely if kept tightly capped.

Preparation and Use Used in making beef tea, gravy and soup, and as a flavouring agent in soups and beef dishes.

Brandy Flavouring

Nutritional Information This is not significant nutritionally; contains significant amounts of naturally occurring salicylates.

Description This is a mixture of vanillin, imitation Jamaica rum, oil of cognac, and various chemicals.

Origin and History An imitation essence.

Buying and Storage Readily available and keeps indefinitely.

Preparation and Use Use sparingly in cakes, biscuits and confectionery.

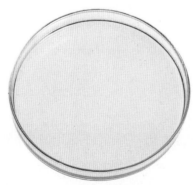

Butterscotch Topping

Major Nutrients Serve Size 20 g

Energy	270 kJ	Sodium	35 mg
Protein	2 g	Potassium	100 mg
Fat	2 g	Calcium	65 mg
Cholesterol	10 mg	Phosphorus	55 mg
Carbohydrate	12 g	Riboflavin	0.15 mg
Total Sugars	12 g		

Nutritional Information A moderate source of calcium, phosphorus and riboflavin.

May contain Food Code Additive Number 150.

Description A rich flavouring made from brown sugar and butter.

Origin and History Butterscotch is a popular hard toffee, possibly of Scottish origin. The imitation flavour is a mixture of oil of lovage, vanillin, oil of lemon, and chemical ingredients.

Buying and Storage Keeps indefinitely in a cool dry place if tightly capped.

Preparation and Use Boil together brown sugar, egg yolk and milk, then add butter and vanilla to make a thick, rich, hot sauce.

Use straight from the bottle over ice cream, waffles and in sundaes.

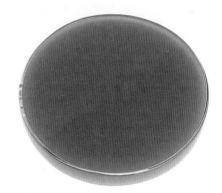

Caramel

Nutritional Information No significant nutritional contribution to the diet.

Food Additive Code Number 150.

Description Caramel is a brown colourant made from controlled heat treatment of carbohydrates such as dextrose, sucrose and malt syrup.

Origin and History There are several kinds: acid-proof caramel which is used in carbonated beverages and acidified solutions; bakers' and confectioners' caramel; dried caramel. Imitation caramel is a mixture of heliotrope, vanillin, alcohol, oil of mace or nutmeg, oil of lemon, oil of orange and chemicals.

Buying and Storage Readily available. It keeps indefinitely.

Preparation and Use Used as a flavouring and colouring agent in soups, gravies, puddings etc. Used commercially in sauces, vinegars, wines, beers, colas and baked products. Also used for coating moulds for a kind of custard pudding, in which case sugar is cooked to an amber colour.

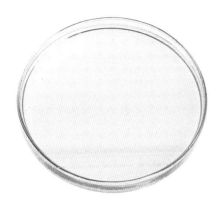

Citrus Fruit Essences

NUTRITIONAL INFORMATION No significant nutritional contribution to the diet.

Food Additive Code Number 330. Contains significant amounts of naturally occurring salicylates.

DESCRIPTION Made from the essential oils found in the peel of the fruit, in the blossoms, leaves, and twigs of the plant.

ORIGIN AND HISTORY The most common citrus fruits used are oranges, grapefruit, lemons, limes, tangerines, mandarins and bergamots.

BUYING AND STORAGE Stocked by specialty food stores, essences keep indefinitely if kept tightly capped.

PREPARATION AND USE A strong flavouring, essences should be used in very small quantities for cakes, pastries, confectionery and soft drinks.

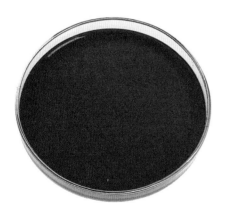

Cochineal

NUTRITIONAL INFORMATION No significant nutritional contribution to the diet.
Food Additive Code Number 120.

DESCRIPTION The cochineal insect is used to prepare a magnificent red dye called carmine.

ORIGIN AND HISTORY In Central America, the female insect is collected between ferti-

lisation and complete development of the egg. It is put into the oven on metal sheets for a few minutes or plunged into boiling water and then dried.

BUYING AND STORAGE Cochineal is purchased in small bottles from food stores and lasts indefinitely if kept tightly sealed.

PREPARATION AND USE Used sparingly as a colouring in cooking, cake making and cake icing.

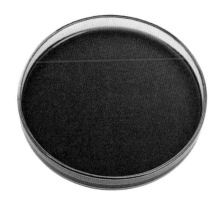

Coffee Essence

NUTRITIONAL INFORMATION No significant contribution to the diet.

DESCRIPTION Concentrated essence extracted from ground, roast coffee.

ORIGIN AND HISTORY The coffee is steeped in boiling water and alcohol, brewed and distilled.

BUYING AND STORAGE The essence will keep indefinitely if tightly capped.

PREPARATION AND USE Used as a flavouring for beverages, baked goods and confectionery.

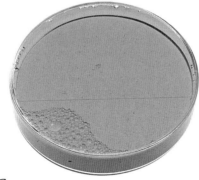

Consomme

MAJOR NUTRIENTS		SERVE SIZE 100 mL	
Energy	55 kJ	Carbohydrate	1 g
Protein	2 g	Sodium	330 mg
Fat	0	Potassium	55 mg

NUTRITIONAL INFORMATION Contains

moderate amounts of sodium if a commercial product is used. Homemade consomme without added salt would have less sodium.

DESCRIPTION Consomme is meat or chicken stock that has been enriched, reduced and clarified.

ORIGIN AND HISTORY In the classic French style, consomme is made twice, once from stock using bones, the second time adding meat to the strained stock. It must be totally clear and naturally coloured by the meat.

BUYING AND STORAGE Available in cans from food stores and keeps indefinitely.

If prepared at home, it must be refrigerated, when it will keep for a few days, or it can be frozen, preferably in small lots.

PREPARATION AND USE Consomme is prepared from basic beef, veal or chicken stock and is further cooked with the meat or chicken that gives the consomme its name, i.e. beef consomme, chicken consomme. These soups may be served either hot or cold. Consomme also forms the basis for many soups bearing the name, such as Celestine with shredded crepes, Madrilene with tomato, and Crécy with carrots. It is added to classic sauces that require a rich base. Consomme can also be further reduced to make aspics.

PROCESSING Made by first simmering bones with vegetables in water until all the goodness is extracted from the bones to make a rich stock. This stock is strained and forms the base for the consomme. Meat and vegetables are cooked in the stock to further enrich it and egg whites are added to clarify it.

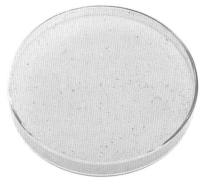

Court Bouillon

NUTRITIONAL INFORMATION Similar to Bouillon Cube.

DESCRIPTION A seasoned, slightly acidulated broth for the cooking of fish but also of meat and vegetables.

ORIGIN AND HISTORY Traditional recipe.

BUYING AND STORAGE Available in solid cubes which keep for several months if stored in a cool dry place.

PREPARATION AND USE Made with water, seasonings, onions, carrots, herbs and wine, vinegar or lemon juice. The food may be cooked in the liquid, or may be boiled with the other ingredients for a given time, then strained.

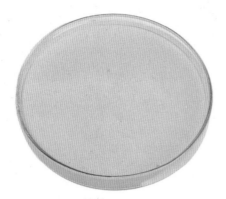

Fish Stock

MAJOR NUTRIENTS		SERVE SIZE 100 G	
Energy	110 kJ	Sodium	650 mg
Protein	4 g	Potassium	110 mg
Carbohydrate	2 g	Niacin Equiv.	1.5 mg

NUTRITIONAL INFORMATION A moderate source of niacin. Contains large amounts of sodium. Homemade stock without added salt would have less sodium.

DESCRIPTION Stock made from whole fish or fish bones.

ORIGIN AND HISTORY A traditional recipe.

BUYING AND STORAGE Commercially available for restaurant use. Store in original container and keep tightly sealed.

PREPARATION AND USE The stock can be homemade from fish bones, vegetables and seasonings. Use as a base for sauces and aspics.

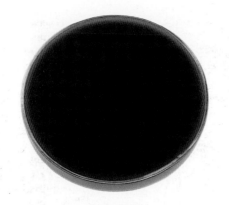

Glacé de Viande

MAJOR NUTRIENTS		SERVE SIZE 10 G	
Energy	110 kJ	Sodium	650 mg
Protein	4 g	Potassium	110 mg
Carbohydrate	2 g	Niacin Equiv.	1.4 mg

NUTRITIONAL INFORMATION This is not used frequently enough to be a primary source in the diet.

DESCRIPTION Strong stock made from meat, poultry or game that is boiled down, or reduced, to produce a brown syrup that becomes a firm jelly when cold.

ORIGIN AND HISTORY A traditional recipe.

BUYING AND STORAGE Can be purchased under commercial names but is usually homemade. Store in the refrigerator and use within a few days.

PREPARATION AND USE A small amount of meat glaze can be added to gravy or sauce to strengthen flavour or it can be dissolved in hot water and used in place of stock. It can also be melted down to be used for brushing over cold tongue etc.

A mock glaze can be made by stiffening a clear brown stock with gelatine.

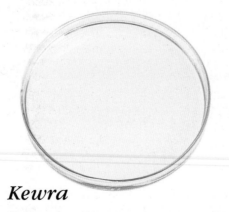

Kewra

NUTRITIONAL INFORMATION No significant nutritional contribution to the diet.

DESCRIPTION A concentrated flower essence.

ORIGIN AND HISTORY Kewra is Hindi for *Pandanus odoratissimus*, a variety of screwpine (see Pandan Leaf in Herbs and Spices). On holidays and special occasions in India, kewra and rose essence are combined in sweet dishes.

BUYING AND STORAGE Sold as a concentrate or essence in specialty Indian food stores, it will keep indefinitely in an airtight container in the cupboard.

PREPARATION AND USE Kewra is so strong only a drop or two is needed for most recipes. The vanilla of the East, it is used mainly in sweet dishes and ice creams; however on festive occasions it flavours colourful rice dishes such as korma pilau and biriani.

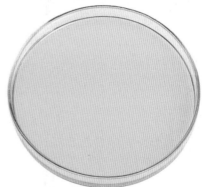

Lemon Essence

NUTRITIONAL INFORMATION No significant nutritional contribution to the diet.

Contains significant amounts of naturally occurring salicylates.

DESCRIPTION Lemon essence is manufactured from the oil expressed from lemon rind, and alcohol.

ORIGIN AND HISTORY A traditional essence.

BUYING AND STORAGE Available in specialty food stores. Keeps indefinitely if stored tightly capped in a cool dark place.

PREPARATION AND USE Most extensively used in bakery products and widely applied in the manufacture of beverages and ice cream.

PROCESSING In the case of the best oil, slices of peel are bent back and the oil which oozes out in drips is collected in a sponge. Every so often the sponge is squeezed and the oil flows into a special container.

Inferior grades of this oil are collected from the peel by pressure, the peel being placed in a press which breaks the oil cells and frees the oil. The cheapest grade is collected by distillation.

a press which breaks the oil cells and frees the oil. The cheapest grade is collected by distillation.

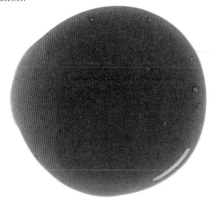

Malt Extract

MAJOR NUTRIENTS		SERVE SIZE 10 G	
Energy	20 kJ	Sodium	10 mg
Protein	0	Potassium	23 mg
Fat	0	Iron	1.1 mg
Carbohydrate	1 g	Zinc	0.9 mg
Dietary Fibre	0	Niacin Equiv.	1 mg

NUTRITIONAL INFORMATION   A good source of iron; moderate source of zinc and niacin. Contains significant amounts of naturally occurring amines.

DESCRIPTION   A dark brown extract.

ORIGIN AND HISTORY   Malt is the name given to barley after it has germinated and the germ has been removed from the grain. The grain starch is converted into sugar known as maltos which results in pure malt.

BUYING AND STORAGE   Available in cans and bottles, it keeps indefinitely.

PREPARATION AND USE   Mainly used for brewing beer and distilling spirits, it also makes a highly nutritious beverage when mixed with hot water. The amber variety is used to make malt extract and various foods for babies and invalids.

VARIETIES
Amber (pale yellow) malt.

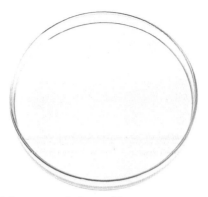

Maraschino Essence

NUTRITIONAL INFORMATION   No significant nutritional contribution to the diet.

DESCRIPTION   Sweet essence made from marasca cherries.

ORIGIN AND HISTORY   The cherry is bleached, pitted, steeped in a syrup of sugar, water, oil of bitter almond, and food colouring, then distilled. Originally made only in Yugoslavia, it is now also produced in Italy and Holland.

BUYING AND STORAGE   Sometimes available in specialty food stores. Keeps well if tightly capped and stored in a cupboard.

PREPARATION AND USE   Used in flavouring certain sweet dishes.

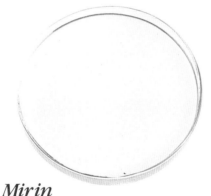

Mirin

MAJOR NUTRIENTS		SERVE SIZE 10 ML	
Energy	40 kJ	Alcohol	1 g
Protein	0	Sodium	0
Fat	0	Potassium	10 mg
Carbohydrate			
	less than 1 g		

NUTRITIONAL INFORMATION   Contains significant amounts of naturally occurring amines.

DESCRIPTION   A sweetened, viscous sherry-like rice wine used in Japanese cooking. It is low in alcohol.

ORIGIN AND HISTORY   Mirin does not have a long or inspired history, it is simply a sweet alcoholic liquor created to add a specific flavour to Japanese cooking. The Japanese are known to favour sweet foods, and a step up from simply adding sugar was to add the aroma and unique taste of a sweet liquor.

BUYING AND STORAGE   Sold in bottles in Japanese food stores, it is rarely stocked in wine or liquor stores. It will keep indefinitely after opening, although in humid climates refrigeration is recommended.

PREPARATION AND USE   It is used to add a rich, sweet flavour and a shiny gloss to sauces and some other Japanese foods. In most instances, the alcohol is burned off by boiling the mirin before use, leaving just the residual sweet flavour. In Japanese cooking it is combined with soy sauce and sugar, and sometimes sake, to give a rich brown sauce or stock with a characteristic Japanese flavour. It can replace Chinese wine in stir-fried dishes, where a little additional sweetness would be appropriate.

SEE ALSO   Rice Wine, Cooking.

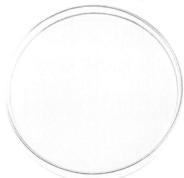

Orange Blossom Essence

also called *Neroli*

NUTRITIONAL INFORMATION   No significant nutritional contribution to the diet. No analysis available.

DESCRIPTION   Essential oil extracted from the blossoms of the bitter orange, *Citrus aurantium* (bigarade, Seville, sour orange). It is yellowish in colour with an intense aroma and a slightly bitter but aromatic flavour.

ORIGIN AND HISTORY   The bitter orange is native to South-East Asia and was introduced to the Arab world in the latter part of the first century AD. It entered Europe by two means — the Moors who entered Spain from AD 712 (hence the Seville orange), and the Crusaders, active from the 11th to 14th centuries.

Perfume was widely used in antiquity in the Far East, Middle East, Greece and Rome, and its use in Europe was revived by the Crusaders. The blossoms of the bitter orange were soon added to the perfumer's list. The name 'neroli' is derived from the Italian princess, Anne Marie de la Tremoille of Neroli, who is said to have discovered it. As with many essential oils used in perfumery, orange blossom essence was adopted as a food flavouring.

Today neroli is mainly produced in southern France, Spain, Italy, Syria, Algeria, Venezuela and Paraguay.

BUYING AND STORAGE Purchase from specialty food stores and pharmacies. Keep tightly sealed and store in a cool place away from direct light.

PREPARATION AND USE Because of its strength, use by the drop until the right flavour balance is achieved. Use for scenting confectionery, pastries, creams, sorbets, custards and pancake batters. It can be used in place of orange flower water in traditional Middle Eastern pastries and puddings, providing it is used in drops rather than by the teaspoonful.

SEE ALSO Orange; Orange Flower Water.

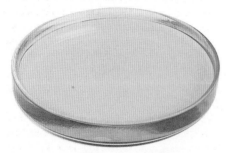

Orange Flower Water

NUTRITIONAL INFORMATION No significant nutritional contribution to the diet.

Contains significant amounts of naturally occurring salicylates.

DESCRIPTION Extracted from orange blossoms by steam distillation to form an aromatic liquid with a subtle orange blossom flavour. The strongly scented flowers of the bitter orange, *Citrus aurantium* (bigarade, Seville, sour orange), are used, but it is also produced from the blossoms of the sweet orange, *Citrus sinensis*.

ORIGIN AND HISTORY The bitter orange, native to South-East Asia, reached Persia and the Arab world via India during the latter part of the 1st century AD. As rose water had long been used from ancient times in the Middle East, the fragrant blossoms of this new fruit were natural candidates for a similar distillation.

Orange flower water is produced and used in Lebanon, Syria, Turkey and Greece,

countries where the orange flourishes. While the bitter orange blossoms are preferred for extraction of the essence, the sweet oranges are more widely grown. As all citrus trees shed a large proportion of their blooms, sheets are spread on the ground to catch the blossoms from the sweet oranges, and these are combined with the bitter orange blossoms for distillation.

BUYING AND STORAGE Orange flower water is available from Middle Eastern and Greek food stores. It is a clear liquid, although some brands are lightly tinged with an orange food dye. The more expensive orange flower waters usually have a better flavour.

Keep tightly sealed in its bottle in a cool place away from direct light.

PREPARATION AND USE Use to flavour syrups, pastries, puddings, ice creams and water ices of Middle Eastern or Greek origin. Orange flower water is a favourite flavouring for Turkish delight. Use by the teaspoonful until the right balance of flavour is achieved — some recipes could use 3–4 teaspoons. However, if orange blossom essence (neroli) is used as a substitute, it must be added in drops because it is so concentrated in flavour.

SEE ALSO Orange; Orange Blossom Essence; Rose Water.

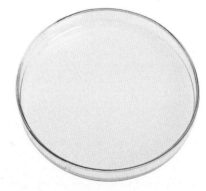

Peppermint Essence

NUTRITIONAL INFORMATION No significant nutritional contribution to the diet.

DESCRIPTION The essence is made from the essential oil of peppermint, distilled from the leaves of the plant.

ORIGIN AND HISTORY Peppermint was used in biblical times.

The high menthol content of peppermint accounts for a characteristic sensation of coolness which invades the mouth after the original pungency has died away. Black peppermint is the kind most grown in the USA because it yields more oil, of which the USA is the world's biggest producer, supplying nearly three-quarters of the total demand.

White peppermint is less hardy and less productive, but its oil has a more delicate flavour and commands a higher price.

BUYING AND STORAGE Available in most food stores, bottled essence keeps a long time stored in a cool dry place.

PREPARATION AND USE Add to sweet confections such as peppermint cream, cake icings and liqueurs. It complements chocolate well.

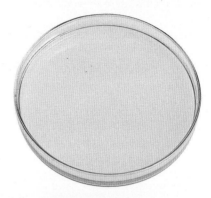

Pineapple Essence

NUTRITIONAL INFORMATION No significant nutritional contribution to the diet.

DESCRIPTION Essence derived from the peel and pulp of the fruit.

ORIGIN AND HISTORY The pineapple is cultivated throughout the tropical regions of the world. Fully ripe pineapples are sliced, mixed with unsweetened pineapple juice and alcohol, then distilled.

BUYING AND STORAGE Available in bottles from specialty food stores, the essence will keep well if tightly capped.

PREPARATION AND USE Used in soft drinks, confectionery and baked goods.

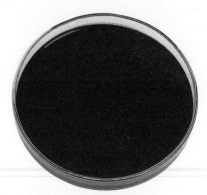

Raspberry Essence

NUTRITIONAL INFORMATION No significant nutritional contribution to the diet. Contains significant amounts of naturally occurring salicylates.

DESCRIPTION Essence made from ripe raspberries.

ORIGIN AND HISTORY Ripe raspberries are sorted by hand and the fruit is washed with care. The juice is expressed from the fruit and immediately processed to yield a concentrate or essence.

Frozen fruit may be used. To prevent deterioration of flavour and for brilliancy of colour, alcohol is added to partially defrosted fruit.

BUYING AND STORAGE Bottled raspberry essence is available from specialty food stores and will keep for a long time if kept tightly capped.

PREPARATION AND USE Use straight from the bottle to flavour drinks, confectionery, baked goods and alcoholic beverages.

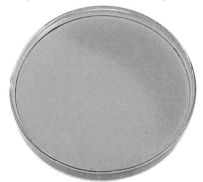

Rice Wine, Cooking

MAJOR NUTRIENTS		SERVE SIZE 25 G	
Fat	0	Sodium	2 mg
Cholesterol	0		

NUTRITIONAL INFORMATION The values of the other nutrients are either not available or nutritionally insignificant.

DESCRIPTION Wine brewed from rice. The Japanese sake is a clear, pure wine, low in alcohol, and with a mild, pleasant flavour, the better quality ones having a slightly lemony flavour. Chinese shao hsing is a golden colour, and has a pungent, brewed flavour rather like malt whisky.

ORIGIN AND HISTORY Sake is Japan's most ancient beverage. Its origins are in the mythological past where it was said it was first made by a miko or shrine maiden who chewed rice until it fermented. In ancient Japanese script the words 'make sake' are synonymous with kasosu, the word for chew. Chewing rice as the first stage of sake making was practised until recently in Tohoku, northern Honshu, and in Okinawa and Taiwan. Sake was originally known as shiroki or white sake, as it was a cloudy unfiltered fermentation that was previously drunk. Kuroki was a greyish-black sake coloured by the ash added to counter its acidic taste.

Sake, shao hsing and other Chinese wines are brewed by fermentation in much the same way as beer is made. Rice is the most commonly used grain, but the Chinese also use wheat and their ancient grain millet, to make a wine known as shu. Even in antiquity there was much attention paid to the brewing of wine. A Later Han dictionary, *Shih-ming*, says that grain wine could be made overnight. This was disputed by the 6th century writing of Chia Ssu-hsieh, stating that the fermentation of a clear wine is a very complicated process and takes a much longer time. A 2nd century writer describes two kinds of wines, li and chiu (the latter the name still applied to Chinese wine). Li was sweet and white, chiu darker and stronger.

Chinese wines have been flavoured and coloured by a wide variety of ingredients including whole birds and exotic animals, various leaves and flowers, fagara pepper, ginger, honey and saffron. At one stage wines were made with water from limestone caves to counter their high acidity. Wisteria seeds were added to some wines to prevent them spoiling.

BUYING AND STORAGE Both sake and Chinese rice wine can be purchased in licensed supermarkets and liquor stores. In hot, humid climates it is advisable to store them in a cool place. They will keep indefinitely, although their intensity of flavour, particularly that of sake, diminishes with age.

PREPARATION AND USE The Japanese technique of sake steaming introduces the unique flavour of sake into solid foods, but the most important use of sake in Japanese cooking is in sauces where it imparts an intense flavour and sweetness, and induces a shiny glaze.

Chinese wines, of which the shaohsing yellow rice wine is probably the best for cooking, are added to marinades and are splashed into the hot wok to add their particular aroma and sweet pungency to most stir-fried dishes. Several Chinese dishes popular in the north are called drunken, because the food is steeped for lengthy periods in wine.

VARIETIES
Sake (Japan); shao hsing chiew (Shao shing rice wine; China).

SEE ALSO Sake.

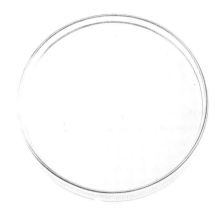

Rose Water

*also called **Attar**, **Golab**, **Ma'el ward***

NUTRITIONAL INFORMATION No analysis available, but makes no significant nutritional contribution to the diet.

DESCRIPTION An essence distilled from fragrant rose petals.

ORIGIN AND HISTORY Rose water is used in Balkan, Middle Eastern and Indian cookery, particularly in sweet dishes, creams and cakes. In Asia and the Middle East it is sprinkled over desserts and fresh fruit and used as a flavouring in the Greek cookies, kourabiedes. It is an important ingredient of Turkish delight.

BUYING AND STORAGE Rose water essence is a concentrate available from chemists. Rose water is available at Middle Eastern and Greek food stores. Both will keep indefinitely but will lose strength on standing. Freshly made rose water will keep for a few days in a cool place or in a refrigerator.

PREPARATION AND USE The essence or concentrate should be used in drops for flavouring both savoury and sweet dishes, including curries and jellies. Add to fingerbowls when serving shellfish or unpeeled fresh fruit. Use to flavour milk drinks.

PROCESSING Fill a pan with fresh, scented petals, preferably from the pink damask rose, barely cover them with water and bring to simmering point for a few minutes. Leave to cool slightly, then strain.

SEE ALSO Turkish Delight.

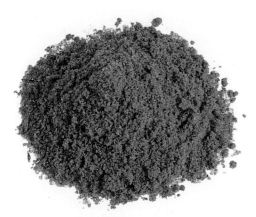

Stock Powder

MAJOR NUTRIENTS　　　　　　SERVE SIZE **5** G

Energy	50 kJ	Carbohydrate	
Protein	2 g		less than 1 g
Fat	0	Sodium	500 mg
		Potassium	70 mg

NUTRITIONAL INFORMATION Contains large amounts of sodium. Sodium based flavour boosters should be used with discretion in sodium-controlled diets. Contains significant amounts of naturally occurring amines.

DESCRIPTION A powder made from a meat, chicken, fish or onion base, flavoured by vegetables, herbs and spices, salt and sugar.

ORIGIN AND HISTORY Sometimes called bouillon, stock powder was originally made for the catering trade.

BUYING AND STORAGE Available in supermarkets and food stores under several commercial brand names, the powder should be kept in the original airtight container in a dry state.

PREPARATION AND USE Always use a dry spoon, as moisture will make the powder go lumpy. Allow 1–2 teaspoons to each 250 mL of hot water.

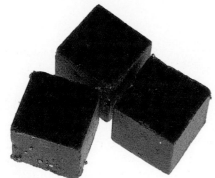

Stock Cube

MAJOR NUTRIENTS　　　　　　SERVE SIZE **5** G

Energy	50 kJ	Carbohydrate	
Protein	2 g		less than 1 g
Fat	0	Sodium	500 mg
		Potassium	70 mg

NUTRITIONAL INFORMATION Contains large amounts of sodium. Sodium based flavour boosters should be used with discretion in sodium-controlled diets. Contains significant amounts of naturally occurring amines.

DESCRIPTION A highly concentrated extract of beef, mushrooms or garlic, prepared with other ingredients such as flavour enhancer, salt, sugar, yeast extract, herbs and spices and natural colouring, and then thickened. The extracts are compounded into a moist cube which is sealed.

ORIGIN AND HISTORY One of the main foods carried by explorers and travellers in early America was 'portable soup', a concentrated stock made from veal trimmings and pigs' trotters, a forerunner of the stock cube.

BUYING AND STORAGE Readily available under several brand names from supermarkets and food stores, the stock cubes should be kept in a sealed container in the cupboard.

PREPARATION AND USE Mix 1–2 stock cubes in 250 mL of hot water. The stock can then be used in soups and stews.

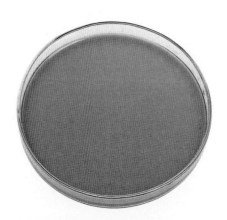

Strawberry Essence

NUTRITIONAL INFORMATION No significant nutritional contribution to the diet.

DESCRIPTION An essence made from ripe strawberries.

ORIGIN AND HISTORY A traditional recipe.

BUYING AND STORAGE Available in small bottles from specialty food stores. Keep tightly capped and store in a cool dark place.

PREPARATION AND USE Use to flavour desserts, confectionery, baked goods and beverages.

PROCESSING The berries are picked in the morning and thoroughly washed. They may be mixed with alcohol either before or immediately after grinding. The juice is expressed by vacuum distillation.

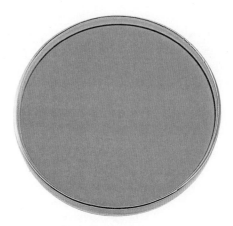

Vanilla Essence

NUTRITIONAL INFORMATION No significant nutritional contribution to the diet.

DESCRIPTION An essence made from the vanilla bean.

ORIGIN AND HISTORY A native of Central America, vanilla was introduced to Europe by the Spaniards in the 16th century. However, it took more than three centuries to learn how to grow the plant outside Mexico. It was thought the spirit of Montezuma had rendered it infertile in the hands of white men. Finally it was discovered that the plant needed the tiny melipona bee to ensure cross-pollination. It was later found that cross-pollination could be done by hand. Now vanilla is mainly produced in Madagascar and Tahiti.

BUYING AND STORAGE Pure vanilla has a delicate, yet mellow aroma. The imitation has a heavy, grassy odour. Keeps indefinitely if tightly capped and stored in the cupboard.

PREPARATION AND USE The pure vanilla essence is very powerful and only a few drops are needed. Its fragrance enhances a variety of sweet dishes, cakes and drinks. Its flavour is detected in chocolate, confectionery and several liqueurs.

PROCESSING Vanilla beans are fermented or cured to develop their characteristic flavour and aroma. During this process, a crystalline substance, vanillin, forms on the outside of the pods.

DRESSINGS AND VINEGARS

This chapter examines accompaniments to foods which are interesting food sources in themselves. Dressings are principally made up of oils and vinegars, with other ingredients such as eggs or flavourings added. They can be used as the base of marinades, poured over food as a sauce or they aid as an incorporating agent in salads.

A national survey of Australians in the 1980s indicated that approximately 40% of salad dressings were consumed as mayonnaise, of which 90% were in a light (lower fat) style. A further 16% were consumed as coleslaw and thousand island style dressings. Of the oil based dressings, 22% were homemade.

Standards for the fat content of dressings are not prescribed in Australia. Many imported dressings contain over 30% fat.

The profile of the fat content can vary, depending on the price and availability of vegetable oils. The dressings found in the United States are generally based on soya bean. The Australasian dressings contain sunflower or cottonseed oil.

The energy content for low energy dressings is on average less than one-tenth of that of conventional dressings. No-oil dressings on average have slightly higher energy levels than low energy dressings.

Sodium content ranges from moderate to very high, in salad dressings. Cholesterol levels vary depending upon whether milk, cheese or eggs are present.

The supermarket shelves carry an ever increasing number of salad dressings. Almost all are made from oils which are predominantly polyunsaturated.

Manufacturers have provided for the consumers who wish to reduce their fat and salt intakes, and when these products carry nutritional labelling they allow the consumer to make an informed choice.

Some of the more exotic vinegars are sufficient to enhance a salad without the use of oils. Although vinegars provide a variety of flavours, they are not of nutritional significance in the diet.

The world annual production of vinegar has been estimated at 10 million hectalitres, about 30% of which is bottled for home use. The major world type, mostly produced in Europe and North America, is distilled vinegar produced from diluted purified ethanol or fusel oils containing crude spirit from grain beer distillations.

Vinegar is used to produce pickles, salad dressings, mustards and mayonnaise and to acidify other foods. Vinegar may be sweetened, spiced and flavoured. There is also an imitation vinegar which is prepared by mixing water and acetic acid.

The nutritional information on the varieties of vinegars is very fragmentary, therefore nutritional information covering cider and distilled vinegars in general is given here, rather than with individual entries.

MAJOR NUTRIENTS — SERVE SIZE 20 G

CIDER		DISTILLED	
Energy	12 kJ	Energy	10 kJ
Protein	0	Protein	0
Fat	0	Fat	0
Carbohydrate	1 g	Carbohydrate	0.6 g
Cholesterol	0	Cholesterol	0
Sodium	0	Sodium	0

NUTRITIONAL INFORMATION Vinegars are 94–96% water and are mostly carbohydrate. Vinegar contains about 5 g of acetic acid per 100 mL. Chinese sweet vinegar probably has a much higher carbohydrate content.

Balsamic Vinegar

DESCRIPTION Balsamic vinegar has a rich mellow flavour and a pleasing aroma. It is made from unfermented Trebbiano (white wine grape variety). The vinegar is similar to sherry and is reddish-brown in colour. Some balsamic vinegars are more viscous than others, depending on the mother vinegar and the age of the vinegar.

ORIGIN AND HISTORY Made in Modena, Italy, it is aged in small wooden barrels for no less than 5 years; some have been aged for more than 150 years. The barrels are stacked in a pyramid with the youngest vinegar at the top and the oldest at the bottom. A system of syphoning is used to transfer the maturing vinegars from the top barrels to the bottom barrels, over a period of years. Theoretically each level of barrels has a little of the next oldest vinegar in it, and all have a little of the oldest vinegar. The quality of balsamic vinegar, and some say it is the best vinegar in the world, depends on the age and the quality of the original wine and the type of barrel or 'vessel' used to hold the vinegar. The vinegar is transferred to barrels made from mulberry, chestnut, juniper, oak and cherry, depending on the stage of maturation of the vinegar. Balsamic vinegar is 20 years old before it is bottled for sale, and will continue to mature in the bottle. The vinegar makers of Modena are very proud of their vinegars, and usually the craft is handed down through the family.

BUYING AND STORAGE The price of balsamic vinegar depends on age and which factory it comes from. It keeps for years and matures like wine.

PREPARATION AND USE Used as an accompaniment with berries, particularly strawberries. Dip each berry in a small bowl of balsamic vinegar. It has a cleansing effect on the palate. Useful for deglazing the pan after cooking meats. Can be used as a salad dressing which should only be added at the table because it discolours the greens.

WINE VINEGAR

BALSAMIC VINEGAR

LEMON VINEGAR

DILL VINEGAR

CIDER VINEGAR

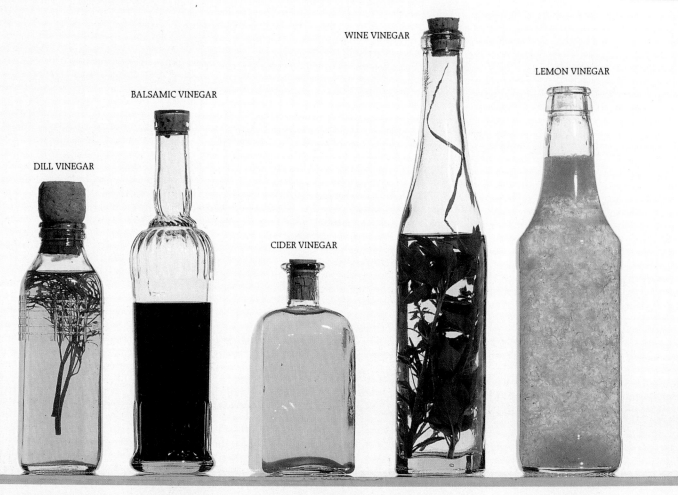

TARRAGON VINEGAR

GARLIC VINEGAR

RASPBERRY VINEGAR

MALT VINEGAR

RICE VINEGAR, WHITE

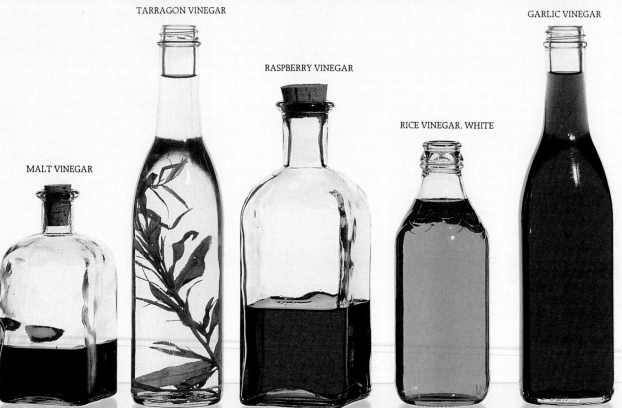

LEMON BALM VINEGAR

ROSEMARY VINEGAR

SWEET VINEGAR, CHINESE

GREEN PEPPERCORN VINEGAR

MAYONNAISE

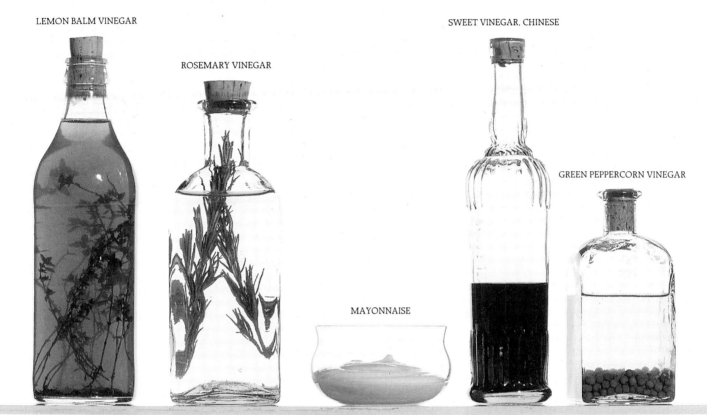

CHILLI VINEGAR

VINAIGRETTE

RED VINEGAR, CHINESE

SHERRY VINEGAR

BLACK VINEGAR

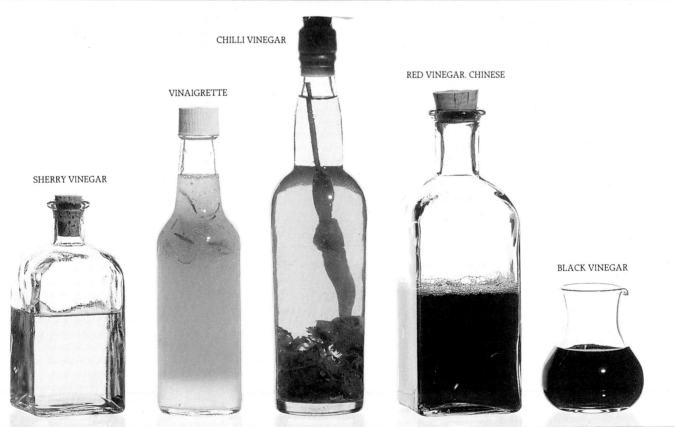

Black Vinegar

DESCRIPTION Chinese black (or brown) vinegar is dark in colour, mild in flavour.

ORIGIN AND HISTORY Like white vinegar, black vinegar has been used as a Chinese seasoning for many centuries. Although some black vinegars are fermented from rice, with colouring added to darken them, they are more often made from glutinous rice, wheat, millet or sorghum which give a more definite flavour. Some of the better dark vinegars have an impressive complexity of flavours ranging from smoky to winelike.

BUYING AND STORAGE Sold in bottles, usually with shaker tops, it can be kept for many months after opening, although the intensity of flavour and aroma will slowly dissipate.

PREPARATION AND USE In central, and parts of northern China, black vinegar is splashed into almost every dish. It gives a special zing to sauces, and a pleasant tang.

Chilli Vinegar

DESCRIPTION White wine vinegar is infused with whole chillies to produce chilli vinegar.

ORIGIN AND HISTORY Chillies arrived in Europe from South America with returning Spanish conquistadors. The vinegar probably originated in Spain, where chillies are an essential ingredient in many dishes.

BUYING AND STORAGE Store in a cool cupboard or pantry. Keeps indefinitely.

PREPARATION AND USE Prepare by infusing 4–6 chillies in white wine vinegar for 5–6 weeks.

Use in a hot spicy salad dressing or in chutneys which are to accompany curries.

Cider Vinegar

DESCRIPTION Cider vinegar has an acidic smell and taste. It is made from cider apples, of which there are many varieties. As apples are fermented, alcohol is produced, which changes to acetic acid on the addition of mother vinegar. Home produced cider vinegar is cloudy, while commercial cider vinegar is clear due to filtering.

ORIGIN AND HISTORY Cider was made by the Anglo-Saxons (who spelt it 'seider'), and was introduced to Britain by the Phoenicians who traded with the Cornish for tin. Cider vinegar almost certainly was made during those times. The Greeks and Romans made cider as well as cider vinegar. It is very popular in North America where many recipes have been developed to enhance the distinctive flavour of cider vinegar. It is said to have curative properties for many illnesses, such as arthritis, and is also thought to be helpful in aiding weight loss.

BUYING AND STORAGE Commercially produced cider vinegar keeps indefinitely because it has been distilled.

PREPARATION AND USE Used in cooking to deglaze pan after cooking pork. It is not as strong in flavour as wine vinegar. Can be used as a substitute for rice vinegar in Chinese cooking. 25 ml cider vinegar to ½ kg flour emulates the flavour of sourdough.

SEE ALSO Apples, Sourdough.

Dill Vinegar

DESCRIPTION Dill vinegar is produced when the flower head of dill is infused in white wine vinegar.

ORIGIN AND HISTORY Dill is one of the oldest known herbs. The Egyptians recorded its use in 3000 BC. Dill vinegar originated in southern and eastern Europe.

BUYING AND STORAGE Store in pantry or cupboard away from light if used for culinary purposes. Strain the dill flower heads from the vinegar through muslin when ready to use. Purchase in specialty stores. For decorative purposes display against window light, although the vinegar can still be used for cooking. Keeps indefinitely.

PREPARATION AND USE Can be made by fusing the bruised flower heads of dill in white wine vinegar. In vinaigrette, it gives an anise flavour. Use in sauces for fish, and in yoghurt and sour cream dressings and sauces. Used for pickling cucumbers.

SEE ALSO Dill.

Garlic Vinegar

DESCRIPTION Whole cloves of garlic are infused in white wine vinegar to produce garlic vinegar. The number of cloves of garlic used, and whether they have been crushed, determines the strength of the vinegar, together with the length of infusion time.

ORIGIN AND HISTORY Garlic was cultivated by the ancient Egyptians and has been used throughout the Mediterranean for thousands of years. Garlic vinegar was made by the ancient Greeks and Romans.

BUYING AND STORAGE Store in a cool pantry. Keeps indefinitely if the garlic cloves are strained from the vinegar. Purchase from specialty food stores.

PREPARATION AND USE For a quick garlic vinegar put 2–3 cloves of crushed garlic in a bottle of vinegar for 24–48 hours.

Used mainly in salad dressings. Use in a marinade for fish and shellfish.

SEE ALSO Garlic.

Green Peppercorn Vinegar

DESCRIPTION Green peppercorn vinegar is made with white wine vinegar and fresh green peppercorns. The flavour and some of the colour from the peppercorns is transferred to the vinegar.

ORIGIN AND HISTORY Green peppercorns are the undried seeds from the plant *Piper nigrum*. The plant comes from tropical areas, but the main source of green peppercorns today is Madagascar.

BUYING AND STORAGE This vinegar keeps indefinitely if stored in a cool dark cupboard or pantry. If kept for a long period of time the peppercorns may disintegrate. Strain the peppercorns from the vinegar before use.

PREPARATION AND USE If fresh green peppercorns are not available, brined green peppercorns can be substituted in preparation.

Use in sauces for fish; in a demiglace with lamb, beef and game; in bearnaise sauce over grilled meats.

SEE ALSO Pepper.

Lemon Vinegar

DESCRIPTION The rind of lemon is used to produce this vinegar. The 'essential oil' of lemon gives the vinegar its pale yellow colour and its flavour.

ORIGIN AND HISTORY Lemons arrived in Persia from Asia in the 6th century BC. They were known in Greece in the 3rd century BC. Lemon vinegar was probably made by the Greeks and Romans.

BUYING AND STORAGE Purchase from specialty stores. Store in cool cupboard or pantry. If storing for more than 1 year, strain the lemon peel from the vinegar through muslin before it disintegrates.

PREPARATION AND USE Use in salad dressings and marinades for fish, shellfish and chicken. Use in place of vinegar in chicken cookery.

Lemon Balm Vinegar

DESCRIPTION Fresh, slightly crushed lemon balm leaves are infused in white wine vinegar to produce lemon balm vinegar. The length of time that the leaves are left in the vinegar determines the strength of the flavour.

ORIGIN AND HISTORY Lemon balm is native to southern Europe. The Romans cultivated it 2000 years ago and introduced it to Britain. Vinegar was made by the Romans and it could be safely assumed that lemon balm vinegar was also made by them.

BUYING AND STORAGE Purchase from some specialty stores. Store in a cool cupboard or pantry until the required flavour is achieved, then strain the leaves from the vinegar through muslin, and rebottle the vinegar.

PREPARATION AND USE In Belgium and Holland it is used as a flavoured vinegar in bottling pickled herrings and eels. Use in salad dressings and when grilling fish.

SEE ALSO Balm.

Malt Vinegar

DESCRIPTION Brown malt vinegar is dark brown with an acid smell and taste. A crude fermented beer is made from fermented malted barley and beech shavings. The addition of the bacterium *Mycodermia aceti*, which lives amongst the floating beech shavings, accelerates the fermentation which changes the alcohol to acetic acid. The acid content of malt vinegar is 4–5%.

White malt vinegar is brown malt vinegar which has been filtered through charcoal to remove the colouring.

ORIGIN AND HISTORY Malt vinegar is of British origin. During wartime it was used with baking soda as a raising agent in cakes and puddings.

BUYING AND STORAGE Keeps well for several years.

PREPARATION AND USE Malt vinegar is generally made commercially and is therefore distilled. Distilling increases the acid content and pasteurises it.

Used as an ingredient in Worcestershire sauce and in pickling where the colour of the vegetables is not important, e.g. pickled onions.

Mayonnaise

MAJOR NUTRIENTS		SERVE SIZE 20 G	
Energy	590 kJ	Carbohydrate	0
Protein	0	Cholesterol	8.6 mg
Fat	15 g	Sodium	70 mg

NUTRITIONAL INFORMATION Mayonnaise is a high fat food. The fat is predominantly polyunsaturated with approximately 14% saturated, 24% monounsaturated and 62% polyunsaturated fatty acids. Other nutrients are present, but not in nutritionally significant amounts. Coleslaw dressing, a more diluted form of mayonnaise, contains less than half the kilojoules and a third of the fat, but proportionately higher sodium (105 mg). The same amount of tartare sauce contains even more sodium (140 mg), and has 450 kJ.

DESCRIPTION This is an emulsion sauce made with the ingredients oil, vinegar or lemon juice, and eggs at room temperature. The unlike ingredients, i.e. oil and egg yolks, are held together in suspension by beating thoroughly, thereby breaking up the oil and water into small droplets no more than 5 microns in diameter, and incorporating air into the mixture. The oil makes up approximately 75% of the volume. This is a pale sauce about the consistency of thick cream, quite dense and savoury in taste when lemon juice or vinegar is added.

Stabilisers are added to commercial mayonnaise to prevent the breakdown of the emulsion. Breakdown can occur if the sauce is kept at too high a temperature or too close to freezing point in the refrigerator. Whole eggs, whose albumen (consisting of long protein molecules) weaves amongst the oil and water droplets, are often used as the emulsifier in recipes requiring the use of a blender. Starches are also used because of their long carbohydrate molecules. Essential oils in mustard also act as emulsifiers. Sugar is sometimes added as a flavouring. The use of stabilisers and thickeners (such as gum tragacanth, gum arabic and carob bean) changes the texture of mayonnaise.

Mayonnaise should contain 50–80% oil, 5–9% egg yolk, and the sugar and mustard content should be lower than that in the variant called salad cream.

ORIGIN AND HISTORY Mayonnaise is said to have been named after Port Mahon, Minorca, Spain. The Duc de Richelieu may have named mayonnaise after he regained the island from the English in 1756. Some say Napoleon's chef named the sauce after his Irish general MacMahon. Others say it derives its name from the French moyeunaise, from the old French word moyeu, meaning the yolk of an egg. The people of Bayonne near the Pyrenees say that it was originally called bayonnaise. It is generally agreed, however, that it originated in the Mediterranean basin where olive oil is plentiful.

BUYING AND STORAGE Store covered in the refrigerator. It should not be kept too close to the freezer section or the emulsion will break down and the oil will 'leak' out of the suspension.

PREPARATION AND USE Basic mayonnaise is made by swiftly beating steady drops of olive oil into an egg yolk flavoured with salt and a little Dijon mustard. More oil is added once the mixture thickens, and it eventually reaches a pale, gelatinous stage. After this, lemon juice or vinegar is usually added.

Mayonnaise is most popular as an accompaniment to eggs (oeufs mayonnaise), fresh salad vegetables, as a dressing for rice and pasta salads, and with cold seafood.

VARIETIES

Aioli Mayonnaise flavoured with garlic.

Coleslaw Dressing Mayonnaise with milk, sugar and water added. Water thins the dressing to a pouring consistency. It has a reduced acid content, therefore requiring refrigeration.

Rémoulade Sauce Mayonnaise with crushed anchovies added.

Salad Cream A commercial dressing which in England and Australia should contain a minimum of 25% edible vegetable oil, with not less than 1.35% egg yolk. In France, however, 50% minimum oil content is required.

Tartare Sauce Another variation using chopped gherkins and capers, with parsley, onions or olives.

Thousand Island Dressing Made with hard-boiled eggs, paprika, parsley and sweet pickles. Sugar is usually added to commercially made sauces.

Raspberry Vinegar

DESCRIPTION Raspberry vinegar, a pale transparent pink colour, is made from fresh raspberries steeped in white wine vinegar.

ORIGIN AND HISTORY This vinegar originated in the cooler, northern parts of Europe, where the raspberry was common. Raspberry vinegar was very popular with the early settlers in New England, America, who picked wild raspberries and infused them in vinegar. Raspberry vinegar was diluted with water to make a refreshing and very popular summertime drink.

BUYING AND STORAGE Store in a cool dark cupboard or pantry. It keeps indefinitely.
Purchase from specialty stores.

PREPARATION AND USE Soak fresh raspberries in white wine vinegar until the required flavour is achieved. Then strain out the raspberries through muslin.

Use as a replacement for vinegar in vinaigrette dressing. Pour a spoonful over sliced strawberries: it accentuates the flavour of the berries. Use in place of lemon when cooking veal or chicken. Served in Yorkshire with Yorkshire pudding as a dessert.

Red Vinegar, Chinese

DESCRIPTION A clear, light, orange-red

liquid with a delicate tart flavour and slight saltiness.

ORIGIN AND HISTORY Developed in wine breweries in coastal China, it remains popular in these areas and in the north.

BUYING AND STORAGE Sold in bottles, usually with shaker tops, it can be kept for several months after opening, although the peak of its flavour is lost within days of opening.

PREPARATION AND USE Red vinegar's main function is as a dip or condiment with seafoods. A tiny dish of red vinegar always appears beside a bowl of shark's fin soup or a plate of braised shark's fin, often accompanied by edible chrysanthemum petals and slivers of crisp pretzel, a cleverly contrived marriage of complementary elements. It can be used similarly with grilled and fried foods, and sprinkled over stir-fries, and it is commonly served as a dipping sauce with fried or steamed dumplings at yum cha.

Rice Vinegar, White

DESCRIPTION Japanese and Chinese white rice vinegars are a clear, very pale yellow in colour, slightly viscous and mild in flavour. They are distilled from fermented rice, using an ancient process of combining rice lees with alcohol.

ORIGIN AND HISTORY Like vinegar making in the West, rice vinegar production is an offshoot of the wine industry. Ancient Chou texts from the 12th century BC in China, make reference to liu, a seasoning that is usually interpreted as vinegar.

BUYING AND STORAGE Sold in small bottles, usually fitted with a plastic shaker cap.
Store in the refrigerator once opened as heat from the kitchen can destroy the flavour.

PREPARATION AND USE It is excellent in dressings and can replace white wine vinegars, but remember that it is mild.

VARIETIES
Japanese; Chinese.

Rosemary Vinegar

DESCRIPTION A sprig of rosemary is infused

in white wine vinegar to produce rosemary vinegar. The leaves are slightly crushed to allow the essential oils from the rosemary to steep into the vinegar.

ORIGIN AND HISTORY Rosemary originated in the Mediterranean region. It was used by the Greeks and Romans. They infused it in vinegar which was used in cooking, and also for dunking their bread during meals.

BUYING AND STORAGE Store in the pantry until the required flavour is achieved. It will keep for up to 1 year.

PREPARATION AND USE Strain the rosemary from the vinegar when ready to use.

Useful for deglazing the pan after cooking lamb. Use in sauces for fish and shellfish, in casseroled kid and rabbit dishes, in vinaigrette dressing and in mayonnaise.

Sherry Vinegar

DESCRIPTION Sherry vinegar is a beautifully mellow vinegar, named for its colour. It is rich and smooth with a slight tartness.

ORIGIN AND HISTORY Sherry vinegars, together with sherry, originated in Spain. The vinegar is aged in wooden barrels.

BUYING AND STORAGE Store in cupboard or pantry where it will keep indefinitely if it is pasteurised. If it is not pasteurised it will continue to mature and become too acidic.

PREPARATION AND USE Use in vinaigrette. It combines well with nut oils.

Sweet Vinegar, Chinese

DESCRIPTION A black-brown, slightly thick rice vinegar resembling dark soya sauce with which it should not be confused. It has a rich, sweet, spicy, caramel aroma, with a suggestion of the Chinese spices, cassia and star anise.

ORIGIN AND HISTORY Developed in southern China, sweet vinegar has a unique place in Chinese cuisine. It could be said that its primary purpose is to flavour a dish which goes under the name 'a gift from the stork' — pork knuckles and young ginger root braised in sweet vinegar. Hard boiled eggs are added to symbolise creation. During the first month after a baby is born to a Cantonese family, this dish is cooked for the confined mother to share with friends, family and relatives. Sometimes the dish is made with chicken, and the new mother is encouraged to eat as much as possible. The ginger has a toning and strengthening effect on her system, weakened by the pregnancy and childbirth.

BUYING AND STORAGE Like other vinegars, sweet rice vinegar is sold in bottles. It keeps indefinitely with no apparent loss of flavour.

PREPARATION AND USE Sweet vinegar is used in large quantities in certain slow-simmered dishes to create a strong, distinctive, sweet and spicy flavour. It goes particularly well with pork, counteracting the high fat content.

PROCESSING A rice ferment is flavoured with sugar and spices and dark vinegar is added for colour. In some, caramel gives a rich dark colour, and enhances the flavour.

Tarragon Vinegar

DESCRIPTION Fresh tarragon is infused in white wine vinegar to produce tarragon vinegar. With the delicate leaves and stem of the tarragon suspended in the pale yellow to pale green vinegar, it is most attractive looking.

ORIGIN AND HISTORY Tarragon is native to western and southern Asia, and was cultivated by the ancient Greeks and Romans. Tarragon vinegar originated with the Greeks. Today it is one of the most popular herb vinegars, particularly in France.

BUYING AND STORAGE Store like any other vinegar in a cool pantry or cupboard, although tarragon and other herbed vinegars look very attractive displayed against the window. For culinary purposes strain the tarragon from the vinegar through muslin after the required flavour is reached (after 1–12 months).

PREPARATION AND USE Slightly bruise the tarragon leaves and place in a bottle, then pour in white wine vinegar.

Use in bearnaise sauce, mayonnaise, marinades for chicken, fish and seafoods. Vinaigrette dressing is enhanced by tarragon vinegar. Use to deglaze the pan after cooking chicken.

SEE ALSO Bearnaise Sauce, Mayonnaise, Tarragon.

Vinaigrette

MAJOR NUTRIENTS		SERVE SIZE 15 G	
Energy	300 kJ	Carbohydrate	0
Protein	0	Cholesterol	0
Fat	8 g	Sodium	1.5 mg

NUTRITIONAL INFORMATION Vinaigrette is a high fat food. The fat in vinaigrette sauce is 50% polyunsaturated, 30.8% monounsaturated, and 19% saturated. Other nutrients are present, but not in nutritionally significant amounts.

DESCRIPTION Vinaigrette is classified as an emulsion. It is a mixture of vinegar and oil, with the usual proportion being 3 parts oil to 1 part vinegar, mixed by shaking them together. The emulsion, or mixture of vinegar and oil droplets, lasts for a short time, then begins to separate with the oil moving to the surface of the vinegar. The addition of mustard or crushed garlic or onion acts as an emulsifier or stabiliser. Vinaigrette is usually made from olive oil and vinegar, although lemon juice can substitute for the vinegar — it gives a sharper, more tangy flavour.

ORIGIN AND HISTORY The name vinaigrette is derived from the French vin aigre — sharp (sour) wine. The sauce originated in the Mediterranean region where olives are grown and vinegar was produced. Garlic vinaigrette originated in the south of France.

BUYING AND STORAGE Purchased vinaigrette is a combination of water, vinegar, wine vinegar and oil with flavourings such as garlic, onion, chives and sugar. After opening, store in the refrigerator because if water has been added, the acetic acid content in the vinegar may not be enough to preserve the garlic or other flavourings.

PREPARATION AND USE Vinaigrette is easily made and the combinations of garlic, chives, mustard, herbs etc. are endless. Used as a salad dressing for lettuce and other salad vegetables. Use with hot asparagus, cauliflower and steamed fish. Add chopped parsley to the sauce along with chopped capers, gherkins, mustard, salt and pepper and serve with cold beef.

SEE ALSO Olive Oil, Vinegar.

Wine Vinegar

DESCRIPTION Wine vinegar is made with the bacterium *Acetobacter aceti*, either naturally or by introduction. This bacterium forms a viscous mass, called the mother vinegar, on the surface of wine, which is either red or white, but does not contain more than 18% alcohol. The vinegar is drawn off from underneath the mother vinegar, usually by a tap in the bottom of a barrel. The bacteria will continue to reproduce and create vinegar for years in the right location, usually in a warm dark place. When vinegar is sealed from the air, the bacteria stop reproducing, therefore keeping the vinegar at a reasonably constant acid level between 4–6% acetic acid. Wine vinegar should not be confused with sour wine, where the wine has 'gone off' before the *acetobacter* has had a chance to grow and produce acetic acid. The acid content of wine vinegar is 5.5–6%.

The flavour of vinegars is not just the acetic acid (which some 'vinegars' are) but the mixture of flavours from the wines, timbers used in the barrels and volatile esters in the mixture. The quality of wine vinegar is entirely dependent on the quality of the wine used.

VARIETIES

Red Wine Vinegar

DESCRIPTION Red wine vinegar is the colour of red wine, the basis of this vinegar. It is sometimes diluted with white wine vinegar for a lighter flavour and colour. If the vinegar has been made in wooden barrels it has a smoky undertaste.

ORIGIN AND HISTORY Vinegars have been made for as long as wine has been made. The ancient Greeks and Romans used vinegars for cooking and for dunking bread during the meal. They diluted it to make a refreshing drink. The Egyptians and Israelites used it regularly. Cleopatra is supposed to have dissolved her pearls in it. It is mentioned in the Bible, and a recipe for pickling peaches comes from Apicius, a Roman gastronome of the 1st century AD.

BUYING AND STORAGE Purchase from specialty food stores. Can be homemade. Unpasteurised vinegars are living foods and they mature with age; therefore if vinegar is homemade, pasteurisation is recommended to prevent the *Acetobacter* from reproducing and making the vinegar too acidic.

PREPARATION AND USE The finest red wine vinegars come from Orléans in France. They are made by slowly allowing the vinegar to get hot, but not so hot as to evaporate the fine flavours from the wine; vinegar is drawn off and more wine is added to the barrel. The making of Orléans vinegar is a slow process, therefore the vinegar is expensive.

Use red wine vinegar in beef, lamb and game cookery. Add to the pan juices for demiglaze. It combines well with olive oil when used in a vinaigrette for a tangy green salad.

White Wine Vinegar

DESCRIPTION White wine vinegar is made with white wine and the bacterium *Acetobacter aceti*, the same way as red wine vinegar. The flavours from the wine and the barrels in which the vinegar is made give this vinegar its subtle flavours. The quality of the vinegar is entirely dependent on the quality of the wine from which it is made. The vinegar looks like white wine — a pale yellow colour. It may also be decolourised by filtering through charcoal or some other filtering system.

ORIGIN AND HISTORY White wine vinegar was made by the Romans, Egyptians and the peoples of Crete.

BUYING AND STORAGE Purchase in specialty stores and supermarkets.

PREPARATION AND USE White wine vinegar is used in mayonnaise and hollandaise sauces, in vinaigrette dressing, and in making herbed vinegars. This vinegar is particularly suited to pickling where the discolouring of malt or red wine vinegar is not desired.

FAST FOODS

The individual items in this chapter give only a small sample of the fast foods available in our cities. Fast foods are widely used and offer plenty of choice to the consumer. Their nutritional value is as varied as the products.

As a group, fast foods are high in fat and salt, and many are energy-dense. Many fried fast foods are crumbed or battered before frying, increasing the absorption of fat.

Fried foods, manufactured meats and foods encased in pastry are easier to handle as fast foods, but it is also possible to buy salads, jacket potatoes, grilled fish, sandwiches, bread rolls, bagels, pita and other breads with low fat fillings. There are leaner meat dishes such as shaslik, or hamburgers on plain bread rolls with salad.

Barbecued chicken has less fat than fried chicken, and if the skin is removed the fat level is further reduced.

Foods such as pizzas and meat pies are variable with respect to nutritional value, and the fat levels range from about 7–16%. When these foods are packaged, they often carry nutritional labelling, which should be checked before purchase.

Asian foods are very popular as fast foods. To reduce fat in these, it is best to choose boiled rice or noodles, and steamed items, like dim sims, rather than fried ones. Vegetable dishes can be eaten along with meat and chicken dishes, and baked whole fish is a nutritious choice. Chicken can be steamed or stir-fried with vegetables, rather than fried.

It is the combination of foods that counts: if one food is fatty, then a meal should include some low fat foods as well. For example, unbuttered bread rolls and salad can be eaten along with fast food.

The fruit shop is in fact a fine dealer in fast food, and fresh vegetable and fruit salads are frequently available from fruit markets and takeaways.

As a beverage to accompany fast foods, it is a good idea to choose milk drinks which are low or reduced in fat, fruit juice, or mineral water.

Fast foods are here to stay, and form a significant part of the diets of many people. It is worthwhile to consider carefully their nutritional value.

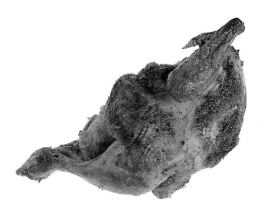

Barbecue Chicken

MAJOR NUTRIENTS		MEAT AND SKIN
	SERVE SIZE: FRONT QUARTER	
Energy	900 kJ	Phosphorus	160 mg
Protein	25 g	Magnesium	20 mg
Fat	12 g	Iron	1 mg
Cholesterol	120 mg	Zinc	1.3 mg
Carbohydrate	1 g	Vitamin A	25 µg
Total Sugars	0	Niacin Equiv.	8.8 mg
Dietary Fibre	0	Riboflavin	0.21 mg
Sodium	70 mg	Thiamin	0.05 mg
Potassium	260 mg		

NUTRITIONAL INFORMATION An excellent source of protein, phosphorus, niacin; good source of iron and riboflavin; moderate source of magnesium and thiamin; contains large amounts of fat and cholesterol.

Total energy content will depend on whether the skin and excess fats are consumed. If fat is not eaten it is a lean, low source of animal protein and associated nutrients. If skin is eaten, product is a major source of fat and therefore kilojoules and cholesterol.

DESCRIPTION Barbecue chickens are usually sold whole, with or without stuffing, or cut into halves or quarters. Cooked on a rotisserie, the chicken has crisp, brown skin. Some outlets coat the chicken with spices and salt before cooking to increase flavour and visual appeal. The chickens are removed to warmed pans after cooking and maintained at 60°C until purchase.

ORIGIN AND HISTORY Reference to chicken as a fast food occurs in a tale of Napoleon, who would often work for several hours before suddenly remembering that he had not eaten. He would demand his dinner instantly, and, to avoid his wrath, his kitchen staff would put a chicken on to roast one hour before dinner time. Every 20 minutes, another chicken would be added to the spit, so that when Napoleon called for his food, there was always one chicken ready for immediate consumption.

BUYING AND STORAGE Barbecue chicken is bought at ready-to-eat temperature, and packaged in a foil-lined bag to keep it hot. It is best eaten within 15 minutes of purchase, as food bacteria thrive in warm conditions. If the chicken has been purchased to be served cold later, use it on the same day, and allow to cool to room temperature before refrigerating. Cooked chicken will remain at its tenderest if it is not refrigerated.

PREPARATION AND USE The main point of takeaway chicken is that the preparation has already been done. It can be served with home-cooked vegetables or allowed to cool and served with salad. Chopped into portions with a cleaver, it can form the basis of such Chinese dishes as sweet and sour or lemon chicken.

PROCESSING Fresh, 9-week-old broilers are used. The cleaned, raw birds are sometimes seasoned with a special stuffing, developed for the fast food outlet. Individual preference governs the treatment of the skin — sometimes the chickens are coated with a salty mixture of herbs, spices and monosodium glutamate to add flavour, colour and crispness. Long rotisserie skewers turn the chickens slowly over a bed of charcoal or under electric elements for approximately 1½ hours until cooked.

VARIETIES
Charcoal chicken.

SEE ALSO Chicken.

Chinese Fast Food

DESCRIPTION Chinese meals are a combination of meat, vegetables and sauces, generally cooked in a wok. Takeaway Chinese food is packed in rigid plastic containers with resealable lids for convenient transport.

ORIGIN AND HISTORY In ancient China, cooking skills were highly esteemed. Lao Tze, the 6th century philosopher, experimented with plants and discovered that the vitality of vegetables was destroyed by improper cooking. Hence his followers (Taoists), based their diet on raw or partially cooked vegetables, which remain a traditional characteristic of Chinese cooking. Although the Chinese formed major ethnic communities in Australia and America during the gold rush days of the mid-19th century, their food was not appreciated until this century, when Chinese restaurants offered the first form of fast, takeaway food. Today, Chinese cuisine is the single largest ethnic food market in Australia, with approximately 27% of all restaurants specialising in Chinese or other Asian food.

BUYING AND STORAGE Chinese food should always be cooked when ordered, especially any food deep-fried in batter. Some outlets have prepared pans of Chinese food, which lose some of the fresh appeal when kept hot for some time. Most restaurants will now prepare meals without monosodium glutamate if they are requested. Although monosodium glutamate occurs naturally in many foods, the high concentration added by some Chinese cooks has been known to cause allergic reactions in asthmatics, and a discomforting condition called 'Chinese restaurant syndrome'. Like other fast foods, Chinese takeaway meals should be consumed as soon as possible after purchase. If the meal begins to cool, it can be reheated by releasing the seal of the lid and microwaving for a short time.

PREPARATION AND USE Chinese meals are fully prepared and ready to eat. It is usual to include one, two or three dishes of varying meats, and serve with fried or steamed rice.

PROCESSING Chinese meals are labour-intensive in the preparation stages, and in many restaurants most of the peeling, slicing and chopping of vegetables and meats is still done manually. Chicken, pork, lamb, beef, fish, shellfish and vegetables can be cooked in many different sauces, such as sweet and sour, black bean, oyster, satay and soya, and with varying seasonings (hence the length of the Chinese menu!). Steamed and fried rice is prepared in large quantities, while individual meal orders are cooked only upon receipt of an order.

VARIETIES
Dishes originate from Canton, Szechuan, Hainan, Shanghai, Peking, Manchuria, Fukien, Hokkien, Hakka. Those given below are mere examples of the rich selection.

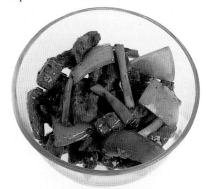

Chicken with Black Bean Sauce

NUTRITIONAL INFORMATION 100 g of cooked lean chicken would provide an excellent source of protein (approximately 27 g). The percentage of carbohydrate present depends on the amount and types of vegetables, the quantity of cornflour and sugar being used. The fat is monosaturated and polyunsaturated depending on the type and amount of fat used. The amount of black beans used per serve is nutritionally insignificant. This dish has a reasonably high sodium content.

DESCRIPTION A Chinese stir-fry dish comprising cubed tender chicken with vegetables — usually celery, onion, carrot and capsicum — in a sauce made from chopped preserved black beans, chilli and garlic.

ORIGIN AND HISTORY Although black beans are one of China's oldest food flavourings, this particular style of dish is a relatively recent innovation. The stir-fry technique required intense heat which could not be achieved with older cooking equipment.

BUYING AND STORAGE Chinese preserved black beans can be purchased whole and will keep indefinitely. Alternatively bottled black bean sauce can be used directly over a finished dish.

PREPARATION AND USE Tender chicken, such as breast or thigh cuts, is cut into small cubes and marinated in a mixture of light soya sauce, Chinese rice wine, salt and sugar. The dried black beans are washed, dried and finely chopped with peeled cloves of garlic and fresh or dried red chillies. The chicken and vegetables are stir-fried in a small amount of vegetable oil in a very hot wok, then the seasoning ingredients added and fried briefly. A sauce is obtained by adding chicken stock and a cornflour thickening, then boiling briefly.

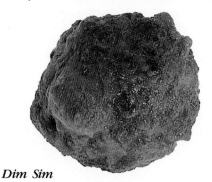

Dim Sim

MAJOR NUTRIENTS			FRIED
			SERVE SIZE 70 G
Energy	660 kJ	Sodium	1200 mg
Protein	7 g	Potassium	105 mg
Fat	6 g	Calcium	45 mg
Cholesterol	5 mg	Phosphorus	80 mg
Carbohydrate	20 g	Iron	1.5 mg
Total Sugars	4 g	Niacin Equiv.	1.5 mg
Dietary Fibre	1 g		

NUTRITIONAL INFORMATION High fat food due to method of preparation. Good source of phosphorus and iron; moderate source of protein, calcium and niacin; contains large amounts of fat and sodium. Energy and fat content much lower if steamed rather than fried.

High sodium level contributed to by additional monosodium glutamate 621. Fried variety cannot be considered as a suitable everyday source of these nutrients.

DESCRIPTION This delicacy is a walnut-sized parcel of meats and cabbage, wrapped in a wonton wrapper and deep-fried until crisp and golden. Often, the fast food variety has a thick, chewy batter, and bears little resemblance to the original.

ORIGIN AND HISTORY Traditionally, the dim sim is one of a range of delicate self-contained foods, including spring rolls and gow gee, referred to as dim sum or dim sim. The literal translation of 'dim sum' is 'snack'.

BUYING AND STORAGE As with most fast foods, dim sims should not be stored. If possible, buy them from a Chinese outlet, as they are more likely to have been made on the premises with good quality ingredients. Many fast food outlets buy frozen, elongated dim sims from a wholesaler, which seldom do justice to the genuine article.

PREPARATION AND USE Like many of the Chinese foods, dim sims are painstakingly assembled by hand, wrapping the pastry around the small balls of meat. They are deep-fried in hot oil until cooked through and golden, and should be well drained to remove excess oil. Frozen dim sims from the supermarket can be cooked in foil-lined bags in the microwave without deep-frying. They are usually served with a soya or chilli dipping sauce.

PROCESSING The dim sims available at fast food outlets are usually manufactured and frozen before distribution to the outlets, where they are thawed before cooking. It is required by law that hot foods be kept at a minimum temperature of 60°C to prevent the growth of bacteria.

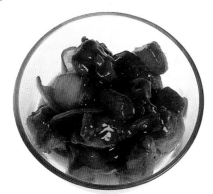

Sweet and Sour Pork

NUTRITIONAL INFORMATION 100 g of cooked lean pork would provide an excellent source of protein (approximately 27 g). The percentage of carbohydrate present depends on the amount and types of vegetables, fruits, the quantity of cornflour and sugar being used. The fat is monosaturated and polyunsaturated depending on the type and amount of fat used.

DESCRIPTION A Chinese dish in which cubes of pork are first coated in a light batter and then deep-fried. A sauce comprising a balanced combination of sweet and sour ingredients is cooked and served separately or may be poured over the meat immediately before serving.

ORIGIN AND HISTORY Sweet-sour dishes are generally regarded as a typical Cantonese (southern China) innovation. However early Chinese history relates that a sour taste was brought to food by a type of native plum, and often sweetened with sugar.

BUYING AND STORAGE Bottled sweet and sour sauce can be used in sweet and sour recipes. It should be kept refrigerated once opened.

PREPARATION AND USE The belly cut of pork, known as 'five flowered pork' by the Chinese because of its alternating layers of pork and fat, is cut into cubes and coated lightly with cornflour. These are then dipped into a batter of cornflour, egg white and water before being deep-fried. The semi-cooked meat is removed from the hot oil and allowed to cool while the sauce is prepared. Immediately before serving, the meat is fried a second time to ensure that the coating is crisp and golden. Sauce comprises shredded vegetables — usually shallots, carrot and celery, but perhaps also cucumber or choko, pineapple and green or red capsicum — and shredded ginger. A mixture of equal parts white vinegar and sugar are boiled together, thinned with water or fruit juice. This liquid is thickened with a mixture of cornflour and cold water, seasoned with salt and pepper, and the shredded vegetables are added and cooked briefly. The red colour characteristic of sweet and sour sauce is achieved by the addition of red food colouring.

SEE ALSO The ingredients mentioned in this entry, and Spring Roll.

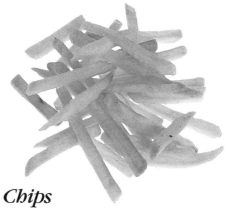

Chips

*also called **French fries, Fries, Potato chips***

MAJOR NUTRIENTS		THIN, FROM FROZEN SUPPLY SERVE SIZE 130 G	
Energy	1420 kJ	Potassium	600 mg
Protein	4 g	Phosphorus	95 mg
Fat	20 g	Magnesium	56 mg
Cholesterol	12 mg	Iron	1 mg
Carbohydrate	38 g	Thiamin	0.15 mg
Total Sugars	1 g	Niacin Equiv.	2.2 mg
Dietary Fibre	5 g	Vitamin C	10 mg
Sodium	200 mg		

NUTRITIONAL INFORMATION An excellent source of phosphorus and vitamin C; good source of magnesium, iron and thiamin. High fat food with over 50% of the energy coming from fats. If chips are cut and left at room temperature for long periods vitamin C level will decrease.

Cholesterol would be present only if animal fat were used for frying.

Larger chips will have a lower fat content and higher percentage energy from carbohydrate. Sodium level will be greatly increased if salt is added at time of serving.

DESCRIPTION Deep-fried potato chips are usually about 1 centimetre square, and as long as the potato from which they came. When cooked, they are a pale golden brown, with the corners and edges slightly darker. The ideal chip is crisp on the outside, and cooked in the middle, with no internal oiliness. French fries are made from julienne strips of potato, usually no thicker than 5 mm.

ORIGIN AND HISTORY Potatoes were brought to Spain from their native South America by conquistadors in 1539. The European population was slow to accept this new food, and the first potato recipes appeared in a German cookbook in 1581. Thomas Jefferson, later third President of the United States, was impressed with French fries during his time as envoy to Paris, and was the first person to serve them with beefsteak in the United States.

BUYING AND STORAGE It is essential that chips are cooked in fresh, very hot oil. Never buy fried foods from a shop that smells of old oil. Ideally, the chips should be deep-fried while you wait, drained well, salted, and eaten straight away.

PREPARATION AND USE The best chips are made with young potatoes. They should be thoroughly dried of all surface moisture before cooking, and cooked in very hot oil, kept at a constant temperature during cooking. This ensures that the outside of the chip seals quickly, preventing oil from permeating the body of the chip.

PROCESSING Commercially produced bulk potato chips, as used in fast food outlets, are dipped in sulphur dioxide to prevent browning. Occasionally, black patches appear on chips — this indicates that they were not thoroughly processed, but are not harmful to health.

SEE ALSO Potato.

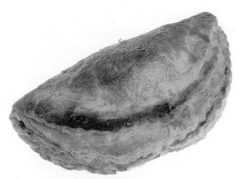

Cornish Pasty

MAJOR NUTRIENTS		SERVE SIZE 150 G	
Energy	1680 kJ	Potassium	210 mg
Protein	10 g	Phosphorus	180 mg
Fat	23 g	Iron	2 mg
Cholesterol	25 mg	Zinc	1 mg
Carbohydrate	33 g	Thiamin	0.1 mg
Total Sugars	2 g	Niacin Equiv.	3.9 mg
Dietary Fibre	2 g	Vitamin C	1.5 mg
Sodium	640 mg		

NUTRITIONAL INFORMATION An excellent source of protein, phosphorus, iron and niacin; moderate source of zinc, thiamin and vitamin C. Contains large amounts of fat, cholesterol and sodium.

Pastry coating is high in fat. This is a high energy snack or meal item with more than 50% of energy coming from fats, generally from animal sources, and high in saturated fats.

DESCRIPTION A pasty is an envelope of shortcrust pastry with a fluted, pinched frill, filled with cubed lamb and vegetables. The vegetable mixture usually comprises potato, carrot and turnip cut into small cubes. Cabbage is sometimes included.

ORIGIN AND HISTORY A traditional food in Cornwall, pasties were used as a compact lunch for flint chippers who worked on the cliff faces. They are also said to have been used in the Cornish tin mines: miners would break away the gritty, dusty pastry and eat the filling. The crescent-shaped pasty was pinched in the middle to divide the filling into two halves — one of savoury meat and vegetable, and the other of sweet apple. Introduced into Australia when the Cornish copper miners migrated to South Australia, pasties still share equal popularity with pies in that State.

BUYING AND STORAGE Fresh hot pasties should be eaten at once. If bought cold, they can be stored in an airtight container under refrigeration for up to 3 days, and reheated in a hot oven.

PREPARATION AND USE Pasties as a fast food need no further preparation. They can be made at home using shortcrust pastry and a filling of cubed lamb or mutton, potatoes and turnip. The potatoes provide a natural thickening agent as they cook, and added thickening is not necessary.

PROCESSING In commercial pasty production, a filling is made by blending a mixture of lightly blanched chopped fresh vegetables and finely minced beef. A 16.5 cm diameter circle of pastry is filled, folded in half, crimped shut, then baked for 15–18 minutes in a hot oven. Semicircular pasties are made by hand, and armadillo-style (crescent shaped) pasties are made by machine.

VARIETIES
Vegetarian pasty.

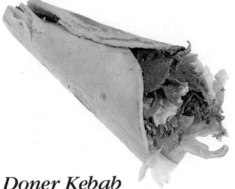

Doner Kebab

*also called **Lebanese Roll, Shavourma***

NUTRITIONAL INFORMATION The nutrient value varies according to whether chicken, beef or lamb is used in the roll. Refer to these roasted meats for nutritional information in the appropriate chapters.

DESCRIPTION The doner kebab is a version of a hamburger, the meat, salad and sauce being wrapped in a round of unleavened bread. Cooked meat is sliced hot from a slow cooking vertical rotisserie, and salad and sauce is added to taste. The bread is then rolled tightly to make a portable meal.

ORIGIN AND HISTORY Being of early Phoenician origin, this method of cooking and preparing meat has become part of the cuisines of Greece, Turkey and Lebanon. Doner kebabs have been introduced to Australian consumers by immigrants.

BUYING AND STORAGE Similar to the hamburger, this hot meat fast food is best assembled while you wait, for maximum freshness. It should not be stored.

PREPARATION AND USE Salads such as tabouli, sliced tomato, sliced raw onion, and lettuce are prepared in advance. The cooked meat is sliced thinly from the rotisserie, spread across the middle of a warmed round of Lebanese bread, topped with hommos, tahini sauce, chilli or barbecue sauce and salad, and rolled tightly.

PROCESSING Sometimes the meat is marinated for two days in wine and spices before being skewered onto the rotisserie for cooking. A whole, peeled onion can be speared onto the top of the rotisserie, so that the onion juices run down over the meat as it cooks. Chicken breasts and lamb or mutton are used. Most lamb kebabs are a combination of 70–80% lamb mixed with 20–30% emulsifier, which is then formed into a large restructured mass. Thin slices are cut from the meat, while the remaining portion continues to cook.

VARIETIES
Beef kebab, Chicken kebab, Lamb kebab.

SEE ALSO Beef, Chicken, Lamb.

Fried Chicken

DESCRIPTION Fried chicken is usually cooked in portions — thighs, drumsticks, breasts or wings — and coated with crumbs prior to frying. According to H. L. Mencken, writing in the 1940s, 'Traditional Southern fried chicken is plump and fried properly in lard or peanut oil (but never butter) in a heavy iron skillet. It may be fried with corn meal, but never with flour or an egg batter.' Chicken nuggets are a highly processed form, made into compact, crumbed shapes using boneless chicken meat.

ORIGIN AND HISTORY This food is undoubtedly as American as apple pie, and is mentioned in early American literature. Fried chicken also became a fast food in the USA and franchised fried chicken outlets are now found around the world.

BUYING AND STORAGE Many fast food outlets have precooked chicken in warmed trays. Because of the danger of bacterial growth, it is best to have the chicken fried while you wait. It can be eaten immediately, or allowed to cool, then refrigerated in an airtight container for later use.

PREPARATION AND USE Methods vary from different food outlets. The Kentucky Fried Chicken chain has developed a method of pressure cooking in oil at very high temperatures, ensuring a maximum retention of moisture and tenderness.

PROCESSING Chickens used in fast food outlets are soaked in a solution of phosphate salts to increase the moisture content, enhancing the tenderness of the meat, and helping to hold the crumb coating together.

VARIETIES

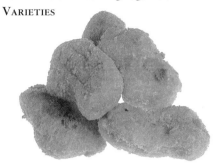

Chicken Nugget A mixture of chicken meat and skin, pressed together, shaped and crumbed, then fried.

MAJOR NUTRIENTS		SERVE SIZE 60 G	
Energy	680 kJ	Sodium	370 mg
Protein	6 g	Potassium	85 mg
Fat	11 g	Phosphorus	45 mg
Cholesterol	17 mg	Iron	0.5 mg
Carbohydrate	11 g	Vitamin A	40 µg
Total Sugars	1 g	Niacin Equiv.	2.3 mg
Dietary Fibre		Vitamin C	2 mg
	less than 1 g		

NUTRITIONAL INFORMATION A good source of niacin; moderate source of protein, phosphorus, vitamin A and vitamin C. Contains large amounts of fat and sodium.

Chicken nuggets are made from mixes of chicken and chicken skin so even before frying in oil they are higher in fat than many chicken cuts. High energy food with more than 65% of energy being supplied by fats. But fat content determines that these should be eaten with discretion.

SEE ALSO Chicken.

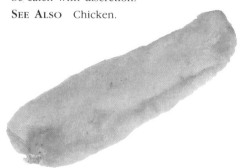

Fried Fish

MAJOR NUTRIENTS		DEEP-FRIED, BATTERED SERVE SIZE 150 G	
Energy	1750 kJ	Calcium	105 mg
Protein	24 g	Phosphorus	255 mg
Fat	127 g	Magnesium	32 mg
Cholesterol	100 mg	Iron	1.5 mg
Carbohydrate	21 g	Zinc	1.5 mg
Total Sugars	0	Thiamin	0.3 mg
Dietary Fibre	1 g	Riboflavin	0.2 mg
Sodium	330 mg	Niacin Equiv.	6.6 mg
Potassium	350 mg		

NUTRITIONAL INFORMATION An excellent source of protein, calcium, phosphorus, iron, thiamin and niacin; good source of zinc and riboflavin; contains large amounts of fat, cholesterol and sodium. If battered coating not eaten fish could be a regular dietary source of these nutrients. Depending on the fish, source can contain significant amounts of vitamin E and folate.

Frying turns a low fat food into a high fat and high energy product. Type of batter will determine just how high in fat the final product is.

DESCRIPTION The average piece of fried fish is about 20 cm long and 10 cm wide, and is usually, but not always, a fillet without bones.

ORIGIN AND HISTORY Some historians believe that deep-fried fish originated in China, where deep-fried battered food has been popular for centuries; it is thought that the process was brought to Britain by traders. The growth of fried fish fillets in the fast food market was greatly assisted in post-war Australia by the fish-on-Friday requirement of the Roman Catholic Church.

BUYING AND STORAGE Precooked battered fish, which is reheated to fill an order, is likely to harbour bacteria. It is better to buy from a shop that coats and fries the raw fillet while you wait. The fish should be white and firm (except for NZ blue cod or hake, which are cream). Fish such as gemfish, flathead and shark are suitable for deep frying. Fish should be eaten while hot and the batter fresh and crisp.

PREPARATION AND USE A good light batter is made using 120 g self-raising flour, 1 egg, and ½ cup of milk beaten together, with salt and pepper. Oil for frying should be maintained at a constant high temperature, to seal the batter quickly and cook the fish right through before the batter burns. The cooked fish should be drained on absorbent paper for a minute or two to soak up excess oil before serving.

PROCESSING Fish should be deep-fried at the time of ordering; no processing is required.

SEE ALSO Cod, Flathead, Gemfish, Hake, Shark.

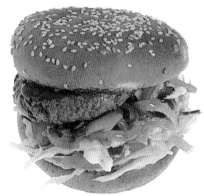

Hamburger

MAJOR NUTRIENTS		PLAIN WITH 45 G PATTY SERVE SIZE 180 G	
Energy	1710 kJ	Phosphorus	235 mg
Protein	11 g	Iron	2.5 mg
Fat	10 g	Zinc	1.1 mg
Cholesterol	47 mg	Vitamin A	130 µg
Carbohydrate	37 g	Thiamin	0.1 mg
Total Sugars	7 g	Riboflavin	0.3 mg
Dietary Fibre	2 g	Niacin Equiv.	4.9 mg
Sodium	1190 mg	Vitamin C	4 mg
Potassium	340 mg		

NUTRITIONAL INFORMATION An excellent source of protein, phosphorus, iron, vitamin A, riboflavin, niacin and vitamin B12; good source of zinc and thiamin; contains large amounts of cholesterol and sodium.

Nutrient content will increase if served with extra egg, cheese or bacon. Depending on how put together may have considerable levels of optional salt added which makes it a high sodium product. This can be avoided.

Balanced total meal with 60% of energy coming from the carbohydrate and 21% energy coming from fat.

DESCRIPTION A hamburger is a self-contained meal within a round, flattish bun. Usually the bun is lightly toasted, and filled with a 1–2 cm thick patty of minced beef about the same size as the bun. The meat patty used in hamburgers is a restructured product using a variety of meat species (i.e. beef, pork, lamb, chicken, turkey, veal or fish), and may include salt, phosphates, water, seasonings, preservatives and soya bean (which aids in binding). Additions of salads, pickles, cheese, pineapple, egg or bacon are optional, and vary with suppliers. It is eaten hot.

ORIGIN AND HISTORY The hamburger appears to be of north American origin and not from the German city, Hamburg. The Brown Derby restaurant in Hollywood has been serving hamburgers since 1926. The popularity of the hamburger took a great leap with the establishment of such hamburger specialty chains as McDonald's and Hungry Jack's, which began around 1950 in the

United States and spread worldwide during the 1960s. The meat was once scraps of beef and less desirable cuts, but the supply of high quality hamburger mince is now a major industry. In Australia, for instance, the McDonald's chain alone used 8600 tonnes of beef during 1987.

BUYING AND STORAGE Whether it comes wrapped in greaseproof paper from the corner shop or packed in a moulded box from one of a chain of franchised specialty hamburger outlets, the hamburger should be eaten as soon as it is made. Any delay will leave lukewarm meat and limp, unappetising salad.

PREPARATION AND USE Hamburgers make a quick, satisfying meal at home. Patties of seasoned minced meat are cooked on a hot plate or in a pan, while salad vegetables (lettuce, tomato, beetroot, onion), are sliced and the split buns lightly toasted. To make a cheeseburger, place the meat on one side of the bun, top with cheese and melt under a hot grill. When melted, finish with salad, sauce, and top of the bun. For an American-style hamburger, use sliced pickles and less salad. Fried onions, egg and bacon are optional.

PROCESSING Hamburgers are made on an 'assembly line' basis, and large containers of the various ingredients are prepared for the beginning of each day's trading. At small fast food outlets, the hamburger is cooked while you wait. The modern clamshell grill used in the large chains cooks both sides of the patty at once. The cooking time is quicker, and the reduced handling produces a neater patty. Up to 12 buns at a time are toasted on their cut sides, to help prevent the juices of the meat from soaking into the bun. The McDonald's meat patty is made of chuck and brisket, with no preservatives, seasonings or binders. The meat is ground coarsely, mixed, and ground again to a finer particle size, when bone and gristle is mechanically removed. The meat is formed into uniform patties before cryogenic freezing and packaging.

VARIETIES

The many additions or variations on the basic hamburger include bacon, cheese, egg, fish, ham and pineapple.

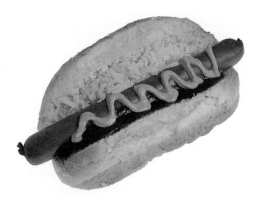

Hot Dog

MAJOR NUTRIENTS		SERVE SIZE 90 G BUN, 80 G FRANKFURTER	
Energy	2220 kJ	Potassium	180 mg
Protein	21 g	Calcium	80 mg
Fat	28 g	Phosphorus	105 mg
Cholesterol	45 mg	Magnesium	42 mg
Carbohydrate	50 g	Iron	3 mg
Total Sugars	2 g	Zinc	2.5 mg
Dietary Fibre	3 g	Thiamin	0.15 mg
Sodium	1185 mg	Niacin Equiv.	4.5 mg

NUTRITIONAL INFORMATION An excellent source of protein, calcium, phosphorus, iron, zinc and niacin; good source of fibre, magnesium and thiamin.

High protein food item where only 36% of the energy comes from carbohydrate and 46% from fat. If bun is buttered the total fat and energy level will increase, resulting in more than 50% of the energy being provided by fats.

DESCRIPTION A hot dog consists of a hot, cooked frankfurter sausage, lying lengthways in a split bread roll. Addition of mustard, sauce and pickles is optional. The roll is specially made for this purpose, and is the length of an average sausage.

ORIGIN AND HISTORY The frankfurter is a traditional snack food in Germany and Switzerland, where it is held between slices of bread. The use of a long roll to cradle the frankfurter has been a North American adaptation, and the hot dog is considered an all-American fast food. The term 'hot dog' was coined in 1906, when American cartoonist T. A. Dorgan depicted a dachshund inside an elongated bun.

BUYING AND STORAGE The ultimate in eat-as-you-go cuisine, hot dogs are often peddled from barrows containing an urn of frankfurters in hot water, a bag of buns, and a selection of sauces and mustards. A hot dog should be consumed at the time of purchase, as storage can promote bacterial growth.

PREPARATION AND USE The preparation of a hot dog has been simplified by the introduction of a heated, pointed rod, which is the

diameter of the sausage, and the length of the bread roll. The unsplit roll is impaled on this rod, left for a moment to warm the bread, then sauce is squirted into the hole, and the sausage snugly inserted into the middle of the roll.

SEE ALSO Frankfurter, White Bread.

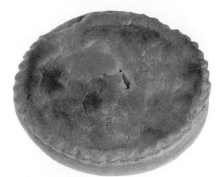

Meat Pie

MAJOR NUTRIENTS		SERVE SIZE 170 G	
Energy	1630 kJ	Magnesium	30 mg
Protein	13 g	Iron	2 mg
Fat	24 g	Zinc	1.5 mg
Cholesterol	34 mg	Thiamin	0.1 mg
Carbohydrate	33 g	Riboflavin	0.25 mg
Sodium	1020 mg	Niacin Equiv.	5.4 mg
Phosphorus	190 mg	Vitamin B12	0.2 µg

NUTRITIONAL INFORMATION An excellent source of protein, phosphorus, iron, niacin and vitamin B12; good source of zinc and riboflavin; contains large amounts of fat, cholesterol and sodium. High amounts of salt may be added to boost the intense taste of the product.

High energy food which has only 32% of energy provided by carbohydrate but over 54% from fats. High fat and energy content indicates that the meat pie should not be consumed on a daily basis as a main meal food, and should only be consumed as a snack food after vigorous activity.

DESCRIPTION A meat pie is usually about the same surface size as a slice of bread, and is either square or round. A base and top of pastry enclose a filling of cooked minced or cubed meat, with a thick, peppery gravy. With a potato pie, the 'lid' of pastry is replaced with a thick layer of mashed potato, browned on top.

ORIGIN AND HISTORY Meat pies were common fare in medieval England. When Archbishop Neville was ordained at York in 1476, records show that 4000 meat pies were consumed. In early days, many people simply did not have enough teeth to chew solid cuts of meat, while pies could be spooned up and eaten with virtually no chewing. The old rhyme of 'four-and-twenty blackbirds baked in a pie' sounds fanciful, but in a cookbook of the 1500s, a recipe begins, 'To make pies that the birds may be alive in and flie out when it is cut up . . .' Unlike the English pork pie, the meat pie should be eaten piping hot.

BUYING AND STORAGE Hot pies should be bought on the day of baking, and eaten soon after purchase. The heavy dose of pepper often found in pie gravies creates the illusion of heat even after the pie has begun to cool. Commercially packaged pies are available from supermarket refrigerators and freezers.

PREPARATION AND USE Fast food pies are ready to eat and require no further preparation. Condiments such as chilli, Worcestershire or tomato sauces are often added. In Adelaide, a meat pie island on a sea of mushy cooked green peas constitutes the famous late-night snack known as 'the Floater'. Although South Australians like to consider it their own, the Floater is also well known in Covent Garden, London.

PROCESSING By legislation, a meat pie must contain not less than 25% meat. An important ingredient is Worcestershire sauce, which boosts both the flavour and the rich dark colour. Cereals are sometimes added to increase the bulk, and industrial caramel is added for colour. The pastry is rolled out in a long sheet, then laid over empty foil containers with a raised cutting edge. After the pastry is pressed into the container (mechanically or manually), the cases are filled with cooked filling. Another sheet of pastry is laid over the top, and a crimper and stamper joins the two sheets of pastry, while the self-cutting edge cuts the pie out of the sheets. A glaze of milk and water or egg and water is brushed or sprayed on the top to prevent a floury finish, and the pies are baked for 12–14 minutes at 230°C.

VARIETIES

Flavours include chicken, curry, mushroom, potato, steak and kidney, steak and onion and 'the Floater'.

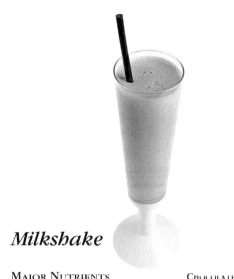

Milkshake

MAJOR NUTRIENTS		CHOCOLATE SERVE SIZE 200 ML	
Energy	710 kJ	Phosphorus	185 mg
Protein	8 g	Magnesium	24 mg
Fat	8 g	Vitamin A	60 µg
Cholesterol	30 mg	Thiamin	0.1 mg
Carbohydrate	22 g	Riboflavin	0.4 mg
Total Sugars	22 g	Niacin Equiv.	1.8 mg
Calcium	230 g	Vitamin B12	0.6 µg

NUTRITIONAL INFORMATION Excellent protein, phosphorus, calcium and riboflavin and vitamin B12; good source of Vitamin A and thiamin; moderate source of folate.

Chocolate and sugars may make the milk more easily digestible for those who have mild lactose intolerance. Fat level will vary if extra ice cream is added.

DESCRIPTION A milkshake is a mixture of milk, ice cream and flavouring, whipped at high speed to make a thick, frothy drink. A long-time favourite throughout the Western world, it is a filling and satisfying light meal for people on the go.

ORIGIN AND HISTORY Although milkshakes as we know them were developed with the invention of milkshake machines in America at the turn of the century, milkshakes actually date back to the 13th century. The Mongol cavalry that rode with Genghis Khan (1162–1227) used to sustain themselves with mares' milk. The milk was dried to a powder in the sun and stored until required. At the beginning of the day, the Mongol horsemen would mix a small quantity of the mares' milk powder with water in a bladder. This was tied to the saddle, and the constant agitation of the day's riding would froth the mixture into a thin porridge, eaten at the end of the day.

Much later in the early 1930s and 1940s in Australia, hundreds of milkbars existed in the cities and country towns. The milkshake has remained popular ever since.

BUYING AND STORAGE A milkshake needs to be consumed as soon as it is made. If left to stand, it soon becomes half a cup of flat, flavoured milk, losing its frothy appeal.

PREPARATION AND USE Small electrical appliances are available for making milkshakes at home. The basic ingredients are 1 scoop of good quality ice cream and a cup of 1–2 day-old milk. Addition of malted milk powder or flavoured syrups is optional. Fresh, soft-textured fruits such as strawberries or other berries, peaches or bananas can be added, but should first be chopped or mashed to assist in integration.

PROCESSING There is a trend towards using soft-serve ice cream in milkshakes. Containing more emulsifiers and thickening agents than standard ice cream, it creates a milkshake with a uniform consistency and smooth creamy texture.

VARIETIES

The numerous variations can be flavoured with a multitude of essences, extracts and fruits.

SEE ALSO Thickshake.

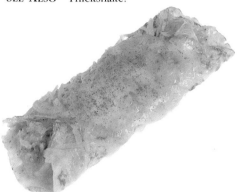

Pancake

also called **Crepe**

MAJOR NUTRIENTS		SERVE SIZE 40 G	
Energy	515 kJ	Carbohydrate	14 g
Protein	2 g	Total Sugars	6 g
Fat	7 g	Calcium	50 mg
Cholesterol	25 mg	Phosphorus	50 mg

NUTRITIONAL INFORMATION A moderate source of calcium and phosphorus. Sodium levels will depend on raising agent used. Pancakes could have a high sodium level.

High fat product with 50% of energy coming from fats. Fat levels will vary depending on the ratio of water to milk used in the recipe. Spreads or toppings commonly used may be high in energy and so change the apparent nutritional uselessness of pancakes.

DESCRIPTION A basic pancake consists of a mixture of eggs, milk, flour and sugar or salt, cooked in a thin layer in a pan. This fairly uninteresting food is 'dressed up' with savoury or sweet fillings, and sometimes topped with a sauce. The idea of the pancake is seen around the world: the Mexican tortilla, the Chinese egg roll, the Russian blini and the French crepe.

ORIGIN AND HISTORY The crepe originated in France, where they are always eaten on Shrove Tuesday (Mardi Gras). Writer Morrison Wood recounts the story of chef Henri Carpentier, who was preparing crepes for Edward VII when the dish accidentally burst into flames. Henri carried the flaming pan to the table, and when the fire had died out, served the little pancakes to the King and his companions. The King named the delicious new dessert Crepes Suzette, in honour of his host's daughter.

BUYING AND STORAGE Ready-to-eat fast food crepes should not be stored. Unfilled crepes or pancakes can be layered between sheets of foil or plastic wrap, then sealed tightly in foil and frozen for later use. Prefilled frozen pancakes are available from supermarket freezers.

PREPARATION AND USE The ideal crepe pan should be made of cast iron, with rounded or low, sloping sides, so that a spatula can be slipped under the cooked batter without tearing the edges. The pan should never be washed, rather wiped out with fresh oil and paper towel for a constant non-stick surface.

Like a pizza, a crepe can be used as a vehicle for any combination of foods, whether it be leftovers from the refrigerator or a gourmet blend of asparagus, herbs and almonds in a creamy cheese sauce. A popular American way of eating pancakes is in a 'stack' of four or six, with maple syrup and whipped butter. This style of pancake is usually thicker, with a smaller diameter, and is not intended to be folded over a filling.

PROCESSING Small specialty crepe outlets make their own batters and cook the crepes in the same manner as home cooking, with individual attention assuring a quality product. High turnover, large scale production such as pancakes at McDonald's outlets is governed by the need for consistency. A dry pre-mix is supplied, requiring only the addition of water to make the batter. This is poured into a dispenser with four legs, which stands on the griddle. A metered amount of batter is released to make each pancake, in much the same way as a dough-making machine dispenses its mixture.

VARIETIES
Seafood, chicken, vegetable, 'Suzette', fruit.

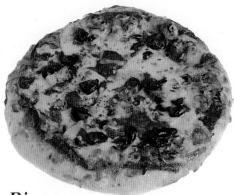

Pizza

NUTRITIONAL INFORMATION The nutrient value of a pizza will depend upon the choice of foods used for the topping. The major nutrients of the dough are similar to those of white bread.

DESCRIPTION The plate-shaped pizza, with its doughy, yeasty base and topping of tomato paste, meats, vegetables and mozzarella cheese, is well known around the world.

ORIGIN AND HISTORY Of Italian origin, the pizza was first introduced to Australian consumers in the early 1950s by an Italian migrant. It evolved as a filling, economical way for Italian country folk to provide a meal using leftovers and a minimum of meat, when tomatoes were a plentiful, cheap resource. Discovered by Allied soldiers during World War II, Italian food, and pizza in particular, has enjoyed immense worldwide popularity in recent years. The home delivery service has made it an ideal convenience and fast food.

BUYING AND STORAGE Individual outlets have their own personal preferences for thick, thin, doughy or dry bases, and some experimenting may need to be undertaken to find your perfect pizza. The topping should be generous and well covered with melted cheese. If not eaten immediately, the pizza should be reheated in a hot oven to restore its crispness.

PREPARATION AND USE For some fast-food outlets, pizza is made in huge slabs, and cut into rectangular pieces which are kept hot in trays until needed. Franchised pizza chains make the pizzas only when an order is received, resulting in a better product that does not really qualify as a fast food. Pizza outlets offering a home delivery service provide a ready-to-eat, made-to-order convenient meal.

PROCESSING Pizzas are made on an assembly line basis. All the topping requirements are prepared and set out in bowls (cheese, onion, chopped meats, capsicum, prawns, pineapple, olives, tomato puree, chillies, etc.). The dough is made some hours

before the outlet opens for business, allowing time for the yeast to have its effect, and set aside in individual balls to rise. Skilled pizza cooks make the base by tossing and spinning the dough until it becomes a round, flat disc. Final assembly is done upon receipt of an order.

VARIETIES
Countless variations on the basic pizza theme are available.

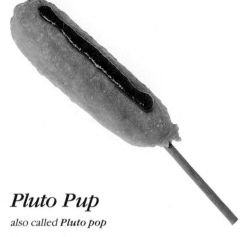

Pluto Pup

also called Pluto pop

MAJOR NUTRIENTS		SERVE SIZE 100 G	
Energy	1260 kJ	Phosphorus	125 mg
Protein	11 g	Iron	1.5 mg
Fat	27 g	Zinc	2 mg
Cholesterol	44 mg	Thiamin	0.1 mg
Carbohydrate	10 g	Niacin Equiv.	2.7 mg
Sodium	580 mg		

NUTRITIONAL INFORMATION An excellent source of protein, phosphorus, iron and niacin; good source of zinc and thiamin; contains large amounts of fat, cholesterol and sodium.

Battered deep-fried coating results in a very high energy and high fat product, with up to 79% of total energy from fats. Lighter batter and higher frying temperature may reduce total fat content.

DESCRIPTION This fast food comprises a frankfurter sausage impaled lengthways on a flat wooden skewer. The sausage is dipped in batter and quickly deep fried until golden brown and crisp.

ORIGIN AND HISTORY The Pluto Pup is a relatively recent addition to the fast food range, being an adaptation of the hot dog. The same hot dog frankfurter is used, and the canine association is continued with the use of the name of Walt Disney's famous dog. These snacks are frequently found in connection with travelling sideshows and mobile food vans.

BUYING AND STORAGE It is preferable to buy Pluto Pups freshly cooked, as cooked food kept in warm places can harbour bacteria. They should not be stored, but eaten at the time of purchase.

PREPARATION AND USE A wooden skewer is pushed lengthways into the frankfurter, until it is holding securely. The frankfurter is then dipped into a batter (see Fried Fish), and deep fried in hot, clean oil. This makes a reasonably filling snack that can be eaten on the move.

SEE ALSO Frankfurter.

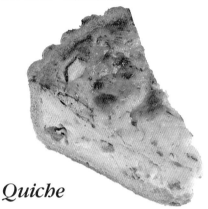

Quiche

MAJOR NUTRIENTS			SERVE SIZE 120 G
Energy	1950 kJ	Phosphorus	290 mg
Protein	18 g	Iron	1.5 mg
Fat	34 g	Zinc	2.2 mg
Cholesterol	160 mg	Vitamin A	290 µg
Carbohydrate	25 g	Thiamin	0.2 mg
Total Sugars	3 g	Riboflavin	0.3 mg
Dietary Fibre	1 g	Niacin Equiv.	3.6 mg
Sodium	820 mg	Vitamin D	1.1 mg
Potassium	230 mg	Vitamin E	1 mg
Calcium	310 mg		

NUTRITIONAL INFORMATION An excellent source of protein, calcium, phosphorus, iron, vitamin A, riboflavin, niacin, vitamin E as well as containing good amounts of zinc, thiamin and vitamin D. In moderation a useful source of these nutrients.

Contains large amounts of fat, cholesterol and sodium. Pastry and egg content results in over 64% of energy coming from fats and only 25% from carbohydrate. Fats also contain significant levels of cholesterol. Nutritional breakdown will vary only slightly with the various filling types.

DESCRIPTION Essentially custard, well-flavoured with cheese and baked in a shortcrust pie shell, a quiche can feature any number of savoury fillings. It is popular as an entrée or a light meal, and when sold as a fast food, is usually in a small individual serving like a meat pie.

ORIGIN AND HISTORY This hot cheese pie originated in France, and has been adopted around the world. The Australians like it with hearty fillings of bacon and onions, the Italians created the Florentine spinach quiche, and the Americans make their own version with clams. In the Alsace-Lorraine region of France, home of the quiche Lorraine, each village has its own jealously-guarded secret recipe, each claiming to be the original one.

BUYING AND STORAGE Quiche can be eaten hot or cold. Wrapped in plastic wrap or sealed in an airtight container, it can be kept in the refrigerator for some days. Quiche can be reheated in a moderate oven if desired.

PREPARATION AND USE Purchased as a fast food, quiche needs no further preparation. It is quickly and easily prepared at home, and recipes are found in many cookbooks.

PROCESSING Many small fast food outlets make their own quiches, or buy them from a local 'cottage industry' supplier. Outlets with higher turnover buy frozen product from wholesale suppliers, who make the quiche using home-cooking methods, but with a crust specially designed for microwave heating. The quiche is cooked before freezing, so that the retailer has only to thaw and reheat it.

VARIETIES

Lorraine, Florentine, crab, chicken, salmon, ham, vegetable, and infinite combinations.

Salad

NUTRITIONAL INFORMATION Vegetable based, non dressed salads are low energy foods. If lettuce/tomato based, excellent source of fibre, vitamin A and vitamin C; moderate source of magnesium, folate and vitamin E. If added to takeaway food can help create a more balanced meal.

DESCRIPTION Fast food salads are presented in cool trays in glass-fronted display units, or prepacked into 250 g or 500 g tubs for sale from refrigerated units. Varieties are usually confined to mixtures including beans, coleslaw, vegetables, tabouli, pasta, rice or potatoes, which have a longer life than leafy salads. Potato salad and coleslaw have the highest volume of sales.

ORIGIN AND HISTORY The use of raw vegetables and herbs in salads in the Western world goes back many hundreds of years. The idea of providing salad bars in supermarkets, delicatessens and fast food outlets is a relatively recent one, originating in the USA.

Ready-made salads were introduced to Australian supermarkets and restaurants in about 1981.

BUYING AND STORAGE Prepacked salads contain no preservatives, although ascorbic acid is added to fruit salad. Always check the use-by date before buying, and refrigerate if not using immediately. Salads sold by weight in supermarket delicatessen sections are made daily.

PREPARATION AND USE Prepared salads are ready to eat and need no further preparation.

PROCESSING Vegetable growers are contracted to produce the requirements for the salads, and the freshly harvested produce is delivered directly to the processors, who subject it to quality control inspection. The vegetables are washed and prepared, using mechanical cutters, corers and shredders. Potatoes are steam-cooked in their jackets to ensure maximum retention of nutrients, then peeled and rapidly cooled before being combined with dressing and fresh herbs. Tossing and blending of salads is done in stainless steel rotating bins. The salads are hermetically sealed with a minimum of retained air, to prevent spoiling. Fresh fruit salads contain vegetable gums (415 and 412) to make the syrup cling to the fruit.

VARIETIES

There are many varieties of prepared salad. Two are listed below as examples.

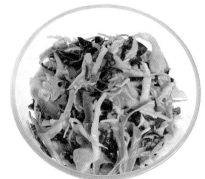

Dressed Coleslaw

MAJOR NUTRIENTS			SERVE SIZE 60 G
Energy	240 kJ	Dietary Fibre	2 g
Protein	1 g	Sodium	160 mg
Fat	2 g	Potassium	95 mg
Cholesterol	7 mg	Vitamin A	40 µg
Carbohydrate	8 g	Vitamin C	12 mg
Total Sugars	8 g		

NUTRITIONAL INFORMATION Final energy level will depend on the amount of dressing and fat content of dressing added. Vegetable content of coleslaw contains excellent amounts of vitamin C if freshly prepared and good amounts of fibre and vitamin A. Fat content will depend on the amount and type of dressing used.

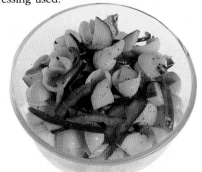

Pasta or Rice-based Salad

MAJOR NUTRIENTS SERVE SIZE 100 G

Energy	680 kJ	Sodium	50 mg
Protein	4 g	Potassium	60 mg
Fat	8 g	Phosphorus	45 mg
Cholesterol	0	Iron	0.5 mg
Carbohydrate	22 g	Niacin Equiv.	1 mg
Dietary Fibre	1 g		

NUTRITIONAL INFORMATION High carbohydrate salads with up to 50% of total energy coming from carbohydrate. Total fat content will depend on the amount and type of dressing used.

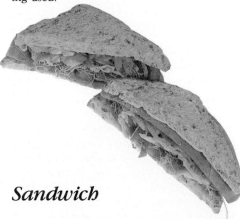

Sandwich

MAJOR NUTRIENTS SERVE SIZE:
TWO SLICES BREAD
30 G ANIMAL PROTEIN SPREAD
SALAD

Energy	1180 kJ	Potassium	250 mg
Protein	15 g	Phosphorus	155 mg
Fat	13 g	Magnesium	40 mg
Cholesterol	25 mg	Iron	2 mg
Carbohydrate	31 g	Zinc	2 mg
Total Sugars	1 g	Vitamin A	100 µg
Dietary Fibre	4 g	Thiamin	0.15 mg
Sodium	290 mg	Niacin Equiv.	4.9 mg

NUTRITIONAL INFORMATION An excellent source of protein, phosphorus, iron, thiamin and niacin; good source of magnesium and vitamin A.

If fats in filling minimised, an excellent complete meal food with at least 40% of energy coming from carbohydrate. Filling will alter some of the nutrient significance but bread will supply significant quantities of magnesium, iron and thiamin. Wholegrain/wholemeal sandwich would contain additional 2.5 g fibre. A cheese filling will provide an excellent source of calcium. A fish filling will provide an excellent source of vitamin E.

DESCRIPTION The basic sandwich is two slices of buttered bread, between which is a filling. This filling can be as mundane as Vegemite, honey or jam, or as exotic as avocado, mayonnaise and capers. The open sandwich has only one slice of bread, and is assembled on a plate and eaten with a knife and fork. A toasted sandwich is buttered on the outside and then browned in a hot pan and served hot. A club sandwich has three or four layers of bread with different fillings that complement each other, and is served in thin fingers trimmed of crust.

ORIGIN AND HISTORY John Montague, the fourth Earl of Sandwich, earned himself a place in history in 1762, when he had his servant bring him a chunk of beef between two slices of bread, so that he could eat without interrupting his gambling, or, as his family always maintained, without interrupting the copious paperwork associated with his position as Secretary of State and First Sea Lord. However, the French insist that their farmers were taking sandwiches of black or wholemeal bread into the fields with them long before the English name was known. During the Depression in America taking a cut lunch of sandwiches to work was referred to as 'brown-bagging', a term which has remained in use.

BUYING AND STORAGE Sandwiches should always be bought from an outlet where they are made to order while you wait. Some cafeterias and fast food outlets have sandwiches already prepared and packaged in airtight wrapping, which should have been made on the day of sale. Plastic wrap keeps sandwiches fresh for up to 12 hours.

PREPARATION AND USE Basic preparation of a sandwich involves 2 slices of bread spread with butter or margarine. Any style of bread can be used, with any choice of filling. Wet fillings such as tuna, tomato and beetroot should not be included in sandwiches not intended for immediate consumption.

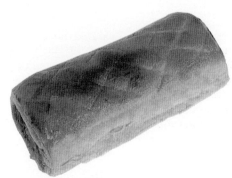

Sausage Roll

MAJOR NUTRIENTS SERVE SIZE 130 G

Energy	1580 kJ	Sodium	845 mg
Protein	10 g	Potassium	120 mg
Fat	23 g	Phosphorus	130 mg
Cholesterol	25 mg	Iron	1.5 mg
Carbohydrate	34 g	Zinc	1.5 mg
Total Sugars	4 g	Thiamin	0.2 mg
Dietary Fibre	1.5 g	Niacin Equiv.	4.6 mg

NUTRITIONAL INFORMATION An excellent source of protein, phosphorus, iron, thiamin, niacin and vitamin E; good source of zinc; contains large amounts of fat and sodium and significant levels of cholesterol. Pastry and sausage together contribute over 53% of energy as fat. Puff pastry varieties may be even higher in fat.

DESCRIPTION The average sausage roll is approximately 15 cm long and 5 cm in diameter. It is made up of a seasoned sausage mixture rolled in puff or flaky pastry and baked.

ORIGIN AND HISTORY Like the Cornish pasty, the sausage roll was initially a portable, compact meal protected and kept warm by the pastry. Once a vehicle for leftovers, all commercial sausage rolls nowadays contain a mince similar to sausages.

BUYING AND STORAGE Hot sausage rolls are available at many snack bars, bakeries and fast food outlets. They are kept warm in special pie ovens which keep them crisp. Sausage rolls for later use can be frozen, sealed in plastic wrap or foil, and reheated in a hot oven when required. Ready-made rolls can be bought frozen in full-size or bite-size form for meals or snacks. Sausage rolls can be heated in a microwave, with the use of proper covering.

PREPARATION AND USE Sausage rolls can be made at home using commercially frozen pastry sheets and sausage mince, or bought frozen, ready to cook in the oven.

PROCESSING The filling for sausage rolls is a finely ground mixture of meat, often mutton, flavours such as tomato and onion, and breadcrumbs. The pastry is rolled out as a large sheet and the raw filling is pumped in rows onto the pastry. A cutting wheel slices the pastry into strips, with the meat on top. The strips are then passed through a device shaped like a plough on both sides, folding the pastry up around the filling, creating a continuous seam along the top. The seam is pressed down flat, and the strips are then cut into lengths, glazed and cooked for about 20 minutes.

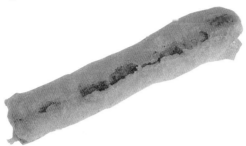

Seafood Stick

also called **Crab stick, Fish stick, Seafood extender**

MAJOR NUTRIENTS		DEEP-FRIED SERVE SIZE 60 G	
Energy	443 kJ	Sodium	360 mg
Protein	5 g	Potassium	110 mg
Fat	4 g	Phosphorus	100 mg
Cholesterol	20 mg	Iron	1 mg
Carbohydrate	13 g	Zinc	1 mg
Dietary Fibre	1 g	Niacin Equiv.	1.1 mg

NUTRITIONAL INFORMATION A good source of phosphorus and iron; moderate source of protein, zinc and niacin.

High fat high salt protein snack. Fat levels are increased due to reheating by frying.

DESCRIPTION About the same size as a frankfurter, a seafood stick is a combination of seafoods, mostly pike, held together with soya protein. The soya protein retains moisture, and helps to give a pleasing texture to the product.

ORIGIN AND HISTORY The fish stick, then known as a crab stick, was introduced to Australia in the early 1980s. Owing to the minimal amount of crab meat contained therein, suppliers were required to change the name. The sticks are manufactured in Japan, Thailand and other South-East Asian countries.

BUYING AND STORAGE Hot seafood sticks are required by law to be kept at a temperature of 60°C to prevent the growth of bacteria. This makes them very hot to handle, and many outlets do not maintain this temperature. The sticks can also be purchased cold and stored in the refrigerator until used.

PREPARATION AND USE Fast food seafood sticks are ready to eat. The sticks may be added to many types of cooking, for example, spaghetti marinara, pizza marinara, and seafood cocktail.

PROCESSING Flaked fish, mostly pike, is mixed with soya proteins, monosodium glutamate, salt, sugar, colour and preservatives, then moulded into sticks.

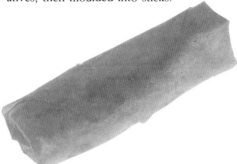

Spring Roll

MAJOR NUTRIENTS		FRIED SERVE SIZE 45 G	
Energy	435 kJ	Dietary Fibre	1 g
Protein	3 g	Sodium	350 mg
Fat	5 g	Potassium	50 mg
Cholesterol	5 mg	Phosphorus	50 mg
Carbohydrate	13 g	Iron	1 mg
Total Sugars	2 g	Niacin Equiv.	1 mg

NUTRITIONAL INFORMATION A good source of iron; moderate source of phosphorus and niacin; contains large amounts of fat and sodium.

High in energy and fats, especially saturated types if non-vegetable oils used in frying. Tasty because of the very high sodium level often in the form of monosodium glutamate. Fat content and energy level will depend on temperature and type of fats used in frying. Often contain monosodium glutamate 621.

DESCRIPTION A spring roll is a paper-thin, pliable pancakelike wrapper, topped with cooked vegetables and meats, rolled up into a neat parcel, and deep-fried until crisp and golden.

ORIGIN AND HISTORY The spring roll is traditional Chinese fare and has its variants throughout Asia. The popiah of Malaysia and Singapore, and the lumpia of the Philippines, are made in the same way except that they are not deep-fried. Deep-frying seals the package and makes it possible for the rolls to be kept warm for some time.

BUYING AND STORAGE The spring roll is one of the few fast foods which can be stored for some hours. It is best not to refrigerate them; however, they can be stored for some hours in an airtight container at room temperature and reheated, uncovered, on a tray in a hot oven. Always buy spring rolls on the day they are needed to ensure freshness. Frozen spring rolls are also available.

PREPARATION AND USE In their 'mini'

form, spring rolls can be used as an entree to a Chinese meal, or as a lunch or snack. Frozen spring roll wrappers are available in supermarket freezers to facilitate cooking at home.

PROCESSING The spring rolls available at fast food outlets are manufactured and frozen before distribution to the outlets, where they are thawed before cooking. It is required by law that hot foods be kept at a minimum temperature of 60°C to prevent the growth of bacteria.

VARIETIES

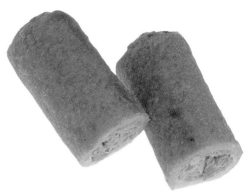

Chiko Roll This is an Australian brand name for a local spring roll.

MAJOR NUTRIENTS		SERVE SIZE 160 G	
Energy	1550 kJ	Potassium	240 mg
Protein	12 g	Calcium	45 mg
Fat	17 g	Phosphorus	175 mg
Cholesterol	11 mg	Magnesium	40 mg
Carbohydrate	45 g	Iron	2.5 mg
Total Sugars	11 g	Zinc	0.5 mg
Dietary Fibre	2 g	Thiamin	0.1 mg
Sodium	1105 mg	Niacin Equiv.	3.9 mg

NUTRITIONAL INFORMATION Deep-fried product high in total fat and therefore energy. An excellent source of protein, phosphorus, iron and niacin; good source of magnesium; moderate source of zinc; contains large amounts of fat, cholesterol and protein. Appealing taste may be due to the very high salt content. Fats used are generally of animal origin so chiko rolls will have a high saturated fat content.

Lumpia Spring roll from the Philippines.

Mini Spring Roll

Popiah Spring roll from Malaysia.

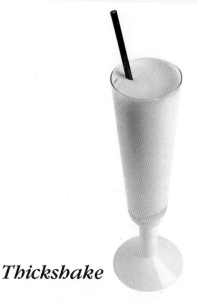

Thickshake

MAJOR NUTRIENTS

SERVE SIZE 200 G

Energy	920 kJ	Potassium	320 mg
Protein	10 g	Calcium	420 mg
Fat	7 g	Phosphorus	330 mg
Cholesterol	20 mg	Magnesium	25 mg
Carbohydrate	30 g	Vitamin A	50 mg
Total Sugars	30 g	Thiamin	0.1 mg
Dietary Fibre	0	Niacin Equiv.	2 mg
Sodium	160 mg	Riboflavin	0.5 mg

NUTRITIONAL INFORMATION An excellent source of protein, calcium, phosphorus, vitamin A and riboflavin; good source of niacin; moderate source of magnesium and thiamin; contains large amounts of fat and cholesterol. Higher fat levels than regular milkshakes with 27% of energy coming from fats.

DESCRIPTION A thickshake is served in the same way as a milkshake, although it is thick enough for a spoon or straw to stand upright without falling to the side. It is made in the same machine as soft-serve ice cream, but has added flavourings and a high proportion of water.

ORIGIN AND HISTORY The thickshake has evolved from the milkshake over the last 20 years, with the advent of soft-serve ice cream machines. An increase in health-conscious consumers has led to the introduction of a yoghurt flavoured thickshake, which many people mistakenly believe to be yoghurt based.

BUYING AND STORAGE Like milkshakes, thickshakes only have appeal when they are freshly made, and should be consumed straight away.

PREPARATION AND USE The equipment needed to make a thickshake is not available for domestic use. However, variations, limited only by the imagination, can be made at home. With 2 scoops of ice cream, a carton of plain or flavoured yoghurt, a little crushed ice and some ripe, soft fruit, a nutritious and filling thickshake can be made in a blender.

PROCESSING Thickshakes are made by the same machines that produce soft-serve ice cream. Although the exact process varies according to different machines, the basic principle is the same: water is added to a powdered pre-mix containing emulsifiers, stabilisers, starches, sugar and flavour and the machine mixes, aerates and freezes the mixture. The addition of air (referred to as overrun) can increase the volume by up to 50% and so improve the operator's profit.

SEE ALSO Milkshake.

CANNED AND PACKAGED FOODS

Some 10 000 years ago, when the seeds of wild grasses were pounded, mixed with water and baked into a crude, flat bread, the search for convenience in food storage and preparation began. Through the ages, by trial and error, methods have been discovered to make food taste better, look more appetising, store longer and become more economical to produce.

Many people bemoan the age of processed foods, fondly recalling homemade apple pies, and feeling obliged to revile the manufacturers of frozen products. The fact is, however, that many other interesting and rewarding pursuits become available to a home cook who can serve a good quality product without having to devote too much time to making it.

Most of the foods we eat undergo some sort of processing, whether the processing is done in a factory or in our kitchens. It is common to blame the food manufacturer for all the nutrition-related health problems in our community, but it rests with the consumer to obtain a knowledge of food and nutrition in order to make the best choices. If the consumer buys wholegrain products, and foods with less fat and salt, the manufacturer will produce them. Without commercially processed foods, in fact, the Western diet would be very much restricted.

When foods are processed (and processing includes home cooking), the greatest loss of nutrients is that of the vitamins. Vitamin C and folate are the least stable, but there is some loss of all vitamins between the harvesting of food and consumption. Losses vary with temperature, exposure to oxygen, and changes in acidity and alkalinity. Nutrients are leached into the cooking medium, whether this is water or fat. High temperatures, and exposure to air and increased alkalinity (for example, with the use of bicarbonate of soda), lead to greater vitamin losses.

Minerals are not destroyed by cooking, but again they may also be leached into the cooking medium. Both vitamins and minerals can be lost from the drippings when meat is grilled or baked.

Proteins, fats, carbohydrates and dietary fibre all undergo changes with cooking and processing, but these changes are less significant than the loss of vitamins. The changes may even improve digestion and absorption: for example, with the cooking of starch.

Many dry foods such as flours, pastas, cereals and biscuits are packaged. For the best results, these foods should be stored in a cool, dry place. The vitamin losses from such foods are small.

All foods with a shelf life of less than two years must be date-stamped. Most of our foods carry a use-by date. When stored correctly, food should be of high quality before the use-by date. After that time food may begin to deteriorate, but the deterioration of most products is slow. The exceptions are foods with a short shelf life, such as milk, which deteriorate quickly.

Most manufactured foods are processed soon after harvesting, which helps to reduce nutrient losses which sometimes occur during the handling of 'fresh' foods.

The labels on packaged foods carry a great deal of information which can assist the consumer to be more informed about nutrition and good food handling practices. A healthy diet can contain a mixture of processed and fresh foods, to suit individual needs and preferences.

CANNED FOOD

The canning industry dates back to 1809, when a French confectioner, Nicholas Appert, was awarded a prize by Napoleon Bonaparte for his invention of a process to keep foods edible for some length of time. He extracted the air from glass jars, and heated food inside the hermetically sealed containers. The following year, an Englishman, Peter Durand, began using tin-plated steel cans instead of jars. When a stamping process was invented in 1847 in the USA the lower cost of canned goods made them more viable for a wide range of foods.

Although canned goods are said to have a shelf life of 2–3 years, they can be stored safely for much longer. An Antarctic expedition not long ago discovered canned food left by Captain Scott 45 years before: the contents were still quite edible. A can of roast veal processed in 1824 was recovered in the 1930s, and was found to be palatable, appetising, and still with its nourishing qualities, including vitamin D.

It is important that a can is sound at the time of buying, and consumers should not accept cans that have bulging lids, rusty seams, dents in the rim or seam or any sign of pitting or corrosion. The ideal storage condition is 15–25°C.

Although the methods of processing canned foods vary depending upon the degree of sophistication of the production line, the actual steps in the process are standard. First the processed (cleaned, blanched, and cut) food is put in the open can. Blemished pieces are removed by hand. Only approved food additives may be used, and preservatives are not required for canned foods. Following cold, warm or hot filling, a puff of steam is shot into the top of the can between the body and the lid before the lid is seamed into place. The steam displaces the air, and upon condensation in the can, leaves a vacuum. The cans are then subjected to heat of over 100°C under pressure, for sufficient time for each product, completely sterilising the contents. A method of aseptic filling, developed in 1948, consists of sterilising a product prior to filling, by a high temperature-short time technique, sterilising the container, and filling under aseptic conditions. No further sterilisation after closing is necessary. Fresh foods for canning are processed as soon as possible after harvest.

When food is canned, it is sealed away from oxygen, and when it is stored in a cool, dry place the vitamin retention is good. Canned fruits and vegetables do not need to be cooked: if they are to be served hot, they only need to be heated just prior to serving. Foods treated in this way are comparable to other cooked foods.

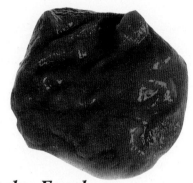

Baby Food

MAJOR NUTRIENTS

		JUNIOR BEEF DINNER SERVE SIZE 125 G	
Energy	410 kJ	Phosphorus	50 mg
Protein	5 g	Iron	1 mg
Fat	2 g	Vitamin A	140 μg
Cholesterol	5 mg	Thiamin	0.1 mg
Carbohydrate	17 g	Riboflavin	1 mg
Sodium	80 mg	Niacin Equiv.	1.9 mg
Potassium	165 mg		

NUTRITIONAL INFORMATION For an 8-month-old baby. An excellent source of protein, phosphorus, vitamin A, thiamin, riboflavin and niacin; good source of iron. There are few nutritional losses as cans are sealed before cooking. Baby food is all prepared under very controlled conditions and strict regulations. It is often lower in fat and sodium than the equivalent home-prepared food and is very convenient and microbiologically safe.

DESCRIPTION Baby food is specially prepared to be easily masticated and digested by infants. It is available with different particle sizes: strained, suitable for 4–8 months old; small particle size, for 8–12 months old; and chewable, for over 12 months. Most baby food is clearly labelled gluten free, salt free or sugar free, and all are free from preservatives, artificial colours and flavours.

BUYING AND STORAGE As with all canned and packaged foods, goods should not be bought if the lids are bulging, or the cans or packages are damaged in any major way. Cans and jars in good condition will last indefinitely if unopened. If less than a whole can is used at one meal, the remainder should be refrigerated in an airtight container. Jars can be re-sealed and refrigerated. A very convenient product for busy mothers is a jar of fruit juice with added vitamin C, which has a lid that can be replaced with a screw-on teat for immediate use.

PREPARATION AND USE Canned and packaged baby food is ready for consumption and requires only warming to a comfortable temperature before use. Rusks and compressed sticks of fruit are packed in airtight foil wraps and are ready for immediate use.

PROCESSING Raw ingredients are subjected to quality control before processing. Vegetables are scrubbed, trimmed by hand and mechanically diced, while fruits are washed, scalded, de-pitted where necessary, and pulped. Chickens and turkeys are cooked whole and then stripped from the bones. Ingredients are measured and mixed together in cauldrons, and for strained food, the mixture is put through a machine and reduced to a puree. It is then steam-cooked rapidly at high temperature, and bottled or canned.

VARIETIES
Canned Main Courses and Desserts, Bottled Gels and Desserts, Packet Rusks, Cereals and Snacks.

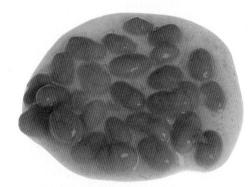

Baked Beans

MAJOR NUTRIENTS

		SERVE SIZE 200 G	
Energy	540 kJ	Calcium	90 mg
Protein	10 g	Phosphorus	180 mg
Fat	1 g	Magnesium	60 mg
Cholesterol	0	Iron	2.8 mg
Carbohydrate	20 g	Zinc	2 mg
Total Sugars	3 g	Thiamin	0.25 mg
Dietary Fibre	10 g	Niacin Equiv.	2.3 mg
Sodium	960 mg	Vitamin E	1 mg
Potassium	600 mg		

NUTRITIONAL INFORMATION An excellent source of protein, fibre, phosphorus, magnesium, iron and folate; good source of calcium, zinc, thiamin and vitamin E. Contains large amounts of sodium, although low sodium varieties are available. The protein does not contain adequate levels of all essential amino acids, but if eaten with a good cereal source, e.g. baked beans on toast, the two sources of protein complete each other.

DESCRIPTION Haricot beans (navy beans) are used for canning. In their tasty tomato sauce, they are a high protein, low cost, nofuss, instant meal. They are popular as a snack served on toast, and as a filling for sandwiches.

ORIGIN AND HISTORY Baked beans were discovered by the Pilgrim Fathers in 1620, when they found Indian squaws soaking beans and then baking them overnight with deer fat and an onion. The Pilgrim women replaced deer fat with pork, and added brown sugar and seasonings. Originally the beans were cooked by the town baker, who called each Saturday morning, took the family bean pot to a community oven, and returned the baked beans with fresh brown bread for Saturday supper. The first canned baked beans were made in 1875.

BUYING AND STORAGE As for canned food in general.

PREPARATION AND USE Baked beans are a fully-prepared product and require only heating. After the cans are sealed, they are cooked in a similar way to pressure cooking, which fully rehydrates the partially dried beans and optimises nutrient retention.

VARIETIES
Baked beans in tomato sauce, baked beans in ham sauce, baked beans in barbecue sauce.

SEE ALSO Haricot Bean.

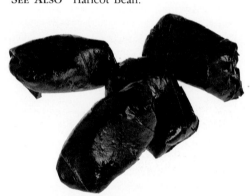

Canned Dolmas

also called Vine leaf rolls

MAJOR NUTRIENTS

		SERVE SIZE 100 G	
Energy	720 kJ	Cholesterol	0
Protein	3 g	Sodium	520 mg
Fat	7 g	Calcium	50 mg
Carbohydrate	24 g	Iron	0.9 mg

NUTRITIONAL INFORMATION Dolmas are a good source of iron; a moderate source of calcium; a high source of fat. There is no vitamin content analysis available. They have a high sodium content.

The analysis is for dolmas without meat. If animal fat is used in cooking, this would contain some cholesterol.

DESCRIPTION These are preserved vine leaf rolls, filled with a rice, pine nut, currant, onion and herb mixture. They are packed in soya oil in cans. There are numerous recipes in Middle Eastern and Greek cooking which carry the same name or slight variations of it, but all are either leaves of some kind, or hollowed out vegetables filled with a stuffing.

ORIGIN AND HISTORY This is one of those dishes which many countries claim as their own. The Turkish word, dolma, comes from the Persian dolmeh, which means 'stuffed'; the early Persians were very advanced in their culinary endeavours, and had a penchant for stuffing foods — fruits in particular.

As to the actual use of grape leaves as a wrapping, Athenaus, in his book, *The Diepnosophists* (AD 200), writes of 'entrees served in vine leaves'. Rice was introduced into Greece in 286 BC, so it might have been included.

The dolmas as described above are used in Armenian, Greek and Turkish cuisines; Orthodox Armenians and Greeks prepared them originally as a fasting food and it is possible that this particular version was adopted by the Ottoman Turks.

BUYING AND STORAGE Dolmas, prepared and packed in Greece, are available in cans from Greek and Middle Eastern food stores and delicatessens. They are also sold loose at delicatessens and takeaway food outlets. Store unopened canned dolmas at room temperature; store loose dolmas in a sealed container in the refrigerator for up to a week.

PREPARATION AND USE Drain excess oil from the dolmas; if they have been refrigerated, bring to room temperature before doing so. As they are packed in soya oil, the dolmas can be given a more authentic flavour if they are sprinkled lightly with a mixture of olive oil and lemon juice after draining. Serve as an appetiser or snack.

SEE ALSO Vine Leaf, in the chapter on Vegetables.

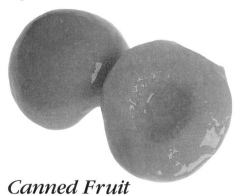

Canned Fruit

MAJOR NUTRIENTS   SERVE SIZE 100 G

Energy	405 kJ	Dietary Fibre	1 g
Protein	less than 1 g	Sodium	less than 5 mg
Fat	0	Potassium	120 mg
Carbohydrate	25 g	Vitamin C	3 mg
Total Sugars	25 g		

NUTRITIONAL INFORMATION A good source of vitamin C. Canning retains the majority of nutrients present in the fresh fruit, so the result is a rich carbohydrate containing significant vitamin C. Canned fruits are often more economical than the fresh variety, when it is not the main season for the fruit.

DESCRIPTION Canned fruits contain halves, pieces or slices of fruit in either a sugar and water syrup, or fruit juice. The consumer demand for low- or no-sugar foods has led to an increase of fruits in natural fruit juice, in both family and snack sizes. Pear juice is usually used, as it does not overpower the flavour of the fruit.

ORIGIN AND HISTORY As for canned food in general.

BUYING AND STORAGE As for canned food in general.

PREPARATION AND USE The fruit is best chilled prior to eating. It can be used as a dessert with ice cream or custard, or to augment a fresh fruit salad. Canned fruits also provide an easy way of decorating sweet flans and fruit tarts, and can replace fresh fruit in cooked desserts. Canned apricot halves can be used in a delicious stuffing for a boned leg of lamb, with herbs, spices and soft breadcrumbs.

VARIETIES
Fruit in heavy syrup, fruit in natural juice, fruit in light syrup.

SEE ALSO Peach.

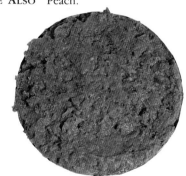

Canned Meal

MAJOR NUTRIENTS

	CANNED BEEF STEAK WITH GRAVY SERVE SIZE 150 G		
Energy	1080 kJ	Phosphorus	150 mg
Protein	22 g	Magnesium	21 mg
Fat	18 g	Iron	3.2 mg
Cholesterol	50 mg	Zinc	5.6 mg
Carbohydrate	1 g	Riboflavin	0.17 mg
Dietary Fibre	0	Niacin Equiv	9.2 mg
Sodium	580 mg	Vitamin C	0
Potassium	360 mg	Vitamin E	1 mg

NUTRITIONAL INFORMATION An excellent source of protein, zinc, iron and niacin; good source of phosphorus. Contains large amounts of sodium, cholesterol and fat.

DESCRIPTION Canned meals usually offer a mixture of meat, carbohydrate in the form of spaghetti or potato, and vegetables. They generally contain TVP to boost the 'meatiness', thickeners, and caramel, Worcestershire sauce or soya sauce to enhance the colour. Although they are savoury meals, most have a small amount of sugar as well as salt and spices.

ORIGIN AND HISTORY As for canned food in general.

BUYING AND STORAGE As for canned food in general.

PREPARATION AND USE Canned pies have a 'lid' of pastry, and, once the top of the can is removed, they are cooked in an oven. Other canned meals are popular with people working or holidaying outdoors, as they can be easily heated in a saucepan and also stored indefinitely as long-term rations. In everyday use, canned meals can be served alone or on toast, used as a pancake or pie filling, or added to vegetables or rice in a casserole.

VARIETIES
Spaghetti in beef sauce, savoury mince, chilli con carne, steak and mushroom pie, chicken pie, vegetables and braised steak, sweet and sour pork.

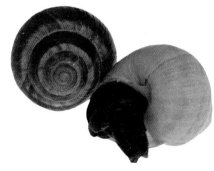

Canned Snails

MAJOR NUTRIENTS   SERVE SIZE 100 G

Protein	16 g	Carbohydrate	2 g
Fat	1.4 g	Iron	3.5 mg

NUTRITIONAL INFORMATION No analysis of other nutrients is available.

DESCRIPTION There are two types of edible snails from France: the Burgundy or French Vineyard variety (*Helix panatis Linnaeii*) and the Little Grey (*Helix aspersa Mullerii*). The *Achitina* swamp snail from Taiwan is tougher than the *Helix* varieties. Snail flesh is chewy, having a delicate flavour with a hint of earthiness. Cans usually contain about 18 snails, and have an over-stocking of mesh which holds cleaned shells.

ORIGIN AND HISTORY Most snail recipes come from the Burgundy, Poitou-Charente, Provence and Languedoc areas of France. Snails in Europe can be bought either fresh or prepared in the shell with garlic butter filling.

PREPARATION AND USE Canned snails are precooked and require only to be carefully placed in the shells and heated for a few minutes. They can be topped with a garlic butter, or served with a wine, garlic or provençale sauce. The snail is eaten with a small fork, or, in robust peasant fashion, sucked from the shell which is held in the fingers.

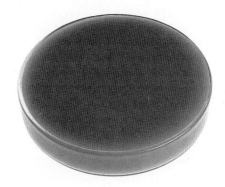

Canned Soup

MAJOR NUTRIENTS TOMATO
SERVE SIZE 200ML

Energy	460 kJ	Sodium	920 mg
Protein	2 g	Potassium	380 mg
Fat	7 g	Phosphorus	40 mg
Cholesterol	35 mg	Iron	0.8 mg
Carbohydrate	12 g	Vitamin A	400 µg
Total Sugars	5 g	Thiamin	.05 mg
Dietary Fibre	0	Niacin Equiv.	1.5 mg

NUTRITIONAL INFORMATION An excellent source of vitamin A; good source of folate; moderate source of phosphorus, thiamin and niacin. Contains large amounts of sodium. Processing reduces vitamin C levels. If diluted with milk rather than water, the nutritional value will be increased. Especially useful if skim milk is used.

DESCRIPTION Canned soups are concentrated to half their made-up volume, and generally have no preservatives, artificial colours or flavours. Although most existing soup ranges contain monosodium glutamate, the makers of Campbells Soups have dropped this flavour enhancer from their entire range of soups, in response to consumer opinion. Cream-style soups contain skim milk powder, whey powder and cream.

ORIGIN AND HISTORY As for canned food in general.

BUYING AND STORAGE As for canned food in general.

PREPARATION AND USE The contents of the can are mixed with equal or varied quantities of water and milk. Because of its milky consistency, a cream-style soup will still have a creamy character if only water is added, although milk is preferable for best results. Canned soups can be used undiluted as a casserole base to which meat and vegetables are added — for example, cream of mushroom or chicken soup with chicken, mushrooms, onions and chicken stock.

VARIETIES
Chicken, tomato, vegetable, mushroom, beef, pea and ham, celery, cream varieties.

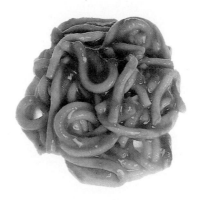

Canned Spaghetti

MAJOR NUTRIENTS SPAGHETTI IN TOMATO SAUCE
SERVE SIZE 200 G

Energy	500 kJ	Sodium	1000 mg
Protein	3 g	Potassium	260 mg
Fat	1 g	Calcium	40 mg
Cholesterol	0	Phosphorus	60 mg
Carbohydrate	24 g	Iron	0.8 mg
Total Sugars	7 g	Niacin Equiv.	1 mg
Dietary Fibre	0		

NUTRITIONAL INFORMATION A good source of phosphorus; moderate source of calcium, iron and niacin. Contains large amounts of sodium. Sodium levels may be lower if no-added or reduced-salt variety is selected. Excellent high complex carbohydrate meal or snack.

DESCRIPTION Long strands of soft, thick spaghetti are canned with a sauce of tomato puree, flavoured with sugar, salt, spices, food acids and cheese. This is a universally popular snack or light meal, served alone or on toast.

ORIGIN AND HISTORY As for canned food in general.

BUYING AND STORAGE As for canned food in general.

PREPARATION AND USE Spaghetti in tomato sauce is a totally prepared food and only requires heating. It can also be used straight from the can as a sandwich filling.

VARIETIES
Spaghetti in tomato sauce with cheese or with cheese and ham.

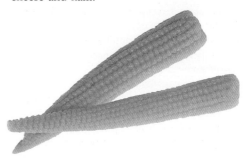

Canned Vegetables

MAJOR NUTRIENTS BABY CORN
SERVE SIZE 100 G

Energy	520 kJ	Phosphorus	120 mg
Protein	8 g	Magnesium	45 mg
Fat	2 g	Iron	0.9 mg
Cholesterol	0	Zinc	1 mg
Carbohydrate	22 g	Vitamin A	60 µg
Total Sugars	2 g	Thiamin	0.2 mg
Dietary Fibre	5 g	Niacin Equiv.	2.9 mg
Sodium	0	Vitamin C	9 mg
Potassium	280 mg		

NUTRITIONAL INFORMATION An excellent source of phosphorus, thiamin and vitamin C; good source of protein, magnesium, iron and niacin; moderate source of zinc. This is a useful high protein vegetable, which is low in sodium when no sodium is added in processing.

DESCRIPTION Essentially fresh vegetables preserved in liquid, some canned vegetables such as carrots, peas and beans tend to have an overcooked consistency, with a high moisture content. Some developments in aseptic packaging are making higher quality vegetables possible because of reduced sterilisation time. Vegetables used in salads, such as beetroot, sweet corn and asparagus, maintain their flavour and texture and are a time-saving convenience for the modern householder.

ORIGIN AND HISTORY As for canned food in general.

BUYING AND STORAGE As for canned food in general.

PREPARATION AND USE Canned vegetables are fully processed and ready for use. Those to be eaten hot need to be decanted into a saucepan or microwave-safe container and heated through prior to serving, but no further cooking is required.

VARIETIES
Tomatoes, beans, sweet corn, mushrooms, asparagus, beetroot, peas.

PACKAGED FOOD

The first processed foods in history were probably chuno, native Andean potatoes, preserved as long as 2000 or 3000 years ago. Pemmican, air-dried venison or buffalo meat, was invented by pre-Columbian American Indians.

In Europe, hot air for drying purposes was introduced in 1795 by Mason and Challet in France, who cut vegetables in thin slices and passed heated air over them. When British soldiers were suffering from scurvy during the Crimean War, it is recorded that shipments of dried carrots, potatoes, and meat powder were sent from England; the soldiers found them most unpalatable.

Both World Wars prompted expansion in food dehydration, but production decreased in peacetime. Onion, garlic, milk, potato and egg dehydration formed the basis of a new 'convenience' food industry. Freeze drying, long assumed too costly for general drying of foods, is now used widely for quality dehydration of red meats, chicken, shrimp, mushrooms, and herbs.

A dried packaged food should be in a pack designed to protect the ingredients from the deteriorating effects of moisture penetration, discoloration from exposure to light, and damage to fragile ingredients from crushing. The use-by date should be checked, and the pack should be inspected for faulty assembly or recent damage. Sachets should not be unevenly wrinkled or distorted, as material can sometimes be trapped between the two layers of the opening when it is sealed, resulting in an inadequate seal. Packets that look damaged are best avoided, as even a minute break in the seal will allow moisture to enter and greatly increase the risk of contamination. Packet dried foods should be stored away from prolonged exposure to moisture or heat. If the entire contents are not used after opening, the top of the packet can be folded down and it can be stored in a screwtop, airtight jar.

Dry foods are blended in stainless steel mixing machines that ensure a consistent, uniform product. Following blending, the dry mixes are packed on a variety of machines, the objective being to achieve the best barrier qualities in the pack while minimising cost. In recent years, laminates comprised of various plastics, nylons, paper, foil and printed or sprayed-on coatings have greatly improved the availability and quality of packaging material.

Aseptic packaging, in containers such as tetrapack cardboard or film, is becoming widely used for foods such as UHT milk, milk drinks, fruit juice, soya beverages, soups and casseroles. Throughout the processing, these foods are handled mechanically to prevent infection and the sterilised, cooled products are put into presterilised containers which are aseptically, hermetically sealed in an atmosphere free of micro-organisms. The vitamin retention of such products is excellent.

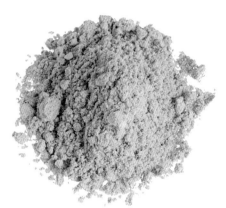

Instant Dried Casserole or Base

MAJOR NUTRIENTS

		INSTANT DRIED CASSEROLE MIX SERVE SIZE 100 G	
Energy	20 kJ	Total Sugars	3 g
Protein	2 g	Dietary Fibre	0
Fat	1 g	Sodium	400 mg
Cholesterol	0	Potassium	500 mg
Carbohydrate	7 g		

NUTRITIONAL INFORMATION Contains large amounts of sodium. Sauce mixes are used to add flavour to base foods, therefore they are often highly seasoned and many will contain monosodium glutamate.

DESCRIPTION Dried casseroles are packed in an airtight moisture-proof pouch, some-times within a cardboard box. They are similar to sauce mixes, and require the addition of meat and liquid to make the casserole. The flavour is usually strongly based on salt, hydrolised vegetable protein, and monosodium glutamate. Although there is a trend towards products which have no added monosodium glutamate, this does not necessarily mean the mix is totally free of it, as it may be contained in small proportions in some of the ingredients.

ORIGIN AND HISTORY A 20th-century phenomenon.

BUYING AND STORAGE Readily obtainable, with a use-by date.

PREPARATION AND USE All brands of packaged casseroles carry instructions. Chopped onion and garlic can be browned in a little oil before adding the other ingredients, and the addition of fresh vegetables during cooking makes the meal a little more 'home-made'. It is advisable to check ingredient listings, as some brands have a high content of dehydrated vegetables while others have none. The meals can be varied by using a different type of meat.

VARIETIES

Beef Stroganoff, chicken, savoury, French onion, Oriental seasoning mixes.

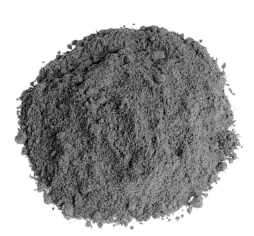

Instant Sauce or Gravy

MAJOR NUTRIENTS

		INSTANT GRAVY SERVE SIZE 50 G	
Energy	130 kJ	Total Sugars	2 g
Protein	1 g	Dietary Fibre	0
Fat	0	Sodium	470 mg
Cholesterol	0	Potassium	100 mg
Carbohydrate	6 g		

NUTRITIONAL INFORMATION Contains large amounts of sodium.

DESCRIPTION Sauce mixes fall into two categories: white sauces — predominantly milk powder, thickening agents, salt and monosodium glutamate; and dark sauces, containing thickeners, hydrolysed vegetable protein, various vegetable powders and pieces, salt, monosodium glutamate and colouring. They are packed in sealed, moisture-proof sachets. When made according to directions, the sauce is smooth, glossy and thick.

ORIGIN AND HISTORY Dates from the 20th century.

BUYING AND STORAGE Available with use-by date.

PREPARATION AND USE The average sauce takes 2–7 minutes to prepare. Water is added to the powder, and it is stirred over heat until it has thickened. The sauce can be enhanced by adding fresh ingredients, such as parsley or mushrooms, or varied to suit individual needs, by adding, for example, grated cheese to the white sauce, and mushrooms and red wine or cream to the beef sauce.

VARIETIES

White, parsley, pepper, chicken, beef, mushroom, onion etc.

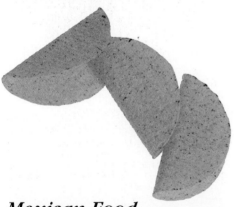

Mexican Food

NUTRITIONAL INFORMATION Although reduced in moisture content, the flour-based Mexican foods are unchanged in nutrient value in their packaged form.

DESCRIPTION Mexican cooking at home has been made possible by the ready availability of all the basic ingredients. Some of the Mexican foods are even marketed as 'kits' that include taco shells, seasoning and sauce. A Mexican meal is based on a thin bread made of finely ground corn (tortilla), sometimes deep fried to make the firm taco shell. Enchiladas are soft tortillas made with various fillings and sauces, then folded. Tamales are similar but made with a more elaborate dough, then steamed.

ORIGIN AND HISTORY Following the advent of dry seasoning mixes, which initially provided a convenient method of preparing

gravies and sauces, manufacturers looked for ways to expand their market by introducing seasonings for preparing a special cuisine at home. In America, the home of processed foods, Mexican food, popular with Californians and Texans in particular, was a logical progression into convenience-based foods.

BUYING AND STORAGE Corn-based products, such as taco shells and corn chips, are prone to insect infestation. Products purchased within the use-by date should be sound, provided the packaging is not split or damaged. To take care after purchasing, avoid storing with other flour-based products, and keep any not immediately used in an airtight container. Follow the same procedures for the dry seasoning mixes and sauces as for any other similar product.

PREPARATION AND USE For tacos, preparation generally involves cooking minced beef with the contents of the seasoning sachet. Vegetables such as lettuce, tomato, cucumber and avocado are sliced or diced, and tasty cheese is grated, each item being put into individual serving dishes. The taco shells are heated in a convection or microwave oven, then filled with the prepared ingredients and topped with sauce or salsa to taste.

PROCESSING See Snack Food for corn chip processing.

VARIETIES

Taco shells, taco seasoning, refried beans, taco sauce, Jalapeno cheese dip, tortillas, corn chips, tamale dip.

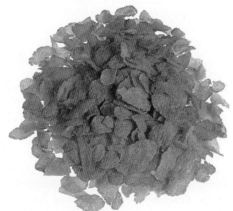

Packet Cereal

MAJOR NUTRIENTS   CORNFLAKES
SERVE SIZE 30 G

Energy	480 kJ	Sodium	350 mg
Protein	2 g	Potassium	30 mg
Fat	less than 1 g	Phosphorus	30 mg
Cholesterol	0	Iron	2.9 mg
Carbohydrate	26 g	Thiamin	0.25 mg
Total Sugars	3 g	Riboflavin	0.50 mg
Dietary Fibre	2 g	Niacin Equiv.	3.5 mg

NUTRITIONAL INFORMATION An excellent source of iron, thiamin, riboflavin and niacin; moderate source of phosphorus. Contains large amounts of sodium, which is added to most commercial cereals during processing. Low sodium varieties or reduced sodium varieties are becoming available. Wholegrain based cereals will have increased levels of fibre and other nutrients.

DESCRIPTION Packet cereals are made from cereal grains that have been processed and reproduced in another form, designed to provide wider appeal to consumers than wholegrain cereals. They are easy to chew, with a light, crunchy texture (not unlike snack foods), and contain added vitamins and minerals. These 'lightweight' cereals are usually high in sugar, although some are specially formulated to be low-joule. Muesli-type cereals have a blend of fruits, nuts, coconut, sugar, oats and oat bran, wheat bran, and seeds, to provide a more wholesome and filling breakfast cereal.

ORIGIN AND HISTORY In Roman times, the goddess of grain was Ceres, from which the word 'cereal' is derived. Cereal was considered so valuable by the Romans that there is a record of discontent among soldiers who were given rations of meat instead of cereal.

In 1866, Mother Ellen Harmon White (spiritual leader of the Adventist Church), founded a health institute in Michigan. Some years later, a Dr John Harvey Kellogg came to manage the institute, changing the name to Battle Creek Sanitarium. To help a patient who had broken her dentures, Dr Kellogg created a breakfast cereal made from thin flakes of corn. These cornflakes began a huge industry, worth billions of dollars worldwide and over $355 million a year in Australia alone.

BUYING AND STORAGE In order to retain their characteristic freshness and crispness, cereals should be packed in moisture-proof bags inside a cardboard box, to prevent the contents being crushed. Check use-by dates and do not buy torn or split packs; also look out for any web, indicating insect activity, near the corners of the box. After opening, fold the inner bag over as many times as possible, or keep the remaining contents in an airtight container to prevent sogginess.

PREPARATION AND USE Most packet cereals are served with chilled or warmed milk, and a sprinkling of sugar is optional. Cereals should not be left to stand after the milk has been added, as this rapidly reduces their crispness. Sliced fruit such as banana rings can be added, and some muesli fanciers like to add extra dried fruits, nuts or bran to suit their own tastes.

PROCESSING Cornflakes are made from maize, off the cob, which initially goes through a 'gritting' process that eliminates the flour component of the grain and leaves hard, glossy sections of maize referred to as 'grits'. Following this, the grits are cooked under pressure with water and flavourings such as malt and sugar. The grain is then left to stand and cool in a 'tempering' stage, while the moisture and flavours evenly disperse and develop through the grits over a number of hours. The dried material passes through mill rolls, making the flakes, which are dropped into a high temperature oven. The heat forms a blister on the flake, drying it and making it crisp. Cereal biscuits such as Weet-Bix are made by compressing the grain at the tempering stage. They are then further cooked and dried out, remaining intact as a biscuit.

VARIETIES
Cornflakes, rice bubbles, Weet-Bix, muesli, bran, oat bran, low-joule cereals.

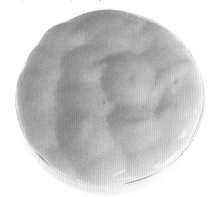

Packet Dessert

MAJOR NUTRIENTS   CUSTARD POWDER
                                   SERVE SIZE 50 ML

Energy	250 kJ	Dietary Fibre	0
Protein	2 g	Sodium	40 mg
Fat	2 g	Potassium	85 mg
Cholesterol	7 mg	Calcium	70 mg
Carbohydrate	8 g	Phosphorus	55 mg
Total Sugars	6 g	Vitamin A	40 µg

NUTRITIONAL INFORMATION A moderate source of calcium, phosphorus and vitamin A. The fat and cholesterol level could be reduced if made with skim milk.

DESCRIPTION In dry-mix desserts, most of the ingredients are included, requiring only the addition of water or milk. They differ from completely homemade products in that they contain emulsifiers, colourings and flavourings to ensure that the end product is of consistent and uniform quality. A sponge pudding mix contains two sachets, one similar to a cake mix, requiring the addition of an egg

and water, and the other a sauce sachet, which is sprinkled over the cake mixture before cooking.

ORIGIN AND HISTORY Largely a 20th century phenomenon, although some prepared mixes were known in the 19th century.

BUYING AND STORAGE Available with use-by date.

PREPARATION AND USE As well as in its traditional presentation, jelly can be used as a topping for flans and cheesecakes, cut into cubes in trifle, used as a filling for hollowed-out orange halves, and poured over fruit before setting. Jelly can be used in many decorative ways, especially in children's food. Using custard powder which already contains eggs, a boiled custard can be made within 10 minutes. Once prepared, it can be used as a pouring custard, mixed with sliced bananas, or included in a trifle.

VARIETIES
Jelly crystals, custard powder, sponge pudding mix, self-saucing puddings.

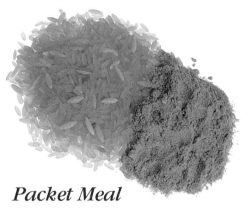

Packet Meal

MAJOR NUTRIENTS   RICE A RISO, COOKED
                             SERVE SIZE 150 G

Energy	800 kJ	Sodium	800 mg
Protein	5 g	Potassium	200 mg
Fat	2 g	Phosphorus	50 mg
Cholesterol	0	Magnesium	45 mg
Carbohydrate	53 g	Iron	1 mg
Total Sugars	1 g	Zinc	2 mg
Dietary Fibre	1 g	Niacin Equiv.	2 mg

NUTRITIONAL INFORMATION A good source of iron and zinc; moderate source of niacin. Contains large amounts of sodium, which gives a strong flavour. Low fat meals with the main nutrients coming from the rice.

DESCRIPTION Popular with people with little time or inclination for cooking, these meals are contained in two moisture-proof pouches within a box. One pouch contains rice or pasta (the bulk of the meal), while the second contains dried meat, vegetables, thickener, hydrolised vegetable protein, and monosodium glutamate. Nearly all packet

meals rely on monosodium glutamate to boost the flavour.

ORIGIN AND HISTORY A 20th century phenomenon.

BUYING AND STORAGE Readily available, with use-by date.

PREPARATION AND USE All packaged meals have cooking instructions on the packet. Macaroni cheese, with the addition of butter and milk, can be made in only 10 minutes using just one saucepan. The more sophisticated two-part meals take about 20 minutes to prepare, and can be enhanced by adding extra vegetables or spices to taste.

VARIETIES
Chicken or prawn curry with rice, macaroni cheese.

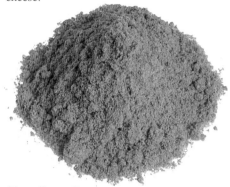

Packet Soup

MAJOR NUTRIENTS   TOMATO
                                   SERVE SIZE 159 mL

Energy	200 kJ	Total Sugars	5 g
Protein	1 g	Dietary Fibre	0
Fat	less than 1 g	Sodium	590 mg
Cholesterol	0	Potassium	130 mg
Carbohydrate	9 g		

NUTRITIONAL INFORMATION Contains large amounts of sodium. The nutrient content would improve if made with milk.

DESCRIPTION Packet soups are comprised of a dry, powdered mixture of thickeners, hydrolised vegetable protein, salt, colourings and flavourings, with a primary ingredient such as mushrooms, split peas, noodles or vegetables. Cream-type soups contain non-fat milk solids and when made up are thick-bodied, smooth and tasty.

ORIGIN AND HISTORY Dates from the 20th century.

BUYING AND STORAGE Available with use-by date.

PREPARATION AND USE Each packet carries specific directions, usually involving the addition of water or milk, and a short simmering time. Individual-serve sachets can be prepared in a mug or cup for extra convenience. Soup mixes can be used in the same way as sauce mixes and casserole bases, and extra recipe ideas are printed on many packets.

VARIETIES

Vegetable, tomato, beef, chicken, pea and ham, mushroom, noodle and cream varieties.

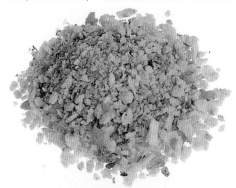

Packet Stuffing

MAJOR NUTRIENTS

		BREADED SERVE SIZE 20 G	
Energy	250 kJ	Total Sugars	1 g
Protein	2 g	Dietary Fibre	
Fat	less than 1 g		less than 1 g
Cholesterol	0	Sodium	1020 mg
Carbohydrate	12 g	Potassium	20 mg

NUTRITIONAL INFORMATION Contains large amounts of sodium. Commercial stuffings rely on high sodium based flavourings.

DESCRIPTION Mostly breadcrumbs, a stuffing mix also contains a herby, salty seasoning with added monosodium glutamate and colour. It requires a moistening agent such as water, butter, egg or wine to make the crumbs soften and cling together.

ORIGIN AND HISTORY Dates from the 20th century.

BUYING AND STORAGE Readily available, with use-by date.

PREPARATION AND USE Instructions for preparation are printed on the packet. The addition of extra chopped onion, garlic and herbs, or more exotic touches such as capers, chopped dried fruit, spices and spirits, can make the mixture more individual. Primarily for use as a poultry and meat stuffing, a breadcrumb mix, combined with a little melted butter, can be used as a crumbly topping for mornays and sauce-topped, oven-baked meals such as moussaka and lasagne.

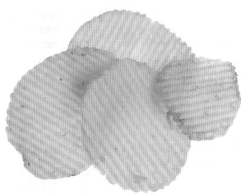

Snack Food

MAJOR NUTRIENTS

		POTATO CRISPS SERVE SIZE 25 G	
Energy	550 kJ	Sodium	120 mg
Protein	1 g	Potassium	300 mg
Fat	7 g	Phosphorus	40 mg
Cholesterol	5 mg	Iron	0.5 mg
Carbohydrate	12 g	Niacin Equiv.	1 mg
Total Sugars	0	Vitamin C	3 mg
Dietary Fibre	1 g		

NUTRITIONAL INFORMATION A good source of vitamin C; moderate source of phosphorus, iron and niacin. Contains large amounts of fat from which over 45% of energy is derived. The large surface area of the thin chips enables maximum fat uptake.

DESCRIPTION Snack foods are bite-size morsels of food, generally based on potato or cereals, which are processed and flavoured. They are consumed with drinks or eaten to take the edge off the appetite while awaiting a main meal. Tending to have a higher savoury flavour profile than whole food, and with a light and crunchy texture, the ratio of flavour to food volume is higher than it is in a meal. Flavours such as vinegar, cheese, tomato, chilli and spices combined with salt and monosodium glutamate make up most of the characteristic snack food tastes.

ORIGIN AND HISTORY The invention of potato chips is generally credited to an American Indian named George Crumb, who was the chef at Moon's Lake House in Saratoga Springs. According to the story, a fussy patron kept sending his French-fried potatoes back to the kitchen, complaining that they were not thin enough. Crumb sliced some potatoes as thin as paper, deep-fried them and sent them out to the guest in a fury. The patron was delighted with the result, and what is now the most popular snack food in the Western world was created.

An American Indian was also the father of popcorn. A brave named Quadequina presented a bushel of popped corn to the Pilgrim Fathers and their Indian guests at the first Thanksgiving in 1621. Today, popcorn stand concessions are a major income earner for American movie theatres. The principle of popcorn applies to snacks such as cheese rings, made with the help of modern technology.

BUYING AND STORAGE Much of the appeal of snack foods comes from the crisp, light, dry, crunchy texture, and it is therefore important that the packaging provides sufficient protection from moisture to prevent sogginess, and that handling does not crush the delicate contents. Because of the relatively short shelf life of snack foods compared to other dry processed foods, check the use-by date. Do not buy packs that are split or crushed.

PREPARATION AND USE Packaged snack foods are ready for immediate use. Corn chips and potato crisps can be served with a dipping sauce, or crushed lightly and used as a topping on mornays and other sauce-covered baked dishes.

PROCESSING Processers contract farmers to grow special low-sugar, low-moisture potatoes for making potato crisps. They are washed, peeled, sliced very thinly, and dropped into oil heated to 184°C for 3 minutes. Extruded snacks such as Twisties are made from a mixture which may contain rice flour, semolina-sized particles of corn, seasonings, or potato, mixed with a minimum of water. This is pushed at extreme pressure through a very hot barrel at high temperature (a process known as extrusion). As it is shot from the end of the barrel, the high internal temperature causes the product to expand rapidly in the cooler air (in the same way that corn pops).

Cheese-flavoured products are immersed in a slurry of oil and cheese, heated to about 40°C. When they emerge, the oil soaks in, and the cheese forms a coating on the outside of the snack food.

Modern popcorn has been improved over the years to have less hull content and more air, so that each kernel expands to forty times its size.

Corn chips are among the oldest kind of fried cereal snacks. The dough, made from a mixture of processed white and yellow corn of the dent type, is formed into large cylindrical loaves. It is then put into a hydraulically powered press with a piston which forces the dough through a die plate with a series of slot-like openings about 1 cm wide. A cutting device severs the extruded strands into pieces of the desired length, and they fall directly into hot cooking oil. The chips are then salted, cooled and packaged. For larger sizes such as taco shells, the dough is rolled out and cut to shape.

VARIETIES

Potato crisps, cheese rings, corn chips, pork skin, popcorn.

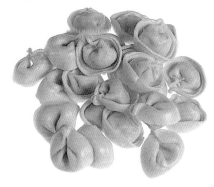

Vacuum Packed Foods

NUTRITIONAL INFORMATION   Vacuum packaging does not alter the nutritional value of any food.

DESCRIPTION   Vacuum packages are made from flexible impermeable materials, either clear or opaque. This packaging removes most of the air from the pack before it is sealed, leaving the characteristic solid block of product. Some foods such as coffee have a longer shelf life when the oxidising effect of prolonged exposure to air is reduced.

ORIGIN AND HISTORY   The first form of vacuum packaging was actually canning, as the air had to be removed before the cans were subjected to heat under pressure to sterilise the contents. In the early days of canning, crude methods involved heating the container until the food began to dribble through a hole in the top (indicating that the air had been expelled), and then closing the hole with a drop of solder. Machines to create a vacuum for canning were developed, consisting of a chamber of about one cubic metre, in which the can was placed with the lid resting on the top of the filled can. A vacuum was drawn in the chamber (and consequently the can also), then the can was spun and a double seam put onto the end to secure the lid.

The first flexible vacuum packs were made of rubber latex. A machine like a vacuum cleaner drew the air out and the rubber was tied off. Modern technology has led to the development of many different films with various barrier qualities, which are used depending upon the application.

BUYING AND STORAGE   Vacuum packs should not be confused with Controlled Atmosphere packs, where the packing is performed in a room with a controlled atmosphere, or Modified Atmosphere packs, where the air is removed and replaced with an inert gas such as nitrogen. Neither of these have the characteristic hard feel of a vacuum pack. True vacuum packs should be almost rock hard; any softness indicates that air has leaked in, either through a faulty seal or damage to the pack. Once opened, vacuum packs should be folded down and stored in an airtight screw-top glass jar to protect the unused contents. Follow the manufacturer's instructions on the label.

PREPARATION AND USE   No special preparation is required for vacuum packed foods. Unless otherwise indicated on the label, instructions for use would be the same as for the particular food if purchased in ordinary packaging.

PROCESSING   Most modern consumer-sized vacuum packs are produced using a machine which has a chamber about 70 cm square and 15 cm deep, with a hinged top-opening lid like a chest freezer. The filled flexible bag is placed in the chamber with the opening lying over a line of heat-sealing wires. The lid is closed and a vacuum is drawn inside the chamber (including the bag). When a pre-set vacuum level is reached, the machine automatically seals the bag (retaining its vacuum) and releases the vacuum in the chamber so that the lid can be opened. In some machines, up to a dozen small bags can be produced at a time. Larger machines that suck the air out of the bag only, without placing it in a chamber, are generally for industrial use only.

VARIETIES

Coffee, meat, smallgoods, grains, nuts, prepared pasta.

FROZEN FOOD

Frozen foods are either fresh foods that have been cleaned, peeled, cut or re-formed in some way prior to freezing, or they are processed foods which have been frozen, and require further cooking or thawing with no further processing. The freezing process takes the temperature down to a level (below −18°C) when micro-organisms cease to be active, and chemical, biochemical and physical reactions act at a much slower rate, thus preserving the food in a condition almost identical to its state just prior to freezing. When food is frozen, the water contained in the cells turns into ice crystals. The longer it takes to freeze a product, the bigger the crystals will become. If the crystals become too large, they damage the walls of the cells, resulting in excess loss of juices when the food is thawed. When quick or 'snap' freezing methods are used, the ice crystals are smaller, and the cell structure is not damaged.

As early as 1000 BC, the Chinese were cutting and storing ice. Man's fascination with ice, and the appreciation of its abilities to preserve food, led to a huge ice-harvesting industry in the mid-19th century in America's northern lakes and rivers, where huge blocks of ice were cut. In an ambitious undertaking in 1833, Frederick Tudor sent his ship *Tuscany* to Calcutta with 180 tons of ice, which remained mostly unmelted for the four month journey. By 1846, 130 000 tons of ice were being transported to more than 50 destinations in the USA as well as the Caribbean, South America, Persia, China, the Philippines, the East Indies and Australia. The icebox (a term coined in America) had become commonplace.

Frozen foods as a commercial product would not have been possible if mechanical refrigeration had not been developed. The English physicist, Michael Faraday, discovered in 1823 that certain gases under constant pressure condense until they cool. Although successive inventors refined mechanical refrigeration, home refrigerators did not appear on the market in America until 1918. By 1937, home freezers had become commercially viable in the USA.

It is important when buying frozen foods to observe how well the retailer handles the goods. Stocks of frozen food in aisles, waiting to be stacked into freezers, are an indication that management is not careful enough. Many frozen and chilled food manufacturers supply handling instructions to supermarkets, and experts in the industry state that tea-breaks and other distractions must all wait until the frozen foods have been correctly stored. Unless these products are properly stored and packed, surface moisture can evaporate, and in extreme cases, the product surface dries out to such a degree that cells and tissues are damaged. This is called 'freezer burn'. Consumers should check the use-by date and, after purchasing, transport frozen food home to the freezer as soon as possible. Insulated containers and bags are useful if frozen foods have to spend more than 30 minutes out of the freezer between the store and home.

Most or all of the preparation of frozen food is done prior to freezing. Frozen vegetables are blanched (that is, plunged briefly into boiling water) before they are frozen, and fully defrosted small vegetables like peas and spinach need only a few minutes in boiling water before serving. Most other frozen vegetables should be cooked in the same way as fresh ones, preferably defrosted before cooking. Meat can be cooked straight from the freezer, allowing about 50% more time than usual, or can be defrosted in the refrigerator for several hours prior to cooking. Although leaving food at room temperature to thaw is a common method, it does give potentially harmful bacteria a chance to develop.

Because of the rigours to which the foods are subjected during freezing, processed foods such as meat pies and cakes often require different flavours and emulsifiers from those normally used in the freshly baked product. Packaging is important, and has a considerable effect on the food when it is thawed. The packaging material must not only be good, it should also be tightly wrapped to prevent loss of quality caused if the packing is not water-vapour proof. It is essential that the temperature of frozen foods be maintained as low as practicable during storage, distribution and retailing. Frozen food, stored at the correct temperature of -18°C or below, has excellent keeping qualities, and the vitamin losses are very small for periods up to 6–12 months. If the temperature is allowed to rise vitamin losses are much higher.

Cooked frozen vegetables are nutritionally comparable to fresh, cooked vegetables, and they may even be superior in comparison with 'fresh' ones which have been stored for several days.

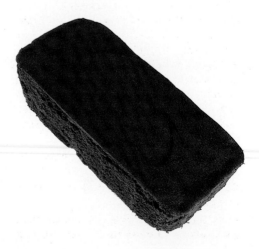

Frozen Cake

MAJOR NUTRIENTS

		CHOCOLATE CAKE SERVE SIZE 50 G	
Energy	770 kJ	Dietary Fibre	0
Protein	2 g	Sodium	100 mg
Fat	11 g	Potassium	55 mg
Cholesterol	70 mg	Calcium	40 mg
Carbohydrate	22 g	Phosphorus	50 mg
Total Sugars	17 g	Vitamin A	140 µg

NUTRITIONAL INFORMATION A moderate source of calcium and phosphorus. Contains large amounts of fat and cholesterol. This cake has a cream filling and chocolate icing, which raises the total fat content. Most frozen cakes tend to have these higher fat fillings.

DESCRIPTION Frozen cakes are generally smaller than the average homemade cake. Reputable brands are made from high quality ingredients, and have a genuine home-cooked flavour. Some varieties are topped with a frosting or icing, and are ready to serve, while others are left plain for further decoration as desired.

ORIGIN AND HISTORY In the late 1940s, Charles Lubin, a Chicago baker, found that demand for his cheesecakes outside his immediate area was increasing. In order to deliver the product in as fresh a condition as possible, he decided to freeze them, and arranged for existing frozen food distributors to transport them. This was so successful that he stopped selling unfrozen cakes altogether, and the well-known Sara Lee company was born. Charles Lubin believed that a cake frozen immediately after baking must always be fresher than a 'fresh' bakery cake, which has already had several hours to begin to stale before being bought.

BUYING AND STORAGE Follow general Frozen Food guidelines.

PREPARATION AND USE Unless further icing or decoration is desired, no preparation is required for frozen cakes. The outer packaging and lid should be removed while the cake is still frozen, and the cake should be left at room temperature for at least thirty minutes to ensure total thawing before using. Uneaten portions can be stored as with fresh cake, or returned to the freezer.

PROCESSING Cakes are fully cooked before freezing, which makes the freezing process relatively simple, and does away with the need for some of the special modified starches and emulsifiers required to keep uncooked or semi-cooked food stable.

VARIETIES
Sultana pound cake, chocolate cake, carrot cake, prefilled sponge sandwich, apple walnut cake, orange cake, banana cake.

SEE ALSO Cakes and Pastries.

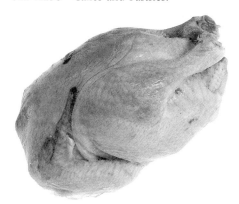

Frozen Chicken

NUTRITIONAL INFORMATION Freezing does not alter the nutrients of poultry.

DESCRIPTION A frozen chicken is a convenience food that can be bought in advance and defrosted on the day that it is to be cooked. Most frozen chickens do not have neck and giblets included, so the weight shown on the pack is the body weight alone.

PREPARATION AND USE The first step in using a frozen chicken is defrosting which can

be done in about thirty minutes on Low or Defrost in a microwave, after first removing any metal clasps from the plastic wrap. A chicken can also be defrosted overnight in the refrigerator, or in a few hours at room temperature. Once thawed, it can be used in exactly the same way as fresh chicken.

PROCESSING Chicken processors have found freezing of surplus production to be the most cost-effective way to meet fluctuations in supply and demand. All fresh chickens are 'deep chilled' until the deep muscle temperature is around three to four degrees Celsius. Those chickens which are additional to the day's requirements for fresh birds are put into freezer bags and 'blast' frozen for three to four hours. As slow freezing forms larger ice crystals (see Frozen Foods, general processing), giving a poorer result, consumers requiring frozen chickens are advised to buy them commercially frozen, rather than purchasing fresh chickens and freezing them in the home freezer.

SEE ALSO Chicken.

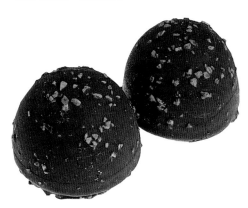

Frozen Dessert

NUTRITIONAL INFORMATION Freezing does not alter the nutrient value of desserts.

DESCRIPTION Frozen desserts are generally of good quality, giving a high degree of convenience for busy householders. The desserts are usually fully cooked, and can be used without further preparation when they are completely thawed.

ORIGIN AND HISTORY A 20th century product.

BUYING AND STORAGE Follow general rules for Frozen Foods. As with all frozen foods, these products should not be allowed to thaw before reaching the home freezer.

PREPARATION AND USE A pie or Danish can be taken from the freezer half an hour before heating in the oven. Always make sure that the oven is fully preheated so that the product heats right through, and the pastry is

crisp. To use a fully cooked dessert cold, allow it to thaw in the refrigerator overnight.

VARIETIES
Apart from ice cream, these include fruit pie, fruit Danish, cheesecake and so on.

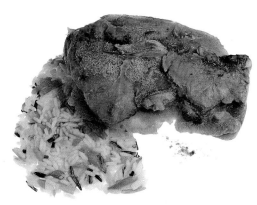

Frozen Main Meal

MAJOR NUTRIENTS		LEAN CUISINE
	ORIENTAL BEEF WITH VEGETABLES	
		SERVE SIZE 245 G
Energy	1090 kJ	Potassium	270 mg
Protein	18 g	Iron	1.5 mg
Fat	8 g	Vitamin A	225 µg
Cholesterol	35 mg	Thiamin	0.15 mg
Carbohydrate	30 g	Riboflavin	0.15 mg
Dietary Fibre	3 g	Niacin Equiv.	2.8 mg
Sodium	1270 mg		

NUTRITIONAL INFORMATION An excellent source of protein, iron, vitamin A, niacin; good source of thiamin and riboflavin. Contains large amounts of sodium and is a significant source of cholesterol. A well balanced main meal with less than 45% of energy coming from complex carbohydrates and less than 30% coming from fat. For people who do not have the time, skills or energy to cook a main meal, these are excellent quick and easy meals that can be stored in the freezer for several weeks.

DESCRIPTION Frozen meals cover a wide spectrum of food styles, from the TV dinner concept of meat and vegetables in a formed foil platter, to foods in separate pouches, which can be heated in boiling water or in a microwave (such as Lean Cuisine and Fish in Sauce). Fierce competition in Australia between suppliers in this convenience food industry has led to some very high quality products for consumers.

ORIGIN AND HISTORY Dates from the 20th century.

BUYING AND STORAGE Follow general Frozen Food guidelines.

PREPARATION AND USE All frozen meal packages carry instructions for preparation. It is important to remember that not all microwave ovens are the same, and microwave instructions should only be considered as a general indication.

VARIETIES
Lean Cuisine, fish in sauce, beef and cheese burgers, roast dinners, chicken Kiev, pasta meals.

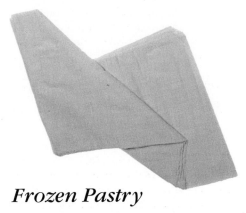

Frozen Pastry

NUTRITIONAL INFORMATION Freezing does not require a change in the formulation of pastry, so fat levels and therefore energy levels depend on the type used.

DESCRIPTION Pastries vary according to the amount of shortening used. Flaky and puff pastries begin in a similar way to shortcrust, and are then folded and re-rolled, with shortening between each layer. Filo is a traditional Greek pastry, almost as thin as a sheet of paper. Most frozen pastry is sold in ready-rolled sheets, ready to use.

ORIGIN AND HISTORY The first frozen pastry was sold in a small block, which needed rolling once it was thawed. This was initially a cost-effective way for pie manufacturers to use excess production capacity. As the market grew, engineering developments made it possible to produce pre-rolled sheets of pastry, which were then frozen. Consumption of frozen pastry is declining, as, in this age of convenience foods, consumers are buying the complete product from the supermarket freezer.

PREPARATION AND USE While they are frozen, sheets of pastry are quite brittle, and it is necessary to thaw them before handling in order to prevent breakages. There are several sheets in a pack, so the required sheets should be carefully peeled away and the remainder sealed in an airtight bag and returned immediately to the freezer. Once thawed, the pastry can be used in exactly the same way as fresh, homemade pastry.

Filo pastry is cooked in several layers, each being brushed with melted butter or margarine, so that as it cooks, each layer separates and becomes light and crisp. During preparation, the filo should be covered with a clean, damp towel to prevent drying out. Unused sheets can be sealed in an airtight plastic bag and returned to the freezer.

VARIETIES
Shortcrust, puff, filo, flaky.

SEE ALSO Cakes and Pastries.

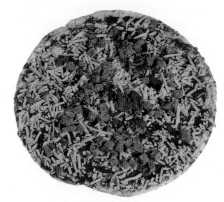

Frozen Pizza

MAJOR NUTRIENTS		SERVE SIZE 150 G	
Energy	1500 kJ	Calcium	240 mg
Protein	21 g	Phosphorus	250 mg
Fat	16 g	Magnesium	30 mg
Cholesterol	27 mg	Iron	1.8 mg
Carbohydrate	40 g	Zinc	2.3 mg
Total Sugars	2 g	Vitamin A	75 µg
Dietary Fibre	3 g	Thiamin	0.10 mg
Sodium	1080 mg	Riboflavin	0.20 mg
Potassium	225 g	Niacin Equiv.	4.8 mg

NUTRITIONAL INFORMATION An excellent source of protein, phosphorus, iron and niacin; good source of zinc and riboflavin; moderate source of magnesium and thiamin. Contains large amounts of fat and sodium and significant amounts of cholesterol. The nutrients will vary slightly with the type of topping. All varieties will be high energy, high sodium products.

DESCRIPTION Frozen pizza is in a partially-cooked state at the time of freezing. Although the pastry base is cooked, the topping is not, and the process of 'finishing off' in the oven at home gives an impression of freshly-cooked, home-baked food with the convenience of a preprepared frozen product.

BUYING AND STORAGE Follow general Frozen Food guidelines.

PREPARATION AND USE Frozen pizzas have instructions on the packaging. The pizza has a close-fitting film of polyester sealed around it, and this must be removed before placing in a hot oven to heat the base and cook the topping. Some brands have microwave directions, and a special tray incorpor-

ated with the packaging is designed to create extremely high temperatures where the pizza base is in contact with the tray. Additional grated cheese and herbs and spices can be added to frozen pizzas prior to cooking to suit individual tastes.

PROCESSING The pizza dough is made in batches by mixing the flour, yeast, oil, salt, seasoning and a certain amount of fresh scrap from previous batches, in a dough mixer. Water is added, and after mixing, the dough is emptied onto a tray to rise or 'proof'. Following the first proof, it is tipped into a pastry extruder and formed into large sheets, which are cut to fit the foil pizza trays. The bases are kept warm for the second proofing period, then baked. After the cooked bases have cooled, tomato-based pizza sauce and cheese are applied, and various garnishes depending upon the type of pizza. More cheese is sometimes added on top of the garnishes, then the pizzas are frozen and packed into polyester film bags within the printed carton.

VARIETIES
Many, including beef, ham and pineapple, cheese and bacon, supreme.

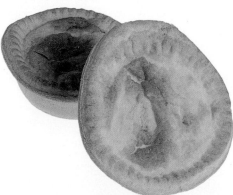

Frozen Snack

NUTRITIONAL INFORMATION Freezing does not alter the nutrients of snacks such as pies, rolls and so on.

DESCRIPTION Frozen snacks are usually small and dry enough to be eaten with the fingers. Pies and sausage rolls are small versions of the usual variety (see Fast Foods). Spinach and meat triangles are Greek-inspired snacks, encased in layers of paper-thin filo pastry. The seafood platter contains a selection of fish fillets, calamari, prawns and scallops which have been crumbed and quickly fried before freezing, so that they achieve a deep-fried finish without extra oil. Chicken nuggets are also processed this way.

ORIGIN AND HISTORY Dates from the 20th century.

BUYING AND STORAGE As with all frozen foods, the out-of-freezer time between the store and home should be as short as possible. The food should not be allowed to thaw until it is to be cooked.

PREPARATION AND USE Chicken nuggets can be reheated in the pan, griller or oven. All frozen snack foods have instructions for heating or cooking. Filo pastry triangles should be kept frozen until they are put into the pre-heated oven, to ensure very dry, crisp pastry. In some ovens, a better result is achieved by spreading the triangles out on a baking sheet instead of leaving them in their foil tray. Frozen Chinese snacks such as dim sims and spring rolls should be quickly deep-fried in very hot oil and drained well before serving. Frozen snacks are particularly useful for buffet parties and for use as hors d'oeuvres.

VARIETIES

Party pies and sausage rolls, spinach and cheese triangles, spicy meat triangles, seafood platter, chicken nuggets, Chinese snacks, crispy pancakes, prefilled vol-au-vent.

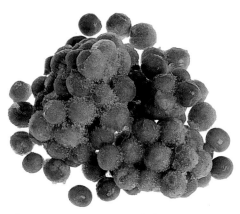

Frozen Vegetables

NUTRITIONAL INFORMATION Freezing does not change the nutrients of a vegetable.

DESCRIPTION With the exception of potato products, frozen vegetables have been cleaned, blanched and rapidly cooled, then frozen with no additives. Potato chips and fries are quickly fried in beef fat before freezing, so that the frozen product is partly cooked and already sealed by the fat. Potato gems are comprised of dehydrated potato flakes and starches, mixed with egg white, vegetable oil and a batter binder. They are formed into balls, fried quickly, and 'blast' frozen.

ORIGIN AND HISTORY The first frozen vegetables went on sale in 1930, under the name of Clarence Birdseye, a scientist from Brooklyn. Due to lack of scientific understanding of the freezing process, he ran into problems caused by the high liquid content of the products, which rapidly shed their moisture on defrosting. Although initially responsive, the buying public soon became disenchanted and transferred their preferences back to canned vegetables for some years. Improved methods and product quality have returned frozen vegetables to popularity.

PREPARATION AND USE Frozen potato chips and gems are partly cooked and should be cooked under a griller or in a hot oven to achieve a 'fried' effect without the addition of more oil. Other vegetables can be added to boiling water direct from the packet; or the required amount can be taken out and thawed first, then cooked in the normal way, with a slightly shorter cooking time than for fresh vegetables.

PROCESSING Vegetables for freezing are contract grown by farmers who deliver the fresh goods directly to the processers. After quality inspections, the vegetables are washed and blanched quickly in boiling water to kill bacteria and enzymes naturally occurring on the surface, and to prevent discolouring when defrosting. Mashed potato products such as 'Pommes Noisettes' are made from dehydrated potato flakes, and have a similar consistency and flavour to instant mashed potato.

VARIETIES

Green beans, butter beans, peas, corn on the cob, mixed vegetables, Chinese vegetables, potato chips, French fries, potato gems.

SEE ALSO Vegetables.

DRINKS

The basis of all drinks, water, is an essential nutrient: without water a human can survive for only a few days. The body of an adult is about 60% water, and about 2.5 litres of water each day is needed to replenish this water content. In a mixed, healthy diet, about half the water needed comes in foods: for example, most fruits and vegetables contain 80% or more water, while lean cooked meats and chicken contain about 60%. A few foods only, such as sugar and oil, do not contain water.

A further 10% of the water needed is produced in the body as an end product of metabolism, while the remaining water (about 40%) must come from drinks.

In an affluent society, plain water tends to be a neglected beverage, most people relying on tea, coffee, fruit juice and other beverages to supply their water needs. Government health bodies in all countries maintain standards for drinking water, which include regulations for levels of minerals and micro-organisms, and for the control of toxic or dangerous contaminants.

Pure or distilled water tastes very 'flat', whereas drinking water from natural sources has a characteristic flavour which is influenced by the level of minerals present. In Australia, for instance, the water supplies in South Australia and Western Australia contain more sodium and other minerals than the waters in the eastern states. The reticulated water supply in many countries is chlorinated, which also affects the taste of the water, but it should be remembered that chlorination does a great deal to eliminate the risk of water-borne diseases such as cholera, typhoid and dysentery.

Another important nutrient which is provided by many reticulated water supplies worldwide is fluoride. Sometimes the fluoride occurs naturally but it is usually added; the fluoridation of water supplies has been an important factor in reducing the prevalence of tooth decay in many societies.

The drinks in this chapter have been chosen to give a representative range of the wide variety of beverages available today. Since it is important to take account of the nutritional differences between non-alcoholic and alcoholic beverages, the chapter has been divided into these two sections.

ALCOHOLIC BEVERAGES

The abuse of alcohol is one of the major health problems in modern times. Although less than 5% of deaths are directly attributable to alcohol in most countries, it can be a factor in about one third of hospital admissions.

Nonetheless, humans have used alcohol for centuries, and they will continue to do so. Education should help to overcome the problems and increase the number of people who drink wisely. Indeed, many people consume alcohol in moderation and it adds to their pleasure and relaxation.

It is important for those who drink alcohol to understand the health hazards linked with alcohol abuse, and to know the meaning of 'safe drinking' and enjoyable drinking.

A standard drink provides approximately 10 g of alcohol, and health recommendations state that women and men restrict their alcohol intake to no more than 2 and 4 drinks daily respectively. It is also recommended that alcohol be avoided on at least 2 or 3 days each week.

Repeated excessive drinking will eventually damage all body tissues, in the brain, liver, heart, muscles, gastrointestinal tract, genitals, lungs, pancreas, nervous system, blood and skin.

Alcohol is produced by the fermentation of sugars from various plant sources. Spirits are produced by distillation, which concentrates alcohol in the liquids so formed. Liqueurs are based on the extraction of essential oils from various fruits and herbs. Fortified wines, such as sherry and vermouth, are produced by adding spirits at the end of fermentation.

The percentage of alcohol in such beverages is as follows: beer 2–6%; table wine 10–12%; fortified wine about 20%; distilled spirits (including liqueurs) 37–45%.

About 10 g of alcohol is normally to be found in the following standard drinks: 425 mL of low-joule beer; 285 mL of regular beer; 120 mL of table wine; 60 mL of fortified wine; 30 mL of spirits.

Drinks are an essential part of our diet. It is important to quench the thirst with water, and use drinks which provide kilojoules in moderation. If alcohol is used, healthy guidelines should be adhered to.

Advocaat

*also called **Advokaat***

MAJOR NUTRIENTS　　　　　SERVE SIZE 30 mL

Energy	370 kJ	Carbohydrate	9 g
Protein	1 g	Alcohol	4 g
Fat	2 g		

NUTRITIONAL INFORMATION This liqueur is unusual because it contains protein, fat and cholesterol. Advocaat contains 13% pure egg yolk, 30–32% sucrose and up to 17% alcohol according to its Australian manufacturers.

DESCRIPTION A thick, yellow liqueur.

ORIGIN AND HISTORY Traditionally made according to a homespun kitchen recipe from the Netherlands, advocaat probably started off as a pleasurable way of using up the plentiful supply of farm eggs, mixed with the native spirits of the area. It has changed little over the centuries, though brandy is now the base spirit and vanilla or other soft aromatic flavours are added. The name stems from the expression 'talking like an advocate or lawyer' — a reference to smooth tongues, perhaps.

BUYING AND STORAGE A generic liqueur that is produced by several distillers to a universal style, it is readily available from liquor stores. Keeps well at room temperature.

PREPARATION AND USE Whipped into cream, advocaat adds a special flavour to trifles. It may be drunk neat or act as the base for long drinks. Add milk, hot or cold, with grated nutmeg on top. It is mixed with gin, cointreau and orange juice for Fluffy Duck and with lemonade for a Snowball.

PROCESSING Egg yolks, sugar, aromatic spirits and brandewijn are blended together, then heated 'au bain-marie' and stirred constantly.

Beer

MAJOR NUTRIENTS　　　　　SERVE SIZE 285 mL

Energy	476 kJ	Phosphorus	86 mg
Carbohydrate	9 g	Sodium	51 mg
Alcohol	11 g	Potassium	3–11 µg
Protein	1 g		

NUTRITIONAL INFORMATION By comparison to other alcoholic beverages, e.g. wine and spirits, ale has a relatively low alcohol content. However, when consumed in quantity, ale can contribute significantly to the energy content of one's diet. It is well known for its diuretic effect although it is unknown which nutrient is responsible for this.

DESCRIPTION Brown, fermented liquid that may form a 'head' of foam when poured.

ORIGIN AND HISTORY It is impossible to say where and when the brewing of beer began, though it was probably discovered by accident when harvested grain became wet and germinated, followed by natural fermentation which produced a crude beer mash. Beer has been made by virtually all people in all stages of civilisation and, as early as 6000 BC, the brewing process was well established in Babylon. All sorts of grains and plants were experimented with. Gradually, however, most countries decided on barley and hops, although potatoes are still used for Strasbourg beer, and wheat is an important element in the famous white beer of northern Germany.

BUYING AND STORAGE Several types of beer are available at liquor stores, including ale, lager, stout and light, in many local and imported brands. Store away from light for no more than three months. In warmer climates, people tend to refrigerate beer for several hours before drinking.

PREPARATION AND USE Serve cold as a drink. Can be added to soups, cheese, batter and meat dishes for flavouring and for tenderising meat.

PROCESSING Brewed from malt, sugar, hops and water and fermented with yeast.

VARIETIES

Ale A type of beer that is usually heavier and slightly more bitter than other beer.

Lager A light-coloured, clear, carbonated beer.

Brandy

DESCRIPTION A light brown spirit.

ORIGIN AND HISTORY Most probable origin of the word brandy is the Dutch brandewijn (burned wine). At one time burning was synonymous with distilling, and the Netherlands was the birthplace of European commercial spirit production, where alchemists spent their time trying to produce gold and an elixir for long life.

BUYING AND STORAGE Made by several distillers, brandy is readily available at liquor stores. It should be stood upright, to prevent the spirit from rotting the cork, and kept at a temperature of between 15–18°C, away from penetrating light and strong odours. Once a brandy is bottled it will not improve further.

PREPARATION AND USE May be served neat, or mixed as a long drink. Adds flavour and distinction to many dishes when used with discretion in the kitchen. Used medicinally for troubled stomachs. Brandy-based cocktails include Brandy Alexander, Sidecar and Brandy Crusta.

VARIETIES

Apricot Brandy Distilled and infused from the kernels and the juicy pulp of ripe apricots. A second liqueur that is distilled from various herbs is added and later enriched with cognac.

Cognac A light brown spirit with the fragrance of wine. The district of Cognac around the town of that name in France is divided into zones of descending prestige: Grande Champagne, Petite Champagne, Borderies, Fins Bois, Bons Bois and Bois Ordinaires. Produced from several grape varieties, the wine is double-distilled in pot stills and matured in oak casks. Some very old and specially fine cognacs are often used for blending with a younger spirit.

Cider

MAJOR NUTRIENTS　　　　　ALCOHOLIC
　　　　　　　　　　　　　　SERVE SIZE 200 mL

Energy	300 kJ	Alcohol	10 g
Carbohydrate	2 g		

NUTRITIONAL INFORMATION Alcoholic ciders are fermented with sacchramices, or wine yeast. Their strength can vary between 6–9% compared to sweet ciders which contain no alcohol. Sweet ciders, as their name implies, contain considerably more carbohydrate (12 g per 100 mL) and 50 more kilojoules per 100 mL, and therefore have very similar nutritional value to apple juice.

DESCRIPTION A pale drink with the scent of apples.

ORIGIN AND HISTORY With wine and beer, cider is one of the oldest fermented beverages. When Julius Caesar landed in Britain in 55 BC he found that cider was already a popular drink. It was made from wild apples growing in the forests and, according to Celtic mythology, the apple was sacred; an apple god is known to have been worshipped.

BUYING AND STORAGE Ciders vary enormously in strength, character and degree of sweetness and may be alcoholic or non-alcoholic. Store in a cool cupboard or cellar.

PREPARATION AND USE May be consumed still or sparkling. Used to flavour soups, main course dishes and desserts.

PROCESSING The fruit is pressed, then fermented either by the addition of acid or naturally in vessels used for the previous batch, and filtered. Draught cider is then matured in wooden barrels.

Alternatively, the cider may be pasteurised or sterilised and stored in aluminium casks (keg cider), or bottled, with or without carbonation.

Clear Spirits

NUTRITIONAL INFORMATION Spirits provide only energy (over 300 kJ in a 30 mL drink) and alcohol (10 g).

DESCRIPTION Any clear, distilled liquor which has an alcohol content of over 37%.

ORIGIN AND HISTORY The Latin 'aqua vitae' (water of life) is the ancient general term for distilled alcohol. Some spirits have a trace of flavour from the material from which they are distilled; others are highly rectified, practically neutral spirits which can be savoured, or tossed down at a gulp, before or at the beginning of a meal, or as a 'nightcap'.

BUYING AND STORAGE Store in a cool dark cupboard or cellar.

PREPARATION AND USE Spirits may be served 'neat', with water or mixes, at room temperature or ice cold, depending on taste and tradition.

PROCESSING Grains, vegetables or fruits are distilled to produce a neutral spirit, which may then be redistilled with other flavourings.

VARIETIES

Aquavit A highly rectified colourless spirit.

Arrack Also called *Arack, Arak, Raki*, this is a straw-coloured spirit.

Calvados A straw-coloured spirit distilled from cider.

Gin A rectified spirit distilled from malted barley, maize and rye, it is flavoured with a choice of or an admixture of juniper berries, coriander seeds, angelica, orris root, cassia bark, almonds, cardamoms, bitter orange peel, fennel and liquorice.

Grappa Sharp, dry, usually colourless, grappa is made from marc — the grape skins, pips etc., left in the wine press after wine is made.

Ouzo This neutral spirit is distilled either once or twice from wine or grain in Greece and Cyprus. Its light green colour becomes opalescent as ice and water are added.

Sake Sake is a doubly fermented brew made from a rice base. Pale amber in colour, with a curious sweet but dry flavour, it is the traditional Japanese beverage taken with meals. It is also drunk to celebrate a marriage and is offered at the shrines of ancestors.

Schnapps Also called *Schnaps, Snaps*, this is a high-alcohol, clear spirit from central Europe, usually flavoured with caraway, though an old custom has recently been revived and myrtle and mixtures of other suitable herbs are used to make schnapps even more bitter.

Slivovitz A clear spirit from fermented plums. In Yugoslavia and other Balkan and Middle European countries it has long been popular as a rather potent home-brew. It has equivalents in other countries, such as the homemade Mirabelle of France.

Tequila Tequila is a clear spirit distilled from the fermented liquid of the crushed, pineapple-like bases of the Mexican succulent, *Agave tequilina*.

Vodka Thought to have originated in the 12th century in Russia and Poland, vodka was the generic name for any spirit drink, whether distilled from grape, grain or potato. The name means 'little water'.

Coffee Liqueurs

DESCRIPTION These are rich, dark liqueurs.

ORIGIN AND HISTORY Made from quality coffee and rum, these liqueurs are popular worldwide.

BUYING AND STORAGE Proprietary liqueurs, readily available from liquor stores, they keep well at room temperature.

PREPARATION AND USE They can be added to desserts, cakes and ice cream, though they are used mainly as a drink. They can be mixed with milk or cream and served in coffee, as a mixed drink with soda or cola, or on their own with ice.

VARIETIES

Kahlua A rich liqueur made in Mexico, and under licence in Denmark.

Tia Maria A Jamaican coffee liqueur, dating from 1655.

Crème Liqueurs

NUTRITIONAL INFORMATION Most cream liqueurs are fully imported and their true recipes are closely kept secrets of their manufacturers. Those made in Australia do not in fact contain any cream (fat), although their name implies this. Their creamy texture is a result of their very high sucrose content, i.e. 30–32%, and of other ingredients providing 'body'. The alcohol level is usually greater than 17%.

DESCRIPTION Liqueurs with a rich, sweet flavour and smooth texture.

ORIGIN AND HISTORY The word 'crème' once designated a drink that had been sweetened, to differentiate it from a dry spirit such as brandy. Nowadays it is used to designate liqueurs that have been heavily sugared to give a cream-like consistency. The word 'cream' on the label can also mean that cream has been added for extra richness.

BUYING AND STORAGE There is a vast list of crèmes, many of which are more syrups than liqueurs, available from liquor stores. May be stored indefinitely in a cool cupboard.

PREPARATION AND USE Serve as an after-dinner drink. Refer to the varieties listed for further use.

VARIETIES

Crème de Bananes A very sweet liqueur with a pleasant banana taste.

Crème de Cacao A brandy-based liqueur using roasted cocoa beans and vanilla.

Crème de Cassis With a blackcurrant flavour.

Crème de Menthe Green or white, and mint-flavoured.

Fortified Wines

Major Nutrients			PORT SERVE SIZE 60 mL
Energy	400 kJ	Alcohol	10 g
Carbohydrate	8 g	Potassium	58 mg

			SWEET SHERRY SERVE SIZE 60 mL
Energy	352 kJ	Phosphorus	6 mg
Carbohydrate	5 g	Sodium	8 mg
Alcohol	9 g	Potassium	100 mg
Calcium	4 mg		

			DRY SHERRY SERVE SIZE 60 mL
Energy	281 kJ	Phosphorus	6 mg
Carbohydrate	1 g	Sodium	6 mg
Alcohol	10 g	Potassium	135 mg
Calcium	4 mg		

			VERMOUTH SERVE SIZE 60 mL
Energy	367 kJ	Alcohol	11 g
Carbohydrate	4 g		

NUTRITIONAL INFORMATION High levels of carbohydrate and alcohol make any fortified wine a high kilojoule drink. The very high potassium content of port and sherry should be noted by those on potassium-restricted diets. Port is also known to contain histamines and natural salicylates which may have side effects such as headache in some sensitive individuals.

DESCRIPTION Fortified wines are golden, rosy red or a deep, tawny brown.

ORIGIN AND HISTORY Mainly enjoyed as after-dinner drinks, the fortified wines are made from grapes, fermented until a point in the wine making process when a spirit is added, to retain the sugar and increase the alcoholic strength.

BUYING AND STORAGE The wines are readily available and keep well at room temperature. Ruby and tawny port may be stored upright but vintage port should be stored on its side and will require decanting.

PREPARATION AND USE Served as an after-dinner drink at room temperature, these wines can also be used in cooking, where the flavours add a richness to soups, meat dishes, sauces and desserts.

VARIETIES

Madeira When Portuguese mariners originally settled on the island of Madeira, they started a fire that lasted seven years. The wood ash deposits that resulted made the soil extremely fertile and when grape vines were planted, they flourished. Madeira, Portuguese for timber, is now the name of one of the finest of fortified wines.

Marsala A sweet fortified wine, originally from the sea port of Marsala on the Italian island of Sicily.

Port The best known of the dessert wines, the true port is made from a variety of grapes grown in the Upper Douro Valley in Portugal.

Ruby is the least expensive and is matured in wood only as long as is required to make it ready for drinking. Tawny is paler and is superior, having spent up to fifteen years in cask. Vintage port is from an exceptional wine and is sold for laying down as it will go on improving virtually indefinitely.

Sherry Also called *Jerez, Sack, Sherris, Xeres*, sherry is a fortified wine produced principally from the Palomino grape. Spanish sherries, unlike many of their imitators, are subject to a very special process of fermentation, ageing and blending which make the product unequalled in the world.

Vermouth Vermouths are aromatised wines which have been fortified. Basic wine is usually of ordinary quality, blended to a set style. Flavouring may include herbs, roots, barks, fruits, flowers, peels, quinine.

Fruit and Nut Liqueurs

NUTRITIONAL INFORMATION No specific data are available, but liqueurs, because of their sugar content, are very high in kilojoules. 10 g of alcohol or more is present in a 30 mL serve.

DESCRIPTION Fruit and nut liqueurs have the mellow colours of the foods from which they are derived, or are refined to a colourless liquid. The texture is usually quite viscous and the taste very sweet, with the high alcohol in the spirit base being easily discernible.

ORIGIN AND HISTORY The recipes for some of these liqueurs are many hundreds of years old, and they have been developed by family companies (and in Europe by religious institutions), to eventually reach markets worldwide.

BUYING AND STORAGE They are readily available, and keep well at room temperature.

PREPARATION AND USE Popular as after-dinner drinks, they may be consumed at room temperature or with ice, depending on preference. They also give character to an endless range of cocktails.

VARIETIES

Amaretto Italian liqueur with a strong almond flavour.

Cherry Brandy The finest quality is made from the juice of ripe dark-red Marasco cherries, which grow in Dalmatia, the coastal area of Yugoslavia. While pressing the cherries to obtain the juice, some of the cherry stones are also crushed to add a touch of attractive bitterness to the very sweet cherry flavour. The most famous comes from Denmark, where Peter Heering started selling it from his shop over 150 years ago.

Cointreau A colourless, viscous liqueur with the tang of oranges. In the middle 1800s, Edouard Cointreau, the son of a French confectioner, visited the West Indies where he tasted the wild orange. He took the dried peel back to France where the family experimented by blending it with other orange peels, steeped them in brandy, then distilled the infusions with various regional herbs and spices. They eventually evolved an outstanding balance of flavours and aromas. The formula for Cointreau, a very fine triple sec, has never been changed.

Curaçao Originally a light rum-based liqueur that was distilled from the dried peel of sweet and bitter oranges on the island of Curaçao, it is now made in the traditional way around the globe, and is available in orange, white and blue.

Grand Marnier A French liqueur, Grand Marnier is an original blend of fine old French cognac from the fine champagne cognac found only in the Charentes region, and an extract of oranges from the peel of the bitter orange.

Kirsch A colourless, fiery liqueur, principally a product of the German Black Forest area, it is distilled from the fermented juice of small, black, very juicy cherries and the crushed kernels of the fruit. It is bottled at a high alcoholic strength and has a strong and penetrating flavour.

Malibu A clear drink based on white rum, with the subtle addition of coconut.

Maraschino This colourless liqueur made in Yugoslavia and Italy has an intense, sweet flavour and a strong aroma of cherries.

Parfait Amour This purple liqueur was created by Bols many centuries ago. Translated, the name means 'Perfect Love'. The exotic aromas and flavours are obtained by the use of curaçao orange peel, vanilla pods, almonds and rose petals.

Van Der Hum A distinctive and popular South African sweet liqueur based on the South African naartjes, a sort of tangerine, and herbs. The name roughly translates from Afrikaans as 'Mr What's His Name' as no one can remember who invented it.

Herb and Spice Liqueurs

NUTRITIONAL INFORMATION No specific data are available, but these liqueurs have a high sugar content and are thus high in kilojoules. 10 g or more of alcohol is present in a 30 mL serve.

DESCRIPTION The addition of herbs and spices to these spirit-based drinks gives rise to a range of brilliant colours, and imparts distinctive aromas to the liqueurs. The texture and sweetness are similar to those of the fruit and nut liqueurs, although some herb liqueurs have an astringent or even slightly bitter taste.

ORIGIN AND HISTORY Many of the recipes for these drinks have been kept secret, and used over centuries in Europe.

BUYING AND STORAGE These liqueurs are readily available and keep well at room temperature.

PREPARATION AND USE Favoured as after-dinner drinks, they may be consumed at room temperature or with ice, as preferred. The bright colours make them especially suitable as ingredients for cocktails.

VARIETIES

Anice A clear, colourless liqueur popular as an aperitif. Derived from aniseeds, including the refined star anise of China, it has a flavour further enhanced by a touch of liquorice.

Anisette This is one of the sweetest liqueurs, distilled from the finest aniseed and a number of other herbs which add depth to the flavour. One of the oldest liqueurs in the world, it is made in many countries, particularly France, Spain, Italy and Holland.

Bénédictine A light brown, aromatic liqueur, that was first compounded by a French monk, Dom Bernard Vincelli, at a monastery at Fécamp in about 1510 from herbs and plants cultivated in the fields and gardens near his abbey. The formula is still a closely guarded secret known to only three people, and is based on fine cognac. The initials DOM stand for 'Deo Optimo Maximo' (to God, most good, most great).

Chartreuse The story goes that an old formula for an elixir of long life was given to the Carthusian monks in Paris in 1605. It was not until a century and a half later, however, that a Carthusian Brother, Jérôme Maubec, sorted out the complicated recipe and actually produced the elixir. The Carthusian Order suffered many ups and downs, including total expulsion from France in 1901, but at all times the monks preserved the secret of their liqueur, and eventually brought it back to its homeland in the Grenoble area. Distilled today from the original recipe involving some 130 herbs, from which five concentrated extracts are derived. These are blended to produce two types of chartreuse, the very strong green chartreuse and the sweet and less strong yellow.

Fiori Alpini This is easily recognisable in its traditional long-necked clear bottle. It is based on alpine herbs and a branch of the herb plant is left in the liqueur. Crystals of sugar are grown on the twigs which add to its dramatic appearance. It has a soft, sweet flavour and is yellow in colour.

Galliano A yellow, viscous liqueur with a distinct aniseed flavour, created in the 1890s by Arturo Vaccari in his laboratory in Leghorn, Italy, Galliano was named after an Italian hero of the Abyssinian campaign of 1895–6. The tall Galliano bottle is one of the few bottles registered as a trademark.

Golwasser Also called Gold Wasser de Danzig, golwasser is a white, orange or gold liqueur made from a variety of imported herbs, seeds and roots. The main ingredient, however, is the curaçao peel, which binds all the components together. It was first known in Germany. The tiny flakes of 22-carat gold floating in the liqueur are part of its ancient tradition and are harmless when consumed.

Kümmel A colourless liqueur, kümmel is flavoured with caraway seeds and other flavours, including cumin. It is popular in Germany, Russia and other Central European countries as both a liqueur and a digestive.

Pastis The general term for a wide variety of aniseed and liquorice-flavoured alcoholic beverages that are made mainly in France and Spain. Though the principal flavour is from the seeds of the anise plant, other herbs are added to give a distinctive flavour.

Pernod A yellow liqueur based on aniseed blended with fifteen herbs distilled together, whose recipe goes back to the late 18th century. The ideal temperature for storing Pernod without risk of crystallisation is over 13°C (crystallisation is the appearance in a solid state of essence of aniseed). If it does occur, put the bottle in a warm place. Never put a bottle of Pernod in the refrigerator.

Sambucca A clear Italian liqueur that is flavoured with a herb very similar to aniseed.

Strega A rich and fragrant Italian liqueur, strega is a combination of more than 70 herbs and spices that are carefully aged in wood.

Mead

NUTRITIONAL INFORMATION No data are available.

DESCRIPTION A smooth, brown liquid with a honey flavour.

ORIGIN AND HISTORY A drink of great antiquity, mead is the oldest fermented drink in the world. It was drunk by the ancient gods and, so the story goes, in order to defeat his father Kronos, Zeus first made him drunk on mead. A kind of fermented honey or honey-flavoured wine was drunk by the Greeks and Romans but mead has been mainly associated with the Britons. Also called methe in the Middle Ages, it was basically made of honey and water with spice added occasionally. Metheglin was fundamentally the same as mead, though it was possibly stronger, with herbs sometimes added to give it flavour. Nowadays essences as well as fresh fruit juices are added, and in fact, mead is frequently promoted as a style of wine.

BUYING AND STORAGE Available at liquor stores, it can be kept at room temperature.

PREPARATION AND USE Served neat as a drink.

Rum

MAJOR NUTRIENTS		SERVE SIZE 30 mL
Energy	290 kJ	Alcohol	10 g
Carbohydrate	0		

NUTRITIONAL INFORMATION Overproof varieties contain 58% alcohol while the so-called 33 OP are 76%, or 76 g per 100 mL. Molasses provides the carbohydrate from which this spirit is distilled, although no free sugars remain after fermentation.

DESCRIPTION A clear or rich brown spirit made from sugar.

ORIGIN AND HISTORY There is controversy over how rum got its name, although it is known that there was a drink called rumbullion or rumbustion in the days of the Spanish Main. It was probably first made by the early Spanish settlers in the West Indies, who introduced the art of distillation. It is made today wherever sugarcane grows freely, including Australia. The white rum of Martinique, with its delicate cane fragrance, is considered to be of superior quality.

BUYING AND STORAGE Distilled in several colours and strengths, it is readily available in liquor stores and keeps well at room temperature.

PREPARATION AND USE Used to flavour ice creams and desserts, rum can be served neat, as a mixed drink or as a basis for cocktails such as Blue Hawaiian, a mixture of light rum, blue curaçao, triple sec, cream and coconut cream.

PROCESSING The molasses that is the end result of sugar production is fermented, then distilled to produce a colourless liquid. As it matures in cask it gradually extracts colour from the wood. Caramel is added for a darker colour.

Stout

MAJOR NUTRIENTS		SERVE SIZE 375 mL
Energy	881 kJ	Sodium	26 mg
Carbohydrate	11 g	Potassium	188 mg
Alcohol	23 g	Riboflavin	0.5 mg

NUTRITIONAL INFORMATION The dark colour results from the effect of increased heat during processing on the roasted malt or barley, producing a caramel. Nutritionally, stouts have a slightly higher alcohol and carbohydrate content than beer, giving them a higher energy content. Guinness has one and a half times the energy of beer and approximately six times the riboflavin (11% RDI).

DESCRIPTION A very dark brown ale that forms a thick, creamy head when poured.

ORIGIN AND HISTORY Stout was developed as brewers attempted to make an even heavier beer than the strongly flavoured porter. The best known stout is Guinness, which originated in Ireland.

BUYING AND STORAGE As for beer in general.

PREPARATION AND USE Stout has a strong flavour and sweet taste. The best known combination is with an equal part of champagne — both beverages, chilled, should be poured into a champagne glass simultaneously — to make Black Velvet.

Whisky

also called **Whiskey**

MAJOR NUTRIENTS		SERVE SIZE 30 mL
Energy	290 kJ	Alcohol	9 g
Carbohydrate	0		

NUTRITIONAL INFORMATION Apart from its energy, whisky has no nutritional value.

DESCRIPTION An amber-coloured spirit.

ORIGIN AND HISTORY The Irish were the first to make whiskey which they called 'uisge beatha', water of life. The soldiers of Henry II took the spirit back to England where the name was changed to whisky. Today it is made in many countries though Ireland, Scotland, America and Canada are the main producers.

Any cereal may be used to make whisky: in Ireland and Scotland barley is the principal ingredient, though wheat and rye may be added. In America maize, rye and corn are used, and in Canada corn is the main ingredient with some wheat and rye.

BUYING AND STORAGE It is readily available and stores well at room temperature.

PREPARATION AND USE Drunk neat, with water or as a mixed drink. Not used to a great extent in the kitchen but goes beautifully with coffee and cream.

PROCESSING Scotch whisky is produced from barley, water and yeast. The barley germinates to produce malted barley which is dried, crushed and fermented with yeast. It is distilled and matured in oak casks for at least three years. Double-malted and specially aged whiskies are popular with connoisseurs.

Whisky-based Liqueurs

DESCRIPTION Rich, brown liqueurs with the aroma of whisky.

ORIGIN AND HISTORY Traditionally the basic elixirs are compounded by the head of a family who alone knows the secret. They are based on fine whiskies, plus ingredients such as honey, herbs and spices.

BUYING AND STORAGE Proprietary liqueurs, they are readily available and may be stored at room temperature.

PREPARATION AND USE As after-dinner liqueurs, they may be enjoyed neat, ice-cold or mixed with other drinks.

VARIETIES

Drambuie A Scots recipe dating from the time of Bonny Prince Charlie.

Irish Mist The origins of Irish Mist go back nearly one thousand years to the days when Ireland was ruled only by warring clans whose favourite drink was known as heather wine. It is now made by the Tullamore Whiskey Distillery.

Southern Comfort The liqueur is based on old Bourbon whiskey flavoured with peaches, oranges and herbs. It is distilled in St Louis, Missouri, from an original French recipe.

Wines

MAJOR NUTRIENTS		DRY WHITE SERVE SIZE 120 mL	
Energy	422 kJ	Alcohol	14 g
Carbohydrate	0		
		SWEET WHITE SERVE SIZE 120 mL	
Energy	448 kJ	Alcohol	13 g
Carbohydrate	5 g		
		RED SERVE SIZE 120 mL	
Energy	432 kJ	Alcohol	16 g
Carbohydrate	0		
		CHAMPAGNE SERVE SIZE 120 mL	
Energy	360 kJ	Sodium	5 mg
Carbohydrate	2 g	Potassium	68 mg
Alcohol	11 g		

NUTRITIONAL INFORMATION Although distinctively different in flavour, sweet and dry white wines are very similar in terms of their carbohydrate and kilojoule content. Red and white wines differ only in their sodium and potassium contents — red wine has twice as much sodium and potassium, although this has no real nutritional significance.

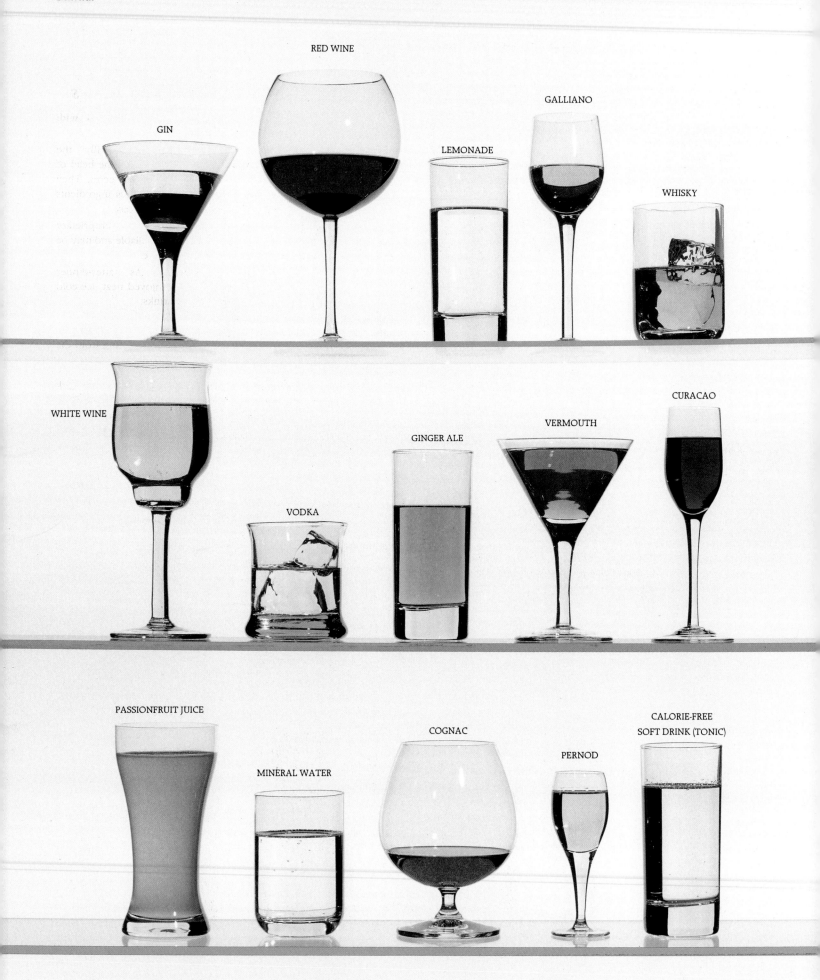

RED WINE

GIN

GALLIANO

LEMONADE

WHISKY

WHITE WINE

CURACAO

VERMOUTH

GINGER ALE

VODKA

PASSIONFRUIT JUICE

CALORIE-FREE
SOFT DRINK (TONIC)

COGNAC

MINERAL WATER

PERNOD

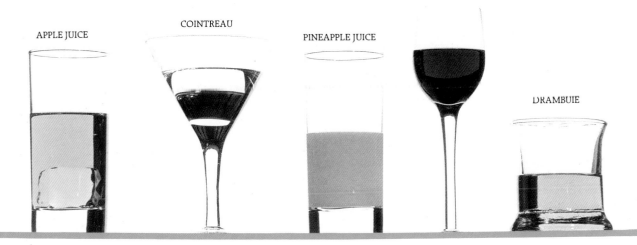

APPLE JUICE

COINTREAU

PINEAPPLE JUICE

CREME DE MENTHE

DRAMBUIE

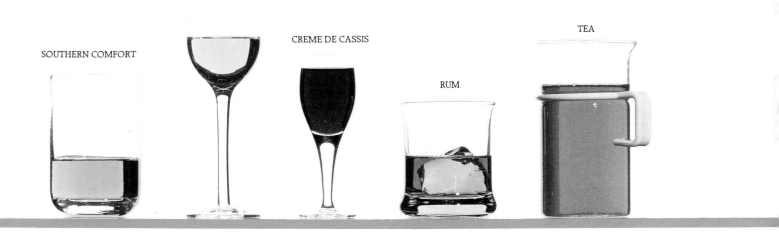

CREME DE BANANES

SOUTHERN COMFORT

CREME DE CASSIS

RUM

TEA

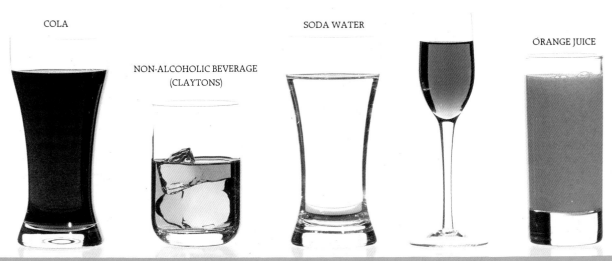

COLA

NON-ALCOHOLIC BEVERAGE
(CLAYTONS)

SODA WATER

PARFAIT AMOUR

ORANGE JUICE

DESCRIPTION Fermented juice of the grape, which when filtered and bottled attains a clear gold or ruby colour and a fragrance characteristic of the wine grape used.

ORIGIN AND HISTORY There are several stories about how wine was first made, and most of them concern women. In Persian mythology, so the story goes, one of the ladies in King Jamshid's harem drank from a jar of fermented, sour grapes that was labelled as poisonous. Instead of dying, she felt so much better she finished off the contents. She shared her secret with her king and so wine making began.

BUYING AND STORAGE Available as red, white or rosé, wines can be labelled according to the grape variety, e.g. Cabernet Sauvignon or Chardonnay, or as a generic variety — such as claret, chablis, moselle, etc. Wine can be bought from liquor stores and winemakers' cellars. Store away from light, ideally at a temperature of 10–13°C. Keep the bottles in a horizontal position to prevent the corks from drying out. White and red wines which are intended to be bottle-aged are marked with the year of vintage on the label.

PREPARATION AND USE Vintage wines can be kept in a cellar until the best time for drinking. White and rosé wines are served chilled, and red is best at room temperature. Used extensively in cooking, wine also adds flavour to most foods.

PROCESSING In the fermentation of red wine, the skins and pips of the grapes are left in to give colour. For white wine, skins are separated from the juice. When rosé is made, only a slight maceration is permitted between juice and skins. Most good red and some white wines are aged in oak casks for some months before bottling.

The 'sweetness' or 'dryness' of a wine is determined during fermentation when the natural grape sugars are converted to alcohol. A 'bone-dry' Chardonnay, for instance, will have no residual sweetness. But the 'late-pick' wines, the dessert wines made from very ripe Rhine Riesling grapes, for instance, will be a deep gold colour, and extremely sweet.

VARIETIES

Champagne A straw-coloured wine suffused with small, energetic bubbles. True French champagne comes only from a designated area in France, though many wine makers worldwide use the Méthode Champenoise for making their sparkling wines, which are available in liquor stores. Champagne does not improve in the bottle and may be drunk immediately. For this reason it is usually stored upright, though, if kept in the cellar, it is stored horizontally. The wines, mainly from chardonnay and pinot noir grapes, are blended in autumn in large vats or casks, then bottled the following spring. The bottles are placed neck down in long racks and turned regularly to ensure that the sediment falls constantly into the neck. After a time the neck of the bottle is plunged into a freezing mixture, and on removal of the cellar cork, the natural gas in the wine forces out the solidified sediment. Sugar is added, plus a tiny quantity of grape brandy, and possibly a little wine to top up. The bottle then receives its final cork, which is wired on.

Green Ginger Wine Fermented with ginger, and with a higher alcohol content than wine.
See also Fortified Wines.

NON-ALCOHOLIC BEVERAGES

Tea and coffee are amongst the most popular non-alcoholic beverages, with an increase in coffee consumption and a drop in tea consumption since 1945.

Except for the delicately flavoured green tea, most teas are made by drying and fermenting the leaves of the tea plant.

A number of these teas have added flavours, such as bergamot or lemon; there are also herbal teas, made from the leaves, seeds, bark, flowers and roots of a variety of plants. These are often drunk in the belief that they are 'healthier' than tea, and unsubstantiated claims are often made about them. In fact, less is known scientifically about these drinks than about tea. Some ingredients of these drinks have been shown to contain drug-like substances: for example, comfrey contains alkaloids which may damage the liver. Like other drinks, they are best used in small amounts in a varied diet.

The infusions of tea and coffee do not provide significant kilojoules, unless milk and/or sugar are added. Cocoa powder and drinking chocolate do provide kilojoules, but only in small amounts. The nutrients provided by these beverages are generally insignificant because of the small quantities used, although tea is a significant source of fluoride.

Tea, coffee, cocoa and cola all contain naturally occurring caffeine which is a mild stimulant to the central nervous system. Caffeine is a stimulant to the heart and respiratory system, and increases the rate of urine production. People react differently to caffeine: some may complain of nervousness, irritability and gastric upsets after ingesting caffeine, while others seem unaffected by it. Most authorities agree that 300 mg daily is a safe and acceptable intake. For those who prefer to avoid caffeine, tea, coffee and cola drinks are available in decaffeinated forms.

Milk is another popular beverage, which is discussed in a separate chapter, Milk Products.

Soya drinks are frequently used as substitutes for milk, but not all these drinks are nutritionally comparable to milk. A soya beverage is free of cholesterol, but its other nutrients should be checked on the nutrition label. It is best to look for the products which have a similar nutrition profile to that of milk.

Many consumers are confused about the differences between various fruit juice products such as fruit juice, fruit juice drinks and fruit juice cordials. Anything labelled 'fruit juice' should not contain any added water, and regulations dictate the levels of added sugar above which the product must be labelled 'sweetened'. All fruit juice products may contain specified additives such as sulphur dioxide, sorbic acid and benzoic acid, but these must be declared on the label.

In many countries, orange, lemon, grapefruit, blackcurrant, pineapple, guava, pawpaw and mango juices must carry a minimum specified level of vitamin C.

Products labelled 'fruit juice drink' contain fruit juice and added water, and may also contain vitamin C and specified additives.

Products labelled 'fruit juice cordials' are subject to regulations stipulating the minimum amount of fruit juice contained. Fruit juice cordial may also contain added vitamin C, but it is not mandatory.

Vegetable juices are not as widely used as fruit juices, but they also may contain a number of specified vitamins and additives.

Minerals and spa waters have been used in many countries for centuries. They were often the safest form of drinking water in countries with a poor water supply. Sometimes they have been promoted as 'miracle cures', but without scientific backing. Some people prefer mineral waters to tap water, while others use them as alternatives to sweetened aerated drinks, alcohol, or caffeine-containing tea and coffee. They are also used as mixers with fruit juice, spirits or wine.

Some mineral waters are 'natural' while others are manufactured; the distinction is unimportant nutritionally. They all contain sodium, potassium, magnesium and calcium salts, and must conform to microbiological standards. Mineral waters (including soda and seltzer water) are helpful as alternatives to sugar-sweetened soft drinks and alcohol, but they have no nutritional advantage over tap water.

Soft drinks are sweetened, with an average sugar content of 10%. Low-joule soft drinks have also been developed, with the sugar content marked on the label. Soft drinks may contain sugar or glucose, flavourings and colourings, food acids, other specified preservatives and additives, and carbon dioxide. Cola-type soft drinks may contain caffeine which, if it is added, must be declared on the label. Bitter drinks, tonic drinks and quinine drinks may contain quinine, in specified proportions.

The consumption of aerated and carbonated drinks has increased markedly since the late 1960s. These include brewed soft drinks, which have specified levels of ethyl alcohol.

Calorie-Free Soft Drink

MAJOR NUTRIENTS   SERVE SIZE 200 mL

Energy	9 kJ	Water	200 mL

NUTRITIONAL INFORMATION Also known as low joule drinks, they are ideal for the weight conscious and suitable for diabetics (after consultation with doctor or dietitian).

Those drinks sweetened with aspartame contain the amino acid phenylalanine, which could affect those with the metabolic disorder called phenylketonuria, but are not harmful otherwise. Saccharin and cyclamate, the so called non-nutritive sweeteners, are used most widely. Since the long-term effect of these sweeteners is unknown, they should be avoided by small children and during pregnancy.

DESCRIPTION Any of a range of commercial products labelled free of calories or kilojoules.

ORIGIN AND HISTORY Soft drinks are usually sweetened with a sugar syrup or honey. However, because of the need for sugar-free foods for diabetics and recent consumer demands for low-calorie soft drinks, some manufacturers have produced drinks using artificial sweeteners.

BUYING AND STORAGE Most carbonated soft drinks and fruit juices are available as low-calorie products from health food stores and supermarkets. Can be stored at room temperature.

PREPARATION AND USE Usually served cold as a beverage.

Cocoa

also called **Hot chocolate**

MAJOR NUTRIENTS   POWDER
                              SERVE SIZE 10 G

Energy	120 kJ	Potassium	150 mg
Protein	2 g	Phosphorus	60 mg
Fat	2 g	Magnesium	50 mg
Cholesterol	0	Iron	0.9 mg
Carbohydrate	1 g	Niacin Equiv.	1.4 mg
Sodium	95 mg		

NUTRITIONAL INFORMATION An excellent source of phosphorus and vitamin E; good source of iron; moderate source of niacin. Over 56% of total energy comes from fat. Contains significant amounts of naturally occurring oxalic acid and amines.

DESCRIPTION A rich, dark brown, opaque drink made from milled cacao beans.

ORIGIN AND HISTORY From the earliest recorded history, a stimulating beverage was made from the seeds of the acuatl or chocolatl tree by the natives in the West Indies and tropical countries of Latin America. There it was mixed with ground annatto and anise seeds, crushed red peppers and cinnamon to produce a sort of hot, spicy chocolate shake. It was not until the 1520s that it was introduced to Europe by the Spanish conquistadors. Instead of mixing chocolate with spices, the Spaniards mixed it with sugar and vanilla essence. When Anne of Austria, a Spanish princess, married Louis XIII in 1615, she introduced drinking chocolate to the French court. It was not long before the taste for chocolate spread throughout southern Europe, and 40 years later, an enterprising Frenchman opened the first chocolate shop in London. In 1824, an English Quaker, John Cadbury, produced Cocoa Nibs, a breakfast beverage, in his tea and coffee business in Birmingham. Four years later a Dutchman, Coenraad van Houten, perfected a method to extract two-thirds of the fat content, leaving a dry powdery cake that we now call cocoa powder.

BUYING AND STORAGE Readily available from food stores in packages, both chocolate and cocoa powder should be stored in a cool dry place.

PREPARATION AND USE To make a beverage, pour boiling liquid (water or milk) on either chocolate or cocoa powder, mix with sugar to taste and stir until blended. Both powders may also be used to flavour cakes, desserts and sauces.

PROCESSING The cacao tree bears clusters of flowers which produce ridged, oval pods. These are stored in boxes in their own pulp until fermentation takes place. They are then dried in the sun and eventually roasted until the shells fall away. What remains are called 'nibs'. Cocoa is obtained by first removing a large part of the fat from the nibs and then powdering the cooled block. Chocolate in any preparation, liquid or solid, is made from the roasted cacao bean.

Coffee

MAJOR NUTRIENTS SERVE SIZE 100 mL

	INSTANT		BREWED
Energy	0	Energy	0
Caffeine	40–100 mg	Caffeine	64–124 g

NUTRITIONAL INFORMATION There is a wide variation in individuals' sensitivity to the alkaloid caffeine, which is present in coffee. Heavy consumption of caffeine-containing beverages can cause nervousness, increased urination, irritability, palpitations etc. The amount of caffeine consumed depends on the length of brewing or standing time and the size of the cup. Caffeine is also found in tea, chocolate products, cola and other soft drinks.

DESCRIPTION A dark liquid made from coffee beans. The word 'coffee' comes from the Turkish kahveh, derived from the Arabic gahwah.

ORIGIN AND HISTORY Coffea arabica, originating in Ethiopia, was the first coffee tree cultivated, about AD 570. Extensive cultivation in Arabia did not begin until the 15th century. From Arabia, coffee cultivation, coffee drinking and the coffee-house spread to Ottoman Turkey. Much of the trade went through the port of Mocha, hence its association with coffee. By the mid-1600s the beverage had reached Europe, and by the late 1600s, North America. Cultivation began in the West Indies, Central and tropical South America early in the 18th century.

BUYING AND STORAGE Available in various roasts and blends, either whole for grinding at home or at point of purchase, or ready-ground in vacuum sealed packs or cans. Purchase only the amount of coffee which would be used within 1–2 weeks and store in a sealed container in the refrigerator.

PREPARATION AND USE Basically coffee is brewed as one brews tea — place coarsely ground coffee in a warmed utensil, pour on boiling water and infuse for 3–4 minutes, strain and serve. Plunger and percolator coffee makers use this principle. For filter coffee, use medium grind and fine grind for espresso. Use about 1 coffee measure (1 tablespoon) coffee per 200 mL water.

For Turkish-style, use 1 heaped teaspoon pulverised coffee per coffee cup (75 mL) water, mix in sugar to taste and bring to the boil.

PROCESSING The beans are fermented and dried, then roasted. During roasting, the colour of the bean changes from green to brown and its characteristic flavour and aroma develop. There are four main types of roast: high roast has a strong, bitter taste; full roast is slightly bitter; medium roast produces a strong tasting coffee and light roast has a delicate taste and aroma.

Spray-dried and freeze-dried instant coffee powders and granules are available in a variety of roasts and blends, including decaffeinated. Coffee and coffee–chicory essences are also available.

Coffee substitutes are the so-called instant cereal beverages, made from such ingredients as barley, rye, chicory, beetroot and dandelion root. They are free of artificial colours and preservatives and are caffeine- and calorie-free.

Cola

MAJOR NUTRIENTS SERVE SIZE 200 mL

Energy	380 kJ	Caffeine	18 mg
Carbohydrate	22 g		

NUTRITIONAL INFORMATION Very popular with young people, possibly because of the addictive effect of the caffeine: some cola type drinks supply a similar amount of caffeine to coffee (2 cans cola contain 70 mg caffeine, while 1 cup of instant coffee contains 60 mg caffeine). Consumed in large quantities, these drinks contribute significantly to sucrose intake, i.e. eight to ten teaspoons per 375 mL can. They are therefore unsuitable for those on kilojoule-restricted diets.

DESCRIPTION A dark brown, clear beverage.

ORIGIN AND HISTORY Two shrubs, the coca from South America and the cola from Africa, were the main ingredients for many soft drinks and gave the name to one that is world famous. Native to Peru and Bolivia, the leaves of the coca plant are a source of cocaine and were chewed by the Indians as a stimulant and narcotic. Coca leaves are no longer used in the manufacture of soft drinks. In the Sierra Leone and Guinea regions of western Africa, cola nuts, a source of caffeine, were chewed as a stimulant, and as a hangover cure. Today cola plants are grown extensively in Brazil and the West Indies.

Two world-famous cola drinks were created in America in the 1890s. John S. Berberton started making Coca-Cola in Atlanta, Georgia, while Pepsi-Cola was made in New Bern, North Carolina, by Caleb Bradham. Both are now made in most countries.

BUYING AND STORAGE Readily available and requires no special care.

PREPARATION AND USE Serve ice-cold and use as a mixer with spirits, especially rum.

PROCESSING A basic syrup of secret formula is bottled, or put into dispensers, with the addition of sugar, water and carbon dioxide.

Cordial

MAJOR NUTRIENTS

NON-ALCOHOLIC, DILUTION, 1:4
SERVE SIZE 200 mL

Energy	234 kJ	Carbohydrate	14 g

NUTRITIONAL INFORMATION The only nutritional benefit derived from cordials is energy, i.e. via their high sugar content. For active children the occasional glass would be acceptable. When consumed on a regular basis, cordials can contribute significantly to sugar and therefore kilojoule consumption.

DESCRIPTION A thick liquid, usually brightly coloured, intended for dilution as a flavoured drink.

ORIGIN AND HISTORY In the southern hemisphere, a cordial is non-alcoholic. It is a sweet, flavoured, concentrated syrup to be mixed with water as a drink. In the northern hemisphere, however, the term cordial may denote an alcoholic drink.

There is some dispute as to whether cordials are the same as liqueurs, since the words are used differently in different countries. Possibly the best distinction between the two is drawn by how they are made. An alcoholic cordial is a beverage compounded from spirits, with fruit or aromatic substances added by a variety of methods such as maceration, steeping, or simply by mixing. In this way, fruit or flavouring is added to a base spirit. A liqueur is a colourless spirit distilled from fruit and/or aromatic substances. Liqueurs and cordials differ from all other spirits because they must contain at least 2½% sugar by weight. The sugar may be beet, maple, cane, honey, corn, or a combination of these. In America, the word 'cordial' is used to designate liquids produced in both the above ways.

BUYING AND STORAGE A wide variety is available under many names. Most cordials keep well at room temperature.

PREPARATION AND USE Can be served alone, with ice and in cocktails. A useful flavouring in the kitchen, cordials have a variety of flavours and aromas that can be added to many dishes.

PROCESSING A fruit syrup is made by dissolving sugar in filtered fruit juice. The resulting liquid is then boiled and strained.

Fruit Juice

MAJOR NUTRIENTS			SERVE SIZE 200 ML
APPLE JUICE, CANNED		ORANGE JUICE, FRESH	
Energy	368 kJ	Energy	368 kg
Carbohydrate	20 g	Carbohydrate	20 g
Calcium	14 mg	Calcium	66 mg
Phosphorus	18 mg	Phosphorus	36 mg
Sodium	2 mg	Sodium	4 mg
Potassium	222 mg	Potassium	336 mg
Vitamin C	2 mg	Vitamin C	100 mg

NUTRITIONAL INFORMATION Many people drink fruit juices believing that they are a healthy alternative to soft drinks. In reality the sugar and energy content is very similar. Because they do not contain any dietary fibre, unlike whole fruit, fruit juices are easy to overconsume, contributing excess kilojoules to the diet. Freshly squeezed juices are rich in vitamin C, therefore would provide an excellent source for those who otherwise consume very little fresh fruit or vegetables.

DESCRIPTION Any juice extracted from fruit.

ORIGIN AND HISTORY Juice has long been extracted from fruit to serve as a drink and, even in ancient times, was served cold with ice from the snow. In China, lychee juice, pawpaw juice, and honey and ginger drinks were served at the formal banquets in the 18th century. It is only in recent times, however, that fruit drinks have been made commercially.

BUYING AND STORAGE A wide range of plain and mixed juices are readily available. Unless the juice is specially treated or has preservatives added, it must be refrigerated. All juices must be refrigerated when opened.

PREPARATION AND USE Can be freshly prepared by extracting the juice either by hand or mechanically in an electric juicer or blender. Extensively used in cooking. Serve ice cold either as a drink or in a punch.

Herbal Tea

also called **Tisane**

MAJOR NUTRIENTS		INFUSION SERVE SIZE 150 ML	
Energy	3 kJ	Potassium	26 mg
Caffeine	n/a		

NUTRITIONAL INFORMATION Caffeine figures not available. Despite the fact that tea provides no more than a trace of kilojoules and no vitamins, many people believe herbal teas are beneficial to good health. Many contain components not yet assessed for safety. Some varieties may have disturbing effects including interfering with the therapeutic value of some drugs if consumed at the same time. Some but not all herbal teas are caffeine-free. Those that are, are usually labelled so.

DESCRIPTION A herbal tea is simply an infusion made by adding boiling water to the leaves or flowers of fresh or dried herbs.

ORIGIN AND HISTORY In many parts of the world, herbal teas have been accepted for their refreshing qualities as well as being used as remedies for all kinds of ailments, from coughs and colds to headaches and sleeplessness.

BUYING AND STORAGE Prepared herbal teas are available from herbal shops, homeopathic pharmacists and health food stores in either sachet form or loose. Can be stored for a few months in a container in the cupboard.

PREPARATION AND USE Tisanes are made in the same way as tea. They can be drunk on their own or with the addition of honey or sugar.

PROCESSING Allow 1 tablespoon fresh herbs per cup or 1 teaspoon of dried. Pour on boiling water, cover cup and leave to infuse for 3–5 minutes. Allow the same amount for making in a teapot, adding 1 more for the pot. Leave to infuse 5–10 minutes, pour through strainer into cups.

VARIETIES These include bergamot, chamomile, dandelion, elderflower, lemon balm tea, lemon verbena, lovage, mint, rose hip, rosemary and yarrow.

SEE ALSO Tea.

Mineral Water

NUTRITIONAL INFORMATION Mineral waters contain only small quantities of mineral salts, e.g. sodium chloride, sodium carbonate and bicarbonate, salts of calcium and magnesium and possibly hydrogen sulphide. The total mineral content is therefore so low that health benefits are questionable. The sodium content varies with each variety, and this should be noted by those on salt-restricted diets.

DESCRIPTION A clear, colourless beverage.

ORIGIN AND HISTORY Natural mineral water has mineral properties from the rocks and soil through which it has passed before emerging in a spring. It has been valued for many years for its reputed curative properties, and was used therapeutically, either internally or externally. Nowadays it is bottled and drunk socially and in countries where the natural water is suspect.

BUYING AND STORAGE Readily available and can be kept at room temperature.

PREPARATION AND USE It is best served chilled and may be used instead of tap water in mixed drinks.

VARIETIES
Mineral waters of many different flavours and colours are available.

Soda Water

MAJOR NUTRIENTS		SERVE SIZE 200 ML	
Energy	0	Sodium	2–34 mg

NUTRITIONAL INFORMATION No detailed nutritional analysis is available. Often used as a mixer with spirits, juices or cordials, soda water can contribute to the total sodium content of the diet. Brands vary in their sodium content: 2–34 mg per 200 ml glass may be significant for those on salt-restricted diets, e.g. for treatment of high blood pressure.

DESCRIPTION A clear liquid, usually carbonated.

ORIGIN AND HISTORY First manufactured towards the end of the 18th century by Jacob Schweppe in England, soda water was originally drunk for health rather than a pleasing additive to spirits. Schweppe retired in 1799 but the firm carried on and finally became a public company a century later.

BUYING AND STORAGE Available under several brand names, it is readily available and may be stored at room temperature.

PREPARATION AND USE An excellent mixer with spirits for long drinks, it is also used in cocktails such as Tom Collins, which originated in England in the late 19th century. Add gin, lemon juice and sugar and garnish with a slice of lemon and a maraschino cherry.

Soft Drink

MAJOR NUTRIENTS   SERVE SIZE 200 mL
Energy   376 kJ Carbohydrate   24 g

NUTRITIONAL INFORMATION Devoid of any vitamins or minerals, soft drinks contribute significantly to sugar intake.

DESCRIPTION A sweetened, flavoured, non-alcoholic drink.

ORIGIN AND HISTORY Soft drinks have always been popular in warm climates. In the earliest days of Western literature the Greek Xenophon in his *Anabasis* noted for the first time how to make them. Later in Europe drinks such as sarsaparilla, fizzy drinks and lemonade were enjoyed by the Spaniards, and Catherine de Medici's cooks introduced to the French a variety of drinks including lemonade and orangeade. By 1789, Nicholas Paul of Geneva had developed a method of manufacturing carbonated waters in bulk.

BUYING AND STORAGE Australians have always been avid drinkers of soft drinks and the range available has been extended to cater for all tastes. They should be drunk soon after being opened.

PREPARATION AND USE Serve chilled, on ice and in mixed drinks with spirits.

PROCESSING Most carbonated beverages are made simply from a mixture of syrup and sparkling water. The tiny bubbles that give fizz to carbonated drinks come from carbon dioxide, either contained in the liquid naturally or added to it artificially.

VARIETIES
Many are available, based on ginger, fruit and other flavours.

Soya Drink

MAJOR NUTRIENTS   SERVE SIZE 200 mL
Energy   320 kJ Carbohydrate   10 g
Protein   6 g   Cholesterol   0
Fat   7 g   Sodium   110 mg

NUTRITIONAL INFORMATION Often fortified with vitamins and minerals to equal milk, although any added calcium will not be as well absorbed as it is from milk. These are the only soya drinks that are suitable for use as a replacement for milk in the diet.

DESCRIPTION Liquid or powdered milk made from soya beans. With certain components extracted, and other ingredients added to give it the properties of cow's milk, soya drink is an excellent substitute for cow's milk.

ORIGIN AND HISTORY Soya drink is one of the latest soya bean by-products to be developed to fulfil a market need for a cow's milk substitute. A particular soya isolate is used as the basis for the drink, with minerals, vitamins, malt extract and sunflower or maize oil usually added to give it the necessary flavour and nutritional composition of cow's milk. Soya oil is bitter when first extracted, and is unstable when exposed to air or high temperatures, hence the use of sunflower or other vegetable oils. Soya milks are also prepared for infant-feeding formulas, as low fat milk, as liquid milk which can be stored at room temperature, and powdered milks of normal or low fat content.

BUYING AND STORAGE Supermarkets and natural food stores stock a wide range of soya drinks, including those above, as well as chilled flavoured drinks. Store chilled drinks in the refrigerator, other liquid milks in a cool place until opened. Unless packed in a can, powdered soya drink should be transferred to a dry, sterilised jar and stored in a cool place away from direct light; retain package directions for use.

PREPARATION AND USE Because of the range of products, follow package directions for preparation. Generally powdered and liquid milks can be used in the same way as cow's milk — as a beverage, poured onto breakfast cereal, for making sauces and custards, and in general cooking and baking.

Spring Water

NUTRITIONAL INFORMATION Spring water, like mineral water, is free of kilojoules. Its mineral water content — sodium, calcium, magnesium etc. — varies depending on its source. Unlike mineral water, spring water is usually sold non-carbonated.

DESCRIPTION Bottled water from a spring, usually alpine.

ORIGIN AND HISTORY Many distilleries and breweries were established at certain locations because of the importance of using clear spring water in the production of high quality products. Because many people suspect tap water, spring water has been bottled, especially in France and Italy.

BUYING AND STORAGE Available under several brand names such as Vichy, Evian and Pellegrino, it is available in specialty food stores and some liquor stores. Can be kept at room temperature.

PREPARATION AND USE Serve chilled and in mixed drinks.

Tap Water

MAJOR NUTRIENTS		SERVE SIZE 1 LITRE	
Energy	0	Magnesium	5 mg
Calcium	8 mg	Sodium	12.5 mg
Chloride		Potassium	1.63 mg
	25 mg (seasonal variation)	Sulphate	7.7 mg
		Iron	0.12 mg
Fluoride	0.91 mg		

NUTRITIONAL INFORMATION Perhaps water can be considered a nutrient itself, since survival time without it is limited to a few days only. Four or more glasses per day is advocated by nutritionists. It is an ideal aid for weight watchers (as a filler), and for the athlete, to replace essential water loss and maintain normal body temperature. Increased intake of water encourages urine flow and therefore decreases the risk of kidney stone development in susceptible individuals.

DESCRIPTION Treated water available through officially controlled Water Boards.

ORIGIN AND HISTORY Provision of water to urban developments has been under continued revision since the first cities grew.

BUYING AND STORAGE Tap water varies greatly in composition, availability and price from one source to another.

PREPARATION AND USE It is usually chemically treated to make it safe to drink, and is thus usually distilled or demineralised before being used in the manufacture of spirits, wines and beers.

Tea

MAJOR NUTRIENTS   INFUSION
SERVE SIZE 100 ML

Energy	0	Caffeine 50 mg
Water	98%	

NUTRITIONAL INFORMATION A cup of tea of average strength provides slightly less caffeine than a cup of instant coffee (50 mg compared to 60–70 mg). Although not everyone may be sensitive to the effects of caffeine, heavy consumption — more than six cups per day — may lead to increased acid production, increased heart rate, dependence and withdrawal effects if stopped suddenly.

DESCRIPTION A light brown, aromatic infusion of leaves.

ORIGIN AND HISTORY Tea, the most universally consumed of all beverages, is derived from the leaves of a small tree that is native to India, China and Japan. It was brought to Europe by the Dutch in 1610, to England in 1644 and arrived in America in the early 18th century. It is now also grown in Sri Lanka, Indonesia, Kenya and Tanzania.

BUYING AND STORAGE All varieties are available in specialty food stores, though the teas sold under brand names are usually blended. Store in a cool cupboard for a few months.

PREPARATION AND USE Always use freshly boiled water. Allow one teaspoonful of tea per person and one for the pot. Rinse teapot with boiling water, measure in the tea and pour in boiling water.

PROCESSING Tea is grown on plantations in the country of origin and exported ready to use. The main stages of manufacture are withering, rolling (also known as curling), fermenting, firing (drying), and sorting.

VARIETIES
Of the over 3000 varieties of tea, most take their names from the area where they are grown. Virtually all the tea drunk in Australia and New Zealand is black tea and is blended from several varieties. The principal types of teas are listed below.

Assam A high-quality Indian black tea that makes a full-bodied, robust brew.

Lapsang Souchong From Taiwan, this has an interesting, smoky flavour.

Darjeeling The finest and most delicately flavoured of the Indian black teas.

Ceylon Black tea that is delicate and fragrant.

Oolong A green tea with a subtle flavour and bouquet.

Japanese Green tea that makes a light, gentle brew.

Tonic Water

MAJOR NUTRIENTS   SERVE SIZE 100 ML

Energy	300 kJ	Carbohydrate 8 g

NUTRITIONAL INFORMATION Tonic water contains quinine, although exact figures are unavailable. In small doses quinine may reduce fever and in large doses it is used to treat malaria. Compared to other carbonated beverages, tonic water supplies about half as much carbohydrate, and is not sugar-free. Low-kilojoule varieties are available.

DESCRIPTION An aerated soft drink; the characteristic flavour comes from quinine, a bitter bark from the cinchona tree.

ORIGIN AND HISTORY Quinine has been used as a medicine for many illnesses including scarlet fever, smallpox and malaria: it was originally added to water and served as a tonic, hence the name.

BUYING AND STORAGE Readily available, it stores at room temperature.

PREPARATION AND USE Served chilled as a refreshing drink, it is used as a mixer, mainly with gin.

Vegetable Juice

MAJOR NUTRIENTS   CANNED
SERVE SIZE 200 ML

Energy	150 kJ	Potassium	456 mg
Carbohydrate	8 g	Vitamin C	14 mg
Sodium	412 mg	Vitamin A	1174 µg

NUTRITIONAL INFORMATION Compared to fruit juices, vegetable juices have a lower energy content (less than half) and approximately one-third the carbohydrate content. However, they also contain up to 100 times more salt and twice as much potassium. Freshly extracted vegetable juices are an excellent source of vitamins C and A.

DESCRIPTION Any juice extracted from a vegetable.

ORIGIN AND HISTORY Juices extracted from vegetables have only become popular since consumers became health conscious.

BUYING AND STORAGE Many varieties are available under several brand names, both canned and packaged, from food stores. Use-by date is given on the container. Store at room temperature unless otherwise specified.

PREPARATION AND USE To make juice from vegetables, rinse well, remove any blemishes, stems and seeds, chop coarsely, and blend in the blender or food processor. Special juice extractor machines are also available. Serve as a refreshing nutritive beverage.

TABLES

RECOMMENDED DIETARY INTAKES OF VITAMINS PER DAY

Group	Age	Vitamin A (µg retinol equivalents)	Thiamin (mg)	Riboflavin (mg)	Niacin (mg niacin equivalents)	Vitamin B-6 (mg)	Total Folate (µg)	Vitamin B12 (µg)	Vitamin C (mg)	Vitamin E (mg alpha-tocopherol equivalent)
INFANTS	0–6 mth									
	Breastfed	425	0	0	4	0‥	50	0	25	2
	Bottlefed	425	0	0	4	0‥	50	0	25	4
	7–12 mth	300	0	0	7	0ß	75	0	30	4
CHILDREN (male and female)	1–3 yr	300	0	0	9–10	0–0	100	1	30	5
	4–7 yr	350	0	1	11–13	0–1	100	1	30	6
BOYS	8–11 yr	500	0	1	14–16	1–1	150	1	30	8
	12–15 yr	725	1	1	19–21	1–2	200	2	30	10
	16–18 yr	750	1	1	20–22	1–2	200	2	40	11
GIRLS	8–11 yr	500	0	1	14–16	1–1	150	1	30	8
	12–15 yr	725	1	1	17–19	1–1	200	2	30	9
	16–18 yr	750	0	1	15–17	1–1	200	2	30	8
MEN	19–64 yr	750	1	1	18–20	1–1	200	2	40	10
	64+ yr	750	0	1	14–17	1–1	200	2	40	10
WOMEN	19–54 yr	750	0	1	12–14	0–1	200	2	30	7
	54+ yr	750	0	1	10–12	0–1	200	2	30	7
PREGNANT		750	1	1	14–16	1–1	400	3	60	7
LACTATING		1200	1	1	17–19	1–2	350	2	60	9

These figures were revised between 1982 and 1987. Note: that mg = 1 thousandth of a gram, and µg = 1 millionth of a gram. The table is supplied by the National Health and Medical Research Council of Australia.

RECOMMENDED DIETARY INTAKES OF MINERALS PER DAY

Subject	Age	Calcium MG	Iron MG	Magnesium MG	Zinc MG	Iodine µG	Sodium MMOL	Sodium MG	Potassium MMOL	Potassium MG	Selenium MCG	Phosphorus MG
INFANTS	0–6 mth			40	3–6	60	6–12	(140–280)	10–15	(390–580)	10	150
	Breast fed	300	0									
	Formula fed	500	3									
	7–12 mth	550	9	60	4–6	60	14–25	(320–580)	12–35	(470–1370)	15	300
CHILDREN (male and female)	1–3 yr	700	6–8	80	4–6	70	14–50	(320–1150)	25–70	(980–2730)	25	500
	4–7 yr	800	6–8	110	6–9	90	20–75	(460–1730)	40–100	(1560–3900)	30	700
BOYS	8–11 yr	800	6–8	180	9–14	120	26–100	(600–2300)	50–140	(1950–5460)	50	800
	12–15 yr	1200	10–13	260	12–18	150	40–100	(920–2300)	50–140	(1950–5460)	85	1200
	16–18 yr	1000	10–13	320	12–18	150	40–100	(920–2300)	50–140	(1950–5460)	85	1100
GIRLS	8–11 yr	900	6–8	160	9–14	120	26–100	(600–2300)	50–140	(1950–5460)	50	800
	12–15 yr	1000	10–13	240	12–18	120	40–100	(920–2300)	50–140	(1950–5460)	70	1200
	16–18 yr	800	10–13	270	12–18	120	40–100	(920–2300)	50–140	(1950–5460)	70	1100
MEN	19–64 yr	800	5–7	320	12–16	150	40–100	(920–2300)	50–140	(1950–5460)	85	1000
	65+ yr	800	5–7	320	12–16	150	40–100	(920–2300)	50–140	(1950–5460)	85	1000
WOMEN	19–54 yr	800	12–16	270	12–16	120	40–100	(920–2300)	50–140	(1950–5460)	70	1000
	55+ yr	1000	7	270	12–16	120	40–100	(920–2300)	50–140	(1950–5460)	70	1000
PREGNANT		+300	22–36	+30	16–21	+30	40–100	(920–2300)	50–140	(1950–5460)	+10	+200
LACTATING		+400	12–16	+70	18–22	+50	40–100	(920–2300)	65–140	(2540–5460)	+15	+200

These figures were revised between 1982 and 1987. Pregnant women should note that the necessary iron intake is not achievable from dietary iron; all pregnant women should thus receive supplemental iron. The table is supplied by the National Health and Medical Research Council of Australia. A millimole (MMOL) is a scientific measurement representing weight in milligrams divided by the equivalent weight.

RECOMMENDED DIETARY INTAKES OF ENERGY AND PROTEIN PER DAY

Subject	Age	Body Weight kg	Energy kJ	Protein g
INFANTS	0– 6 mth	Variable	See note	2g/kg body weight
	7–12 mth	Variable	460–420 per kg	1/kg body weight
CHILDREN	1– 3 yr	13	5400	14–18
BOYS	4– 7 yr	19	7200	18–24
	8–11 yr	28	9200	27–38
	12–15 yr	41	12 200	42–60
	16–18 yr	61	12 600	64–70
GIRLS	4– 7 yr	18	7200	18–24
	8–11 yr	27	8800	27–39
	12–15 yr	42	10 400	44–55
	16–18 yr	55	9200	57
MEN	19–35 yr		11 600	55
	36–55 yr	70	10 400	55
	55–75 yr		8800	55
WOMEN	19–35 yr		8400	45
	36–54 yr	58	7600	45
	54 + yr		6400	45
PREGNANCY 2nd & 3rd trimester	18–35 yr	+ 12kg	9000	51
	35 + yr		8200	51
LACTATION	18–35 yr	58	10 900	61
	35 + yr		10 100	61

The figures for energy are under review, last revised in 1970. Those for protein were revised in 1988. In the INFANTS column, it is assumed that a breastfed infant with a satisfactory growth rate is receiving an appropriate amount of food energy. This table is supplied by the National Health and Medical Research Council of Australia.

THE HEALTHY DIET PYRAMID

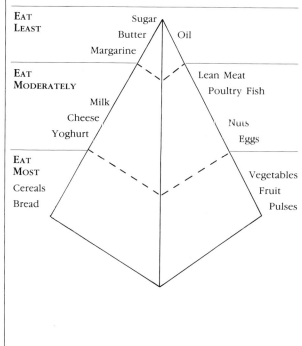

VITAMINS IN THE DIET

Vitamin	Functions	Food Sources
VITAMIN A (Retinol equivalents) Comes as preformed vitamin A or retinol in animal foods and beta-carotene in plant foods. Beta-carotene is converted to vitamin A in the body.	Action in night vision in the formation of visual purple with changes in light intensity. Essential for healthy mucous-secreting epithelial tissue, lining the gastrointestinal tract and respiratory tract. Infections are more likely to occur when these tissues are damaged. Essential for normal reproduction and growth and the development of the skeletal tissues. In third world countries where deficiencies may be extreme, much of the blindness is due to vitamin A deficiency.	Preformed vitamin A. Liver, fish liver oils, kidneys, butter, table margarine, reduced-fat spreads, full cream dairy products, egg yolk. Beta-carotene (converted to vitamin A in the body) Green leafy vegetables, broccoli, yellow and orange vegetables and fruit.
THIAMIN	Acts as a co-enzyme in the metabolism of nutrients such as carbohydrate. In the absence of thiamin, these nutrients cannot be used by the body to produce energy. Extreme deficiency leads to beri beri and Wernicke-Korsakoff syndrome. The former occurs mainly in third world countries and the latter amongst alcoholics in affluent countries such as Australia. Mild deficiencies are associated with poor appetite, tiredness and irritability.	Bread and cereals are the main source in the Australian diet. The levels are highest in wholegrain products such as wholemeal bread, wholegrain breakfast cereals, oatmeal and wheatmeal porridge, wheat germ, breakfast cereals with added thiamin. White bread does contribute thiamin to the diet but brown, mixed grain and wholemeal bread contribute more. Yeast extracts (Marmite, Promite, Vegemite) are excellent sources. Meat, particularly liver, kidneys and lean pork and vegetables, are important sources. Milk and milk products contribute about 10% of the thiamin in the diet.
RIBOFLAVIN	A co-enzyme associated with the release of energy from nutrients in body tissues. Deficiencies are rare in societies where milk is drunk. The common features of deficiency are: cracks at the corner of the mouth; swollen, cracked lips; a magenta-coloured tongue; and a rash at the junction of the nose and face.	The main sources in the western diet are milk and milk products, meat and meat products, bread and cereals including cereals with added riboflavin. Eggs and yeast extracts (Marmite, Promite and Vegemite) are excellent sources, and vegetables contain small amounts.

TABLE3

VITAMIN	FUNCTIONS	FOOD SOURCES
NIACIN (niacin equivalents) Niacin can also be produced in the body from the amino acid, trypto-phan. The sum of the latter niacin and preformed niacin is referred to as niacin equivalents.	Along with thiamin and riboflavin, niacin is essential for the production of energy in the body tissues. Niacin is required for the manufacture of fatty acids in body tissue. Extreme deficiency leads to pellagra, a disease seldom seen in western countries.	Meat and poultry are the most important sources. Bread and cereals, particularly wholemeal and wholegrain varieties and breakfast cereals with added niacin, are excellent sources. Yeast extracts are excellent sources. In a National Dietary Survey of Adults, 1983, in Australia, approximately 8% of the niacin equivalents in the diets came from both vegetables and milk and milk products. Meat and meat products provided almost 45% and bread and cereal products almost 20%.
VITAMIN B-6	Acts in many systems involving the metabolism of amino acids (the units in protein) in the body. Requirements are related to dietary protein.	Widespread in foods, occurring in meat (particularly liver), poultry, fish, bread and cereals (particularly wholemeal and wholegrain varieties), pulses and eggs. Most fruits and vegetables contain small amounts, but avo-cados and bananas are excellent sources.
VITAMIN B-12	With folate, this is essential for the production of red blood cells. Essential in maintaining the myelin in the nervous system. Assists in detoxifying cyanide from foods and cigarette smok-ing. Deficiency leads to pernicious anaemia.	Vitamin B-12 is synthesised by micro-organisms, and animals obtain their vitamin B-12 from these bacterial sources. All ani-mal foods provide some vitamin B-12, and fermented foods such as miso contain varying amounts. Most meats are excellent sources, and liver and kidneys are particularly rich sources. Eggs and cheese are an excellent source and milk a good source. Fish is an excellent source and sardines, oysters and pilchards are rich sources.
FOLATE	Essential for the proliferation of all cells. There is an interde-pendence of folate and vitamin B-12 in the formation of red blood cells.	Widely distributed in foods. The most important sources are liver, kidneys, eggs, wholemeal bread, wholegrain cereals, wheat germ, green vegetables, corn, nuts — particularly peanuts — legumes, yeast extracts, oranges, bananas, avocados.
VITAMIN C	Aids in the formation of collagen, the fibrous connection tis-sue which holds the cells of body tissues together. Essential for the metabolism of certain amino acids in the body and for the formation of some hormones. Improves the absorption of iron from plant foods such as cereals and vegetables by reducing ferric to ferrous iron. With vitamin E and selenium, it acts as a free radical scavenger, counteracting free radicals, which are produced in the body by oxidative processes and radiation, and are highly reactive substances, damaging to tissues. Suppresses the formation of nitrosamines, which are carcinogenic. Acts to detoxify certain drugs and chemicals produced in the body. Cigarette smoking, the taking of oral contraceptives and exposure to certain atmospheric pollutants increase vitamin C requirements. Requirements are increased during pregnancy and lactation, following infection, and following trauma such as injury or surgery. Extreme deficiency results in scurvy.	All fruits and vegetables contain some vitamin C. Frozen and canned products retain much of the vitamin, but losses are high with dehydration. Losses are increased in an alkaline medium, for example, when sodium bicarbonate is added to vegetables. Exposure to heat, light and oxygen also increases loss. To preserve vitamin C when cooking, add fruits and vege-tables to sufficient boiling water to prevent burning. Cook in a receptacle with a well fitting lid, until just tender. Microwaving and stir-frying are good methods of maximising the retention of vitamin C. In Australia, in a National Dietary Survey of Adults, 1983, fruit juices, fruits and vegetables each contributed approximately 32% of the vitamin C. Orange juice and citrus fruits were the biggest contributors, but potatoes contributed more than 10%. Guavas, black currants, capsicum, kiwifruit and pawpaw are excellent sources. Human milk contains more vitamin C than cow's milk. Liver and kidneys are the only meats with significant amounts of vitamin C, much of which is lost during storage and cooking.
VITAMIN D	Acts to regulate the absorption of calcium from the gut, to maintain a constant level of calcium in the blood, and to con-trol the deposition of calcium and phosphorus in the bones.	The most important vitamin D for people who spend some time out of doors is that formed in the skin by the ultraviolet light from the sun. The ultraviolet light acts on 7-dehydrocholesterol in the skin and converts it to vitamin D. Housebound and institutionalised people who cannot get out of doors may need a supplement. Fatty fish (sardines, tuna, salmon, mackerel, herrings) table margarine, fish liver, oils and egg yolk are excellent sources. Butter is a good source.

VITAMIN	FUNCTIONS	FOOD SOURCES
VITAMIN E	Acts as an antioxidant protecting the fats (phospholipids) in the cell walls from damage. With vitamin C and selenium it acts as a scavenger in the control of free radicals (see vitamin C).	The richest sources are the polyunsaturated seed oils (safflower, sunflower, maize, cottonseed, soyabean) and wheatgerm. Polyunsaturated margarine and reduced-fat spreads are excellent sources. Egg yolk and tuna, avocados, asparagus and broccoli are excellent sources.
VITAMIN K	Essential for the manufacture of the blood clotting factor.	Vitamin K is produced by micro-organisms in the human gut. Green leafy vegetables and liver are excellent sources.

Additional vitamins

Biotin and pantothenic acid are two additional vitamins. They are very widespread in foods and deficiencies are unlikely to occur.

MINERALS IN THE DIET

MINERAL	FUNCTIONS	FOOD SOURCES
CALCIUM	99% of the calcium in the body is in the skeleton and teeth. Ionised calcium (electrically charged atoms) in the blood is important for blood coagulation, muscle contraction and relaxation and conduction of nerve impulses. When there is insufficient calcium in the skeleton, conditions such as rickets, osteomalacia and osteoporosis may occur. These conditions occur because too little calcium is deposited in the skeleton or too much is withdrawn. A deficiency of dietary calcium is only one factor. More important in the case of rickets and osteomalacia is a lack of vitamin D and therefore a poor absorption of calcium. In the case of osteoporosis, hormonal changes are important.	Milk, cheese and yoghurt, including reduced fat and low fat varieties, are the major sources. The absorption of calcium from these foods is very good. Canned fish with edible bones such as sardines and salmon are excellent sources. Broccoli, dried peas and beans, almonds and wholegrain cereals are moderate sources. The absorption from wholegrain cereals is inhibited by the phytates in cereals, but it is better from wholemeal bread because the phytates are partially destroyed in preparation.
CHROMIUM	Chromium occurs in the body in the glucose tolerance factor (GTF) which acts with insulin in carbohydrate metabolism.	Brewer's yeast is the food in which chromium was first identified. It also occurs in flesh foods, particularly liver, in oysters, wholegrain cereals, yeast extracts and egg yolk.
COPPER	Copper is involved in the production of haem in haemoglobin. It is incorporated in a number of enzymes in the body. Deficiencies with adults have not been reported. Rare cases of deficiencies have been reported in infants who were premature or on formulae with a low copper content.	The richest sources are shellfish and other seafoods and offal. There are small amounts in meat, wholegrain cereals, pulses and other vegetables.
FLUORINE	Fluorine is an essential nutrient. It is incorporated into the hydroxyapatite in the bones and teeth, thereby strengthening these structures.	Fluorine is not widely distributed in foods. Tea and seafoods are moderate sources. The main source is water. In some cases the water contains fluoride as a natural ingredient, but in many countries 1 part per 1 million fluoride is added to the reticulated water supply. This is usually followed by a drop of 50% in the prevalence of dental caries. It is also believed to have a role in preventing osteoporosis.
MAGNESIUM	Magnesium is widely distributed in the body in a number of enzymes and as ions (electrically charged atoms). It is involved in the synthesis of protein, fats, complex carbohydrates and nucleic acid. It is also involved in the transmission of nerve impulses and in muscle contraction. Magnesium also occurs in the bones and teeth.	The main sources in the Australian diet are cereals and cereal products, which contribute about 30% of the magnesium, and then vegetables, contributing 15% and meat 12%. In green vegetables magnesium occurs as a constituent of chlorophyll. Nuts and pulses are also valuable sources. The absorption from plant foods is better than from animal foods.

TABLE3

MINERAL	FUNCTIONS	FOOD SOURCES
IODINE	Occurs in 2 hormones produced in the thyroid gland, thyroxine and triiodothyronine. These hormones control the metabolic rate in the body. In children they are essential for growth and the development of the central nervous system. Goitre and cretinism are the result of extreme deficiencies. Cretinism is characterised by stunted growth and arrested mental development.	Seafoods are the best source. Smaller quantities occur in fresh water fish, meat, milk, cheese and cereals. The amounts vary according to the iodine level of the environmental soil. Milk and milk products become valuable sources when iodophors are used as sanitising agents in dairies.
IRON	About 95% of the iron in the body is combined with protein in the haemoglobin in the blood and the myoglobin in the muscles. These combine with oxygen and carry it to the tissues for release. Iron also occurs in a number of body enzymes which are involved in processes such as the generation of energy and the synthesis of DNA. Iron deficiency results in nutritional anaemia and low body stores of iron. Anaemia is accompanied by tiredness and impaired work capacity and possibly impaired intellectual capacity in children.	Lean meat is the most important source in the diet, and liver, kidneys and heart are particularly rich sources. Chicken, fish, also contain iron, but in lower concentrations than in red meat. The iron in flesh foods — haem iron — is well absorbed. The non haem iron in cereals and vegetables is less well absorbed but absorption is improved by including vitamin C rich foods and small amounts of meat in the meal. Cereals and cereal products contribute significant amounts of iron to the diet and many breakfast cereals have added iron. Green vegetables and pulses also provide iron.
PHOSPHORUS	85% of the phosphorus in the body is in the skeleton, where its main function is as a constituent of calcium salts, which provide rigidity for the bones. It occurs in all cells of the body, where it is a constituent of compounds essential in the release of energy from carbohydrate. Compounds containing phosphorus have a role in maintaining the acid/base balance of the body. Deficiencies in humans are rare and they are usually associated with disease conditions which result in abnormal metabolism. Very high intakes of phosphorus can inhibit the absorption of calcium.	Because it occurs in all cells it is present in all natural foods. Dairy foods, meat, chicken, fish, nuts, eggs, wholemeal bread and wholegrain cereals are rich sources, but most foods, other than highly processed foods such as sugar and oils, contain phosphorus.
SELENIUM	Interest in selenium has been stimulated by research into disease states which were found to be associated with a dietary deficiency of selenium linked to a deficiency of selenium in the soil. Keshan's disease in China is one such disease, which affects the muscles of the heart. The main function of selenium in the body is as an antioxidant, protecting the polyunsaturated fatty acids in the cell walls from oxidation. In this it interacts with vitamin E.	The amounts in foods are related to the levels in the soil in which they are produced. Cereals, seafoods and offal are the best sources with eggs, meat and vegetables and fruits also providing some selenium. Dairy products are not a significant source.
SODIUM AND POTASSIUM	The functions of sodium and potassium are interrelated in the body. They both occur as ions (electrically charged atoms). Most of the sodium is in the extra-cellular fluids (the fluids outside the cells) and most of the potassium is within the cells. The balance is maintained within normal limits by the kidney. They assist in maintaining acid/base balance, in regulating fluid balance, blood volume and blood pressure and in controlling muscle contraction and relaxation. Sodium also has a role in transporting glucose across the intestinal wall. The human race evolved on a diet high in potassium and low in sodium. The modern diet has reversed this, most of our sodium coming from added salt (sodium chloride). This has been linked to the high prevalence of high blood pressure.	Most naturally occurring foods have a high ratio of potassium to sodium. As food is processed and refined, potassium is removed. As salt and other sodium compounds such as sodium bicarbonate and sodium benzoate are added, sodium is increased. The aim should be to increase the potassium intake by eating some fresh fruits and vegetables and wholegrain cereals. At the same time the sodium intake should be reduced by not using the salt shaker, cooking without salt and using more foods processed without salt.
ZINC	Zinc occurs in more than 90 enzymes in the body. One of its roles is in the production of protein in the body. Symptoms of deficiency include a poor sense of taste, anorexia, growth retardation, poor wound healing, lack of hair and impaired function of the testes and ovaries.	Meat contributes about half the zinc in the diet. Cereals, milk and vegetables each contribute between 10 and 20%. The absorption from animal foods is better than from cereals and vegetables.

FOOD ADDITIVES

A food additive is a substance intentionally added to food in order to improve its keeping quality or stability, reduce waste, make the food more attractive by enhancing flavour, colour or consistency, or to maintain nutritional quality. Examples of food additives used in the home are baking powder, vinegar, flavouring essences, pectin, gelatine, tartaric acid, and food colours such as cochineal.

The use of additives by the food industry is regulated by standards which specify permitted additives, the foods in which the additives may be used, and the maximum levels permitted.

Some additives are extracted from naturally occurring substances, or they are made in the laboratory to be 'nature identical'. For example, egg yolk contains lecithin: in the home we use egg yolk to make mayonnaise, while in the factory lecithin or another purified emulsifier may be used. Vitamins C and E are used as antioxidants and beta-carotene is used as a food colour.

Among the substances used as additives which occur naturally in foods, are salicylates and monosodium glutamate. Additives such as tartrazine, sulphur dioxide, sodium carboxymethylcellulose and butylated hydroxyanisole, however, do not occur naturally in food.

Any adverse reactions to either naturally occurring substances or synthetic additives are dose-related: that is, small amounts may be well tolerated, but when large amounts are consumed, reactions may occur. For example, at Christmas time more people report reactions as a result of eating a lot of dried fruits, which are preserved with sorbic acid and sulphur dioxide. In the stone fruit season some people report reactions because of the salicylates naturally occurring in stone fruit. Such adverse reactions occur in only a minority of consumers.

All additives used must be listed on the label either by specific name or by the official numbering system, based on international standards.

The use of additives is of concern to many consumers. It is true that the unnecessary use of additives should be avoided, but it should also be remembered that additives can help to make food safe: by preventing or slowing down the growth of micro-organisms, many additives improve the keeping quality of food and help to stabilise food prices. Consumers who wish to avoid specific food additives can do so by reading food labels and avoiding those foods which contain the additives.

Listed below are the approved class names used on food labels, which reflect the functions performed by food additives:

ANTI-CAKING AGENTS are added so that products such as salt will flow freely when poured

ANTIOXIDANTS are added to prevent foods that contain fats and oils from becoming rancid

ARTIFICIAL SWEETENING SUBSTANCES are used to sweeten low-joule foods

BLEACHING AGENTS are used to whiten foods, e.g. flour

COLOURS are added to restore losses during processing and storage and give a uniform colour to the finished product

EMULSIFIERS are added to keep oil and water mixtures from separating into layers

ENZYMES break down foods, e.g. milk into curds and whey

FLAVOUR ENHANCERS are added to bring out the flavour of the food without imparting a flavour of their own

FLAVOURS are added to restore losses during processing and maintain uniformity

FLOUR TREATMENT AGENTS improve flour performance in bread making

FOOD ACIDS maintain a constant acid level in food despite variations in the acid level of ingredients

HUMECTANTS prevent foods from drying out

MINERALS are added to certain foods to supplement dietary intake

MINERAL SALTS are added to maintain the texture of goods such as processed meats, which might lose fats and meat juices

PRESERVATIVES are added to prolong the shelf life of foods

PROPELLANTS are used in aerosol containers

THICKENERS and VEGETABLE GUMS are used to maintain constant consistency in food products

VITAMINS make up for losses in processing and storage and are added to certain foods to supplement dietary intake

Listed below are Australian approved food additive numbers as at June 1988:

No.	Food Additive
100	Curcumin
100	Turmeric
101	Riboflavin
101	Riboflavin 5'-phosphate sodium
102	Tartrazine
107	Yellow 2G
110	Sunset yellow FCF
120	Carmines
120	Cochineal (Cl 75470)
122	Azorubine
123	Amaranth
124	Ponceau 4R
127	Erythrosine
129	Allura red AC (Cl 16035)
132	Indigotine
133	Brilliant blue FCF
140	Chlorophyll
142	Food green S
150	Caramel
151	Brilliant black BN
153	Activated vegetable carbon
153	Carbon blacks
155	Brown HT
160	Carotene, others
160	β-apo-8' Carotenoic acid methyl ester
160(a)	β-Carotene
160(b)	Annatto extracts
160(e)	β-apo-8' Carotenal
160(f)	β-apo-8' Carotenoic acid ethyl ester
161	Xanthophylls
161(g)	Canthaxanthin
162	Beet red
163	Anthocyanins
170	Calcium carbonate
171	Titanium dioxide
172	Iron oxide black
172	Iron oxide red
172	Iron oxide yellow
181	Tannic acid
200	Sorbic acid
201	Sodium sorbate
202	Potassium sorbate
203	Calcium sorbate
210	Benzoic acid
211	Sodium benzoate
212	Potassium benzoate
213	Calcium benzoate
216	Propylparaben
218	Methylparaben

No.	Food Additive
220	Sulphur dioxide
221	Sodium sulphite
222	Sodium bisulphite
223	Sodium metabisulphite
224	Potassium metabisulphite
225	Potassium sulphite
228	Potassium bisulphite
234	Nisin
235	Natamycin
249	Potassium nitrite
250	Sodium nitrite
251	Sodium nitrate
252	Potassium nitrate
260	Acetic acid, glacial
261	Potassium acetate
262	Sodium acetate
262	Sodium diacetate
263	Calcium acetate
264	Ammonium acetate
270	Lactic acid
280	Propionic acid
281	Sodium propionate
282	Calcium propionate
283	Potassium propionate
290	Carbon dioxide
296	Malic acid
297	Fumaric acid
300	Ascorbic acid
301	Sodium ascorbate
302	Calcium ascorbate
303	Potassium ascorbate
304	Ascorbyl palmitate
306	Tocopherols concentrate, mixed
307	*dl*-α-Tocopherol
308	γ-Tocopherol
309	δ-Tocopherol
310	Propyl gallate
311	Octyl gallate
312	Dodecyl gallate
317	Erythorbic acid
318	Sodium erythorbate
319	*tert*-Butylhydroquinone
320	Butylated hydroxyanisole
321	Butylated hydroxytoluene
322	Lecithin
325	Sodium lactate
326	Potassium lactate
327	Calcium lactate
328	Ammonium lactate
329	Magnesium lactate

No.	Food Additive
330	Citric acid
331	Sodium acid citrate
331	Sodium citrate
331	Sodium dihydrogen citrate
332	Potassium citrate
332	Potassium dihydrogen citrate
333	Calcium citrate
334	Tartaric acid
335	Sodium tartrate
336	Potassium acid tartrate
336	Potassium tartrate
337	Potassium sodium tartrate
338	Phosphoric acid
339	Sodium phosphate, dibasic
339	Sodium phosphate, monobasic
339	Sodium phosphate, tribasic
340	Potassium phosphate, dibasic
340	Potassium phosphate, monobasic
340	Potassium phosphate, tribasic
341	Calcium phosphate, dibasic
341	Calcium phosphate, monobasic
341	Calcium phosphate, tribasic
343	Magnesium phosphate, dibasic
343	Magnesium phosphate, tribasic
350	DL-Sodium hydrogen malate
350	DL-Sodium malate
351	Potassium malate
352	DL-Calcium malate
353	Metatartaric acid
354	Calcium tartrate
355	Adipic acid
357	Potassium adipate
365	Sodium fumarate
366	Potassium fumarate
367	Calcium fumarate
375	Niacin
380	Triammonium citrate
381	Ferric ammonium citrate
400	Alginic acid
401	Sodium alginate
402	Potassium alginate
403	Ammonium alginate
404	Calcium alginate
405	Propylene glycol alginate
406	Agar
407	Carrageenan
410	Locust bean gum
412	Guar gum

No.	Food Additive
413	Tragacanth
414	Acacia
415	Xanthan gum
416	Karaya gum
420	Sorbitol
421	Mannitol
422	Glycerin
433	Polysorbate 80
435	Polysorbate 60
436	Polysorbate 65
440(a)	Pectin
441	Gelatine
442	Ammonium salts of phosphatidic acid
450(a)	Ammonium phosphate, dibasic
450(a)	Ammonium phosphate, monobasic
450	Potassium metaphosphate
450	Potassium polymetaphosphate
450	Potassium pyrophosphate
450	Potassium tripolyphosphate
450	Sodium acid pyrophosphate
450	Sodium metaphosphate, insoluble
450	Sodium polyphosphates, glassy
450	Sodium pyrophosphate
450	Sodium tripolyphosphate
460	Cellulose, microcrystalline
460	Cellulose, powdered
461	Methylcellulose
464	Hydroxypropylmethyl cellulose
465	Methyl ethyl cellulose
466	Sodium carboxymethylcellulose
469	Sodium caseinate
471	Glyceryl monostearate
471	Mono- and di-glycerides of fat-forming fatty acid
472(a)	Acetic and fatty acid esters of glycerol
472(b)	Lactic and fatty acid esters of glycerol
472(c)	Citric and fatty acid esters of glycerol
472(d)	Tartaric and fatty acid esters of glycerol
472(e)	Diacetyltartaric and fatty acid esters of glycerol
473	Sucrose esters of fatty acids
475	Polyglycerol esters of fatty acids

No.	Food Additive
476	Polyglycerol esters of interesterified ricinoleic acid
480	Dioctyl sodium sulphosuccinate
481	Sodium stearoyl lactylate
482	Calcium stearoyl lactylate
491	Sorbitan monostearate
492	Sorbitan tristearate
500	Sodium bicarbonate
500	Sodium carbonate
501	Potassium bicarbonate
501	Potassium carbonate
503	Ammonium bicarbonate
503	Ammonium carbonate
504	Magnesium carbonate
507	Hydrochloric acid
508	Potassium chloride
509	Calcium chloride
510	Ammonium chloride
511	Magnesium chloride
514	Sodium sulphate
515	Potassium sulphate
516	Calcium sulphate
518	Magnesium sulphate
519	Cupric sulphate
526	Calcium hydroxide
529	Calcium oxide
536	Potassium ferrocyanide
541	Sodium aluminium phosphate, acidic
542	Bone phosphate
551	Silicon dioxide
552	Calcium silicate
553(b)	Talc
554	Sodium aluminosilicate
556	Calcium aluminium silicate
558	Bentonite
559	Kaolin
570	Stearic acid
572	Magnesium stearate
575	Glucono δ-lactone
577	Potassium gluconate
578	Calcium gluconate
579	Ferrous gluconate
620	L-Glutamic acid
621	Monosodium L-glutamate
622	Monopotassium L-glutamate
623	Calcium di-L-glutamate
624	Monoammonium L-glutamate
625	Magnesium di-L-glutamate

No.	Food Additive
627	Disodium guanylate
631	Disodium inosinate
636	Maltol
637	Ethyl maltol
900	Dimethylpolysiloxane
901	Beeswax, white
901	Beeswax, yellow
903	Carnauba wax
904	Shellac, bleached
905	Mineral oil, white
905	Petrolatum
920	L-Cysteine monohydrochloride
924	Potassium bromate
925	Chlorine
926	Chlorine dioxide
928	Benzoyl peroxide
931	Nitrogen
932	Nitrous oxide
965	Hydrogenated glucose syrups
967	Xylitol
1200	Polydextrose
1201	Polyvinylpyrrolidone
1202	Polyvinylpolypyrrolidone
1400	Dextrins
1403	Bleached starch
1404	Oxidised starch
1405	Enzyme-treated starches
1410	Monostarch phosphate
1412	Distarch phosphate esterified with sodium trimetaphosphate
1412	Distarch phosphate esterified with phosphorus oxychloride
1413	Phosphated starch phosphate
1414	Acetylated distarch phosphate
1420	Starch acetate esterified with acetic anhydride
1421	Starch acetate esterified with vinyl acetate
1422	Acetylated distarch adipate
1440	Hydroxypropyl starch
1442	Hydroxypropyl distarch phosphate
1450	Starch sodium octenylsuccinate
1505	Triethyl citrate
1510	Ethyl alcohol
1517	Glycerol diacetate
1518	Triacetin
1520	Propylene glycol

INDEX

Photographs in this book occur with entries, and are therefore not specifically listed in the index. The exceptions, photographs which appear on a different page from the food entry, are indicated below by numbers in italics.

A

aamchur 339, 352
abalone 148, 167
    mushroom, see oyster mushroom
abbaye, see port salut
abi, see abiu
abiu 46
acetic acid 233
achar 404
achiote, see annatto
adlay, see millet
aduki bean, see adzuki bean
advocaat 455
adzuki bean 302
aerosol cream 262, 264
African brown bean, see brown bean
African horned melon, see kiwano
agar agar 233–34
agnolotti 221
aguacate, see avocado
aioli 384, 425
aji-no-moto, see monosodium glutamate
ajowan, see ajwain
ajwain 339
albacore 165, 186
albumen 234
alcohol 11, 242, 246, 454
ale 455
Alessandria 121
alexanders 340
alfalfa sprouts 15
algue rouge, see dulse
alligator pear, see avocado
allspice 340
almond 312–13
    essence 413
    jelly 313
    oil 324
Alpina salami 121
amaranth 14, 200
amaretto 457
amber malt 417
amchoor, see aamchur
American cheddar, see colby
American lobster 170
ammonium carbonate 234
amsamgelugor, see tamarind
anari 281
ancho pepper 345
anchovy
    butter, see patum peperium
    canned 175
ancient egg, see thousand-year egg
andouille sausage 92
anelini 221
angel cake 244
angelica 340
    stems, candied 340, 372
angelot 278
angkak 398
angostura bitters 413
anice 458
animal shortening 334
anise 340–41
    seed 313
aniseed, see anise
    stars, see star anise
anisette 313, 341, 458
annatto 279, 283, 290, 341
ansgar 299
appenzeller 274
apple 46–47
    dried 76–77
apple
    cucumber 27
    juice 461
    puree 254
    and rhubarb crumble 254
    sauce 385
    snow 253
    strudel 251
apricot 47
    dried 77

apricot
    brandy 455
    conserve 382
    kernel oil 324
    soufflé 260
aquavit 456
arachis nut oil, see peanut oil
araruta, see arrowroot
arborio 209
Ardennes ham 132
Arles 121
arrack 456
arrowhead, see water chestnut
arrowroot 234–35
artificial sweeteners 364
    see also individual names
asafoetida 341
asatuki, see garlic chives
ascorbic acid, see vitamin C
Asian wheat noodle 228–29
asparagus 15
    bean 16
aspartame 365
aspic 235, 415
assam powder, see tamarind, cream of
assam tea 467
Athole Brose 206
Atlantic salmon 148
atta flour 214
    brown coarse 214
attar, see rose water
aubergine, see eggplant
Australian frankfurter 115
Australian salmon 161
avgotaraho, see botargo
avocado 46, 48
    oil 324–25
awabi, see abalone
azuki bean, see adzuki bean

B

baba 188
    au rhum, see baba
babaco 48, 67
baby blue pumpkin 37
baby cabbage, see Brussels sprout
baby food 442
bacalao, see cod, dried and salted
bacalhau, see cod, dried and salted
back bacon, see Canadian bacon
backsteiner 291
bacon 126–28
    bones 91
badian, see star anise
bagel 188–89
bagnes, see raclette
bagoong 398
baharat 338
bakaliaros, see cod, dried and salted
baked beans 442
baked custard 256
baked Virginia ham 132
baker's flour 214
baking powder 233, 235
baking soda, see bicarbonate of soda
baklava 258
Balleron 112
balm 341–42
Balmain bug 167
balsam pear, see bitter melon
balsamic vinegar 421
balut 143
bamboo
    fungus 81
    mustard cabbage 22
    shoot 15–16
bamee, see Asian wheat noodle
banana 49
    caramel 253
    chocolate-coated 254
    dried 77
banana
    passionfruit 67
    pumpkin 37
bangers 116
    and mash 116
banh trang rice paper wrapper 229
bantam egg 143
bap 189
barbecue
    chicken 429–30

pork, Chinese 128
barley 10, 200, 201
    popped 201
barley
    flakes 201
    flour 214–15
    grits 201
    sugar 371
    water 201
barleycorn, see barley
barramundi 149
Bartlett pear 68, 69
basderma 128–29
basil 342
Basmati rice 208
bass, Australian 149–50
bastard cinnamon, see cassia
batter 433
bau yeu, see abalone
bavariablu, see Bavarian blue
Bavarian blue 274
bay leaf 342
    crumbled (nutrients) 339
    oil 328
bay lobster, see Moreton Bay bug
bay rum berry, see allspice
bay salt, see sea salt
Bayonne ham 132
bean
    fritter 303
    herb, see savory
    paste
        Chinese hot 399
        sweet 399
    sauce 385–86
    shoot, see bean sprout
    sprout 15, 17
bean, green 16–17
beancurd, see tofu
béarnaise sauce 386
Beaufort, see gruyère
bechamel sauce 386
bêche-de-mer, see sea cucumber
bee balm, see bergamot
beef 88–91
    roast 136
    smoked 136
beef
    bacon 126
    extract 413
    sausage 116
    Wellington 135
beefsteak plant, see shiso
beer 455
    salami 121
beet, see beetroot
beetroot 17–18
bel paese 275, 299
Belgian endive 28
belimbing asam, see carambola
belimbing manis, see carambola
bell capsicum 23
bellelay 275
belly bacon, see kaiserfleisch
beluga 176
bénédictine 342, 362, 458
Bengal gram, see chickpea
Bengal isinglass, see agar agar
beni shoga 404–5
benne, see sesame seed
bentong, see kecap manis
bergamot 342–43
    oil of 342
Berliner fleischwurst 110
Berliner sausage 112
Bermuda arrowroot, see arrowroot
besan 215, 306
beta carotene 12, 14, 46
Beurre Bosc pear 68
bi-sun, see rice noodle, dried
biarom 285
bicarbonate of soda 236, 441
bierschinken 110
bierwurst 110
big eye 126
biji, see annatto
bilimbi, see carambola
billy goat plum, see green plum
biltong 129
biltongue, see biltong
biotin 12, 471
bird's foot, see fenugreek
biryani 356, 360
biscuits 244
bishop's weed, see ajwain
bitter almond 313
bitter gourd, see bitter melon
bitter melon 18

blachan 399
black bean, salted 303
black bean sauce 386
black carp, see carp
black cumin, see nigella
black-eyed bean 303
black-eyed pea, see black-eyed bean
Black Forest ham 132
black kidney bean 303
black lovage, see alexanders
black nightshade 50
black olive 407, 408
black pot-herb, see alexanders
black pudding 110–11
black raspberry 73
black rye bread 198
black sapote 50
Black Velvet 459
black vinegar 424
blackberry 49
blackcurrant 54
blackfish 150, 154
blacklip abalone 167
blacklip mussel 171
bladder leaf seaweed, see hijiki
blade 90
blanket tripe 105
blended shortening 334
bleu, see blue vein
bleu de Bresse 275
blini 203
bloc tunnel de foie gras truffé 131
blood sausage 111
bloodwort, see yarrow
bloodwurst 111
Bloody Mary 396
blue castello 275, 282
blue catfish 152
blue cheese, see blue vein
blue cheshire 280
blue cod 433
blue grenadier 150
Blue Max pumpkin 37
blue moki, see trumpeter
blue pea 304
blue shropshire 275–76
blue stilton, see stilton
blue swimmer crab 168, 169
blue threadfin 150
blue vein 276
blue wensleydale 300
blueberry 50
bluefin tuna 165, 186
bluefish, see tailor
bluff oyster 172
blushing ginger, see beni shoga
boar, wild 108
boarfish 151
boar's head 94, 108
bocconcini 276, 292
bockwurst 111
boiled pudding 260–61
boiled sweets 370–71
boiler (hen) 140
bok choy 22, 345
boletus 81–82
bollito misto 115
bologna 112
bolognaise, see bolognese sauce
bolognese sauce 387
Bombay duck 151
bomeloe, see Bombay duck
bonavist, see hyacinth bean
bonbel 298
bone-in leg ham 133
boneless leg ham 132
bones 91
bonito 165
    flake 175
Bonox 413
boomla, see Bombay duck
borage 343
borecole, see kale
borlotti bean 304
Botany Bay spinach, see warrigal greens
botargo 175–76, 402
bottarga, see botargo
bottle gourd 18, 406
boudin
    blanc 112
    noir 112
bouillabaisse 358
bouillon cube 414
bouillon, see stock powder
bounce berry, see cranberry
bouquet garni 338, 342, 352, 357, 362

boursin 294
Bovril 414
bow ties, see farfalle
boysenberry 50–51
bracken
    root 18–19
    tip 19
Bradenham ham 132
brains 91–92
bramble, see blackberry
bran 202–3
brandy 455
    flavouring 414
bratwurst 112–13
    cooked in beer 113
brawn 94, 129
Brazil nut 314
Brazilian guava, see feijoa
Brazilian tree grape, see jaboticaba
bread
    brown 187, 195
    fibre-increased 192
    flavoured 192–93
    mixed grain 187, 195
    rye 198–99
    sourdough 199
    white 187, 188
    wholemeal 187, 188
bread and butter custard 256
breadcrumbs 189
breadfruit 19
breakfast rashers, see big eye
breakfast sausage 116
bream 151
breast, of chicken 140
bresaola 130
Bresse bleu, see bleu de Bresse
brewer's yeast 242
brie 277
    de coulommiers, see coulommiers
brinjal aubergine 28
brioche 189
brisket 90, 130
broad bean 19–20
    dried 304–5
broadleaf Batavian endive 28, 29
broccoli 20
brown bean 305
brown bread 187, 195
brown onion 34
brown rice 207
brown sugar 365
Brunswick salad 118
Brussels sprout 20–21
bu thei, see bottle gourd
buah keras, see candle nut
bucatini 221–22
buckweizen, see buckwheat
buckwheat 203
buetten 289
buffalo 92
buffalo herb 15
buffe 137, 147
buffet 137, 147
bulgur, see burghul
bull's eye 371
bully beef 130
bulrush millet, see millet
bultong, see biltong
bummalow, see Bombay duck
bun pho, see rice noodle, fresh
bunderfleisch 129
bunya bunya pine nut 314
burdock root 21
burghul 212
burpless cucumber, see European cucumber
bush damper, see damper
butt (beef) 88
butter 323, 325
    bean, see lima bean
    filling 246
    pumpkin 37
butterfish, see jewfish
butterflies, see farfalle
butterhead lettuce 31
buttermilk 262–63, 264
butternut pumpkin 37
butterscotch 371
    topping 414
button mushroom, see cultivated mushroom
buttons, see tansy

C

cabanossi 113
cabbage 21–23

cacao butter, see cocoa butter
Cacciatore 121
caerphilly 277
caffeine 462, 464
caimito, see star apple
caimo, see abiu
cake flour, see sponge flour
cake, frozen 450–51
calabash, see bottle gourd
Calabrese 20, 122
calamansi, see kalamansi
calamondin, see kalamansi
calcium 12, 148, 262, 471
    hydroxide, see slaked lime
calf
    lungs 99
    sweetbreads 104
calf's liver 99
calico bean, see lima bean
Calrose rice 208
calthrop, see water chestnut
calvados 456
Cambridge sausage 116
camembert 277–78, 296
Canadian bacon 126
canbra oil, see rapeseed oil
candied fruit 371–73
candied peel 372
candle nut 314
candy sugar, see coarse sugar
cane syrup 365
canistel 51
cannellini bean 305
canneloni 222
canola oil, see rapeseed oil
canteloupe melon 73
Cantonese sausage, see lap
    cheong
cape gooseberry 51
capelli di angelo 222
capellini 222
capers 343
capon 140
cappelletti 222
Cappicola 122
caprice des dieux 300
caps, see cultivated mushroom
capsicum 23
carambola 51–52, 60
caramel 373, 414
    bananas 253
caraway seed 315
carbohydrates 11, 12, 187, 301
carbonate of ammonia, see
    ammonium carbonate
cardamom 343–44
    pods/seeds, see cardamom
Cardinal grape 57
carob 373–74
    powder 374
Carolina rice 208
carom, see ajwain
carp 152
carrageen 182
carrot 24
    cake 243, 245
casaba melon 59
Casalingo cacciatore 122
cashew nut 315
cassava 24
cassia 344
    bark, see cassia
cassis 54
cassoulet 114, 125
caster sugar 365
cataplana 120
catfish 152
catjang, see black-eyed bean
cattle pumpkin 37
cauliflower 24–25
cavatappi, see tortiglioni
Cavendish banana 49
caviar 148, 176
cayenne, see chilli pepper
celeriac 25
celery 25
    cabbage, see napa cabbage
    knob, see celeriac
    root, see celeriac
    salt 239, 316
    seed 239, 315–16
Celestine 415
cellophane noodle 229
cep 82
cepe, see cep
cereal
    beverage 464
    dessert 252–53
cereals, packaged 446–47
cervelas, see cervelat

cervelat 113
cervelatwurst 122
Ceylon moss, see agar agar
Ceylon tea 467
cha gio 229
cha siew 128
    pow 128
chaat masala 352
champagne 462
champignon, see cultivated
    mushroom
chanterelle 82
chaource 281–82
chapatti 190, 214
chappati, see chapatti
chard, see leaf beet
Charentais melon 59
chartreuse 342, 458
chasoba noodle, see soba noodle
chaumes 278
chaurice, see chorizo
chayote 26
cheddar 273, 278
    American, see colby
    reduced fat 283
cheedam 279
cheerio 115
cheese 273–74
    blue, see blue vein
    cottage 280–81
    cream 282, 293–94, 300
    dietary modified 283
    goat 287
    matured, see cheddar
    processed 296
    tasty, see cheddar
cheese
    salami 122
    spread 279
chelou kebab 360
cherimoya 52–53
cherry 53
    brandy 457
    tomato, see Tom Thumb
        tomato
chervil 344
cheshire 279–80
chester 279, 280
chestnut 312, 316
chevres, see goat cheese
chicharrones, see crackling
chicken 139–40
    barbecue 429–30
    cuts of 140–41
    free-range 140
    fried 432–33
    frozen 451
    smoked 136
chicken
    with black bean sauce 430
    liverwurst 133
    loaf, see chicken roll
    nugget 433
        frozen 452–53
    roll 130
chickpea 215, 306, 400
    spread, see hommos
chicory, see Belgian endive and
    curly endive
chiko roll 439
chiku, see sapodilla
chilitepines, see chilli pepper
chilli
    bean paste, see bean paste,
        Chinese hot
    oil 328
    pepper 23, 344–45, 393
    sauce 387
    vinegar 424
China root, see galangal
Chinese bacon 126–27
Chinese barbecue sauce, see
    bean paste, sweet
Chinese black moss 183
Chinese broccoli 20
Chinese chard, see Chinese
    white cabbage
Chinese cherry, see lychee
Chinese flowering white
    cabbage 21
Chinese gooseberry, see
    kiwifruit
Chinese kale, see Chinese
    broccoli
Chinese mushroom, see oyster
    mushroom and shiitake
    mushroom
Chinese mustard cabbage 22
Chinese parsley, see coriander

Chinese pea, see snow pea
Chinese pepper 345
Chinese red date 53
Chinese sausage, see lap cheong
Chinese sesame paste, see tahini
Chinese sweet pickles, see chow
    chow pickle
Chinese water chestnut 43
Chinese white cabbage 22, 23
chipolata 114
    with tomatoes 114
chips 431
    frozen 453
chitlins, see chitterlings
chitterlings 92
chives 345
    fresh chopped (nutrients) 339
    garlic 345, 349
    onion, see chives
chocolate 374, 387, 464
    cooking 374
    white 374–75
chocolate
    bar 374
    cake 245
    chips 374
    flake 374
    pudding fruit, see black sapote
    sauce 387
    soufflé 260
chocolate-coated banana 254
chocolate-coated crunch
    bar 374
chocolate sauce pudding 259
chok wo, see arrowroot
choko, see chayote
cholesterol 46, 87, 139, 148,
    243, 262
chorizo 92, 114
choux pastry 248
chow chow pickle 405
Christmas
    cake 245–46
    melon 59
    pudding 260–61
chromium 12, 471
chuck 90–91
chuk gai choy, see bamboo
    mustard cabbage
chump 97
chuno 445
chutney 405
cider 455–56
    vinegar 424
cilantro, see coriander
cinnamon 345–46
citric acid 236
citron 53–54
citronella, see lemon grass
citrus fruit essences 415
clam 148, 168
    chowder 168
claytons 461
clementine 64
clingstone nectarine 65
clingstone peach 68
clobassy 114–15
clotted cream 263, 265
cloud ear fungus 82
clove flowers, see star anise
cloves 346
club sandwich 438
coarse sugar 365
cob nut, see hazelnut
cochineal 415
cockle 148, 168
cockney bream 162
cocktail avocado 48
cocktail frankfurter 115
cocoa 374, 463–64
    butter 326
coconut 316
    desiccated 316
coconut
    barfi 375
    cream 316
    fudge, see coconut ice
    ice 375
    milk 316
    oil 323, 326
cod 152–53
    dried and salted 176
    smoked 176–77
codfish, see cod
coffee 464
    crystals 365
    essence 415
    ice cream 255
    liqueurs 456
coffee sauce pudding 259

cognac 455, 460
cointreau 457, 461
cola 461, 464
colby 280
cold cuts 109
coleslaw 21
    dressed 437–38
coleslaw dressing 421, 425,
    425–26
colewart 21, 25
colic root, see galangal
collard, see kale
coloured sugar crystals 365–66
colza oil, see rapeseed oil
common balm, see balm
common mushroom, see
    cultivated mushroom
common tomato 75
compound butter 325
comte, see gruyère
conchiglie 222
conchigliette 222
conchiglione 222
condensed milk 263, 264
Conference pear 68
confit 135
    d'oie 145
congee 120, 143
congo pea, see pigeon pea
conpoy 177
conserve 381
    apricot 382
consomme 415
continental flour 215
continental frankfurter 115
continental lentil, see lentil
continental liver sausage 133
cooking margarine 330
Cooktown salmon, see blue
    threadfin
copha, see coconut oil
Coppa ham 132
copper 12, 471
coquille Saint Jacques, see
    scallop
coral cod, see coral trout
coral crab 169
coral trout 153
cordial 464–65
Corella pear 68
coriander 346
    seed (nutrients) 339
Corinth grape 77
corn 26
    see also maize
corn
    chips 448–49
    meal 204
    oil 326–27
    starch, see cornflour
    syrup, see glucose
corned beef 130
corned silverside, see corned
    beef
cornflakes 446, 447
cornflour 215–16
Cornice pear 68
Cornichon grape 57
Cornish pasty 432
cos lettuce 31
cotechino 115
Cotswold cheese 284
cottage cheese 280–81
cotto 281, 283
cottonseed oil 323, 327
coulommiers 281–82
country-style pork sausage 116
courgette, see zucchini
court bouillon 415–16
couscous 212–13, 389
cowpea, see black-eyed bean
cow's horn, see fenugreek
cow's milk 265, 266
crab 148, 169–70
    canned 177
crab-apple 47
crab stick, see seafood stick
cracked wheat 213
crackling 92–93
cranberry 54, 388
    bean, see borlotti bean
    sauce 388
craneberry, see cranberry
crawfish, see lobster
cray, see crayfish
crayfish 148, 169
cream 265, 266
    aerosol 263, 264
    canned reduced 263, 264
    clotted 263, 265

long life 264, 268
    mock 265, 269
    sour 264, 270–71
    thickened 264, 271
    whipping 271
cream
    cheese 282
    low fat, see neufchâtel
    triple 300
    mixture, see cream, thickened
of tartar 236
Crécy 415
crème
    brûlée 256
    caramel 257
    Chantilly 265, 266
    de bananes 456, 461
    de cacao 456
    de cassis 456, 461
    de menthe 456, 461
    fraîche 265, 266–67
    pâtissière 246
Crenshaw melon 59
crepe, see pancake
Crepes Suzette 436
cress 26–27
creste di gallo 222
crispbread 190
crisphead lettuce 31
crocodile 93
crocus, see saffron
croissant 190–91
croquembouche 248
Crown Prince pumpkin 37
crucian carp, see carp
crumble-topped pudding 254
crumpet 191
crustaceans 148
crystallised fruit 373
csabai 122
cube sugar 366
cucumber 27
culatello 122
cultivated butter 325
cultivated mushroom 82–83
Cumberland sauce 388
cumin 346–47
    seed, see cumin
cumquat 54
cups, see cultivated mushroom
curaçao 457, 460
curd cheese, see cottage cheese
curly endive 28, 29
curly kale, see kale
curly-leaved lettuce 31
currant 54–55
    dried 77
curry powder 346, 347
custard-apple 52
custard powder 236, 447
custard squash 32
cuttlefish 148, 169–70
cyclamate 366

D
d'Agen sugar plum 79
dahi, see yoghurt
dai gai choy, see Swatow
    mustard cabbage
daikon 38
Dairy Blend 327
dalo, see taro
damper 191
danablu, see Danish blue
danbo 298
Danish blue 282
Danish ham 132
Danish pastry 191–92
Danish salami 122
darjeeling tea 467
dark chocolate icing 246
dark rye bread 198
dasheen, see taro
dashi no moto 175
dashi stock 184
date 55, 56
    dried 78
date plum, see persimmon
daun ketumber, see coriander
daun limau perut, see lime leaves
Delicious apple 47
demerara, see raw sugar
dent corn 26
desi chickpea, see chickpea
desserts
    frozen 451
    packaged 447
devil's dung, see asafoetida
Devon 130

Devonshire cream, *see* cream, clotted
dhansak masala 352
dhu-fish, Western Australia 153
diamantini 222
dibs roman, *see* grenadine
dietary fibre 11, 13, 14, 46, 81, 187, 200, 243
dietary modified cheeses 283
Dijon mustard 396
dill 347
   pickles 347
   seed 317
   vinegar 424
   water 347
dillisk, *see* dulse
dim sim 430-31
   frozen 453
dip 384, 385, 400
ditalini 222-23
dock, *see* sorrel
dolmas 43
   canned 442-43
doner kebab 432
dory 153-54
double gloucester 283-84
doughnut 192
Dover sole 163
dow see, *see* black bean, salted
dragon's eyes, *see* longan
drambuie 459, *461*
drabart 284
dried apple 76-77
dried apricot 77
dried banana 77
dried black fungus, *see* cloud ear fungus
dried currant 77
dried date 78
dried duck 130-31
dried fig 78
dried mullet roe, *see* botargo
dried nectarine 78
dried peach 78-79
dried pear 79
dripping 323, 327-28
drummer 154
drumstick (chicken) 141
drumstick vegetable 27
dry onion 34
Dublin Bay prawn, *see* Norway lobster
duck 141-42
   dried 130-31
duck egg 143
   salted 143
duckling 142
dulse 183
durian 55-56
durum 212, 213, 220
Dutch brown bean, *see* brown bean
Dutch cheese, *see* cottage cheese

E

e-fu noodle 229
ear shell, *see* abalone
earthnut oil, *see* peanut oil
Easter bun, *see* hot cross bun
eastern rock lobster 170-71
easy-cut leg ham 132
edam 273, 284
edible tallow, *see* dripping
eel 148, 154
   smoked 149, 177
egg
   fruit, *see* canistel
   mushroom, *see* chanterelle
   noodle 229-30
   roll wrapper, *see* wonton wrapper
   tomato, *see* Roma tomato
   white mix, *see* albumen
eggplant 27-28, 46
eggs 139, 142-44
   pickled 406
Egyptian brown bean, *see* ful medami
elicoidali, *see* tortiglioni
emmental 284-85
emmer 202-3, 212
emperor 154-55
emu egg 143
endive 28-29
English bacon, *see* gammon
English country pork sausage 116
English liver sausage 133
English mustard 396

powder 396-97
   wholegrain 397
enokitake mushroom 83
entrammes, *see* port salut
Epicam ham 132
escarole, *see* broadleaf Batavian endive
esrom 285, 295
Eureka lemon 61
European carp 152
European cucumber 27
European noodle 230
European sole 163
evaporated milk 263, *265*, 267
Evian water 466
extra virgin olive oil 332

F

fa ts'ai, *see* Chinese black moss
faa goo, *see* shiitake mushroom
fabada 112, 114
fagara, *see* Chinese pepper
falafel 306
fancy meats, *see* offal
farfalle 223
farfallini 223
farm butter 325
farm cheese, *see* cottage cheese
farm-style sausage 113
fat back, *see* crackling
fats 11, 12
fava, *see* ful medami
fava bean, *see* broad bean *and* broad bean, dried
fedelini, *see* capellini
feet, of chicken 141
feijoa 56
Felinetti 122
fennel 29, 347
   giant, *see* asafoetida
fennel
   bulb 347
   flower, *see* nigella
   leaves 347
   seed 317, 347
   stems 347
fenugreek 348
ferule perisque, *see* asafoetida
fesonati, *see* mafalde
feta, *see* fetta
fetta 285
fettuccine 223
fibre-increased bread 192
fiddlehead fern, *see* bracken tip
field mushroom 83
fig 56
   dried 78
filbert, *see* hazelnut
   oil, *see* hazelnut oil
file fish, *see* leatherjacket
fillet
   beef 88
   pork 101
fillings, for cakes 246
filo pastry 243, 248-49
   frozen 452
   triangles 452-53
fines herbes 338, 344, 345, 359, 362
finger millet, *see* millet
fingerlings 161
fiocchetti, *see* farfallini
fiore sardo 295
fiori alpini 458
fish
   ball, Chinese 177-78
   maw 178
   sauce 10, 388
   stick, *see* seafood stick
   stock 416
fish, fried 433
five corners fruit, *see* carambola
five spice 338, 360
flageolet bean 308
flake 161
flaky pastry 249
flapjack 171
flathead 155
flats, *see* cultivated mushroom
flavoured breads 192-93
flavoured milk *265*, 267
flavoured oils 328, 329
flint corn 26
'Floater, the' 435
Floating Island 258
Florida mustard 397
flounder 155, 163
flour 214-19
flour corn 26
Fluffy Duck 455

fluoride 148, 454, 462
fluorine 12, 471
focaccia 193
foie gras 131
folate 14, 46, 87, 200, 441, 471
fondant 375
   uncooked 375
fonduta 286
fontal, *see* fontina
fontina 285-86
fontinella 286
food
   additives 13, 109, 412, 473
   groups 13
   pyramid 13, 469
foot-long frankfurter 115
forequarter
   lamb, whole 98
   pork 103
   veal 107
fortified wines 454, 457
fourme
   d'Ambert 286
   de Montbrison, *see* fourme d'Ambert
   de Pierre-sur-Haute, *see* fourme d'Ambert
frankfurter 115, 434, 436-37
free-range chicken 140
free-range egg 143
freestone nectarine 65, 66
freestone peach 68
French artichoke, *see* globe artichoke
French bean 16
French Bordeaux mustard 397
French fries, *see* chips
French herb salami 122
French pepper salami 122
French shallot, *see* shallot
French tarragon, *see* tarragon
freshwater perch, *see* bass, Australian
frizzes 122
frog 93
frogs' legs 93
fromage fondu, *see* gourmandise
frosting 246
frozen yoghurt *265*, 267-68
fruit
   candied 371-73
   canned 443
   crystallised 373
   dried 76-80
   flambéed 253
   glacé 371, 373
   poached 253
   toffee-glazed 254
fruit
   bread 193
   cobbler 254
   compote 253
   coulis 253-54
   drop 371
   jelly 381, 382
   juice *460*, *461*, 462-63, 465
      cordial 463
      drink 463
   paste 375-76
   pudding 254
   roly-poly, baked 254
   salad 253, 437
   soufflé 253
fruit dessert
   cooked 253
   uncooked 253-54
frumenty 256
fu kwa, *see* bitter melon
fudge 376
Fuerte avocado 48
fufu 241
ful medami 306
fusilli 223
   bucati 223

G

gado gado 393
gai laarn, *see* Chinese broccoli
gajus, *see* cashew nut
galangal 348
galantine 131
Gallia melon 73
Galliano 458, *460*
game 93
gammon 127
ganselandleberwurst 134
ganseleberwurst 134
garam masala 352
garbanzo bean, *see* chickpea

garden burnet, *see* salad burnet
garden pea 35
garden thyme, *see* thyme
garfish 155-56, 179
gargaut, *see* galangal
gari, *see* beni shoga
garlic 348-49, 399
   butter 325
   chives 345, 349
   loaf 192
   oil 328
   powder 239
   salt 239
   sausage 116-17
   vinegar 424
gasleverkorv 134
gekochte schinkenwurst 125
gelatine 91, 100, 237
gemfish 156
Genoa salami 122
Genoa torta 121
gentleman's relish, *see* patum peperium
German bologna 112
German liverwurst 134
German mustard 397
German salami 122
ghee 92, 328-29
gherkin 406
   cucumber 27
ghi, *see* ghee
giant granadilla 67
giant king crab 169
giant white cabbage, *see* napa cabbage
giant white radish 38, 410
giblets, of chicken 141
'gift from the stork' 426-27
gin 350, 456, *460*
gingelli, *see* sesame seed
ginger 349, 404-5
   ale *460*
   pudding 261
ginkgo nut 317-18
ginnie pepper, *see* chilli pepper
girolle, *see* chanterelle
gjetöst 286, 293
glacé de viande 416
glacé fruit 371, 373
glacé icing 246
glamer schabzieger, *see* sapsago
globe artichoke 29
globe eggplant 28
glucose 366, 372
gluten 216
glutinous rice 208-9
glycerine 237
glycerol, *see* glycerine
gnocchetti sardi 223
gnocchi 204, 224
   di patate 224
   verdi 224
goanna 93-94
goat 94
   cheese 287
goat's milk *265*, 268
gobo, *see* burdock root
Goettinger 113
golah, *see* rose water
golden berry, *see* cape gooseberry
golden celery 25
golden gram 17
   see also mung bean
golden granadilla 67
golden nugget pumpkin 37
golden syrup 366
golwasser 458
gomser, *see* raclette
goober, *see* peanut
goose 144-45
   egg 143
gooseberry 56-57
gorgonzola 287
Goteborg 113
Gothaer 113
gouda 287-88
Gould's squid 174
gourmandise 288
gourmet oils, *see* flavoured oils
gow choy, *see* garlic chives
graham, *see* wholemeal flour
grain sprout 15
gram flour, *see* besan
gramigna 224
   rigata 224
grana, *see* parmesan
granadilla, *see* passionfruit
Grand Marnier 457
Granny Smith apple 47

granulated sugar 366-67
   see also white sugar
grape 57
grapefruit 57-58, 71
grapeseed oil 329
grappa (spirit) 456
grappe (cheese) 288
grass carp, *see* carp
grass mushroom, *see* straw mushroom
gravy 389
Great Northern bean, *see* cannellini bean
Greek hayseed, *see* fenugreek
green asparagus 15
green bacon 127
green bean, *see* bean, green
green dill, *see* dill
green ginger wine 462
green gram 17
   see also mung bean
green olive 407, 408
   cracked 408
green onion 34
green pea, *see* garden pea
green pepper, *see* capsicum
green peppercorn 424
   mustard 398
   vinegar 424
green plum 58
green ridge cucumber 27
green sprouting broccoli 20
green zucchini 45
greenlip abalone 167
greenlip mussel 171
grenadine 71, 367
   molasses, *see* grenadine
greyerzer, *see* gruyère
gripe water, *see* dill water
grissini 193
groper 156
ground cherry, *see* cape gooseberry
groundnut, *see* peanut
   oil, *see* peanut oil
grouper, *see* groper
grouse 145
groviera, *see* raclette
gruyère 288
guacamole 381, 384
guava 58
   green 60
gudeg 60
gugelhupf 194
guinea corn, *see* millet
guinea fowl 145
   egg 143
Guinness 459
gula jawa, *see* palm sugar
gumbo, *see* okra
gunga pea, *see* pigeon pea
gurnard 156
gutsleberwurst 134
guy lan, *see* Chinese broccoli
Gyulai 122

H

haam suen choy, *see* mustard greens, pickled
haddock, smoked 178
haew, *see* water chestnut
haggis 41, 117, 206
hair vegetable, *see* Chinese black moss
hairtail 156-57
hairy lychee, *see* rambutan
hairy orange aubergine 28
hake 156, 433
haldi, *see* turmeric
halloumi, *see* haloumy
haloumy 288-89
halva 322, 376-77
ham 127, 131-33
   canned 132
ham
   bologna, *see* schinkenwurst de luxe 132
   spec, *see* speck
   steak 132
ham-style bologna 112
Hamburg parsley root 356
hamburger 433-34
Hamwich 133
hamwurst, *see* schinkenwurst
hana-katsuo, *see* bonito flakes
hare 94
   jugged 94
hare's lettuce, *see* sow thistle

harhardal, *see* split pea
haricot bean 16, 306–7
harissa 120, 389
hartshorn 234
Hass avocado 48
hausmacher leberwurst 134
havarti 289, 299
Hawaiian granadilla, *see* golden
  granadilla
hazelnut 318
  oil 329
head cheese, *see* brawn
head, of chicken 141
heads 94
health bar 377
hearts 95
hearts of palm, *see* palm hearts
hed hunu, *see* cloud ear fungus
heeng, *see* asafoetida
herb
  of grace, *see* rue
  oil 328
herbal tea 465
hergard elite 284
herrgardsöst 284
herring 148, 157
  kipper 179
  matjes 178
  rollmop 178–79
hervé 291
high-ratio cake flour, *see* sponge
  flour
hijiki 183
hilba 389
hiratake, *see* oyster mushroom
ho yo jeung, *see* oyster sauce
hobelkäse, *see* sapsago
hock (pork) 101
hog maw 95, 105
hogget 95, 97
hog's pudding 117
hoisin sauce 389, 399
hollandaise sauce 390
Holsteinerwurst 113
holvshki 230
hominy 204
  grits 204
hommos 306, 322, 399–400
hon dashi 175
honey 367, 370
honeycomb 377
  tripe 105
honeydew melon 59
hong dow, *see* adzuki bean
hoong joh, *see* Chinese red date
horse parsley, *see* alexanders
horsemint 391
horseradish 349–50
  sauce 349, 390
hot bean sauce, *see* bean paste,
  Chinese hot
hot chocolate, *see* cocoa
hot cross bun 194
hot dog 115, 434
hot water pastry 249
hou goo, *see* oyster mushroom
hoy sum, *see* sea cucumber
hu gwa, *see* bottle gourd
Hubbard pumpkin 37
hummus, *see* hommos
Hungarian salami 122
hurka 117
hussar 157
hyacinth bean 307

I

Iberian moss, *see* carrageen
ice cream 252, 255
icicle radish, *see* giant white
  radish
icing sugar 367
icings 246
imlee, *see* tamarind
inanga, *see* whitebait
Indian corn, *see* corn *and* maize
Indian date, *see* tamarind
Indian fig 59
Indian chilli sauce, *see*
  sambal ulek
injera 205
instant dried casserole/base 445
instant oats 206
instant sauce/gravy 445–46
iodine 148, 472
Irish ham 132
Irish Mist 459
Irish moss, *see* carrageen
iron 12, 87, 472
isinglass 182
Italian cucumber 27

Italian rice 209
Italian salami 122
Italian-style pork sausage, *see*
  cotechino
Italian tomato, *see* Roma tomato
ito, *see* lotus

J

jaboticaba 60
jack cheese 274, 292
jackfruit 60
Jaffa orange, *see* sweet orange
jagdwurst 118
jaggery, *see* palm sugar
jam 238, 381–82
  roly-poly 260
Jamaica pepper, *see* allspice
jamar kuping, *see* cloud ear
  fungus
Japanese aubergine 28
Japanese loquat, *see* loquat
Japanese medlar, *see* loquat
Japanese moss, *see* agar agar
Japanese plum pickle, *see*
  umeboshi
Japanese tea 467
jarlsberg 289
Jarrahdale pumpkin 37
jasmine rice, *see* Thai rice
jellied confectionery 377–78
jelly (dessert) 255–56, 447
  whip 256
jelly beans 378
jelly mushroom, *see* straw
  mushroom
jellyfish, dried 179
jerez, *see* sherry
jerked beef 129
Jerusalem artichoke 30
Jesuit's nut 43
jewfish 157–58, 163
jewie, *see* jewfish
Jews' mallow, *see* melokhia
jiang 386
Jindivick Supreme 300
Job's tears, *see* millet
John Dory 153–54
Johnny cakes 191
jollytails, *see* whitebait
Josephine pear 68
jubes 378
jugged hare 94
jujube, *see* Chinese red date
juk soon, *see* bamboo shoot
juniper berries 350
junket 256, 257

K

kaala chana, *see* chickpea
kaasdoop 288
kabana 113
kabanos, *see* cabanossi
kabli chana, *see* chickpea
kadaif, *see* kataifi pastry
kaffir corn, *see* millet
kahlua 456
kai laarn, *see* Chinese broccoli
kaiserfleisch 127
kakee, *see* persimmon
kaki, *see* persimmon
kalamansi 60–61
kalbs 134
kale 30
kamaboko 179–80
kamoteng kahoy, *see* cassava
kampyo 406
kan ts'ao 351
kangaroo 96
kanten, *see* agar agar
karcom, *see* saffron
karela, *see* bitter melon
Karlsbader ham 132
kasha 201, 205
  see also buckwheat
kashmiri masala 353
Kasseler 132
kasseri 289–90
kataifi pastry 249–50
kathal, *see* jackfruit
katsuo-bushi, *see* bonito flake
katzenkopf, *see* edam
kecap asin 391
kecap manis 390–91
keem 184
kelp 183
kemiri, *see* candle nut
Kentucky ham 132
keta-red caviar, *see* salmon roe
ketjap, *see* kecap manis
kewra 416

Key lime, *see* Mexican lime
kezuri-bushi, *see* bonito flake
kha min, *see* turmeric
khanun, *see* jackfruit
khoubiz, *see* pita
kibbled wheat, *see* cracked
  wheat
kidney 87, 96
kielbasa 118
  salad 118
kikurage, *see* cloud ear fungus
kimchee 406–7, 410
kina, *see* sea urchin
kinako, *see* soya flour
king threadfin 150
kingfish 158
kipper, canned 179
kirsch 457
kishk 212
kitchen salt 240
kitron, *see* citron
kiwano 61
kiwifruit 61
knackwurst 118
knight's milfoil, *see* yarrow
kochu chang 400
kohlrabi 30
kohlkasa 41
kolbasa 119
kolkas 41
kolokassi 41
kombu 183–84
konafa, *see* kataifi pastry
kong syin ts'ai, *see* watercress
kosher salt 240
kourabiedes 419
kransky 119
kadju, *see* kuzu
kugelhoff, *see* gugelhupf
kumara 41
kümmel 315, 458
kumquat, *see* cumquat
kunyit, *see* turmeric
kuping tikus, *see* cloud ear
  fungus
kuwai, *see* water chestnut
kuzu 180, 237
kvass 210
kway tiow, *see* rice noodle,
  fresh

L

lablab, *see* hyacinth bean
labu air, *see* bottle gourd
lachsschinken, *see* ham de luxe
lady fingers banana 49
lady's fingers, *see* okra
lager 455
lamb 96–99
  leg of, stuffed with
    apricots 443
lamb's
  brains 92
  fry 99
  head 94
  heart 95
  kidney 96
  lettuce, *see* leaf lettuce
  sweetbreads 104
lamington 243
lancashire 290
landgang 293
Landjäger 113
langoustine, *see* scampi
laos, *see* galangal
lap cheong 119–20
lapsang souchong tea 467
lard 323, 329–30
lasagne 224
  verde 224
lasagnette 224
lat yu, *see* chilli oil
latkhan, *see* annatto
Latvian liverwurst 134
lavash 194
Le Pitchou 287
leaf
  beet 18
  lettuce 31
leatherjacket 158
Lebanese cucumber, *see*
  European cucumber
Lebanese roll, *see* doner kebab
leberkäse 133
leberstreichwurst 134
leberwurst 134
lecithin 310, 335
leek 31
leg
  ham, on the bone 133
  lamb 97

pork 101
  veal 106
legumes, *see* pulses
leicester 290
leiden, *see* leyden
lemon 61–62
  balm, *see* balm
  balm vinegar 425
  barley water 201
  essence 416–17
  grass 350
  meringue pie 259
  mousse 260
  sole 163
  sorbet 255
  thyme 362
  verbena 350
  vinegar 425
lemonade 460, 466
lentil 307–8
leong goo, *see* shiitake
  mushroom
leopard cod, *see* coral trout
lesser galangal 348
lettuce 31
leveret 94
leverkorv 134
leverwurst 134
leyden 288, 290–91
lichee, *see* lychee
light rye bread 199
lights 99
lillypilly 62
lima bean 308
limbourg, *see* limburger
limburger 291
lime 62
  dried 407
  leaves 351
limewater 241
limu omani, *see* lime, dried
ling 158
ling-bye, *see* carrageen
ling gok, *see* water chestnut
lingcod 158
linguiça 120
linguine 224–25
link sausages 116
liptauer 281
Lisbon lemon 61
Lismore salami 122
litchee, *see* lychee
litchi, *see* lychee
litchie, *see* lychee
little Bertie 278
livarot 278
liver 87, 99, 100
  cheese, *see* leberkäse
liverwurst 133
lo-chol cheese 283
lobby, *see* lobster
lobe-leaf seaweed, *see* wakame
lobster 148, 170–71
locust bean, *see* carob
loganberry 62
loh bok 38
loin
  lamb 97
  veal 106
lokum, *see* Turkish delight
lollipop 371
long life cream 264, 268
long life milk 264, 268
long rice, *see* rice noodle, dried
longan 63
longaniza, *see* linguiça
loomi besra, *see* lime, dried
loquat 63
lotus 32
lotus root
  flour, *see* lotus root starch
  starch 237–38
loukanika 120
loukoum, *see* Turkish delight
lovage 351
  sauce, for fish 351
  soup 351
love apple, *see* tomato
love-in-a-mist, *see* nigella
low fat
  cream cheese, *see* neufchâtel
  milk 268–69
low salt butter 325
lower salt bacon 127–28

lubia, *see* hyacinth bean
lucerne sprouts, *see* alfalfa
  sprouts
luderick 150
lumache 222
lump sugar, *see* cube sugar
lumpfish roe 180
lumpia 439
lungan, *see* longan
lungs, *see* lights
lupin 308
lychee 63–64
Lyoner 125
lysine 11, 301

M

ma t'ai, *see* water chestnut
macadamia nut 318
  butter 318
  oil 330
macapuno 316–17
macaroni 225
  cheese 447
mace 355
mackerel 148, 158–59
  smoked 180
Madagascar bean, *see* lima bean
madeira 457
Madrilene 415
ma'el ward, *see* rose water
mafalde 225
mafueng, *see* carambola
magnesium 12, 148, 471
mahlab 352
mahlepi, *see* mahlab
Maibowle 363
maidenhair tree, *see* ginkgo nut
main meals, frozen 451–52
maize 200, 203–4
  see also corn
maize
  oil, *see* corn oil
  starch, *see* cornflour
malibu 457
malt
  extract 417, *and see* malt
    flour
  flour 216–17
  vinegar 425
mamaliga 204
manbollen, *see* edam
Manchurian bean oil, *see* soya
  bean oil
mandarin 64
mandioca, *see* tapioca
manga, *see* mango
mangel-wurzel, *see* mangold
mangetout, *see* snow pea
mango 64
  chutney 405–6
  coulis 253–54
  mousse 260
  squash, *see* chayote
mangold 18
mangosteen 64–65
mangrove crab 168, 169
manioc, *see* cassava *and* tapioca
mantua, *see* parmesan
maple syrup 367
maranta starch, *see* arrowroot
marasca cherry 417, 457
maraschino 457
  essence 417
marchpane 413
margarine 323, 330–31
marinade 421
marinara 391
marjoram 352
marmalade 381, 382
  fruit, *see* canistel
Marmite 383
marron 169
marron glacé 373
marrow (bone) 91
marrow (vegetable) 32
marsala 396, 457
Marsh grapefruit 58
marshmallow 370, 378
maryland 141
marzipan 378
  uncooked 378–79
marzoline 287
masala 352–53
mascarpone 282, 291, 300
masoor dal, *see* lentil
mast, *see* yoghurt
mastic 353
masticha 353
matar dal, *see* split pea
matjes herring 178

matrimony vine 14
matsutake mushroom 83
matured cheese, see cheddar
matzah, see matzo meal
matzo 194, 205
  meal 204–5
mawa 416
mayonnaise 384, 421, 425–26
mazum, see yoghurt
mead 458
meals
  canned 443
  packaged 447
meat
  paste 383
  pie 434–35
mee, see Asian wheat noodle
mein, see Asian wheat noodle
mekabu 184
Melba sauce 391
mellowfruit, see pepino
melokhia 32–33
Melton Mowbray pie 249
merguez 120
meringue 257–58
metelt 230
Mettwurst 123
Mexican food, packaged 446
Mexican lime 62
Mexican oregano 355
Mexican strawberry, see pinto
  bean
Meyer lemon 62
mid-loin
  lamb 97–98
  pork 101–2
middle cut bacon 128
mie, see Asian wheat noodle
Milano salami 123
military herb, see yarrow
milk 262
  condensed 263, 264
  cow's 265, 266
  evaporated 263, 265, 267
  flavoured 265, 267
  goat's 265, 268
  long life 264, 268
  low fat 264, 268–69
  powdered 265, 269
  sheep's 265, 270
  skim 264, 270
milk pudding 256–57
milkshake 263, 267, 435
milkweed, see sow thistle
millet 10, 200, 205
mineral water 460, 463, 465
minerals 11, 12–13, 187, 441
  RDI 468
  see also individual names
minnows, see whitebait
mint 353
  jelly 391
  julep 353
  sauce 391–92
mirin 417
mirliton, see chayote
miso 301, 400
Mississippi nut, see pecan nut
mistki, see mastic
miswa noodle 228
mixed grain bread 187, 195
mixed spice 346
mizithra 291–92
mock cream 265, 269
molasses 367–68
  sugar 365
molbo 284
molluscs 148
mona lisa 284
monkey nut, see cashew nut and
  peanut
  oil, see peanut oil
monosodium glutamate 233,
  238, 412
montasio 284
Monterey jack 292
moong dal, see mung bean
moor fowl, see grouse
moor's head, see edam
morcilla blanca 112
morel 83–84
Moreton Bay bug 171
morille, see morel
mornay sauce 386, 395
mortadella 112, 120–21
morue, see cod, dried and salted
mountain yam 44
mousse 259–60
moutarde de Meaux 398
mouth/mowth dal 309

mozzarella 276, 292
mu erh, see cloud ear fungus
muesli 446
muffin
  American 195
  English 195–96
mulato pepper 345
mulberry 65
mullet 159
mulloway, see jewfish
Münchner weisswurst 125
mung bean 308–9
  sprouts 17
Murray crayfish 169
Murray perch 160
Muscat grape 57, 79
muscovado 365
  see also raw sugar
mushroom, common, see
  cultivated mushroom
mushroom soy 394
mushy peas 304, 435
musk melon, see rockmelon
mussel 148, 171
  canned 180
mustard
  cress 27, 354
  greens, pickled 407
  oil 331
  pickle, see piccalilli
  seed 354
mutton 96, 97, 99–100
mutton fish, see abalone
mycella 292–93
myrtle 354
mysore-pak 377
mysöst 286, 293

N
naan 196
nago imo, see mountain yam
nam pla, see fish sauce
nam prik 28
nameko 84
nangka, see jackfruit
nannygai, see redfish
napa cabbage 22–23
Napoli salami 123
nashi 65
Nassau groper 156
native capers, see wild orange
native grape 57
natto 310
Navel orange 66
navy bean, see haricot bean
neck (veal) 107
neck chops (lamb) 98
nectarine 65
  dried 78
needlefish, see garfish
neeps 41
neroli, see orange blossom
  essence
nettle 14
neufchâtel 282, 293–94
New England sausage 112
New Zealand spinach, see
  warrigal greens
ngopi, see blachan
niacin 12, 87, 148, 470
nigella 354–55
nimbin 274, 283
nira, see garlic chives
nitre, see saltpetre
non-alcoholic beverages 461,
  462–3
noodles 227–32
noomi, see lime, dried
nori 184
Norway lobster 170
nose bleed, see yarrow
nougat 379
nouilles 230
noyau 413
nudeln 230
nuka 410
nuoc mam, see fish sauce
nutmeg 355
  ground (nutrients) 339

O
oak-leaved lettuce 31
oat
  bran 202
  fibre, see oat bran
  flakes 205–6
  flour 217
oatmeal 206
oats 10, 200, 205–6
oboro konbu 183

ocean perch 160
ocean trout 148
octopus 148, 171–72
oden 179
oeufs mayonnaise 425
offal 100
Ogen melon 59
oil of dill 317
okra 33
olive 407–8
  oil 12, 331–32
onion 33–34
  pickled 408–9
onion
  and liver sausage 134
  seed 354
onionwurst 134
oolong tea 467
open sandwich 438
opossum, see possum
orange 66
  juice 461
orange blossom essence 417–18
orange flower water 418
orange roughy 159
orecchiette 225
oregano 355
Oregon pea 17
ormer, see abalone
oseille, see sorrel
osetra 176
osso buco 91, 107
ostrich egg 143
ou fen, see lotus root starch
ouzo 341, 456
ox
  kidney 96
  tongue 105
Oxford sausage 116
oxtail 100
oyster 148, 172
  canned 180
oyster mushroom 84
oyster sauce 392

P
Pacific oyster 172
packet
  cereal 446–47
  dessert 447
  meal 447
  soup 447–48
  stuffing 448
Packham pear 68
paddy-straw mushroom, see
  straw mushroom
pai pah guor, see loquat
pak chai, see Chinese white
  cabbage
pak chee, see coriander
palm
  heart 34
  nut 318–19
  oil 323
  sugar 368
pancake 435–36
pancetta 134
panch phora 338, 347, 348, 354
pandan leaf 356
  cake 356
paneer 281
panettone 196
pannarone 287
pantothenic acid 12, 471
papain 48, 67
papaw, see pawpaw
papaya, see pawpaw
pappadum 196, 339
paprika 356
  ground (nutrients) 339
paprika
  salami 123
  sausage 116
parakeelya 34–35
parasol mushroom 84
parata, see paratha
paratha 196–97
parboiled rice 209
pare, see bitter melon
Parfait Amour 458, 461
pariser 110
Parma ham 133
parmesan 294
parmigiano reggiano, see
  parmesan
parr 161
parrot fish 159–60
parsley 356–57
  dried (nutrients) 339
parsley fern, see tansy

parsnip 35
partridge 145–46
Pascal celery 25
pasilla pepper 345
passionfruit 66–67
  butter 67
  juice 460
pasta 220–27
  made with eggs 221
  vegetable flavoured 221
  white 221
  wholemeal 221, 227
  with fillings 221
pasteli 379
pastille 379–80
pastina 221
pastis 458
pastorello 294–95
pastourma, see basderma
pastrami 134
pastry 248
  frozen 452
pâté 135, 383
  de foie gras truffé en
    croûte 131
patis, see fish sauce
patna rice, see Carolina rice
patty pan squash 32
patum peperium 400–1
pau t'sai, see Chinese white
  cabbage
paua, see abalone
paunch 105
pavlova 257–58
  mix, see albumen
pawpaw 67
pea 35–36
  aubergine, see Thai pea
    aubergine
  bean, see haricot bean
peach 67–68
  dried 78–79
peanut 312, 319, 393
  butter 319, 381, 383
  oil 319, 332
pear 68–69
  dried 79
pear moss, see carrageen
pearl barley 201, 215
pecan
  nut 319
  oil 332
pecorino 295
pectin 238, 382
  sugar 368
Peking cabbage 22–23
Peking duck 142
pelemeni 230
Pellegrino water 466
pemmican 388, 445
penne 225
pepino 69
pepita, see pumpkin seed
pepper 357
  dulse 183
  oil 328
peppermint 353, 418
  essence 418
pepperoni 123
perch 152, 160
peria, see bitter melon
Perigord truffle 86
periwinkle 148
pernod 341, 458, 460
Persian lime, see Tahiti lime
Persian melon 73
persimmon 69
pesto 392
petit brie, see coulommiers
petit pois 35, 36
petticoat tails 244
pfälzer 134
pfeffer plockwurst 121
pheasant 146
  egg 144
Philadelphia cream cheese 282,
  295
phosphorus 12, 262, 472
phyllo pastry, see filo pastry
piccalilli 409
pickled cabbage, see mustard
  greens, pickled
pickling onion 34
picnic rashers, see big eye
pide, see pita
pie 258–59
  canned 443
  frozen 452–53
  meat 434–35
Piedmontese truffle 86

pigeon 146
  pea 309
pigface 69–70
pignolia, see pine nut
pig's head 94
pig's trotters 100
pike 160
pilau rice 207
pilchard, see sardine
  canned 180–81
pimento, see allspice
pimento, pickled 409
pimiento 356
pine
  mushroom, see matsutake
    mushroom
  nut 320
pineapple 70
  essence 418
  guava, see feijoa
  juice 461
Pink Gin 413
pink ling 158
pinon nut, see pine nut
pinto bean 309
pinze, see focaccia
pipis 148
pirogi 230
piroshki 230
  see also buckwheat
pirozkki 230
pistachio nut 320
pita 197
pitta, see pita
pizza 123, 197, 251, 292, 436
  frozen 452
pizza
  cheese, see mozzarella
  sausage 115
plaice 155
plantain 70
pligouri, see burghul
plockwurst 121
pluck 100
plum 70–71
  pudding 260, 261
  sauce 392
  tomato, see Roma tomato
Pluto Pup 436–37
pocket bread, see pita
poe 41
poi 41
pointed head cabbage 23
polenta, see corn meal
Polish salami 123
Polish sausage, see kielbasa
polka sausage, see plockwurst
pomegranate 71
pomelo 71–72
pommarola 'n coppa 226
pommes noisettes 453
pont l'evêque 278
Pontiac potato 36
popcorn 26, 206–7, 448
  cheese, see cottage cheese
popiah 439
poppy seed 320–21
porgy 160
pork 101–3
  roast 136
  sweet and sour 431
pork
  pie 135
  sausage 116
  spring 102
port 457
port salut 295
  see also biarom
possum 103
pot cheese, see cottage cheese
potassium 12, 46, 472
  acid tartrate, see cream of
    tartar
  bitartrate, see cream of tartar
  nitrate, see saltpetre
potato 36, 431
  chips, see chips
  crisps 448
  flour 238
  gems 453
  starch, see potato flour
pound cake 243
pourgouri, see burghul
poussin 140
powdered milk 265, 269
pozole, see hominy
Prager ham 133
prawn 148, 172–73
preserving sugar 368
pressed duck, see dried duck

pressure pack cream, see aerosol cream
presswurst 135
pretzel 197
prickly custard-apple, see soursop
prickly pear, see Indian fig
processed cheese 296
profiteroles 248
prosciutto 133
protein 11–12, 14, 87, 148, 200, 301
provahira 296
provolo 296
provolone 296
prune 71, 79
puff pastry 250
puha, see sow thistle
pulled sugar 371
pullet egg 144
pulses 301
pumpernickel 197–98
pumpkin 37
  pie 37
  seed 37
  oil 333
pure olive oil 332
puri 198
purple broccoli 20
purple granadilla 67
purslane 14
pyridoxine, see vitamin B6

Q
quail 146–47
  egg 144
quark, see cottage cheese
quatre epices 338, 354
Queensland blue pumpkin 37
Queensland nut, see macadamia nut
quiche 437
  Lorraine 437
quick cooking oats 206
quince 72
quinine 467
quinnat salmon 161
quinoa 200, 207

R
raajma, see red kidney bean
rabbit 103–4
raclette 296
radish 38
ragi, see millet
ragnit 299
rahat lokum, see Turkish delight
rainbow trout 148, 164
raisin 79–80
raki 353, 456
rambutan 63, 72
ramen, see Asian wheat noodle
rampe, see pandan leaf
rapeseed oil 333
raspberry 72–73
  essence 418–19
  vinegar 426
ratafia 72
ratatouille 45
rattlesnake 104
ravioli 221, 225–26
raw sugar 368
ray 160–61
rebung, see bamboo shoot
recommended dietary intake (RDI) 13
  of energy and protein 469
  of minerals 468
  of vitamins 468
red bopple nut 321
red bream 162
red cabbage 21, 23
  pickled 409
red cheshire 280
red date, see Chinese red date
red emperor 154, 155
red globe onion 34
red-grained truffle 86
red gram dal, see pigeon pea
red hots 115
red kidney bean 309–10
red leicester, see leicester
red lentil, see lentil
red pepper, see capsicum and chilli pepper
red pickled ginger, see beni shoga
red radish 38
red raspberry 73
red rice, see sekihan

red salmon 161
Red Spanish pineapple 70
red sweet potato 41
red vinegar, Chinese 423, 426
red wine 460, 462
  vinegar 423, 427–28
red yeast 242
redcurrant 54, 55
redfish 161
reduced cream, canned 263, 264
reduced fat cheddar 283
refined olive oil 332
relish, see chutney
remoudou, see hervé
rémoulade sauce 426
rempah 393
renkon, see lotus
rennet 256, 257, 269–70
rhubarb 38–39
rib chops (lamb) 98
rib eye
  beef 91
  lamb 98
rib loin (pork) 102
ribbon-fish, see hairtail
riboflavin 12, 262, 470
ribs
  beef 91
  lamb 98
rice 10, 200, 207–10
  bran 202
  oil 323, 333
  desserts 252–53
  flour 217
  noodle
    dried 228, 230
    fresh 230–31
  pudding 253
  stick, see rice noodle, dried
  vinegar, white 426
  wine 419
Rice Imperial 253
rich shortcrust 251
ricotta 286, 292, 297
ridder 298
ridged gourd 14
rigani 355–56
rigatoni, see macaroni
ripened butter 325
risotto 209
  nero 170
rissoni 226
roast beef 136
roast pork 136
roaster (chicken) 140
Robinson potato 36
rock
  cake 247
  carp 152
  ling 158
  lobster 170, 171
  salt 240
rocket 39
rockmelon 73
Rocky Road 374
rodsallat, see dulse
roe 148
  botargo 175–76
  lumpfish 180
  salmon 181
  soft herring 157
roker, see ray
rokka, see rocket
rolled oats 206
rollmop herring 178–79
roly-poly pudding 254, 260
Roma tomato 75
romadur 291
Roman/o bean, see borlotti bean
romano, see parmesan
roquefort 297
rose hip syrup 368
rose water 419
rosé wine 462
rosemary 357
  vinegar 426
roti 190
roucou, see annatto
rough puff pastry 250
round
  beef 89
  pork 102
round, smooth head cabbage 23
roux 395
royalp 299
rue 357–58
rum 459, 461
rump

beef 89
pork 102
rump and loin 89
runner bean 16
rush leeks, see chives
rusks 442
rutabaga, see swede
rye 10, 200, 210–11
  bread 198–99
  flakes 210
  flour 217
  meal 211

S
saccharin 368–69
sack, see sherry
safflower oil 333–34
saffron 358
sage 358
sago 211
sahlab, see salep
Saint Claire 285
St John's bread, see carob
Saint Marcellin 287
Saint Otho 283
Saint Paulin 295, 298
sake 419, 456
salad 437–38
  burnet 358–59
  cream 426
  seaweed, see wakame
salad, pasta/rice-based 438
salade de mâche, see leaf lettuce
salame de Felino 122
salami 10, 121–23
salep 238–39
salitre, see saltpetre
salmon 148, 161
  canned 181
  smoked 149, 181
salmon
  roe 181
  trout 162
salsa di pomodori 395
salsiccie 124
  casalinga, see salsiccie
salt 12, 109, 239–40, 243, 273, 274
salt beef 130
salt cod 176
saltpetre 240–41
saluggia bean, see borlotti bean
sambal ulek 393
sambar masala 353
sambucca 458
samsoe 293, 298
sand whiting 166
sandwich 438
sansho, see Chinese pepper powder
Santa Claus melon 59
santol 60
sao mai, see wonton wrapper
sapodilla 73
sapsago 273, 298
sar hor fun, see rice noodle, fresh
sardenaira, see focaccia
sardine 148, 162
  canned 181–82
sarsaparilla 466
sashimi 148, 165, 401, 403
satay sauce 383, 393
satsuma 64
satura 245
saucisson 124
  au foie de porc 134
  fumé, see saucisson
  fumé aux herbes, see saucisson
sauerkraut 10, 21, 409–10
sausage, fresh 115–16
sausage roll 438–39
  frozen 452–53
saveloy 124
savarin, see baba
savory 359
savoury shortcrust 251
savoy cabbage 21, 23
scalded cream, see clotted cream
scallion, see green onion
scallop 148, 173
scallopine 32
scampi 148, 173–74
schiacciata, see focaccia
schinken
  jagdwurst 118
  kalbfleischwurst 125
  plockwurst 125

schinkenbrot 198
schinkenwurst 124–25
schmierkäse, see cottage cheese
schnapps 456
school prawn 173
Scottish bap, see bap
screwpine, see pandan leaf
sea cucumber 182
sea ear, see abalone
sea egg, see sea urchin
sea moss, see carrageen
sea parsley, see lovage
sea perch, see orange roughy
sea salt 240
sea urchin 174
seafood
  platter, frozen 452–53
  stick 439
seagull egg 144
seakale, see silverbeet
seam tripe 105
seaweed 182–84
  noodle 231
seeng, see drumstick vegetable
seet gnee, see snow fungus
sekihan 209
selenium 472
self-raising flour 214, 218, 219
self-saucing pudding 259, 447
semolina 213
serai, see lemon grass
sesame seed 321–22
  oil 334
  wafer, see pasteli
Seville orange 66
sevruga 176
sha gu, see water chestnut
shaddock, see pomelo
shallot 39
Shanghai noodle 231
shank (lamb) 99
shao hsing 419
shark 148, 162
shark's fin 184–85
  braised 185
shark's fin soup 185
Sharon persimmon 69
Sharwil avocado 48
shavourma, see doner kebab
sheep's kidney 96
sheep's milk 265, 270
sherbet 255
sherry 454, 457
  vinegar 426
shichimi 338
shiitake mushroom 84–85
shimeji, see oyster mushroom
shin beef 89
shiraita kombu 183
shirataki noodle 231
shirokikurage, see snow fungus
shiso 359
short loin 97–98
shortbread 244
shortcrust pastry 250–51
shortening 243, 328, 330, 334
shoulder
  lamb 98
  pork 103
  veal 107
shovel-nosed lobster, see Balmain bug
shoyu 394
shrimp, see prawn
  canned 185
shrimp sauce 393
shropshire blue, see blue shropshire
shu yu, see yam
Sicilian sumac, see sumach
sieva bean, see lima bean
silver carp, see carp
silver dory 154
silver drummer, see drummer
silver fungus, see snow fungus
silver jew, see jewfish
silver pin noodle 231–32
silver salmon 161–62
silverbeet 39–40
silverside
  beef 89
  pork 102
singhara nut 43
sirloin 89–90
siwalan, see palm nut
skate, see ray
Ski Queen 286
skim milk 264, 270
skin, of chicken 141
skinless sausages 116

skirt steak 90
slaked lime 241
slave fruit, see okra
slivovitz 456
sloe gin 71
Smithfield ham 133
smoked beef 136
smoked chicken 136
smoked frankfurter 115
smoked ham spec, see speck
smoked liverwurst 134
smoked pork loin, see Canadian bacon
smoked turkey 137
smolt 161
Smooth Cayenne pineapple 70
snack food 448
  frozen 452–53
snails, canned 443–44
snake 104
  bean 16–17
  squash 32
snapper 162–63
snow fungus 82, 85
snow pea 35, 36
Snowball 455
soba noodle 203, 232
soccerball leg ham 133
soda water 461, 465–66
sodium 12, 13, 46, 187, 233, 243, 472
  bicarbonate, see bicarbonate of soda
sodium-free baking powder 235
soft drink 463, 466
  calorie-free 463
soft herring roe 157
soisson, see haricot bean
sol, see dulse
sole 163
soluum, see dulse
somen noodle 228–29
Soppressa salami 123
sorbet 255
sorghum 205
sorrel 360
soubise 386
soufflé 259–60
soup
  canned 444
  packet 447–48
sour cream 264, 270–71
sour finger carambola 51, 52
sourdough bread 199
soursop 52–53
southern calamari 174
Southern Comfort 459, 461
southern rock lobster 171
sow thistle 40
soya
  drink 466
  flour 217–18
  milk 466
  sauce 10, 390, 393–94
soya bean 301, 310, 311, 386
  curd, see tofu
  oil 335, 466
  paste, see tempeh and miso
  sprouts 17
spa water 463
spaghetti 226
  canned 444
spaghetti squash, see vegetable spaghetti
spalen 298
Spam 130
spangled emperor 154, 155
Spanish melon 59
Spanish onion
  red 33, 34
  yellow 34
Spanish orange, see sweet orange
spanner crab 169
spare ribs 91
spatchcock 140
spätzle 230
spearmint 353
spec, see speck
speck 137
spegelpoelse 122
spetsofagi 120
spiced English sausage 116
spiced French sausage 116
spinach 40
  see also silverbeet
spiny lobster 170, 171
spirits, clear 454, 455, 456

split pea 311
sponge
    cake 247
    flour 218
    mushroom, see morel
spotted jewfish 157–58
spread 383
spring bamboo shoot 15–16
spring chicken 140
spring greens 23
spring onion 34
spring roll 430, 439
    frozen 453
spring roll wrapper 232
    frozen 439
spring water 466
Springerle 244
Sprinkles 374
spun sugar, see pulled sugar
squid 148, 174
    dried 185
squire 162
star anise 360
star apple 73–74
    see also carambola
star fruit, see carambola
starch 215–16, 441
staunchweed, see yarrow
steak and kidney pudding 251
steamed pudding 260–61
steel-cut oats 206
stilton 299
stinking gum, see asafoetida
stirabout 205
stock
    cube 420
    powder 420
stout 459
stracchino 299
strassburg 137
straw mushroom 85
strawberry 74
    toffee-glazed 254
strawberry
    essence 420
    guava 58
    tomato, see cape gooseberry
streaky bacon 128
strega 458
striped trumpeter, see trumpeter
strudel 258
    pastry 251
stuffed goose (sausage) 95
stuffing, packet 448
sucrose 369
suet 323, 335
    crust pastry 251
Suffolk ham 133
sugar 11, 364
    brown 365
    caster 365
    coarse 365
    cube 366
    granulated 366–67
    icing 367
    lump, see sugar, cube
    molasses 365
    palm 368
    pectin 368
    preserving 368
    pulled 371
    raw 368
    white 369
sugar
    bananas 49
    beet 18, 364
    pea, see snow pea
    snap pea 35, 36
sugarcane 364, 368
sultana 80
    grape 57
sulze 129
sum-sum, see pasteli
sumach 339, 360–61
summer sausage 113
summer savory 359
summer squash, see marrow
sunchoke, see Jerusalem
    artichoke
sunflower
    meal 322
    oil 322, 335–36
    seed 322
suprême de foie gras truffé 131
surf parrot fish 159, 160
sushi 148, 184, 359
sveciaöst 288
svenbo 298
swamp cabbage 14
Swatow mustard cabbage 22

swede 40–41
sweet and sour pork 431
sweet basil, see basil
sweet corn, see corn and maize
sweet granadilla, see golden
    granadilla
sweet orange 66
sweet pickle, see piccalilli
sweet potato 41
sweet shortcrust 251
sweet vinegar, Chinese 426–27
sweetbreads 104
sweetlip emperor 154, 155
Swiss chard, see silverbeet
Swiss mushroom 83
Swiss roll 243
swordfish 148
Sydney rock oyster 172
Szechuan pepper, see Chinese
    pepper

T

Tabasco sauce 394
table margarine 331
    low salt 331
    polyunsaturated 331
tabouli 212
taco 199
tagliarini 226
tagliatelle 226
tahini 322, 400, 401
Tahiti lime 62
tahu, see tofu
tailor 163
takenoko, see bamboo shoot
takuan 410
talo, see taro
tamari 394, 401
tamarillo 74
tamarind 361, 410
    cream of 361
tamarind water 361
tandoori masala 353
tandoori paste 401–2
tangelo 64, 74
tangerine, see mandarin
tansy 361
tap water 466
tapioca 24, 211
    meal 211
    starch 24, 211
tarama 402
taramosalata 176, 381, 384, 402
taro 41–42
    starch 42
tarragon 361–62
    vinegar 427
tart 258–59
tartare sauce 426
tartaric acid 241
tartrazine 341, 412
tarwhine 151–52
Tasmanian trumpeter, see
    trumpeter
tasty cheese, see cheddar
tea 461, 467
teawurst 137–38
teewurst, see teawurst
teff, see millet
telemes, see fetta
tempeh 10, 301, 402
tempura 359
tequila 456
teraglin 163–64
terrine, see pâté
terung engkol 28
tête de maure, see edam
tête de moine, see bellelay
tête de mort, see edam
Texan pink grapefruit 58
textured vegetable protein 311
Thai aubergine 28
Thai pea aubergine 28
Thai rice 210
theobroma oil, see cocoa butter
thiamin 12, 200, 470
thickened cream 264, 271
thickshake 440
thigh, of chicken 141
Thompson grapefruit 58
thousand island dressing 421,
    426
thousand-year egg 144
thuringer 113–14
    bockwurst 111
thyme 362
    oil of 362
thymol, see thyme, oil of
Tia Maria 456
tick bean, see ful medami
tientsin red bean, see adzuki

bean
tilsit 299
Timboon Triple Cream 300
tisane, see herbal tea
toasted sandwich 438
toffee 380
    glazing 253, 254
tofu 10, 301, 302
Tom Collins 466
Tom Thumb tomato 75
tomatillo, see cape gooseberry
tomato 75
    paste 402–3
    sauce 394–95
tomme fraîche 300
tongue 105, 138
tonic water 460, 467
topside
    beef 90
    pork 102–3
tororo 183
tortellini 221, 226
tortiglione 226
tortilla 190, 199
toor dal, see pigeon pea
Toscana salami 123
Toulouse sausage 125
tournedos Rossini 131
trag, see teraglin
trasi, see blachan
treacle 369
treccia 292
tree ears, see cloud ear fungus
tree melon, see pepino
tree tomato, see tamarillo
trenette 227
trevally 164
tripe 105
triple cream cheese 300
triticale 212
trombone pumpkin 37
trout 148, 164
    smoked 149, 185–86
truffle (confection) 374
truffle (tuber) 86
trumpeter 164
tsao, see Chinese red date
tsu ts'ai, see nori
tubetti, see macaroni
tuna 148, 164–65
    canned 186
tung ku, see shiitake mushroom
turkey 147
    smoked 137
turkey
    bologna 112
    ham 133
    salami 123
Turkish delight 380, 419
turmeric 354, 362
turnip 42
turnip-rooted celery, see
    celeriac
turtle bean, see black kidney
    bean
tuscarora, see wild rice
TVP see textured vegetable
    protein
Twisties 448
two-horned water chestnut 43
two-tooth, see hogget

U

ubi kayu, see cassava
udon noodle 229
ugli fruit 64
UHT cream, see long life cream
UHT milk, see long life milk
umbrella mushroom, see parasol
    mushroom
umeboshi 359, 392, 411
umeshu 411
unbleached flour 218
unsalted butter 325
upo, see bottle gourd
upside-down pudding 254
urucu, see annatto

V

vacherin fribourgeois 288
vacuum packed foods 449
val, see hyacinth bean
Valencia orange 66
Van der Hum 458
vanaspati 336
vanilla 362–63
    beans/pods, see vanilla
    essence 420
vanillin 363
variety meats, see offal

vc-tsin, see monosodium
    glutamate
veal 106–7
    knuckle 107
Vegemite 381, 383
vegetable
    gelatine, see agar agar
    ghee, see vanaspati
    juice 467
    oil, blended 336
    pear, see chayote
    shortening 334, 336
    spaghetti 42
vegetable-flavoured pasta 221
vegetables
    canned 444
    frozen 453
velouté 395
Veneto salami 123
venison 107
verjuice 396
vermicelli, see capellini
vermouth 454, 457, 460
Vichy water 466
Villa Franca lemon 62
vinaigrette 427
vindaloo paste 403
vine leaf 42–43, 411
    rolls, see dolmas, canned
vinegar 10, 233, 421
violet truffle 86
virgin olive oil 332
vitamin
    A 12, 46, 148, 469
    B1 12
    B2 12
    B3 12
    B5 12
    B6 12, 46, 470
    B12 12, 87, 148, 470
    C 12, 14, 46, 87, 441, 470
    D 12, 470
    E 12, 14, 471
    K 12, 471
vitamins 11, 12, 441
    RDI 468
    see also individual entries
vodka 456, 460
Vogel bread 195

W

wakame 184
waldmeister, see woodruff
walnut 322
    pickled 411
walnut oil 337
Waltham Cross grape 57, 79
warrigal greens 43
wasabi 403
water 11, 13, 454; see also tap
    water
    ice, see sorbet
    spinach 14
water chestnut 43
    powder 241
    starch, see water chestnut
    powder
watercress 43–44
watermelon 75–76
Weet-Bix 447
weisslacker bierkäse 291
weisswurst 125
wensleydale 300
West Indian lime, see Mexican
    lime
western king prawn 173
Westphalian ham 133
wheat 10, 200, 212–13
    bran 202
    noodle
        raw 228
        steamed and dried 228
        steamed and fried 228
    starch, see cornflour
wheatgerm 213
wheatmeal, see wholemeal flour
    flour, see wholemeal flour
Wheeney grapefruit 58
whelk 148
whey 264, 271
whipping cream 271
whisky 210, 459, 460
white asparagus 15
white bread 11, 187, 188
white cabbage 21, 23
white currant 55
white flour 11, 218
    self-raising 218
white fungus, see snow fungus

white Hungarian salami 122
white mustard cabbage, see
    Chinese white cabbage
white onion 34
white pasta 221
white rice 207, 208
white rum 459
white sauce 395
    see also bechamel sauce
white stilton 299
white sugar 369
white sweet potato 41
white wensleydale 300
white wine 460, 462
    mustard 398
    vinegar 428
whitebait 148, 165–66
whiting 166
whole dried pea, see blue pea
whole wheat flour, see
    wholemeal flour
wholemeal bread 187, 188
wholemeal flour 218–19, 243
    self-raising 219
wholemeal pasta 221, 227
wholemeal pastry 251
Wiener, see frankfurter
wild boar 108
wild onion seed, see nigella
wild orange 76
wild rice 210
Williams pear 68, 69
Windsor bean, see broad bean,
    dried
Windsor black pumpkin 37
wine 459, 460, 461, 462
    vinegar 427–28
wing, of chicken 141
winter bamboo shoot 15–16
winter melon 14
winter mushroom, see shiitake
    mushroom
winter savory 359
winter squash, see pumpkin
witchetty grubs 108
witloof, see Belgian endive
woderberry, see black
    nightshade
wombok, see napa cabbage
wonton wrapper 232
woo kok 42
woo la gua, see bottle gourd
wood ear fungus, see cloud ear
    fungus
woodruff 363
Worcestershire sauce 395–96,
    410
wrasse 166

X

Xeres, see sherry

Y

yabbie 148, 169
yabby, see crayfish
yam 44
    flour 241
    starch, see yam flour
yama no imo, see mountain yam
yarrow 363
yeast 242
    extract 381, 383
yellow bean sauce, see bean
    sauce
yellow mushroom, see boletus
yellow pepper, see capsicum
yellow raspberry 73
yellow zucchini 45
yellowfin bream 151
yi noodle, see e-fu noodle
yoghurt 265, 271–72
    frozen 265, 267–68
York ham 133
you erh, see cloud ear fungus
yu chee, see shark's fin
yu lu, see fish sauce
yucca, see tapioca
yufka, see filo pastry

Z

zabaglione 396
zabaione, see zabaglione
zabalin, see lemon grass
za'tar 338, 361
zieger, see goat cheese
Ziger 297
ziltoni, see macaroni
zinc 12, 87, 148, 472
zucchini 45, 46
zungenwurst 138
zwiebelwurst 134

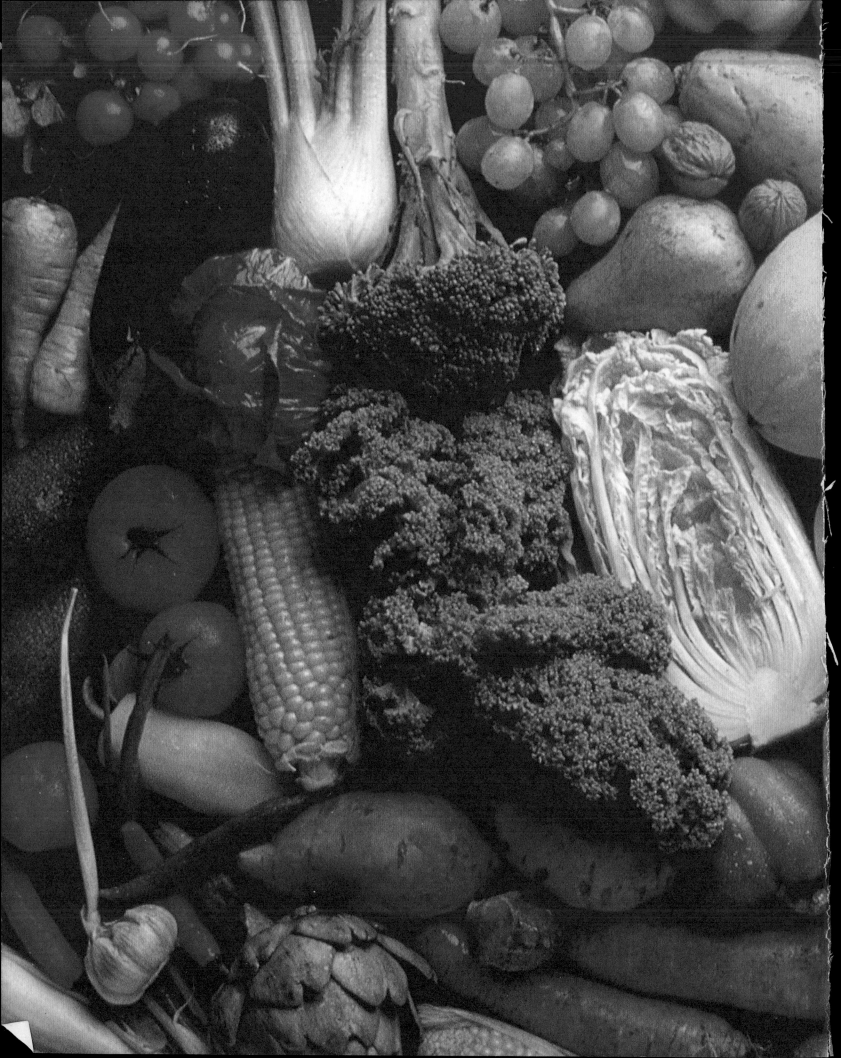